Living Well

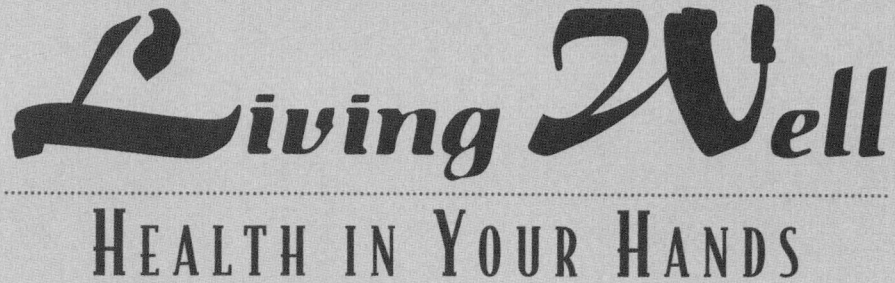

Living Well

HEALTH IN YOUR HANDS

Second Edition

CURTIS O. BYER
Mt. San Antonio College

LOUIS W. SHAINBERG
Mt. San Antonio College

■ HarperCollinsCollegePublishers

Executive Editor: Bonnie Roesch
Developmental Editor: Karen Trost
Project Editorial Manager: Melonie Salvati
Design Manager: Lucy Krikorian
Text and Cover Designer: John Callahan
Cover Photo: © David Young-Wolff/PhotoEdit
Art Studio: Vantage Art Inc.
Photo Researcher: Mira Schachne
Electronic Production Manager: Su Levine
Desktop Administrator: Laura Leever
Manufacturing Manager: Willie Lane
Electronic Page Makeup: Laura Leever
Printer and Binder: R. R. Donnelley & Sons Company
Cover Printer: The Lehigh Press, Inc.

For permission to use copyrighted material, grateful acknowledgment is made to the copyright holders on pp. C-1–C-6, which are hereby made part of this copyright page.

Living Well: Health in Your Hands, Second Edition

Library of Congress Cataloging-in-Publication Data
Byer, Curtis O.
    Living well: health in your hands / Curtis O. Byer, Louis W. Shainberg.—2nd ed.
    p.   cm.
    Includes index.
    ISBN 0-673-52337-3
    1. Health.   I. Shainberg, Louis W.   II. Title.
RA776.B962   1994
613—dc20   94-3413
                                               CIP

95 96 97 98   9 8 7 6 5 4 3 2 1

BRIEF CONTENTS

DETAILED CONTENTS

UNIT FIVE AGING AND DEATH   369

CHAPTER 12 AGING   370

CHAPTER 13 DYING AND DEATH   402

CHAPTER 19 SEXUALLY TRANSMITTED DISEASES 584

PREFACE

Personal Health may be one of the most important courses students will take during their college years. For many, it will be the first time that they are systematically exposed to the basic concepts of wellness, health promotion, and disease prevention. We believe that the textbook they use should be an essential tool for empowering them with the information and motivation necessary to develop and maintain a healthy life-style. We have written the second edition of *Living Well: Health in Your Hands* with an increased focus on individual responsibility for wellness, cultural diversity, and effective interpersonal communication. These three integrated themes provide a framework for the text and offer your students a manageable and enjoyable exploration of the subject matter while at the same time encouraging them to consider carefully what changes and adaptations they can and should make as they strive towards a healthier life.

Long established habits die hard. Many students find that maintaining new, more healthful habits for the long term is simply not easy. In writing this book, we have recognized that motivation and desire are key to effective, enduring change. We also recognize that basic conditions must exist in order for your students to seek changes in their habits and attitudes. Students must have a basis of fact on which to choose a particular behavior as more desirable than others. They must be able to expect attainable and worthwhile rewards for making healthful life-style choices. And most importantly, they must care enough about themselves to feel that they deserve the best that life has to offer. Our goal for this revision of *Living Well* is to provide your students with the *knowledge, insight,* and *decision-making* skills needed to inspire them in setting and reaching their personal health goals.

INTEGRATED THEMES

INDIVIDUAL RESPONSIBILITY

Each of your students is to a great extent responsible for the quality of his or her own health. Only when an individual feels personally involved can he or she be motivated to adopt a wellness life-style. As the subtitle of the text indicates, we want your students to understand that health is "in your hands." This theme of individual responsibility is expressed throughout the text material. Chapter outlines indicate what the student can expect to gain—in terms of factual knowledge, personal insight, and ability to make informed decisions. *In Your Hands* behavioral inventories help the student to evaluate the healthfulness of various behaviors and to use this knowledge as a basis for any changes that need to be made.

CULTURAL DIVERSITY

Cultural diversity influences the attitudes and behaviors that affect every area of wellness. There is no one single healthful life-style. "Health" means many different things to different cultures. A text that presented only a single cultural view of health would not serve any of its readers well. We have made a great effort to ensure that *Living Well* reflects the multicultural richness of North America and its colleges and universities. Rachel Spector, author of *Cultural Diversity in Health and Illness,*

3rd edition, reviewed the entire draft of the manuscript. Her insights and suggestions were immensely helpful to us in portraying the wealth of differences we all encounter in our daily lives.

EFFECTIVE COMMUNICATION

Effective communication is one of the cornerstones of healthful living. Good communication skills enable us to speak with confidence, listen critically, and respond appropriately. These skills can improve your students' success in maintaining a wellness way of life by giving them the tools needed to make choices and to express to others their goals. In this second edition of *Living Well*, we have introduced a new chapter (2) that overviews the basics of human communication. In addition, most chapters include boxes, "Communication for Wellness," that discuss specific aspects of communication related to the chapter content.

NEW TO THIS EDITION

This second edition of *Living Well* has been revised extensively to reflect new information as well as changes in emphasis within the personal health course. Each chapter has been completely updated to include the latest information on each topic. The new emphasis on cultural diversity is reflected in the text discussions as well as in the revised illustration program.

In addition, the pedagogy of this edition has been expanded. We have added chapter objectives, and have replaced chapter opening vignettes with factual case studies related to each topic.

The 24 chapters of the text are grouped into 8 units. The first five units deal with concepts and topics in which students have an opportunity to apply good health promotion practices and take their health into their own hands as a result of their understanding of content. The content of the final three units guides students in confronting some of the challenges, such as disease prevention, that can arise in the pursuit of healthful living. While this organization provides a positive and natural progression of information that works well in the classroom, each unit is designed to be free-standing, so the text may be successfully presented in any sequence to fit the needs of your individual course.

The following content descriptions highlight some of the exciting changes to this edition within each unit:

Unit One, Introduction to Wellness

Chapter 1, Introduction to Wellness, has entirely new sections on cultural diversity, locus of control, judging health research, and the Healthy People 2000 goals for the nation. Chapter 2, Communication for Wellness, is a completely new chapter, introducing the principles of effective communication and their applications to health and wellness.

Unit Two, Mental Health and Stress Management

Chapter 3, Positive Emotional Wellness, has new sections on happiness and boosting self-esteem. Chapter 4, Stress Management and Other Mental Health Challenges, has new sections on stress and college and on serious mental illness.

Unit Three, Sexuality

Chapter 5, Sexual Relationships and Lifestyles, includes new sections on communication in relationships and on Sternberg's components of love. Chapter 6, Sexual Biology and Behavior, includes a new section on the reproductive life plan and expanded coverage of PMS and premature ejaculation. Chapter 7, Contraception, has been completely reorganized, updated, and expanded to include the most current information. Chapter 8, Pregnancy and Parenting Decisions, includes new sections on advances in fertility, teratogens and pregnancy, Kegel exercises, genetic disorders, low birthweight infants, bonding and the newborn, and the responsibilities of parenthood.

Unit Four, Food and Fitness

Chapter 9, Nutrition, has been heavily revised, with new sections on lactose intolerance, artificial sweeteners, fat substitutes, vegetarianism, the new food groups, daily values, the food pyramid, eating right, new food labels, food allergies, and food additives.

Chapter 10, Weight Management, has also been heavily revised, with new sections on body mass index, waist to hip ratio, healthy weight, choosing a weight goal, body fat ideal, obesity, fats, dietary books, very-low calorie diets, and weight cycling. Chapter 11, Turning on to Fitness, includes new sections on wellness, fitness potential for popular sports, exercise readiness, cardiovascular exercise, exercise-related problems, and myths about exercise.

Unit Five, Aging and Death

Chapter 12, Aging, includes new sections on the six types of aging, multicultural perspectives on aging, programmed versus stochastic aging theories, dietary restrictions and aging, and overmedication of older persons. Chapter 13, Dying and Death, includes a new section entitled, Why Study Death? and expanded coverage of multicultural perspectives on death.

Unit Six, Substance Use and Abuse

Chapter 14, Drugs in American Families and Society, is an all new chapter reflecting the new direction of this unit from one about detailed knowledge of how drugs work towards strategies for winning the war on drugs through drug education. This new chapter takes a family and social approach to substance abuse, emphasizing how substance abuse affects families and society and how families and society can either promote or deter substance abuse. Chapter 15, Psychoactive Drugs, is completely restructured and examines the basic biology of psychoactive drugs—entrance into the body, distribution through the body, action, and elimination from the body—and surveys the drugs currently in common use. Chapter 16, Tobacco, contains expanded coverage of the risks of passive smoking and a new section on the effectiveness of different smoking control strategies. Chapter 17, Alcohol and Health, contains a new section examining physical dependency on alcohol and the forms of alcohol withdrawal, and a new feature addressing the health benefits versus the risks associated with alcohol use.

Unit Seven, Diseases

Chapter 18, Communicable Diseases, includes new coverage of psychoneuroimmunology, prevention of diseases, bacterial pneumonia, and tuberculosis. Chapter 19, Sexually Transmitted Diseases, has been completely updated with the latest information and statistics, a thorough discussion of AIDS, and includes a new section on bacterial vaginitis. Chapter 20, Cardiovascular Health, has been almost completely rewritten, including new coverage on women and heart disease, diagnostic tests, and a rewritten section on risk factors including those you can modify, those you cannot change, and contributing risk factors. Chapter 21, Cancer and Other Chronic Disorders, has new coverage of lung, breast, skin, and prostate cancers, the occurrence of cancers in various ethnic groups, cancer research, diabetes, multiple sclerosis, seizure disorders, Alzheimer's disease, emphysema, cystic fibrosis, and back problems.

Unit Eight, Consumer Action and Environmental Health

Chapter 22, Health for the Smart Consumer, includes new information on taking charge of your health, prescription and nonprescription drugs, generic drugs, multiple drug use, hair dyes, products for the skin and teeth, and do-it-yourself test kits. Chapter 23, Health Care Systems, includes new information on mainstream and alternative health care providers, health insurance, and National Health Care Reform. Chapter 24, Environmental Health, includes new sections on indoor air pollution, water pollution, lead poisoning, irradiation of food, population dynamics, personal responsibility for environmental quality, and the Federal Clean Air Act.

LEARNING AND MOTIVATIONAL AIDS

To ensure student interest and success, a number of learning and motivational aids are built into the text. Many are retained from the first edition, having been well received by students. Several new additions have been included to enhance the already successful pedagogical strategy.

CHAPTER OUTLINES

The headings reflecting the key topics to be discussed are listed at the beginning of each chapter giving the students a preview of the text to come.

LEARNING OBJECTIVES

New to this edition, each chapter opens with a list of learning objectives which have been divided into three categories: *knowledge,* covering basic factual learning; *insight,* showing students how they can extrapolate and apply the material in the chapter to their own lives; and *decision-making,* illustrating the types of informed decisions that students will be prepared to make upon learning the material in the chapter.

OPENING CASE STUDIES

Newly written for this edition by Dr. David White of East Carolina University, each chapter now opens with a brief case study examining a relevant, interesting and controversial topic related to the chapter's topic. These case studies highlight contemporary health issues, and are designed to create interest in the topic as well as to stimulate critical thinking about the issues discussed.

IN YOUR HANDS

At least one behavioral inventory for self-assessment of related health habits is included in each chapter. By completing these inventories, students can gain insight into their own health behaviors or attitudes, and, based on the results of these self-assessments, set tangible goals for improving their own well-being.

COMMUNICATION FOR WELLNESS

New to this edition, these boxes reinforce the text's emphasis on the importance of communication as a tool in promoting good health. Found in most chapters, coverage include such topics as "Talking About Birth Control," "Fitness as a Social Activity," "Drugs as a Substitute for Communication," "Issues on Regulation of Tobacco Advertising," and "22 Ways to Say No to a Drink."

FEATURE BOXES

A popular feature of the last edition, these special boxed essays in each chapter address high-interest, controversial, and contemporary issues.

CHECKPOINT QUESTIONS

Another popular feature of the first edition, these in-text review questions appear throughout each chapter, allowing students to assess comprehension of material that they have just covered before moving on to other topics.

MARGINAL GLOSSARY

Each key term is printed in bold-face type at its first appearance in the text; its definition appears in the bottom margin on that page as well as in the end-of-text glossary.

PRONUNCIATIONS

Phonetic pronunciation guides for new and difficult words are given throughout the text.

CHAPTER SUMMARY

Each chapter ends with a brief summary of its important concepts for student review.

REFERENCES AND SUGGESTED READINGS

The facts throughout each chapter are documented by the numbered references presented in the References Section. The Suggested Readings provide other resources of interest on the topics contained within the chapter.

ANCILLARY MATERIALS

This text is a part of a complete package of materials designed to facilitate a dynamic, interesting, and effective health course. The materials included in this package are described below.

INSTRUCTOR'S MANUAL/TESTBANK

Cathy Kennedy and Vanna West of Colorado State University have compiled a comprehensive manual that includes detailed lecture outlines and teaching tips, as well as additional activities and suggested resources for enhancing your classroom presentation. A complete testbank with more than 1750 questions is included in a separate section of the manual. The testbank is also available on *Testmaster* for use with IBM or Macintosh computers.

QUIZMASTER

Quizmaster is a new program that coordinates with the *Testmaster* test generator program. *Quizmaster* allow students to take timed or untimed tests created with *Testmaster* at the computer. Upon completing a test, a student can see his or her test score and view or print a diagnostic report that lists the topics or objectives that have been mastered or that need to be restudied. When *Quizmaster* is installed on a network, student scores are saved on disk and instructors can use the *Quizmaster* utility program to view records and print reports for individual students, class sections, and entire courses.

STUDENT WORKBOOK

Dee Crary, our respected colleague, has prepared an extraordinary student workbook to accompany this text. Full of valuable, self-directed activities, it is designed to reinforce and expand on concepts from the text. Students will find it fun and interesting to use.

TRANSPARENCIES

A set of 75 full-color acetates, incorporating illustrations, tables, and other material from the text, is available to all adopters of the text.

VIDEOS

A selection of videos is available to qualified adopters. Please contact your local HarperCollins College representative for further information.

HEALTHDESK

HealthDesk is an information management and education tool designed to help students take a more active role in managing their health. Available for use with IBM computers, *HealthDesk* provides general information about the human body and health and helps students track information about their personal medical history and health related activities. Please contact your HarperCollins College representative for further information.

ACKNOWLEDGMENTS

We are very grateful to all of the highly competent personnel at HarperCollins who worked so hard on the preparation and production of this book. Special thanks to Bonnie Roesch, Executive Editor, Karen Trost, Developmental Editor, Melonie Salvati, Project Editor, and Mira Schachne, Photo Researcher.

We would also like to express a special thank you to Rachel Spector for all her expertise in helping us implement an enhanced multicultural focus in the book and to David White for writing the introductory case studies for each chapter.

In addition, we wish to thank all of the following people for their extremely valuable reviews of the manuscripts for this text.

FIRST EDITION REVIEWERS

Judy Baker, East Carolina University; Kenneth Becker, University of Wisconsin—LaCrosse; Fay Biles, Kent State University; Elaine Blasko, West Liberty State College; Debra Boehme, Western New Mexico University; Annette Caruso, Pennsylvania State University; Don Chamblee, Longview Community College; Donna Clark, North Carolina State University; Ted Coleman, Utah State College; Janine Cox, University of Kansas; Thomas Crumb, Triton College; Dorothy Downey, West Texas State University; Michael Gadell, Del Mar College; Janet Gleason, Corning Community College; John Gratton, Bee County College; Steven Hafen, Cantonsville Community College; Jack Hansma, Baylor University; Charlotte Hendricks, University of Alabama; Bill Hyman, Sam Houston State University; Gordon James, Weber State College; Georgia Keeney, University of Minnesota—Duluth; Cathy Kennedy, Colorado State University; Michael McAvoy, New College of San Francisco; Nancy McNames, Kellogg Community College; Thomas Nicholson, Western Kentucky University; Linda Olasov, Northern Kentucky University; Fred Pearson, Ricks College; JoAnn Pederson, Kean College of New Jersey; Eleanor Prueske, Northeastern Illinois University; Richard Riggs, University of Kentucky; James Rothenberger, University of Minnesota; Laurna Rubinson, University of Illinois; Michael Savage, Purdue University; Vicki Staggs, Eastern New Mexico State University; Jeannette Tedesco, Western Connecticut State University; Mitchell Twardowicz, Essex Community College; Charles Underhill, Brevard Community College; and Michael Young, University of Arkansas.

SECOND EDITION REVIEWERS

Marigold Edwards, University of Pittsburgh; Helaine Alessio, Miami University of Ohio; Sandra Bargainnier, Plymouth State College–New Hampshire; Rick Barnes, East Carolina University; Rosie Barretta, Salisbury State University–Maryland; Elaine Blasko, West Liberty State University; Susan Burge, Cuyahoga Community College; Marsha Campo, Modesto Junior College; Reece Carter, Western Kentucky University; Jonathan Coron, University of Florida; Marigold Edwards, University of Pittsburgh; Kathie Garbe, Youngstown State University; Stephen Goodwin, University of Delaware; Robert Harper, Indiana Wesleyan University; Andrina Jones, Nassau Community College; Catherine Kennedy, Colorado State University; Nancy LaCur-

sia, Southern Illinois University; Dan McBride, East Los Angeles College; David Moore, Valdosta State University–Georgia; Shirley Morgan, East Tennessee State University; Pat Raguse, Ventura College–California, Walt Rehm, Cuesta College–California; Janet Reis, University of Illinois; James Robinson, University of Northern Colorado; John Sciacca, Northern Arizona University; Lee Scott, University of Maine at Farmington; Kevin Simms, University of California at Riverside; John Smith, Springfield College–Massachusetts; Sunas Speece, Anderson University; Lois Thompson, Slippery Rock University; and Vincent Zuccala, New Hampshire College

Curtis O. Byer
Louis W. Shainberg

LIVING WELL
Health in Your Hands
Second Edition

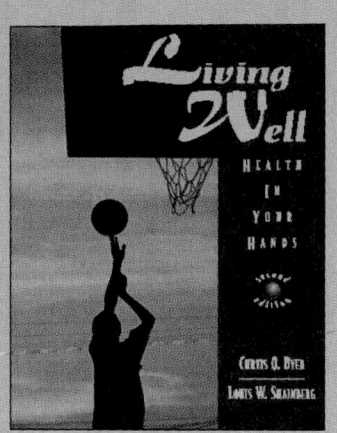

Curtis O. Byer
Mount San Antonio College

Louis W. Shainberg
Mount San Antonio College

ISBN 0-673-52337-3

What does it take to promote a healthier life-style and maintain well-being? A text that imparts the knowledge, motivation, and desire needed to obtain wellness.

The thoroughly revised second edition of *Living Well: Health in Your Hands* provides students with the *knowledge, insight,* and *decision-making* skills they need to make informed, healthy decisions now, and for the rest of their lives. While the core theme continues to focus on self-responsibility for achieving good health, this second edition's broadened coverage encompasses two new related issues: *cultural diversity* and *communication.*

Chapter 4   Stress Management and Other Mental Health Challenges

IN YOUR HANDS
A STRESS-MANAGEMENT ASSESSMENT

Each of us must develop effective ways of managing our stress level and coping with the day-to-day challenges of life. How well are you handling your stress? Circle the appropriate number of points for each statement.

	Often	Sometimes	Seldom
1. I am happy.	0	1	2
2. I assume responsibility for my own happiness and emotional well-being.	0	1	2
3. I feel hopeless and discouraged.	2	1	0
4. I can cope successfully with stressful periods without using alcohol or other drugs.	0	1	2
5. If I were experiencing an unusually stressful period, I would be willing to seek professional help.	0	1	2
6. I tend to feel sad.	2	1	0
7. I spend time wishing I were someone else.	2	1	0
8. I spend time wishing I were somewhere else.	2	1	0
9. I tend to get upset easily.	2	1	0
10. Of the 37 warning signs of excess stress listed on page 88, the number of those signs that apply to me is _____.			

Total points for items 1–10: _____.

INTERPRETATION

0–3 points: You appear to manage stress effectively and cope well. You are probably quite happy.

4–7 points: Your methods for coping with stress are about average. You can benefit by carefully reading this chapter.

8 or more points: You are showing definite signs of difficulty in coping and stress management. If you don't initiate more effective coping and stress-management methods as described later in this chapter, you are at risk of severe health problems.

HOW STRESS CAUSES ILLNESS

Stress, by modifying almost every body function, is capable of producing illness in a number of ways. We will next consider a few of the leading examples.

HEART DISEASE

Stress contributes to heart disease in many ways. During periods of stress, the blood pressure rises and pulse increases, placing an added burden on the heart. Stress induces changes in blood chemistry, such as elevated cholesterol levels, that promote atherosclerosis. Finally, the coronary arteries that supply blood to the heart muscle itself constrict, reducing the amount of oxygen available to the heart muscle. These problems are discussed in greater detail in Chapter 20. Also discussed in Chapter 20 is the Type A–Type B personality dichotomy. Some, though not all, heart experts associate the Type A personality (compulsive, competitive, impatient, hard driven) with a higher rate of heart disease than is found in the more relaxed Type B personality.

INFECTIOUS DISEASES

Psychoneuroimmunology is the study of the relationships that exist among the nervous system, the hormonal system, and the immune system. Excessive stress reduces the effectiveness of the immune mechanism and thereby increases the risk of infectious disease.[5] For example, many people find that they experience colds mostly during stressful periods. Similarly, both oral and genital

....

psychoneuroimmunology the study of the relationships that exist among the nervous system, the hormonal system, and the immune system.

INDIVIDUAL RESPONSIBILITY THEME

In Your Hands self-assessment feature.
The text's primary theme of individual responsibility throughout its narrative is augmented by "In Your Hands" self-assessment boxes. With at least one box in each chapter, these sections help students gain insight into their health and health-related habits, attitudes, and behaviors, while helping them set tangible goals for improving their own well-beings.

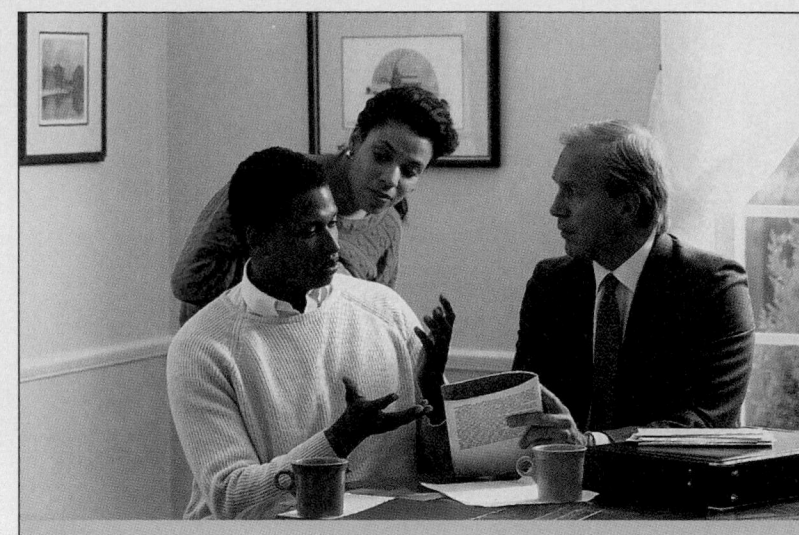

EMPHASIS ON EFFECTIVE COMMUNICATION

Communication Chapter:
For students to understand their own health and their future goals, they must be able to express themselves to others. The text now features a new communication chapter (Chapter 2) which introduces the principles and significance of effective communication and their applications to health and wellness.

2
COMMUNICATION FOR WELLNESS

UNIT SIX   Substance Use and Abuse

COMMUNICATION FOR WELLNESS:
FAMILY COMMUNICATION AND SUBSTANCE ABUSE

As the text points out, dysfunctional family life is frequently associated with chemical dependency and growing up in a healthy, strong family is the best prevention for substance abuse. What characterizes a healthy family? Every expert who studies this issue concludes that the number one trait of a healthy family is the ability to communicate.

Children in dysfunctional families do not feel free to talk to their parents about difficult subjects such as using alcohol or other drugs, or about sexual issues. Instead of relying on their parents for help, they turn to equally confused peers or just try to work things out on their own. Efforts to communicate with parents turn out unhappily. Some parents turn a "deaf ear" to their children's concerns, while others interrupt their children with angry and judgmental responses, quickly ending the possibility of any effective interaction. Parents jump to conclusions and overreact on the basis of incomplete information. Following their example, the children jump to their own conclusions and overreactions. Soon everyone is yelling and nobody is really listening to anyone else.

Healthy families gather around the table at mealtime and talk and really listen to each other. In addition to the day's events, feelings and concerns are shared. Children feel free to be open because they are confident that they will receive an understanding and supportive response. Parents listen in a way that encourages more communication. Instead of jumping to conclusions they listen attentively and draw out more information.

When parents communicate there is a sense of equality. They don't bully their children or force children into a position of subordination or submission. Members of healthy families don't use silence as an expression of hostility or a means of punishment. When disagreements occur, as they will in any family, communication continues. Issues are talked out, feelings are explored, and a mutually acceptable conclusion is reached. Children growing up in such families feel worthy and competent. They might "sample" drugs with their friends, but their self-esteem and sense of responsibility will almost always protect them from the overwhelming drug involvement characteristic of so many children of unhappy families.

COMMUNICATION FOR WELLNESS BOXES

Reinforcing the text's new emphasis on communication, these boxed features found in most chapters relate the importance of communication to each chapter's topic.

BROAD MULTICULTURAL FOCUS

By presenting a broad cultural focus, the authors convey how different cultures have their own concepts of health and illness. This is particularly important in the United States where cultural differences have an ever growing influence on individuals' personal decision making about their own health and life-styles.

HEALTH AND CULTURAL DIVERSITY

Culture is all of the customs, beliefs, values, knowledge, and skills that are shared by a specific group of people. The United States is a nation of many cultures. America's early immigrants were mostly from Europe. As recently as 1960, less than 15 percent of the U.S. population were of anything other than European ancestry. At that time, prevailing American attitudes toward health quite naturally reflected the European influence. Health was defined and health care delivery systems were designed mainly by people of European background and reflected European concepts of health and illness. Health care providers tended to reject other approaches to health as being backward and unscientific.[1]

Since 1960, the non-European population in the United States has more than tripled, reaching 64.3 million people by 1992 (see Table 1.1). If these 64.3 million people lived in an independent country, it would be the thirteenth largest in the world, more populous than Great Britain, France, Italy, or Spain. By 2050 the non-European ethnic groups will represent almost half of the U.S. population.[2]

Health and *illness* mean different things to people of different ethnic groups. Even health care providers (physicians, nurses, etc.) can be viewed as a separate group with their own culture. Their professional socialization teaches them a set of beliefs, practices, likes, dislikes, and rituals that influence how they relate to their clients. They tend to view health and illness in strictly scientific terms, with little emphasis given to supernatural or spiritual issues. They expect their patients to follow the orders given them. They are likely to feel some hostility toward patients whose culture gives them a different view of health and illness.[3]

Throughout this text we will try to incorporate the health views and concerns of the nation's many ethnic groups. Let's start by briefly surveying some meanings of health to several groups. *Please understand that space limitations require us to generalize for each group but by no means do we wish to stereotype or to imply that all members of a group hold certain beliefs or follow certain practices.* Also, we know that by discussing a few specific ethnic groups, we risk offending many others by their omission. If your ethnic group is not included it would be quite productive for you to interview several older members of your group to find out what health beliefs prevail and how these beliefs may have influenced your own views of health, illness, and wellness. Finally, we hope that we do not seem to advocate the European ways of looking at health and illness as the standard by which other cultures should be judged. That is not our intention.

NATIVE AMERICANS

At the time Europeans "discovered" North America the continent was already populated by over 200 nations of Native Americans, each with its own well-developed society and culture. After the native populations had been weakened by diseases introduced by the Europeans and had been disrupted and demoralized by the intrusions of the better-armed Europeans, treaties were signed forcing the Native Americans to give up most of the continent to the Europeans and establishing "reservations" for Native Americans, primarily in the western portion of the continent. Today about half of the country's Native Americans live on reservations or in rural areas while about half live in cities.

Traditional health beliefs varied among the nations as does the degree to which those beliefs are still followed by contemporary Native Ameri-

Table 1.1
U.S. Population by Race and Ethnicity, 1992

Group	Number	Percent
Total U.S. Population	254,922,000	100
Non-Hispanic		
White	190,604,000	75
African American	30,372,000	12
Asian/Pacific Islander	7,937,000	3
Native American	1,873,000	1
Hispanic*	24,136,000	9

*Hispanic origin is considered an ethnic identity rather than a race. Hispanic people list their race as white (about half of Hispanics), black (3 percent), Asian (1 percent), Native American (1 percent), and "other" (43 percent).

Source: U.S. Bureau of the Census, Current Population Reports, P-25, No. 1090 (1992).

culture all of the customs, beliefs, values, knowledge, and skills shared by a specific group of people.

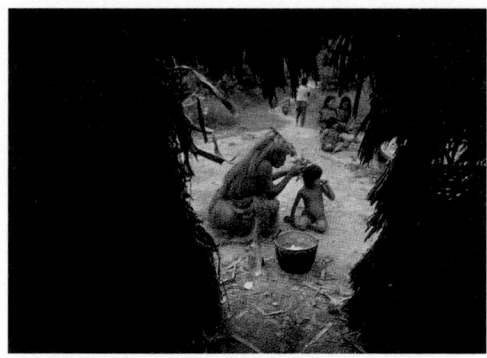

Health and illness mean different things to people of different cultures. Different concepts of illness lead to different forms of healing.

cans. To generalize somewhat, the traditional Native American belief about health emphasizes living in harmony with nature. In order to maintain health, the Native American must maintain his or her relationship with nature. The forced movement of Native Americans from their historical home areas often made this difficult or impossible.

Many Native Americans believe that there is a reason for every illness, that illness is a price to be paid for something that happened in the past or that will happen in the future. Illness is something that *must be*. Illness may be viewed as the best possible price to be paid for past or future events. Illness is not thought to result from infection by microbes or by physiological disorders.[4] Motivating healthful behavior, as healthful behavior is defined by scientific medicine, is difficult for those who hold this point of view.

Some Native American nations associate illness with evil spirits. The evil spirit responsible for a certain illness is identified by the "medicine man," and the remedy for the illness involves treating the evil spirit. Other causes of illness include displeasing holy people, annoying nature, disturbing plant or animal life, breaking a taboo, misusing a sacred ceremony, or suffering the effects of witches.[5] Again, people holding these beliefs will have little motivation to engage in what others would call healthful behavior.

Native Americans even today often favor traditional healers and remedies over physicians and hospitals. The medicine man determines the spiritual cause of an illness by using methods such as meditation, stargazing, chanting, and listening for sounds. Treatments then prescribed can include chanting, ceremonies to rid the sick person of evil spirits, and a wide range of herbal remedies.

Native Americans often avoid the services of physicians and hospitals because physicians tend to interpret and treat illness differently, are perceived as being disrespectful, and are thought to pry too much. The client prefers the medicine man's way of deducing or divining the problem over the physician's asking many personal questions.[6]

CHINESE AMERICANS

Traditional Chinese medicine views health as a state of spiritual and physical harmony with nature. This **holistic** concept (the philosophy that people function as complete units that cannot be reduced to the sum of their parts) of health has two main components.[7] These concepts, although thousands

holistic relating to the philosophy that people function as complete units that cannot be reduced to the sum of their parts.

ILLUSTRATION PROGRAM

A strong illustration program, which includes clearly drawn, full-color illustrations and up-to-date photographs, helps clarify coverage and enhances the text's overall appearance. It also reinforces the multicultural focus by reflecting the diversity of the human population.

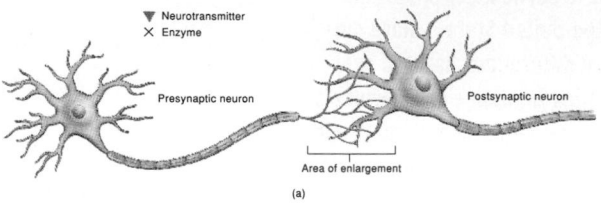

Portion of cell membrane with receptor sites

Natural body chemicals

Drug molecules

Figure 15.1
Receptor Sites
Many psychoactive drugs mimic normal body chemicals and occupy receptor sites on the surface of brain cell membranes intended for the body chemicals. (a) A portion of cell membrane illustrating microscopic receptor sites. (b) Natural body chemicals intended to react with each receptor site; note their complementary shapes. (c) Psychoactive drug molecules; note how the shapes of the drug molecules closely resemble those of the natural body chemicals.

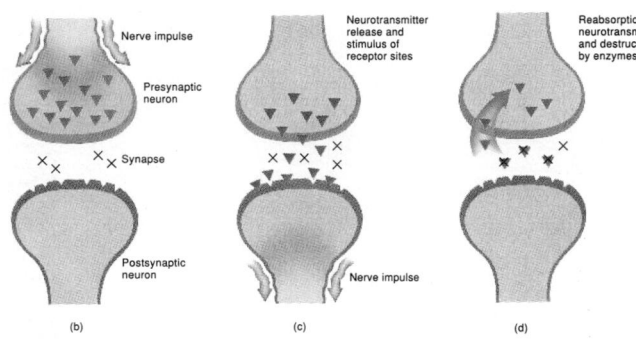

▼ Neurotransmitter
✕ Enzyme

Presynaptic neuron

Postsynaptic neuron

Area of enlargement

(a)

Nerve impulse

Presynaptic neuron

Synapse

Postsynaptic neuron

Neurotransmitter release and stimulus of receptor sites

Reabsorption of neurotransmitter and destruction by enzymes

Nerve impulse

(b) (c) (d)

Figure 15.2
The Synapse
A synapse, the junction between two neurons (nerve cells). When a nerve impulse reaches the end of the first neuron, ...nsmitter substance that simulates an impulse to start down the second neuron. The neu-...estroyed by enzymes (Xs in sketch).

FEATURE 3.1
HUMAN EMOTIONS

If someone asked you how many different emotions a human can feel, how would you answer? Every language contains many words that describe emotions and, in many cases, there are no exact translations from language to language. Here are some words in the English language for common emotions. You may wish to add some of your own to this list.

anger	joy	excitement
contempt	sadness	hostility
distress	anxiety	loneliness
guilt	depression	shame

| boredom | fear | love |
| disgust | interest | surprise |

Each of these emotions can form a continuum of degrees of intensity, such as:

slight bother → annoyance → severe irritation → anger → rage

When potentially destructive feelings are addressed at lower levels of intensity, they are less likely to escalate to more intense levels at which severe physiological changes and/or destructive behaviors occur.

identical situations may react very differently. Some of these differences are thought to be genetically determined, while some are culturally learned.

In recent years, increased emphasis has been placed on the *genetic basis* of human emotions and behavior. Starting from birth, infants respond dif-ferently from one another. Some babies are happy, while others are irritable and cry at the slightest provocation. Studies of adult identical twins, raised separately from birth in different environments, have demonstrated many similarities in their emotional reactions.

Emotions are characterized by overt expression and are usually betrayed by facial expressions and body postures. Often a particular emotion can be induced by assuming its characteristic posture and facial expression.

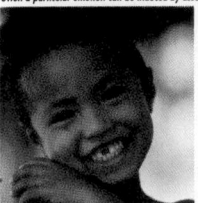
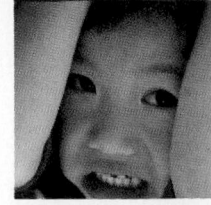
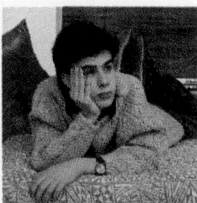
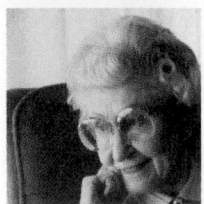
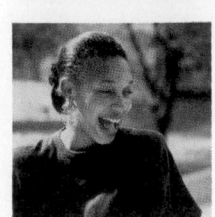
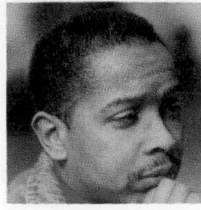

CHAPTER OBJECTIVES

Each chapter opens with a list of learning objectives which help inspire students in setting and reaching their personal health goals. These fall into one of three categories: *knowledge* objectives that cover basic factual learning; *insight* objectives that ask students to extrapolate and apply the material in the chapter to their own lives; and *decision-making* objectives which illustrate the types of informed decisions students should be prepared to make after learning the chapter material.

CHAPTER OBJECTIVES

Upon completion of this chapter you will be able to:

KNOWLEDGE

- Define the terms *ecology, ecosystem,* and *biosphere.*
- List the interrelationship that governs us humans as members of the global community.
- List the six most common kinds of pollutants.
- Define the term *air pollution.*
- Discuss the stratospheric ozone layer and how human activities are affecting it.
- Define the term *solid waste.*
- Name some hazardous wastes.
- Contrast sound and noise.
- Give the present United States and world population totals.
- List five slow-growth countries and five rapid-growth countries.

INSIGHT

- Identify the principles that you might include in an Environmental Bill of Rights.
- Describe ways in which you might be inadvertently affected by lead poisoning.
- Discuss your feelings on the use of nuclear power plants as an energy source.
- Identify your expectations on the number of children you anticipate having and why.
- List some ways in which you can respond responsibly to environmental problems.

DECISION MAKING

- Decide if your community is the ideal place for you to live.
- Identify what you are going to do to improve the quality of the air in the house in which you live.
- Outline steps you plan take to reduce the amount of urban garbage that is being hauled to landfills.
- Outline ways in which you are going to increase the amount of recycling you do.
- Decide how you intend to commit yourself to protecting the health of the environment.

The lifetime of Arthur Ashe was characterized by triumphs over situations in which he faced huge odds. As a youngster, growing up in segregated Richmond, Virginia, he excelled at tennis, a sport that was almost exclusively played by whites. At only 37 years of age, while he was at the top of his professional tennis career, he suffered from the first of several heart attacks. He was able to overcome all of these problems. He could not overcome AIDS, however, at the age of 49, he succumbed to that disease.

The cause of Arthur Ashe's HIV infection was a tainted blood transfusion that he received after his second coronary bypass operation in 1983. Nine years later, in 1992, he stunned people who watched as he announced, under the pressure of a possible newspaper story, that he had AIDS. Yet Arthur Ashe was not the type of person to withdraw or expect pity. Soon after that announcement, he became active in promoting AIDS research and set up an AIDS foundation. He spoke at many gatherings about his disease and about other issues of importance, such as race relations.

Less than one year after announcing that he had AIDS, Arthur Ashe died. Blood supplies are now screened and blood and blood products are tested to ensure that HIV is not transmitted. Sadly, these techniques were not available when Ashe received his transfusion. The world will miss this great man whose graceful style on and off the court was combined with a strong dedication to improving life for others.

Source: Time February 15, 1993, p. 70.

OPENING CASE STUDIES

Each chapter also opens with a new, intriguing case study which highlights contemporary health issues and shows students how the concepts relate to their lives. In-text questions correlate closely to the cases to help stimulate critical thinking about the issues covered, helping students to make informed decisions regarding their own life-styles.

FEATURE BOXES

Special boxed essays in each chapter address high-interest, controversial, and contemporary issues, such as AIDS, the environment, substance abuse, and health care. These encourage students to contemplate the many different factors that affect their personal health.

FEATURE 19.3
HOW HIV IS *NOT* TRANSMITTED

A certain amount of hysteria has surrounded the HIV epidemic, just as it has surrounded every disease epidemic in history. The fact that today's scientific knowledge makes the methods of transmission of HIV much better understood than were the transmission of earlier epidemics such as plague, smallpox, and polio has not eliminated myths and misconceptions regarding HIV transmission. We want to clarify some ways that HIV is *not* acquired:

- HIV is *not* acquired through the air. There is no need to fear working with, attending school with, or other non-sexual contact with infected people.
- HIV is *not* acquired while donating blood. All equipment used to collect blood from donors is perfectly sterile. There is no risk of HIV infection from donating blood.

- HIV is not acquired by eating food that has been cooked or served by an HIV-infected person. Even though virus could theoretically contaminate food if the food handler got cut and bled on the food, the digestive tract is a very poor portal of entry for HIV. There is no known case of someone acquiring HIV in this way.
- HIV is *not* transmitted by mosquito bites. Mosquitoes are effective vectors for some viruses, such as yellow fever, but are not capable of carrying most viruses. For example, there is no mosquito transmission of colds, influenza, polio, rabies, measles, chicken pox, and hepatitis B (which has the same modes of transmission as HIV). Even though some of the places where HIV is most prevalent have plenty of mosquitoes, there has never been a single known case of mosquito-borne HIV.

HIV (see Table 19.2). The most efficient mode of sexual transmission appears to be anal intercourse. The rectal lining is not well suited to withstand the wear and tear of intercourse and abrasions allow entry of HIV. The most likely path of transmission is from the male whose penis is inserted to his sexual partner. Vaginal intercourse has also been documented as a method of transmitting HIV, from either male to female or female to male. The greater risk of transmission, however, is from male to female. Oral sex has not been identified as a major risk factor in studies of either homosexual or heterosexual populations, though there are cases where it has been the method of transmission. It is advisable to avoid oral sex with an infected person or anyone whose HIV status is unknown.[4]

It must be emphasized that not everyone who is infected with HIV will display symptoms. *Even when infected people are not presently experiencing any symptoms, they are capable of infecting others.* Consequently, the potential for the spread of the disease is considerable. One person who is sexually promiscuous or who shares needles could infect many people over a period of years.

FIVE SIGNIFICANT TIME PERIODS

There are five significant time periods related to HIV infection.[5]
They are:

1. The time from when the virus enters the body until it is circulating in the blood in quanti-

ties that make the infection *contagious to others*. This takes only one to three weeks, following which the virus remains contagious to others for the remainder of the infected person's life. We want to emphasize that many people who are capable of infecting others with HIV are totally free of symptoms and appear and feel quite healthy.

2. The time from when the virus enters the body until a *short-term illness* (Stage I HIV infection) develops. This period ranges from one to eight weeks. The illness may be mild and mononucleosis-like (fever, fatigue, and enlarged lymph nodes) or more severe.

3. The time from when the virus enters the body until an *HIV antibody test* (the standard blood test for HIV infection) would become positive. This is usually about two to three months, but may be a year or longer.

4. The time from when the virus enters the body until the onset of any *longer-lasting symptoms*. This period may range from one week to many years, but is often about two years.

5. The time from when the virus enters the body until the development of AIDS (Stage 6 HIV infection). This ranges from 6 months to more than 15 years and averages about 10 years.

TYPICAL PROGRESSION OF HIV INFECTION TO AIDS

Symptoms of Stage 2 to Stage 5 HIV infection include enlarged lymph nodes, loss of appetite,

---

be vaccinated against rubella. Rubella antibodies in the blood, either from vaccination or contact with the disease, indicates an immunity to the disease. Congenital defects can also be caused by a mother drinking alcohol or using drugs such as cocaine during pregnancy.

Congenital heart defects can be treated with medicine or surgery. The surgery is designed to repair the defect as completely as possible. Some congenital heart conditions do not require surgery, but respond to medical treatment. Many congenital heart defects are correctable, and treatment can restore the child to a normal life.

CHECKPOINT

1. List the five major cardiovascular diseases described by the American Heart Association.

2. How do cardiovascular diseases rank as a cause of death in the United States?

3. Describe atherosclerosis and explain what happens to the arteries in this disease.

4. What are the causes and effects of hypertension?

5. Define the terms *myocardial infarction, ischemia, angina pectoris,* and *coronary thrombosis.*

6. List the symptoms of a heart attack.

7. What is a stroke? What is its major cause?

8. Describe arrhythmia, congestive heart failure, and rheumatic heart disease.

RISK FACTORS IN CARDIOVASCULAR DISEASES

The United States Public Health Service has, since 1948, been following the cardiac history of more than 10,000 residents of Framingham, Massachusetts. An intent of the Framingham Heart Study has been to identify risk factors in the incidence of cardiovascular diseases. The study has documented that a person's overall risk of cardiovascular disease is increased as the severity of these factors increases, and that the risk also increases as the number of factors present increases.

Risk factors are grouped into two categories: major risk factors and contributing risk factors. Major risk factors are those definitely associated with a significant increase in the risk of cardiovascular diseases. Contributing factors are those associated with increased risk of cardiovascular disease, but whose significance and prevalence have not yet been precisely determined. Some major risk factors can be changed, others cannot.[21]

MAJOR RISK FACTORS THAT YOU CAN MODIFY

Major risk factors that result from life-style habits that can be modified are cigarette smoking, high blood pressure, high blood lipid levels, and physical inactivity.

Cigarette Smoking

The Surgeon General has identified smoking as the most dangerous cardiovascular disease risk factor

CHECKPOINT QUESTIONS

These in-text review questions appear throughout each chapter, allowing students to assess their comprehension of the material they have just read before they move on to other topics.

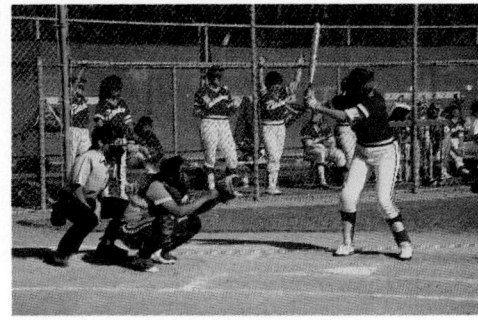

Exercise such as softball, that involves sudden bursts of muscle activity, is an anaerobic activity. In such activities the sudden vigorous activity may momentarily outstrip the ability of the body to maintain the needed supply of oxygen.

cles work they consume oxygen and give off carbon dioxide. Any activity, whether it is sleep or running, depends upon the cardiovascular and respiratory systems. Also referred to as **aerobic capacity**, this consumption of oxygen is the most important of the fitness components.[11]

Aerobic exercise is a method of conditioning the cardiorespiratory system by performing activities that increase the demand by muscles for oxygen over a period of time. This kind of exercise improves the cardiovascular and respiratory systems' capacity to deliver oxygen to and remove carbon dioxide from working muscles. As continuous exercise trains the heart, it is able to pump more blood per beat than the untrained heart. The more strenuous the exercise and the longer it is sustained over time, the higher the body's capacity. Assess your cardiorespiratory endurance by testing yourself according to the Modified Step Test in Feature 11.1.

Improving CRE Through Exercise

There are two types of exercise, aerobic and anaerobic. **Aerobic** (*a-rṓ'bik*), meaning "with oxygen," is exercise using energy that requires oxygen for continuous exertion. **Anaerobic** (*an-ā-er-ṓ'bik*),

meaning "without oxygen," is exercise that uses energy stored by the body for fast bursts of speed.

The energy that cells use is stored in a compound called **adenosine triphosphate (ATP)** (*a-den'ō-sēn trī'fos'fāt*). ATP is found in all cells, particularly muscle cells, and stores energy derived from carbohydrates, fats, and proteins. Cells have only a small reserve of ATP on hand; this is just enough to last for a few seconds of intense activity.[12] Muscle cells have an additional reserve material, which with ATP can supply energy without oxygen for 15–20 seconds. The release of further energy requires a supply of oxygen.

Continuous rigorous exercise lasting more than two minutes, such as jogging, long-distance swimming, bicycling, and cross-country skiing, brings about an aerobic training effect. Because aerobic exercise is rhythmic in nature, using large muscle groups and elevating heart rate for prolonged periods of time, the cardiovascular system is challenged to deliver oxygen to muscles.[13, 14] Muscles produce energy efficiently when oxygen is present. A small amount of ATP can be extracted from glucose stored within the muscle cells, without oxygen, during anaerobic exertion, but oxygen is needed to extract the maximum amount of ATP from glucose.

---

aerobic in the presence of oxygen; such exercise requires oxygen for continuous exertion.

anaerobic without oxygen; such exercise uses energy stored by the body for fast bursts of speed.

adenosine triphosphate (ATP) an enzyme found especially in muscle cells which, when split, releases stored energy.

RUNNING GLOSSARY

Each time a key term is first presented, it is printed in bold-faced type and its definition appears in the bottom margin of that page, as well as in the text's glossary.

SUMMARY

Communicable diseases are caused by microscopic parasites, called pathogens, that invade the body. Pathogens are classified into five major categories: viruses, bacteria, fungi, protozoa, and parasitic worms. Of these, viruses are most difficult to control with medications because their simplicity presents few vulnerabilities for drugs to attack.

The source of a pathogen is called its reservoir. For many diseases this is an asymptomatic human carrier. Pathogens leave an infected host by a specific portal of exit and reach a new host by either direct contact, indirect contact, droplets, common vehicle transmission, airborne transmission, or by a vector such as an insect. The portal of entry is where the pathogen enters its new host. It must enter in an infective dosage large enough to overcome body defenses in order to establish infection.

Following infection, the course of a disease progresses through the symptomless incubation period, the prodromal period of early symptoms, the typical illness period, and the convalescence period. Following recovery, some people remain active carriers of the pathogen. Others become carriers without experiencing symptoms. Even in the absence of symptoms, carriers are able to infect other people.

Nonspecific body defenses, collectively called resistance, include unbroken skin and mucous membranes, respiratory cilia, stomach acid, phagocytic white blood cells, inflammation, and interferons. Highly specific body defenses, collectively called immunity, are stimulated by the presence of an antigen, usually a substance that is foreign to the body.

Specific immune responses are carried out by special white blood cells called T lymphocytes and B lymphocytes. T lymphocytes produce cell-mediated immunity, attacking pathogens and abnormal body cells, and also regulate the function of the B lymphocytes. B lymphocytes release antibodies (immunoglobulins) to circulate with the blood. This is humoral immunity.

Active immunity is produced upon exposure to an antigen, either as part of a pathogen or in a vaccine. Active immunity is slow in developing, but it is long term. Passive immunity is produced by passively receiving preformed antibodies from outside of the body. It is instant, but not long term.

Immune deficiency can result from radiation, chemicals, or viruses, such as HIV (discussed in Chapter 19). Immune deficiency leads to frequent and/or severe infections and increased risk of cancer.

An allergy or hypersensitivity is an immune response against an otherwise harmless substance. Anaphylactic shock is a severe allergic reaction that can be fatal if not treated promptly.

Autoimmune disorders are immune responses against part of your own body. The result is a gradual, progressive degeneration of tissues or organs.

Communicable diseases are prevented through maintaining a healthful life-style, immunization, and public health efforts (education and enforcement of sanitation guidelines). They are treated with antimicrobial drugs such as antibiotics. Drug resistance, however, is reducing the ability of drugs to control many pathogens.

The chapter concluded with a survey of some important communicable diseases. Although communicable diseases are not currently among the top causes of death in the United States, they remain ever-present threats to your health and well-being. Keeping pathogens under control requires ongoing efforts by public health workers and each of us as individuals. *You* must take responsibility for maintaining your own health through practicing healthful living habits and taking advantage of all known precautions, such as getting immunizations, avoiding exposure to contagious pathogens, and obtaining prompt treatment for diseases before serious complications develop.

REFERENCES

1. Stine, G. *Acquired Immune Deficiency Syndrome.* Englewood Cliffs, NJ: Prentice-Hall, 1993.
2. Talaro, K., and Talaro, A. *Foundations in Microbiology.* Dubuque, IA: Wm. C. Brown, 1993.
3. Tortora, G., Funke, B., and Case, C. *Microbiology,* 4th ed. Redwood City, CA: Benjamin/Cummings, 1992.
4. Ibid.
5. Ibid.
6. Benjamini, E., and Leskowitz, S. *Immunology: A Short Course,* 2nd ed. New York: Wiley-Liss, 1991.
7. Ibid.

CHAPTER SUMMARIES

Each chapter concludes with a brief summary of important concepts which students can use to test their understanding of the chapter material.

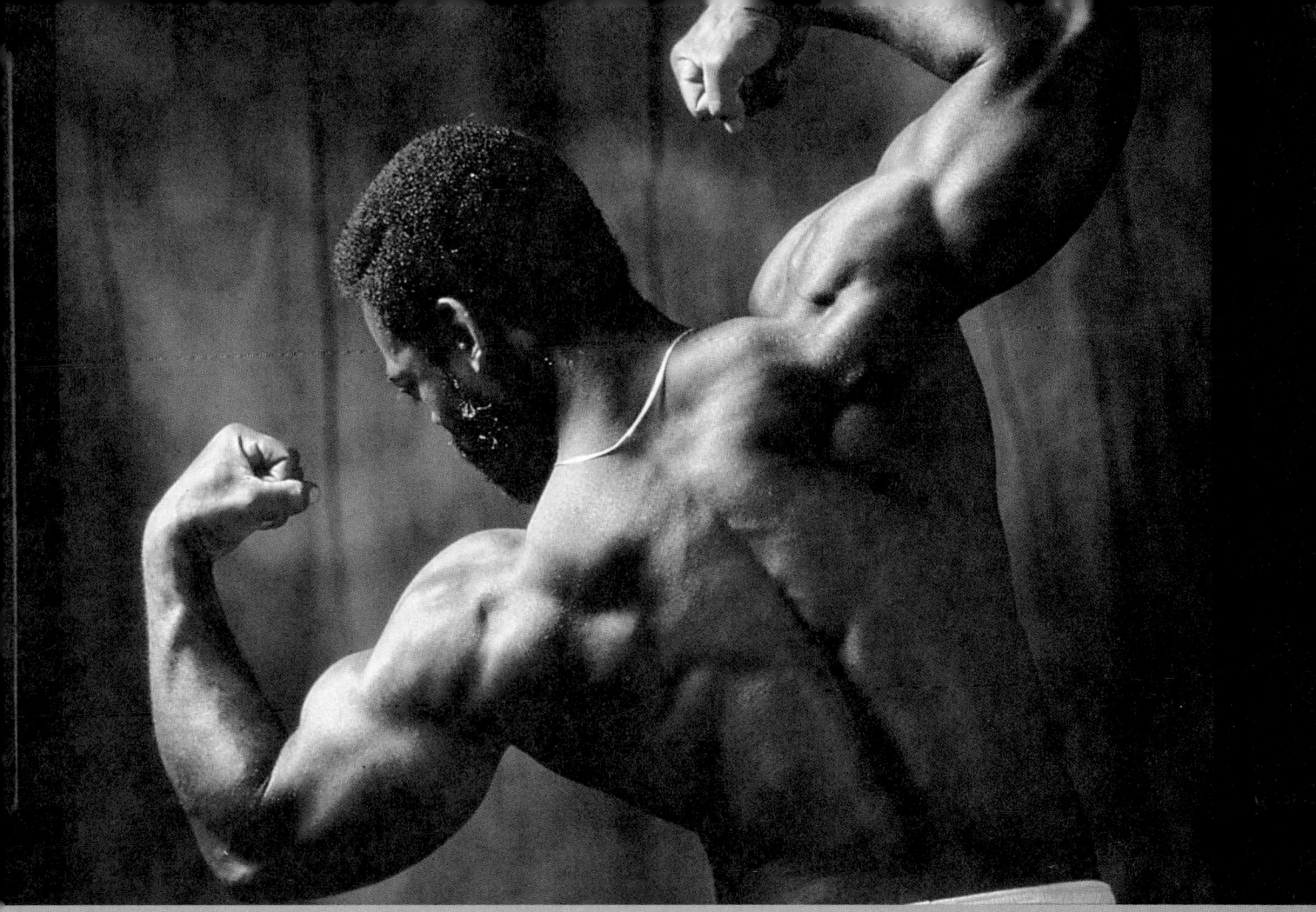

ONE

INTRODUCTION TO WELLNESS

Living Well: Health in Your Hands has been written to help and encourage you to enjoy a long life at a high level of wellness. It reflects the philosophy that life can be a joyful adventure for those who apply the principles of healthful living. There are several themes in this book:

- Developing healthful habits requires factual knowledge, self-knowledge (insight), and the motivation to make decisions to improve one's life-style. Thus, each chapter opens with chapter objectives for knowledge, insight, and decision making.

- The well-being of the mind, body, and spirit are interdependent, meaning that each affects the others. A problem with any one of them will have an impact on the others.

- Each individual is personally responsible for his or her own health-related behavior. This is why this book is subtitled "Health in Your Hands."

- Different cultures have different concepts of health and illness that influence how they define healthful behavior.

- Effective communication contributes to wellness in many ways, such as by improving our relationships and self-esteem, and our effectiveness as health care consumers.

Chapter 1 of *Living Well* introduces us to wellness, cultural diversity, health research, and how to make and keep the commitment to a wellness life-style. Chapter 2 introduces the principles of effective communication as they apply to the wellness life-style. Effective communication relates to every topic discussed in this book.

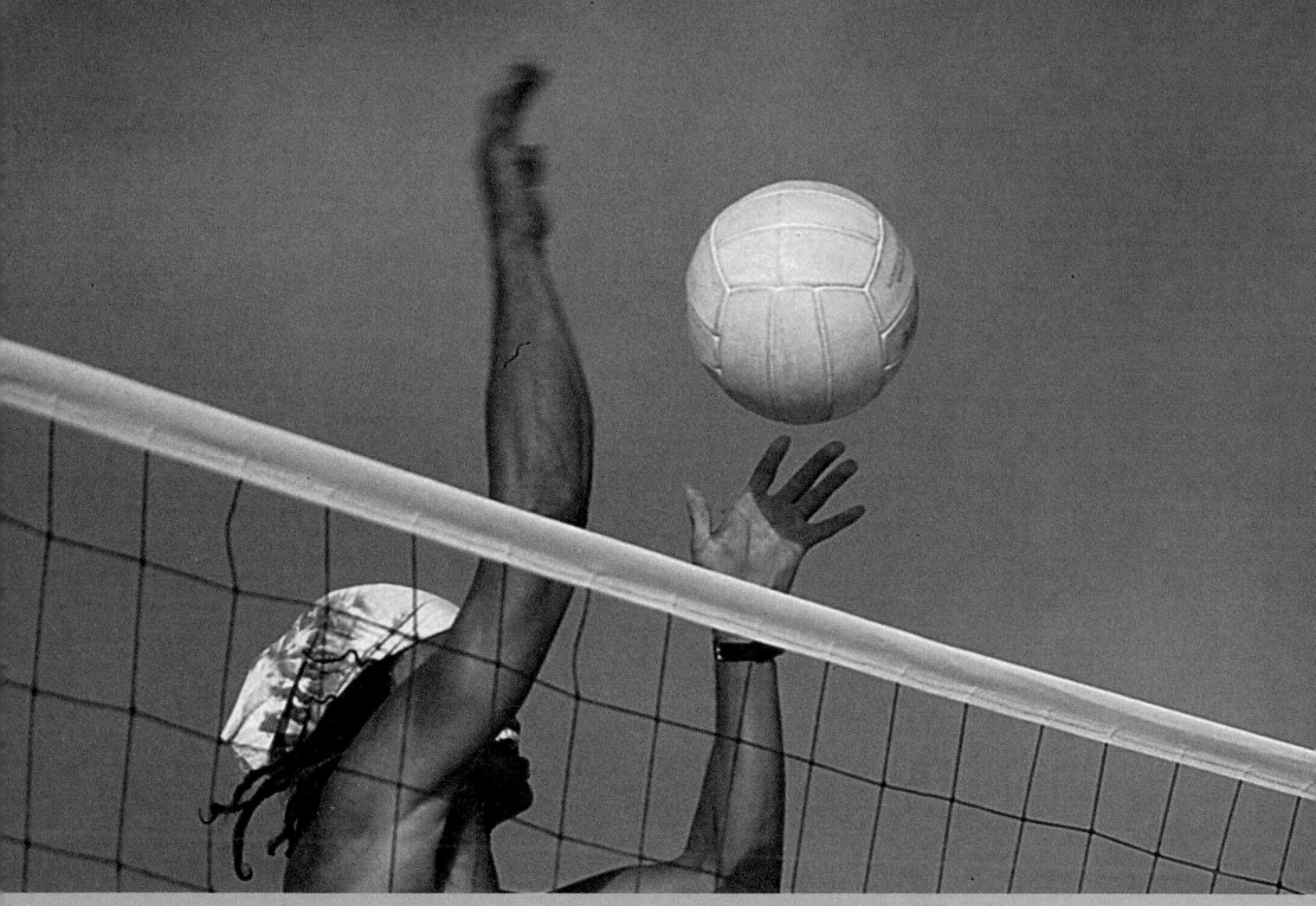

1
HEALTH AND WELLNESS

KNOWLEDGE

- Explain why in the multicultural United States there can be no single definition of health that is acceptable to everyone.
- Explain how the concept of wellness goes beyond conventional definitions of health.
- Explain the attitudes that promote wellness.
- Explain the traditional views of health and illness of Native Americans, Chinese Americans, African Americans, European Americans, and Hispanic Americans.
- List the components of wellness and explain how each affects wellness.
- Explain the holistic view of wellness.
- Judge the validity of the new health research reported in the media.

INSIGHT

- Explain how your ethnic background has influenced your concepts of health and illness.
- Explain how your attitudes have worked for or against your wellness.
- Identify where you currently fit on the continuum of wellness.

DECISION MAKING

- Apply new, more positive attitudes in your daily life.
- Integrate the scientific view of health and illness with your cultural views.
- Commit to a wellness life-style and keep that commitment.

I n spite of—or possibly because of—his tremendously busy schedule and the immense pressures he faces, in his daily activities President Bill Clinton reflects an understanding of the importance of health and wellness. In fact, President Clinton's health-promoting habits have been part of his life for many years. While at Yale in 1971, he followed the advice of his future wife, Hillary Rodham, and began running. He has been running for more than 20 years. With a family history of heart disease and a tendency toward overweight, he recognized that he should make regular exercise a priority in his life. Mr. Clinton has also revealed that his daily jog is an important stress reducer and a time to get away and think.

He knows that he must also watch his diet. It is no secret that Bill Clinton has a tendency to gain weight and has a taste for high-calorie foods, such as fast foods, doughnuts, and chocolate chip cookies. However, at the White House, he and his family have made changes in the type of foods served and the way they are prepared. There is an emphasis on lowering fat and calories and including more fruit and vegetables. Mr. Clinton could probably have not chosen a better vegetable—broccoli—to be his favorite; it is an excellent source of Vitamin A, Vitamin C, and fiber. There are aspects of President Clinton's personal life other than diet and exercise that reflect his dedication to a wellness life-style. He has a strong family life and always sets aside time to spend with his wife and daughter.

Clinton's original choice for Surgeon General, Jocyelyn Elders, reflects his understanding of the importance of health promotion. Dr. Elders believes that the emphasis in health care should be on "keeping Americans healthy rather than worrying about how to care for them once they get sick." Both Clinton and Elders are applauded by a variety of groups for their views on health promotion and education.

Others, though, find Dr. Elders to be too outspoken and offensive in her ideas. In late 1994, she was forced to resign because of a statement about masturbation and sexuality education. This political controversy, however, does not change the emphasis on health education and disease prevention that Clinton supports as a component of health care reform.

The evidence continues to mount regarding the impact a health-promoting life-style can have, not only on the quantity of life but also on the quality of life. Obviously, President Bill Clinton realizes how important it is to incorporate health-promoting behaviors into his daily life and those of the American people.

■   ■   ■

Welcome to your college health course. Regardless of your major, this will be the most valuable college course you will ever take. It will help you achieve high-level *wellness,* the quality of physical, mental, social, and spiritual well-being that you need to find success in college and to fulfill your personal and career goals.

Throughout this book you will be reading about ways in which to practice wellness. Wellness affects every aspect of your life, including career success and social and personal fulfillment. But what is wellness and how can you begin to enjoy it?

DEFINITIONS OF HEALTH AND WELLNESS

Health is a cultural concept, and it is defined differently in different cultures. Thus, the word *health* means different things to different people. To most people, and as defined in many dictionaries, it means the absence of illness. This definition dates back to before the twelfth century A.D., when lives were short and people were fortunate to be free of disease. Infectious diseases such as smallpox, tuberculosis, malaria, and plague were rampant, and their prevention was largely beyond the individual's control. In some parts of Africa, Latin America, and Asia such is the situation even today.

Another historic definition of health was having a long life. This, too, made sense when the average life expectancy was about 40 years, which was the case into the twentieth century. But today we have higher expectations for the quality of our lives and just being alive isn't equated with health.

The definition of health as merely the absence of disease or having a long life is inadequate in most nations today. Now you can aspire to a higher level of well-being than simply the absence of disease. A revised view of health was first formally defined by the World Health Organization back in the 1940s. At that time, vaccines, antibiotics, and improved sanitation were reducing the threat of many diseases. The

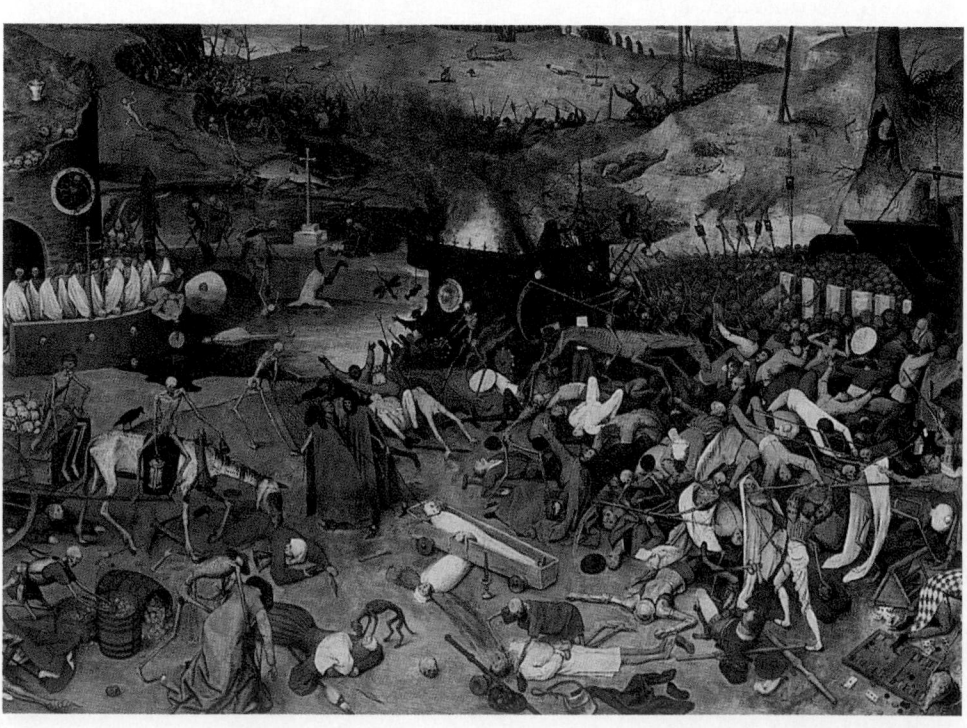

During the fourteenth century, the plague destroyed about one-fourth of the total population of Europe. When such diseases raged uncontrolled, being free of disease was a far-reaching goal. As we have gained control over many diseases, our definition of health has evolved to encompass more than just the absence of disease.

FEATURE 1.1

HOW TO ACHIEVE WELLNESS

Your attitudes and outlook on life profoundly influence your health and wellness. If you adopt healthful attitudes, you can expect to enjoy an enhanced level of physical, emotional, and spiritual well-being. Some of these attitudes include the following:

- The three C's:

  1. Develop a feeling of being in *control* of your own life and destiny (see p. 12). The feeling of having no control eliminates any motivation or sense of personal responsibility for healthful living. It is also highly stressful to feel that your life is not in your hands.

  2. Feel a sense of personal *commitment* to what you are doing in life. Believing in the worth of what you do enhances self-esteem, which contributes to wellness in itself and is essential for motivating healthful behavior.

  3. Have the *courage* to face new challenges in life. You live in an ever-changing world in which people who view changes as new opportunities thrive. Also, many health-promoting behaviors, such as developing intimate relationships, require some risk-taking.

- Assume personal responsibility for the quality of your own health. Recognize that your life-style greatly influences your level of wellness.

- Maintain a positive, optimistic view of life. Love life and aspire to all of the rewards that it offers. Studies have shown that optimistic people enjoy better health than pessimists.[a]

- Be tolerant of imperfection in yourself and in others. Demanding perfection of yourself means setting an impossible goal, dooming yourself to failure. Demanding perfection of others creates difficulties in relationships.

- Be other-centered, rather than self-centered. Self-centered people tend to focus their attention on every minor discomfort. They risk becoming handicapped by minor problems other people just ignore.

- Hold the expectation of health, rather than of illness. Positive expectations tend to be self-fulfilling and negative expectations are equally self-fulfilling.

[a]Peterson, C., and Bossio, L. "Healthy Attitudes: Optimism, Hope, and Control." In D. Goleman and J. Gurin (eds.), *Mind Body Medicine.* Yonkers, NY: Consumer Reports Books, 1993.

World Health Organization's constitution thus defines **health** as a state of complete *physical, mental, and social well-being,* and not merely the absence of disease. This definition is also now viewed by many people as being inadequate.

The definition of health has evolved further. Today we think of health in terms of **wellness,** which is an ongoing, *active process,* a life-style that emphasizes such health-promoting behaviors as following a healthful diet, avoiding harmful substances, enjoying regular exercise, and cultivating self-esteem (Feature 1.1). Wellness means taking charge of your own health and well-being.

Wellness means reducing the risk of premature death or disability. It means making full use of

physical and mental abilities and preserving these abilities through healthful living habits and accident prevention. Wellness is not a substitute for medical care when it is needed. It does not mean rejecting the services of physicians and other health care providers in favor of fad diets and unproven remedies. Wellness does, however, reduce dependency on physicians by eliminating much of the need for their services.

The goal of wellness is to live a long, healthy, active, and rewarding life. All you need is the *desire* to do so, the *belief* that you have considerable control over your life, and the factual *information* on which to act. This book is intended to help provide that desire, belief, and information.

health as defined by the World Health Organization, a state of complete physical, mental, and social well-being.

wellness a life-style that emphasizes such health-promoting behaviors as eating a healthful diet, avoiding harmful substances, enjoying regular exercise, and cultivating self-esteem.

CHECKPOINT

1. What is an old definition of health and why is it inadequate today?

2. What is wellness?

3. Why do we say that wellness is an ongoing process?

HEALTH AND CULTURAL DIVERSITY

Culture is all of the customs, beliefs, values, knowledge, and skills that are shared by a specific group of people. The United States is a nation of many cultures. America's early immigrants were mostly from Europe. As recently as 1960, less than 15 percent of the U.S. population were of anything other than European ancestry. At that time, prevailing American attitudes toward health quite naturally reflected the European influence. Health was defined and health care delivery systems were designed mainly by people of European background and reflected European concepts of health and illness. Health care providers tended to reject other approaches to health as being backward and unscientific.[1]

Since 1960, the non-European population in the United States has more than tripled, reaching 64.3 million people by 1992 (see Table 1.1). If these 64.3 million people lived in an independent country, it would be the thirteenth largest in the world, more populous than Great Britain, France, Italy, or Spain. By 2050 the non-European ethnic groups will represent almost half of the U.S. population.[2]

Health and *illness* mean different things to people of different ethnic groups. Even health care providers (physicians, nurses, etc.) can be viewed as a separate group with their own culture. Their professional socialization teaches them a set of beliefs, practices, likes, dislikes, and rituals that influence how they relate to their clients. They tend to view health and illness in strictly scientific terms, with little emphasis given to supernatural or spiritual issues. They expect their patients to follow the orders given them. They are likely to feel some hostility toward patients whose culture gives them a different view of health and illness.[3]

Throughout this text we will try to incorporate the health views and concerns of the nation's many ethnic groups. Let's start by briefly surveying some meanings of health to several groups. *Please understand that space limitations require us to generalize for each group but by no means do we wish to stereotype or to imply that all members of a group hold certain beliefs or follow certain practices.* Also, we know that by discussing a few specific ethnic groups, we risk offending many others by their omission. If your ethnic group is not included it would be quite productive for you to interview several older members of your group to find out what health beliefs prevail and how these beliefs may have influenced your own views of health, illness, and wellness. Finally, we hope that we do not seem to advocate the European ways of looking at health and illness as the standard by which other cultures should be judged. That is not our intention.

Table 1.1
U.S. Population by Race and Ethnicity, 1992

Group	Number	Percent
Total U.S. Population	254,922,000	100
Non-Hispanic		
White	190,604,000	75
African American	30,372,000	12
Asian/Pacific Islander	7,937,000	3
Native American	1,873,000	1
Hispanic[a]	24,136,000	9

[a]Hispanic origin is considered an ethnic identity rather than a race. Hispanic people list their race as white (about half of Hispanics), black (3 percent), Asian (1 percent), Native American (1 percent), and "other" (43 percent).

Source: U.S. Bureau of the Census, Current Population Reports, P-25, No. 1090 (1992).

culture all of the customs, beliefs, values, knowledge, and skills that are shared by a specific group of people.

NATIVE AMERICANS

At the time Europeans "discovered" North America the continent was already populated by over 200 nations of Native Americans, each with its own well-developed society and culture. After the native populations had been weakened by diseases introduced by the Europeans and had been disrupted and demoralized by the intrusions of the better-armed Europeans, treaties were signed forcing the Native Americans to give up most of the continent to the Europeans and establishing "reservations" for Native Americans, primarily in the western portion of the continent. Today about half of the country's Native Americans live on reservations or in rural areas while about half live in cities.

Traditional health beliefs varied among the nations as does the degree to which those beliefs are still followed by contemporary Native Ameri-

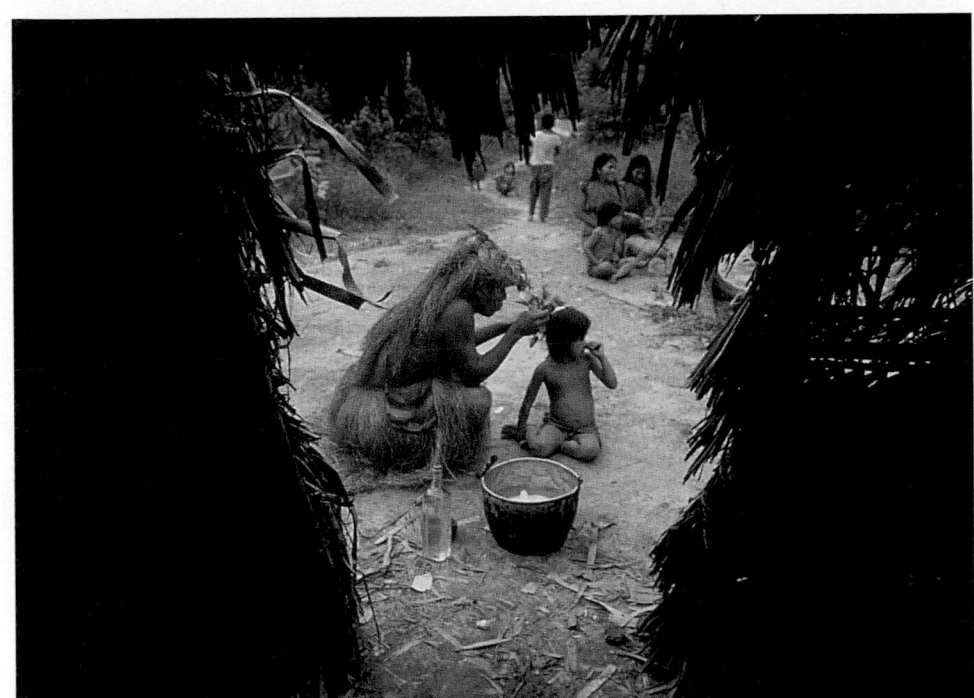

Health and illness mean different things to people of different cultures. Different concepts of illness lead to different forms of healing.

cans. To generalize somewhat, the traditional Native American belief about health emphasizes living in harmony with nature. In order to maintain health, the Native American must maintain his or her relationship with nature. The forced movement of Native Americans from their historical home areas often made this difficult or impossible.

Many Native Americans believe that there is a reason for every illness, that illness is a price to be paid for something that happened in the past or that will happen in the future. Illness is something that *must be*. Illness may be viewed as the best possible price to be paid for past or future events. Illness is not thought to result from infection by microbes or by physiological disorders.[4] Motivating healthful behavior, as healthful behavior is defined by scientific medicine, is difficult for those who hold this point of view.

Some Native American nations associate illness with evil spirits. The evil spirit responsible for a certain illness is identified by the "medicine man," and the remedy for the illness involves treating the evil spirit. Other causes of illness include displeasing holy people, annoying nature, disturbing plant or animal life, breaking a taboo, misusing a sacred ceremony, or suffering the effects of witches.[5] Again, people holding these beliefs will have little motivation to engage in what others would call healthful behavior.

Native Americans even today often favor traditional healers and remedies over physicians and hospitals. The medicine man determines the spiritual cause of an illness by using methods such as meditation, stargazing, chanting, and listening for sounds. Treatments then prescribed can include chanting, ceremonies to rid the sick person of evil spirits, and a wide range of herbal remedies.

Native Americans often avoid the services of physicians and hospitals because physicians tend to interpret and treat illness differently, are perceived as being disrespectful, and are thought to pry too much. The client prefers the medicine man's way of deducing or divining the problem over the physician's asking many personal questions.[6]

CHINESE AMERICANS

Traditional Chinese medicine views health as a state of spiritual and physical harmony with nature. This **holistic** concept (the philosophy that people function as complete units that cannot be reduced to the sum of their parts) of health has two main components.[7] These concepts, although thousands

....

holistic relating to the philosophy that people function as complete units that cannot be reduced to the sum of their parts.

of years old in Chinese medicine, have been largely ignored in American medicine until recent years. They are as follows:

1. The human body is recognized as functioning as a unit. A diseased condition of one organ is considered in conjunction with the functioning of all the organs and tissues of the entire body.

2. Special attention is given to the integration of the human body with the external environment. The development of illness is considered in relation with geographic, social, and other environmental factors.

Chinese medicine incorporates the theory of yin and yang, two universal forces that are in opposition yet in unison. Their balance affects everything in the universe. Traditional Chinese medicine defines health as a balance between yin and yang. The attraction between them creates an energy known as *qi* (pronounced *chee*), which is similar to the Western concept of vitality or life force. *Qi* flows to all parts of the body through 14 major *meridians,* theoretical channels that run along the surface of the body and branch into its interior. The meridians, which do not correspond to nerves or any known anatomical structures, are important in acupuncture, discussed in the following.[8]

When yin and yang are balanced, the person lives in peaceful interaction with the mind and body in proper order. Disease is seen as being caused by an upset in the balance of yin and yang, causing an excess or deficiency of *qi* in some part of the body. Heat, cold, wind, fire, dampness, dryness, emotional factors, diet, and sexual and physical activity are all thought to affect the balance of yin and yang.

Disease is diagnosed by inspection of the body and by feeling the pulse in six different places on each wrist. Each pulse point is specifically related to certain organs and there are over 15 possible types of pulses at each site, each associated with specific conditions such as pregnancy or impending death.

Acupuncture, a well-known healing and pain relief method of Chinese origin, is gaining acceptance and popularity in the United States. The body is punctured with thin metal needles at specific points on or near the meridians to treat specific symptoms. The Chinese view this treatment as a way to restore the balance of yin and yang. Western research reveals that acupuncture causes release of endorphins (natural pain relievers; discussed in Chapter 15) and other measurable physiological changes.[9] Herbal remedies are also important in Chinese medicine, with a wide range of herbs used to combat or prevent specific conditions (see Feature 1.2).

Chinese people sometimes have difficulty accepting American health care practices. They may feel that too many diagnostic tests are performed and take special exception to the frequent

---

FEATURE 1.2

TOXIC REACTIONS FROM HERBAL PRODUCTS

In North America, Chinese herbal products are widely available as nonprescription remedies for a variety of ailments. At least 3 percent of the total U.S. population and higher percentages of people within many ethnic groups, such as African Americans, Asian Americans, and Hispanic Americans, make use of herbal remedies. Many consumers falsely assume that because herbs are "natural" products they will always be safe to use. Some of these remedies are in fact both safe and effective, but some are ineffective and/or toxic. Because the marketers of herbal products maintain that these products are dietary supplements rather than drugs, they generally are not subject to standard testing for safety and effectiveness.

Sometimes problems arise from the use of herbal products. In 1993, six cases of life-threatening illness were reported as resulting from use of the traditional Chinese herbal product Jin Bu Huan, sold in health food stores and herbal shops as a sedative and pain reliever. Three children developed severe respiratory depression and slow pulse; three adults developed severe liver damage. All recovered after the use of Jin Bu Huan was discontinued. Chemical analysis of the Jin Bu Huan product showed it to be mislabeled both in the identity and the percentage of its active ingredient.

If you choose to try herbal remedies, be alert for any new symptom that may be caused by the herbal product. You will want to discontinue use of the product immediately if that occurs. If you seek medical attention be sure to mention your use of the herbal product and take a sample to be analyzed if possible. Inaccurate labeling of herbal products can impede the proper treatment of adverse reactions until the true identity of the product is known.

Source: Centers for Disease Control and Prevention. "Jin Bu Huan Toxicity in Adults—Los Angeles, 1993." *Morbidity and Mortality Weekly Report,* Vol. 42, No. 47, December 3, 1993.

blood tests. Blood is seen as the source of life for the entire body and some Chinese people believe that it is not regenerated. They also believe that a good physician should be able to make a diagnosis simply by examining a person. Believing that it is important to die with their bodies intact, many Chinese refuse to undergo surgery.[10]

AFRICAN AMERICANS

The majority of black people living in the United States trace their ancestry to Africans brought here as slaves between 1619 and 1860. Smaller numbers have voluntarily immigrated from African, Caribbean, and other nations. Current African American health practices blend African traditions with those of the whites and Native Americans among whom they have lived for so long.

In Africa, life is viewed as a process rather than a state. The nature of a person is viewed in terms of energy rather than matter. All things, whether living or dead, are believed to influence each other. Health is a state of harmony with nature; illness a state of disharmony. Death is described as passing from one realm of life to another, better realm. These health traditions do not separate the mind, body, and spirit.[11]

Illness (disharmony with nature) is attributed to a number of causes, including demons and evil spirits. Some African Americans continue health practices derived from ancient beliefs in voodoo (hoodoo). Illness or bad luck is believed to result from the placing of a *fix, hex,* or *spell* by one person onto another. Various charms, symbols, oils, and powders, collectively called *gris-gris* (pronounced *gree-gree*) are used to ensure luck and remove hexes.

The most common method of treating illness is prayer. Many African Americans believe in the healing powers of religion and in the power of special faith healers within their community. Also, many folk remedies using everyday items and substances, such as turpentine, herbs, and garlic, are popular.

There is often a reluctance to visit physicians and hospitals until symptoms are advanced and severe. This has been attributed to low income levels, lack of insurance, tendency to self-treat illness, and the feeling that receiving health care will be a degrading and humiliating experience.[12] A health care provider may not intend to be insulting, but

his or her impersonal treatment, actions, or words may be interpreted as being disrespectful.

Many African Americans are practicing Muslims, who may have strict health practices. Emphasis is placed on cleanliness. An individual is purified by sharing his or her wealth with those who are in need. Dietary restrictions prohibit pork products and beans. Each year there is one month of fasting, Ramadan. No food is consumed between dawn and sunset and other restrictions apply. Most Muslims avoid any use of alcohol because of the belief that it dulls the senses and causes illness.

EUROPEAN AMERICANS

The non-Hispanic, European American population is far from uniform in its origins and culture. It includes a mixture of people with roots in such diverse nations as Germany, Italy, Great Britain, Ireland, Austria, Hungary, Poland, Russia and indirectly from Europe by way of Canada and South America.

With such diversity, we can only generalize about the health beliefs of European Americans. In general, there is acceptance of the "scientific" view of health and illness. Illness results from either infection by pathogens (germs) or by degenerative processes within the body itself. Health is maintained by combating pathogens through measures such as proper sanitation and immunization. The importance of good diet, exercise, and other healthful behaviors is accepted, but such behaviors are not always practiced. Most European Americans place little emphasis on spiritual forces as causes of health or illness, but many will pray for supernatural intervention when they are ill.

European Americans use home remedies, but also readily turn to physicians and hospitals when they are ill. Some have a high degree of expectation that the physician will be able to restore their health and may become indignant when this does not occur.

HISPANIC AMERICANS

Hispanic is a rather broad term covering people of Mexican, Puerto Rican, Central and South American, Cuban, Spanish, and other origins. As indicated in Table 1.1, Hispanic people can be of any race.

As is true with African Americans, Asian Americans, and European Americans, the specific health beliefs and practices of Hispanic people vary somewhat by their country of origin. Some Hispanic people view health as purely a matter of luck and thus tend to take a rather passive role in maintaining their own health. Some believe that good health is a reward from God for good behavior and try to maintain their health by pleasing God rather than by engaging in what scientists might consider to be healthful behavior. Illness is prevented by good behavior, prayer, wearing religious medals, and keeping religious items in the home. Still other Hispanic people view health as a matter of balance within one's body. Foods consumed together, for example, may be carefully balanced in terms of hot and cold, wet and dry, and sweet and salty.[13]

Folk healers, called *curanderos,* are a part of many Hispanic cultures. A *curandero* is a holistic healer who has received the ability to heal in one of three ways. Some are "born to heal," some learn by apprenticeship, and some receive a supernatural "call" to begin healing. Treatments involve herbs and massage and also include many religious elements such as penance, confession, and lighting candles. A close personal relationship develops between the client and the *curandero.* Many Hispanic people prefer to visit a *curandero* rather than a physician because communication with a Spanish-speaking *curandero* is easier than with an English-speaking physician, the cost is lower, the experience is more comfortable and personal, and such visits are more convenient.

C H E C K P O I N T

1. What is culture?

2. How can cultural beliefs influence health practices?

3. What is the traditional view of health held by Native Americans, Chinese Americans, African Americans, European Americans, and Hispanic Americans? How would those members of each group who hold the traditional view of health act to maintain their own health?

COMPONENTS OF WELLNESS

Social, physical, intellectual, career, emotional, and spiritual factors and *personal health habits* all play a part in achieving high-level wellness. Each of these components of wellness will be examined in this book.

SOCIAL COMPONENTS OF WELLNESS

Humans are social beings and our social structure influences our wellness in many ways. A society promotes high-level wellness when it encourages and facilitates effective social interaction, provides adequate opportunities for **self-actualization** (making full use of one's abilities), and ensures adequate housing, education, and health care.

Rewarding relationships are essential to wellness.[14] Each of us must work to develop effective ways of relating to other people. We need to enhance and nurture our capacity to enjoy mature, mutually-rewarding, intimate relationships. We must also be assertive enough to expect mutual respect of our rights and needs, and accept nothing less.

CULTURAL COMPONENTS OF WELLNESS

Culture, as previously defined, is all of the customs, beliefs, values, knowledge, and skills that are shared by a specific group of people. As discussed earlier in this chapter, some members of some ethnic groups believe that health and illness are results of external forces rather than one's own physiology or behavior. For these people, "healthful behavior" might mean praying or taking care not to offend nature or spirits rather than choosing nutritious foods or exercising regularly.

PHYSICAL COMPONENTS OF WELLNESS

Physical factors influence wellness on a very basic level. Some examples of physical factors are heredity, the healthfulness of our environment, regular exercise, and the quality of our nutrition.

New research is placing increased significance on the genetic basis of human health. Heredity is now thought to influence almost every aspect of our physical and mental health. This does not excuse us from taking responsibility for our own health. On the contrary, knowing that we may have inherited a tendency to some problem, such as alcoholism or diabetes, increases our responsibility to act in ways that minimize the possibility of that problem actually developing.

....

self-actualization making full use of one's abilities.

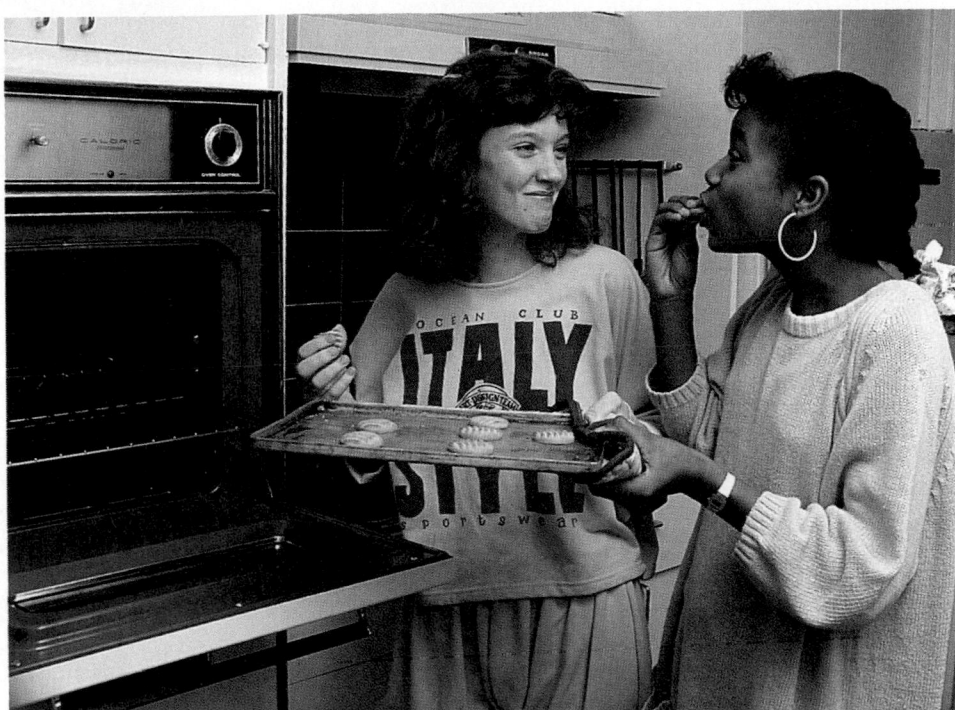

Rewarding relationships are essential to wellness. Humans are social beings and depend on each other for some of their need fulfillment.

Our physical environment also influences wellness. Even the most healthful living habits cannot entirely compensate for the impact of polluted air and water and other harmful environmental forces. Each of us is responsible for reducing our own adverse impact upon the environment and encouraging our friends and the nation's politicians and corporations to show concern and take active steps toward maintaining a healthful environment.

INTELLECTUAL COMPONENTS OF WELLNESS

How can we behave healthfully if we don't know which behaviors are healthful? Though knowledge alone does not motivate healthful behavior, knowing the factual basis for healthful behavior does help us to make healthful choices. One of the roles of this book is to provide this knowledge.

CAREER COMPONENTS OF WELLNESS

One's career can have a great impact on his or her wellness. Rewarding work under good working conditions can build self-esteem and contribute to self-actualization, as well as providing the more obvious rewards of income and security. Poor working conditions, or a career that is not suited for the individual, can be stressful, degrading, de-

pressing, and generally damaging to all aspects of health.

EMOTIONAL COMPONENTS OF WELLNESS

Even though our personalities are genetically and environmentally influenced, each of us has the potential to deal with life situations in a variety of ways. Whether we learn how to cope with life effectively or try to avoid dealing with life by abusing alcohol or other drugs is ultimately our own responsibility.

Certain attitudes promote wellness.[15, 16] Prominent among these are the feeling of being in control of your life (but not expecting to have total control of all circumstances at all times), maintaining a generally positive outlook on life, and having the expectation of good health.

SPIRITUAL COMPONENTS OF WELLNESS

Whether or not you hold or practice any religious beliefs, spirituality is an important component of wellness.[17] It involves seeing yourself as a part of a larger "scheme of things," having a sense of a purpose on earth, and feeling concern for the well-being of other people.

Figure 1.1

A Continuum of Health and Wellness

Levels of health may fall anywhere along a continuum ranging from death at one extreme to high-level wellness at the other. Note that a decline in health, as represented by one step on this scale, would take you from (a) average health to illness, while in (b), a similar decline from a state of high-level wellness would not result in illness. This is only one of many benefits of high-level wellness.

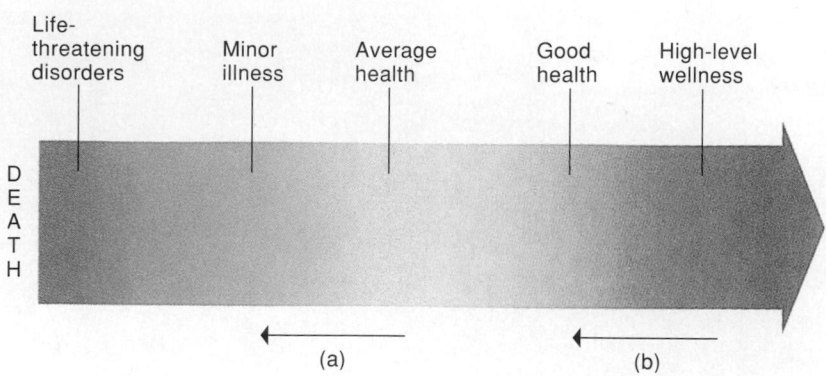

CHECKPOINT

1. What is self-actualization?

2. Give an example of how each type of component—social, cultural, physical, intellectual, career, emotional, and spiritual—is part of wellness.

CONTROL AND WELLNESS

Hundreds of studies have shown that having a sense of being in control over your life is beneficial to your health.[18] The phrase **locus of control** means one's sense of where the control over one's life lies. An **internal locus of control** means having the feeling of being in control of your own life, while an **external locus of control** means believing that your life is under the control of other people or powers.

The benefits of an internal locus of control fall into at least two categories. First, having the feeling of being in control of your own life is immensely rewarding in and of itself. Second, and especially important, is the fact that there can be little motivation to make healthful behavior choices if you believe that your health is controlled by people or forces outside of yourself and beyond your control. As we have mentioned, this concept creates a dilemma for those who seek to motivate more healthful

....

locus of control one's sense of where the control over one's life lies.

internal locus of control having the feeling of being in control of your own life.

external locus of control believing that your life is under the control of other people or powers.

behavior among members of ethnic groups that view health as not being subject to direct individual control.

LEVELS OF WELLNESS

Levels of health and wellness fall along a **continuum** (*kun-tin'ū-um*) (a progression of infinite degrees of some characteristic between two extremes) ranging from high-level wellness down through good health, average health, minor illness, life-threatening disorders, and eventually, to death. Note that the wellness side of the continuum (Figure 1.1) is open-ended. Throughout your entire life you can continue to grow, develop, and achieve ever-higher levels of wellness.

Every chapter of this book will include a health behavior and/or attitude assessment called In Your Hands. The first of these, General Health Behavior and Attitude Assessment, is general in scope. Take a moment to complete it at this time. Those in the following chapters will be more specific.

CHECKPOINT

1. What are some benefits of having an internal locus of control?

2. What is a continuum?

THE STATUS OF AMERICA'S HEALTH

Where does the average American fall along the continuum of wellness? While recent years have

....

continuum a progression of infinite degrees of some characteristic between two extremes.

IN YOUR HANDS

A GENERAL HEALTH BEHAVIOR AND ATTITUDE ASSESSMENT

Health behavior inventories called In Your Hands will appear in each chapter of this book. These inventories will help you to identify areas in which your health behaviors might need improvement. This first inventory is quite general; the remaining inventories will deal with the specific topics of each chapter.

NOTE:

Questions 1 and 2 on this assessment reflect European American views of health. They may not be valid for people in cultures holding other views on health. An alternate scoring for those who choose to skip the first two questions will be presented.

Circle the number of points (to the right of each entry) that represents each of your responses.

1. To what extent do you believe that the quality of your health is under your own control?

not at all	0
to a slight degree	3
somewhat	5
considerably	10

2. Which most closely fits your definition of wellness?

absence of illness	3
having a long life	3
enough energy to get through the day	5
a state of complete physical, mental, and social well-being	7
a life-style that emphasizes health-promoting behaviors	10

3. How many people in your life can you go to with any kind of a problem and feel assured of a supportive response? _____ × 3 points each =

4. How often do you feel that there is just too much stress in your life?

never	10
seldom	7
sometimes	5
often	3
usually	0

5. How comfortable do you feel with your sexuality?

completely	10
mostly	7
somewhat	5
not very	3
very uncomfortable	0

6. If you are currently sexually active, how consistently do you use a birth-control method?

always, no exceptions	10
usually	7
sometimes	5
seldom	3
never	0

7. To what extent do you either practice sexual abstinence or follow the safer-sex guidelines?

always, no exceptions	10
usually	7
sometimes	5
seldom	3
never	0

8. How many servings of fruits and vegetables do you consume on an average day?

7 or more	10
5 or 6	7
3 or 4	5
1 or 2	3
none	0

9. How does your weight compare to the ideal for your height and sex?

more than 30 percent over	0
21 to 30 percent over	3
11 to 20 percent over	6
within 10 percent	10
11 to 20 percent under	6
21 to 30 percent under	3
more than 30 percent under	0

10. How many days a week do you exercise vigorously for at least 20 consecutive minutes?

3 days or more	10
1 or 2 days	5
none	0

11. How comfortable do you feel about the fact that you are growing older?

completely	10
mostly	7
somewhat	5
not very	3
very uncomfortable	0

12. How comfortable do you feel about the fact that you will eventually die?

completely	10
mostly	7
somewhat	5
not very	3
very uncomfortable	0

13. Do you use recreational (street) drugs?

never	10
seldom	7
sometimes	5
often	0

14. How often do you use tobacco in any form?

never	10
very rarely	5
occasionally	3
daily	0

15. How much alcohol do you consume?

none	10
not over 1 drink a week	8
2 or 3 drinks a week, but never more than 2 a day	6
4 to 6 drinks a week, but never more than 2 a day	4
4 to 6 drinks a week, and sometimes over 2 a day	2
over 6 drinks a week	0

16. Are you certain that you have had all necessary immunizations?

I'm certain	10
I think so	7
Not sure	5
I think not	3
Definitely not	0

INTERPRETATION FOR THOSE COMPLETING ALL QUESTIONS:

144 or more points: your health behaviors and attitudes seem to be excellent.

128–143 points: your health behaviors and attitudes are very good, but there is room for improvement.

112–127 points: your health behaviors and attitudes are about average; many improvements could be made.

111 points or less: your health behaviors and attitudes are severely deficient; you deserve to be treated much better than you are treating yourself.

ALTERNATIVE INTERPRETATION FOR THOSE SKIPPING QUESTIONS 1 AND 2:

124 or more points: your health behaviors and attitudes seem to be excellent.

108–123 points: your health behaviors and attitudes are very good, but there is room for improvement.

92–107 points: your health behaviors and attitudes are about average; many improvements could be made.

91 points or less: your health behaviors and attitudes are severely deficient; you deserve to be treated much better than you are treating yourself.

seen a major surge of interest in health and wellness, many Americans have done very little to improve their health. Many still view their health as a matter of luck and make little commitment to achieving a high level of wellness.

There are several commonly used indices of the quality of a nation's health, such as life-expectancy and infant-mortality rates. None of these accurately reflects today's view of wellness as a process of healthful living and attitudes, but they do give some indication of the general health of a nation. Table 1.2 compares some health statistics for five nations, while Table 1.3 presents the leading causes of death in the United States.

Table 1.2
Health Indicators for Five Nations

	Annual Health Cost per Person[a]	Hospitalized Days per Person (avg)	Infant Deaths per 1000 Live Births[b]	Life Expectancy for Males[c]
United States	$2354	1.3	10.0	71.5
Britain	$836	2.0	9.0	72.4
Canada	$1683	2.0	7.2	73.0
Germany	$1232	3.5	7.6	71.8
Japan	$1035	4.1	4.8	75.5

[a]In U.S. dollars, 1989.
[b]Deaths during first 12 months of life.
[c]In years. Female life expectancy is 7–8 years longer.

Source: Medical World News, July 1993.

Table 1.3
Leading Causes of Death in the United States, 1992

Cause	Rate per 100,000	Percent of All Deaths
All cardiovascular diseases	418.0	49.0
Heart diseases	282.2	33.0
Strokes	56.3	6.6
Cancers, all types	202.6	23.7
Chronic obstructive pulmonary disease	35.5	4.2
Accidents, all types	34.3	4.0
Pneumonia and influenza	29.8	3.5
Diabetes	19.9	2.3
AIDS	12.0	1.4
Suicide	11.3	1.3
Homicide	10.6	1.2
Liver disease	10.3	1.2

Source: National Center for Health Statistics, Monthly Vital Statistics Report, 41(7), December 16, 1992.

Another measure of a nation's wellness is its *premature death rate,* defined by the U.S. government as deaths before age 65. This is a conservative estimate, because most of us aspire to live longer than 65 years. By subtracting a person's age at his or her time of death from 65, the government calculates *years of potential life lost* (YPLL). Figure 1.2 illustrates the years of potential life lost in one year by various causes of death in the United States. Accidents emerge as the most significant

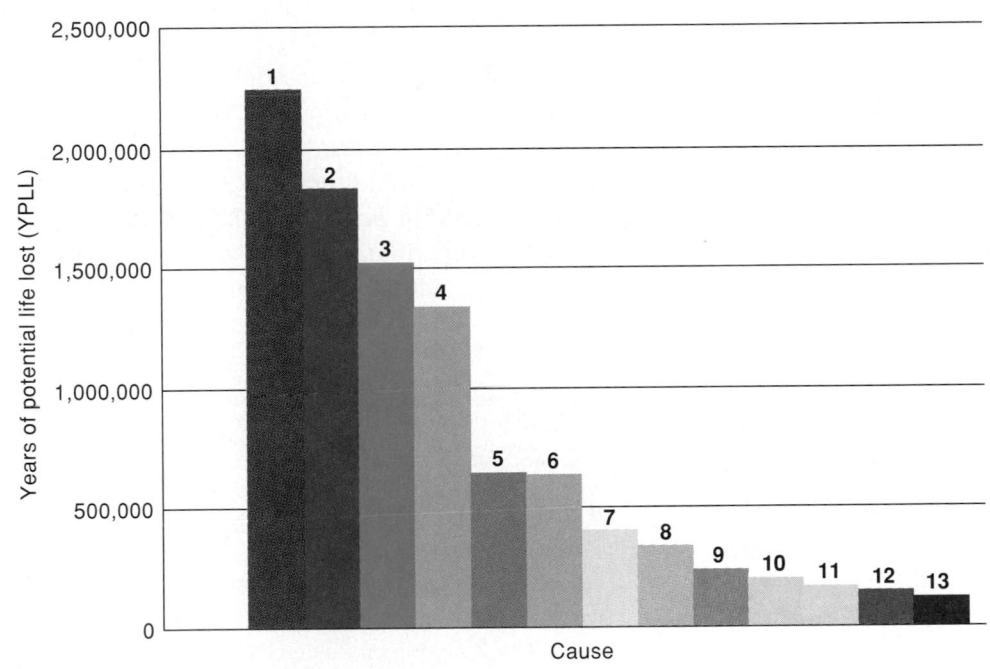

Figure 1.2
Years of Potential Life Lost

Years of potential life lost (YPLL) during 1990 by major causes of death in the United States. YPLL is calculated by subtracting the age at the time of death from 65. Someone who dies at age 24 represents 41 YPLL; someone who dies at age 64 represents 1 YPLL. On this basis, accidents, though causing only about 4 percent of all deaths, are number one in terms of YPLL.

Source: Centers for Disease Control. Morbidity and Mortality Weekly Report 41 (18), May 8, 1992, pp. 313–315.

1. Accidents (all kinds): 2,247,094 YPLL
   Healthful Behavior: many accidents are preventable by safety awareness and maintaining good emotional health

2. Cancers (all kinds): 1,839,900 YPLL
   Healthful Behavior: many cancers are preventable by healthful living habits and are curable if detected and treated early

3. Suicide and homicide: 1,520,780 YPLL
   Healthful Behavior: most suicide and much homicide relates to emotional health problems; maintain good emotional health

4. Heart Diseases (all kinds): 1,349,027 YPLL
   Healthful Behavior: much heart disease can be prevented by regular exercise, good diet, and stress management

5. Birth Defects: 644,651 YPLL
   Healthful Behavior: many birth defects can be prevented by avoiding harmful substances during pregnancy and receiving adequate prenatal care

6. AIDS: 644,245 YPLL
   Healthful Behavior: risk of infection by human immunodeficiency virus is reduced substantially by not sharing injection equipment and by practicing safer sex guidelines

7. Premature Births: 415,638 YPLL
   Healthful Behavior: obtain adequate prenatal care

8. Sudden Infant Death Syndrome: 347,713 YPLL
   Healthful Behavior: unknown at this time

9. Strokes: 244,366 YPLL
   Healthful Behavior: many strokes can be prevented by regular exercise, proper diet, stress management and control of blood pressure

10. Chronic Liver Disease and Cirrhosis: 212,707 YPLL
    Healthful Behavior: avoid heavy drinking or other drug abuse; avoid hepatitis B (vaccine is available)

11. Pneumonia and Influenza: 165,534 YPLL
    Healthful Behavior: much pneumonia and influenza can be avoided by immunization and by maintaining good resistance

12. Diabetes: 143,250 YPLL
    Healthful Behavior: much diabetes can be prevented by maintaining normal weight and its effects can be minimized by early detection and treatment

13. Chronic Obstructive Pulmonary Disease (COPD): 127,464 YPLL
    Healthful Behavior: much COPD can be prevented by not smoking

cause of lost life, because the average person killed by an accident is much younger than the average heart attack or cancer victim.

As this century comes to an end, it is revealing to compare today's leading causes of death with those as the century began. At that time, life expectancies were much shorter, with many lives prematurely ended by infectious conditions. Tuberculosis, pneumonia, and intestinal infections, for example, were numbers one, two, and three on the list of causes of death. Today, with infectious conditions better controlled, degenerative conditions such as cardiovascular disorders and cancers have emerged as the leading killers.[19]

What needs to be done now is to gain a higher degree of control over today's killers. Part of the need is for increased knowledge of the causes and, thus, the preventions of these conditions. But even applying today's limited knowledge can result in a significant decrease in premature deaths from cardiovascular disorders and cancers. The U.S. Public Health Service has set some goals for the health of the nation by the year 2000. Feature 1.3 lists some of these goals, along with the current status of the nation.

At the same time, we cannot assume that the infectious disorders are a thing of the past. The pathogens are still with us and in many cases are increasing in their deadliness. Resistance to existing drugs is making some diseases as difficult to cure as they were many years ago, before antibiotics became available. We cannot let our guard

FEATURE 1.3

HEALTHY PEOPLE 2000: GOALS AND CURRENT REALITIES

The United States Public Health Service has set many health-related goals for the United States to meet by the year 2000. Here are some examples, along with the current statistics.

1. Infant mortality rate (deaths in first year of life)
   Year 2000 target: 7 per 1000 live births
   Current rate: nearly 9

2. Death rates of people 15–24 years of age
   Year 2000 target: 85 per 100,000 per year
   Current rate: about 100

3. People who engage in at least 30 minutes of exercise 5 or more times a week
   Year 2000 target: 30 percent of the population
   Current rate: about 24 percent

4. People age 20 or over who smoke
   Year 2000 target: 15 percent
   Current rate: about 26 percent

5. Average age of first use of alcohol
   Year 2000 target: 14.1
   Current age: about 12.6

6. Fifteen-year old females who have had sexual intercourse
   Year 2000 target: 15 percent
   Current rate: about 45 percent

7. People with adverse health effects from excessive stress
   Year 2000 target: 35 percent
   Current rate: about 41 percent

8. Homicide rate (per 100,000 per year)
   Year 2000 target: 7.2
   Current rate: about 10.1
   Current rate for African American males 15–34 years: about 130

9. Breastfeeding of infants under 5 months of age
   Year 2000 target: 75 percent
   Current rate: about 53 percent

10. Obesity
    Year 2000 target: 20 percent of population
    Current rate: about 28 percent

11. Coronary heart disease deaths
    Year 2000 target: 100 per 100,000 people per year
    Current rate: about 122

12. Cancer deaths
    Year 2000 target: 130 per 100,000 people per year
    Current rate: about 135

13. Diabetes-related deaths
    Year 2000 target: 34 per 100,000 people per year
    Current rate: about 38

14. Condom use at last intercourse for sexually active females age 15–19
    Year 2000 target: 60 percent
    Current rate: about 38 percent

15. Condom use at last intercourse for sexually active males age 15–19
    Year 2000 target: 75 percent
    Current rate: about 54 percent

Source: National Center for Health Statistics. *Health United States 1992 and Healthy People 2000 Review.* Hyattsville, MD: U.S. Public Health Service, DHHS Publication No. (PHS) 93-1232, August 1993.

down and ignore immunization and sanitary precautions or the massive epidemics that killed millions in the past will rage once more.

In this book we will provide information that will help you become motivated to practice healthful living. Ultimately, the choice is yours: Each of us, to a very great extent, controls the quality of our own health and therefore, the quality of our lives. High-level wellness (Feature 1.4, p. 18) results from ongoing individual commitment and effort.

CHECKPOINT

1. What are the three leading causes of death in the United States?

2. What is the leading cause of years of potential life lost (YPLL) in the United States?

3. Based on *your* life-style, which factors in Figure 1.2 might relate to YPLL for you?

4. How do today's causes of death in the United States compare with those as this century began?

HIGH-LEVEL WELLNESS: THE HOLISTIC VIEW

Many people believe that high levels of wellness can best be achieved through the holistic approach, which emphasizes the interaction among the mind, body, and spirit. They are all **interdependent** (two or more entities each being dependent upon the other[s])—none can function well unless all do (Figure 1.3). A problem in any one affects the other two. We cannot isolate the function of the physical body without considering the influence of the mind and spirit, nor can we understand the function of the mind without considering its biological basis.

Physical illnesses that are thought to result largely from a person's mental state are sometimes termed **psychosomatic** (pertaining to the relationship of the mind and the body). Although they may originate in the mind, these are not imaginary dis-

....

interdependent   two or more entities each being dependent upon the other(s).

psychosomatic   pertaining to the relationship of the mind and the body.

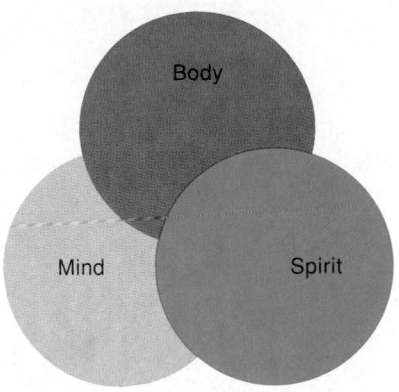

Figure 1.3
The Holistic Approach to Wellness

The holistic approach to wellness emphasizes the interdependence of mind, body, and spirit. The relative size of the circles varies throughout life, as does the degree of their overlap.

eases. They are very real, objectively measurable, disorders of the physical body. From a holistic perspective, a disease can never be purely of the body or the mind. This partitioning of the human being is impossible; thus no disease is limited to only the body or the mind.

The holistic approach to wellness emphasizes personal responsibility for health and well-being. This responsibility includes maintaining excellent emotional health by adopting a positive outlook on life, eating nutritious foods, exercising regularly, practicing effective stress-management techniques, and partaking of recreational and social activities. Using alcohol, tobacco, and other harmful substances is discouraged. The holistic approach also views us in a larger, spiritual context that gives a sense of purpose to our lives.

PERSONAL RESPONSIBILITY FOR HEALTH AND WELLNESS

Each of us determines, to a large extent, the degree of our own health and wellness. The best efforts of our physicians and public health workers cannot guarantee our health. No one can exercise for us, relax for us, control our alcohol and other drug use, or ensure that we eat correctly. For most of us, the quality of life is largely in our own hands.

This is a European view of health. People who hold the traditional health views of other cultures may not feel that they have this much direct control over their health. For them, assuming personal responsibility for health may involve living in har-

FEATURE 1.4

HIGH-LEVEL WELLNESS

What is it like to experience high-level wellness? Here are some highlights from a typical day of someone who has achieved a high level of wellness. This could be you.

- You wake up feeling good, refreshed, alert, and confident in your ability to deal with the challenges of the day.

- Looking in the mirror, you notice that you look much better these days than you did before you changed some of your habits. What ever happened to those bags that used to be under your eyes?

- You enjoy your breakfast of unsweetened, whole-grain cereal with milk, fresh fruit, and fruit juice. It carries you through until lunch.

- You arrive at school or work a little early, giving yourself time to relax and get organized.

- Your colleagues drag themselves in a little late. Some complain of hangovers; some have colds or coughs. Some don't arrive at all. You haven't been ill one day in months.

- The day goes well. There are plenty of challenging situations, but you deal with them appropriately.

- Even though you are busy, you take the time for a good lunch and a relaxing walk.

- After work or school, you usually enjoy some vigorous physical activity, followed by a fairly light dinner.

- In the past, you would have spent the evening drinking, but now you like the way you feel without drinking more than the way you felt when you used to drink.

- Using some of the money you have saved since you stopped smoking, you take a friend to see a movie that has received good reviews. You enjoy the film and remember that you used to fall asleep at the movies.

- After the movie, you go to bed and immediately fall into a restful sleep.

High-level wellness allows us to enjoy long, full, rewarding days. It provides the physical stamina and the mental alertness to deal with the challenges of the day and still have plenty of energy left over for an evening of pleasure. Does this appeal to you? It's an attainable goal. In recent years, millions of people of all ages have raised their level of wellness and are enjoying their lives more than ever.

mony with nature or praying to their supernatural powers.

PERSONAL RESPONSIBILITY FOR SOME ILLNESS

While many of us can accept the concept of personal responsibility for our own health, we may feel uncomfortable accepting personal responsibility for our illnesses. Yet, if we are responsible for our health, then we must be responsible, to some degree, for some of our illnesses. This does not imply that a person should feel guilty about being ill; that would be dwelling on the past, which is rarely productive. Of far more value is looking at our life-style and finding ways to live more healthfully, in order to avoid future illnesses.

There are still diseases that are out of our control and for which there is no known avoidance behavior. For example, many diseases have a strong hereditary element, over which we have no control. Further, the specific behaviors that may help prevent some illnesses, such as Alzheimer's disease, are not yet known. But when these preventive behaviors are learned, it will become our responsibility to practice them.

Again, this is a European view of illness. In many non-European cultures, there is no concept of personal responsibility for illness because the locus of control for illness is seen as lying totally outside of the individual.

EMPHASIS ON PREVENTION

An old approach to health (and one that some people still follow) was not to worry too much about preventive health behavior but to look for a good doctor when one became ill. There are many flaws in this approach. First, as we have already seen, wellness is far more than the mere absence of illness. People who want to live high-quality lives know that there are levels of wellness that go far beyond just not being sick and want to enjoy such high-level wellness.

Second, illness is not always easily curable and some conditions can be prevented but cannot be cured at all. Even when a condition can be totally cured, there is a period of reduced quality of life that most of us would just as soon avoid.

Finally, it is economically advantageous to prevent, rather than cure, illness. Treating illness is almost always more expensive than preventing it. For example, heart disease can often be prevented at little or no cost through proper diet and appropriate exercise, while coronary bypass surgery is extremely expensive. Most health insurance plans now recognize this fact and place a great emphasis on keeping their clients healthy through education, immunization, and emphasis on healthful life-styles.

Throughout this text we emphasize the prevention of illness. Though the methods for preventing some conditions are not yet known, the majority of health problems can now be prevented in ways that this book will describe. Most of these preventive behaviors, however, require motivation. We hope that this book will help you become motivated to apply the known healthful behaviors to your own life-style.

CHECKPOINT

1. Why is preventing illness better than curing it?

2. What are the basic concepts in the holistic view of wellness?

JUDGING HEALTH RESEARCH

Virtually every newspaper, magazine, and TV newscast includes items on new health research. How reliable is this information? Some is quite valid; some is very faulty. Here, very briefly, are some common types of research and information on how to judge each.

EXPERIMENTAL RESEARCH

In experimental research, an experiment is performed to test a **hypothesis** (a tentative assumption made prior to experimental testing). Typically, in an experiment, two groups of subjects (people or animals) are compared under conditions that are

....

hypothesis a tentative assumption made prior to experimental testing.

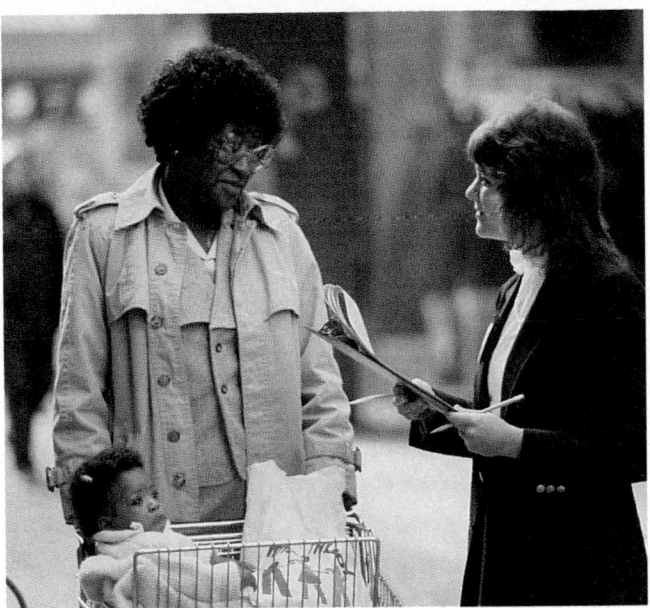

Almost every newspaper, magazine, and TV newscast includes items on new health research. Some is of excellent quality; some is poorly done. Some is valid, but is misrepresented or exaggerated by the media. Each of us needs to be able to judge the validity of health research for ourselves.

identical in every way except for one variable factor. The validity of experimental research depends upon its having a good experimental design. As an example, we will consider a possible experiment to test the hypothesis that a certain new drug will cure the common cold.

- For validity, there must be two groups of subjects. One group, called the experimental group, will receive the new drug. The other group is the **control,** the standard against which observations or conclusions must be checked in order to establish their validity. For example, the control group in this case would include people who have not been given the new drug taken by the experimental group. Members of the control group will receive a **placebo** (an inert substance). Some medical research is flawed by the lack of a control group.

....

control in an experiment, the standard against which observations or conclusions must be checked in order to establish their validity; for example, a person who or animal that has not been exposed to the treatment or condition being studied in the other people or animals.

placebo an inert substance.

- The subjects belonging to each group need to be comparable. This is accomplished by **random assignment,** in which each person or animal has an equal chance of being assigned to either group. For example, slips of paper with subjects' names might be drawn from a paper bag to determine who will be assigned to each group or a computer might make random assignments.

- The larger the number of subjects in each group, the more reliable the results will be. Typically, once initial, small-scale testing has been performed, a new drug is tested using thousands of subjects and controls.

- Validity is increased by using the **double-blind method** (experimentation in which neither the subject nor the evaluators know which subjects are in the experimental group and which are in the control group). This means that neither the subjects nor their evaluators know which people are receiving the drug and which are receiving the placebo. This is essential because the power of suggestion will affect the course of a disease (illustrating the powerful influence of the mind over the physical body).

- The results need to be analyzed to reveal the probability, if any, that the differences between the two groups of subjects are significant. For example, maybe the people receiving the new drug recovered in a mean (average) time of 2.7 days while the controls recovered in a mean time of 3.1 days. A statistical analysis can tell us the probability that this is a significant difference.

SURVEY RESEARCH

Carefully designed and conducted surveys can be useful in revealing health-related attitudes, beliefs,

....

random assignment experimentation in which each person has an equal chance of being assigned to either the experimental or the control group.

double-blind method experimentation in which neither the subject nor the evaluators know which subjects are in the experimental group and which are in the control group.

and behaviors. People may complete questionnaires or be personally interviewed. In deciding how much credence to give to a particular survey, consider these questions:

- How were the participants selected? Do they truly represent the entire U.S. population or do they mainly represent a certain age group, educational level, ethnic group, or socioeconomic level? Do they include urban, suburban, and rural dwellers?

- What about the people who chose not to participate in the survey? Does their absence skew the results?

- How were the questions worded? By skillful phrasing of questions, almost any desired answer can be obtained.

CORRELATIONS

A relationship between two variables is a **correlation.** In a *positive* correlation, high values for one variable are associated with high values for the other. For example, high intake of animal fats correlates with high serum cholesterol levels. In a *negative* correlation, high values for one variable are associated with low values for the other. For example, higher levels of exercise correlate with lower blood pressures. Correlations are constantly being suggested between various health-related behaviors and conditions. Correlations must be evaluated very carefully. Just because two variables appear to show a correlation does not necessarily prove a cause-and-effect relationship. There may easily be other, unrecognized and unaccounted for, variable factors.

Prospective Versus Retrospective Studies

Prospective studies look ahead. They take a group of people, assess them in some respect, and then follow this group of people over a period of (usually) years to see whether the development of some condition correlates to the original assessment. For example, the personality traits of a group of people might be evaluated, then over a

....

correlation a relationship between two variables.

period of 20 years the rates of heart attacks, cancers, alcoholism, or other conditions could be compared to the personality assessments for any possible correlations.

Retrospective studies look back. They look for past factors that might correlate to current health conditions. For example, people who have experienced heart attacks and otherwise comparable people who have not had heart attacks might be interviewed regarding their eating and exercise habits to see if any correlations exist.

CHECKPOINT

1. Define the terms *hypothesis, placebo, random assignment,* and *double blind.*

2. What is the purpose of the control group in medical research?

3. Why does a correlation between two variables not necessarily prove cause-and-effect relationship between them?

MAKING THE COMMITMENT TO WELLNESS

Motivating other people to behave in healthful ways is a difficult, if not impossible, task. One can *inspire* motivation, but cannot motivate another person. Thus, it is difficult for physicians to motivate their patients, for drug abuse counselors to motivate their clients, and for health educators to motivate their students. *Knowing how* to behave healthfully is one thing; *doing* it is quite another.

Behavioral theories suggest that we tend to repeat behavior that is rewarded and avoid behavior that is punished. Unfortunately, the effects of healthful or unhealthful behavior often seem unrelated to the actual behavior. The rewards of healthful behavior are usually not immediately apparent and neither are the harmful effects of unhealthful behavior. In fact, unhealthful behaviors are often quite pleasurable in the short term. Choosing healthful behavior often requires a high level of motivation. How can one find that motivation?

In a general sense, finding the motivation for any form of behavior requires two perceptions: The goal must be perceived as *worthwhile* (re-

warding) and it must be perceived as *attainable.* Relating this to health, at least four factors can be identified as essential for motivating healthful behavior:

1. A sound, factual knowledge of which forms of behavior are beneficial to our well-being and why.

2. A sense of being in control of our lives—the belief that healthful behavior will, in fact, produce beneficial results.

3. A strongly positive approach to life—a view of life as a celebration to be savored.

4. A strongly developed sense of self-esteem—a feeling of being worthy of enjoying the best life has to offer.

How can you make the behavioral changes necessary to achieve high-level wellness?

CHECKPOINT

1. In terms of reward and punishment, why is it difficult to motivate healthful behavior?

2. What are four factors that are essential for motivating healthful behavior?

MAKING BEHAVIORAL CHANGES

One of the goals of this book is to help you develop the motivation to raise your level of wellness. This may be a real challenge for many students because most health habits are deeply ingrained and difficult to change. Some ways to improve the chances of success in meeting this challenge follow.

SET SPECIFIC, REALISTIC GOALS

Through the In Your Hands health inventories, in each chapter, you can identify those health areas you may want to improve. Set realistic and modest goals that avoid failure, and that provide you with the confidence to move forward. A lofty goal that is never achieved reduces your confidence in meeting any health goals.

Break up major health goals into small incremental goals, such as losing 5 pounds. Then reward yourself when each incremental goal is achieved.

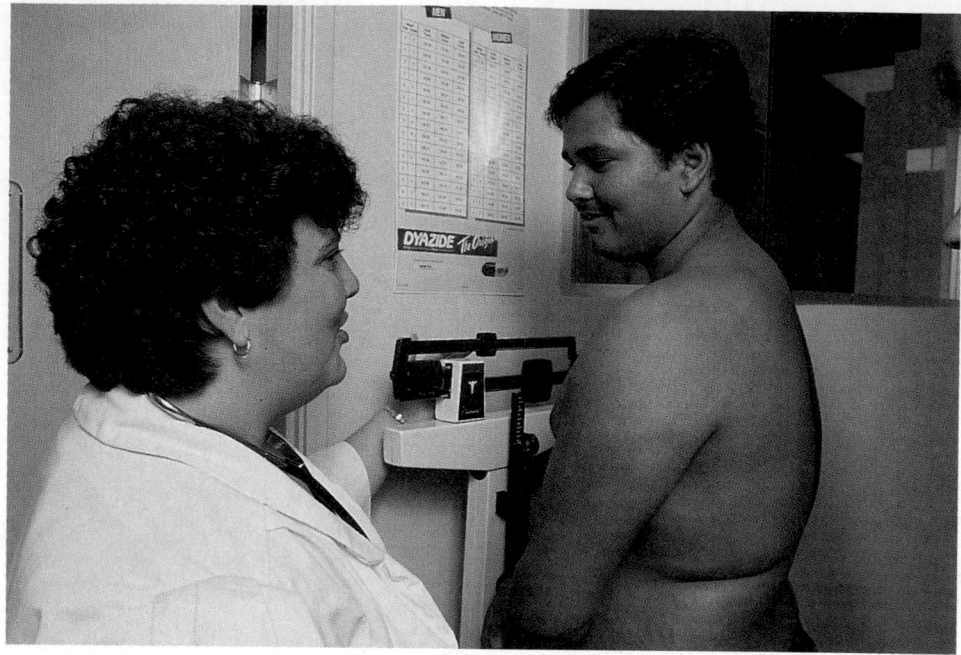

Break major goals up into small increments. If, for example, you need to lose a lot of weight, set a goal to lose 5 pounds, which should not seem (or be) too difficult to achieve. When you meet that goal, set the next goal to lose 5 more pounds, and so on. In all human endeavors, success motivates success.

PROGRESS TAKES TIME

You should expect some difficulty in reaching any worthwhile goal. If you take two steps forward and one step back, you are still moving forward and you will eventually get to where you are going. If you view that one step back as a failure, you may give up hope of ever reaching your goal. If you understand that very few people achieve any goal without some steps back you can still feel good about your progress. Remember, perfection is an unattainable goal.

REWARD YOURSELF

One of the most basic principles in the behavioral theory is that behavior that is rewarded is repeated. Of course, healthful behavior carries its own built-in rewards; but as we have mentioned, these rewards are too far removed from the desired behavior to act as reinforcements. One might be rewarded for quitting smoking by not getting can-

cer ten years later, but this is not the kind of reward that best motivates changing a behavior.

Tie your rewards to modest incremental goals—5 pounds lost, a week of regular exercise, a month without alcohol—so that you will be frequently rewarded for the desired behavior. A reward should be something you enjoy, but it doesn't have to be big or expensive. It might be a new compact disk or book, a movie, an item of clothing, or anything else you really enjoy. For major milestones in your progress, you may want to plan larger rewards.

KEEPING THE COMMITMENT TO WELLNESS

All of us know people who have had short-term success with improved health behaviors, only to fall back to their old ways. How can we maintain our commitment to high-level wellness over a long period of time?

CONCENTRATE ON FEELING GOOD

Foremost in helping keep the commitment can be the wonderful new feeling of well-being as a result of improved health habits. Think often about how much better you feel now that you exercise more, eat more carefully, and avoid harmful substances. Take pride in your accomplishment!

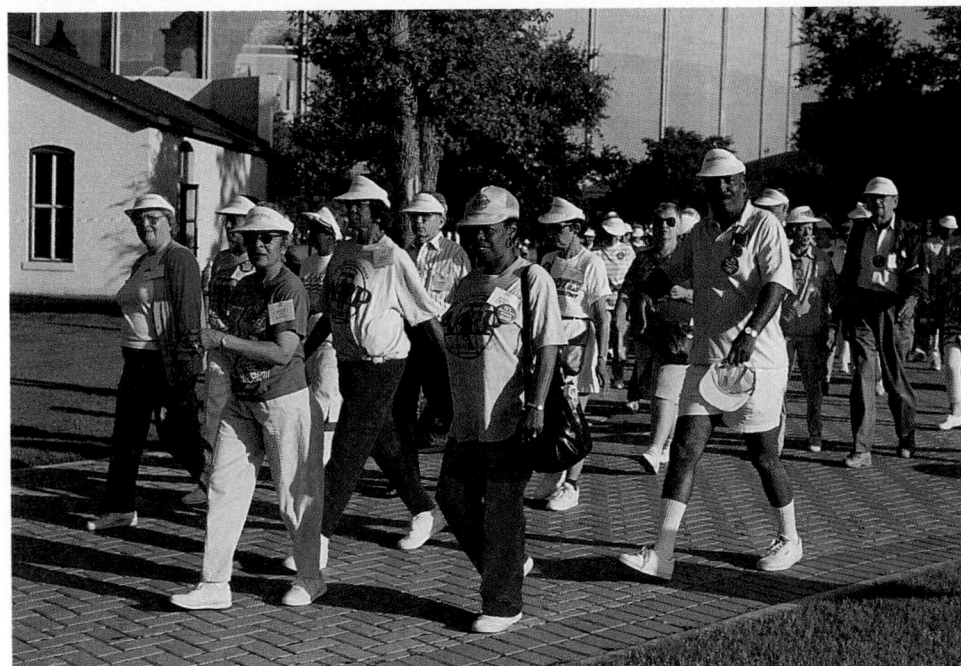

Group effort makes it much easier to stay motivated and maintain a commitment to wellness.

USE POSITIVE PEER PRESSURE (REINFORCEMENT)

Many of our undesirable habits can be traced back to peer pressure. Very few people are alone when they take their first drink, smoke their first cigarette, or first use other drugs. These behaviors are usually a response to peer pressure. With today's emphasis on wellness, peer pressure can serve a more constructive purpose by helping people to overcome unhealthful behaviors. The encouragement and support of friends, family, and others can provide effective **positive reinforcement** (any stimulus that increases the probability that a behavior will occur) of desirable behavior.

An ideal way to use peer pressure is to find one or more of your friends who are interested in working on the same health behavior, such as quitting smoking, losing weight, or exercising more. The group effort makes it much easier to stay motivated as you support each other.

Finally, tell your family and friends about your health plan. You will find most people to be very supportive. Their support will give you a sense of pride and accomplishment that will further motivate you to achieve your goal.

....

positive reinforcement any stimulus that increases the probability that a behavior will occur.

CHECKPOINT

1. Why is it often better to set small, incremental goals in health behavior?

2. What small rewards might you consider in motivating healthful behaviors?

3. Which of your family and friends provide you with encouragement to change?

✓

SUMMARY

Health is a cultural concept that is defined differently in different cultures. The prevailing definition of health has evolved from the "absence of illness" to the broader term, wellness, with its definition as "a life-style that emphasizes such health-promoting behaviors as eating a healthful diet, avoiding harmful substances, enjoying regular exercise, and cultivating self-esteem." The goal of wellness is to live a long, healthy, active, and rewarding life.

America's health attitudes and delivery systems have reflected the primarily European origins of the population. Non-European Americans often view health and illness differently from European Americans. These different views lead to different approaches to maintaining health and treating illness when it occurs.

Wellness has social, cultural, physical, intellectual, career, emotional, and spiritual components. All of these components are interdependent.

Having a sense of control over your health is an important part of the European concept of wellness. Without a feeling of control, there is little motivation to behave in healthful ways.

When this century began, most deaths were from infectious conditions. As it ends, most deaths are from degenerative conditions, such as cardiovascular disorders and cancers. The germs (pathogens) of infectious diseases are still with us, however, and are developing resistance to the drugs that we have depended upon to control them.

The holistic view of wellness holds that the mind, body, and spirit are all interdependent, that each of us is responsible for our own health and illness, and that illness often serves a function for the individual. Prevention of illness, as opposed to cure, is emphasized.

It is helpful to be able to judge health research. Experimental research tests a hypothesis. Valid experiments include a control group of subjects (standard against which observations are checked), determined by random assignment, and apply the double-blind method, in which neither subjects nor evaluators know which people are in the experimental group and which are in the control group. Validity of survey research depends on how participants are selected and how questions are phrased. A relationship between two variables is a correlation. Just because two variables appear to show a correlation does not necessarily prove a cause-and-effect relationship.

Attaining a high level of wellness requires commitment and motivation because the rewards for healthful behavior are not always immediate, whereas the rewards for unhealthful behavior are usually instantaneous. You can help maintain motivation by rewarding yourself when you attain your health goals and by involving your family and friends as reinforcers of your desired behavior.

REFERENCES

1. Spector, R. *Cultural Diversity in Health and Illness,* 3rd ed. Norwalk, CT: Appleton & Lange, 1991.
2. O'Hare, Wm. "America's Minorities—The Demographics of Diversity." *Population Bulletin* (December 1992), 1–47.
3. Spector, op. cit.
4. Primeaux, H. "American Indian Health Care Practices: A Cross-Cultural Perspective." *Nursing Clinics of North America* (March 1977), 57.
5. Spector, op. cit.
6. Bilagody, H. "An American Indian Looks at Health Care." In R. Feldman and D. Buch (eds.). *The Ninth Annual Training Institute for Psychiatrist-Teachers of Practicing Physicians.* Boulder, CO: WICHE, 1969.
7. Spector, op. cit.
8. "Acupuncture." *Consumer Reports,* Vol. 59 (January 1994), 54–59.
9. Ibid.
10. Spector, op. cit.
11. Jacques, G. "Cultural Health Traditions: a Black Perspective." In M. Branch and P. Paxton (eds.). *Providing Safe Nursing Care for Ethnic People of Color.* New York: Appleton-Century-Crofts, 1976.
12. Spector, op. cit.
13. Ibid.
14. Hafen, B., et al. *The Health Effects of Attitudes, Emotions, Relationships.* Provo, UT: EMS Associates, 1992.
15. Ibid
16. Peterson, C., and Bossio, L. "Healthy Attitudes: Optimism, Hope, and Control." In D. Goleman and J. Gurin (eds.). *Mind Body Medicine.* Yonkers, NY: Consumer Reports Books, 1993.
17. Hafen, op. cit.
18. Peterson and Bossio, op. cit.
19. National Center of Health Statistics. "Births, Marriages, Divorces, and Deaths for 1991." *Monthly Vital Statistics Report* Vol. 40, No. 12 (15 April 1992).

SUGGESTED READINGS

Goleman, D., and Gurin, J. (eds.). *Mind Body Medicine.* Yonkers, NY: Consumer Reports Books, 1993.

Hafen, B., et al. *The Health Effects of Attitudes, Emotions, Relationships.* Provo, UT: EMS Associates, 1992.

Spector, R. *Cultural Diversity in Health and Illness,* 3rd ed. Norwalk, CT: Appleton & Lange, 1991.

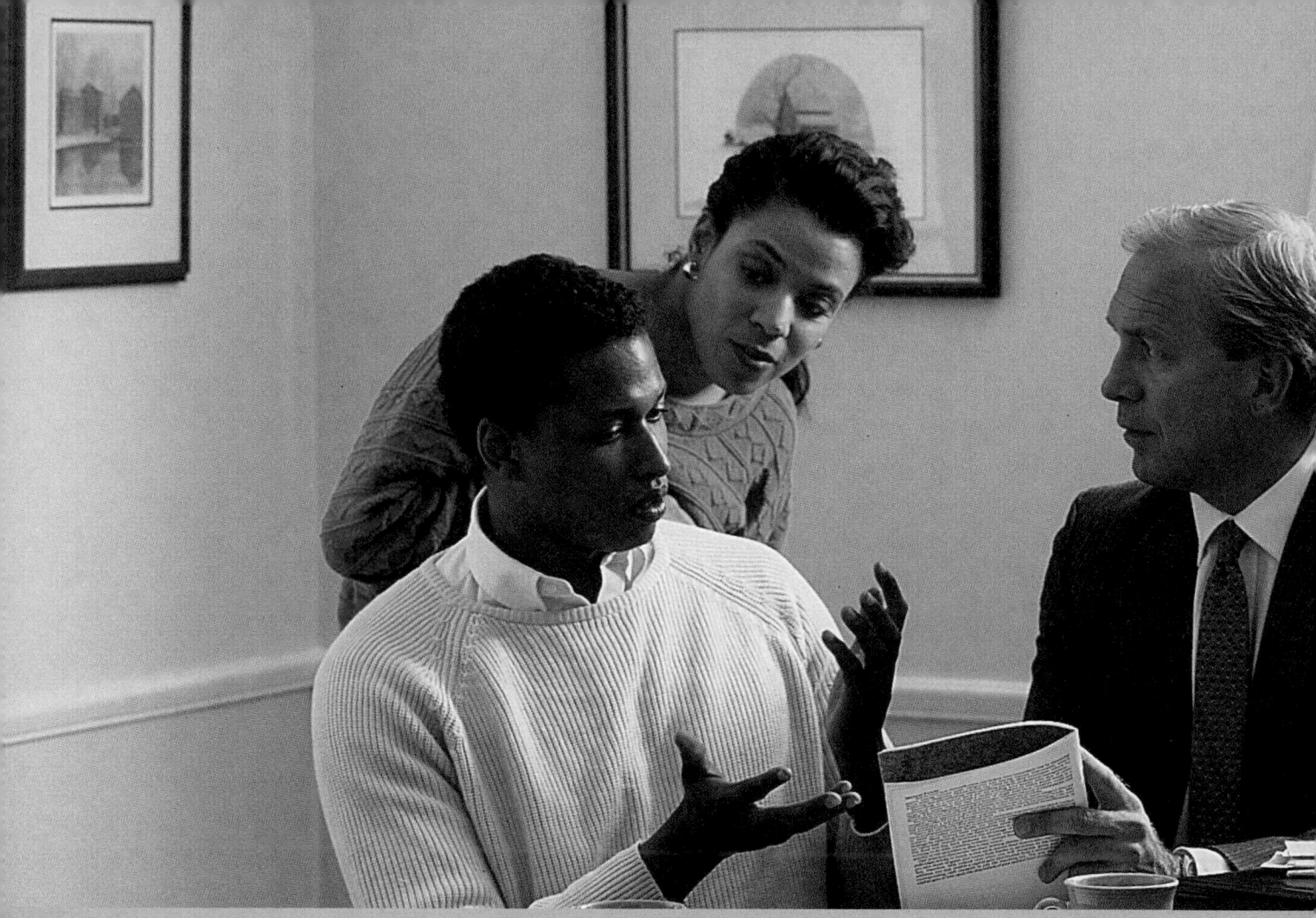

2
COMMUNICATION FOR WELLNESS

Upon completing this chapter, you will be able to:

KNOWLEDGE

- Define cultural diversity and explain how it affects communication.
- List and explain seven elements that contribute to the success of communication.
- List and explain six principles that affect all interpersonal communication.
- Describe seven ways to improve listening skills.
- Explain how we communicate nonverbally and how people of different cultures use different nonverbal signals.
- Explain "I" statements and "you" statements.
- Contrast passive, assertive, and aggressive behaviors.
- Explain common styles of handling conflict in relationships.
- Explain how the mass media can positively or negatively affect health attitudes and behaviors.

INSIGHT

- Understand how your own cultural values influence how you interact with people of different cultures.
- Identify areas in which you can improve the effectiveness of your speaking and listening skills.
- Analyze your communication habits for the excessive use of "you" statements.
- Analyze your behavior for patterns of passiveness, assertiveness, and aggressiveness.

DECISION MAKING

- Make a commitment to accept the communication differences between different cultures without feeling that you must judge which one is "better" or "right."
- Make a commitment to work toward more effective communication in your relationships.
- Make a commitment to improve how you respond to the ideas expressed by others.
- Make a commitment to deal with the conflicts in your relationships in more effective ways.

There has been much criticism of the way politicians have used brief, 10–15 second TV commercials to communicate certain positions or portray an opponent as being easy on crime or favoring drug use. However, through televised debates, these same politicians can be studied intensely as they attempt to portray the characteristics that people want in their leaders. The communication techniques used during these debates, both verbal and nonverbal, are analyzed carefully. Almost everyone would agree that people communicate through body language, the nonverbal language of physical movements and eye contacts. Freud once said, "If his lips are silent, he chatters with his fingertips."

There is probably no more well-rehearsed and well-studied setting for nonverbal communication than a debate among presidential candidates. After one of the debates during the last presidential campaign, the body language of the three candidates— Bill Clinton, George Bush, and Ross Perot—was evaluated in several different areas. These included "presidentialness" (composure, clarity in movements, and response to stress); "likability" (interactions with others and signs of hostility or fear); and "leadership style" (evidence of initiative in movement or repetitive, stylized patterns of gesture).

After analyzing one of these debates, it was determined that George Bush's body language revealed a much different person than the one portrayed in his "kinder and gentler" campaign in 1988. He scored high in "presidentialness," but his forceful gestures and repetitive hand movements caused him to lose points in "likability." Bill Clinton's scores were also mixed, showing some flashes of high scores in all categories. His tendency to listen with his mouth slightly open and shaped so that it had slight upturns at the end of his lips left something to be desired. Although he still did not outperform either Clinton or Bush, in this particular debate Ross Perot gave his best performance in terms of communicating effectively through body language. For example, he reduced the number of times he pointed forcefully with his hand above his shoulders, movements that had previously caused him to lose "likability" points.

Since Bill Clinton eventually won the election, perhaps he improved his communication through body language to persuade the American public that he did possess "presidentialness," "likability," and "leadership style." Whether one is running for president, or simply working to maintain a positive relationship with a friend, communication is certainly a key to success and a healthy life-style.

Source: Washington Post, *October 13, 1992, p. WH9.*

■   ■   ■

Placing communication first among the topics in this text reflects the significance of effective communication in wellness. Communication has many associations with wellness:

- Communication skills help you to develop and maintain rewarding relationships with people of diverse cultures, for your personal, social, and career benefit.

- Communication skills contribute to rewarding, smooth-functioning relationships, which are essential to wellness.[1] Intimate relationships, which are defined in terms of open communication, are highly beneficial to your emotional wellness.

- Effective communication helps you resolve conflicts in your relationships. Ongoing conflicts are very stressful and stress management requires finding satisfactory ways to resolve such conflicts.

- Communication skills enable you to explain your problems and needs clearly to your health care providers and to understand their messages to you. Too often, people are reluctant to communicate information that is necessary for a correct diagnosis of their problems.

Example: In complaining of a urinary discharge, Kevin neglects to mention a recent new sexual partner.

In this chapter we will explore communication and cultural diversity, some basic concepts of communication, effective speaking and listening, nonverbal communication, assertive communication, communicating our emotions, and effective ways of resolving conflicts.

COMMUNICATION AND CULTURAL DIVERSITY

More than through any other characteristic, the nature of a culture is revealed through its traditions of communication. In fact, one definition of culture is as a "metacommunication system." Communication doesn't just reveal culture; it *is* culture. Effective communication, and thus understanding, between people of different cultures involves much more than simply speaking the same language.

Cultural diversity refers to people with a variety of histories, ideologies, traditions, values, life-styles, and languages living and interacting togeth-

....

cultural diversity people with a variety of histories, ideologies, traditions, values, life-styles, and languages living and interacting together.

er. The United States is increasingly a nation with large populations of people representing many different ethnic groups. Communication difficulties between ethnic groups may involve language barriers, but also may reflect basic cultural differences that impair communication even when language differences are not a factor. In culture A, for example, communication may tend to be very direct and to the point. In culture B, the same topics may be approached very obliquely and indirectly, with allusions and inferences made, but without actually stating the message in any direct way. Members of culture A will probably not understand what members of culture B are trying to say, while members of culture B will perceive members of culture A as being overbearing or rude.

In many occupations, an understanding of cultural differences in communication habits is essential. In the classroom, for example, students representing some ethnic groups are reluctant to challenge the opinions of the professor or even to

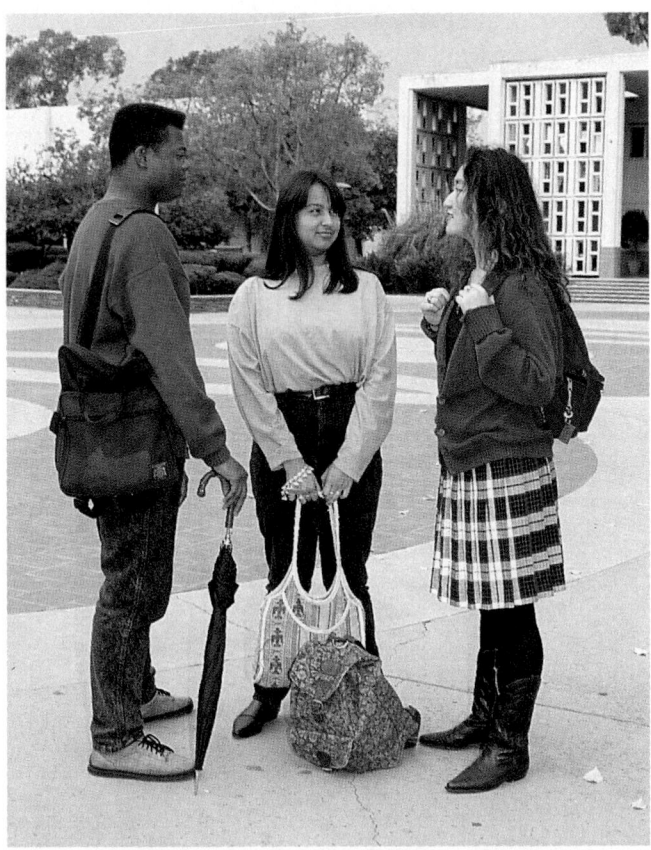

Even when people of different ethnic groups are fluent in the same language, cultural differences in communication can lead to misunderstandings. The identical statement can be interpreted quite differently by people of different cultures.

ask for clarification of unclear statements. For another example, health care workers often have clients from ethnic groups other than their own. Unless those involved in health care receive special training regarding ethnic communication differences, serious misinterpretations can occur.

Example: Chinese patients in U.S. hospitals rarely complain about what bothers them. The hospital food may seem strange and be served in an unfamiliar manner. The only indication of a problem may be an untouched food tray and the silent withdrawal of the patient. This silence may be regarded by health care workers as reflecting good behavior. Such misunderstanding can cause the patient a great deal of suffering and may delay recovery.[2]

Even those of us who have little occupational need to sharpen our intercultural communication skills may have frequent personal and social opportunities for communication across ethnic lines. Schilling and Brannon have compiled the following suggestions to enhance communication between members of different cultures:[3]

- Develop an understanding of your own cultural values and biases. Most of us tend to be somewhat ethnocentric, assuming that the ways of our own culture are "best" and judging other cultures by how closely they approximate our own.

- Develop an understanding of the cultural values, beliefs, and customs of other ethnic groups with which you interact.

- Be respectful of, interested in, and nonjudgmental about cultures other than your own. When two cultures are different, it is not necessary to judge which one is "better" or "right," we can simply accept them as being different. We can learn to enjoy and appreciate the richness that ethnic diversity brings to our classrooms and our communities.

- Speak in a way that promotes understanding and shows respect for someone from a different ethnic group. Be especially careful to avoid statements such as "She's really very (smart/tall/beautiful/etc.) for a (fill in the ethnic group)." Even though the intention may be good, such statements are certain to offend the subject and to reveal the speaker's biases.

- Avoid using slang or idioms that might be misunderstood by someone from a different ethnic group. Many of the everyday phrases instantly understood within one ethnic group may have no meaning or a totally different meaning to someone from a different group.

- Remember that the same gestures can carry different meanings in different cultures. Avoid body language that might be offensive or misunderstood. Observe closely the use of gestures by people in different cultures; it could save a major embarrassment.

Example: the hand gesture that means "perfect" in the United States refers to sexual intercourse in the Philippines.

To these suggestions, we might add:

- If you are conversing in English with someone who is fairly new at speaking it, listen very carefully to what she or he says. If you don't understand a word, you might ask to have it spelled or written out for you and encourage him or her to make the same request. The correct pronunciation of English words is very unpredictable and there are many exceptions to the rules of pronunciation.

- Don't assume that someone who speaks less-than-perfect English or speaks English with an accent is not intelligent or has nothing important to say. Remember that he or she speaks at least two languages, even though one is spoken with an accent.

One of the many benefits of the college experience is that it can help you to develop and maintain an awareness of, an appreciation of, and a sensitivity to, the many different histories, traditions, values, ideologies, life-styles, and languages that exist among people from different areas of the world.

Now answer the In Your Hands assessment, How Well Do You Communicate? As pointed out in its introduction, this assessment reflects the communication values of the dominant European American culture. People belonging to some other cultures tend not to be as open or assertive in their communication, especially with health care providers or in sexual situations.

ELEMENTS AND PRINCIPLES OF COMMUNICATION

Understanding the basics of communication can help us to develop more effective communication skills. Seven important elements contribute to the success or failure of our communication efforts:

1. The *medium*. The medium is how a message is carried. In personal communication, it might be a face-to-face discussion, a telephone call, or a note or letter. Some of us communicate best face-to-face, some by telephone (perhaps the distance makes us feel more comfortable), and some by writing notes or letters in which we have time to choose our words more carefully and can make our meaning more precise. The mass media, such as magazines, newspapers, radio, and especially television, can be very effective means of conveying health information and influencing people's attitudes and behaviors.

2. The *message*. In your personal communication, is it always clear to you just what you want to communicate? First we have to *understand* our feelings, needs, and desires, then we can effectively communicate them. Sometimes we don't come right out and say what we would like to say. We talk all around the subject, hoping that our listener will somehow understand our desires. Communication usually needs to be direct to be effective.

Directness of communication is culturally influenced. People of some cultures communicate very directly, so directly that people of other cultures may view them as being blunt. People of some other cultures tend to communicate very indirectly, implying rather than specifically stating their message. People accustomed to direct communication will probably not understand the message.

3. The *speaker*. Do you deliver your messages in a clear and effective way? Misunderstandings occur when the speaker lacks adequate vocabulary or phrases ideas in ambiguous ways. In communi-

IN YOUR HANDS

HOW WELL DO YOU COMMUNICATE?

Communication skills contribute to wellness in many ways. For example, effective communication is essential if we are to have successful relationships and adequate need fulfillment.

NOTE:

As we have discussed, communication patterns are highly cultural and people of different cultures can be expected to communicate differently. This assessment is more valid for people of European ancestry than for those of non-European ethnic groups. Preface each statement with "Compared with others in my ethnic group. . . ." Members of non-European ethnic groups may wish to compare their answers with other members of their ethnic group and ignore the interpretation given. For each statement, circle the appropriate number of points:

	Usually	Sometimes	Seldom
1. I find it easy to express my needs and feelings to others.	2	1	0
2. I am sensitive to the needs and feelings expressed by others, and especially their nonverbal expressions.	2	1	0
3. My relationships with other people are pleasant and rewarding.	2	1	0
4. When a conflict arises in one of my relationships, it is resolved with ease.	2	1	0
5. I find it easy to communicate with a physician, counselor, or other health care provider.	2	1	0
6. I find it easy to communicate with people of both genders.	2	1	0
7. I can communicate effectively with people of various ethnic groups.	2	1	0
8. I can find the right words to express the ideas I want to convey.	2	1	0
9. I am good at interpreting nonverbal messages from other people.	2	1	0
10. I try very hard not to interrupt someone who is speaking to me.	2	1	0
11. I try very hard to be nonjudgmental in my responses when people share their ideas and feelings with me.	2	1	0
12. When a discussion is causing me to feel uncomfortable, I try hard not to withdraw from the discussion or change the subject.	2	1	0
13. I try to help people open up by asking open-ended, rather than yes-or-no type questions.	2	1	0
14. When I want to express my feelings, I try to phrase them as "I" statements, rather than "you" statements (see p. 40).	2	1	0
15. I feel that I am adequately assertive.	2	1	0
16. I let someone know when they are not respecting my rights or feelings.	2	1	0
17. I find it easy to say no to pressure for unwanted sexual activity.	2	1	0
18. I find it easy to say no to pressure for unwanted use of alcohol or recreational drugs.	2	1	0
19. When conflicts arise in my relationships I am, if necessary, willing and able to make a compromise in order to resolve the conflict.	2	1	0
20. When conflicts arise in my relationships I try to find a resolution that satisfies the needs of both persons involved.	2	1	0

Total points: _____

INTERPRETATION

36–40 points: You have developed highly effective patterns of communication and assertiveness.

32–35 points: You have above-average communication and assertiveness skills.

28–31 points: You have about average communication and assertiveness skills. Sharpening these skills will improve your relationships and need-fulfillment.

27 points or less: It would be very rewarding for you to improve your communication skills. Your relationships would function much better and you would experience much greater need-fulfillment.

Seven elements—the medium, the message, the speaker, the listener, feedback, interference, and the context—contribute to the success or failure of our communication efforts. Does it look like this conversation is going to succeed?

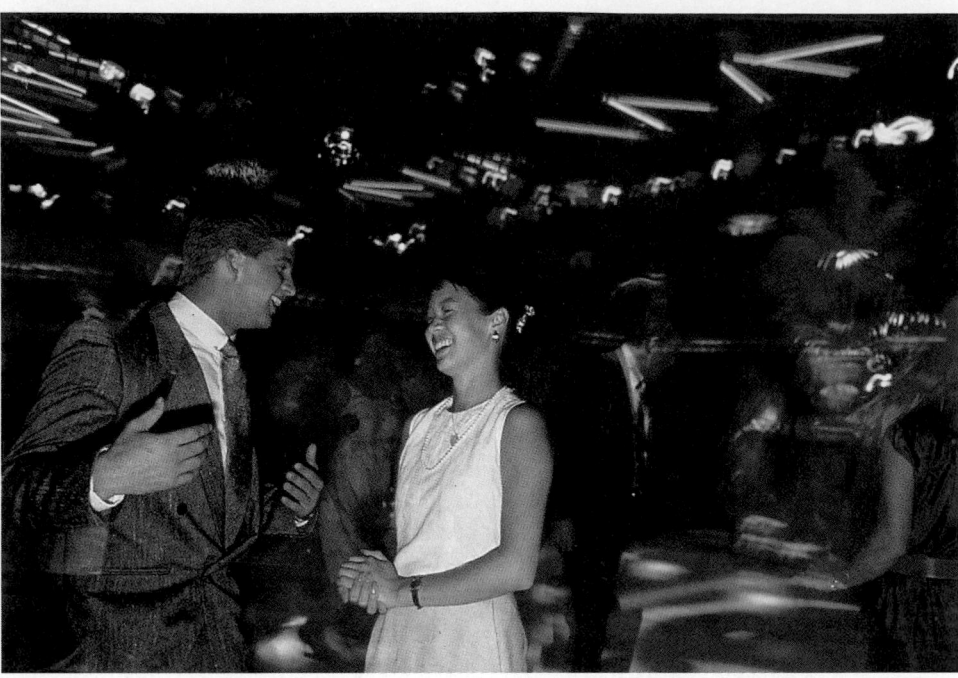

cation between people of different cultures misunderstanding can easily occur because each culture gives subtle shades of meaning to a particular word. Even though a dictionary may list several words as synonyms, in reality, each may carry a slightly different meaning. Someone who is new at speaking a certain language or who comes from a different culture but speaks the same language may not yet understand these subtleties.

4. The *listener*. Do you devote full attention to a speaker? Effective listening, discussed later in this chapter, can be even more difficult than effective speaking.

5. *Feedback*. Do you give a true indication of your reaction to the speaker? It is very frustrating to a speaker when the listener shows no response and gives no opportunity to correct or clarify misunderstood statements.

6. *Interference*. Messages often fail to get through or the content becomes confused because of interference:

- *External interference* is noise and other interruptions. If you sense that you are not "getting through" to your listener, suggest conducting your conversation at another time or place.

- *Internal interference* is within the listener. Does the listener have something else on his or her mind or have prejudices or precon-

ceptions that alter perception of the message? It takes skillful, direct communication to overcome this kind of interference.

7. The *context*. No two situations in communication are ever exactly the same. The effectiveness of the communication depends on the time, place, and context in which it occurs. Sometimes a discussion is better delayed until both participants are in a more receptive frame of mind or there is less interference.

PRINCIPLES OF COMMUNICATION

Understanding the principles of communication can help us to improve our communication habits. Richard Weaver has identified some principles that affect all interpersonal communication:[4]

- *Communication can be verbal or nonverbal.* The words we use convey only part of our message, often the smallest part. Nonverbal communication includes such behaviors as facial expressions, posture, and gestures. Further, the same words can take on very different meanings conveyed by voice qualities such as volume, pitch, speed, and inflection.

  Example: The phrase "I love you, too" can have an entirely different meaning if spoken sincerely than it does when spoken in anger.

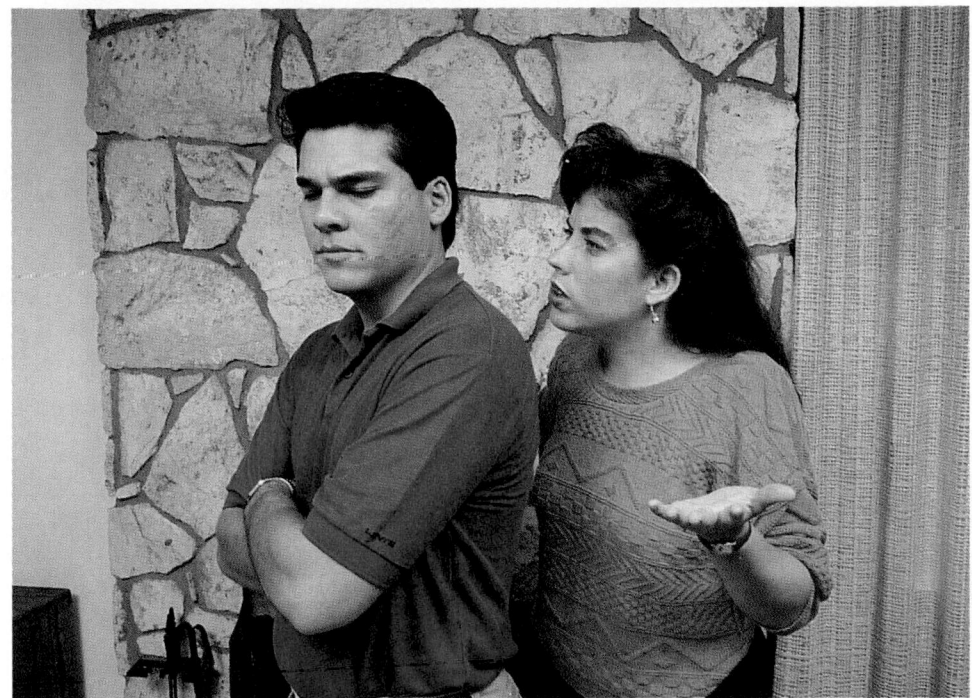

We cannot not communicate. Even without making any sound, we reveal more about ourselves than we may realize.

- *We cannot not communicate.* Communication is more than just the exchange of words. Even without making any sound, we communicate through our body language—our facial expression, posture, manner of dress, grooming, and other visible clues. Even our silence can carry a powerful message. A single touch can communicate a lot. Without opening our mouths, we reveal far more about ourselves to others than we may realize.

  Example: Gazing for even a second longer than our culture considers "normal" can convey sexual interest, curiosity, anger, or other nonverbal messages depending on the accompanying facial and bodily expressions.

- *Every communication contains information and defines relationships.* The *content* dimension of communication involves the information presented. The *relationship* dimension involves the feelings conveyed both through words and our many nonverbal symbols.

  Example: A message can be stated in a very factual way, which in many circumstances would be interpreted as being "cold." The same message could be stated more "warm-

ly" by changing a facial expression or putting a different inflection on a word or two.

- *Communication in relationships develops over time.* Patterns of communication within a relationship gradually change over a period of time as changes occur in the way the participants think of each other and define the rules governing their relationship. Over a period of time, unwritten rules and understandings develop to govern what is discussed, what is left unsaid, and the choice of terms used. Each person involved learns the meaning of a particular tone on a certain word, and the meaning of a particular facial expression or gesture. Even a simple raised eyebrow can convey a huge meaning to a knowing person. Conversely, some couples maintain a communication (or perhaps we should say noncommunication) style that depends mainly on mind reading and guessing. Every couple is unique from all other couples and, over time, their style of communication becomes similarly unique.

  Example: For a couple who know each other well, a single raised eyebrow at a party can say, "This is boring, let's get out of here."

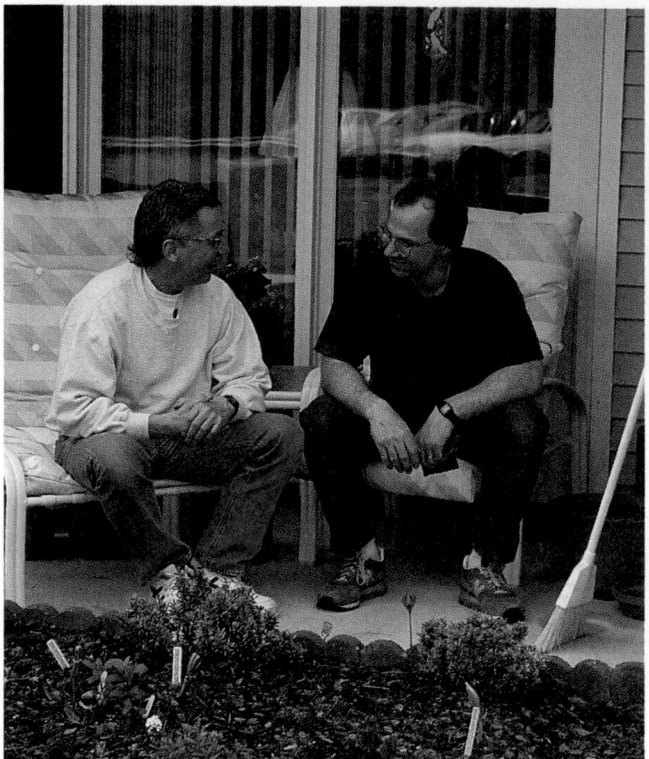

Communication in relationships develops over time. In successful relationships, communication gradually becomes more and more effective as each person learns to understand the other's facial expressions and the meaning of inflections placed on certain words.

- *Communication is an ongoing process.* Our communication experiences are cumulative; each is influenced by what has preceded it. To understand any single communication fully, we need to know all that has come before it. A casual observer could easily misinterpret a conversation taking place between two long-term friends.

- *Communication is irreversible.* It's very old advice, but the admonition to "think before you speak" remains very important if we are to develop and maintain valuable relationships. Is there anyone who has never, in anger or frustration, said something that he or she later wished had remained unsaid? But remarks can never be taken back and you can't totally undo the damage done by a careless remark, no matter what you say or how much you apologize later.

When the inevitable occasional slip does occur, every effort should be made to minimize its impact. A sincere, honest explanation of the frustration, anger, or other feeling

that motivated the remark can lead to a productive conversation.

Example: "I feel really bad about what I said to you today. Nothing had gone right at school all day long and I guess I just had to take my frustration out on someone. I chose you because I feel the most comfortable with you. I guess you always hurt the one you love. I hope you will be able to forgive me."

CHECKPOINT

1. What seven elements in communication have been identified?

2. What are six principles of interpersonal communication?

3. Explain the following: "We cannot *not* communicate." ✓

EFFECTIVE SPEAKING

Do you ever feel that people don't seem to understand what you are saying or, worse still, just aren't interested in what you have to say? Being an interesting, effective speaker is a characteristic that anyone can develop and one that contributes greatly to the quality of your relationships.

For starters, you need to *have something interesting to say.* This means having familiarity with a broad range of topics and being sensitive to the interests of the listener.

Even though the pressures of school or work may dictate where much of your attention is directed, you need to reserve time to broaden your interests and expand your awareness of a variety of subjects. If you are highly knowledgeable about your major field, but have little awareness of other subjects, there will be relatively few people who find you a stimulating conversational partner.

If you find yourself being misunderstood, you may need to *improve the exactness of your communication.* Vocabulary building may be necessary. Communication is often handicapped by a lack of the precise word to express a particular idea or feeling. It can be very frustrating to know what you want to say, but to lack the words that would convey that thought. Many colleges offer vocabulary-building courses. Books, tapes, computer programs, and other media are also available to help expand your vocabulary.

When communicating with someone from another ethnic group, remember that you may use a word or phrase to convey a particular meaning but it may only have that meaning to someone with your own background. Even people from different regions of the United States may interpret the same phrase differently.

In health-related communication, vocabulary is especially important. Many problems arise in communication between health care providers and their clients when the clients are unable to describe symptoms or concerns adequately or the providers speak above or below the ability of the client to comprehend.

Example: Some people describe any pain between their neck and their crotch as a "stomachache."

If this book seems to use a lot of terminology, it's because precise communication does require

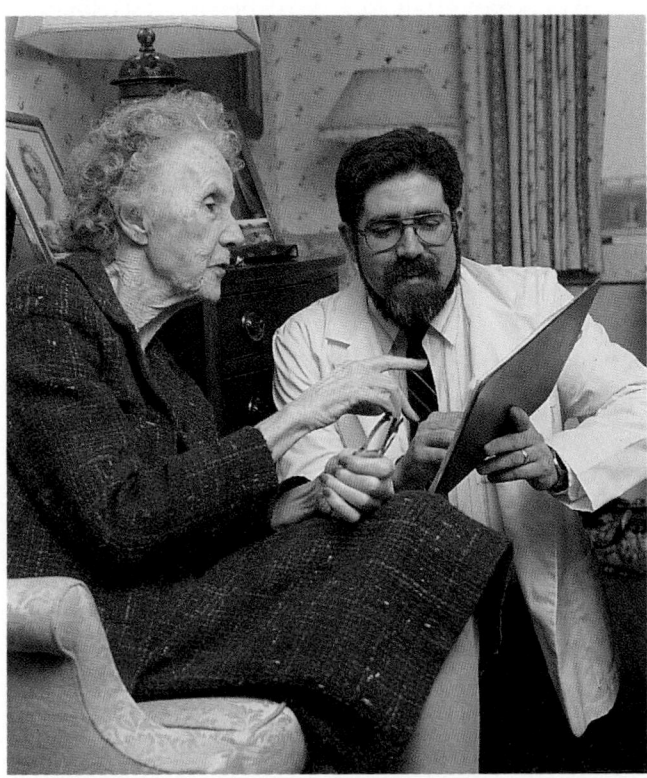

In health-related communication, vocabulary is especially important. Problems arise when clients are unable to describe their symptoms or concerns adequately or when care providers speak above or below the ability of the client to comprehend.

using the proper term. Too often, health-related communication suffers from inadequate vocabulary. One unfortunate result of inadequate vocabulary is that sometimes, not knowing which word to use, we simply fail to communicate at all.

To ensure the clarity of your communication, *think through what you intend to say before you say it*. Even though this may cause a slight pause in the flow of the conversation, it reduces the risk of your being misinterpreted. To further reduce this risk, when you have something important to say, repeat it several times, phrasing it in different ways. Of course, don't go overboard with repetition. It can get annoying!

Be very alert to the verbal and nonverbal feedback you get from your listener and use this feedback to guide your communication. For example, you may sense the need to speak more slowly or to rephrase your message.

CHECKPOINT

1. What are four guidelines for effective speaking?

2. Do you feel that you have an adequate vocabulary for most communication situations?

3. What do you usually do when someone seems not to understand what you are saying?

EFFECTIVE LISTENING

An effective listener is just as actively involved in communication as the speaker. In fact, effective listening requires greater effort and concentration than speaking. Your attention must remain focused on the speaker and not wander. Any momentary inattention can cause you to miss the meaning of what is being said.

In any important discussion, it is essential to minimize distractions so that your full attention can be focused on the speaker. Turn off the TV or stereo; close the door; suggest moving to a less distracting location; ask the other person to speak louder. If you can't eliminate distractions, at least make every effort to concentrate on the discussion.

Often the speaker's nonverbal communication reveals more than his or her actual words. Be very alert to posture, gestures, facial expressions, eye movements, and the tone and inflection in the speaker's voice.

Listeners often misinterpret what they hear. For instance, people sometimes interpret messages as being hostile or critical when they were not intended that way. Major misunderstandings can develop when you fail to ask for clarification of some vague or seemingly hurtful statement. If you have any doubt about the meaning of what you have just been told, immediately ask for clarification.

When someone makes a statement that causes you to feel hurt, angry, or defensive, it is often productive to reveal your feelings (see p. 40), allowing the misunderstanding or conflict to be worked out *at that time*. Otherwise, hostility builds up and will be expressed eventually, often in a nonproductive manner, which can severely damage or even destroy a relationship.

In summary, Eugene Raudsepp has identified seven ways to improve your listening abilities:[5]

1. *Take time to listen.* Sometimes people aren't sure just what they need to say or how best to express their message. They think as they speak and may modify their message as they go. Though you may wish they would hurry up and get to the point, effective listening requires you patiently to allow the speaker to finish his or her message, and reassure him or her on that point.

Example: "Take your time. I'm listening to you. There's no rush."

2. *Don't interrupt.* Even though you think you know what the speaker is leading up to and you are impatient for him or her to make a point, resist the temptation to interrupt and finish sentences (see Feature 2.1). Doing so implies a sense of superiority and may break down communication. Interruptions often confuse the speaker and there is a possibility that your assumptions may be wrong.

Example: "I know what you are going to say and I think you're wrong. You think that. . . ."

If you have the habit of interrupting, as many of us do, Raudsepp suggests breaking that habit by making yourself apologize every time you interrupt. After a few apologies, you'll think twice before interrupting someone.

Example: "Excuse me for interrupting you. It's a habit I'm trying to break, so let me know whenever I do it."

3. *Teach yourself to concentrate.* One reason we sometimes have trouble concentrating on a speaker is that we can think much faster than a person can speak. We get bored and begin to think about something else. To remain focused on the speaker, keep analyzing what he or she is saying.

4. *Disregard speech mannerisms.* Don't focus on a person's accent, speech impediment, or delivery style; you will lose track of his or her message.

5. *Suspend judgment.* We tend to listen to the ideas we want to hear and to shut out others. We unconsciously do this because ideas that conflict with our own are threatening. But by listening to what others have to say, we can come to under-

FEATURE 2.1

PLEASE DON'T INTERRUPT ME

Interruptions are a leading cause of communication breakdown in families, at work—whenever and wherever people need to resolve issues. First one participant in the discussion interrupts the other and then he or she is in turn interrupted. Neither gets to communicate an idea or a concern completely. Both are talking and neither is listening to the other. Soon the discussion degenerates to yelling, maybe to hitting, and the issue remains unresolved.

There is a better way! Try this the next time you have a serious issue to discuss with someone, especially if your previous communication with that person has been difficult. Here are the rules:

1. Each person gets to speak, in turn, without being interrupted, for five minutes. A timer is very useful so that no one has to watch the clock.

2. During each five-minute period the listener must focus his or her entire attention on the speaker. The listener's eyes must remain on the speaker, although the speaker does not have to look into the listener's eyes.

3. Absolutely no interruptions are allowed.

4. Turns continue until each has said all that he or she cares to say.

Following the five-minute communication periods, if the participants wish, they can converse normally, but the rule against interrupting still holds. Each party gets to finish making his or her point before the other party responds.

Try it. You might be surprised to hear what someone will say if they are just given the chance.

stand our own line of reasoning better and may even change our mind.

6. *Listen between the lines.* Much of the important content in the messages we receive is unstated or only indirectly implied. Focusing only on the message actually verbalized leads us to miss most, if not all, of the true message. Be sensitive to what the speaker is feeling and the true message may become evident.

> *Example: Lori says, "I've heard that that's a good place to get a sandwich." Lori means, "I'm hungry!"*

7. *Listen with your eyes.* Pay attention to the speaker's nonverbal signals, as discussed on p. 39. Rarely can the full message be gained from words alone.

> *Example: "How are you feeling today?" "I'm fine." "Well, the sad look on your face and the way you're wringing your hands tells me that something is bothering you. Would you like to talk about it?"*

CHECKPOINT

1. List seven suggestions for improving listening abilities.

2. In addition to being rude, what implications does interrupting a speaker carry?

RESPONDING TO COMMUNICATION (FEEDBACK)

When we receive any message, our first response is internal. Our emotions, knowledge, and past experiences cause us to feel a particular way in response to what we have just heard. Our own particular style of feedback will then determine how or whether we communicate this feeling back to the speaker. Weaver has identified some common styles of feedback.[6]

WITHDRAWING

The withdrawing response may occur when the topic of discussion creates uncomfortable feelings. The listener just ignores what the speaker has said or perhaps changes the subject of the discussion. Withdrawing from an unpleasant topic does not contribute to a rewarding relationship or help resolve a problem. Withdrawing tends to be taken as evidence of callousness or lack of concern.

> *Example: A good friend is trying to tell you that she or he thinks you have been drinking too much, but you quickly change the subject.*

JUDGING

One of the quickest ways to cut off open communication is to make a judgmental response. By

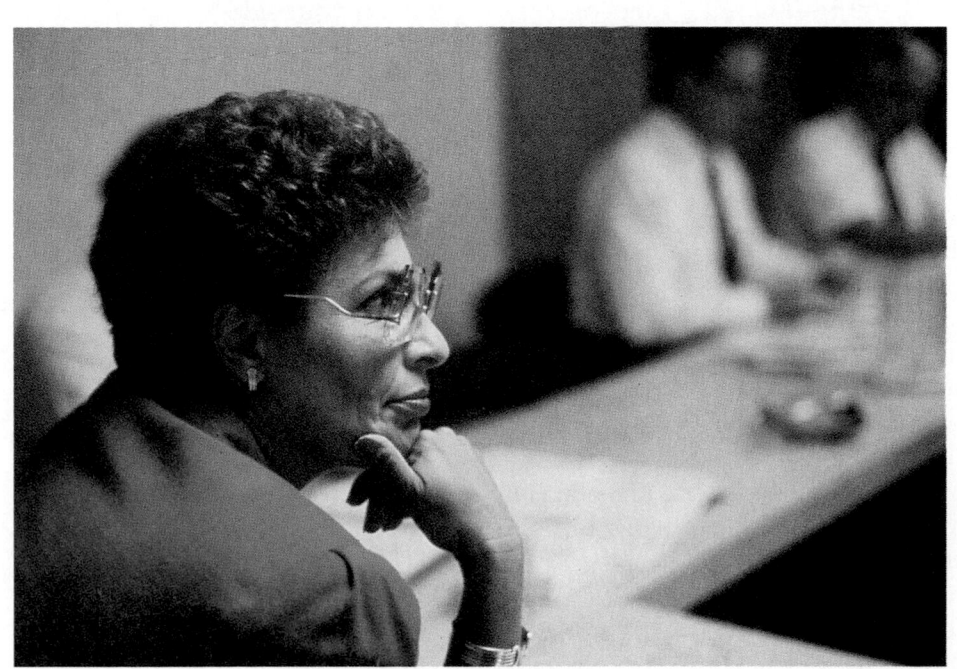

Listen with your eyes. Watch closely for nonverbal signals; they may reveal far more than a speaker's words.

bluntly telling someone that her or his idea or action is good or bad, we imply that we know more than she or he does. By making a judgment, one takes control of the communication and causes the other to feel that there is no point in continuing the discussion. The judging person seems to have already made up his or her mind and seems uninterested in hearing the whole story.

Judgmental responses can be very damaging to relationships, especially when someone is judged in a negative way. The judged person is placed in the position of having to defend his or her opinion, belief, or behavior. This leads to rejection of and resistance to the "judge." A common result is terminating the communication, if not the entire relationship.

> *Example: "You've got it all wrong. How could you be so stupid. Anyone with half a brain could see it's not like that."*

ANALYZING

Analyzing is very similar to judging. It is when we explain to someone why they feel, believe, or act as they do. Once again, we have set ourself up as the expert, the superior person. And the results are the same: People are made to feel defensive and become less likely to reveal their thoughts and feelings.

> *Example: "The reason you believe that way is because you just haven't been around very much."*

QUESTIONING

Depending on one's choice of questions, asking questions can either enhance or inhibit communication. Helpful questions are those that are neither threatening nor judgmental. They encourage a person to express ideas and feelings and often to gain insights that they had previously overlooked. Damaging questions express a negative value judgment and force a person into a defensive position. Weaver suggests that "why" questions are best avoided for that reason. *"Why did you do that?" really means "You shouldn't have done that."* Helpful questions tend to begin with "what," "where," "when," "how," or "who." These questions encourage people to open up, rather than to try to defend themselves.

Try to avoid questions that can be answered with a simple yes or no. These are closed-ended questions that don't usually lead to very revealing answers. The same is true of either/or questions. Better to ask open-ended questions that encourage self-disclosure. Where would you expect each of these questions to lead?

- "Do you drink too much?" (closed-ended)
- "Tell me about your drinking patterns. Where and when do you drink and about how much?" (open-ended)
- "Do you think I'm too fat?" (closed-ended)
- "What do you think would be an ideal weight for me?" (open-ended)
- "Do you want hamburgers or tacos for lunch?" (either/or)
- "What would you like to have for lunch?" (open-ended)

You can see that, in each case, the open-ended question is more likely to lead to a productive discussion than a yes/no or either/or question.

REASSURING

One important thing that friends do for each other is to provide emotional support. This often takes the form of reassuring a friend who is feeling upset that he or she has someone who cares and who shares his or her concerns. A reassuring response acknowledges the validity of the other person's feelings. It says "I'm on your side."

> *Example: "I'm really sorry to hear about your miscarriage. You must be feeling so much loss right now."*

When appropriate, it includes pointing out more positive ways of viewing the troubling situation. Care must be taken, however, not to imply that the friend should not feel as he or she does, because that would be a judging response.

PARAPHRASING

Paraphrasing is an effective listening device. **Paraphrasing** is simply restating what has just been

....

paraphrasing restating what someone has said, putting the message into one's own words.

said, and putting it into the listener's own words. It shows the speaker that the listener has really heard what has been said and gives the speaker a chance to correct any misconception that may have occurred. Paraphrasing makes certain that we have understood what has been said. It encourages the other person to expand and clarify her or his message. And it assures the other that we are hearing and understand and truly care about what he or she is saying.

Example: Maria says, "I just feel the need for a little more space right now. I still want to be your friend." Carlos responds, "You're saying that you don't want to spend as much time together as we have been, but you still want to spend some time together."

CHECKPOINT

1. What are six common styles of response to a speaker as identified by Weaver?

2. What is the likely outcome of each style of response?

NONVERBAL COMMUNICATION

Effective communication requires alertness to the many nonverbal signals we receive from others. Nonverbal communication includes what we commonly call "body language," meaning posture, gestures, and facial expressions. It includes how we speak—the tone, force, tempo, and inflection given to each word. It even includes how a person dresses and how close to someone a person stands while speaking.

We tend to reveal much through our nonverbal communication, often more than we reveal through our words. Even information we might prefer not to reveal is readily conveyed nonverbally.

Nonverbal communication is influenced by numerous factors. It reflects the personality of the individual, how he or she feels in respect to others present, and to a surprising degree, his or her cultural or ethnic background. The better we know an individual, the better we are able to read his or her nonverbal signals. Close friends often carry on complex exchanges of information without the use of a single word.

When people are less familiar with each other, and especially when they represent different cultures, misperceptions can easily occur. Some expressions and gestures take on very different meanings within different cultures, as many politicians and businesspersons who travel a great deal have learned to their dismay.

One area in which misperceptions occur is in the use of touching as a form of nonverbal communication. Usually touching is a positive gesture, such as a pat on the back, a hug, a high five, a handshake, or a kiss. A simple touch can convey affection, caring, joy, empathy, sympathy, and many other emotions. Humans have a basic need for the touch of other humans and touching is considered important for maintaining emotional health.

Occasionally, touching is, or is interpreted as, an expression of power or domination over a person. Different people may respond quite differently to the same touch. One person might appreciate it as a symbol of closeness or caring, while another might view it as an invasion of his or her private space. Like most nonverbal communication, being touched is interpreted differently by people of different cultures.

INTERPRETING BODY LANGUAGE

Understanding the messages of other people depends very much on our ability to interpret the nonverbal elements of their communication. As we have mentioned, we are best able to do this with people we know well and with whose culture we are familiar.

As you talk with people, evaluate their overall posture. Do they sit or stand confidently erect or is their head bowed and their shoulders slumped forward? Are they looking you in the eye or are they looking at the ground or who knows where?

How close does the person stand as you talk? In general, moving closer to you indicates an interest in you or the discussion. Keeping a distance may indicate uncertainty about you or a dislike of or disinterest in the topic of discussion. Bear in mind, however, that some people just naturally prefer more space under any circumstance.

Watch the person's hands as you interact. Even though he or she may seem calm, nervousness is often revealed through hand activity. Watch also for the classic sign of arms folded across a person's chest. This often means that he or she is feeling defensive and you may need to back off somewhat in your approach. Of course, it could also just mean that the person feels cold, showing how easily body language can be misinterpreted.

Perhaps the most important signs to watch are found in facial expressions. Watch for smiles at inappropriate times. Genuine emotions usually cause a quick smile. If someone is faking an emotion, they often hold the expression too long. Further, a genuine smile goes up into the eyes and involves the whole face. A false smile usually just involves the bottom of the face.

Keep in mind that body language is easily misinterpreted. If you are not sure what a person is saying or feeling, getting clarification could prevent your discussion from ending in a misunderstanding.

WHEN VERBAL AND NONVERBAL MESSAGES CONFLICT

We have all had the experience of talking to someone whose nonverbal messages clearly contradict their words. Which message are we to believe? With only rare exceptions, the nonverbal message will be the more accurate. It is easy to control our choice of words, but more difficult to control our tone of voice, facial expression, posture, and other nonverbal signals.

C H E C K P O I N T

1. What are the components of nonverbal communication?

2. Why might the same gesture made by different people have different meanings?

3. How can you distinguish a genuine smile from a faked one?

SHARING EMOTIONS

Emotions are mental states that include feelings, physiological changes, and a pattern of overt expression. Even people who fail to express their emotions verbally can seldom avoid expressing them through their facial expressions and body language. Though the perception of emotions is highly subjective, they are real, valid, and important. Emotions are a big part of what it means to be human.

....

emotions mental states that include feelings, physiological changes, and a pattern of overt expression.

One of the more difficult forms of communication, at least for some of us, is the sharing of emotions. We are embarrassed to reveal that much of ourselves. We have been taught to keep our feelings to ourselves. We just don't know what words to use. Yet, there can be significant benefits to sharing emotions. Sharing emotions with others can help solve personal problems, reduce stress levels, resolve interpersonal conflicts, and contribute to intimacy in relationships.

Before we can communicate our emotions we have to understand just what it is that we are feeling. Often our emotions, especially those involving our closest relationships, are intense, but unclear. We can, for example, feel a mixture of emotions such as jealousy, anger, fear, and sadness, which can be difficult to express in words until we sort out just what we are feeling.

In sharing emotions, it is more effective to use "I" statements, rather than "you" statements. **"I" statements** are expressions of your own feelings, emotions, or other responses. **"You" statements** are those that judge another's behavior and place responsibility for your emotions on that other person. "You" statements place blame and tend to force the listener into a defensive position, while "I" statements encourage discussion. Consider the likely response to each of the following statements:

- You really made me mad when you let him stay overnight at your place.
- I felt hurt when I came to your apartment and found him there.

- You never talk to me; you always go running to someone else.
- I felt rejected when you called her instead of talking over your feelings with me.

- You must not love me if you want to talk to other women.
- I feel unloved when you talk to other women.

....

"I" statements expressions of your own feelings, emotions, or other responses.

"you" statements statements that judge another's behavior and place responsibility for your emotions on that other person.

In each case, the "you" statement is an accusation or placement of blame. It closes the door to a meaningful sharing of feelings and encourages an angry response and escalating hostility. The "I" statement reveals feelings without placing blame for causing those feelings.

C H E C K P O I N T

1. Why are "you" messages seldom helpful?
2. In addition to the book's examples of "I" messages, write down several examples that might be useful in your current life situation.

ASSERTIVE COMMUNICATION

Assertiveness is a highly culture-sensitive topic. What might be considered proper behavior in one culture might be considered very passive or overly aggressive in another culture. Further, members of different cultures tend to be assertive in different areas. For example, by European-American standards, the members of a particular culture might be considered very assertive, even aggressive, in business situations, but considered quite passive in dating situations. Thus, readers need to interpret this section in terms of their own ethnic traditions.

Assertiveness is making our needs and desires known to others and, when necessary, defending our rights. Rather than passively sitting back and wishing that other people would recognize and help fulfill our needs, we actively work toward fulfilling our own needs. Most of us have, at times, allowed someone to take advantage of us in some situation and later on, felt extremely resentful for letting it happen. Other times we act aggressively and try to dominate a situation, but end up fearing retaliation from those who were repressed.

We need to be able to distinguish among three types of behavior in ourselves:

1. **Passive behavior** is when we deny our own needs and rights. We fail to express our true feelings and desires. We allow others to make choices for us. As a result, we fail to reach our goals or to fulfill our needs. We feel resentful to-

ward others, but even more resentful toward ourselves for being so passive. As a result, our self-esteem is reduced and our relationships with others may become strained. We are exhibiting passive behavior when we:

- seldom speak up in groups
- avoid taking a stand on issues
- allow others to make decisions for us
- avoid forming friendships because we fear rejection
- speak in a soft voice and avoid making eye contact when speaking
- just agree with other people in order to avoid a confrontation
- consider ourselves weaker and less capable than others
- avoid assuming responsibilities

    Example: Someone in one of your classes is seriously cheating on the exams. You study hard and take your tests honestly. The professor grades on a curve and the cheater is raising the curve. Also, your anger over the situation is interfering with your own work in the class. But you don't say anything to either the cheater or the professor because you don't want a confrontation.

2. **Aggressive behavior** is an attempt to accomplish our goals or fulfill our needs at the expense of others' rights, needs, or feelings. Aggressive behavior may hurt or humiliate others, or it may put them on the defensive. Aggressive behavior alienates other people, who, in reaction to our aggressive behavior, may go out of their way to see that we don't achieve our goals. Internally, we feel guilt, remorse, fear of retaliation, and personal anxiety. Aggressive behavior does not contribute to rewarding relationships; in fact, it can ruin relationships. We are being aggressive when we:

- interrupt others before they finish speaking
- try to force our position on others
- make decisions for other people

passive behavior denying our own needs and rights by failing to express our true feelings and desires.

aggressive behavior attempting to accomplish our goals or fulfill our needs at the expense of others' rights, needs, or feelings.

FEATURE 2.2

ON BECOMING MORE ASSERTIVE

Many of us could be happier and have our needs better fulfilled if we were more assertive. For even the shyest of us, this is not an impossible goal. The biggest step is deciding that we are going to become assertive; this can be a very threatening idea for a nonassertive person.

In all things in life, success builds upon success. Becoming assertive is a gradual process—start with small acts of assertiveness, then, after seeing how well they work, move on to progressively more assertive actions.

Assertiveness skills can be developed through attending special classes, seminars, or minicourses offered on most college campuses. Another option is to work with one of the many assertiveness training books, which are available at most bookstores. Some basic steps in developing assertiveness skills are the following:

1. Learn to distinguish between passive, assertive, and aggressive behavior.

2. Observe and analyze your own behavior for passiveness, assertiveness, and aggressiveness.

3. Identify situations in which you might act more assertively than you would normally act.

4. Think about ways in which you might be more assertive in those situations. Observe how other people act in similar situations.

5. Try assertive behaviors in role-playing situations with a friend, teacher, or counselor.

6. Evaluate the results and ask for feedback from the other person.

7. Try assertive behavior in real-life situations, perhaps starting with minor matters.

8. Continue to evaluate and develop your assertiveness. Talk to friends about how you handled a particular situation. Build upon your success.

Long-established behavior patterns do not change overnight. With the reinforcement of success, however, assertive behavior can become increasingly spontaneous and effective. In time, you will be able to be assertive, without hesitation, in any situation.

Source: Alberti, R., and Emmons, M. *Your Perfect Right*, 6th ed. San Luis Obispo, CA: Impact, 1990. (This is a good resource for anyone who wants to develop their assertiveness.)

- take advantage of friendships by using people
- speak loudly and say or do things to call attention to ourselves
- have little regard for the feelings of others
- aren't always honest with other people
- act as if we are superior to other people

Example. It is the first week of the term and there is a long line at the cashier in the bookstore. Instead of going to the end of the line, you look for someone you know who is near the front of the line. You walk up, start a conversation, and pretty soon you are paying for your books. The people behind you are giving you hard looks and you leave with an uncomfortable feeling.

3. **Assertive behavior** (Feature 2.2) is when we make our needs and desires known to others and when we stand up for our right to have our

....

assertive behavor making our needs and desires known to others and, when necessary, defending our rights.

needs fulfilled. We make our own choices and achieve our goals without infringing upon the rights of other people. As a result, we feel good about ourselves and others, and others respect us. Assertive behavior results in maximum need-fulfillment, increased self-esteem, a feeling of autonomy, good feelings about others, and healthy interpersonal relationships. Assertive behavior is sometimes confused with aggressive behavior, but there are distinct differences. We are being assertive when we:

- allow others to complete their statements without interrupting them
- stand up for our beliefs
- think for ourselves
- enjoy meeting people and forming new friendships
- are comfortable speaking to others and make eye contact with them
- try to understand the feelings of others and make our own feelings clear to them
- face problems and confidently make decisions
- consider ourselves equal to other people

Example: The person who sits behind you in one of your classes constantly chews gum, making distracting smacking and popping sounds. You tell him that these sounds are making the class unpleasant for you and ask him to either not chew gum in class or to chew it very quietly. He apologizes, says he didn't realize he was making noise, and doesn't chew gum in class again.

Why are some people too passive or too aggressive? Part of the answer may be found in the conflicting messages we get from our culture. On the one hand, tact, diplomacy, politeness, modesty, and self-denial are often praised. On the other hand, "getting ahead" is also valued and in some circles it is considered necessary to "step on" or exploit others in the process. As a result, some people have never learned to distinguish among the three types of behavior.

CHECKPOINT

1. Contrast passive, aggressive, and assertive behavior.

2. What are the most likely outcomes of each?

3. Judging by the discussion in this section, is your behavior more often passive, aggressive, or assertive?

4. What factors have contributed to your being as you are regarding assertiveness?

RESOLVING CONFLICTS

Conflict is any situation in which our wants, needs, or intentions are incompatible with the wants, needs, or intentions of another person. If one person has his or her way, the other does not. Conflict is a part of every relationship. In even the best relationships, there are inevitably some periods of conflict. No two people can have exactly the same desires, tastes, and ways of doing things.

....

conflict any situation in which our wants, needs, or intentions are incompatible with the wants, needs, or intentions of another person.

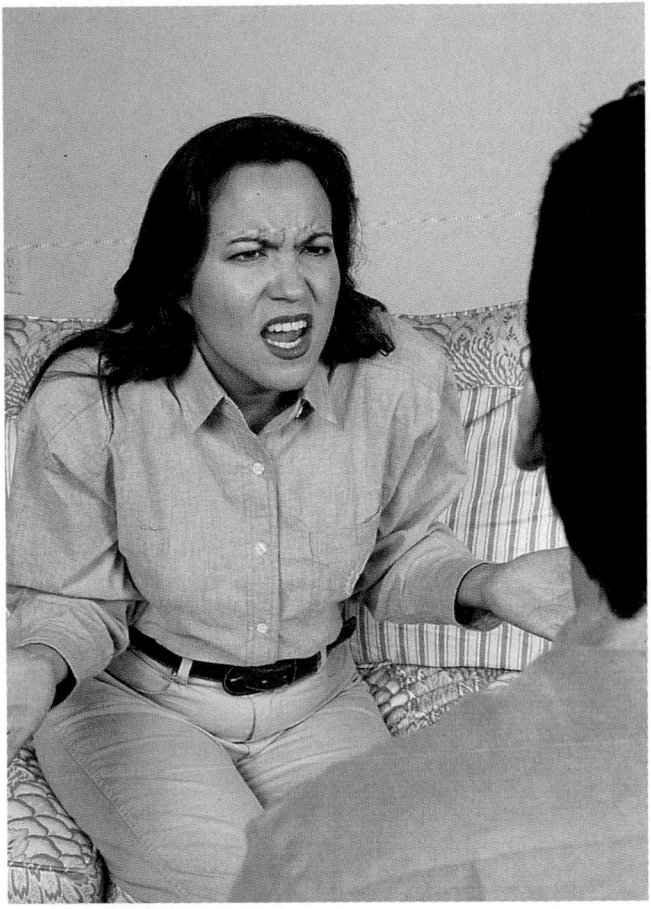

Conflict is a part of every relationship. It can be handled in ways that build the relationship or destroy it. Constructive ways of dealing with conflict avoid putting either party into a defensive position and tend to use "I" statements rather than "You" statements.

It may seem that conflicts destroy relationships, and they certainly do have the potential to do so. The needs and tastes of some people are so different that they really are incompatible with each other. But more often it is not conflict itself, but how conflict is handled that destroys a relationship.

Conflict can be either constructive or destructive, depending on how we deal with it. In destructive conflict, neither person listens to the other. Both talk and scream at the same time. Reactions are highly emotional. Name-calling can escalate to shoving and other physical abuse. But none of this is necessary.

In constructive conflict, the key to resolving a situation successfully is to avoid forcing either person to have to defend him- or herself. In one approach, each party, in turn, using "I" language, expresses his or her feelings about the situation while the other quietly listens without interrupting.

By emphasizing feelings as being the problem there is less need or likelihood for anyone to take a defensive posture.

STYLES OF HANDLING CONFLICT

Conflict is often handled in one of five common ways, reflecting differing degrees of passive, aggressive, or assertive, and competitive or cooperative behavior. Think about the most recent time you were in a conflict situation. Which of the following seems to describe most closely what took place?

Avoiding

Avoiding is behavior that is both passive and uncooperative on the part of one or both parties. There is no attempt to resolve the conflict or to address each other's needs and concerns.

> *Example: Tom and Tina are both busy in their careers and spend little time in shared activities. Each feels neglected by the other, but neither mentions it. Lately Tina has started seeing a man she met at work, while Tom retreats further into his job.*

Avoidance may be acceptable as a temporary measure until there is time to discuss a conflict or the means of dealing with it. But conflicts that go unresolved over a long period often destroy or damage a relationship. Even though conflicts are not discussed, they influence how the partners feel about each other and may even have physical effects. For example, an unresolved conflict over how a couple manages their money or disciplines their children may lead to high blood pressure, asthma attacks, ulcers, or any of dozens of other physical disorders.

Accommodating

Accommodating behavior is cooperative, but passive. One person gives up the satisfaction of his or her needs in order to accommodate the conflicting needs of the other. If the yielding person really isn't too concerned about the situation, this may be fine. But if one partner is frequently accommodating the needs of the other, this is likely to lead to resentment, loss of self-esteem, and even loss of respect by the other partner.

> *Example: Tony loves to have fast food for dinner every night. Anita prefers home-cooked food, but goes along with Tony "to keep the peace." While eating her fast-food dinner, however, Anita sits quietly, saying little to Tony, mostly thinking about the weight she can't seem to keep from gaining on her fast-food diet.*

Competing

Competing takes place when both partners are aggressively trying to fulfill their own needs, but cooperating little to ensure the need fulfillment of each other. Power becomes an ever-present issue, with each person doing everything possible to assert power over the other. Competition consumes a lot of energy and, except for the few relationships that seem to thrive on competition, tends to eliminate the possibility of any true intimacy.

> *Example: Lisa and Ray are sales reps for different product lines. Each likes to make more money than the other does. On a morning when one has an important presentation to make, it can be predicted that the other will start a fight about some trivial complaint. They often go to work tired and upset.*

Compromising

Compromising requires a moderate degree of both cooperativeness and assertiveness by each person. A mutually acceptable solution to the conflict is found, but it only partially satisfies each person's needs. Though it is not ideal, a compromise may be

avoiding behavior that is both passive and uncooperative.

accommodating behavior that is cooperative, but passive.

competing when both partners are aggressively trying to fulfill their own needs, but cooperating little to ensure the need-fulfillment of each other.

compromising when a mutually acceptable solution to a conflict is found, but it only partially satisfies each person's needs.

the best solution to a conflict. Any ongoing relationship requires a certain amount of compromise.

Example: Tony and Anita, of the fast-food conflict, agree to eat home-cooked food on alternate nights. They also agree to take turns with the shopping, cooking, and cleanup. Both lose some excess weight.

Collaborating

Collaborating means working together. It satisfies the needs of both partners through a maximum use of both cooperation and assertiveness. Weaver identifies a series of steps that enable collaborative conflict resolution:[7]

1. Acknowledge that there really is a conflict (no avoidance).
2. Clearly define what the conflict is (some couples fight for years without knowing what their basic conflict really is).
3. View the conflict as a joint problem (the only approach that can lead to a win-win resolution).
4. Identify and acknowledge each person's needs.
5. Identify a number of possible resolutions for the conflict.
6. Speculate on the likely consequences of each resolution for each person.
7. Reach a mutually acceptable decision on which alternative best meets the needs of each party.
8. Implement the decision and set a date to review its effectiveness.
9. Evaluate the results and if either party is dissatisfied, return to Step 5 or possibly even Step 2.

This is a time-consuming process that cannot be carried out if either partner is rushed or upset. It may be advantageous to set a time, ideally within 24 hours of when the conflict emerges, to talk. When the couple sits down to talk, there must be no distractions—no TV, no music, no phone calls, and so forth. If the discussion is not going well,

either partner should feel free to call a time-out. Stop talking about the conflict and set another time to continue to talk, again within 24 hours.

If one person absolutely refuses to talk, the relationship may be deeply troubled and in need of the help of a qualified counselor. Ideally, both partners will visit the counselor, but if one refuses, the other should feel free to consult a therapist alone.

CHECKPOINT

1. Name and briefly characterize five styles of handling conflict.
2. Which of the five described styles of handling conflict fits most closely with your style?
3. Can you see any ways to resolve current conflicts in your life more effectively?

THE MASS MEDIA AND WELLNESS

As we will discuss in specific subject matter chapters, the popular media have a powerful ability to influence public attitudes and behavior. Media executives recognize that power only selectively. While they deny that their glorification of alcohol and drug abuse and irresponsible sexuality affects public behavior, they sell their advertising time and space on the promise that it *will* affect public behavior. Are we to believe that the ads affect behavior, but the programming does not?

Television in particular, being both auditory and visual, has the ability to motivate people toward either healthful or unhealthful behaviors. Some of the disturbing messages, apparent in both programming and ads, are the following:

- association of drinking with status, glamour, fun, and sexual conquest
- the need to prove masculinity, femininity, or maturity through sexual activity
- casual sexual activity with no concern for preventing disease or pregnancy
- violence as acceptable behavior

Programs featuring healthful life-styles can influence attitudes and behaviors in a very positive way and still achieve high ratings. The extremely successful and long-running *Cosby Show* is a case in point.

collaborating working together.

People are always interested in the latest health research and new findings are often presented in the media. Unfortunately, the popular media do an uneven job of presenting health research. Many stories compete for time and space in the media. In general, the more sensational topics will be presented while the less "exciting" research, though it may be quite important, is ignored. We need to evaluate critically the health research that is presented in the media, using the criteria described in Chapter 1.

SUMMARY

Effective communication promotes wellness in many ways: It contributes to rewarding relationships and helps you express emotions, interact with health-care providers, relate to people from various ethnic groups, and resolve conflicts.

Cultural diversity means people with a variety of histories, ideologies, traditions, values, life-styles, and languages living and interacting together. Communication among people of different cultures may face difficulties beyond language barriers. Cultural differences can lead to misinterpretation of messages. To enhance your communication with people of different ethnic groups you can do the following: develop an understanding of your own cultural values and biases; develop an understanding of the cultures of other ethnic groups with which you interact; be respectful of, interested in, and nonjudgmental about cultures other than your own; speak in a way that promotes understanding and shows respect for someone from a different ethnic group; avoid using slang or idioms that might be misunderstood; and remember that the same gesture can carry different meanings in different cultures.

Seven elements of communication include the medium, the message, the speaker, the listener, feedback from the listener to the speaker, internal and external interference, and the context.

Among the principles of communication are the following: communication can be verbal or nonverbal, you cannot not communicate, every communication contains information and defines relationships, communication in relationships develops over time, communication is an ongoing process, and communication is irreversible.

To be an effective speaker you must have something interesting to say and the vocabulary to convey your true meaning. You must think through what you are going to say and be alert to your listener's verbal and nonverbal feedback.

To be an effective listener you must give full attention to the speaker. You can improve listening by taking time to listen, not interrupting, teaching yourself to concentrate, disregarding speech mannerisms, suspending judgment, listening between the lines, and listening with your eyes.

Listeners provide feedback to speakers in various ways, including withdrawing, judging, analyzing, questioning, reassuring, and paraphrasing.

Effective communication requires being alert to the many nonverbal signals you receive from others. They include posture, gestures, facial expressions, tone and inflection of words, how a person dresses, and how close they stand to you. Nonverbal communication reflects the personality of the individual and his or her culture. When people are unfamiliar with each other and especially when they represent different cultures, misperceptions can easily occur.

Emotions are real, valid, and important. Sharing them can help solve personal problems, reduce stress levels, resolve conflicts, and contribute to intimacy in relationships. In sharing emotions, "I" statements are more effective than "you" statements.

Assertiveness is making your needs and desires known to others and defending your rights. It can be contrasted to passive behavior, when you fail to communicate your feelings, needs, and desires, and aggressive behavior, when you attempt to accomplish your goals or fulfill your needs at the expense of others' rights, needs, or feelings.

Conflict is any situation in which your wants, needs, or intentions are incompatible with the wants, needs, or intentions of another person. Conflict is a part of even the best relationship. Conflict can be handled in constructive or destructive ways, which include avoiding, accommodating, competing, compromising, and collaborating.

The mass media have a powerful ability to influence public attitudes and behavior in positive or negative ways. Some of the messages in the media do not promote the wellness life-style. Further, the media do an uneven job of reporting new health research.

REFERENCES

1. Hafen, B., et al. *The Health Effects of Attitudes, Emotions, Relationships*. Provo, UT: EMS Associates, 1992.
2. Spector, R. *Cultural Diversity in Health and Illness,* 3rd ed. Norwalk, CT: Appleton and Lange, 1991.
3. Schilling, B., and Brannon, E. *Cross-cultural Counseling, a Guide for Nutrition and Health Counselors*. Alexandria, VA: U.S. Department of Health and Human Services, Nutrition and Technical Services Division, 1986.
4. Weaver, R. *Understanding Interpersonal Communication,* 5th ed. Glenview, IL: Scott, Foresman/Little, Brown, 1990.
5. Raudsepp, E. "Seven Ways to Cure Communication Breakdowns." *NursingLife* 4(1) (January/February 1984).
6. Weaver, op. cit.
7. Weaver, op. cit.

SUGGESTED READINGS

Alberti, R., and Emmons, M. *Your Perfect Right,* 6th ed. San Luis Obispo, CA: Impact, 1990.
Elgin, S. *Genderspeak*. New York: Wiley, 1993.
Glass, L. *He Says, She Says*. New York: Perigree, 1993.
Spector, R. *Cultural Diversity in Health and Illness,* 3rd ed. Norwalk, CT: Appleton and Lange, 1991.
Tannen, D. *You Just Don't Understand*. New York: William Morrow, 1990.
Tannen, D. *Talking from 9 to 5*. New York: William Morrow, 1994.
Weaver, R. *Understanding Interpersonal Communication,* 5th ed. Glenview, IL: Scott, Foresman/Little, Brown, 1990.

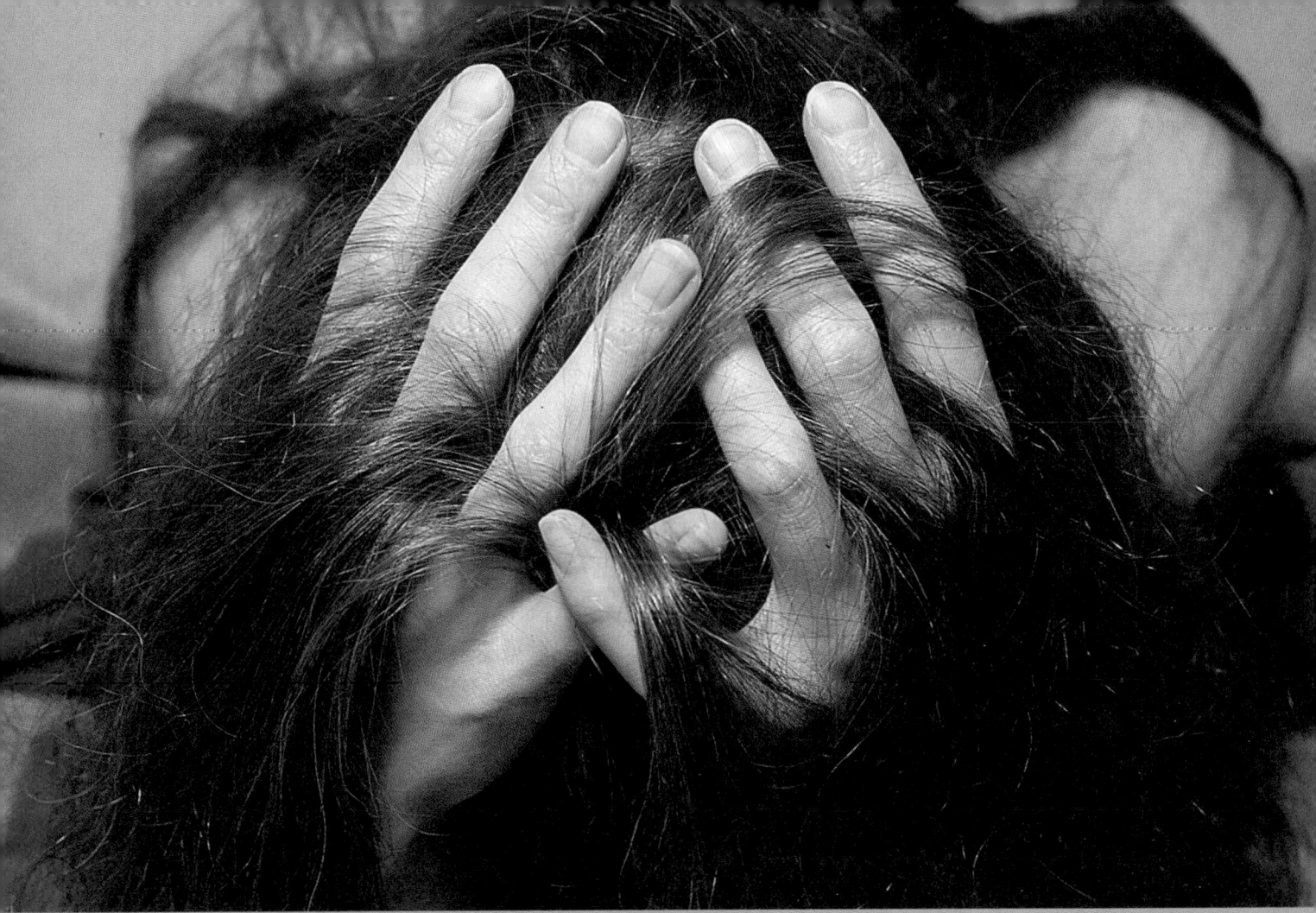

TWO

MENTAL HEALTH AND STRESS MANAGEMENT

Our discussion of mental health has been positioned early in this book because mental health is basic to all aspects of health. Your mental health influences the quality of your life in many ways:

- the quality of your relationships with others
- your ability to succeed in college
- your level of productivity
- your sense of fulfillment in life
- your body's physical functioning and, thus, the physical aspects of your wellness
- the kinds of coping devices you use in dealing with life
- your self-esteem, an important element in your mental health

Mental health affects physical health in many ways that will become apparent in almost every chapter of this text. For example, people with well-developed coping abilities are better able to control stress effectively and are less likely to make excessive use of alcohol and other harmful substances. The topic of self-esteem will appear repeatedly in this text, as it greatly influences how healthfully we behave. The better we feel about ourselves, the better we tend to take care of ourselves. A well-developed sense of self-esteem is needed to motivate healthful behavior; people who lack self-esteem tend to behave in many self-destructive ways. Excessive stress levels are very destructive to physical health. Effective stress management, an outgrowth of good mental health, leads to better physical health.

This unit consists of two chapters: Chapter 3 examines some of the basics of emotional wellness, while Chapter 4 considers stress management and other common mental health challenges.

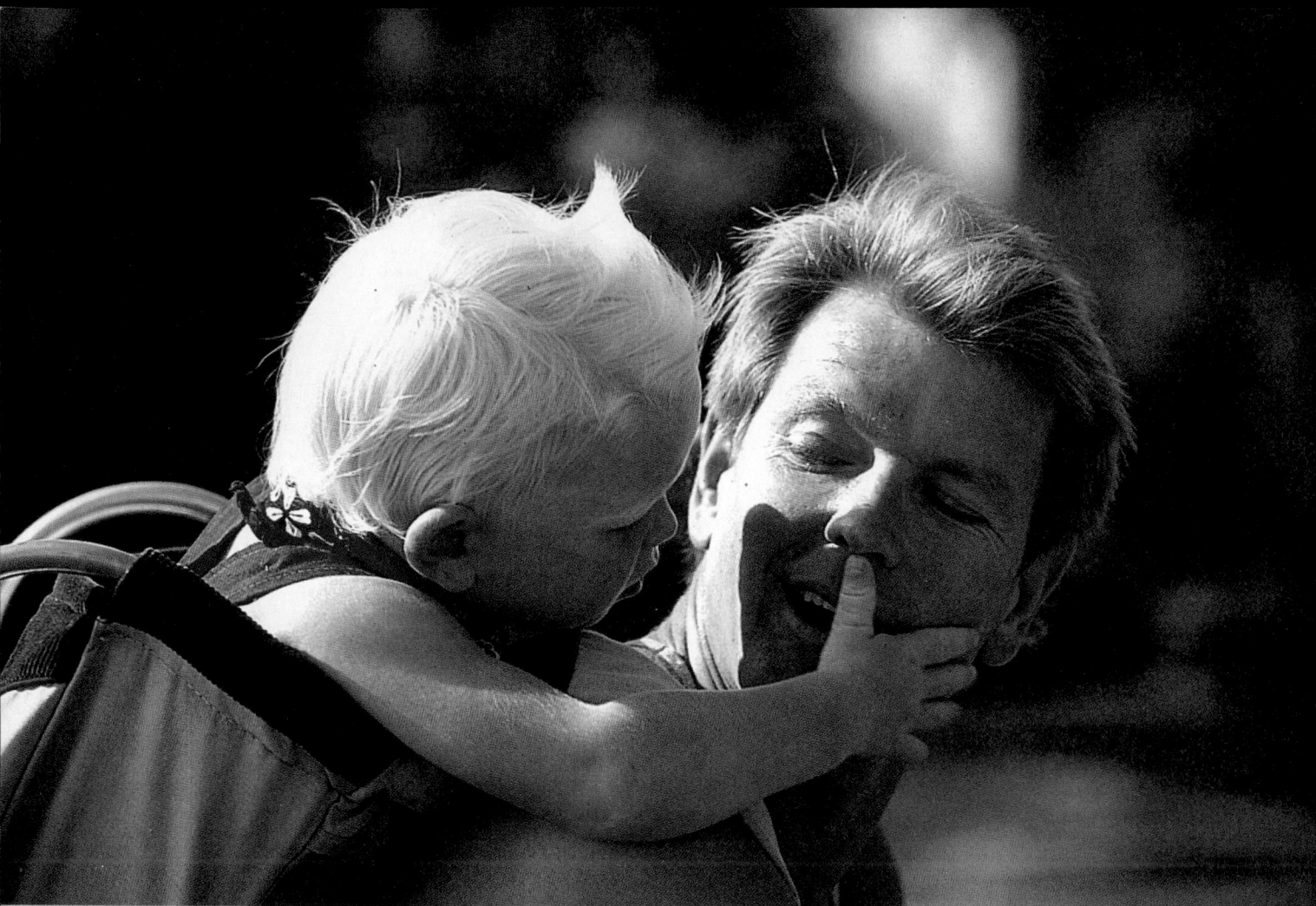

3
POSITIVE EMOTIONAL WELLNESS

KNOWLEDGE

- Explain the relationship between the terms *mental* and *emotional.*
- Explain the factors that contribute to the emotions we feel.
- Define personality and explain psychoanalytic, behavioristic, developmental, and humanistic theories of personality development.
- Explain Maslow's progression of human needs.
- Explain why some people make humiliating remarks (put-downs) to other people.
- Define repression, suppression, denial, displacement, projection, regression, rationalization, reaction formation, and sublimation.
- List six factors that contribute to a person's happiness.
- List 13 other characteristics of emotional wellness.
- Explain the relationships of identity, self-esteem, and intimate relationships to emotional wellness.

INSIGHT

- Explain what factors have contributed to your own emotional characteristics.
- Explain where you stand in Erikson's progression of developmental tasks.
- Relate your feelings and behavior to Maslow's hierarchy of human needs.
- Evaluate the appropriateness of your personal use of defense mechanisms.
- Evaluate your happiness in terms of the six factors mentioned in this chapter.

DECISION MAKING

- Decide to take personal responsibility for your own emotional well-being.
- Make a commitment to build your emotional health by working on problem areas you have identified through reading this chapter.

The Reverend Dr. Norman Vincent Peale was probably one of the most influential people of the twentieth century. His writings on the importance of a positive self-concept and positive thinking have helped millions of people. He has helped many of us to realize that state of mind has a great impact on the course of our public and personal lives. The Power of Positive Thinking, *Dr. Peale's most famous book, sold millions of copies and was probably responsible for the emerging popularity of self-help books and movements designed to help us learn more about ourselves.*

Dr. Peale was active as a writer and a minister virtually up to the day of his death at age 95 in December 1993. Born in Ohio, he decided at a young age to follow his father into the ministry. It was his father who taught him that the best way to reach people was through simplicity. This lesson must have made quite an impression on him because his books are full of simple guidelines and steps to success that anyone can follow. As a young minister, counseling the many that came to him for help, he realized that there was a need to combine the principles of psychiatry with those of ministry. Thus, he began to work with a psychiatrist, Dr. Smiley Blanton, who had studied under Freud in Vienna, and began in earnest to combine the principles of spirituality with those of positive self-image.

He began writing books and appearing on radio and television in an attempt to reach as many people as he could with his teachings. Dr. Peale's work focused on such basic ideas as not accepting defeat, maintaining high expectations of yourself and of others, and believing in yourself. His work is filled with such guidelines as, "The secret of a better and more successful life is to cast out those old dead unhealthy thoughts" and "To make your mind healthy, you must feed it nourishing, wholesome thoughts." He often spoke of "confidence concepts" and "energy-producing thoughts."

Dr. Norman Vincent Peale was a powerful positive role model throughout his life. His actions demonstrated the power of positive thinking and the importance of positive mental health. He was truly a leader in helping us to realize the role that positive emotional health can play in our lives.

Source: New York Times, *December 26, 1993, p. 14.*

■   ■   ■

Mental health is central to the quality of our lives. It influences personal happiness, career success, interpersonal relationships, and every aspect of our physical health. Our emotions directly affect most body functions and powerfully influence our level of wellness. Mentally healthy people feel good about themselves and are motivated to take good care of themselves.

What exactly is the relationship between the terms *mental* and *emotional?* Of the two words, **mental** is the more general, and means of or related to the mind, and encompasses *all* of an individual's sensory perceptions, thought processes, and emotional responses. All thoughts, memories, emotions, dreams, perceptions, and beliefs fall under the umbrella of "mental health." The word **emotional** means of or related to the emotions. Psychologists usually define emotions as mental states that include three components:[1]

1. *A characteristic feeling or subjective experience.* Joy, sadness, fear, and anger all can be used to describe the subjective component of emotions. Though emotions are subjective feelings, they are very real.

2. A pattern of physiological arousal. Emotions invariably trigger involuntary changes in body function, serving to prepare your body for whatever type of activity (such as mating or fighting) a particular emotion may make appropriate.

3. A pattern of overt expression. Emotions are usually betrayed in facial expressions and body postures. The relationship between emotions and corresponding expressions and postures is so strong that a particular emotion can often be induced by assuming its characteristic posture and facial expression.

In reality, the mind and the emotions are interrelated and interdependent. Emotions do not exist independently of our mental functions and our mental functions are affected by our emotional state. Thus, in many circumstances, one might correctly speak of mental health or emotional health interchangeably.

THE NATURE OF EMOTIONS

Though the perception of emotions is highly subjective, they are real, valid, and important. Emotions (Feature 3.1) are a major part of what it means to be human. They include the joy, fear, and sadness of living. Emotions play important social and personal functions.[2] For example, if we had no potential for feeling sorrow or shame, why would anyone hold back from harming others? If we felt no fear, what would motivate us to protect ourselves from danger?

The importance of emotions extends beyond how we feel and act, because every emotion influences body functions. Have you ever been so nervous you could barely breathe? Or have you ever felt your heart pounding from excitement or fear? Have you ever blushed? All of these common reactions illustrate how emotions affect body functions. When we are feeling calm and peaceful, our body relaxes and allows our energy to be restored.

INDIVIDUAL DIFFERENCES IN EMOTIONS AND THEIR EXPRESSION

There are marked individual differences in how we experience and express emotions. Two people in

---

mental of or related to the mind.

emotional of or related to the emotions.

FEATURE 3.1

HUMAN EMOTIONS

If someone asked you how many different emotions a human can feel, how would you answer? Every language contains many words that describe emotions and, in many cases, there are no exact translations from language to language. Here are some words in the English language for common emotions. You may wish to add some of your own to this list.

anger	joy	excitement
contempt	sadness	hostility
distress	anxiety	loneliness
guilt	depression	shame

boredom	fear	love
disgust	interest	surprise

Each of these emotions can form a continuum of degrees of intensity, such as:

slight bother → annoyance → severe irritation → anger → rage

When potentially destructive feelings are addressed at lower levels of intensity, they are less likely to escalate to more intense levels at which severe physiological changes and/or destructive behaviors occur.

identical situations may react very differently. Some of these differences are thought to be genetically determined, while some are culturally learned.

In recent years, increased emphasis has been placed on the *genetic basis* of human emotions and behavior. Starting from birth, infants respond differently from one another. Some babies are happy, while others are irritable and cry at the slightest provocation. Studies of adult identical twins, raised separately from birth in different environments, have demonstrated many similarities in their emotional reactions.

Emotions are characterized by overt expression and are usually betrayed by facial expressions and body postures. Often a particular emotion can be induced by assuming its characteristic posture and facial expression.

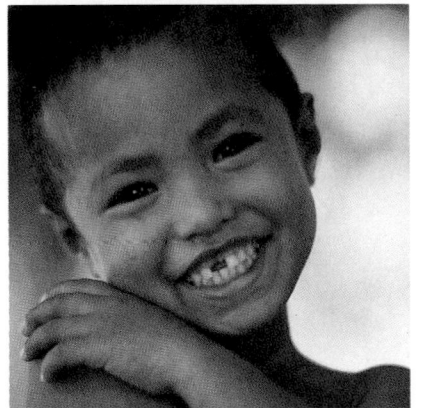
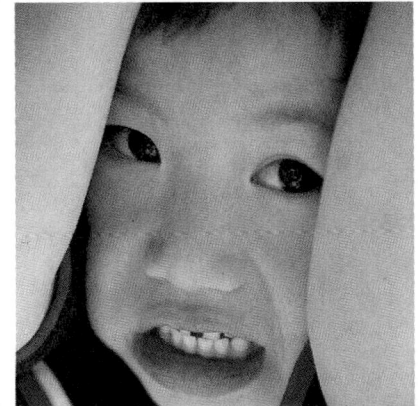
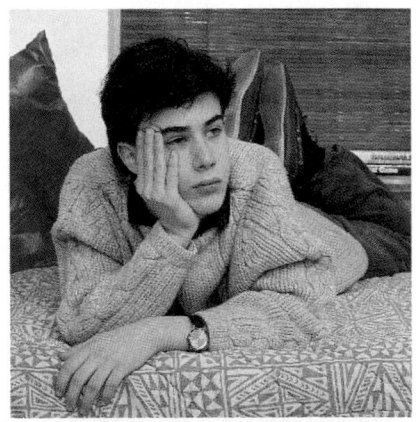
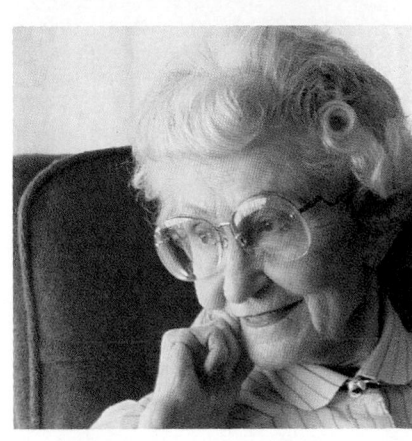
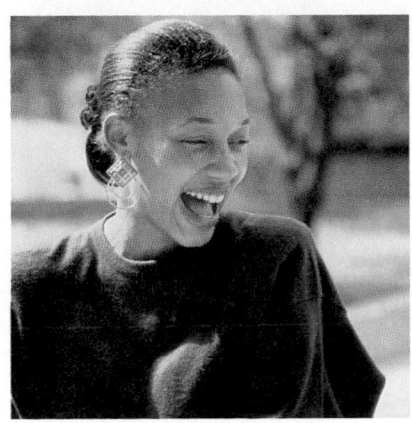
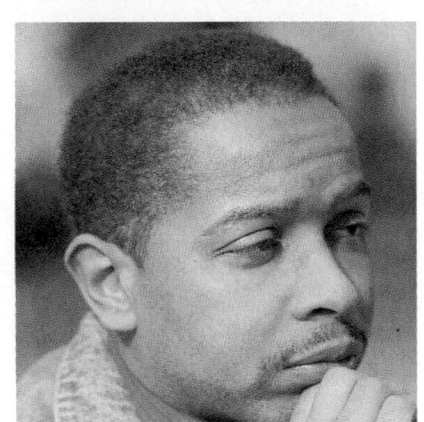

Cultural factors also play an important role in how we deal with our emotions. Many of our fears and joys are culturally determined, learned responses. People of different cultures, because of the learned expectations of their cultures, respond with different emotions to the same situation. Further, the same emotion will be expressed (or not expressed) differently by people of different cultures. Some cultures are noted for their open display of emotions, while others have a reputation for keeping emotions hidden from view.

Because of *individual childhood experiences,* some people have intense emotional reactions to objects or events that leave other people entirely unmoved. For example, one person who sees a cat may feel joy, while another may not react at all, and still another may feel frightened. Some people learn to suppress most outward signs of emotion while others learn to be quite expressive.

Emotions can be physically exhausting and create considerable stress; however, they are also desirable and useful. Emotions make us human, make our lives more interesting, and help us to function more effectively in our environment. Take a minute now to complete In Your Hands: An Emotional Wellness Assessment.

IN YOUR HANDS

AN EMOTIONAL WELLNESS ASSESSMENT

In this inventory, you have the opportunity to evaluate your level of emotional wellness as it relates to your self-image and need-fulfillment. Circle the number that most closely matches your reaction to each statement.

As with certain other assessments, some of these items reflect cultural values and this assessment may not be valid for people of every ethnic group.

	Strongly Agree	Somewhat Agree	Strongly Disagree
1. I have many friends.	2	1	0
2. People seem to like me.	2	1	0
3. I feel proud of the way I have lived my life so far.	2	1	0
4. I find it easy to adjust to sudden, unexpected changes.	2	1	0
5. I feel that I am mostly in charge of my life.	2	1	0
6. I find it easy to feel love for other people.	2	1	0
7. I enjoy the work I do.	2	1	0
8. I find it easy to express my feelings.	2	1	0
9. I am usually happy.	2	1	0
10. I enjoy most of the people I meet.	2	1	0
11. I feel that I am someone whom people would want to know.	2	1	0
12. There aren't many things about myself that I would want to change.	2	1	0

Total Points: _____

INTERPRETATION

20–24 points: You are enjoying positive emotional wellness. You have a fine sense of your own identity, well-developed self-esteem, effective ways of fulfilling your needs, and are enjoying life.

16–19 points: You are probably fairly happy, but could develop more effective means of need-fulfillment. You may have some doubts about your identity and are possibly unsure of your value as a person.

15 points or less: You appear to have many unfulfilled needs. Read this chapter carefully for suggestions on improved need-fulfillment. You could be enjoying life much more than you have been.

C H E C K P O I N T

1. What are the three characteristics of an emotion?
2. Why do different people respond to the same situation with different emotions?

☑

PERSONALITY AND ITS DEVELOPMENT

When we first meet people, we often base our impression on their personality. But what exactly is a personality? How can we define it? Personality is so complex that the English language has over 18,000 different words to describe personality traits.[3] All of us possess some personality traits and lack others. Our particular combination of traits is what makes each of us unique.

Personality can be defined as the overall response of a person to his or her environment. This includes how a person thinks, feels, and relates to people and situations. How did each of us come to have our own unique personality?

Psychologists once believed that the period of early childhood set the course for the rest of one's life. After the first few years of conditioning, they thought, one simply acts out a personality script that was written earlier. If this were true, there would be no point in studying personality in a college health course—it would be too late for us to make any significant changes in our lives. Today, though, human development is viewed as a process that continues throughout life. We continue to be able to profit from new experiences, to learn, and to change for as long as we live.

Over the years, many mental health experts have attempted to explain personality development. In the following sections we will discuss some of the milestones in this effort.

FREUD'S PSYCHOANALYTIC THEORY

The most famous of all views of personality is Sigmund Freud's **psychoanalytic theory.** This theo-ry assumes that unconscious forces influence human behavior. A key idea in Freud's theory of personality is that all humans possess a basic energy, called **libido** *(li-bē'dō),* directed at maximizing pleasure. Many of the acts that might bring pleasure, however, would cause conflict with other people, so must be suppressed. For example, we suppress most of our sexual impulses because to act upon them would cause problems for us.

Freud strongly believed in the importance of the unconscious portion of the mind. In fact, Freud was the first to suggest the now well-accepted idea that the conscious portion of the mind is small in comparison with all of the mental activity taking place in the unconscious mind, which he saw as having powerful effects on our emotions and behavior.

Freud's concept of the human personality and mind included three major parts: the id, ego, and superego. Freud viewed the **id,** which is in the unconscious mind and consists of the libido and aggression, as the most basic and primitive of the three parts.

The **ego** is what Freud called the conscious part of the mind that develops as we grow. The ego must deal with the demands of the id. When the id's demands can be satisfied in some reasonable way, the ego permits satisfaction. When the id's demands threaten to have us rejected by society, the ego uses **repression,** a process by which unacceptable thoughts, memories, desires, or motives are excluded from consciousness and left to operate in the unconscious mind. The ego tries to provide more socially acceptable substitutes.

The **superego** is our conscience, or our sense of right and wrong. While the ego decides what

· ·

libido in psychoanalytic theory, a basic energy directed at maximizing pleasure.

id in psychoanalytic theory, the unconscious part of the human mind containing the libido and aggression.

ego in psychoanalytic theory, the conscious part of the mind.

repression a process by which unacceptable thoughts, memories, desires, or motives are excluded from consciousness and left to operate in the unconscious mind.

superego in psychoanalytic theory, our conscience or our sense of right and wrong.

· ·

personality the overall response of a person to his or her environment.

psychoanalytic theory the theory that assumes that unconscious forces influence human behavior.

helps us avoid social disapproval, the conscience tells us what we "should" do. Like the id, the super-ego is largely unconscious and influences our behavior far more than we realize.

Freud believed that the three parts of the mind are often in conflict. Results of the conflict among the three personality elements include anxiety, inability to enjoy sex or give affection, vague and unwarranted feelings of guilt and unworthiness, and an unconscious need for punishment.

Freud's theory has had many critics, and today few people fully accept it in its original form. No one has been able to prove the existence of an id, ego, or superego. Most of today's authorities also feel that Freud overemphasized the role of sexual motivation of behavior. Few deny, however, that the unconscious mind does influence human emotions and behavior.

THE BEHAVIORIST VIEW OF PERSONALITY

Behaviorism, founded in 1913 by John Watson, a professor of psychology at Johns Hopkins University, is a philosophy of psychological study holding that only measurable behavior is a proper subject of psychological study. Early behaviorists studied human behavior much as one might study physics or chemistry. All behavior was seen as conditioned response to stimuli. Behavior that resulted in a reward would be repeated. Behavior that resulted in no reward or in a punishment would not be repeated. Emotions, feelings, thoughts, and the unconscious mind were ignored. Few psychologists today take such a narrow view. Even those with a strong interest in behaviorism recognize the importance of emotions and thought processes.

One unfortunate behavioral implication for wellness is that unhealthful behavior sometimes carries an immediate, tangible reward while healthful behavior may not. For example, eating a box of donuts (which could be considered an unhealthful behavior) carries an immediate reward: It tastes good. Not eating all of those donuts (a more healthful behavior) carries rewards such as long-term weight management and overall health, but

behaviorism a philosophy of psychological study holding that only observable behavior is a proper subject of psychological investigation.

these rewards are not immediate. Similar examples are abundant in many health areas, such as sexuality and substance abuse.

One way to motivate yourself to behave in healthful ways is to create your own more immediate rewards for desirable behaviors. For example, you might reward yourself for a week without junk food by purchasing a new tape or compact disk. Even a gold star on your calendar can serve as a reward.

ERIKSON'S THEORY OF PSYCHOSOCIAL DEVELOPMENT

Erik Erikson, a prominent personality theorist, characterized the human life-cycle as having eight phases, each presenting us with a specific development task or challenge (Table 3.1). Each of these tasks must be resolved in some way before we can proceed to the next level of development.[4] The success with which each task is resolved has last-

Table 3.1
Erikson's Developmental Tasks

Erik Erikson described the developmental challenges that occur at each stage of life. Maturing successfully requires meeting each challenge.

Stage	Challenge	Favorable Outcome	Unfavorable Outcome
Early infancy (first year)	Trust vs. mistrust	Faith in future	Suspicion, fear of future
Late infancy (second year)	Autonomy vs. doubt	Sense of self-control and adequacy	Feelings of shame and self-doubt
Early childhood (ages 3–5)	Initiative vs. guilt	Ability to initiate own activities	Sense of guilt and inadequacy
Middle childhood (6–puberty)	Industry vs. inferiority	Ability to understand and organize	Feelings of inferiority
Adolescence	Identity vs. confusion	Well-developed sense of identity	Confusion over who and what one really is
Early adulthood	Intimacy vs. isolation	Ability to form intimate relationships	Inability to form close relationships
Middle adulthood	Generosity vs. self-absorption	Concern for family and society in general	Concern only for self
Late adulthood	Integrity vs. despair	Feeling that one's life has been valid; able to face death	Dissatisfaction with life; despair over prospect of death

Source: Erikson, E. Childhood and Society, 2nd ed. New York: Norton, 1963.

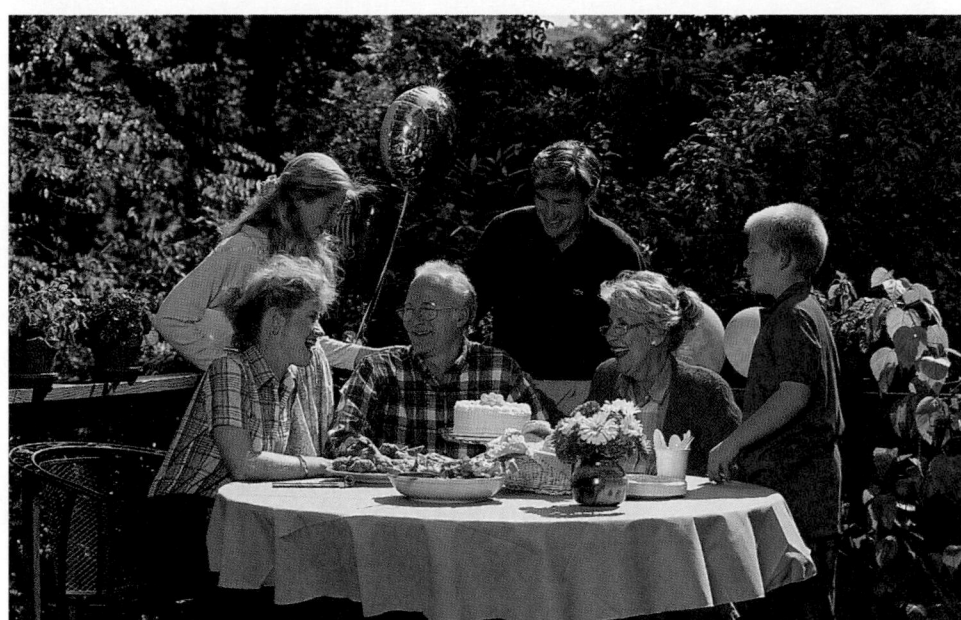

Every age, from birth to death, presents us with psychosocial developmental tasks. Erik Erikson described eight of these challenges, summarized in Table 3.1. If we are unsuccessful in meeting any of these challenges, we could have lingering problems as a result.

ing effects on our personality. If we meet these challenges, we emerge with greater maturity and richer personalities.

Erikson has formulated each stage of development in terms of psychological contrasts that represent the two extremes of successful and unsuccessful task resolution or personality development. The actual outcome in an individual is always somewhere between the two extremes for each of the eight developmental tasks.

Each development step builds on the successful completion of the previous steps. Thus, unsuccessful development at an early stage can interfere with later development. Many people, as adults, must deal with development tasks that would ideally have been resolved during infancy or childhood. For all of us, these tasks are never completely resolved, but continue to be worked on during successive stages in our development. Personality development is considered to be a lifelong process.

CHECKPOINT

1. What did Freud mean by the id, ego, and superego?

2. In behaviorist terms, why is it difficult to motivate healthful behavior?

3. What did Erikson see as the main developmental task for each of the eight phases of the human life-cycle?

HUMANISTIC THEORIES OF PERSONALITY

Humanism is a philosophy of psychological study that emphasizes the whole person and the importance of each person's subjective experience. Humanists believe that human nature is basically good and that the core of personality is the desire to use and perfect our skills and to find peace and happiness. This view contrasts sharply with Freud's view of people as being driven by sexuality and aggression. Humanistic theories tend to be optimistic, concentrating on human strengths, rather than weaknesses. Humanists believe that all people want to grow in positive ways and will do so if they have the chance and the proper encouragement. We will discuss the work of two humanistic theorists—Abraham Maslow and Carl Rogers.

Maslow's Progression of Need-fulfillment

Abraham H. Maslow, in his classic book, *Motivation and Personality*,[5] described personality development as progressive need-fulfillment. He characterized need-fulfillment abilities as being learned or developed, rather than innate or inborn.

humanism a philosophy of psychological study that emphasizes the whole person and the importance of each person's subjective experiences.

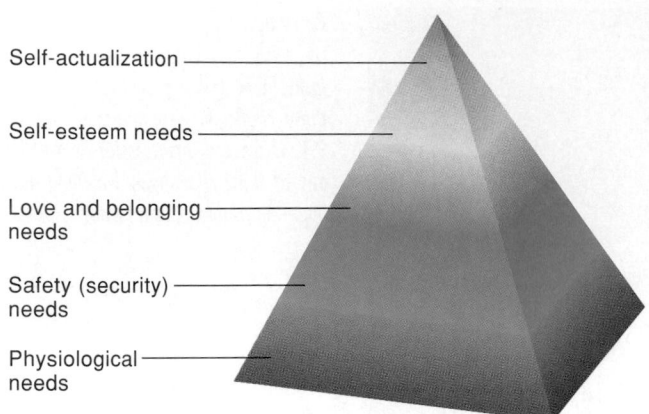

Self-actualization

Self-esteem needs

Love and belonging needs

Safety (security) needs

Physiological needs

Figure 3.1

Maslow's Hierarchy of Needs

This humanistic view of personality emphasizes progressively felt needs, ranging from the basic physiological needs, to self-actualization, making full use of one's potential.

Maslow arranged the various human needs in sequence from the most basic to the highest. The higher needs (Figure 3.1) are progressively felt as the lower needs are fulfilled, but not before. Maslow saw human behavior as motivated by our desire to fulfill our needs.

At any given time, the lowest unfulfilled need is viewed as the most powerful motivator of behavior. An individual may move up and down the hierarchy during the same day, but will tend to focus more energy on some needs than others. As in Erikson's developmental progression, a person can remain focused on any level of need-fulfillment. Thus, many people go through life struggling to fulfill low-level needs.

Briefly, Maslow's progression of human needs is as follows:

1. *The physiological needs.* The most basic human needs are physical needs, such as food, water, shelter, sleep, and sexual satisfaction. When physiological needs are unmet, as in a starving person, all other needs seem relatively unimportant. When these most basic needs are satisfied, other needs emerge and dominate thinking and behavior.

2. *The safety needs (security, order, and stability).* People of all ages feel the need to survive and to protect themselves. The safety needs are most easily seen when infants and children react to something with fear. Adults often attempt to hide or inhibit these reactions. Thus, when as adults we feel our security threatened, we may not react in a visible manner, but rather with masked anxiety and such physical changes as rapid pulse and other stress responses (which will be discussed in Chapter 4).

3. *The need for love and belonging.* As soon as the physiological and safety needs are met, we feel a strong need for friends and, often, for a mate. We feel the need for belonging and group acceptance, and the need to love and be loved.

4. *The need for self-esteem.* At this point in the hierarchy of needs, we begin to assess our **self-esteem**—our subjective sense of personal value or worth, success, achievement, self-respect, and confidence in facing the world. This is often the need level at which people in industrialized societies get stuck, and go through life trying to find fulfillment, but with only limited success.

5. *The need for self-actualization.* Self-actualization, attainable only by people with adequate self-esteem, means making full use of our abilities and working toward achieving our full potential as human beings. Self-actualization is an ongoing *process,* not a goal. According to Maslow, few people live on this level; most of us are still struggling to fulfill lower needs, such as the need for love or self-esteem. Many others have little opportunity for self-actualization due to their circumstances, such as living in poverty or under a dictatorship.

Carl Rogers and the Role of Self-concept

Carl Rogers, like Maslow, was a humanistic psychologist. Rogers emphasized the importance of our **self-concept,** which is the way we perceive ourselves as functioning human beings.[6] Our self-concept includes our judgments about our appearance, abilities, accomplishments, and relationships with other people.

Our self-concept does not necessarily represent reality. Many people who are considered successful, and are highly respected by others, perceive themselves as failures. How can this be? To a great extent, our self-concept depends on how we have been accepted by other people, particularly during

....

self-esteem one's subjective sense of personal worth.

self-concept the way we perceive ourselves as functioning human beings.

our childhood. We are much more likely to have a positive self-concept if we have grown up in a family in which we have been accepted, loved, valued, trusted, and respected.

According to the Rogers theory, in order to raise children to have a positive self-concept, we want to treat them with what Rogers called *unconditional positive regard*. This means that even when they do things we disapprove of, we want to make it clear that we disapprove of the specific *behavior,* not of the child.

What about those of us who were not treated with unconditional positive regard? Are we doomed to always underestimate ourselves? Fortunately, we are not. By understanding how self-concept develops (as we now do) and by consciously working toward developing a more positive self-concept it is possible to overcome negative thoughts about ourselves. Recommendations include the following:

- Make the conscious decision that you are going to attempt to improve your self-concept.
- Whenever you catch yourself thinking negatively about yourself, immediately replace the negative thought with a positive thought about yourself, perhaps remembering a recent success or compliment.
- Accept the compliments and respect you receive from others. People with a poor self-concept usually automatically discount or disregard anything that conflicts with their self-image.
- Accept the validity of your achievements and successes. Give yourself the credit. People with a poor self-concept discount their successes, attributing them to chance, luck, or to someone else.
- Understand the psychology of put-downs and learn how to deal with them (Feature 3.2).

Rogers believed that maladjustment and problem behavior are caused by people's failure to integrate all of their experiences, desires, and feelings into their self-concept. Maladjusted people tend to regard any experience that is not consistent with their self-concept as a threat. This includes achievements and successes of people who have a negative image of themselves. As a result, some

---

FEATURE 3.2

COPING WITH PUT-DOWNS

A put-down is a humiliating remark or degrading gesture directed at some aspect of one's self, job, values, possessions, or religious, ethnic, or other affiliation. It is usually not difficult to distinguish a put-down from a well-intentioned suggestion.

How we deal with put-downs makes a statement about our self-concept and self-esteem. If we accept as valid the negative remarks people make, our self-concept and self-esteem are going to suffer. Understanding the basis of put-downs will help us to deal with most of them successfully.

Put-downs reveal much more about their source than their target. People who put you down seldom know why they do it, but they are usually motivated by one of the following feelings, working at an unconscious level:

- First and foremost is *low self-esteem.* People of low self-esteem try to devaluate other people so that they can feel superior by comparison.
- Feelings of *powerlessness.* Sometimes put-downs are an effort to put the recipient into a weaker position by destroying his or her self-confidence.
- Feelings of *dependency.* A person who feels dependent, which is an uncomfortable feeling, may use put-downs to "equalize" the relationship.

- Feelings of *envy.* People often react to their envy by knocking the thing or person they would actually like to have for themselves.

You must keep in mind that when someone makes a disparaging remark to you, it does not reflect your own inferiority or inadequacy, but the unhappiness of the person who made the statement. He or she is trying to feel better by feeling superior to you. It usually doesn't work. Putting someone down only further lowers self-esteem by adding to feelings of guilt and shame.

So how do you deal with put-downs? Above all, keep in mind that they reflect negatively on the person saying them, not on you. If it's just an occasional put-down from someone who plays only a minor role in your life, it's usually best to just let it pass. If you are put down frequently by someone who plays an important role in your life, such as your boss, mate, parent, or child, however, you may wish to discuss your feelings with that person. Avoid "you statements," such as "You always say that." Use "I statements," such as "I feel hurt when people say things like that and I would appreciate it if you wouldn't say that again." You may or may not be successful in getting the person to stop, but you will have the satisfaction of knowing you made the effort and in doing so, will have boosted your self-esteem.

people sabotage their own success. For example, a student with a low self-concept may be doing very well in a course and be going into the final exam with an "A." Because this "A" conflicts with his or her self-concept, it causes anxiety. To spoil the success, such a student might "forget" to show up for the final or might get drunk the night before or otherwise act to ensure failure. If our student still manages to get an "A," it will be necessary to banish the conflicting experience from his or her conscious thoughts by "forgetting" what grade he or she got.

Rogers used the phrase "fully functioning person" for someone who sees all of his or her experiences as consistent with his or her self-concept. When there is substantial inconsistency between the self-concept and reality, serious psychological problems can result. As reality becomes further removed from self-concept, more elaborate defenses must be set up and more tension results. Based on these theories, Rogers developed a widely used form of therapy, called client-centered therapy.

C H E C K P O I N T

1. How do humanistic views of personality differ from psychoanalytic and behaviorist views?

2. What is the progression of human needs, as seen by Maslow, and where are you in that progression?

3. What are self-concept, self-esteem, and self-actualization?

4. How can a poor self-concept interfere with success in life?

DEFENSE MECHANISMS

Defense mechanisms are unconscious psychological techniques we use to try to protect ourselves from uncomfortable feelings. The use of defense mechanisms—which mechanisms we use and to what extent we use them—is a major component of personality.

Defense mechanisms are recognized by most psychologists as necessary and potentially valuable

....

defense mechanisms unconscious psychological techniques we use to protect ourselves from uncomfortable feelings.

in dealing with stressful situations. Kagan and Segal[7] call them the "gray area" between successfully coping with stress by eliminating its sources and failing to deal with stress at all. (Stress management will be discussed in Chapter 4.)

The use of defense mechanisms expends a great deal of emotional energy, and overuse can cause emotional problems. Used in moderation and in the proper circumstances, a defense mechanism might be of great value. The same mechanism, used to excess or in inappropriate situations, might be undesirable and could be symptomatic of emotional illness. We will discuss some, though not all, of the commonly used defense mechanisms.

REPRESSION

Repression is the process of restricting a stress-producing memory, thought, or feeling to the unconscious mind. An example of repression is when people "forget" a dental appointment because they are afraid of the visit. More complex examples deal with how we repress memories of accidents, attacks, or other frightening events in our lives and how we repress socially unacceptable thoughts and feelings.

Repression is mentioned first among the defense mechanisms, because it is the underlying force of most other defense mechanisms, which are various ways of applying repression. *Example:*

Lydia was sexually molested by her stepfather for several years during her childhood. She has been unable to enjoy sex as an adult, but cannot recall the molestation.

SUPPRESSION

Suppression, related to repression, is when a person *consciously* avoids thinking about something that would cause stress or anxiety. Repression, in contrast, is an unconscious process. *Example:*

Shondale knows that she will be taking her history final exam in three days and has studied very little for it. Whenever the thought of this

....

suppression consciously avoiding thinking about something that would cause stress or anxiety.

exam comes to her mind, she says, "I'm just not going to think about it right now."

DENIAL

Denial is keeping anxiety-producing realities out of one's conscious awareness. It is refusing to admit the reality of or to acknowledge the existence of something that would cause an unpleasant feeling. *Examples:*

Lupe is pregnant but refuses to accept the reality of her pregnancy. As a result, she fails to make a decision as to whether to abort the pregnancy or to begin prenatal care. She does neither.

Dan has a serious drinking problem, but denies that his drinking is a problem. Year after year he continues to drink while his marriage, career, and health go down the drain.

DISPLACEMENT

Displacement is transferring an emotion such as aggression, anger, or hostility from the person or situation with which it was originally associated to a new person or situation. *Example:*

Phuong had a terrible day at school. He got a C- on his speech and a D on his biology exam. When he got home he yelled at everyone there, even though they had nothing to do with his difficulties at school.

PROJECTION

Projection is a mechanism by which people bolster their own self-images by unconsciously attributing their own unacceptable characteristics,

....

denial keeping anxiety-producing realities out of one's conscious awareness.

displacement transferring an emotion such as aggression, anger, or hostility from the person or situation with which it was originally associated to a new person or situation.

projection attributing one's unacceptable characteristics, behaviors, or urges to others.

behaviors, or urges to other people. When we use projection, we accuse others of doing exactly what we are doing or would like to be doing. *Examples:*

People who feel guilty about lying, cheating, or stealing may want to believe that everyone lies, cheats, or steals.

People who have low self-esteem are usually convinced that everyone else holds a low opinion of them too.

A married person who is having an affair, or would like to have one, accuses his or her spouse of having an affair.

REGRESSION

Regression is when we retreat by using behaviors that were used at earlier times in our lives. We tend to regress during times of stress. When we regress, we unconsciously remember our more carefree, less responsible childhood and attempt to return to those days.

Regression is quite common. For example, people often act immature and "silly" when they are under stress. Part of the satisfaction gained from sucking on a cigarette has been attributed to regression—the cigarette is seen as a replacement for a mother's breast. *Examples:*

Just before a major exam, a group of students start acting very goofy and childlike.

An extreme example is the emotionally ill person who curls up, mute and withdrawn, into the fetal position.

RATIONALIZATION

Rationalization is making up socially acceptable excuses for our behavior rather than exposing the true reasons. People who rationalize really believe what they are saying or thinking. They use this

....

regression retreating to a more immature form of behavior during times of stress.

rationalization making up socially acceptable excuses for our behavior rather than exposing the true reasons.

mechanism to protect their self-esteem, not just to influence the opinions others have of them. *Examples:*

Anthony failed English because he rarely went to class and completed few of the assignments. He blames the professor for failing to motivate him.

Rosina gets a ticket for driving 50 in a 35 zone. She blames the officer for hiding behind a large van where she couldn't see her.

Back to Dan the denial-using drinker for a moment. He blames his drinking on his boss, who Dan says is always on his case.

REACTION FORMATION

Reaction formation is used to mask a trait that is unacceptable to ourselves or others by assuming an opposite attitude or behavior. Reaction formation often results in exaggerated behavior. *Examples:*

Bich is basically very shy, but forces herself to be very outgoing.

Jerome, who has a great fear of death, has taken up skydiving.

Carol is sexually inhibited, but she dresses very seductively and flirts constantly.

SUBLIMATION

Sublimation is redirecting socially undesirable urges into socially acceptable behavior. For example, instead of expressing our aggressive impulses toward others through destructive behaviors, we can act them out in various forms of acceptable competition, such as through sports, politics, and business.

....

reaction formation masking an unacceptable or distressing trait by assuming an opposite attitude or behavior.

sublimation redirecting socially unacceptable urges into socially acceptable behavior.

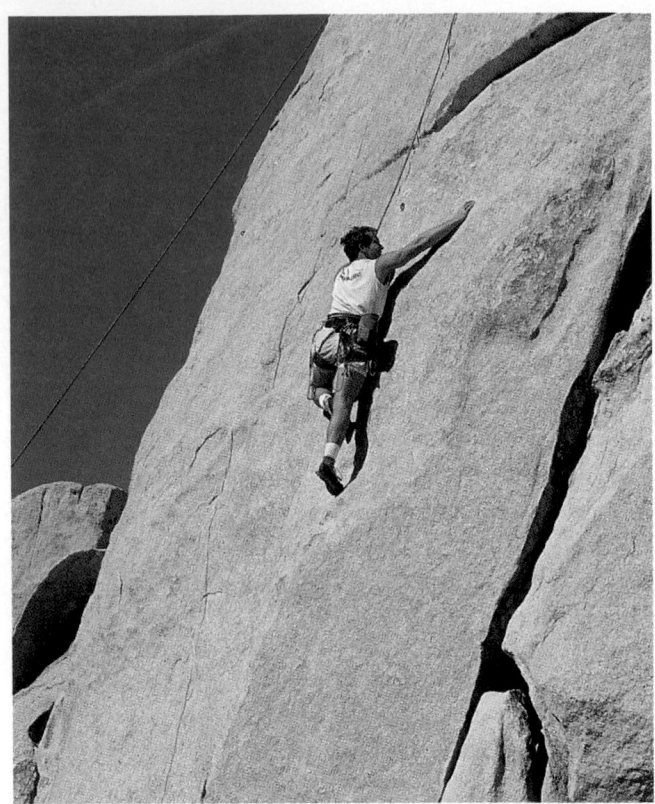

Reaction formation is assuming an attitude or behavior that is opposite to one's true characteristic. For example, sometimes a person who is afraid of death performs "death defying" acts.

The term sublimation is also used when we substitute the satisfaction of higher needs for fulfillment of lower needs. Sublimation is considered by many authorities to be among the most constructive of the defense mechanisms. *Examples:*

Tyrone has a tendency to discharge his stress by becoming violent, but has redirected his violence into his hobby of boxing.

Elda has been known as a very aggressive person, but now she directs most of her aggression into her successful career in computer sales.

CHECKPOINT

1. What is the function of defense mechanisms? Is their use always undesirable?

2. Define the following terms: *repression, suppression, denial, displacement, projection, regression, rationalization, reaction formation,* and *sublimation.*

HAPPINESS

Happiness is a state of emotional well-being and contentment. The fact that happiness is a subjective condition and not readily measurable by scientific instruments makes it no less important. Happiness is a prominent feature of emotional wellness.

We all know of some people who almost always seem to be happy and some who, though equally fortunate, almost never seem happy. What is the difference between these people? How can *we* achieve and maintain a state of joy?

Before we get specific we need to mention that the same formula won't bring the same level of happiness to everyone. Because we all carry different sets of genes, and have all had different sets of life experiences, no two of us can be expected to respond in exactly the same way. But certain factors are commonly associated with a high level of happiness.

HAVING REALISTIC EXPECTATIONS

We tend to feel happy when the realities of our lives measure up fairly well to our expectations for our lives. We don't mean that the key to happiness is to hold very low expectations. But we do mean that some people doom themselves to unhappiness by having goals (such as becoming a millionaire by age 30) that are unlikely to be achieved. Similarly, perfection is an unattainable goal and anyone who measures the reality of their life against the goal of perfection is going to be disappointed and unhappy.

HAVING A POSITIVE OUTLOOK

Each of us has been conditioned by our life experiences to view the world with some degree of optimism or pessimism. Those who take the optimistic view are far happier than those who always expect the worst. We want to emphasize the word "conditioned." If our positive or negative response is a conditioned response and if we have been conditioned to see life negatively, then we can recondition ourselves to see life more positively.

....

happiness a state of emotional well-being and contentment.

How can we do this? We can start by making the conscious decision and the commitment to become more positive in our outlook. Then, whenever we find ourselves thinking negatively, we can push that negative thought out of our mind, replacing it with a more positive thought. In time, the positive thought will come automatically. And since positive and negative expectations tend to be self-fulfilling prophecies, we will find that our optimistic views are reinforced by positive outcomes in most of our life experiences.

HAVING REWARDING RELATIONSHIPS

The happiness of most people is quite dependent on the quality of their relationships with other people. As social beings we need each other for the fulfillment of many of our human needs. Every one of us, for example, needs to feel loved and accepted as the person we are in order to be happy. We need the emotional support and the sharing of life's high and low points that can only occur within intimate relationships. Without intimate friends, even the most successful person feels that something is missing from his or her life.

ASSUMING RESPONSIBILITY FOR OUR OWN HAPPINESS

Even though we depend on our relationships to contribute to our happiness, the happiest people are those who understand that each of us is ultimately responsible for her or his own happiness. We can't let someone else determine whether or not we are happy. We can become self-sufficient enough not to need to be constantly entertained by someone else. We can become secure enough in ourselves that the occasional cruel or unthinking comment from someone important to us can't spoil our whole day.

HAVING A REWARDING CAREER

A rewarding career can make a huge difference in a person's happiness. Abundant research has shown that people who are unemployed or underemployed are among society's least happy people. Also unhappy are people whose work is poorly matched with their abilities or personalities. The right career can provide many rewards:

Happiness is a prominent feature of emotional wellness. Traits associated with happiness include having realistic expectations, a positive outlook, and rewarding relationships, assuming responsibility for one's own happiness, having a rewarding career, and having spirituality.

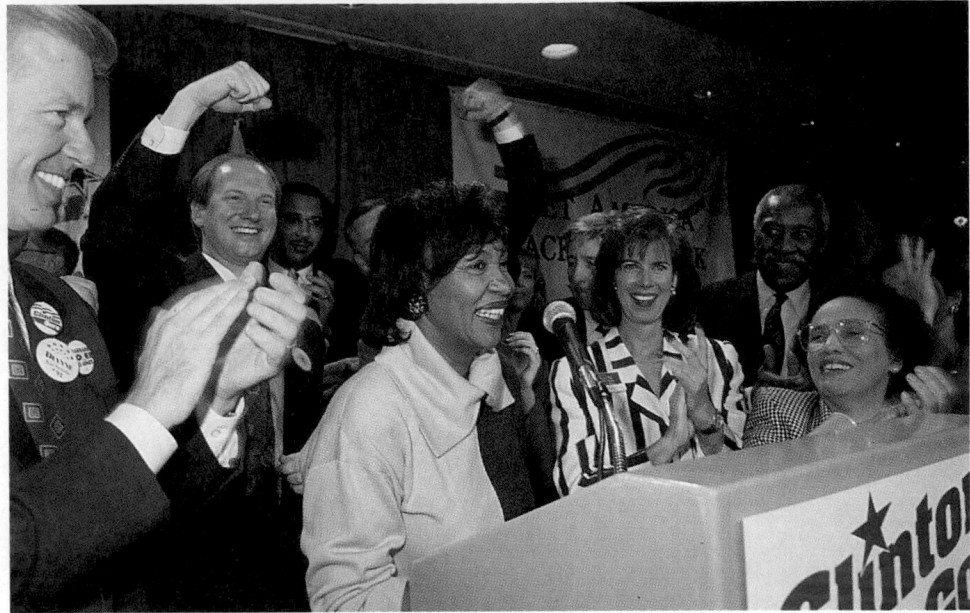

- *The intrinsic enjoyment in doing interesting work.* You know that you have found the right job for yourself when you enjoy your work so much that you wake up in the morning looking forward to the day's challenges.

- *Sense of purpose in life.* The right job gives you the feeling that you are doing something of value to society. You are proud of the work you do.

- *Economic security.* Someone has said, "Money is only important when you don't have any." Though money certainly doesn't guarantee happiness, the lack of it pretty well guarantees unhappiness. The right job may not pay a huge salary, but it should pay enough and provide sufficient benefits so that the costs of food, shelter, health care, and educating your children are not constant worries.

- *Self-esteem.* Being employed, and especially being employed in enjoyable work, is a great boost to your self-esteem and thus, to your happiness.

- *Self-actualization.* As discussed earlier in this chapter, self-actualization is making full use of one's abilities. People are happiest when they are working at about the level of their abilities. People working at a job that makes little use of their abilities or people who are working at a job that is poorly

matched to their abilities are not likely to be very happy.

HAVING SPIRITUALITY

Happy people, though enjoying strong self-esteem, do not think of themselves as the center of the universe. They do not live for "me first." They have a sense of selflessness and a caring for others. They are willing to do more for others than for themselves. They live by a set of principles or ethics based on something larger and stronger than themselves. This may or may not involve traditional religious beliefs. Some experts believe that spirituality is the most happiness-producing quality a person can possess.[8]

Spirituality brings happiness in many ways. For example:

- It acts as the unifying force that integrates the physical, emotional, and social aspects of our lives, bringing them into a meaningful whole.

- It brings focus and meaning to our lives. Without spirituality our lives make little sense and we proceed aimlessly, perhaps straying into chemical dependencies or other substitutes for a meaningful existence.

- Because spirituality transcends the individual, it can form a common bond between people. With this common bond, we can unselfishly share our love, warmth, and compassion with other people. We find happiness in putting the interests of another person ahead of our own. We find joy and fulfillment in helping others experience spiritual growth and when we do so we grow ourselves.

CHECKPOINT

1. What are six characteristics that are typical of happy people?

2. How can a career contribute to one's happiness?

3. How does spirituality contribute to happiness?

OTHER CHARACTERISTICS OF POSITIVE EMOTIONAL WELLNESS

Degrees of mental health can fall anywhere along a continuum ranging from extreme mental disturbance to very high levels of positive emotional wellness. Most of us have some strong and some weak areas in our personalities, and find that our overall level of emotional wellness varies from day to day.

In the next few sections, we will discuss some characteristics associated with positive emotional wellness. If you find that you don't rate very highly in one or more of these areas, it does not mean that you are mentally ill. It may indicate, however, an area where you could focus your efforts for self-improvement.

POSITIVE SELF-CONCEPT AND SELF-ESTEEM

Self-esteem is the portion of one's self-concept that includes confidence and satisfaction about oneself. Emotionally healthy people feel good about themselves. They feel up to facing life's challenges and feel a strong sense of personal worth. They accept themselves as they are, and understand that perfection is an impossible goal; they accept their imperfections as part of being human. They don't spend their time wishing that they were smarter or better looking, or feeling sorry for themselves because they're not. (Ways of building self-esteem are discussed later in this chapter.)

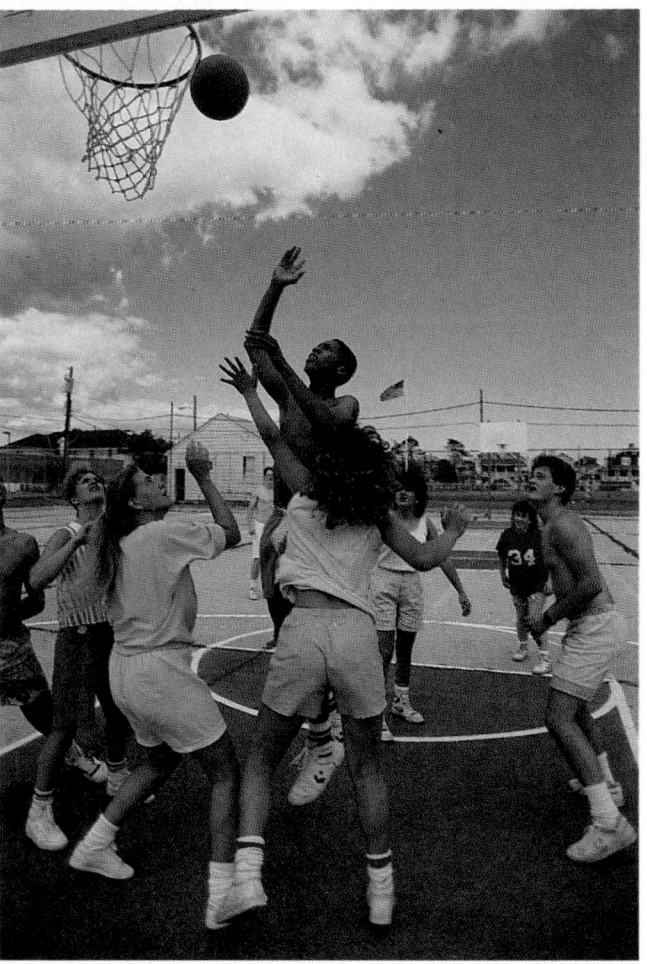

Emotionally healthy people feel good about themselves. They carry a positive self-image and have well-developed self-esteem. They feel competent and worthy of the respect of others.

PSYCHOSOCIAL DEVELOPMENT APPROPRIATE TO AGE

Emotionally healthy people have successfully achieved Erikson's developmental goals (see Table 3.1) as appropriate to their age group. Although these developmental tasks are never completely resolved, they are worked out progressively during successive stages. Because the nature of emotional wellness is never finite, there is always the possibility of improving our emotional responses.

EFFECTIVE METHODS OF NEED-FULFILLMENT

We are not born with the ability to fulfill our needs, but must *learn* effective methods of need-fulfillment through experience. Many of these methods, such as assertiveness, communication skills, and developing intimate relationships, are discussed in this and the following chapter.

It helps to know what our needs really are. People often confuse superficial goals such as wealth or status with the underlying needs such as security or self-esteem. When they achieve their goals, they wonder why they still feel unfulfilled.

Another barrier to need-fulfillment is denying that we have particular needs.

Example: Some people deny that they need the love and acceptance of other people.

In reality, they do feel this need, but fear possible rejection. In essence, they reject others first, thus avoiding any possibility of being rejected by others. By behaving this way, an important human need goes unfulfilled.

COPING WITH UNFULFILLED NEEDS

Regardless of how skilled we become at fulfilling our needs, there will inevitably be times when some of our needs will not be met. Invariably, external factors such as the unpredictability of the weather, the unreliability of machines, and the frailty of human beings will serve as obstacles to our need-fulfillment.

Emotionally healthy people develop effective and appropriate ways of dealing with the frustra-tion of their needs. Like need-fulfillment, this is a *learned* ability that develops with maturity. Mature people understand that no one can have all of their needs met at all times. They maintain a positive outlook on life, knowing that their frustration is just temporary. They focus on the positive aspects of each life situation, instead of the negative ones. They have learned to talk about their frustrations, rather than bottle them up inside and let them fester. Mature people "work off" their frustrations by being active, rather than by sitting and brooding or by attempting to escape from their frustrations with alcohol or other drugs or, even more commonly, overeating.

Example: You have blown an exam. Rather than spending the evening all depressed, you go to the gym, work out, and feel a lot better.

ADEQUATE ADAPTABILITY

One of the basic rules of biology is that every organism is faced with a constantly changing environment and must adapt if it is to survive. Human beings are no exception; because the world is constantly changing, we must constantly adapt to these changes. Although the familiar gives us a sense of security, seeing change should spark in us a sense of excitement about the future. When we feel secure enough to look forward to the future with

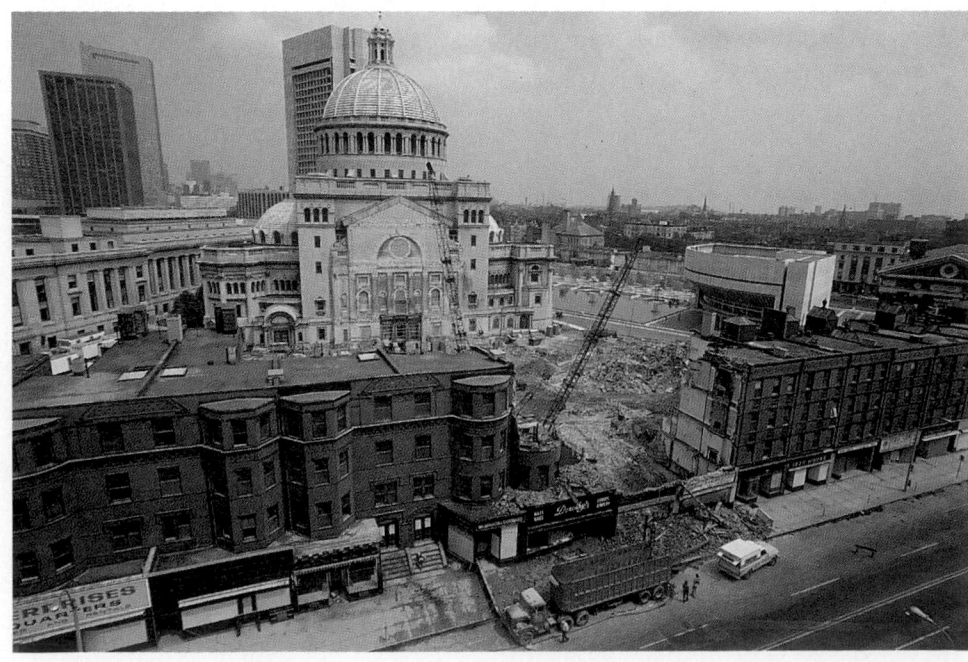

Emotionally healthy people understand that we live in a constantly changing world and look forward to the future with interest and confidence, rather than with fear.

interest and confidence, rather than with fear, we have achieved a high level of emotional wellness.

Example: A relationship that has been important to you is broken off by the other person. Instead of moping around for months, you soon begin dating again.

REASONABLE DEGREE OF INDEPENDENCE

People with positive emotional wellness can function independently. They can think for themselves, make decisions, plan their lives, and follow through with their plans. Conversely, people who have difficulty making decisions are often immature and insecure. They are afraid to face the consequences of the decisions they make, so they make as few decisions as possible. Growth involves making mistakes as well as achieving success. Our mistakes are best viewed as learning experiences. We must take some risks (see the next section) in order to live our lives most fully.

Example: Jim's parents were very domineering. Now that he is away at college he is having trouble making decisions for himself, living in fear of making a bad choice.

Everyone needs a certain degree of dependency too. The goal of total independence is unrealistic since it denies the importance of others in fulfilling our human needs.

Example: A love relationship involves mutual dependency, and without this dependency a very basic need would be unfulfilled.

APPROPRIATE RISK-TAKING

Almost every human activity that carries potential rewards also carries some physical, emotional, or financial risk. Emotionally healthy people weigh the potential benefits of an activity against its potential risks and are willing to take reasonable risks in order to live full, rewarding lives. They understand, for example, that relationships involve emotional risk, but the benefits outweigh the risk. They understand that participation in any sport involves some risk, but they take appropriate precautions and go ahead and enjoy sports.

Example: You could break your leg skiing, but with proper instruction and equipment the risk is minimized.

Less healthy people, in contrast, may pass up many rewarding activities out of fear of being emotionally or physically hurt. Conversely, they may expose themselves to unnecessary risks by failing to take appropriate precautions for an activity or engaging in very dangerous activities that present risks that are greater than their potential benefits.

Example: Having sex without taking precautions to prevent pregnancy and/or disease is taking unnecessary risk and indicates lack of concern for yourself and your partner.

REASONABLE EXPECTATION FOR CONTROL

Positive emotional wellness is associated with a sense of being *mostly* in control of your own life. It is not emotionally healthy to feel as if you have *no* control over your life—there is no sense of security for someone who feels helpless and frightened. At the same time, it is unrealistic to try to have *total* control over your life, as it can't be done. There are certain aspects of our lives that are simply beyond our control. If we strive for total control at all times, we are setting ourselves up for frustration and a high degree of stress.

Example: Someone who attempts to live on an extremely tight schedule will often be stressed when conditions beyond his or her control make it impossible to stay on schedule.

EFFECTIVE STRESS MANAGEMENT

Contemporary life can be highly stressful; yet many people live extremely busy, rewarding lives without experiencing stress-related problems. These are the people who have developed effective stress-management techniques (discussed in the next chapter). Those who do not manage stress well are subject to crippling physical and emotional disorders and are at high risk of abusing alcohol and other life-threatening chemicals.

CONCERN FOR OTHERS

A sign of emotional wellness is the ability to feel a genuine concern for other people's well-being. Humans are inherently social; in fact, sociobiologists say that we are genetically "programmed" to care about each other. We are also programmed to take care of our own needs first. People whose own needs are largely unfulfilled tend not to show much concern for the rights and happiness of others.

Example: The rude, uncaring, or self-centered person is typically an unhappy person with many unfulfilled needs that are given precedence over anyone else's needs.

REWARDING RELATIONSHIPS WITH OTHERS

A good measure of emotional wellness is the quality of one's relationships with others. Emotionally healthy people like and trust most people and expect that people will like and trust them. Their relationships with others are satisfying and lasting, and these people have enough self-confidence to be able to feel a part of a group. They feel accepted and make others feel accepted.

THE ABILITY TO LOVE

Before people can love others, they must be able to accept, respect, and love themselves. This love for others is more than sexual love; it is a love for all people and a love for humanity. Many people are unable to express love, even for those who are closest to them. This inability to love often is based on low self-esteem, inability to trust, and the feeling of being unworthy of being loved. For one individual to have the ability to love another, he or she has to have *received* acceptance, respect, and love first. The nurturing or lack of nurturing is then mirrored back to others.

Example: Someone who, as a child, received little display of affection from his or her parent(s) will often have difficulty displaying affection in adult relationships.

WORKING PRODUCTIVELY

The ability to work productively and effectively, whether at a job, at school, or at household tasks, is an often-cited indicator of emotional health. The inability to be productive results from emotional conflicts that occupy our attention and sap our energy. It is impossible to concentrate on school-

Positive emotional wellness includes a genuine concern for the well-being of other people. Uncaring, self-centered people are typically unhappy people with many unfulfilled needs that take precedence over the needs of anyone else.

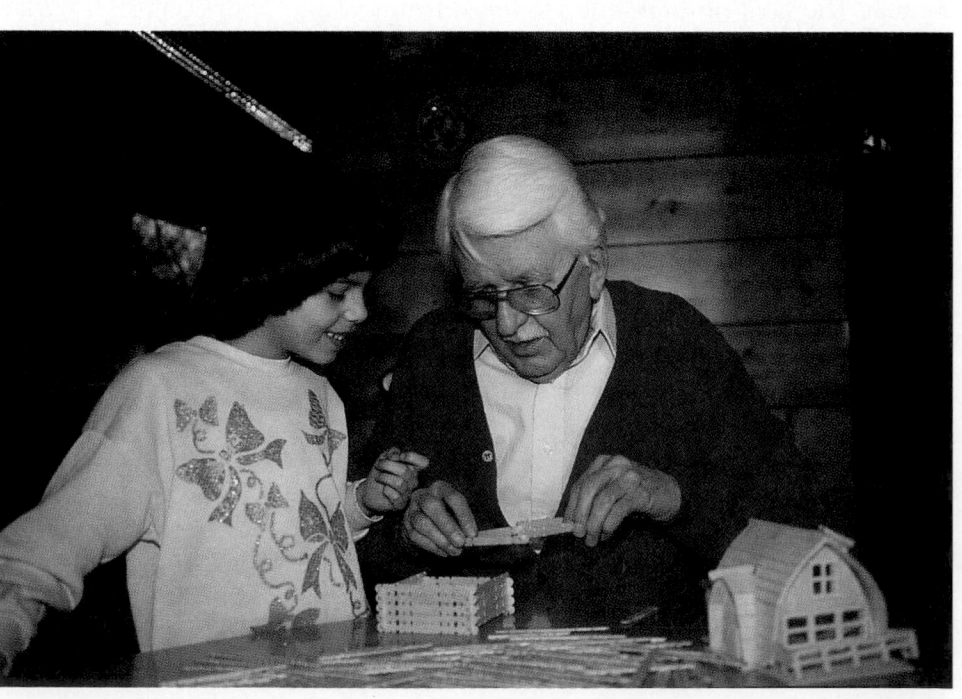

work or any complex task if we are preoccupied with problems.

Lack of self-confidence or low self-esteem can also lower productivity. If one has little confidence that he or she can successfully complete a task, he or she is less motivated to try.

Example: Some unemployed or underemployed people do not feel confident that they can get a good job or perform challenging work satisfactorily; therefore, they may go through life working far below the level of their abilities.

CHECKPOINT

1. What is the most emotionally healthy view of independence and control over one's life?

2. Why are some people unable to love others?

3. What are some barriers to working productively?

BUILDING EMOTIONAL WELLNESS

High-level emotional wellness is the result of years of learning effective ways of living and coping with reality. These skills are not innate; they must be learned. Keys to emotional wellness include having a well-developed sense of identity, strong self-esteem, and the ability to form intimate relationships, all discussed here. Also important are having effective communication skills and being adequately assertive, which were discussed in Chapter 2. Finally, effective ways of meeting the day-to-day challenges of living are the subject of Chapter 4.

DEVELOPING IDENTITY

Erik Erikson associated the task of developing **identity,** one's concept of who he or she is, with adolescence, but many people continue to struggle for a more clearly defined identity well beyond adolescence. We all undergo a constant, lifelong

identity one's concept of who he or she is.

evolution in our sense of identity as we grow and mature. At any age, we may find ourselves wondering who we really are in relation to the rest of the world.

In the United States, more than in some other countries, our identities revolve around our occupation. Americans often view people largely in terms of what they do for a living. Although our occupation is certainly part of our identity, it is only one of many parts. We gain a very incomplete view of ourselves and of others if we think only in terms of occupation.

Our complete identity integrates many characteristics: age, gender, ethnic group, religion, occupation, talents, leisure pursuits, and relationships with others. Each of us must successfully integrate all aspects of ourselves into one overall identity.

What if one does not feel comfortable with his or her identity? In some areas of identity—age, gender, and ethnic group, for example—we are what we are and simply need to learn to feel comfortable with ourselves by working on our self-esteem. In other areas of identity—occupation, religion, and leisure pursuits, for example—we can try out different identities, keeping those we like and dropping those we don't.

BOOSTING SELF-ESTEEM

Our self-esteem affects almost every aspect of our lives. It influences our happiness, our relationships, and our health-related behavior. Low self-esteem is very prevalent in our society because of the high standards set by society and especially by the role models presented by the media. Also, the parenting style of many has lasting detrimental effects on the self-esteem of their children. Fortunately, we all have the potential to raise our self-esteem. Following are some suggestions of ways to do this:

- Gain an understanding of how your self-esteem may still be influenced by your childhood experiences and how those experiences do not mean that you are not a valuable and worthy person.

- Don't judge yourself against the unreal, perfect image of celebrities in the media. In real life, many of them have their own self-esteem problems.

- Develop the habit of thinking positively about yourself. Don't put yourself down. When you need a boost, make a list of ten good things about yourself.

- Find things you can do well. Success breeds success—each success gives you the increased confidence that leads to further success. Try out some new activities to see where your talents lie. Everyone has areas in which she or he can excel.

- Ensure success in the things you do. Prepare thoroughly for exams, speeches, job interviews, and other activities. Don't set yourself up to fail simply because of inadequate preparation. Doing well on an exam because you prepared thoroughly for it does much more for your self-esteem than failing an exam because you were not prepared. If you need to do fewer things in order to do them well, then evaluate your priorities and eliminate some nonessential uses of your time.

- Develop a support network of good friends. Choose friends who have enough self-esteem to be able to boost yours. Other people with low self-esteem will often put you down as they attempt to feel better about themselves (review Feature 3.2).

- Accept compliments graciously with a "thank you" and a smile.

- Assume responsibility for your own emotions and happiness.

- Don't be a perfectionist. No one can be perfect, so the goal of perfection is impossible to achieve and only sets you up to feel like a failure.

- Keep yourself well-groomed and wear clothing that enhances your appearance. When you make a good appearance you automatically feel better about yourself. Also, other people respond to you much more positively when you are dressed attractively and are well-groomed, and the positive way that they relate to you further builds your self-esteem.

DEVELOPING INTIMATE RELATIONSHIPS

Intimate relationships are friendships characterized by close emotional, intellectual, social, and spiritual bonds. Intimate relationships include caring and sharing. Sex may or may not play a role, just as sexual relationships may or may not include intimacy. Intimacy can develop between friends, lovers, relatives, neighbors, or co-workers.

Freedom of communication is essential to developing an intimate relationship. Thoughts, feelings, and needs can be freely expressed without fear of being judged.

Intimate relationships are important in our need-fulfillment and overall emotional wellness. Intimate relationships are characterized by close emotional, intellectual, social, and spiritual bonds and by open communication of feelings.

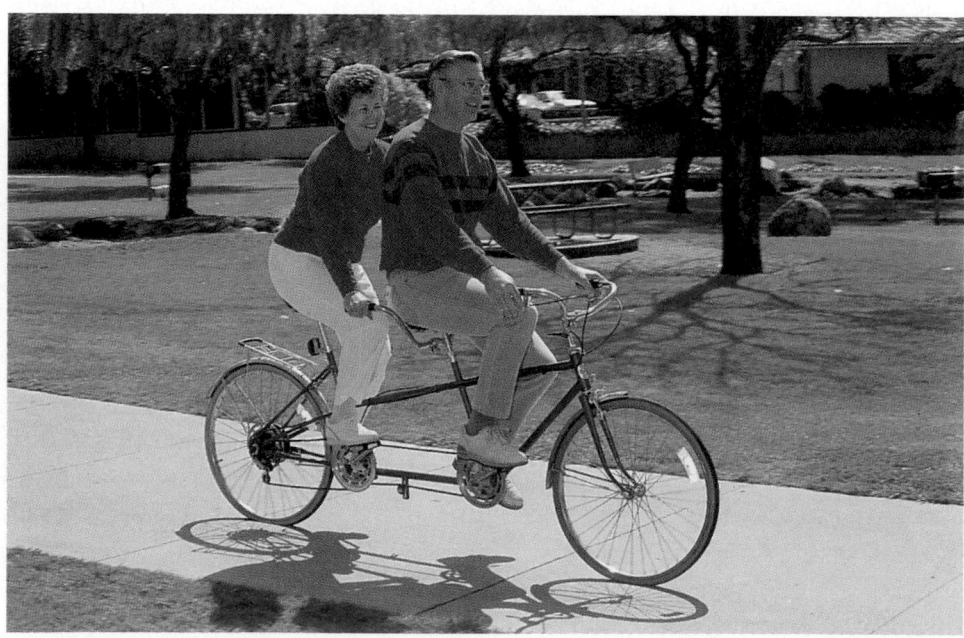

COMMUNICATION IN INTIMATE RELATIONSHIPS

Intimate relationships are important in building and maintaining positive emotional wellness. Intimate relationships are, in turn, based upon open and effective communication. In intimate relationships we communicate our most personal *feelings*. We don't stick with the "safe" subjects such as sports and the weather, but we reveal much of our innermost selves.

Revealing so much of ourselves requires *risk-taking*. We may feel quite vulnerable when we begin establishing intimate relationships, especially if this has not been our habit in the past. We must let down some of our defenses and expose more of ourselves than we may feel comfortable doing. But without this risk-taking there is no way to enjoy the rewards offered by intimate relationships.

Example: You have always been a very private person who has rarely revealed your feelings, either happy or unhappy. You take a chance and tell your friend how much you enjoy spending time with him or her.

Intimacy evolves gradually. *Trust* is a major element in an intimate relationship and takes time to develop. First we must reveal something about ourselves. This gives our friends permission to reveal something about themselves. Then we reveal something further about ourselves and the relationship gradually becomes one in which each party feels free to share feelings.

Example: You tell your friend about something that you have recently done about which you feel quite embarrassed, trusting that your friend won't take advantage of your vulnerability and tell you how dumb you were to do what you did.

Relationships proceed to intimacy only as long as both parties remain *supportive and nonjudgmental*. If you reveal something about yourself that is ridiculed, minimized, or ignored, you feel humiliated and immediately pull back from further exposure of your feelings. This arrests the development of intimacy, as least for the time being.

Example: When you told your friend about your embarrassing episode, your friend said not to worry, everyone does similar things, and told you about an even more embarrassing thing he or she had recently done. Then you both had a good laugh together.

In summary, the communication skills necessary for the development of intimate relationships include:

- open communication of our feelings
- carefully listening to the feelings expressed by our friends
- being nonjudgmental and supportive of the thoughts and feelings expressed to us.

Intimate relationships allow us to feel very comfortable. We are able to relax and be ourselves, knowing that our true self is "good enough" and is accepted, for better and for worse. Intimate relationships help build self-esteem because they confirm our right to be who we are. Conversely, if we put on a false front, for which we win the approval of others, that acceptance doesn't mean much since it is not our true self that is being accepted.

Intimate relationships are essential to positive emotional wellness because they help to fulfill some of our needs by providing us with a support system that helps us through our most difficult times.[9] The lack of intimate relationships results in emotional isolation. Lack of intimacy is often a symptom of unhappiness and severe emotional problems.

Some people choose to avoid intimate relationships, either for fear of being hurt or from a sense of pride in being able to "go it alone" in life. In either case, these people are depriving themselves of need-fulfillment and emotional support that could come from intimacy.

How can someone who lacks intimate relationships begin to develop close friendships? Some of the elements in developing intimacy include:

- *Risk-taking.* We are vulnerable when we begin establishing intimate relationships. We must let down some of our defenses and expose more of ourselves than we may feel comfortable doing. Although we risk rejection, without risk-taking, we may forfeit badly needed intimacy.

- *Effective communication.* In intimate relationships we communicate our *feelings,* not just "safe" topics. We must be in touch with our feelings, accept them as valid, and communicate them effectively. (Refer to Communication for Wellness: Communication in Intimate Relationships.)

- *Sharing oneself.* Intimacy evolves gradually. Trust is a major element in an intimate relationship and takes time to develop. First we must reveal something about ourselves. This gives our friends "permission" to reveal something about themselves. Then we reveal something more about ourselves. This is the start of open communication.

- *Being nonjudgmental and supportive.* Relationships proceed to intimacy as long as both parties remain supportive and nonjudgmental. If we reveal something about ourself that is ridiculed, minimized, or ignored, we feel humiliated and begin to withdraw; this arrests the development of intimacy, at least for the time being.

Our intimate relationships help satisfy our need to belong, to give and receive affection, and to develop self-esteem. They also enable us to keep our problems in perspective; when others share their troubles with us, our own problems may not seem so monumental. Sometimes, just by listening to us in a nonjudgmental manner, our friends help us to reduce our emotional stress level by allowing us to verbalize our internal conflicts and, by doing so, sorting out possible solutions. It may take some courage to establish intimate relationships, but our efforts are well rewarded.

CHECKPOINT

1. What are some major elements in a person's sense of identity?

2. How can one raise his or her self-esteem?

3. How would you characterize an intimate relationship?

4. Why are intimate relationships important to emotional wellness?

SUMMARY

Emotions are mental states that include characteristic subjective feelings, patterns of physiological arousal, and patterns of overt expression. Emotions are real, valid, and a major part of what it means to be human. Because every emotion influences physical body function, emotional wellness relates directly to physical wellness.

Personality is a person's total response to his or her environment. Because of the complexity of personality, it has been studied in many ways. Psychoanalytic theorists such as Freud have emphasized the importance of the unconscious portion of the mind. Behaviorists such as Watson have explained all behavior as a conditioned response to an external stimulus. Developmentalists such as Erikson have emphasized the need to meet successfully the psychosocial challenges typical of each stage in our lives. Humanists such as Maslow have emphasized the whole person and the importance of emotions and need-fulfillment. Maslow's hierarchy of human needs includes the physiological needs, the safety needs, the need for love and belonging, the need for self-esteem, and the need for self-actualization. Rogers, another humanist, has emphasized the importance of self-image in personality development.

Defense mechanisms, an important part of personality, are unconscious psychological techniques we all use to protect ourselves from uncomfortable feelings. They include repression, suppression, denial, displacement, projection, regression, rationalization, reaction formation, and sublimation.

Happiness is a subjective state of emotional well-being and contentment. Factors commonly associated with a high level of happiness include having realistic expectations, having a positive outlook, having rewarding relationships, assuming responsibility for your own happiness, having a rewarding career, and having spirituality.

Other characteristics of positive emotional wellness include a positive self-concept and self-esteem, psychosocial development appropriate to your age, effective methods of need-fulfillment, ability to cope with unfulfilled needs, adequate adaptability, a reasonable degree of independence, reasonable risk-taking, a reasonable expectation for control of your life, effective stress-management techniques, a concern for others, rewarding relationships with others, the ability to love, and the ability to work productively.

Keys to emotional wellness include having a well-developed sense of identity, strong self-esteem, the ability to form intimate relationships, having effective communication skills, being adequately assertive, and having effective ways of meeting the day-to-day challenges of living.

REFERENCES

1. Crider, A., Goethals, G., Kavanaugh, R., and Solomon, P. *Psychology,* 4th ed. New York: Harper-Collins, 1993.
2. Kagan, J., and Segal, J. *Psychology,* 7th ed. San Diego: Harcourt Brace Jovanovich, 1992.
3. Ibid.
4. Erikson, E. *Childhood and Society,* 2nd ed. New York: Norton, 1963.
5. Maslow, A. H. *Motivation and Personality,* 2nd ed. New York: Harper & Row, 1970.
6. Rogers, C. *Client-Centered Therapy: Its Current Practice, Implications, and Theory.* Boston: Houghton Mifflin, 1951.
7. Kagan and Segal, op. cit.
8. Hafen, B., et al. *The Health Effects of Attitudes, Emotions, Relationships.* Provo, UT: EMS Associates, 1992.
9. Ibid.

SUGGESTED READINGS

Coon, D. *Introduction to Psychology.* St. Paul, MN: West, 1992.
Elgin, S. *Genderspeak: Men, Women and the Gentle Art of Verbal Self-Defense.* New York: Wiley, 1993.
Pettijohn, H. *Psychology, a Concise Introduction,* 3rd ed. Sluice Dock, CT: Dushkin, 1992.
Most larger bookstores carry a huge selection of books on every aspect of psychology. See also the excellent psychology texts mentioned in the References list.

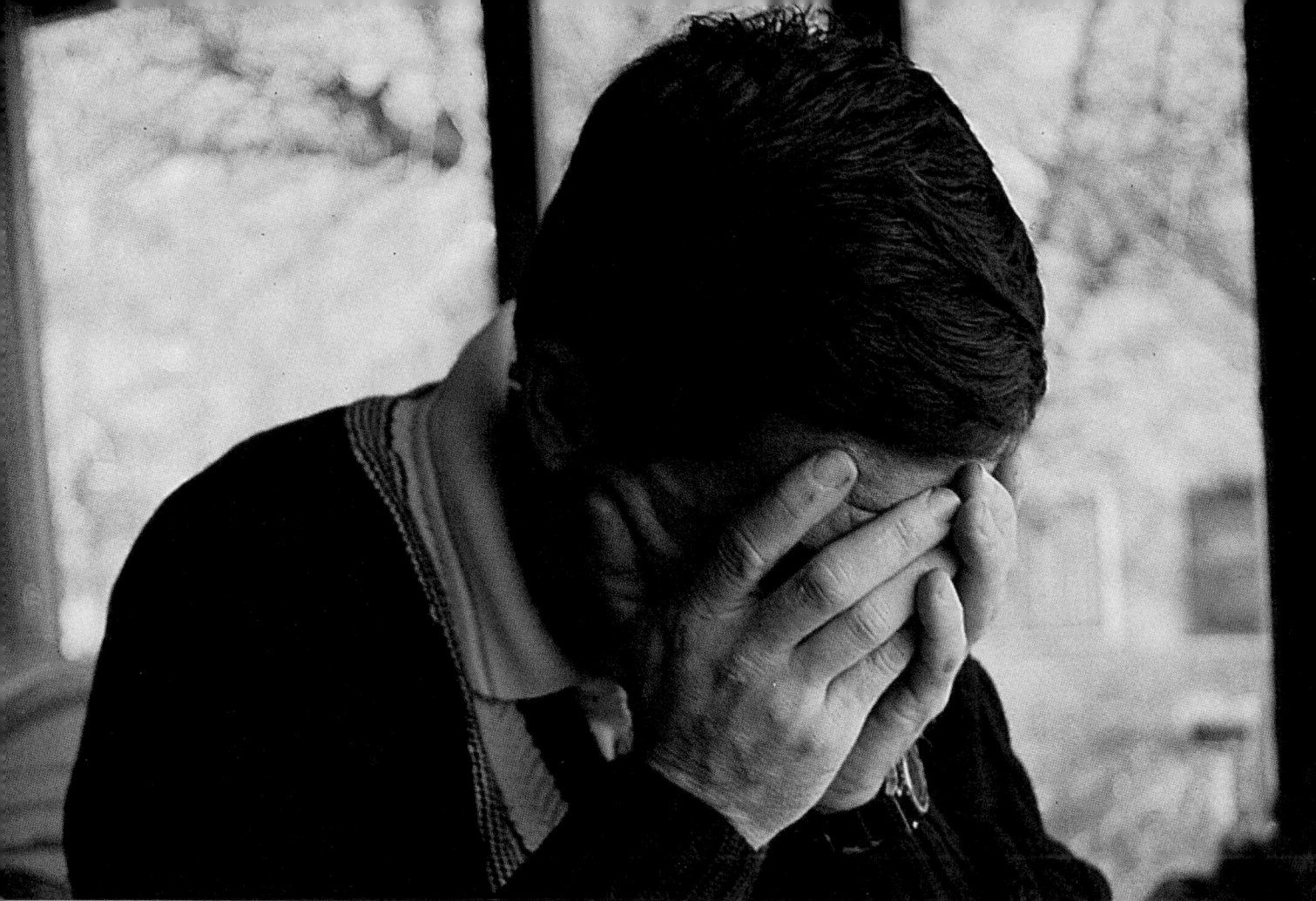

4

STRESS MANAGEMENT AND OTHER MENTAL HEALTH CHALLENGES

KNOWLEDGE

- Explain the stress response and how it may be beneficial or damaging.
- Explain the concept of locus of control.
- Explain the roles of the hypothalamus, pituitary gland, and autonomic nervous system in the stress response.
- Explain how college students can deal with their special stressors.
- Explain the principles of stress management.
- Describe the causes, symptoms, and ways of dealing with moderate anxiety and depression.
- Explain how some major depression has a biochemical basis and how such depression is often treated.
- Identify the characteristics associated with high suicide risk.
- Explain how to intervene when someone appears suicidal.
- Describe the training of psychiatrists, clinical psychologists, psychoanalysts, and clinical social workers.
- Contrast psychodynamic therapies, behavior therapy, humanistic therapy, and Gestalt therapy.

INSIGHT

- Recognize your own warning signs of excess stress.
- Evaluate your own stress level and need for improved stress management.

DECISION MAKING

- Make a commitment to design and implement a personal stress-management program.
- Decide to take a nonjudgmental view of mental illness and emotionally disturbed people.

Dick Cavett has long been noted for his intellectual and witty television interviews of world leaders, entertainers, and many others. Since 1968, he has hosted talk shows on ABC, CBS, PBS, and cable's CNBC with such apparent ease that he left the impression that his work was effortless. The truth is that his performances were far from effortless. In fact, he has revealed that sometimes it took every bit of his energy and willpower to make himself sit in front of the camera and talk with his guests. The reason is that for much of his life, Dick Cavett has suffered from clinical depression.

He remembers his first bout with serious depression during 1959, soon after he had graduated from college. He recalls feeling that he had some fatal disease, and now recognizes this hypochondria as a symptom of his depression. When he experienced a bout of depression, even deciding what to wear would completely stonewall him. He could not concentrate at all, except on his "terrible qualities and shortcomings." Cavett notes that his feelings of depression also had a physical presence; he often had what he described as horrible anxiety attacks. He would experience difficulty in breathing, tightness in his chest, and an overriding sense of doom. His cycles of depression lasted for years. Most of the time he would be functional and feel fine, then, for no reason, he would slide into depression.

Finally, with the encouragement of his wife, he sought the help of a psychiatrist. He was treated with antidepressants and, after one of his most serious episodes of depression in 1980, he was carefully treated with electroconvulsive therapy. Cavett believes that this type of therapy is seriously misunderstood, because it helped him a great deal.

Dick Cavett takes his medication daily and visits his therapist weekly, and feels that he is back into life. He knows that while he may never be cured, there are ways that he can get out of his depression if it occurs. Depression is one of the most common ailments of our society; it is thus very important to realize that there is help available and that clinical depression can be treated very successfully.

Source: People, *August 3, 1992, pp. 88–90.*

Life requires constant adjustments, be they major or minor, to our ever-changing environment and selves. Each day presents us with new opportunities and challenges. Maintaining our physical and mental health requires countless adjustments as well. How successfully we adapt depends largely on how we view the challenge. Those who enjoy positive emotional health see most changes as interesting, exciting, and as offering new opportunities. They are able to cope with even the more unfortunate changes, such as accidents, illness, and the loss of loved ones or possessions, better than those who do not have the same degree of emotional health. This chapter offers suggestions on how we can develop more effective ways of coping with life's challenges.

STRESS: STIMULUS AND RESPONSE

Stress means different things to different people. Many, for example, use the term to refer to anything that requires us to make adjustments. In this text, we will follow the precedent of Hans Selye (*sel'yā*) and define **stress** as a group of bodywide,

nonspecific defense *responses* induced by any of a number of stressors.[1] The key concept in Selye's definition is that stress is the body's *response*.

STIMULUS: STRESSORS

A **stressor** is any situation or event that elicits the stress response. There are many potential stressors, such as:

changes (vacation, marriage, divorce, new job, and so on)

emotional conflict

any intense emotion

fear

fatigue

physical injury

surgery

temperature extremes

noise

crowding

disease agents

illness

Change is one of the most powerful stressors. Any kind of change in our lives, even a positive one, requires us to adapt to a new set of circumstances. Getting married, getting divorced, entering college, and graduating from college all require us to adapt, and so are all stressors. Even winning $10 million in the lottery requires adapting to a new status and is a stressor.

The effects of stressors are cumulative. The more stressors we have in our lives at any given time, the higher our stress level will be.

EVERYDAY STRESSORS

No two of us are exactly alike in which aspects of our daily lives increase our stress levels. The identical life situation might be quite pleasant to one

stress a group of bodywide, nonspecific defense responses induced by any of a number of stressors.

stressor any situation or event that elicits the stress response.

person while extremely stressful to another. In a general sense, a situation will be a stressor if it is perceived as threatening our well-being or requiring our adjustment in any way. We want to emphasize that it is our *perception* of each situation that makes it either stressful or not stressful, so almost *any* event or situation can be a stressor. In the following paragraphs we will discuss some of the more common stressors. Ways of dealing with these stressors are described in the section of this chapter entitled Stress Management.

Negative Outlook

As we have mentioned, the same life situation can be perceived very differently by different people. Those with a positive outlook know that there are few situations with which they can't deal. They expect that everything will turn out all right and it usually does. Those with a negative outlook focus on the possible adverse outcomes of any situation and develop stress over problems that are not very likely to occur.

External Locus of Control

Locus of control, a person's perception of the amount of control he or she holds over his or her life, is influenced by one's culture and life experiences. People with an *external* locus of control

believe that, relative to other people in their ethnic group, they have very little control over their lives. This belief is associated with high stress levels. People with an *internal* locus of control believe that they have a considerable amount of control over their lives, a belief associated with lower stress levels. For someone with an external locus of control a first step in stress management is accepting that people do have considerable control over their lives and beginning to assume more control over and responsibility for his or her own life.

Relationships

For many of us, our relationships with people are unquestionably our greatest cause of stress. Some of us spend much of our adult lives trying to come to terms with one of our parents. Some of us suffer great stress over our relationships with our spouses or significant others. And, of course, roommates have caused their share of stress.

If one certain person is a major cause of your stress, you might check Feature 4.1 Dealing with Difficult People (p. 78). If your relationships with many different people are stressful, perhaps *you* are a difficult person. If you suspect that you may be hard to get along with, try asking several close friends, "Please be honest with me. Am I difficult to get along with? Because if I am, I really would like to change."

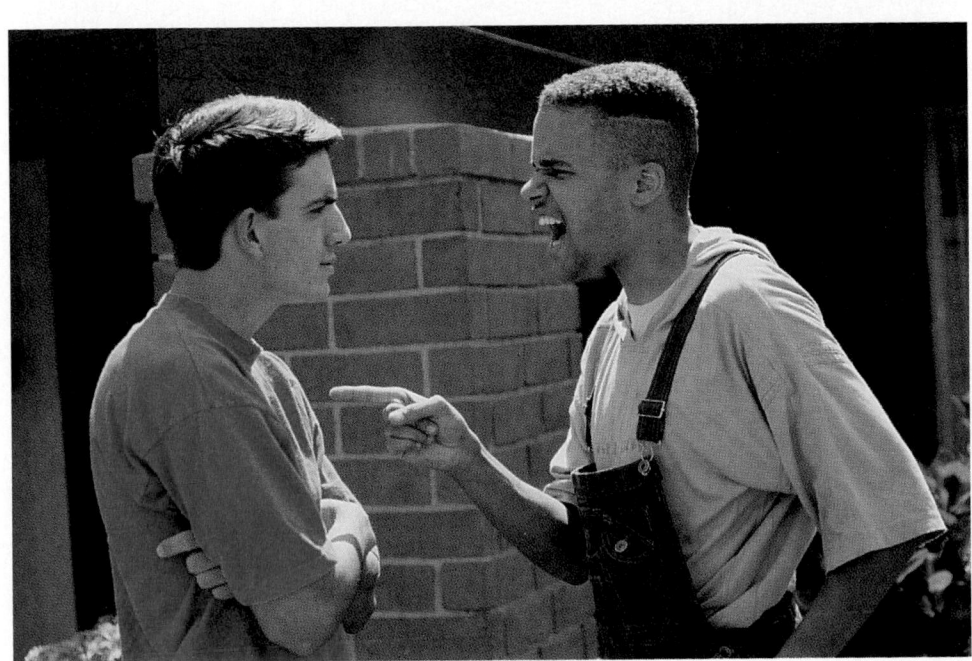

For many people, relationships stand unchallenged as their greatest cause of stress. Stress management requires developing excellent relationship skills.

FEATURE 4.1

DEALING WITH DIFFICULT PEOPLE

Much stress originates in our relationships with other people and certain people can cause far more than their share of difficulty for us. If someone routinely makes your life miserable, remember that *you* are responsible for your emotional well-being and your health and happiness are too important to sacrifice for someone else. Take some definitive action to deal with your difficult person.

Books are available to help you learn to deal with difficult people. Some good ones are *Dinosaur Brains,* by Albert Bernstein and Sydney Rozen (Wiley, 1989); *Neanderthals at Work,* by Albert Bernstein and Sydney Rozen (Ballantine, 1992); *Coping with Difficult People,* by Robert Branson (Doubleday, 1981); *Nasty People,* by Jay Carter (Contemporary Books, 1989); and *Don't Let the Jerks Get the Best of You,* by Paul Meier (Thomas Nelson, 1993). Some of the kinds of people these books teach you how to deal with are:

THE INVALIDATOR

Problem: Boosts own ego by destroying the self-esteem of everyone else. Openly or subtly ridicules you. Will embarrass you in front of other people. Makes you feel tiny and insignificant.

Cause: Invalidator feels inferior because he or she has personally experienced invalidation.

Dealing with an invalidator: Identify the problem for the invalidator; explain how he or she affects you; describe the behavioral changes you expect and set a time limit for change.

THE COMPLAINER

Problem: Complains constantly, but never tries to do anything to fix what he or she complains about.

Cause: Feels powerless or refuses to take responsibility.

Dealing with a complainer: Listen to his or her complaints, but don't agree with or apologize for the situation. Try to move the complainer to a problem-solving mode.

THE CLAM (SILENT AND UNRESPONSIVE)

Problem: Makes no response to questions or requests.

Causes: Way of avoiding dealing with a problem; way of controlling others.

Dealing with a clam: Ask open-ended questions that can't be answered with a yes or a no; wait quietly for a response; don't fill up the silence with your conversation; if still no response, inform the clam what you must and will do, since no discussion has occurred.

THE KNOW-IT-ALL

Problem: Acts and feels superior. Believes and wants you to recognize that she or he knows everything that is worth knowing. Condescending, imposing, pompous; makes you feel like a fool.

Cause: Strong need to feel in control; belief that knowledge forms a strong foundation in an unstable world; no faith in the abilities of anyone else.

Dealing with know-it-alls: To get them to consider alternative views, make adequate preparations; question and suggest; don't put them on the defensive by challenging them; leave them a way to change their position without losing face.

THE NEGATIVIST

Problem: Automatic response to any proposal is no.

Cause: Feels little power over own life, but gets some sense of power by stopping others from acting.

Dealing with a negativist: Don't be dragged down into his or her despair; discuss a situation thoroughly before making your proposal; indicate your plans to take action on your own if necessary.

Performance Anxiety

Many of us experience stress when we are called upon to perform in some way. Taking examinations, giving speeches, or even having sex can be stressful. Our stress in these cases derives from our fear of failure. No one likes to fail in any way, but for many of us, especially those who are struggling to maintain a sense of self-esteem, failure is very painful. Unfortunately, one's high stress level can itself interfere with one's performance, thus ensuring the failure that we so dread. Every professor can tell of students whose only reason for failing exams is their fear of failing. Every sex therapist can tell of clients whose only reason for sexual dysfunction is their fear of sexual failure. If, as a college student, you experience test anxiety, almost every college has programs available to deal with this problem.

Money

Money (or actually the lack of it) is a major source of stress for many people. In a sense, this is one of the most "valid" stressors because so many of our basic survival needs require money. Anyone struggling to survive on a small income is likely to feel plenty of stress. But money has significance beyond its obvious value as a medium of exchange. Even some of the wealthiest people become stressed over money-related issues. To some people, wealth is a measurement of human value and their self-esteem is based on their material assets. Stress management for such people requires taking an objective look at the role money plays for them.

Sex

"Sex relieves stress." That's true in many cases, yet sex can also be a stressor. Like money, sex carries symbolic values beyond its obvious purposes. When one's self-esteem revolves around being sexually attractive, the lack of a partner or rejection by a sexual partner can be quite stressful. Conversely, being pressured for unwanted sex is very stressful. Sex accompanied by fear of pregnancy or disease, or by physical or emotional abuse is stressful. People who have not come to terms with their sexuality may find that sex arouses stress-producing feelings of guilt, fear, and shame. And as previously mentioned, people who place too much emphasis on their sexual performance may become highly stressed during sex, which, ironically, impairs their sexual abilities.

Lack of Organization

It might seem that the least stressful life-style would be very laid-back and free-form. But actually, being disorganized is stressful. Without a certain amount of organization, much time and effort is wasted. Without adequate planning and preparation everything goes wrong. What is more stressful than facing a deadline for which you are totally unprepared?

Inflexibility

The least stressful life-style is well organized, yet flexible enough to be able to deal with life's little surprises. Even with the best organization, unforeseeable problems (and opportunities) arise. People and machines fail to do their jobs. Natural disasters occur. People who lack the flexibility to adapt to sudden challenges experience great stress and miss out on great opportunities.

Noise and Stress

Noise, perhaps the most neglected form of environmental pollution, is one of the most troublesome stressors for many people. Trying to sleep, work, study, or relax in a noisy place mobilizes the body's stress response, with measurable increases in blood pressure, heart rate, and muscle tension.[2] Even though we seem to "get used to" a certain noise, it can still be causing physical changes.

RESPONSE: THE GENERAL ADAPTATION SYNDROME

The stress response includes hundreds of measurable physiological changes, which Selye referred to as the **General Adaptation Syndrome** (GAS).[3] Selye emphasized that all stressors result in essentially the same response. We don't have a lot of different kinds of stress, just different degrees of the same stress response, regardless of the nature of the stressor. The General Adaptation Syndrome is thus the response to any stressor and has three stages: alarm, resistance, and exhaustion.

The stress response is controlled by the **hypothalamus** (*hī-pō-thal'a-mus*), a small structure located deep in the brain (Figure 4.1, p. 80). The hypothalamus is an important link between mental and physical function and constantly adjusts numerous body functions according to our emotional state. The hypothalamus produces the stress response by the way it regulates the pituitary gland and the autonomic nervous system.

The Pituitary Gland

The tiny **pituitary** (*pi-tū'i-tā r'ē*) **gland,** sometimes called the body's "master gland" because it controls the levels of many of the body's hormones, is in turn, controlled by the hypothalamus. The pituitary gland is suspended from the hypothalamus. Releasing factors travel from the hypothalamus to the pituitary gland, causing the release of specific pituitary hormones. Most of these pituitary hormones then stimulate the functioning of other glands.

....

General Adaptation Syndrome the body's response to a stressor, made up of the stages of alarm, resistance, and exhaustion.

hypothalamus a portion of the brain that controls the stress response and regulates the pituitary gland and the autonomic nervous system.

pituitary gland the body's "master gland" which controls the levels of many of the body's hormones through the effects of pituitary hormones on other glands.

Figure 4.1

Functions of the Hypothalamus and Pituitary Gland in Stress Response

The hypothalamus, with the associated pituitary gland, plays a major role in bringing about the physiological changes that make up the stress response. Upon stimulus from the cerebral cortex, the hypothalamus directly activates the sympathetic nervous system and through its control over the pituitary gland, the hypothalamus regulates the levels of many of our hormones.

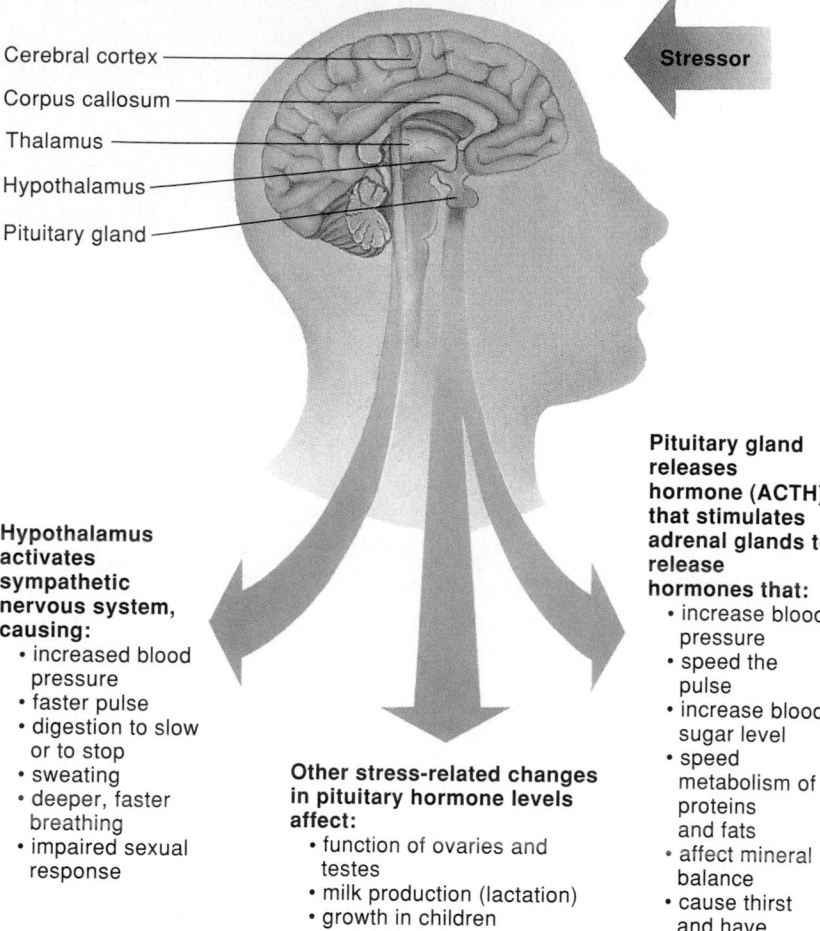

Cerebral cortex
Corpus callosum
Thalamus
Hypothalamus
Pituitary gland

Stressor

Hypothalamus activates sympathetic nervous system, causing:
- increased blood pressure
- faster pulse
- digestion to slow or to stop
- sweating
- deeper, faster breathing
- impaired sexual response

Other stress-related changes in pituitary hormone levels affect:
- function of ovaries and testes
- milk production (lactation)
- growth in children
- thyroid function

Pituitary gland releases hormone (ACTH) that stimulates adrenal glands to release hormones that:
- increase blood pressure
- speed the pulse
- increase blood sugar level
- speed metabolism of proteins and fats
- affect mineral balance
- cause thirst and have many other effects

Hormones from the pituitary gland control the following functions:

- body growth and metabolism
- function of the thyroid gland
- function of the adrenal glands
- function of the ovaries or testes
- milk production and release

Any or all of these functions can be modified in the stress response.

The Autonomic Nervous System

The hypothalamus also regulates the autonomic (involuntary) portion of the nervous system. Autonomic nerves control glands and involuntary muscles, such as the muscles in the heart, blood vessels, and digestive system.

There are two opposing branches of the **autonomic nervous system,** contrasted in Table 4.1. The **sympathetic nervous system,** mobilized by emotions such as fear and anger, prepares the body for emergency action. The **parasympathetic nervous system,** mobilized by feelings of well-being, acts to restore and conserve energy. The

autonomic nervous system the portion of the nervous system that controls glands and involuntary muscles.

sympathetic nervous system the branch of the autonomic nervous system that prepares the body for emergency action.

parasympathetic nervous system the branch of the autonomic nervous system that acts to restore and conserve energy.

Table 4.1
Sympathetic Versus Parasympathetic Nervous System

Sympathetic Nervous System	Parasympathetic Nervous System
Activated by fear, anger, anxiety, hostility.	Activated by sense of well-being.
Acts to prepare body for emergency action (fight or flight). Diverts blood from internal organs to muscles of movement.	Acts to restore and conserve energy.
Speeds pulse (felt as "pounding" of heart).	Slows pulse.
Raises blood pressure (cannot be felt).	Lowers blood pressure.
Causes "cold sweat."	No opposite effect.
Shuts off most digestive juices, causing dry mouth and indigestion. Stomach acid is not shut off, accumulates and contributes to ulcers.	Stimulates digestion.
Blocks male and female sexual arousal. Stimulates male ejaculation, making control difficult.	Produces sexual arousal.

balance of power between these two branches varies from moment to moment as our emotional states fluctuate.

Activation of the sympathetic nervous system is an important part of the stress response, especially in the alarm reaction. Prolonged high levels of sympathetic activity can be quite damaging; it can contribute to heart disease, ulcers, sexual difficulties, and other health problems. Study Table 4.1 carefully so that you will be able to identify when your sympathetic nervous system is activated. By becoming familiar with these signs, we can recognize when our stress level is adversely affecting our physical selves. Remember that these responses are involuntary and can only be consciously controlled to a limited extent. They can be controlled indirectly, however, by applying stress-management techniques in order to reduce the amount of sympathetic activity.

STAGES IN THE GENERAL ADAPTATION SYNDROME

Selye divided the General Adaptation Syndrome into three stages: the alarm reaction, the stage of resistance, and the stage of exhaustion.[4]

The Alarm Reaction

The **alarm reaction** is our immediate response to a stressor. This reaction prepares the body for emergency action. We respond with increased alertness and activation of the sympathetic nervous system. Heart rate and blood pressure increase, digestion slows, and blood moves from other organs to the body muscles. In an emergency, such as being in a burning building, the alarm reaction can be extremely useful. When the emergency has passed, we move into the stage of resistance.

The Stage of Resistance

After the initial alarm stage of the GAS, our stress level drops to a lower, more sustainable, level. When we are in the stage of **resistance,** we have an increased long-term ability to tolerate stressors. We are in a state of improved physical and mental health, better able to fight off germs and deal with emotional challenges. If, however, our stress level is too high for too long, we progress to the third stage, the stage of exhaustion.

The Stage of Exhaustion

High stress levels consume considerable energy and create physiological conditions that, if prolonged, exhaust our resistance to stressors. In this state of **exhaustion,** illness is likely to occur. The immune system becomes less effective, increasing our susceptibility to infectious diseases and cancer. Selye emphasized that any one stressor has the potential to exhaust resistance to all stressors. Thus, people in the state of exhaustion often suffer complete physical and mental collapse.

EUSTRESS

Despite all of the negative things we hear about stress, it is not always harmful. On the contrary, the human mind and body function best under a moder-

alarm reaction immediate response to a stressor, in which the body is prepared for emergency action.

resistance a sustainable level of stress in which the resistance to stressors increases.

exhaustion following prolonged high stress levels, the body's resistance to stressors is lost and illness or death occurs.

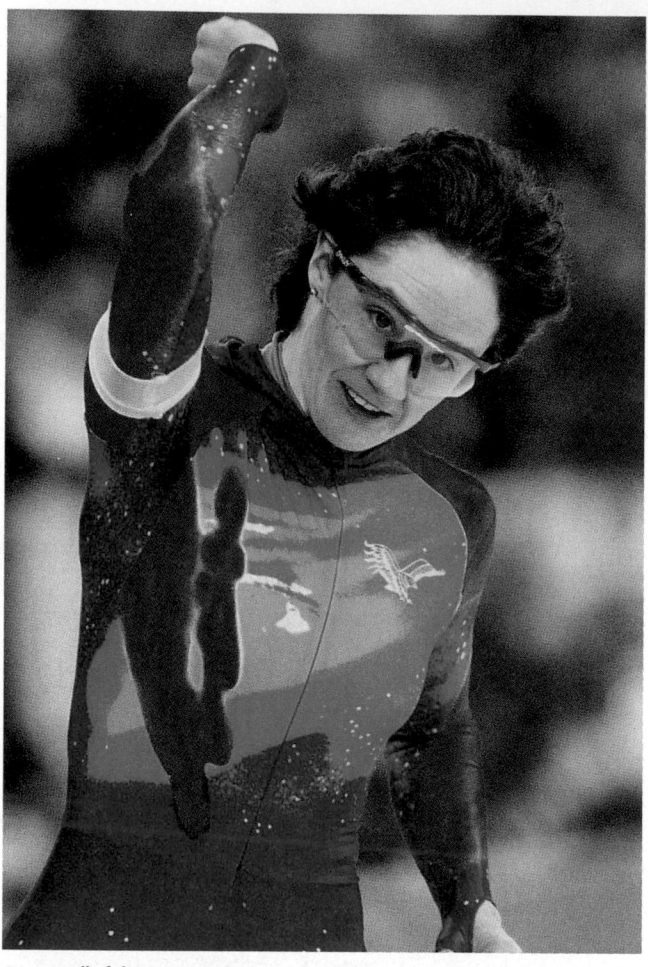

Despite all of the negative things we hear about stress, it is not always harmful. An example of eustress is an athlete or performer of any kind who is "up" for a competition or performance and doing a spectacular job.

ate amount of stress. Selye used the term **eustress** (*ū'stress*) to describe stress as a beneficial force. Eustress (*eu* is the Greek for good or true) prepares the mind and body for optimum functioning. As stress levels increase, they remain beneficial for shorter periods of time. A high stress level might remain beneficial for only a very short time. An example of eustress is an athlete or a performer being "up" for the competition or performance and doing a spectacular job. Another example is when a student studies hard for an exam and does well on it.

DISTRESS

Distress is stress that has harmful effects. An athlete may be so highly stressed that his or her per-

....

eustress stress that has beneficial effects.

distress stress that has harmful effects.

formance suffers. Most students have, at some time, felt so much stress over an exam that it hurt their performance. You may find that during the exam you can't remember anything, but as soon as you turn in the paper and walk out the door, you remember everything. The act of turning in the paper reduces your stress level, which allows you to think normally again.

Stress also becomes distress if it leads to illness. Many people who have not learned effective stress-management techniques live with very high stress levels day after day. Table 4.2 cites just a few examples of the kinds of problems that can result from prolonged high stress levels. Take a minute right now and complete In Your Hands: A Stress-Management Assessment.

CHECKPOINT

1. Define *stressor, stress,* and *General Adaptation Syndrome.*

2. What is locus of control and how does it relate to stress?

3. What are some common everyday stressors?

4. What are some signs that a person's sympathetic nervous system is active?

5. Contrast eustress and distress.

Table 4.2
Some Problems That May Be Stress-related

Each of the conditions on this list is often caused or aggravated by excessive stress. Though each can also have causes other than stress, anyone whose stress level is very high for an extended period can expect to experience one or more of these problems.

Allergies	Inability to concentrate
Arthritis	Indigestion
Asthma	Infertility
Backaches	Insomnia
Cancers	Menstrual disorders
Colds	Muscle spasms
Headaches	Skin disorders
Heart disease	Sleep disorders
High blood pressure	Ulcers
Impaired sexual response	

IN YOUR HANDS
A STRESS-MANAGEMENT ASSESSMENT

Each of us must develop effective ways of managing our stress level and coping with the day-to-day challenges of life. How well are you handling your stress? Circle the appropriate number of points for each statement.

	Often	Sometimes	Seldom
1. I am happy.	0	1	2
2. I assume responsibility for my own happiness and emotional well-being.	0	1	2
3. I feel hopeless and discouraged.	2	1	0
4. I can cope successfully with stressful periods without using alcohol or other drugs.	0	1	2
5. If I were experiencing an unusually stressful period, I would be willing to seek professional help.	0	1	2
6. I tend to feel sad.	2	1	0
7. I spend time wishing I were someone else.	2	1	0
8. I spend time wishing I were somewhere else.	2	1	0
9. I tend to get upset easily.	2	1	0
10. Of the 37 warning signs of excess stress listed on p. 88, the number of those signs that apply to me is _____.			

Total points for items 1–10: _____.

INTERPRETATION

0–3 points: You appear to manage stress effectively and cope well. You are probably quite happy.

4–7 points: Your methods for coping with stress are about average. You can benefit by carefully reading this chapter.

8 or more points: You are showing definite signs of difficulty in coping and stress management. If you don't initiate more effective coping and stress-management methods as described later in this chapter, you are at risk of severe health problems.

HOW STRESS CAUSES ILLNESS

Stress, by modifying almost every body function, is capable of producing illness in a number of ways. We will next consider a few of the leading examples.

HEART DISEASE

Stress contributes to heart disease in many ways. During periods of stress, the blood pressure rises and pulse increases, placing an added burden on the heart. Stress induces changes in blood chemistry, such as elevated cholesterol levels, that promote atherosclerosis. Finally, the coronary arteries that supply blood to the heart muscle itself constrict, reducing the amount of oxygen available to the heart muscle. These problems are discussed in greater detail in Chapter 20. Also discussed in Chapter 20 is the Type A–Type B personality dichotomy. Some, though not all, heart experts associate the Type A personality (compulsive, competitive, impatient, hard driven) with a higher rate of heart disease than is found in the more relaxed Type B personality.

INFECTIOUS DISEASES

Psychoneuroimmunology is the study of the relationships that exist among the nervous system, the hormonal system, and the immune system. Excessive stress reduces the effectiveness of the immune mechanism and thereby increases the risk of infectious disease.[5] For example, many people find that they experience colds mostly during stressful periods. Similarly, both oral and genital

....

psychoneuroimmunology the study of the relationships that exist among the nervous system, the hormonal system, and the immune system.

herpes attacks (see Chapter 19) tend to develop during periods of high stress. Finally, the relationship of stress to mononucleosis and meningitis is well established (see Chapter 18).

Stress is believed to impair immunity by raising the level of adrenal hormones, such as epinephrine, which damage the immunity producing lymphocytes (discussed in Chapter 18). The immune system is extremely complex and is likely to be influenced by stress in many ways that are not yet known.

STRESS AND CANCER

As with infectious diseases, excessive stress increases your risk of cancer by reducing the efficiency of your immune system. Many cancer experts believe that in every person, from time to time, cells become cancerous (see Chapter 21). If the immune system is working properly, these cancerous cells are usually destroyed quickly. When your immunity is impaired, however, there is increased risk of cancer becoming a life-threatening problem.

STRESS AND DIGESTIVE DISORDERS

As indicated in Table 4.1, the sympathetic nervous system, which is activated during periods of stress, reduces production of most digestive juices, except for stomach acid. Food lies in the stomach, the acid builds up in response to the presence of the food, causing indigestion, and, in time, this acid can erode the wall of the stomach or intestine, causing an ulcer. Indigestion is a very common sign of excessive stress. Further, many people overeat or undereat during stressful periods, contributing to weight-management problems.

STRESS AND SKIN DISORDERS

The impact of excessive stress on human skin has long been recognized. Two very obvious effects are the appearance of rashes ("breaking out") and premature aging. Stress produces rashes by modifying the activity of the immune mechanism. Premature aging of the skin results from stress-induced constriction (narrowing) of the small blood vessels supplying food and oxygen to the skin cells. People who have lived stressful lives often appear years older than their true age.

CHECKPOINT

1. What are some effects of stress on the immune system?

2. What is believed to be the relationship between stress and cancer?

3. What are the effects of excessive stress on one's skin?

STRESS AND COLLEGE

Despite the public image of college students as carefree and funloving, some experts believe that the college years are the most stressful in our lives.[6] Although this generalization isn't true for every college student, it certainly applies to many. College is stressful both for students of "traditional" college age and for those returning to college at some later time.

Younger college students have their special stressors, such as adjusting to the very different demands of college as compared to high school, resolving identity issues, being shy and lonesome in the college setting, making new friends, satisfying the expectations of parents, and dealing with the whole arena of dating and mating, with its emotional high and low points.

Older college students often must contend with the necessity of balancing the demands of work and school, helping children with their schoolwork, initially feeling out of place in college, reestablishing study habits, finding time and a quiet place to study, and in many cases dealing with the same dating and mating problems as the younger students (if they have time for any social lives at all).

New college students of any age have many adjustments to make. Remember that change is one of the biggest stressors and entering college is one of the biggest possible changes in a person's life. Problems shared by all college students include the pressures to make acceptable grades and the near-universal shortage of time.

TIME MANAGEMENT

One of the most common reasons for poor grades is inadequate time-management skills. During the busy college years and throughout our lives, the effective use of time-management techniques can greatly increase our productivity while providing adequate time for recreational activities. Jerrold Greenberg[7] describes an effective time-management plan:

- *Assess how you spend your time now.* Keep a diary of how your time is spent for a week. (Be honest!) You might be surprised where your time is going.

- *Set goals.* Effective time management requires having goals for each day, week, month, and year. This is a must in time management; there is no way to allot your time effectively without having clear goals.

- *Prioritize.* Rate each goal as either an A (must do), a B (want to do or should do), or a C (wouldn't matter if you never do).

- *Schedule your day.* Base your day's schedule on your priorities. Don't forget to include some physical activity, some relaxation, and some recreation.

- *Just say no.* Don't let people manipulate you. Don't be pressured into activities that use up your time but don't mean much to you.

- *Delegate.* When possible, without exploiting other people, get other people to do some of the things that need to be done.

- *Work efficiently.* Look for ways to streamline what you do. For example, when you open a piece of mail, act on it immediately; handle each piece of paper just once.

- *Limit interruptions.* People who apparently have very little to do can be quite insensitive to your time needs. Lock your door. Unplug your phone. Firmly but politely say, "I'm sorry, I just can't talk right now; I've got some deadlines to meet."

- *It takes time to save time.* It does take a little time to set up a time-management program. Don't say "I'm too busy to keep a time diary for a week." The small amount of time you invest setting up a time-management program will pay for itself many times over in better use of your time over the months and years to come.

OVERCOMMITMENT

In the authors' experience, one of the most common stressors for today's college students is attempting to do more than is humanly possible. Our society gives the superachiever a lot of approval, so many students attempt to do what only a very few can do. They try to take too many courses and work too many hours at their jobs, while trying to carry out all of their family and personal obligations. The result is almost always the same: frustration, low grades, problems in relationships, physical health problems, and loss of self-esteem. They end up feeling like failures when the only thing they did wrong was set unattainable goals for themselves. *Moral of the story:* Don't set yourself up to fail. Your grade point average doesn't need it and your self-esteem doesn't need it.

WORK-RELATED STRESS

Work-related stress has increased significantly in the last few years.[8] People are spending more hours at work and bringing more work home with them. Job security has decreased in almost every industry. Pay, for many, has failed to keep up with the cost of living. Women are subject to exceptionally high stress levels as they try to live up to all of the expectations placed upon them (Feature 4.2, p. 86). Finally, many people feel that they are trapped in jobs they hate, but can't escape.

More specific causes of job-related stress can be attributed to either the worker or the job. Worker characteristics that increase stress include the following:

- negative view of the job or of work in general
- poor decision-making skills
- inactive life-style; lack of exercise
- feeling of inadequacy to perform job
- feeling that job is not challenging enough
- abuse of alcohol or other drugs
- lack of skill in interpersonal relations
- narrow focus on job; inadequate outside interests

Research has revealed many characteristics of jobs that make them stressful to workers. Some of these include the following:[9]

- ambiguity or lack of clarity about the scope of workers' responsibilities
- workers' lack of authority

Work-related stress has increased in the United States in recent years as working hours have lengthened, leisure time has decreased, and considerable job security has been lost.

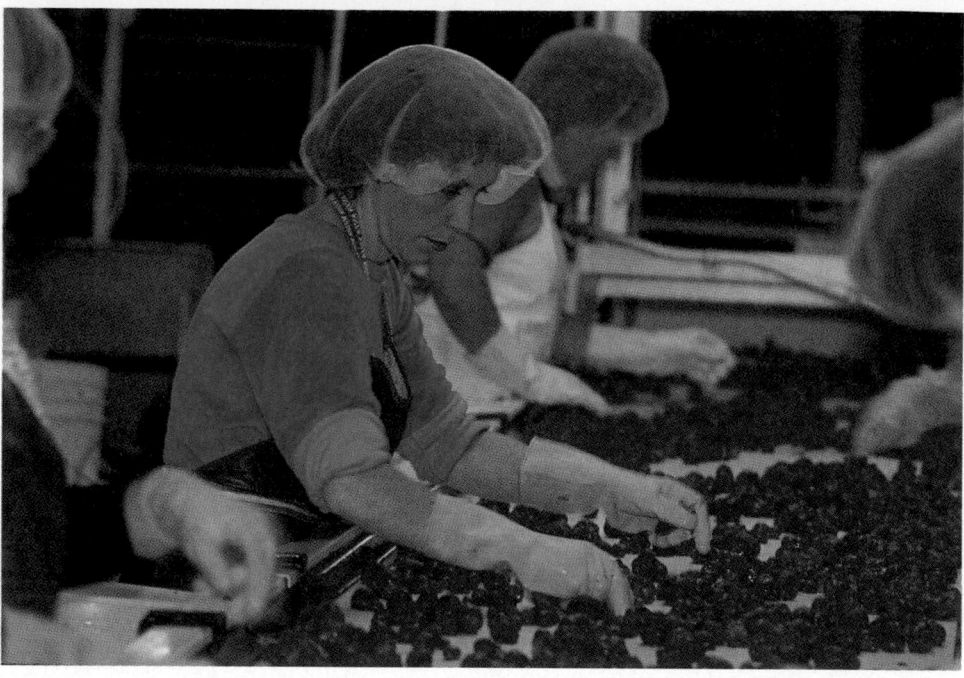

- conflict of job responsibilities with judgment or values
- long work hours
- poor work environment
- too much work *or* too little work
- little chance for promotion
- low pay

- inadequate display of appreciation of workers by management

Job-related stress usually falls into five stages.[10] In the *first stage,* people suffer from anxiety, anger, and tension. The *second stage* occurs when stress is chronic. The responses are mostly psychological and include depression, feelings of fatigue, and alienation. In the *third stage,* physiological changes

---

FEATURE 4.2

WOMEN OF THE NINETIES: FEELING THE PRESSURE

Career woman, mother, daughter, wife, lover, homemaker, and friend . . . just a few of the roles many women of the nineties are trying to fit into their lives. While the expectations for and of women have changed, the day is still only 24 hours long. When do women have time for themselves?

Our society has created the image of the "superwoman," who does it all. Many women are trying hard to conform to this image, but often with limited success. For some, the consequences are divorce, career burnout, stress-related health problems, and guilt or lowered self-esteem over not being able to hold everything together.

What can women do to control their stress levels in the 1990s?

- They can make certain that their goals are their own and not a reflection of media "superwoman" hype.
- They can separate some of their goals in time; for example, they can concentrate on career at one period in their lives and parenthood at another.

- They can, in many cases, elect to have a modified work schedule that balances their professional and domestic needs.
- They can encourage their employers to establish on-site child-care facilities for preschool children.
- They can encourage any man who may be a part of their life to do his share of household duties. Many men apparently still view household chores as "woman's work." As recently as 1988, it was found that when both spouses in a marriage are employed full-time, the wives still do 70 percent of the housework.[a]
- They can apply the stress-management suggestions presented in this chapter.

[a]Grant, E. "The Housework Gap." *Psychology Today,* January 1988, p. 10.

start to occur. Blood pressure rises and the stomach is constantly in knots. In the *fourth stage,* health damage becomes evident. Common problems include ulcers, heart disease, asthma attacks, sexual dysfunction, chemical dependency, and many other disorders. In the *final stage,* productivity falls off and the worker may be fired or demoted.

Whether excessive stress comes from a job, school, personal life, or any other source, it lowers the quality of life and eventually leads to severe health problems. Effective stress-management skills are a must for all of us.

Some specific suggestions for dealing with job-related stress include the following:

- View your job positively. Don't get caught up in the negative attitudes of co-workers. Negative thinking can be contagious, but so can positive thinking.
- Make sure that your job is only one aspect of your life. Have plenty of other interests and activities.
- Maintain good general health habits: plenty of exercise, good diet, avoid alcohol and other drugs.
- Practice stress-management techniques as described in the following section of this chapter.

C H E C K P O I N T

1. What employee characteristics increase work-related stress?

2. What job characteristics increase work-related stress?

3. How can an individual decrease his or her work-related stress?

STRESS MANAGEMENT

Each of us has our own optimum stress level, which is influenced by heredity and other factors. Some people thrive at stress levels that would quickly lead others to the state of exhaustion. How can we tell if we are stressed beyond our optimum level? Sometimes it is obvious; but, more often we fail to associate the symptoms we experience with their cause. In Feature 4.3 we discuss some of the more common clues that indicate when our stress is above the optimum level. Note that different people respond to stress differently. For example, one person might gorge him- or herself with food while another might lose his or her appetite. One person might have trouble falling asleep at night while another person might sleep most of the time. Take a minute right now to see how many of the signs listed in this feature apply to you. If you are experiencing one or more of the warning signs listed in Feature 4.3 (p. 88), it is time to implement some effective stress-management techniques.

GENERAL GUIDELINES FOR STRESS MANAGEMENT

1. *Adopt a new way of looking at life.* Stress management begins with adopting the philosophy that you, as an individual, are basically responsible for your own emotional and physical well-being. You can no longer allow other people to determine whether or not you are happy. You have little control over the behavior of anyone but yourself, and your emotional well-being is too important to trust to anyone but yourself. Your goal should be to develop such positive emotional wellness that nobody can ruin your day.

2. *A positive outlook on life.* This is absolutely essential to successful stress management. Your perception of events, not the events themselves, is what causes stress. Almost any life situation can be perceived as either stressful or nonstressful, depending on your interpretation. A negative view of life guarantees a high stress level. People who habitually view life negatively can recondition themselves to be more positive. One way is by applying a thought-stopping technique: Whenever you catch yourself thinking negatively, force yourself to think about the positive aspects of your situation. Eventually you will just automatically begin to see life more positively.

3. *A regular exercise program.* Exercise is an excellent tension reliever. In addition to the physical benefits, exercise is also good for the mind. Participating in at least three aerobic exercise sessions a week for at least 20 minutes each can greatly reduce stress. Daily stretching exercises provide relaxation and improve flexibility and posture. Participate in leisure activities that keep you physically active.

4. *Be reasonably organized.* Disorganization, sloppiness, chaos, and procrastination may seem

FEATURE 4.3

SOME WARNING SIGNS OF EXCESS STRESS

Everyone has certain warning signs they experience when they are stressed above their optimum level. Not everyone, however, has learned to recognize these warning signs in themselves and to associate them with the need to reduce stress. If you are experiencing one or more of these symptoms, your stress level is probably too high. If that is the case and you don't reduce your stress level, you can expect to develop serious health problems.

- difficulty in thinking clearly, making decisions, or solving problems
- feeling nervous
- vague anxiety
- strong impulse to hide or to cry
- loss of joy of living
- tendency to tire easily
- no energy
- sighing
- irritability, criticizing others
- feeling helpless
- feeling hopeless
- trouble sitting still or relaxing
- itching, skin rashes
- headaches
- difficulty sleeping
- nightmares

- wanting to sleep much of the time
- feeling weak or dizzy
- increased use of alcohol, tobacco, or other drugs
- loss of appetite
- eating too much
- digestive problems such as indigestion, diarrhea, or belching
- menstrual problems
- loss of sexual interest
- compulsive sexuality
- impaired sexual response
- tendency to be easily startled
- pounding heart
- dry mouth
- nervous tics or twitches
- trembling
- tooth grinding
- cold sweat
- back pain
- chest pain
- hyperventilation (rapid breathing)
- frequent accidents

very relaxed, but they are stressful. Set short-term, intermediate-term, and long-term goals for yourself. Every morning list the things you want and need to accomplish that day. Assign each item an A, B, or C priority (see p. 85). Take care of the most urgent matters first. Be realistic; don't expect too much of yourself. Perhaps some C priority items don't really have to be done.

5. *Learn to say no.* Some people accept too many responsibilities. If you spread yourself too thin, not only will you be highly stressed, but important things will be done poorly or not at all. Know your limits and be assertive. If you don't have time to do something or simply don't want to do it, don't. Practice saying no effectively. Try, "I'm flattered that you've asked me, but given my commitments at this time, I won't be able to. . . ."

6. *Learn to enjoy the process.* Our culture is extremely goal oriented. Many of the things we do

are directed toward achieving a goal, with no thought or expectation of enjoying the process. You may go to college for a degree, but you should enjoy the process of obtaining that degree. You may go to work for a paycheck, but you should enjoy your work. Happiness can seldom be achieved when pursued as a goal. It is usually a by-product of other activities. In whatever you do, focus on and enjoy the activity itself, rather than on how well you perform the activity or what the activity will bring you.

7. *Don't be a perfectionist.* Perfectionists set impossible goals for themselves, because perfection is unattainable. Learn to tolerate and forgive both yourself and others. Intolerance of your own imperfections leads to stress and low self-esteem. Intolerance of others leads to anger, blame, and poor relationships, all of which increase stress.

8. *Look for the humor in life.* Humor can be an effective part of stress management. Humor results

in both psychological and physical changes. Its psychological effects include relief from anxiety, stress, and tension, an escape from reality, and a means of tolerating difficult life situations. Physically, laughter increases muscle activity, breathing rate, heart rate, and release of brain chemicals such as catecholamines and endorphins. Following laughter, muscle tension, breathing, pulse rate and blood pressure drop to below-normal levels as you enter a state of relaxation.[11]

We want to emphasize that humor is not always appropriate. In grave or critical situations, for example, efforts at humor are out of place. And *any attempt at humor that stereotypes, degrades or humiliates another person or group of people is never appropriate.* To be avoided at all times are jokes based on ethnicity, race, or religion; gender or sexual orientation; disability; age, or any other personal characteristic.

What forms of humor, then, are appropriate in stress management? Look for the humorous aspects of a stressful situation. Look for absurdity, exaggeration, and incongruity. Look for the unexpected and the ironic. And don't be afraid to laugh at yourself.

9. *Practice altruism.* **Altruism** is unselfishness, placing the well-being of others ahead of one's own. Altruism is one of the best roads to happiness, emotional health, and stress management. As soon as you start feeling concern for the needs of others, you immediately feel less stressed over the frustration of your own needs. Invariably, the most selfish people are the most highly stressed as they focus their attention on the complete fulfillment of their own needs, which can never happen.

Not only does doing for others divert your attention away from whatever frustration of your needs you may be feeling, it directly helps you fulfill those same needs. You gain a sense of self-esteem and self-actualization through your good deeds. You feel more loved and even more secure as you build up a pool of goodwill among those you help.

How can a busy, broke college student do much for anyone else? Consider these examples:

- You can tutor a struggling classmate. Incidentally, the grades of the tutor usually go

up as well as those of the tutee, as tutoring forces you to really understand your subject.

- You can do volunteer work. Most communities offer many opportunities to help the homeless, the sick or disabled, the old and the young.

10. *Let go of the past.* Everyone can list things in the past that he or she might have done differently. Other than learning through experience and trying not to make the same mistakes again, there is nothing to be gained by worrying about what you did or didn't do in the past. To focus on the past is nonproductive, stressful, and robs the present of its joy and vitality. An exception to this rule is those forms of psychotherapy that explore a person's past in order to understand present behaviors and attitudes. Such directed examination of the past can be quite productive.

11. *Eat a proper diet.* How you eat affects your emotions and your ability to cope. When your diet is good you feel better and deal better with difficult situations. Try eating more carefully for two weeks and feel the difference it makes.

There is no unique stress-reduction diet, despite many claims to the contrary. The same diet that helps prevent heart disease, cancer, obesity, and diabetes (low in sugar, salt, fat, and total calories; adequate in vitamins, minerals, and protein) will also reduce stress.

12. *Get adequate sleep.* Sleep is essential for successfully managing stress and maintaining your health. People have varying sleep requirements, but most people function best with seven to eight hours of sleep per day. Some people simply don't allot enough time to sleep, while others find that stress makes it difficult for them to sleep. It is easy to become trapped in a cycle in which stress makes sleep difficult and lack of sleep further increases stress. Feature 4.4 (p. 90) outlines some suggestions for overcoming sleep problems.

13. *Avoid alcohol and other drugs.* The use of alcohol and other drugs in an effort to reduce stress levels actually contributes to stress in several ways. In the first place, it does *not* reduce the stress from a regularly occurring stressor such as an unpleasant job or relationship problems. Further, as alcohol and other drugs wear off, the rebound effect makes the user feel very uncomfortable and more stressed than before (see Chapter 14). Also,

---

altruism placing the well-being of others ahead of one's own; unselfishness.

FEATURE 4.4

A GOOD NIGHT'S SLEEP

Adequate sleep, in terms of both time and quality, is essential to stress management and your general health and effectiveness. Here is a checklist of common barriers to sleep, with some suggested remedies.

ENVIRONMENTAL PROBLEMS:	SUGGESTIONS:
Too much noise	Earplugs
Too much light	Sleeping mask
Too hot or cold	Adjust bedding
Uncomfortable bed	New mattress

BEHAVIORAL PROBLEMS:	SUGGESTIONS:
Erratic sleep routine	Establish regular bedtime
Using bed to eat, read, watch TV or study	Use bed for sleep and sex only
Lack of exercise	Regular exercise program
Too much alcohol or other drugs use	Reduce or eliminate alcohol and other drugs

DIETARY PROBLEMS:	SUGGESTIONS:
Obesity causes sleep apnea (periodic failure to breathe) or discomfort	Lose weight
Too much caffeine	No caffeine in the evening
Heavy meal close to bedtime	Eat earlier and/or more lightly
Eating the wrong foods	Avoid foods that disagree with you

MENTAL PROBLEMS:	SUGGESTIONS:
Can't turn off thoughts	Apply relaxation techniques from this chapter (see pp. 90–91)
Sexual tension	Try masturbation if no available partner
Sex is too stimulating	Have sex in the morning
Worry about insomnia	Get out of bed and read, work, or watch TV

heavy use of alcohol or other drugs invariably creates problems that further increase stress levels. Eliminating or minimizing alcohol and other drug use is essential to stress management.

Don't overlook the possibility that excess caffeine intake is contributing to your stress. Caffeine is a powerful stimulant that, by itself, produces many of the physiological manifestations of stress. Plus, its effect of increased "nervous" energy contributes to more stressful, rushed behavior patterns. Remember that not only coffee and tea, but chocolate and many soft drinks contain caffeine.

CHECKPOINT

1. Why might two people in the same situation experience very different stress levels?

2. What is meant by "learn to enjoy the process"?

3. In what ways can being other-centered help reduce stress?

INSTANT STRESS RELIEVERS

All of us, from time to time, have especially stressful periods during which we feel the need for in-

stant relief from tension. The following suggestions, used as supplements to the general guidelines for stress management that we have discussed, can help you to relax quickly and reestablish normal body function.

1. *Physical exercise.* One of the best instant stress relievers is physical activity. Take a break from whatever you are doing and walk, run, bike, dance, swim, or play tennis.

2. *Deep breathing.* Concentrating on the process of breathing removes sources of stress from your mind temporarily and may help put those stressors back into their proper perspective. One deep breathing technique is explained in Feature 4.5.

3. *Body relaxation techniques.* These techniques are good for falling asleep or relaxing at any time. Here are three variations:

- Lie or sit down and close your eyes. Starting with your toes and working to the top of your head, concentrate on relaxing each body part, one by one. When you are completely relaxed, sit or lie quietly, enjoy the moment and discover how your body feels in the absence of tension.

FEATURE 4.5

DEEP BREATHING FOR STRESS RELIEF

A few minutes spent doing the following exercise can result in several hours of relaxation.

1. Lie or sit comfortably. Close your eyes. If sitting, sit upright so you can breathe freely.

2. Inhale slowly and deeply through your nose. Breathe with both diaphragm and ribs (your stomach should push out, not pull in).

3. Exhale slowly and fully through your mouth.

4. While breathing, *either:*

Count slowly to about 6 or 8 while inhaling and to about 8 or 10 while exhaling (a longer count for exhalation); *or*

During each inhalation say slowly to yourself, "I am," and during each exhalation say very slowly "relaxed"; *or*

Breathe in deeply and slowly while silently saying HOLD, 2, 3, 4, 5, 6. Then exhale slowly while silently saying RELAX, 2, 3, 4, 5, 6.

5. Repeat about 8 times or as long as is comfortable.

6. Breathe normally and rest quietly for a few minutes, enjoying the feeling of total relaxation.

• Lie down and close your eyes. Again, working from your toes to the top of your head, first contract the muscles of each body part for about 5 to 7 seconds, then let that body part relax for 20 to 30 seconds. This technique effectively relaxes tense shoulder and neck muscles and is great for falling asleep.

• Take a hot bath or shower (some people find cold showers more relaxing).

4. *Breaks from reality.* Even though the first characteristic of emotional wellness is being in touch with reality, stress management often requires taking a brief break from your day-to-day world. There are both appropriate and inappropriate ways to do this. Inappropriate methods include using alcohol or other drugs as escape routes or daydreaming when full attention is essential. Here are some more appropriate breaks from reality:

• *Vacations and weekends away.* A day or two away from your everyday routine provides a refreshing break, helps put day-to-day concerns into their proper perspective, and greatly relieves stress. Like other stress-management techniques, this may seem to consume valuable time, but ultimately, taking a badly needed break will increase your productivity and creativity to a degree that compensates for the time used.

• *Films, TV, videos, and books.* A good film, television program, or book can provide a relaxing and enjoyable break from reality.

Even reading a short story or magazine article can provide a brief, relaxing break.

• *Imagery.* You can use your imagination as a means of relaxation or as a method of "rehearsing" more effective ways of dealing with stressful situations. For example, as a rehearsal, you can visualize yourself assertively confronting someone who is causing some of your stress. After having gone over your presentation several times in imagery, you will feel more confident in the actual confrontation.

To use imagery to relax, sit or lie comfortably, close your eyes, and imagine a pleasant, peaceful scene. It might be a lake, meadow, beach, forest, stream, desert, or any place your really enjoy. Envision yourself in that scene. Concentrate on all of the details and all of your senses—the colors, the sounds, smells, and feelings. Some people like to add a companion, such as a person or an animal, to the scene. Continue the imagery for several minutes. This will relax your mind and body and will have a residual relaxing effect that will last for some time after the image is gone.

• *Meditation.* There are many varieties of **meditation,** a method of producing a

meditation a method of producing a relaxed state of consciousness by focusing one's thoughts.

Stress management may require taking a brief break from one's everyday world. There are many constructive ways to do this, such as taking a vacation or weekend off; immersing oneself in a good film or book; using imagery; and meditating. If personnel policies permit, one can break up a vacation day and leave work two hours earlier on four different days.

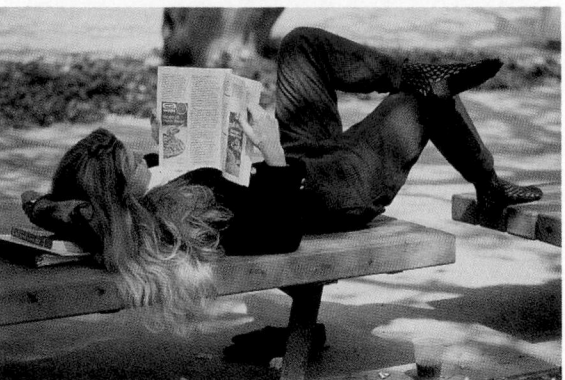

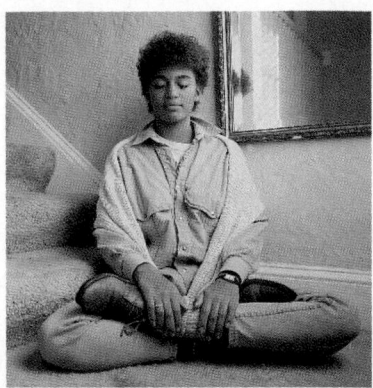

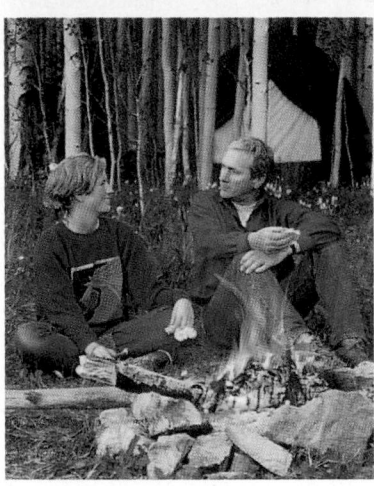

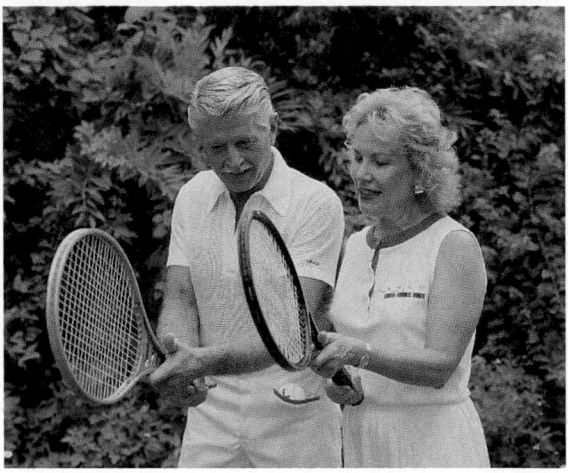

relaxed state of consciousness by focusing one's thoughts. Practiced regularly, meditation can help bring about feelings of well-being and inner peace.

Virtually all forms of meditation involve three common features: assuming a comfortable body position, maintaining physical immobility, and focusing attention on some object, sound, or bodily process. When you do these things, by definition, you are meditating. Some people meditate with their eyes closed, while other people gaze at a visually soothing object such as a flower or a picture. The aim is to focus on an object, rather than on yourself or your problems. Don't be concerned about how well you are meditating; this defeats the purpose of meditation.

Many people meditate by focusing on a *mantra,* a word or several words. Dr. Herbert Benson, author of *The Relaxation Response,* suggests the word *one.*[12] Close your eyes, relax, clear your mind of all concerns, and focus on your breathing. Silently repeat your mantra with each cycle of inhalation and exhalation: "I am . . . relaxed" or "inner . . . peace."

Some people like to meditate twice a day for about 10–20 minutes each time, but the frequency and length of meditation are up to the individual.

5. *Biofeedback.* Stress includes many measurable changes in body function. **Biofeedback** is a method of learning voluntary control over measurable body functions that are usually involuntary, as a way of reducing stress. As a training method, biofeedback makes use of instruments that record sweating, the contraction of muscles, skin temperature, and other stress-related body functions.

Biofeedback instruments provide either an audible or a visible "feedback" of your success in either relaxing a muscle, reducing skin sweating, or warming your skin or altering other stress-related

biofeedback a technique of taking voluntary control over body functions that are usually involuntary, as a way of reducing stress.

functions. For example, in response to your slower pulse rate, a light might grow dimmer or brighter as you relax. After a series of biofeedback sessions in which you learn the kinds of thought patterns that contribute to relaxation, you can often duplicate the relaxation without further use of the biofeedback equipment.

6. *Hypnosis.* **Hypnosis** is a psychological state, induced by a ritualistic procedure, in which the subject experiences changes in perception, memory, and behavior in response to suggestions by the hypnotist. Hypnosis has been studied and debated for over 200 years[13] and is sometimes used as a form of therapy for excessive stress, as well as smoking, eating disorders, and other behavioral problems.

The hypnotic procedure consists of two stages: *hypnotic induction,* in which the subject is hypnotized (induced into the hypnotic state), and *hypnotic suggestion,* in which suggestions for behavior modification are made. Such suggestions are technically known as *posthypnotic suggestions,* because, although received under hypnosis, they are carried out after the subject is no longer in the hypnotic state.

Techniques used to induce hypnosis vary among hypnotists, but typically include narrowly focusing the attention of the subject, under the guidance of the hypnotist, until the subject enters a state of relaxed alertness. Then the posthypnotic suggestions are made. In the case of stress management, these suggestions would relate to relaxation.

7. *Massage.* Massage is among the most relaxing of the stress-reducing activities. Receiving a massage by a mate or a good friend is extremely fulfilling and can serve as a means of sharing affection. Self-massage of many parts of the body such as the head, neck, shoulders, or sole of the foot is also easy to do and can provide instant relief.

8. *Slowing down.* One of the simplest ways to reduce stress is simply to slow down. Much of our stress is the result of trying to do too much, too quickly. Rushing is stressful. You can instantly reduce stress by just slowing down whatever you are doing.

....

hypnosis a psychological state, induced by a ritualistic procedure, in which the subject experiences changes in perception, memory, and behavior in response to suggestions by the hypnotist.

9. *Cutting back.* Many people try to do more than is humanly possible. Not only do they experience high stress levels in trying to achieve unrealistic goals, but they also set themselves up for failure, which causes further stress. It is more rewarding to do fewer things, and do them well, than to do many things poorly. If you are always racing to catch up, but falling further and further behind, it is time to evaluate your priorities. Perhaps you are expending a lot of time and energy on goals that are not really that important to you, to the detriment of attaining goals that are important.

Now, since the majority of the stress most of us experience relates to emotional causes, let's examine some of the psychological ways in which we try to avoid the conscious perception of being in a state of stress. We will also look at some common and severe emotional problems, ranging from mild anxiety to suicidal depression. Then, we will complete this chapter with an exploration of how to deal with emotional disorders.

CHECKPOINT

1. What is biofeedback and how can it contribute to stress management?

2. What are the two stages in the hypnotic procedure?

3. How do "slowing down" and "cutting back" contribute to stress management?

COMMON EMOTIONAL PROBLEMS

All of us can expect to experience some periods of emotional difficulty during our lives. For most of us, these difficult periods will be relatively brief and in response to unusual challenges to our coping abilities. For some of us, however, the difficult periods may be longer or more severe, or not associated with any unusually stressful life events. If symptoms are persistent or severe enough to interfere with your joy of living, your effective functioning, your physical health, or your relationships with others, it should be taken as a sign that you should consider seeking help. For example, if you lose a valued job, you can expect to go through a period of depression. But if you become so deeply depressed that searching for another job is impossible or that all joy of living is lost, then you should consider professional help in dealing with your depression.

We will now explore two of the more common emotional problems: anxiety and depression.

ANXIETY

Anxiety is a vague feeling that something bad is going to happen. Anxiety is related to, but different from fear. Fear is a response to an immediate, real danger, while anxiety is a response to a vague, obscure, or imagined danger. Fear is what you feel when you walk in tall grass and almost step on a rattlesnake. Anxiety is what you might feel on your first day in a new job before you have any idea what lies ahead. Symptoms of anxiety include worry, tension, "nervousness," and being ill-at-ease.

Circumstances that evoke anxiety vary from person to person, but anxiety is likely to arise whenever the future is clouded by uncertainty and doubt. Kagan and Segal[14] identified five common situations in which you are likely to feel anxiety:

1. You have conflicting motives, such as wanting to spend more time studying to improve your grades, but also wanting to spend more time socializing.

2. Your behavior is in conflict with your values (you are doing something you believe to be wrong).

3. You are in a new situation and are not sure what is expected of you, such as during your first few days on a new campus.

4. You are faced with events for which the outcome is unpredictable and beyond your control.

5. You face the possible loss of a loved person, such as when a close friend or relative is very ill, or the loss of a job, status, or possessions.

Within limits, anxiety can be beneficial. It can alert you to threats and dangers and can motivate you to take appropriate action. Recognizing the

sources of your anxiety can enable you to devise improved methods of coping with stress. In contrast, excess anxiety not only makes you unhappy, but it can also prevent you from taking any useful action. Severe, disabling anxiety is called **panic.**

Anxiety can be either specific or general. Most of us have a few specific anxieties, such as stage fright or, among students, *test anxiety*. Some people, though, experience general anxiety, feeling anxious most of the time, regardless of where they are or what they are doing.

Both specific and general anxiety can feed on themselves. When we become anxious, we are aware of the physical signs of anxiety such as rapid pulse, sweaty palms, rapid breathing, and "butterflies" in the stomach. This awareness increases the amount of anxiety.

We can usually deal with minor anxiety using the self-help methods discussed under stress management. Other forms of relaxation training, such as meditation, yoga, hypnosis, and biofeedback can also be valuable. Severe, disabling anxiety, however, warrants professional help, which involves getting at the basic source of the anxiety, relaxation training, and possible short-term use of tranquilizers.

DEPRESSION

Depression, a feeling of sadness and apathy, can vary in severity. A depressed person shows little emotion or interest in life. Most minor and even some major depression has a psychological basis.[15] Depression in the absence of any of the psychological causes we will now describe is likely to be associated with a disorder of the brain chemistry. Such biochemically caused depression is discussed later in this chapter in the section on serious mental problems.

Loss, whether actual or anticipated, is the most common psychological cause of depression. Depression is commonly associated with any form of loss, such as loss of a job, money, or friend, or the failure to achieve a desired goal. Loss-associated depression is usually fairly short-term, but it can be prolonged, as in a midlife crisis, during which someone is depressed over failing to achieve career or personal goals. Divorce or the death of a

anxiety a vague feeling that something bad is about to happen.

panic severe, disabling anxiety.

spouse can also precipitate a prolonged period of depression.

Sometimes depression develops when feelings of anger and hostility toward another person are displaced and turned inward. This commonly occurs in nonassertive people. If someone takes advantage of them or fails to respect their needs or rights, rather than confronting that person, they direct their anger at themselves. Loss also plays a role in this depression because there is loss of self-esteem and of other need-fulfillment.

Dwelling continually on negative thoughts is a habit that can also promote depression. Everyone has some negative aspects to their lives and emotionally healthy people constantly work toward improving their lives. But if an unpleasant circumstance is not amenable to change, there is no point in dwelling on it. Negative thinking is a habit that can be overcome by intentionally redirecting your thoughts in a more positive path, as described earlier in this chapter in the section on Stress Management.

Depression that results from a feeling of lack of control over one's life is referred to as **learned helplessness.** When people are placed in situations over which they have no control, they develop the expectations that their behavior will have no effect on improving their situation. This expectation of lack of control then transfers to other life situations where it may not be true. Learned helplessness causes people to act passively in situations where they could otherwise take control.

Finally, the lack of intimate relationships is associated with depression. We depend upon our close friends as our emotional support network. We need to be able to share our joys, our sorrows, and our problems with others. Without intimate friends we feel alone in the world. In this situation, it is easy for negative thoughts to prevail.

Dealing with Minor Depression

Depression can form a "vicious circle" in which it feeds upon itself, leaving a person depressed year after year. You can break the cycle of minor, psy-

chologically based depression by doing exactly those things a depressed person least wants to do:

- *Increase your exercise level.* Exercise helps to counteract depression; in addition to the mood-raising physiological effects of exercise, activity breaks the pattern of just sitting and brooding.

- *Increase your social contact.* Depressed people usually want to be alone, but their isolation magnifies their depression.

- *Develop intimate friends.* Your close friends are your support network that help you replace your negative thoughts with more powerful positive thoughts.

- *Focus on the positive.* Depressed people often block out all positive thoughts, wallowing in their negative thoughts of hopelessness and helplessness. A conscious effort is necessary to redirect thoughts toward the positive.

- *Do something constructive.* Depressed people feel helpless. Accomplish something in order to regain some feeling of power and control over your life. It doesn't have to be any major accomplishment—clean out your room, mow the lawn, bake a cake, just *do something.*

Any prolonged or severe depression should receive professional treatment. Some depression, discussed in the following, has origins in our brain chemistry and can be controlled only by prescribed medication.

CHECKPOINT

1. What is anxiety and what are some of its causes?

2. What are some psychological causes of depression?

3. When would you suspect that depression might be of biochemical origin?

SERIOUS MENTAL ILLNESS

Mental illness has not been easy to define. Each of us has many different areas of our mental health, with infinite degrees of wellness possible in each

---

learned helplessness a feeling of lack of control over one's life; a condition in which previous inability to make changes in situations is transferred to other situations in which changes could be made.

of those areas. All of us have our stronger and weaker areas and day-to-day ups and downs. There is no clear line dividing mental health and mental illness, and different cultures define mental health differently. For example, in some cultures, it is considered normal to hear voices. As a working definition for a recent survey of the extent of serious mental illness, however, the National Institute of Mental Health defined serious mental illness as "any psychiatric disorder present during the past year that seriously interfered with one or more aspects of a person's daily life."[16]

Based on that definition, during a recent one-year period about 3.3 million people aged 18 or older in the *noninstitutionalized, home-dwelling* population of the United States had a serious mental illness.[17] Of this group, about 2.6 million have one or more specific limitations in work, school, personal care, social functioning, concentrating, or coping with day-to-day stress.

When all adult Americans are included, the number who are seriously mentally ill jumps to 4–5 million people, or 2.1–2.6 percent of the adult population. In addition to those living at home, it is estimated that 200,000 seriously mentally ill people are homeless on any given day. An additional 1 to 1.1 million are residents of nursing homes, 50,000–60,000 are patients of mental hospitals, and about 50,000 are inmates of state prisons.

We have mentioned ability to work as a characteristic of good mental health. In the survey, about 1.4 million noninstitutionalized, home-dwelling people ages 18–69 were unable to work at all or were limited in the work they could do because of mental conditions. Of these people, 82 percent had had their work limitation for a year or longer.

Clearly, mental illness is a major problem in the United States. In economic terms, the lost productivity of several million people, the cost of care for those who are institutionalized, outpatient treatment for others, plus the disability payments many of the mentally ill receive, adds up to billions of dollars. In human terms, the loss of quality of life for the mentally ill and those close to them is incalculable.

It is beyond the scope of this book to detail every form of serious mental illness, but several examples include:

- **panic disorder** (repeated attacks of severe, disabling anxiety)
- **agoraphobia** (intense fear of places or situations from which it would be difficult or embarrassing to escape)
- **major depression** (a severe mood disorder in which a person experiences major depressive episodes) is the most common condition reported in the survey just described and is discussed further in the following section
- **bipolar disorder** (formerly *manic depression*) (a mood disorder characterized by extreme mood swings from deep depression to exaggerated joy)
- **schizophrenia** (a mental disorder characterized by severe disruptions in thinking, perception, and emotions, in which people are out of touch with reality)

Recent research points to a genetic, biological basis for many of these severe disorders. Thus, their treatment usually includes medications to normalize a disrupted brain chemistry. About 68 percent of the surveyed mentally ill people who had seen a health professional for their condition were taking one or more prescription medications. Unfortunately, many mentally ill people do not seek treatment, refuse to accept treatment, or are unreliable in taking prescribed medications. Many "fall through the cracks" in the mental health system and are unable to receive the treatment that they need.

....

panic disorder repeated attacks of severe, disabling anxiety.

agoraphobia intense fear of places or situations from which it would be difficult or embarrassing to escape.

major depression severe mood disorder in which a person experiences major depressive episodes.

bipolar disorder (formerly manic depression) mood disorder characterized by extreme mood swings from deep depression to exaggerated joy.

schizophrenia mental disorder characterized by severe disruptions in thinking, perception, and emotions, in which people are out of touch with reality.

MAJOR DEPRESSION

Major depression implies a severe and relatively persistent depressed (sad, helpless, and hopeless) mood that interferes with daily functioning. Severely depressed people are sad most of the time and tire easily. They have little interest in anything and have problems with sleeping and eating. They often have feelings of guilt, worthlessness, and inadequacy; the future looks hopeless to them. Many are unable to hold a job. Major depression carries a high risk of suicide. A diagnosis of major depression is usually based on the presence of at least four of the following symptoms:[18]

- change in appetite
- change in sleep

Depression is a feeling of sadness and apathy. It can have psychological or biological causes. Major depression carries a high risk of suicide and, by affecting the immune system, increases the risk of physical illness.

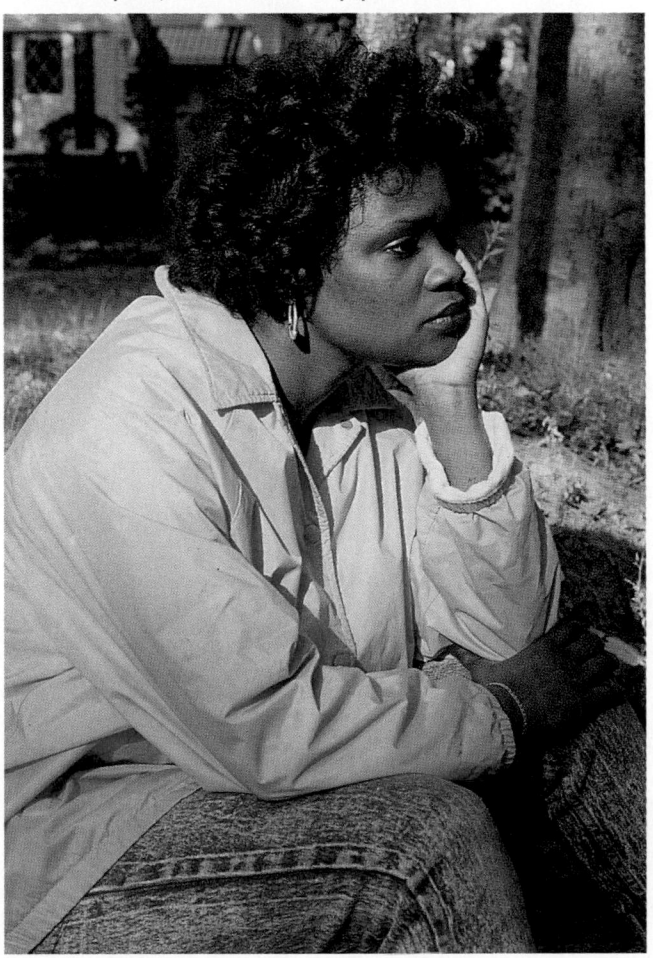

- increased or decreased activity level (psychomotor agitation or retardation)
- loss of interest in usual activities
- decrease in sex drive
- increased fatigue
- feelings of guilt or worthlessness
- slowed thinking or impaired concentration
- a suicide attempt or suicidal thoughts

Biochemical Basis of Major Depression

Although some major depression has psychological origins, most major depression has biochemical causes. Biochemically caused depression has been associated with low levels of the neurotransmitters, norepinephrine and serotonin, within the brain. The tendency toward this form of depression is inherited.

Treating Major Depression

Because major depression is usually biochemical in origin, its successful treatment usually requires medication to normalize the brain chemistry. It is often treated with drugs that raise norepinephrine and serotonin levels.

An earlier class of drugs, the tricyclics, includes Elavil and Tofranil. They are effective in about 70 percent of patients, but must be taken for two to four weeks before they become effective and can be fatal if an overdose is taken. Clients must be encouraged to continue to take what at first seems to be an ineffective drug. Further, if the client is suicidal, as depressed people often are, the supply of the drug must be carefully regulated.

A newer drug is fluoxetine (Prozac). Following its 1987 introduction, the drug was a huge success, used by over 5.5 million people in its first five years. Prozac offers advantages over tricyclics such as quicker action and fewer unpleasant side effects. But within two years of its introduction questions began to emerge about Prozac. Prozac was blamed for the suicides or attempted suicides of some of its users and in at least 20 cases defendants on trial for violent crimes attempted to use their taking of Prozac as a defense.[19] Defenders of Prozac point out that depression itself can cause suicide and violence and no treatment, including Prozac, has more than an 80 percent success rate, so some suicides and violent behavior would be expected among the large number of Prozac users.

Any major depression should receive professional treatment, since the suicide risk for a depressed person is about twenty-five times that of the general population.[20] Only a physician can prescribe the medications needed to regulate biochemically caused depression.

CHECKPOINT

1. In terms of millions of people, and in percentage of the population, how many Americans have serious mental illness during any given year?

2. Define panic disorder, agoraphobia, major depression, bipolar disorder, and schizophrenia.

3. What causes most major depression and how is it often treated?

SUICIDE

Suicide is a leading cause of death among Americans.[21] Each year in the United States, approximately 12 suicides are reported for every 100,000 people. The actual suicide rate is possibly double this number since many suicides are not recognized as such.[22] For example, many one-car accidents and drug overdoses are, in reality, suicides. Only about one-third of the persons who commit suicide leave notes telling of their intent.[23]

RISK CHARACTERISTICS

No category of people is entirely free of the risk of suicide, but certain people are at a higher-than-average risk of suicide. Characteristics associated with high suicide risk include:

- prior suicide attempts
- current or previous severe emotional disturbances
- major depression
- lack of intimate relationships
- alcoholism
- other drug dependency
- violent behavior
- chronic illness
- blaming self for illness
- recent personal losses
- unemployment
- financial problems
- confusion about one's sexuality

Which of these people are at risk of suicide? The risk is higher among those with severe depression, lack of intimate friends, chronic illness, chemical dependencies, alcoholic parents, or those who are unemployed or who are recently divorced, separated, or widowed.

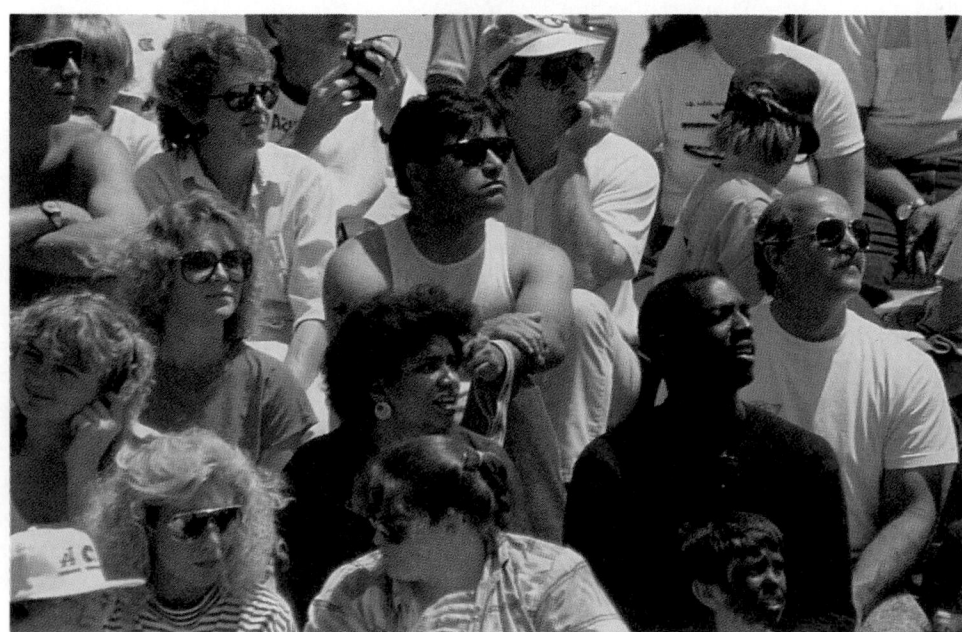

- child of alcoholic(s)
- recent loss of spouse through divorce, separation, or death

Nearly 60 percent of all suicides involve chemically dependent people. Of this group, the majority (84 percent) have abused both alcohol and other drugs.

Suicide rates vary with age, sex, and ethnic affiliation. In general, rates increase with age, are higher for males than for females, and are higher among European American people than among African American people, who have the lowest rate of any American ethnic group. Rates in other ethnic groups are relatively low, except for a very high rate among young Native Americans.

For African American males and females and for European American females, suicide rates peak in early to middle adulthood and then decline over the life span. In contrast, the suicide rate for Euro-

pean American males continues to increase over the entire life span. Further, at any age, the suicide rate for European American males is higher than for African American males or African American or European American females (see Figure 4.2).[24] Many factors influence the suicide rates of different ethnic groups, such as each group's incidence of depression, its attitudes about suicide, its religious beliefs, and its ability to support distressed members.

CAUSES OF SUICIDE

Psychologists have difficulty explaining suicide, because it conflicts with one of our strongest drives: the will to live. Suicide can have many motives, and in any given case there is seldom one single cause, but several causes that act together.

People who attempt suicide are almost always severely depressed and often lack intimate rela-

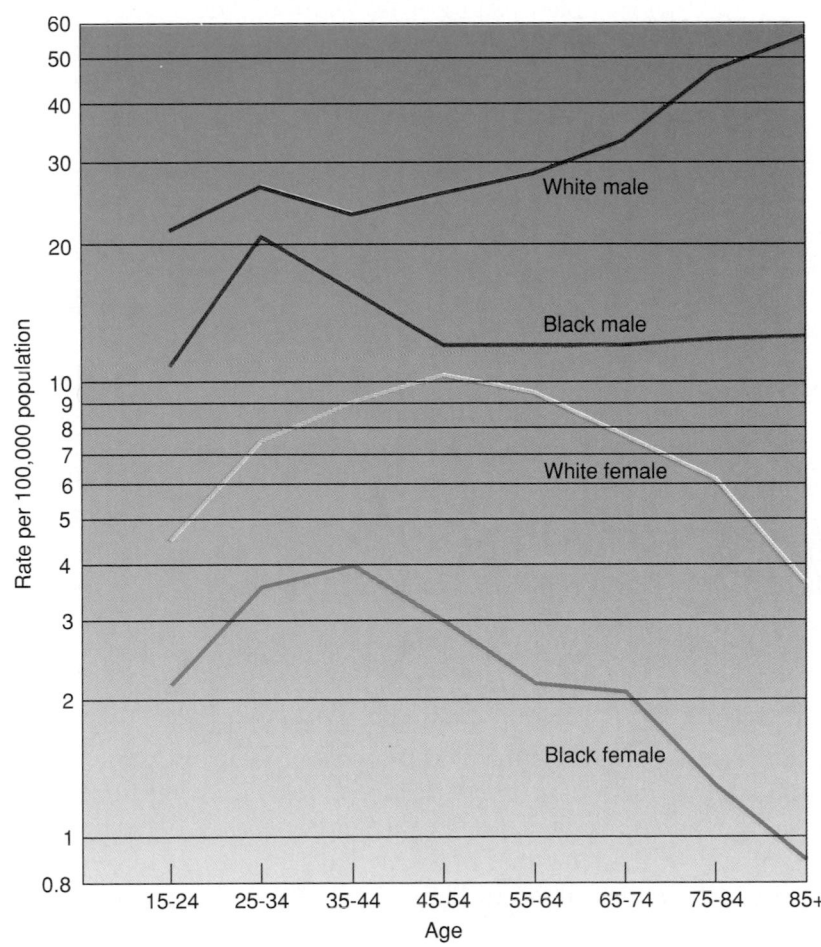

Figure 4.2

Suicide Versus Age (By Gender and Race)

Suicide death rates in the United States, 1982.

Source: Data from Mental Health, United States 1985, Department of Health and Human Services Publication No. ADM 85-1378.

tionships. They are unable to deal adequately with stress and feel they have no other alternative.

Nearly 80 percent of suicide victims give some kind of warning before the act.[25] During "psychological autopsies," in which those who knew suicide victims are interviewed, it has become evident that many suicides are preceded by the victim saying things such as "I would be better off dead" or "The world would be better off if I were dead." There may have been prior discussion of death or suicide methods, or overt suicide threats. Ironically, if someone who has seemed suicidal suddenly appears happy, that may be the gravest danger sign of all. It could indicate a feeling of relief at having made the decision to die.

SUICIDE AMONG YOUNGER PEOPLE

Suicide is rare below age 14, but the rate increases sharply during adolescence and the early twenties. In the last 30 years, the suicide rate for the 15–24 age group has nearly tripled. Though it is impossible to say with certainty why this increase has taken place, speculation regarding its causes has included the following:

- the increased number of divorces among parents
- decreased availability of parents at home for emotional support
- increased abuse of alcohol and other drugs by young people
- increased complexity of society
- depersonalization of life as technology increases
- increased difficulty in becoming established in a career

Psychologists often say that the two most important factors in positive mental health are feeling loved and feeling satisfied with one's work. Many young people develop a sense of hopelessness in both areas; they may feel that they will never enjoy a stable relationship or a successful career. Alcoholism and other forms of drug abuse also contribute to the mental chaos and confusion of many young people.

Which specific young people are at risk of suicide? There appears to be no one type of suicidal young person. They can be from any socioeconomic level, for example. They can be from troubled families or model families. They can be academic underachievers or superachievers or anywhere in between.

The young person at greatest risk of suicide is a white male. Although four to eight times as many young women *attempt* suicide, about 80 percent of successful suicides in the 15–24 age group are males.[26]

In addition to the suicide risk characteristics listed on p. 98, some additional factors associated with suicide in young people are:

- a prior suicide or suicide attempt within the family or the suicide of a close friend (see the following discussion of cluster suicides)
- serious problems among other family members, such as family conflict, alcoholism or other drug abuse, parental depression, and physical abuse
- a long history of traumatic experiences, losses, and poor family relationships
- the loss of a parent through either death or divorce, or the breakup of an intense relationship with a boyfriend or girlfriend

SUICIDE AMONG COLLEGE STUDENTS

Compared to nonstudents of the same age, the suicide rate among college students is somewhat higher. Why is this so? For one thing, among the younger college students who commit suicide (ages 18–22), a common thread is the inability to separate themselves from their family and to solve problems on their own. College presents many of these younger students with the challenge of having to be independent in many ways while remaining dependent on family in other ways, such as financially and emotionally.

Several other characteristics of the college experience may relate to suicide. A great emphasis is put on attaining high grades and the significance of grades may be blown out of proportion. A student may come to perceive grades as a measurement of his or her total worth as a person, rather than just one of many ways a person can be evaluated. If a student is unable to achieve expected grades, there may be a total loss of self-esteem and loss of hope for any success in life.

In the college setting, where self-esteem can be tenuous, the end of a relationship can also be devastating. A student who has recently lost a close friend or lover can become so deeply depressed that suicide becomes an attractive alternative. The problem can be compounded when depression interferes with coursework and grades slip.

The college suicide problem can be attacked on many levels. Most colleges' student health services are quite concerned over the problem and offer counseling for troubled students. A more general awareness of the fact that grades are not the total measurement of a person would be helpful. And anything that can help make college a more human and humane experience should reduce the incidence of college suicide. Those of us who are students can develop a network of intimate friends and social contacts. Those of us who are professors can see our students as total persons whose lives are or should be much larger than just going to class and studying for exams.

CLUSTER SUICIDES

First Paul shot himself in the head. Six weeks later, his close friend Sean did the same thing. Then another friend, Wesley, hanged himself. Soon these suicides of three Texas 19-year-olds had triggered three more "copycat" suicides of younger teenagers—Darren, Lisa, and Gary, 14, 15, and 16 years old, respectively—all in the same small town. What causes such cluster suicides among young people?

Public attention to a suicide in a community may take away some of the taboo associated with suicide. It can give someone else the idea that suicide is acceptable, in effect, giving permission to commit suicide. Further, there may be an emotional identification with someone who has committed suicide. For many young people, suicide may not seem real. Often, young people do not appreciate the finality of death and may perceive suicide as just another adventure or attention-getting device. Finally, suicide may be used as the ultimate revenge against parents, a former boyfriend or girlfriend, or society in general. Seeing how another

person's suicide has made people feel really sad may give one the idea to do the same thing.

Peer pressure can also be an effective preventive against suicide. Psychologists advise us that, should we sense that a friend seems at risk of suicide, we should listen to his or her problems, discuss the topic of suicide openly, remove weapons or medications if possible, and insist that he or she get help from a health professional, as discussed in the following section.

SUICIDE INTERVENTION

The role of a friend or family member in a suicide crisis is much the same as in any first-aid situation: to preserve life until professional help can be obtained. It is not to attempt to "play doctor" and solve the underlying problems. Every case is unique, so there is no uniform way to prevent suicide. The following steps, though, often prove valuable:

1. Establish a dialogue with the person and maintain contact. As an opening line, you might ask, "Are you thinking of killing yourself?" This may seem quite abrupt or even rude, but during crisis intervention communication must be open and direct.

2. Remain calm and convey your genuine concern. Let the person know you're there to help.

3. Most suicidal people have some ambivalence about dying. Build a sound case for why the person should want to keep living. Most suicidal people still have an underlying will to live; they just do not wish to live as they are, for they see their lives as being the same or worse than death. Even as suicidal impulses become almost overwhelming, the will to live is still there and can be used for suicide prevention, a thin "thread" by which the suicidal person can be, figuratively or literally, "pulled in from the ledge."

4. Getting suicidal people to *promise* not to commit suicide before seeing a counselor often is successful.[27]

5. Talk with the suicidal person about how he or she feels. Be very positive in telling the person that, with help, things can get much better.

6. *Go with the person* to get help. A counseling center, hospital emergency room, or police head-

quarters are places where professionals will know how to handle the situation. Over 200 cities have 24-hour telephone suicide-crisis hotlines listed in the phone book.

7. Follow through and be certain that professional help is obtained. Suicidal impulses recur, and it is dangerous to assume that there will be no further attempts.

8. As many friends and relatives as possible should be enlisted to provide emotional support. The chance of suicide is reduced through social interaction.

C H E C K P O I N T

1. What are some personal characteristics associated with high risk of suicide?

2. How do the suicide rates of white males differ from those of black males and black or white females?

3. What are some special factors associated with suicide of college-age people?

4. If a close friend of yours appeared to be suicidal, how would you deal with the situation?

☑

RESOLVING SERIOUS EMOTIONAL PROBLEMS

At one time or another, many of us (about one in three, according to the National Institute of Mental Health)[28] experience emotional problems serious enough to merit professional attention. We have discussed the extreme condition of becoming suicidal. Short of this extreme are problems ranging from feeling unhappy and unfulfilled to being severely disturbed and out of touch with reality. We will briefly examine the professions dedicated to helping people with these problems, and some of the methods used.

MENTAL HEALTH PROFESSIONALS

A person's choice of a mental health professional is critical to the success of the therapy. In addition to the type and amount of the professional's training, his or her own personality traits will influence the progress of the client's recovery. First, we will explore the main types of therapists and how to select a therapist. Then we will discuss some types of therapies.

Psychiatrists

Psychiatrists are physicians who have been trained to specialize in mental disorders. They treat patients both within hospitals and as outpatients, using any of the approaches discussed in the following. Depending on the severity of the illness, a patient may be seen once or several times weekly. Psychiatrists are the only therapists who can prescribe drugs. They tend to think of emotional problems as illnesses and commonly use the term *patient* rather than *client*.

Clinical Psychologists

Clinical Psychologists usually hold a Ph.D. or master's degree from a graduate program in psychology and have special expertise in assessing psychological problems and treating people with emotional or behavioral problems by using psychological techniques. They are likely to use the term *client* rather than *patient*. The client is typically seen once a week for an extended period of time. Clinical psychologists do not prescribe drugs, so they would usually not treat disorders that are caused by abnormal brain chemistry, such as some types of major depression.

Psychoanalysts

Psychoanalysts are therapists who use intense exploration of the patient's unconscious mind in order to bring out repressed conflicts. Most psychoanalysts are psychiatrists who have received several more years of training at a psychoanalytic institute and have gone through a full analysis

....

psychiatrist a physician who has taken further training to specialize in mental disorders.

clinical psychologist person who has special expertise in assessing psychological problems and treating people with emotional or behavioral problems by using psychological techniques.

psychoanalyst therapist who uses intense exploration of the patient's unconscious mind in order to bring repressed conflicts up to consciousness.

themselves. A few hold Ph.D. rather than M.D. degrees. Most analysts use a variation of Freudian theory or the theories of later psychoanalysts, such as Carl Jung, Alfred Adler, or Karen Horney. Psychoanalysis can require one or more sessions per week for many years.

Clinical Social Workers

Clinical social workers have a master's (M.S.W.) or doctorate (D.S.W.) in social work and can counsel clients with emotional problems. Their help is especially appropriate in problems with relationships, social situations, or arranging for needed health care or social services.

Counselors and Others

Most counselors have extensive schooling, including a master's degree and hours of supervised training; however, in some states, almost anyone can use the title "counselor." Marriage and family therapists should have special training, such as internships in dealing with problems that involve family relationships. Other professionals include psychiatric nurses, clinical nurse specialists in mental health, psychiatric social workers, and members of the clergy.

Members of some ethnic groups rely heavily on lay or folk practitioners, such as *santeros* or *curanderos,* for help with mental health problems. In the context of the beliefs held by people in these ethnic groups, such practitioners may be quite successful in restoring emotional health.

SELECTING A THERAPIST

The best way to find a therapist is through a recommendation from a knowledgeable physician, school counselor or nurse, member of the clergy, or community mental health service agency. Ask thorough questions about the credentials of a therapist you are considering. Even though a therapist may be well qualified, he or she may not be right for you. After a few sessions, ask yourself the following questions:[29]

- Is the therapist someone I can trust and depend on?
- Does the therapist treat me with respect or inhibit me and put me down?
- Does the therapist seem sincere and genuine?
- Does the therapist seem to be helping me?
- Does the therapist seem to understand my problems?
- Does the therapist listen well?
- Do I have confidence that the therapy will work?

If the answer to any of these questions is no, you might want to discuss your concerns with your prospective therapist. If that doesn't help, the two of you may not be a good match. Look for another therapist. If the therapist is unprofessional in his or her conduct, report this to the organization that has certified him or her.

SOME COMMON TYPES OF THERAPIES

There are two general types of therapy for mental disorders—**biological therapy** (treatment of mental problems through biological methods such as medications) and **psychotherapy** (treatment of emotional disorders using psychological, rather than biological, methods).

Psychotherapy

Of the more than 200 different kinds of psychotherapy being practiced today, most can be categorized as primarily psychoanalytic, behavioral, or humanistic in their approach. Many therapists are trained in several approaches and may combine more than one to make treatment more effective.

Psychodynamic (Psychoanalytic) Therapy
Psychodynamic therapies are the most prevalent

clinical social workers people who have a master's degree (M.S.W.) or doctorate (D.S.W.) in social work and can counsel clients with emotional problems.

biological therapy treatment of mental problems through biological methods such as medications

psychotherapy treatment of emotional disorders using psychological, rather than biological, methods.

psychodynamic therapies therapies that assume that unconscious forces influence human behavior.

of all approaches. They include psychoanalysis and its offshoots that explore the role of unconscious conflicts and early experiences in determining behavior.

Classic (Freudian) psychoanalysis is relatively rare today. It involves four to five sessions a week for several years. The patient lies on a couch without making eye contact with the analyst, who offers clarifications and interpretations of the patient's recollections of childhood and more recent experiences.

Far more common today is psychoanalytic psychotherapy, which involves more active participation by the therapist, including more dialogue and face-to-face contact. There are usually two or three sessions per week. Less emphasis is placed on a thorough reconstruction of the childhood experiences contributing to the patient's difficulties and more emphasis is placed on issues arising from his or her current interactions with others.

Behavior Therapy (Behavior Modification)

Behavior therapy is based on the assumption that our actions are learned responses to stimuli and that new, more desirable, responses to the same stimuli can be learned by providing reinforcement for the desired behavior. No attempt is made to explore the unconscious mind or to increase awareness. Behavior therapy is used mainly as a short-term therapy to modify a specific unwanted behavior pattern. It is most successful in treating fear of flying or other phobias, such as agoraphobia. It can also be used to treat sexual disorders, overeating, gambling, smoking, and other compulsive behaviors.

Humanistic Therapy

Humanistic theories of personality, with their emphasis on self-actualization and emotional well-being, are reflected in the many humanistic approaches to psychotherapy. **Humanistic therapy** is based on the belief that people will grow in constructive ways if they can be helped to explore and make use of their existing hidden potential. Techniques vary widely and do not conform to a rigid set of procedures. This type of therapy focuses on exploring the client's inner experience solely from the client's perspective and encouraging personal responsibility, freedom, and self-determinism.

One of the most prominent examples of the humanistic approach is Carl Rogers's *client-centered or person-centered therapy*. Client-centered therapists help their clients gain understanding of and control over their lives. The process has three steps:

1. Clients begin to experience, understand, and accept feelings and desires (such as sexuality and hostility) that they had previously denied.

2. Clients begin to understand the reasons behind their behavior.

3. Clients begin to see how they can use more positive forms of behavior.

Gestalt therapy (a theory of psychotherapy that rejects the analysis of emotions and behavior into discrete events of stimulus, perception, and response, but emphasizes awareness of the whole of a person's being) is another commonly used humanistic approach. Frederick (Fritz) Perls (1894–1970) developed this therapy in the 1940s. The gestalt theory holds that the whole of a person is greater than the sum of his or her parts. Each aspect of a person's functioning is part of his or her **gestalt** (*ga-shtalt'*), which is the German word for shape or form, and has meaning only in relation to the whole. When the physical or mental parts of a person are considered individually, they lose meaning.

Gestalt therapy focuses on our here-and-now emotional responses to life situations. Clients are encouraged to express or dramatize their feelings. Awareness of self is emphasized. Sessions are typically held once a week and can be very intense and emotionally draining.

---

behavior therapy therapy based on the assumption that our actions are learned responses to stimuli and that new, more desirable, responses to the same stimuli can be learned.

humanistic therapy therapy based on the belief that people will grow in constructive ways if they can be helped to explore and make use of their existing hidden potential.

gestalt therapy a theory of psychotherapy that rejects the analysis of emotions and behavior into discrete events of stimulus, perception, and response, but rather emphasizes awareness of the whole of a person's being.

gestalt shape or form.

Biological Therapy (Chemotherapy or Psychopharmacology)

Biological therapy for mental problems consists primarily of administering medications or, rarely, of electroconvulsive therapy or psychosurgery. **Chemotherapy** is a very general term that encompasses any use of drugs in treating any kind of disease. More specifically, **psychopharmacology** refers to the science of using drugs that affect emotional states and behavior. Drugs play a major role in today's treatment of emotional problems. These drugs fall into several basic groups. Tranquilizers (antianxiety agents) are used to calm anxiety; sedatives to combat overactivity, anxiety, and insomnia; antidepressants to help raise the mood of severely depressed people; and antipsychotics to reduce symptoms such as hallucinations and help bring people into contact with reality.

Psychopharmacology is not the answer for every emotional problem and it carries the potential for abuse. It is considered an abuse, for example, to use drugs alone for someone who really needs psychotherapy. Also, some nursing care homes have been accused of keeping their elderly patients heavily sedated simply to make them more easily manageable. Drug treatment, however, may be appropriate and very beneficial in at least three situations:[30]

1. *Mental disorders resulting from abnormalities in the brain chemistry.* Many cases of severe depression fall into this category as do many cases of bipolar disorder, in which moods swing between depression and euphoria. Biologically caused depression and bipolar disorder are basic disorders involving the neurotransmitter substances (see p. 464) in the brain's synapses and no amount of psychotherapy can cure them. Appropriate drug dosages can often normalize the brain chemistry and bring the disorder under control.

2. *Severe emotional disturbances.* Some people become so agitated or so withdrawn that productive psychotherapy is impossible. In the past,

. . . .

chemotherapy the treatment of disease using drugs.

psychopharmacology the science of drugs that affect emotional states and behavior.

these people might have spent many years in mental hospitals as "hopeless" cases. Today, treatment with drugs can often calm agitated patients or bring out the withdrawn so they can participate in effective psychotherapy.

3. *Temporary situational stress.* Many people encounter life experiences that challenge even the best coping skills. Divorce, death of a loved person, or loss of a job are transitory situations that may prove so stressful that one is unable to cope effectively with life. In such cases, the *temporary* use of a tranquilizer or other prescribed sedative may be quite helpful. Long-term use of tranquilizers as a substitute for effective everyday coping skills, however, is not recommended.

CHECKPOINT

1. Distinguish between a psychiatrist, a psychoanalyst, and a clinical psychologist.

2. What is the basic premise of psychodynamic therapies? Of behavior therapies? Of humanistic therapies?

3. For what kinds of emotional problems is psychopharmacology appropriate?

SUMMARY

A stressor is any situation or event that elicits the stress response. Examples include life changes, emotional conflicts, fear, fatigue, physical injury, surgery, temperature extremes, crowding, disease agents, and illness. Stressors in our everyday lives include a negative outlook, external locus of control, difficult relationships, performance anxiety, financial issues, sexual problems, lack of organization, inflexibility, and noise.

Stress is the body's response to any stressor and, in moderation, can act to increase our resistance to stressors. Stress includes many physical changes collectively called the General Adaptation Syndrome and controlled by the hypothalamus of the brain. Stages in the General Adaptation Syndrome include the alarm reaction, resistance, and exhaustion.

Eustress is beneficial stress; distress is excessive stress that has harmful effects. Excessive stress contributes to heart disease, infectious diseases, cancers, digestive disorders, skin disorders, and many other problems.

For some students, college is very stressful. Adjustments, time management, and overcommitment of time are major stressors for college students.

Work-related stress has increased in recent years. Some causes of job-related stress can be attributed to the workers and some to the job. Women are subject to especially high work-related stress levels. Suggestions include the following: view your job positively, make sure that your job is only one aspect of your life, maintain good general health habits, and practice stress-management techniques.

Stress management can be divided into general guidelines, mainly concerned with your outlook on life and general health habits, and instant stress relievers you can apply during especially stressful times.

Common emotional problems include anxiety and depression. Anxiety is a vague feeling that something bad is going to happen. Severe, disabling anxiety is panic. Depression is a feeling of sadness and apathy. Its cause can be psychological or biochemical. Psychological depression is commonly associated with any form of loss. Serious mental illness affects 2.1–2.6 percent of the adult U.S. population (4–5 million people) at some time during each 12-month period. Major depression is the most common serious condition; others include panic disorder, agoraphobia, bipolar disorder, and schizophrenia. Biochemical depression is associated with inherited low levels of norepinephrine and serotonin in the brain. It is best treated with medications that normalize brain chemistry. Uncontrolled depression carries a high risk of suicide.

Suicide is a leading cause of death. The official rate is about 12 suicides each year per 100,000 people; the actual rate is possibly double this. Certain characteristics are associated with high suicide risk; nearly 60 percent of all suicides involve chemically dependent people. White males have an especially high suicide rate. Suicides of college students often relate to difficulty in becoming independent, grades, end of relationships, and depression. The role of suicide intervention is to preserve life until professional help can be obtained.

Mental health professionals include psychiatrists, clinical psychologists, psychoanalysts, clinical social workers, counselors, and others. The best way to select a therapist is through a recommendation from a knowledgeable person. Some common therapies include psychodynamic therapy, behavior therapy, humanistic therapy, and drug therapy.

REFERENCES

1. Selye, H. *The Stress of Life,* rev. ed. New York: HarperCollins, 1976.
2. Greenberg, J. *Comprehensive Stress Management,* 4th ed. Dubuque, IA: Brown & Benchmark, 1993.
3. Selye, op. cit.
4. Ibid.
5. Greenberg, op. cit.
6. Ibid.
7. Ibid.
8. Forman, J., and Myers, C. *The Personal Stress Reduction Program.* Englewood Cliffs, NJ: Prentice Hall, 1987.
9. Ibid.
10. Ibid.
11. Greenberg, op. cit.
12. Benson, H. *The Relaxation Response.* New York: Morrow, 1975.
13. Crider, A., Goethals, G., Kavanaugh, R., and Solomon, P. *Psychology,* 4th ed. New York: HarperCollins, 1993.
14. Kagan, J., and Segal, J. *Psychology, an Introduction,* 7th ed. San Diego: Harcourt Brace Jovanovich, 1992.
15. Pettijohn, T. *Psychology, a Concise Introduction,* 3rd ed. Sluice Dock, CT: Dushkin, 1992.
16. National Center for Health Statistics. "Serious Mental Illness and Disability in the Adult Household Population: United States, 1989." *Advance Data* No. 218 (16 September 1992).
17. Ibid.
18. American Psychiatric Association. *Diagnostic and Statistical Manual of Mental Disorders, 3rd ed., revised (DSM-IIIR).* Washington, DC: American Psychiatric Association, 1987.
19. Schwartz, J., and Cohn, B. "'The Drug Did It': A Tough Sell in Court." *Newsweek* (1 April 1991), 66.
20. Crider et al., op. cit.
21. Centers for Disease Control, U.S. Public Health Service. "Operational Criteria for Determining Suicide," *Morbidity and Mortality Weekly Report* 37, No. 50 (23 December 1988), 773–780.
22. Ibid.
23. Ibid.
24. Weed, J. "Suicide in the United States." In *Mental Health, United States, 1985* (Department of Health

and Human Services publication No. ADM 85-1378). Washington, DC: Government Printing Office, 1985.

25. Pettijohn, op. cit.
26. Weed, op. cit.
27. Davison, G., and Neale, J. *Abnormal Psychology: An Experimental Approach,* 5th ed. New York: Wiley, 1990.
28. Goode, E. "For a Little Peace of Mind." *U.S. News & World Report* (28 September 1987), 98–102.
29. Goode, op. cit.
30. Pettijohn, op. cit.

SUGGESTED READING

Alberti, R., and Emmons, M. *Your Perfect Right,* 6th ed. San Luis Obispo, CA: Impact, 1990.
Greenberg, J. *Comprehensive Stress Management,* 4th ed. Dubuque, IA: Brown & Benchmark, 1993.
Enger, J., and Goleman, D. *The Consumer's Guide to Psychotherapy.* New York: Fireside, 1992.
Holmes, D. *Abnormal Psychology,* 2nd ed. New York: HarperCollins, 1994.
Any good, current, psychology text should have further information on the topics in this chapter.

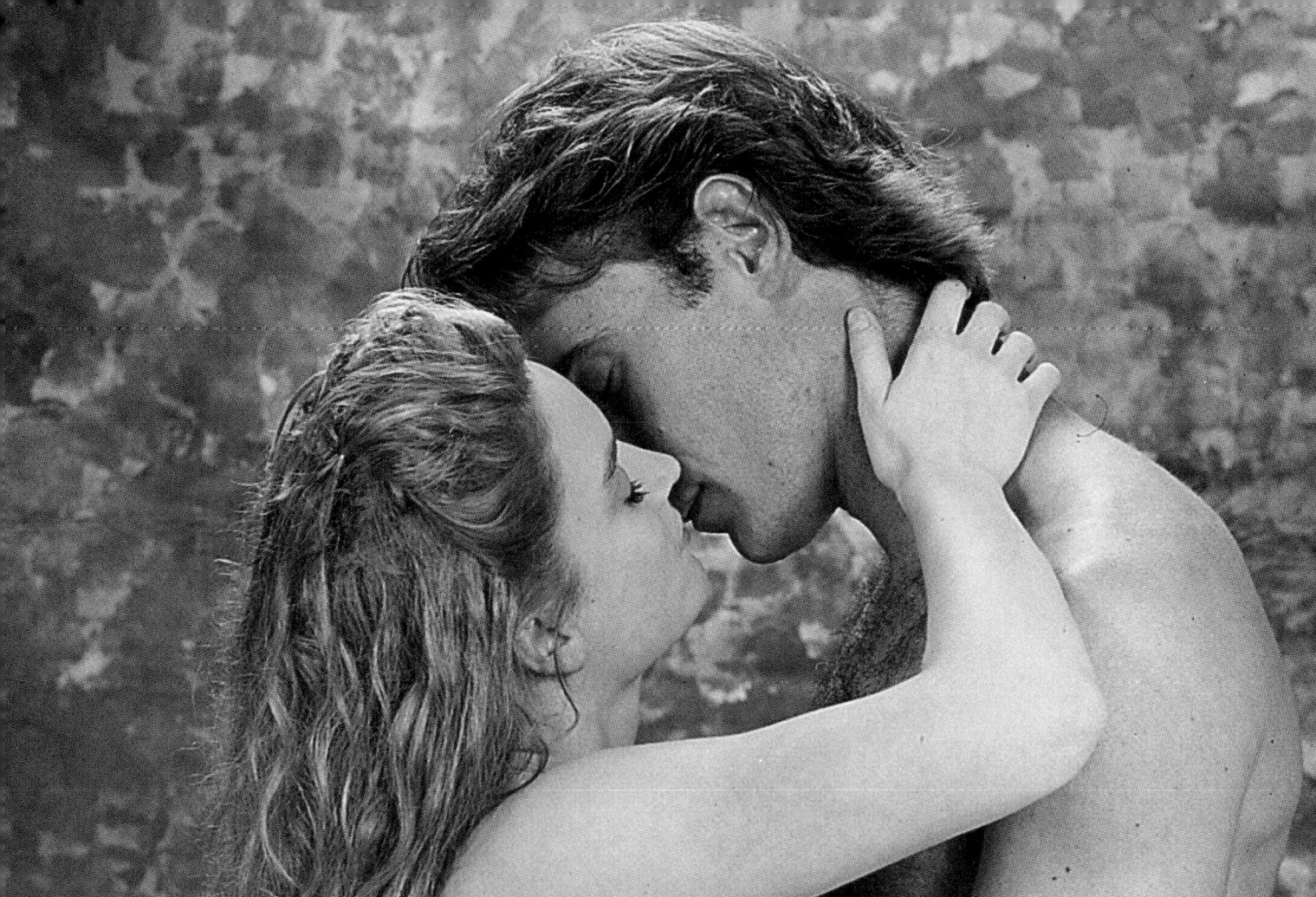

THREE
SEXUALITY

In our society, the sexual climate is currently undergoing dramatic changes. While behaviors that were once condemned as immoral by many have gained greater acceptance, there is increased concern regarding the consequences of sexual behaviors. Society has become more relaxed in its views of sexuality, but fear of sexually transmitted diseases and the emergence of AIDS as a health crisis have forced a reexamination of values. A new conservatism, marked by increased personal responsibility, has taken hold.

Humans are sexual beings. This sexuality may be expressed in a variety of ways, many of which are neither inherently right nor inherently wrong. Healthy sexuality involves decision making. Unfortunately, people are often ill equipped to make rational decisions regarding their sexual behavior. This unit on sexuality addresses the choices—of roles, life-styles, values, responsibilities, and consequences—involved in healthy sexual interaction.

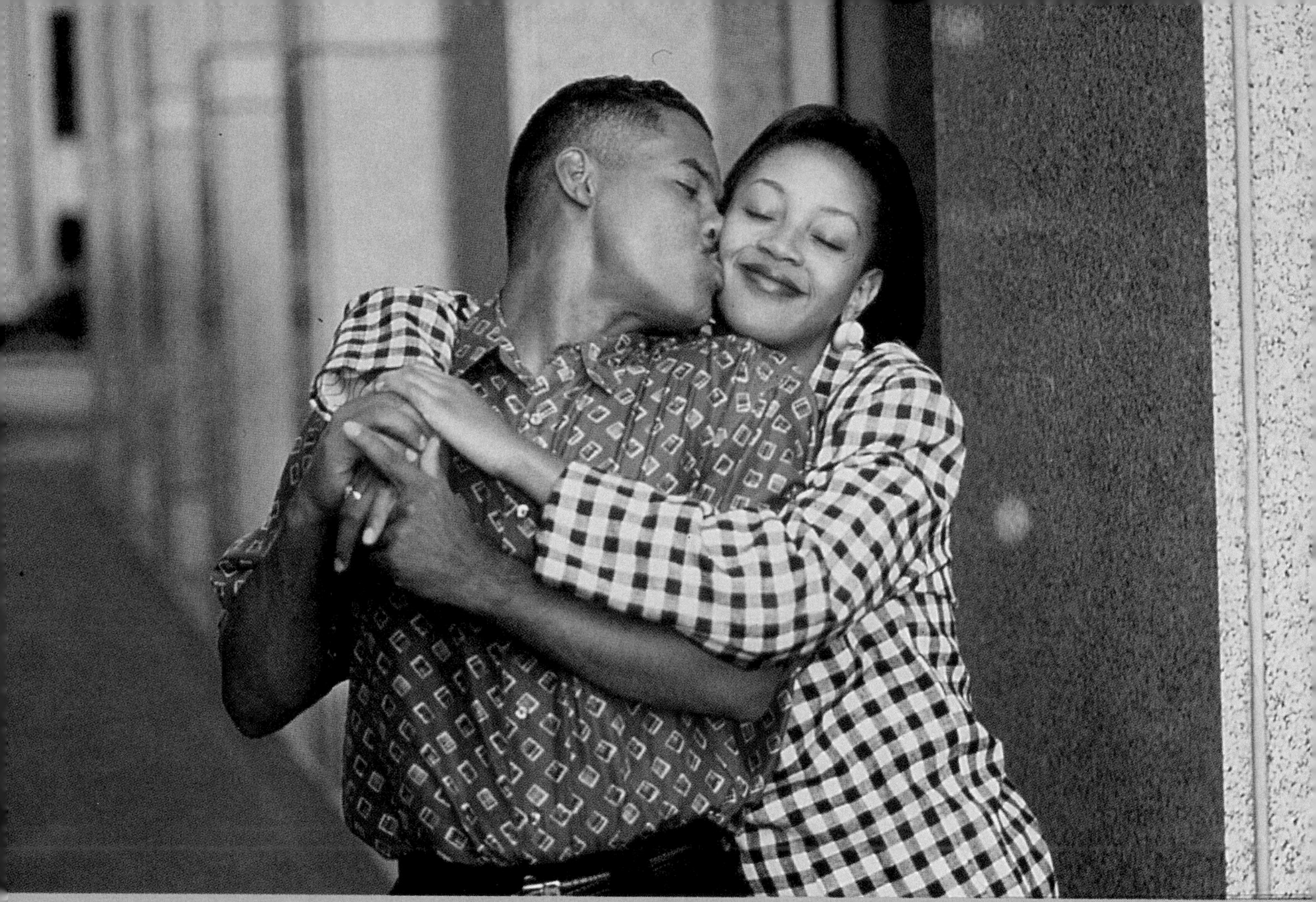

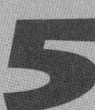

5

SEXUAL RELATIONSHIPS AND LIFE-STYLES

CHAPTER OBJECTIVES

Upon completing this chapter, you will be able to:

KNOWLEDGE

- Compare moral conduct with immoral conduct.
- Define emotional intimacy.
- Distinguish between romantic love and mature love.
- List the factors affecting sexual life-styles.
- Explain why there is such a large number of singles in the population.
- Define monogamy.
- Describe a "no-fault" divorce.
- Compare pandering and pimping.
- Explain why pornography is a form of sadism.
- Define sexual harassment.

INSIGHT

- Identify some of your own sexual values.
- Identify what you think might be an ideal age for a couple to marry and why.
- Discuss the reasons why a divorce might be emotionally devastating for you.
- Explain how you might feel if your sister were a victim of rape.

DECISION MAKING

- Identify the criteria you might use in deciding on the morality of your sexual activities.
- Decide if you think both partners in a marriage should have their own careers.
- Explain the advantages of a person with a homosexual orientation "coming out."
- Explain what you can do to avoid giving confusing social signals that might be interpreted by an acquaintance as being sexually enticing.

With the increase in the incidence of sexually transmitted diseases, discussion about the importance of monogamous relationships has intensified. Webster defines monogamy as "the practice of marrying only once during a lifetime, or, the state or custom of being married to one person at a time." Modern discussions of monogamy relate more closely to a sexual life-style than to the practice of marriage. Mutual monogamy has been recommended to reduce the spread of diseases, such as AIDS. Engaging in promiscuous escapades like those of former professional basketball star Wilt Chamberlain, who stated in his memoirs that he slept with 20,000 women over a 40-year span, is becoming less and less something to brag about in this day and age. However, the term monogamy has a variety of meanings and may be interpreted in a variety of ways, somewhat like a monogamy continuum.

One end of the monogamy continuum is an individual having sexual intercourse with only one person over the course of a relationship. When that relationship is over, and another relationship begins, the person has sexual intercourse with only the new partner. This type of "serial" monogamy is consistent with *the ideal of being faithful to one's partner. However, with each new relationship comes the well-known risks associated with multiple sex partners.*

The other view of the monogamy continuum is an individual having sexual intercourse with only one person in a lifetime. Assuming that neither is infected with any sexually transmitted disease, this is absolutely "safe sex." For many, safe sex in a monogamous relationship has become the only choice for a healthy sexual relationship. While there are many other factors involved in making this choice, the Casanova-type sexual life-style of previous years is quickly being replaced by sexual relationships that include serious consideration of the concept of monogamy.

■   ■   ■

From its inception, a relationship involves decision making. The opening scenario illustrates the claims of a well-known athlete regarding his decisions on sexual life-styles. Rather than being a sport, sexual relations reflect our basic values.

Students today receive a wealth of information to help them make decisions about their future. This chapter explores some of the issues concerning emotional and sexual needs and examines how sexual values, love, and intimacy contribute to a healthy relationship.

SEXUAL VALUES

Values are principles, or standards, by which we evaluate the worth of something. Values serve as guides for our behavior, giving our lives direction. As children, we tend to adopt our parents' values. As we grow and gain experience in the world, though, we learn to appraise our goals, beliefs, and relationships for ourselves. We may assign worth to achieving an academic degree, to a relationship, to a certain set of beliefs, or to parenthood. Our values then influence our aspirations and guide our actions.

As social beings, humans interact with each other continually. Consequently, much of our judgment of right and wrong is dictated by our relationships with others. **Moral values** are those val-

values the principles or standards by which we assign worth.

moral values values that guide us in our conduct with and treatment of other people.

ues that guide us in our behavior or conduct with and treatment of other people. Morality is about treating people fairly and lovingly. In relationships, conduct that enhances growth, builds trust, and helps an individual to reach his or her potential is **moral.** In contrast, behavior that reduces self-esteem and self-worth, breaks down the capacity for communication with others, or results in exploitation is **immoral.**

Ethics are systems of moral values. Professionals, for example, often establish sets of moral standards known as **codes of ethics.** In our personal lives, sexuality is dictated by a code of ethics, which determines how our sexuality will be expressed. These are our **sexual values.** Sexual values vary widely among people and groups in our society.

Many factors contribute to a mature, healthy relationship. Love, commitment, and respect are but a few of the qualities valued by many people. Sexual values can guide an individual's behavior in an intimate relationship, promoting actions that are consistent with the well-being of both partners.

CHECKPOINT

1. Define the term *moral value.*
2. Contrast moral with immoral behavior.
3. Explain the meaning of the term *code of ethics.*

RELATIONSHIPS

One of the most basic human needs is the need to "belong." Human beings need close interpersonal relationships, and devote a considerable amount of time and effort fulfilling this need. Almost instinctively, we know that building relationships will

moral conduct that enhances growth, builds trust, and helps a person reach his or her potential.

immoral conduct that reduces self-esteem and self-worth, breaks down the capacity for communication, or results in exploitation.

ethics systems of moral values.

code of ethics a set of moral standards.

sexual values a sexual code of ethics that determines how our sexuality is expressed.

SHARING SEXUAL FEELINGS WITH A PARTNER

Sharing sexual feelings with a partner requires tact and practice. In our culture, with its idealized sexual images and partnerships, it is common for people to internalize their sexual feelings, especially if they perceive themselves as being less than perfect. To learn to share such feelings takes courage. Yet, few of us have training in everyday communication skills, let alone those dealing with sexual feelings.

In order to communicate successfully, we need to talk. Nonverbal communication takes us only so far. Yet, talking about sex may not be easy. Partners differ in their ability to talk about sex. They sometimes differ in their feelings of tenderness, fears, or admission of ignorance. Both need to feel approval for talking openly about feelings and sexuality. A vocabulary is needed that is neither too vulgar nor too clinical. Both need to feel that it's acceptable to express sexual feelings and inhibitions accurately and candidly, and to encourage the same honesty and tolerance in the partner.

In addition, there are three skills you need to learn and practice for sensitive communications:

1. *Neutrality.* You must take responsibility for your own feelings and not assume or blame anything on your partner. "I wish," "I think," or "I'm afraid" are more acceptable than "You think," "You need," or "You're afraid."

2. *Mutual intent.* You must both want to improve the relationship. All sexual communication needs to be motivated by a concern for both partners. Self-centeredness limits intimacy and growth in a relationship.

3. *Managed conflicts.* You need to view relational differences as conflicts to be managed through ongoing communication. Few problems are fully resolved by blunt, sudden decisions. Successful problem solving requires sufficient time to evaluate what's really going on.

Revealing your true feelings does not come easily to those who have been trained to protect themselves and others from uncomfortable communications. Differences in feelings are a part of any relationship. Using nonthreatening language, within a framework of caring, allows room to air conflicts and keep alive the process of learning and discovery.

---

enhance our lives. Often, however, our quests for intimacy are unsuccessful. While music and literature are rich in their descriptions of the exhilaration of love and the despair of loneliness, they rarely describe how to build and maintain relationships. By learning how intimacy develops, we can be better prepared to fulfill our needs in a constructive manner. The development of such intimacy hinges on skills in communication. Communication for Wellness: Sharing Sexual Feelings with a Partner reviews steps necessary for effective sexual communication.

LIKING

The earliest stages of a relationship follow a subtle progression. Initially, you must become aware of another person's presence. This may seem obvious, but people can work in the same classroom or office for weeks before becoming aware of one another. Chances are, you have experienced such a situation. Have you ever attended classes faithfully all semester, only to see someone at the final exam whom you did not recognize?

Awareness of a new person may lead to curiosity. You may wonder what the person's name is, where he or she lives, whether he or she is dating someone, and so on. Upon learning the answers to these questions, personal concern may develop. If

both people respond well to curiosity and concern, they may grow to feel affection for—or like—each other.

Inherent in the human need for belonging is a need for esteem. If we have high self-esteem, we believe that we deserve to be liked and that people *will* like us. All humans wish to feel good about themselves and seek relationships in which others affirm their views and behavior. It is not surprising, then, that people of similar backgrounds and viewpoints tend to be attracted to one another. In relationships with those who are most like us, we receive the affirmation that we need in order to develop self-esteem. People with healthy self-esteem become more open to people who are different from themselves. Similarly, people with low self-esteem are often convinced that they are not worthy of the affection of others. They may question the motives of people who like them, and often reject the very affection that they need in order to develop healthy self-esteem.

Standing in contrast to liking is **infatuation.** This is a state of strong sexual attraction to someone based mainly on his or her resemblance to a lover fantasy. This fantasy may be based on past

....

infatuation an attraction based on similarity to an idealized partner.

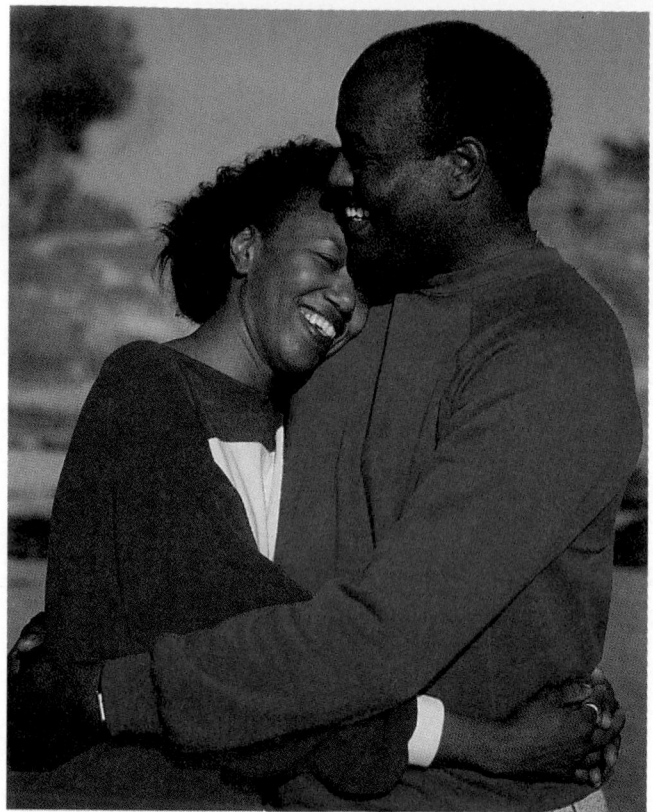

We are often attracted to people with interests similar to our own. People who are the most like us help to affirm us and help us develop self-esteem.

love experiences, on family we love, or on images of the ideal lover shaped by imagination and by the media. If that person notices us, we feel more sexually attractive. Such infatuation over time may or may not develop into a love growing out of rewarding emotional experiences. It is a beginning of love, but requires the development of an inner commitment to the other person before it can be considered genuine love. Infatuation may provide the spark of interest to ignite a relationship; however, a committed love provides the fuel that can sustain the relationship.

INTIMACY

Many people view **emotional intimacy** as an essential component of a sound relationship. In an

emotional intimacy an essential component of a sound relationship characterized by open communication and sharing of innermost feelings, needs, and desires.

emotionally intimate relationship, the partners encourage each other to communicate their thoughts, feelings, needs, and desires. A couple can then evaluate their relationship and determine which areas require attention.

A prerequisite of true intimacy, then, is that each partner be aware of his or her expectations of the relationship. By identifying emotions, wants, and needs, an individual becomes able to share with another. People may withhold their emotions for a variety of reasons. They may disguise their emotions by hiding behind their work, social activities, other people's problems, or drugs in order to keep their true feelings from surfacing. If one or both partners do not contribute to a shared intimacy, the relationship may not endure. Intimacy often carries a risk of rejection. This vulnerability may prevent people from sharing themselves. However, trust develops through intimacy. As each partner gains trust, more is shared, and intimacy is heightened. Just as betrayed trust can destroy a relationship, trust that is honored leads to stronger feelings and a deeper sense of commitment.

In an intimate relationship you feel free to communicate your feelings, desires, and thoughts with your partner.

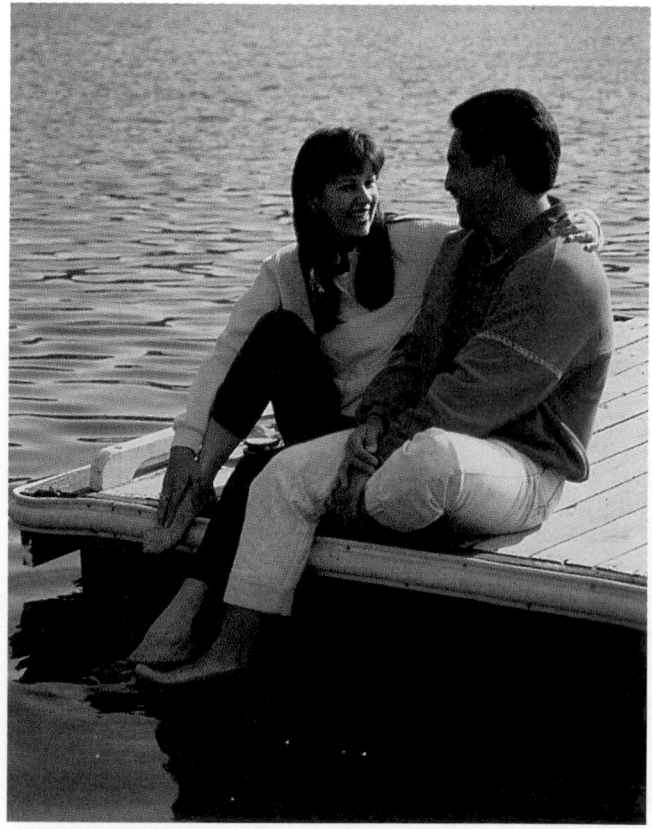

There are many ways to express intimacy: intellectually, as with the sharing of ideas; or spiritually, as when exploring the meaning of life. When using the term *intimacy,* many people think of physical intimacy, in which there is affirmation through touch, or sexual intimacy. These expressions of intimacy may all be a part of a healthy relationship.

LOVE

Intimacy is a precursor to and accompanies feelings of love. In an intimate relationship, **love** is an intense feeling of affection characterized by a deliberate choice to act in the best interests of another person. This is demonstrated by the caring and respect that one partner shows to the other. Love involves intentional, conscious decisions, not a surrender to infatuation.

Two basically different forms of love can be identified. In *A New Look at Love,* passionate love is distinguished from companionate love.[1]

Passionate Love

The stages in which love progresses may vary from person to person. Many people fondly recall the early stages of a relationship, when they felt a kind of emotional intensity. During **passionate love,** which is sometimes called infatuation, you may be "swept off your feet" over your sexual excitement for the other person. You idealize the person in a noncritical way in which faults, or traits, you later see as undesirable, are overlooked. Commonly there arc feelings of possessiveness and jealously. Such feelings by your lover may initially prove flattering and provide a sense of security, but may become restricting and stressful. You may have a sense of relief when such an experience is over. Passionate love is often based on a false verbal or physical intimacy, without a revelation of the true self. With such love there may be strong sexual attraction, with or without true companionship or emotional support. Passionate love as we know it in our culture is not universally practiced. Among

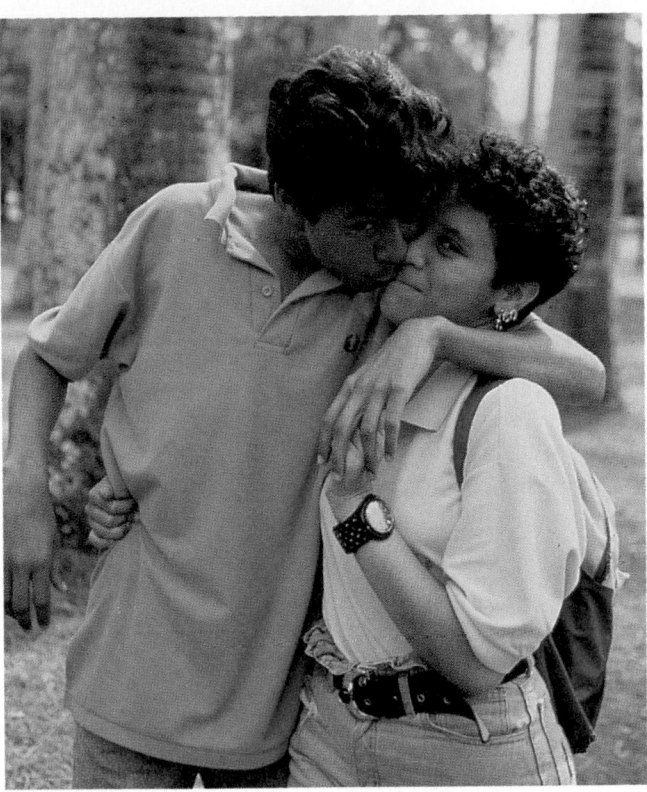

A first love is an awakening of the realization that someone prizes me above all others.

the Mehinaku people of Brazil, passionate love is viewed as absurd, and seen as being in bad taste.[2]

Companionate Love

Passionate love may mature into a **companionate love,** which is more predictable and secure than early infatuation. Companionate love is less possessive and allows both partners space and independence to live their own lives. In such a relationship the partners encourage each other to reach their own goals even if the goals reached by one partner may appear more meaningful than those reached by the other partner. Companionate love is also based on commitment. An inherent part of mature and lasting relationships, a commitment is a promise that responsible persons make and keep. It is a promise in which another person can place trust. A **commitment** is an assurance, or

love an intense feeling of affection characterized by a deliberate choice to act in the best interests of another person.

passionate love early, idealistic, noncritical love; infatuation.

companionate love mature, predictable, and secure love.

commitment a pledge or assurance to stay true to a promise.

pledge, that a person will stay true to regardless of fluctuations in feelings, and it provides security in both good times and bad. Commitments are "islands" of certainty in an "ocean" of uncertainties.

Because the foundation of mature love is strong, the relationship of the partners is resilient. With managed emotions and imaginative input on ways to improve the relationship, many mature love affairs flourish for decades.

LOVE WITHOUT SEX

Love can exist between partners without culminating in sexual activity. There are many points along the continuum of increasing sexual intimacy. Activities such as closeness, touching, holding hands, kissing, caressing, dancing, and fantasy can give a person pleasure and the relationship meaning. At the same time, they do not require the emotional intensity that occurs with sexual intercourse, nor do they involve the risk of contracting HIV, the virus that causes AIDS, or the prospect of an unplanned and unwanted pregnancy. Refraining from penis-in-vagina intercourse is called **abstinence.** Sexual abstinence until marriage is a growing sexual practice among young people in the United States.[3] While it may amount to saying no to intercourse, it can be seen as saying yes to a broad range of low-risk, but highly enjoyable, sexual activities.

Couples may abstain from sex for a variety of reasons. For example, they may decide to wait until marriage for personal, social, or religious reasons; they may not wish to risk disease or pregnancy; or they may face geographical separation. Some agree to abstain from sex for a period of time to reduce a preoccupation with sex and to focus their attention on other aspects of their relationship.

Psychologist Robert Sternberg has conceived of love as the interaction of the three important components of *intimacy, passion,* and *commitment* (see Figure 5.1).[4, 5] Structured as a triangle, his model shows the importance of the three elements for a complete, lasting, adult relationship. According to Sternberg, intimacy refers to emotional closeness and bonding. The component of passion in the triangle includes the expression of one's needs and desires, such as self-esteem, nurturance,

....

abstinence refraining from sexual intercourse.

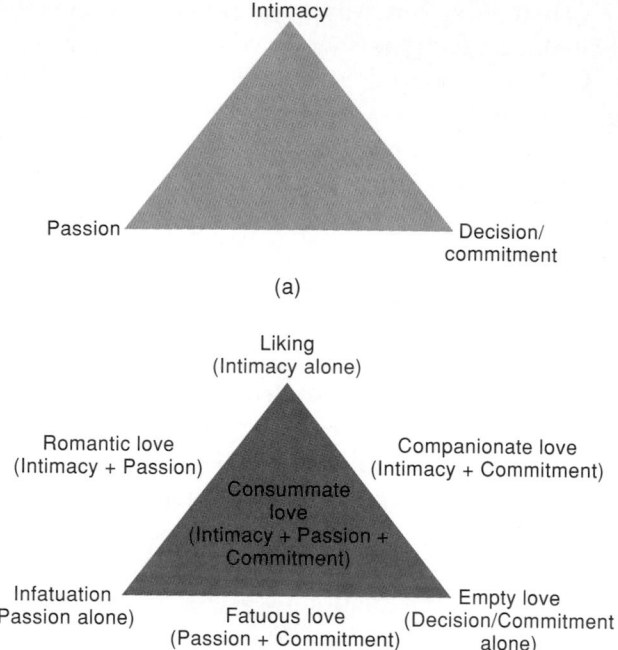

(a)

(b)

Figure 5.1
The Triangle of Love

The triangle of love, as conceived by Robert Sternberg: (a) the three components of love, (b) the kinds of loving as different combinations of the three components of love.

and belonging. The commitment component of the love triangle consists of two phases: One is the decision to love another person, and the other is the commitment to maintain that love. The commitment component not only interacts with both intimate involvement and passionate attraction, but keeps the relationship alive even if intimacy and passion may fade. Commitment helps see it through until the return of good times.

LOVE AND SEX

Though love and sex may accompany one another, they are independent. By itself, sexual desire needs only sexual activity in order to achieve satisfying sexual release; love, on the other hand, places sexual satisfaction secondary to the feelings of caring and respect for the other person. People who mistake sex for love often develop relationships in which relational needs go unmet. While they receive ego affirmation and sexual release, they do not achieve intimacy or love.

Today, sexual intercourse outside of a marital relationship is common. Many individuals find

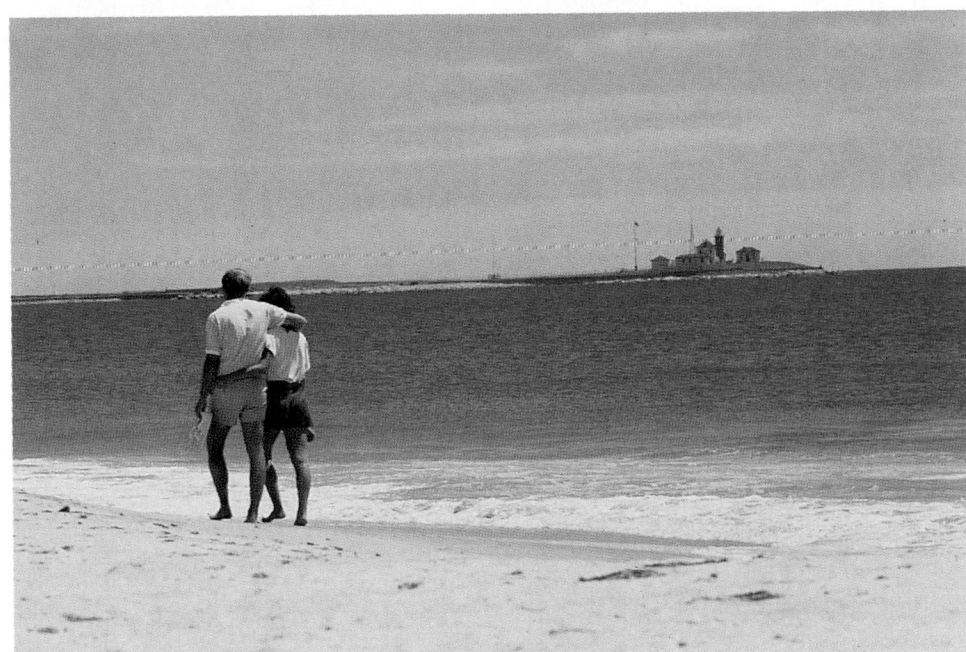

Sexual activities such as closeness, hugging, and caressing are low risk sexual activities that can be highly enjoyable and give meaning to a relationship.

such activity exciting and pleasurable to some degree. For some, nonmarital sex is thrilling because it serves as a statement against parental values. Even with society's sexual permissiveness, such premarital sex may still have an aura of intrigue for some.

Within a healthy, intimate relationship, sexual activity can enhance the feelings that the partners share. Problems arise, however, when the partners have divergent expectations of the relationship. Fears of whether or not a person's sexual performance "measures up" to a partner's anticipations may fuel uncertainties that later develop into sexual performance problems. Entering into sexual intimacy in the hope it will lead to love or that it will "trap" a partner into a relationship he or she may not yet be ready for often results in a weak relationship. Prematurely entering into sexual intimacy while still confused about the roles of love and sex in the relationship can be damaging to both partners.

The prevalence of sexually transmitted diseases and unplanned pregnancies make it imperative that partners discuss the health and social consequences of their actions before entering into a sexual relationship. When partners share similar expectations and approach sexuality in an open, informed manner, sexual intimacy can be a healthy and rewarding way for people to express themselves.

At this time you should complete In Your Hands: Relationship Vulnerability Scale (p. 118).

This is an assessment of your chances of being hurt in a relationship.

CHECKPOINT

1. Describe the significance of liking other people and being liked by them.

2. What is emotional intimacy? What are the risks and rewards that go with it?

3. Explain love and its relationship to sexual activity.

4. Compare romantic love with companionate love.

SEXUAL LIFE-STYLES

Traditionally, many Americans marry in their early twenties, conceive their first child shortly after marriage, and live together until the death of one spouse. Many others, on the other hand, do not follow this pattern. Many adolescents and young adults are sexually active without the expectation of commitment. Today in the United States, 43 percent of all adolescent girls will have been pregnant at least once by age 20. Cutting across ethnic lines, teenage pregnancy rates are increasing faster for Hispanics and whites, although the rates are highest for black teens.[6] Many single women choose to bear children outside of marriage. Today, nearly a

RELATIONSHIP VULNERABILITY SCALE

PURPOSE:

People begin and continue relationships for a variety of reasons. Sometimes these motives are not mutual. A person can be taken advantage of and eventually hurt in the process. Relationships can sometimes evolve into a situation where one member plays a dominant role and the other a submissive role, without either person realizing it. This inventory is designed to help you evaluate your relationship and determine, to some degree, your chances of being in a vulnerable situation.

DIRECTIONS:

Read each question carefully while reflecting on your present or most recent relationship. Place a check in the True or False column as either relates to your situation.

	TRUE	FALSE
1. Is your partner often unavailable for phone calls at home or at work?	_____	_____
2. Does he/she ask about the amount of money you earn or your parents earn, or try to get involved with your financial planning?	_____	_____
3. Does your partner ever belittle your efforts and/or ideas?	_____	_____
4. Has your partner ever disappeared for any length of time (overnight, several days, a week) and not informed you of his/her whereabouts?	_____	_____
5. Does he/she live with you and contribute little or nothing to household maintenance?	_____	_____
6. Does your partner borrow money and seldom bother to repay it, or frequently ask you to buy him/her things, or always use your car?	_____	_____
7. Has he/she had one or more tragic misfortunes that needed your financial assistance?	_____	_____
8. Has your partner told you early in your relationship that he/she would like to be married and described a life of love and luxury for both of you, but made no definite steps in that direction?	_____	_____
9. Do you stop your present activity or postpone your plans when he/she calls to do something on the spur of the moment?	_____	_____
10. Is he/she the only person in your life?	_____	_____
11. Do you allow your partner to take the "upper hand" in your affairs?	_____	_____
12. Have you ever noticed any discrepancies concerning what your partner has told you in regard to his/her name, job, background, family, and so forth?	_____	_____
13. When you are away and he is out by himself does your partner avoid socializing with his/her or your family and friends?	_____	_____
14. Do you usually wait for others to introduce you to potential partners instead of taking the initiative to meet new people on your own?	_____	_____
15. When your partner describes his/her future goals, does it seem unclear as to where you fit into the future?	_____	_____
16. Do you feel that you should be married to be happy?	_____	_____

Scoring: Give yourself one point for each true response to the questions.

13–16: You are very vulnerable to being in a lopsided relationship, which may result in hurt feelings in the future. You should seriously examine the contour and direction of your relationship with your partner. For you to continue with your present situation is almost certain to be a waste of time and energy.

9–12: You are vulnerable to being taken advantage of. Stop and ask yourself if you are getting out of this relationship what you are putting into it.

5–8: You are somewhat vulnerable to being hurt. Your relationship probably has potential but needs to be evaluated. You and your partner should discuss your future to determine what type of life-style you both desire.

1–4: You do not seem vulnerable to being dominated in your relationship. Keep the statements to which you responded "true" in mind and openly discuss them with your partner.

Source: "Relationship Vulnerability Scale" from *Your Sexuality: Your Personal Inventory* by R. Valois and S. Kammerman. Copyright © 1984 McGraw-Hill, Inc. Reprinted by permission of McGraw-Hill, Inc.

quarter of unmarried women become mothers.[7] A growing number of couples live together prior to, or without the expectation of, marriage. About one-third of all people cohabit, or live together in a sexual relationship as unmarried persons, at some time in their lives. This, along with other factors, accounts for the rise in the average age of partners entering into a first marriage.[8]

Clearly, there are many sexual life-styles in our society. Individuals may be heterosexual or homosexual, married or single. They may live alone, or together. A healthy individual's sexual life-style reflects his or her values, desires, and needs.

FACTORS AFFECTING SEXUAL LIFE-STYLES

The dramatic change in sexual life-styles over the past 30 years can be attributed to a combination of sociological, biological, psychological, and technological factors.

Sociological Factors

Several major influences affect life-styles. People are attending school longer, are more independent in their thinking, and are less tradition minded. Women, especially, are the benefactors of more education and of increased capability of economic security. Not having to marry for economic stability, women are more apt to accommodate marriage to their own interests and preferences. At the same time, others are postponing marriage due to economic uncertainties. To postpone dealing with commitment, many singles, both never married and previously married, have decided simply to live together. Because society is more tolerant of nonmarital sex, many people feel that they need not marry in order to ensure a sexual partner. Along with this, the current economic climate makes it more comfortable for divorced and single individuals to support themselves. The consequence is that more young adults are spending a longer period of time in singlehood.[9, 10]

Biological Factors

During the past century, the average age of puberty for girls has dropped from 17 to 12. Heredity, family size, and improved nutrition have contributed to this phenomenon.[11] In addition, life expectancy has increased by nearly three years in the past decade. The combination of these factors has increased the time available for reproduction and sexual activity.

Psychological Factors

Our society has become more permissive in its attitudes toward sexual intimacy. Activities previously condemned are now tolerated by many. For example, there is increasing evidence that the double standard, in which different sexual standards applied to males and females, is less tolerated today.[12] This increased sense of sexual freedom has contributed to the change in sexual life-styles in our society.

Technological Factors

Advances in contraceptive technology have, if used correctly, reduced the chances of unwanted pregnancy occurring as a result of sexual intercourse. Greater access to birth control and abortion services have also reduced the risk of unwanted births. Many consider the greatest risk associated with sexual activity to be pregnancy; the removal of this risk has resulted in freer expression of sexual intimacy.

BEING SINGLE

Obviously, everybody spends part of his or her life as a single person. Traditionally, it was common that as adolescents entered adulthood, they felt compelled to find both jobs and marriage partners. Today, expectations and goals are changing. As an adolescent moves through high school, and perhaps college, he or she faces a number of decisions regarding the future. Marrying right after school is no longer a top priority for many, and the social stigma against remaining single is rapidly disappearing. In fact, single adults are now one of the fastest-growing factions in the United States; in the past two decades, the number of singles has more than doubled, and now represents more than one-fourth of all households (see Figure 5.2, p. 120).[13, 14]

Many singles who are well-educated professionals may choose to remain unmarried. They often enjoy the freedom to spend their earnings as they wish and to pursue job opportunities.

While some choose to remain unmarried, many single people do wish to marry eventually. Although the median age for those entering into

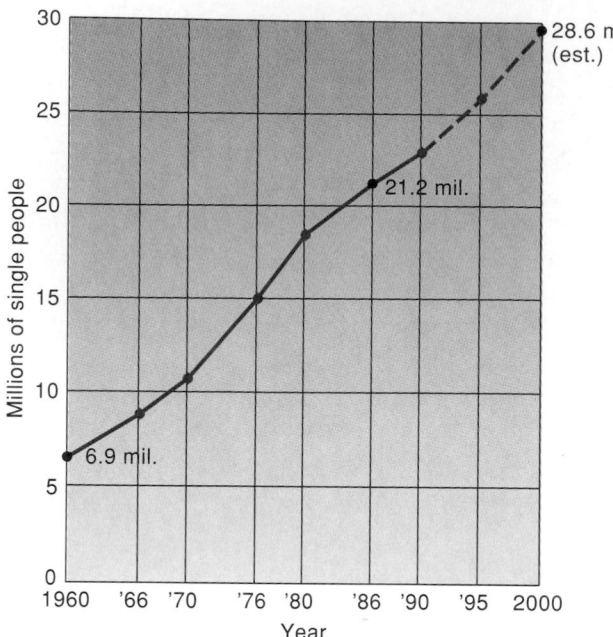

Figure 5.2

Singles Count: A Dramatic 40-Year Increase

Over the past 30 years, the number of Americans living alone has more than tripled.

Source: McGrath, A., et al. "Living Alone and Loving It." U.S. News & World Report, 3 August 1987, pp. 52–57; Hoffman, M. (ed.). World Almanac and Book of Facts 1993. New York: Pharos, 1992; U.S. Bureau of the Census. Statistical Abstracts of the United States 1993, 113th ed. Washington, DC: 1993.

first marriages has risen to its highest level since 1900 (see Figure 5.3),[15] approximately 90 percent of the single population does marry at some point.[16]

Individuals who are widowed or divorced make up about 60 percent of the single population.[17] Although divorce may represent a release from an unfortunate marriage, many divorced people would like to remarry. Widowed individuals often remarry as well, though as they age the number of unmarried widows who are unable to find new spouses far exceeds the number of widowers who remain unmarried due to fewer available widowers.[18]

Both single life and married life have unique rewards and disadvantages. Many single people cherish the opportunity to develop the skills of managing a household independently and the freedom to pursue their own interests. At the same time, singles are statistically more likely to be lonely and unhealthy than are those who can share their stresses with a partner.[19] Yet, singles who have well-established networks of friends and family, and who have a well-defined sense of worth, often find life as rich and interesting as their married counterparts.

INTIMATE RELATIONS

People are social creatures whose lives take on meaning when they are in relationships with other people. People need people with whom to share experiences, frustrating and happy. Although some people seem to thrive on solitude, many others experience loneliness when they are without a partner. The question is how to go about discovering and retaining likable partners.

Finding a Partner

As anyone who has participated in the dating ritual knows, finding the perfect partner can seem to be impossible. The initial goal is to find someone with whom you can share a mutual attraction. Complications arise, however, when people construct images of the perfect partner. One may envision a partner with certain physical, economic, and personality traits, and become disillusioned when he or she finds that such a person does not exist. The search for a partner can be difficult, intimidating, and discouraging, especially when undertaken with unrealistic expectations.

When looking for a partner with whom to have a serious relationship, a person is most likely to seek someone who shares a similar background, interests, and intellect. The statistical likelihood that a relationship will endure tends to improve when the partners' values converge and their race and religion are the same.

Dating allows you to try out your interpersonal skills. It provides a forum in which you can be open and honest about your feelings. It provides a setting in which you can experiment with reconciling your interests and behavior with another, inevitably different person. It provides an activity in which you can disclose your likes, strengths, and weaknesses, without fear of vulnerability. When you fully reveal yourself to another and find that he or she accepts, better yet, approves of you, it boosts your self-esteem.

Intimacy in dating may or may not lead to sexual interaction. Satisfying partner relations commonly create feelings of sexual attraction. Yet, it's important to recognize that what may appear as a sexual need may actually be a need for compan-

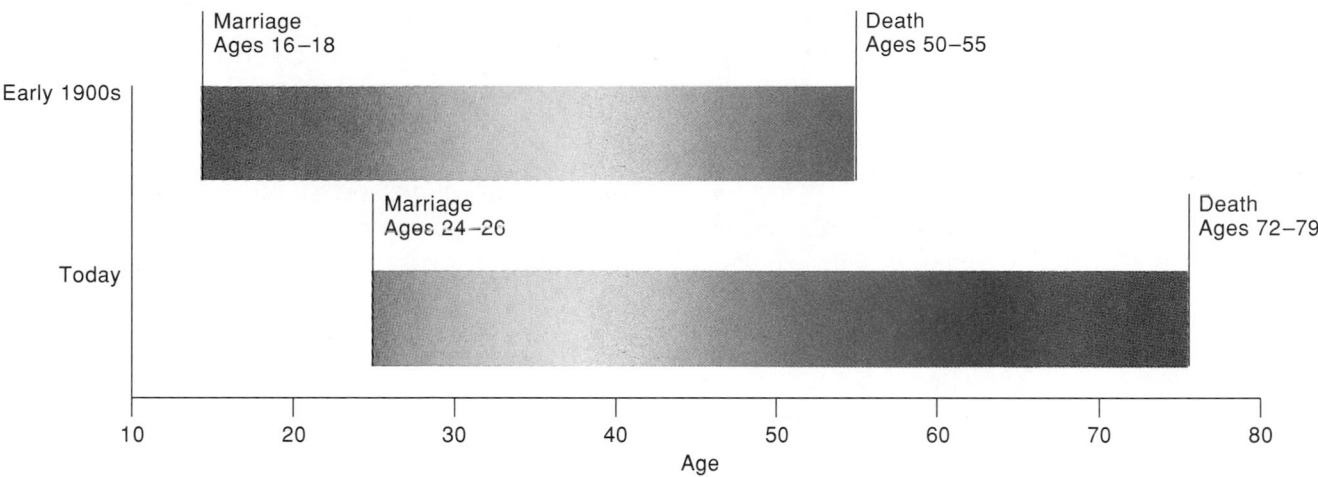

Figure 5.3
Marriage and Increasing Life Expectancies

As shown in the figure, couples are getting married later and are living significantly longer than in 1900. A young couple entering into marriage today faces a considerably longer commitment than at the turn of the century.

Source: U.S. Bureau of Census, Statistical Abstracts of the United States 1993, *113th ed. Washington, DC, 1993; Population Reference Bureau,* 1993 World Population Data Sheet. *Washington, DC, 1993; Hoffman, M. (ed.),* The World Almanac and Book of Facts, *1993. New York: Pharos, 1992.*

ionship, self-esteem, or security. Any interest in having sexual intercourse needs to be predicated on both partners feeling that it is the right thing to do. A concern for the mutual sexual enjoyment between partners excludes coercive acts. Any genuinely caring relationship allows for hesitations or saying no without jeopardizing the relationship. The ability to delay sexual intercourse until both you and your partner feel ready enriches respect, as well as enhances your positive feelings about yourself and the other person if and when sexual activity begins.

Sustaining a Relationship

Human relationships present many opportunities for developing satisfying qualities within a person and bonding between persons. You must first learn to like yourself and sustain self-love. There needs to be self-acceptance before there can be an acceptance of other people. There is the challenge of establishing positive relationships with people within a person's social circles—family, peers, teachers, fellow employees, and employers. There is the opportunity for intimate relationships with certain friends; for some people, this may move into an ongoing committed relationship. Commitment may lead to a desire and decision to marry.

As for essential ingredients in a lasting love relationship, some of the many facets include self-acceptance, liking each other, shared interests, commitment, acceptance of each other, fair expectations, and handling conflict effectively. There needs to be a deliberate attempt to cultivate these traits and to act in your partner's best interest, even when emotionally you may not want to. Some of the same rules that apply to a happy marriage apply as well to a happy nonmarital relationship. In a study of 300 happily married couples[20] the reasons given for success in marriage, from the greatest to least frequently mentioned, were:

1. seeing one's partner as a best friend
2. liking each other as persons
3. seeing marriage as a long-term commitment
4. viewing marriage as sacred
5. agreeing on aims and goals
6. seeing each other as growing persons
7. desiring that the relationship succeed

Before entering into a sustained commitment, such as a marriage, it is necessary that both you and your partner assess your willingness to respond to the interests of the other person. Applying what you learn after reviewing Feature 5.1 can help you to assess your readiness for such a commitment.

MARRIAGE

When two people marry, they affirm their commitment to each other by entering into a formal, legal, social, and spiritual agreement. Marriage represents one of our society's frameworks for love, friendship, and support in physical, emotional, intellectual, and spiritual matters. In marriage, the couple may share all major responsibilities, such as finances, property, and children. When a couple marries, both partners, in essence, endorse a social institution. In many cases this institution becomes

---

FEATURE 5.1

CONSIDERATIONS FOR COUPLES PLANNING TO COHABIT OR MARRY

Each person planning to marry or live with another person should be aware of his or her own feelings and those of the partner in a variety of areas relevant to a partnership. Both participants should be aware of areas of general agreement and disagreement. Perfect agreement is unlikely and not even necessarily desirable. However, disagreement on a large number of important topics suggests that a couple may be in for some rough sledding.

We suggest that each of you respond to these questions separately first, before you share your responses. On a separate piece of paper, indicate the importance to you of each item. Then indicate how important this particular issue is to you by placing a number to the right of the response, using the following scale:

1 = not at all important
2 = not very important
3 = somewhat important
4 = important
5 = extremely important

1. Who should be responsible for the economic support of the household?

2. Who should be responsible for the physical maintenance of the household (meal preparation, dish and clothes washing, housecleaning, grocery shopping, and so forth)?

3. Who should be responsible for paying bills?

4. How neat and clean do you want the house to be?

5. In general, would you characterize yourself as paying bills and then spending whatever is left as you choose, or spending money as you choose and then paying bills with whatever is left?

6. Do you approve of the use of intoxicants (liquor, nicotine, marijuana, tranquilizers, and so forth)? How do you feel about your partner using intoxicants?

7. Do you intend to confine sexual intimacy to your partner while you are together?

8. How would you respond to the knowledge that your partner had been sexually intimate with someone else?

9. Do you believe that couples should always inform each other of everything they do, where they go, whom they see?

10. Do you believe that couples should take vacations together, or do you think separate vacations are occasionally acceptable?

11. If you and your partner were invited to a party and you didn't feel well, would you find it acceptable for your partner to attend the party without you?

12. How do you and your partner feel about having children? If you want children, how many do you want?

13. In the event that you have children, who should take primary care of them?

14. In the event that you don't want children, who would be responsible for birth control?

15. If you and your partner both had rewarding jobs and one of you was offered a promotion that involved moving to another city, whose job would take precedence, assuming that you wanted to continue to live together?

16. If one of you felt more sexually adventurous (in terms of variations in coital positions, kinds of stimulation, for example) than the other, how would you resolve conflicting desires?

17. Do you believe that holidays should be spent with relatives? If you disagreed with your partner on this issue, how would you resolve differences on whether or not to visit relatives, and whose relatives to visit?

18. How do you feel about your partner's attending conferences, meetings, conventions, and so forth without you?

19. How important is religion to you?

20. Do you like to entertain friends at your house frequently, occasionally, or rarely?

Source: Allgeier, E., and Allgeier, A. *Sexual Interactions,* 3rd ed. Lexington, MA: Heath, 1991.

the basis for the biological family and provides the dynamics of the relationship.

One of the bases of a successful marriage is trust. Trust can be defined as the degree of confidence one has in the relationship in terms of predictability, dependability, and faith. Without trust, intimacy will not develop and the relationship may fail.[21]

Another basis for the success of a marriage is the ability to communicate. Effective communication of thoughts, needs, desires, feelings, and preferences is essential in the smooth working of a marital partnership. The partners each have important expectations on a wide range of matters, such as which TV programs to watch, who chooses the brands of cereals, how household duties are shared, who pays the bills, how leisure time is spent, and many more. Even with good communication all differences are unlikely to be resolved, but without it the relationship is headed for serious trouble.

Legal Commitment of Marriage

Marriage is a legal contract. Before entering into marriage, a couple must, by law, satisfy a series of requirements. Blood tests and medical exams are required in many states, and laws limit who can marry. States refuse to grant licenses for marriage between close relatives, when one partner is already married, and when one partner is judged to be mentally ill. In addition, a marriage contract will not be issued, or will be annulled, if the court discovers that intentional misrepresentation or force is used.

The institution of marriage has been impacted upon by the greater acceptability of divorce, the presence of more married women in the work force, and an increase in cohabitation. Most people do wish to be married, and 90 percent eventually do marry.[22]

Getting and Staying Married

In the United States today, people still seem to be dedicated to getting married. Marriage rates, or the number per 1,000 people, for those 15 years of age and over have shown a decline over the last 20 years. The marriage rate in 1992 for unmarried men was 62.8 and was 53.3 for women, a reflection of the fact that in 1992 there were about 7 million more unmarried women 15 years of age and over

in the United States. Overall, there were 2.362 million marriages in the United States in 1992, or a rate of 9.3 marriages per 1000 people. The American divorce rates, after rising for nearly 20 years, peaked in 1981. Since then, divorce has declined slightly, to its present rate of 4.8 divorces per 1000 people in 1992. In actual numbers, for the most recent year for which statistics are available, this amounts to 1.215 million divorces.[23]

Marriage counselors report a renewed interest in maintaining marriage relationships. In *How to Stay Married*, Kantrowitz[24] reports that the words *commitment* and *responsibility* are taking on more important roles in contemporary marriages and notes that couples are more likely today to try to solve marital problems than to abandon their relationships. Those couples who resolve problems early in marriage are especially likely to have enduring relationships.

People in the United States expect more out of marriage than members of many other cultures. The qualities most admired by partners in healthy marriages include integrity, caring, sensitivity, and a sense of humor. Spouses in successful marriages regard their partners as the kind of person they would want as a friend even if they were not married. People seek romance and excitement, as well as security and companionship, in a marriage relationship. Despite some unrealistic expectations, many achieve successful marriages.

Being a Faithful Spouse

Marriage is practiced by most cultures, yet its practice among them takes on different forms. The marriage ideal as generally defined in our society includes elements of legality, permanence, heterosexuality, sexual and emotional exclusiveness, and **monogamy,** an exclusive sexual involvement with only one partner at a time. Some societies allow or expect marriages between one man and several women (polygamy), such as in some regions of Nigeria,[25] or less commonly, between one woman and several men (polyandry).

Even in our society, monogamy is variously interpreted. Some see it as sacred to a marriage, while others view it less seriously. To them,

....

monogamy an exclusive sexual involvement with only one partner at a time.

monogamy is a commendable ideal if it is achieved but should this not happen, they would not be surprised. Some couples see marriage as an experiment in which, if the marriage becomes rocky, one or both spouses would feel free to go outside the marriage for sexual activity.

Surveys in the early 1980s indicated that about 50 percent of men and 35 percent of women reported having extramarital sexual relationships. By the end of the 1980s there was evidence of a decline in extramarital sex. Some of this may be due to the fear of contracting HIV.[26]

While extramarital affairs are common, they can be very damaging to a relationship. Although husbands are more commonly involved in extramarital affairs than are wives, husbands are more likely to perceive of them as destructive if the wife is unfaithful. Many find the deception and violation of trust as more difficult to accept than the actual act of extramarital sex itself. While a marriage can sometimes survive infidelity, it may be severely damaged and is often destroyed. There is a consensus among many authorities that even an occasional act of extramarital sex is harmful.[27]

Guidelines that couples can follow to avoid extramarital affairs include the following:

- Discuss your views of extramarital sex before marriage. Since being unfaithful is a matter of choice, not having settled on your views may make an affair harder to resist if an opportunity for infidelity arises.
- Know your emotional limits and end relationships that seem to be progressing toward unwanted sexual involvement.
- Talk to your partner about his or her friendships. Avoid concealing friendships from one another.
- Avoid prolonged absences from your partner.
- Discuss the consequences of infidelity. Tell your partner how you would feel and what you would do if he or she were unfaithful.
- Tell your spouse how much his or her faithfulness means to you.

Two-Career Couples

One of the realities of our society is the prevalence of two-career couples. Among couples without children it is usual for both partners to be employed. In couples with children under the age of 18, almost all fathers and three-quarters of all mothers work outside the home.[28] Aside from economic reasons, both partners may pursue careers in order to fulfill personal needs, such as a need for accomplishment, to establish identity, to use professional training, or for social contact.

For some two-career couples, the employment of both persons will require nontraditional assignment of roles. Both persons will need to share equitably in the many household tasks—grocery shopping, cooking, bill paying, laundering, cleaning, doing yard work, and financial decision making. Beyond these tasks, both need some time for leisure activities—which may or may not be engaged in together.

The prospect and/or presence of children places stress on any couple, but especially on two-career couples. In the past, many career mothers lacked job protection when they became pregnant. As of 1993, the Family and Medical Leave Act has provided unpaid leave from work for the birth or adoption of a child and for the care of a seriously ill child, while protecting the job of the parent. Applying to companies with 50 or more employees, the law provides 12 weeks of unpaid leave per year and guarantees that a worker can return to the same or a comparable job. Where available through an employer, maternity leave provisions are of significant help to the mother, and to the father, in adjusting to a new child. (While not common, some employers provide parental leave provisions for new fathers.) Access to acceptable child care becomes crucial, both for the child and for the parents. Facing up to the financial costs of child rearing, as well as the time demands, often places unexpected stresses on a couple.

There are advantages and disadvantages to both parents pursuing careers. For many, the need for the combined income is a stark necessity in order to provide for the costs of essential housing, food, and clothing. For couples for whom this is not so, their careers may provide for sufficient fulfillment to compensate for the extra duties they must perform when they come home. For others fortunate enough to have their basic needs met through a single income, the couple may wish to assess their priorities more carefully. One parent may choose to work part-time in order to provide more time with the child or to take over some of the household chores shared by both partners after coming home. Other couples make the choice to forego certain expenditures or to do without some things in order for one parent to be able to stay home with their children, especially during their preschool years. Although the stresses may be great for two career parents, they can be that much greater for single parents, on whom all of the responsibilities for the home and family fall (see section on Single Parents, p.127).

ALTERNATIVES TO MARRIAGE

Some people choose not to marry. Remaining single, however, does not preclude the desire for intimate relationships. Alternatives to marriage, such as cohabitation, provide this intimacy and are discussed in this section.

Cohabitation

When two adults with a sexual relationship share a household without benefit of marriage, it is referred to as **cohabitation.** The percentages of adults who have cohabited at some time in their lives range from 18 percent to 49 percent, the numbers varying with different surveys.[29, 30]

The increasing economic status of women, a greater acceptance of sex outside of marriage, and an increasing emphasis on personal satisfaction in close relationships bear on how we live, with whom we live, and in what settings. For some, cohabiting is a natural first step toward marriage. Living together allows unmarried couples to share their lives together without being bound by the social and legal expectations that are inherent in marriage. This arrangement may also appeal to couples who want an intimate relationship without entering into the formality of marriage, or to people who have been married and divorced, and are hesitant to enter into a legally binding contract again, but still want to share their lives with someone. Some people are unable or unwilling to face up to the issue of commitment, so they postpone it by living together.

....

cohabitation living together in a sexual relationship as unmarried persons.

Living together presents its own kinds of problems. The relationship of living together may be more tentative and guarded, with less sense of security than is expected in a marriage. It may not protect the rights and possessions of each partner in the same way a marriage does. Sometimes, families with traditional values may oppose this lifestyle, and the couple may have to defend their living arrangements. Studies show that people who cohabit may have different values than couples who don't. Those who live together tend to be more independently minded, more self-protective, and are more likely to view relationships as breakable if they are not personally satisfying, rather than believing in the permanence of relationships. Studies conducted by researchers at the University of Wisconsin and Johns Hopkins University found that couples who live together before marriage have a higher divorce rate than those who did not cohabit. This tends to contradict the belief by some that living together before marriage helps to iron out potential marital problems.[31]

The dissolution of a cohabitation relationship may be especially problematic. The partners may not have equal claim to property or income acquired during the relationship, or one partner may forfeit his or her right to an equal share of community property. If the partners are not able to reach an amicable arrangement, or if they have not drawn up a contract addressing the distribution of property in case of dissolution of the relationship, resolution of property issues is defined by the laws of the state in which the couple resides.

To live together successfully, each partner must know where he or she stands in the relationship. Therefore, open communication is essential (see Communication for Wellness: Sharing Sexual Feelings with a Partner). Both partners may not share the same view of the relationship; for their protection, any differences must be revealed (see Feature 5.1). Research indicates that males often view living together as a more casual relationship than do females; females appear to have a greater desire for security and eventual marriage. Yet, only about 60 percent of those who live together eventually marry their partners.[32] Some of the causes for failure of cohabitation relationships are similar to those causing divorce. Living together before marriage, therefore, does not necessarily result in a more successful marriage.

Breaking Up a Relationship

Whenever a relationship is ended, regardless of the reasons, both partners are affected emotionally. Initial disbelief may evolve into anger, and then into resignation and grief. Even after the partners have physically separated, the emotional separation may take longer to resolve. Depression, insomnia, physical illness, and loneliness are common after a partner has left. Research has shown that, as a rule, men have more difficulty adjusting to the loss of a partner than do women.[33]

A large number of marriages end in divorce. Currently, over 40 percent of marriages are dissolved. With teenage marriages, about 50 percent end in divorce. Statistically, there are about 9.3 marriages per 1000 people in the United States, and 4.8 divorces.[34] Although a couple marries with the expectation that their relationship will endure, there is, unfortunately, no guarantee of permanence. Some marriages are condemned to fail from the outset for a variety of reasons. A couple may marry before they know enough about their partners and themselves; they may select their partners for the wrong reasons; they may be led into marriage by romantic love instead of mature love; or they may have divergent expectations for their lives together.

After marrying, some couples discover that their communication skills begin to deteriorate; they may stop talking and listening to each other. As a result, misunderstandings grow and lead to feelings of hostility. At this point couples may become convinced that they are incompatible. The emotional separation may become accelerated as one or both partners find themselves attracted to other people who offer to meet their needs.

No-fault divorce laws, which require no finding of misconduct, have been adopted by nearly every state since 1970. Under these laws, grounds previously cited for divorce, such as adultery and cruelty, were replaced by a finding of irreconcilable differences. In some cases, these new laws have created economic hardship for women and their children by redefining family assets in favor of men (see Feature 5.2).

Children of a Broken Marriage Relationship

Ending a marriage may be a relief to mismatched partners, but it can be difficult for their children. Recent studies indicate that the effects of divorce on children range from mild to disabling. Ten years after their parents' divorces, a majority of children, especially boys, express a sense of powerlessness, vulnerability, and guilt. They view their parents' divorces as the central experience in their lives, and

Singlehood, whether from a life choice, divorce, or death involves many opportunities for personal growth.

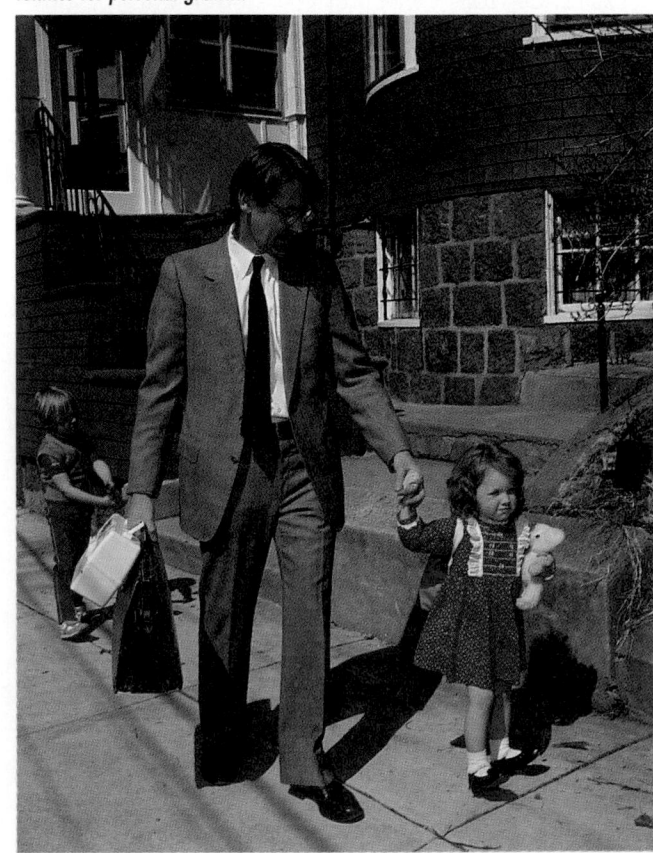

FEATURE 5.2

WOMEN (AND CHILDREN) AND NO-FAULT DIVORCE

According to sociologist Lenora Weitzman of Stanford University, no-fault divorce laws can economically damage women and their children. In her book, *The Divorce Revolution: The Unexpected Social and Economic Consequences for Women and Children in America* (New York: Free Press, 1985), she describes how shifting the focus in divorce from a legal determination of fault to economic issues can force women to assume an economic burden. Some examples of the economic impact of no-fault divorce on women include the following:

- In some states, marital property is supposed to be divided equally. While this may seem fair on the surface, what is not obvious is that the woman, who most often gets custody of any children, must share her half of the assets with her children.

- Since 60 percent of divorcing couples have less than $20,000 in combined net assets, most have to sell the family home and divide the assets. For children, this often means a change in neighborhood, schools, and friends.

- Since settlements address the division of fixed assets and property only, women may lose valuable assets such as health insurance, pensions, and recognition of her lower earning capacity.

- Courts often do not require equal division of property, and women may receive no alimony, or be awarded alimony for a limited time only.

- More than one-half of all fathers do not comply with court orders for child support, forcing women to assume the burden of providing for their children alone.

- Child support often covers only a fraction of the actual costs of raising a child, and often does not provide for day care. This is significant for the woman who must return to work or school, as day care represents a significant expense.

- In the first year following divorce, the standard of living improves for almost one-half of divorced men, but falls for almost three-quarters of divorced women and their children.

express intense concern about their own present and future relationships.[35] Children of divorced parents show more dependency, irrelevant talk, withdrawal, blaming, inattention, and unhappiness than children of married parents.[36] Negative effects of divorce can be reduced if parents do not express overt hostility toward their ex-partners, and if they make efforts to address their children's emotional needs.

Single Parents

Single parents, whether as a result of divorce or death of a partner, face a unique set of demands. A single mother with custody of her children may return to work or school, and thus have less time to spend with her children. A father with custody may find himself preoccupied with both his work and household duties that are new to him. The parent who does not have custody must satisfy him- or herself with seeing the children only on specified occasions. The difficulties inherent in being either a custodial or noncustodial parent make daily life more complex, at best. In fact, only 10 percent of divorced individuals with children report an improvement in their lives as a result of divorce.[37]

For divorced people, developing new social contacts becomes important. Developing a rela-

tionship with a new partner while children are in the home is, however, a delicate matter. Some parents wish to conceal their sexuality from their children. Other parents want to bring their new partners into the home, yet are reluctant to send mixed messages about sex and relationships to their children. Most parents are very cautious in these situations to prevent the upset in family dynamics that can occur when a new person is introduced.

Another group of single parents is comprised of single women who become mothers, either intentionally or unintentionally. The number of young women bearing unwanted children is becoming epidemic in the United States. Many of these women fail to use available contraception. Many of these mothers choose to keep and raise their children. Dealing with an unexpected pregnancy can be difficult under even the best of circumstances. Often, a lack of education, financial problems, and immaturity make it especially hard for the unmarried mother to cope. There are serious concerns for both the parent and the child.

Some adult single women intentionally choose to conceive and give birth alone. Some of these women are impregnated by a male friend, while others are artificially inseminated by donor semen (see Chapter 8). Some of these women are single professionals who desire the companionship of a child and a biological heir. Others may be lesbians—singles or couples—who wish to bring up a child.

Remarriage

The majority of younger divorced or widowed people find new partners. These new marriages often succeed because the partners, having learned from their previous "failures," are sensitive to what makes a relationship work. Divorced men are more likely to remarry, and do so sooner than women.[38] A divorced parent with custody of his or her children is more apt to remarry than to cohabit with a new partner. Today, a new family is emerging, in which both partners bring together children from previous marriages. These "blended" families are often highly successful.

Older widowed or divorced people are less likely to remarry. The great majority of these are women, because of their greater life expectancy. Older live-alones tend to seek companionship among friends and family.

CHECKPOINT

1. Compare the statistical incidence of marriage to that of divorce in the United States.

2. Explain the meaning of no-fault divorce.

3. What are some of the needs of children living with single parents?

4. Describe several changing trends in the remarriage of divorced persons.

HOMOSEXUAL RELATIONSHIPS

Sexual attraction, be it to people of the same sex, other sex, or both sexes is defined as sexual orientation. Being attracted primarily to people of one's own sex is **homosexuality.** According to survey results of the National Opinion Research Center at the University of Chicago, 2.8 percent of men and 2.5 percent of women report exclusively homosexual activity.[39]

There is little consensus on the origins of homosexual orientation. Such orientation may develop as early as childhood, or it may appear in adulthood. It may grow out of nonerotic affection between two people of the same sex, or it may develop after two individuals determine that same-gender affections are acceptable. Some experts see homosexual orientation as being largely due to social learning, or overly strong or weak authority figures; others consider biological factors, such as hormone levels, to be definitive (see Chapter 6).

An awareness of a homosexual or heterosexual orientation may occur at various ages. The type of adolescent sexual activity a person has had may or may not relate to that person's sexual orientation. Many eventually heterosexual adolescents have had some same-sex experience that may or may not relate to a homosexual attraction or predict an adult homosexual orientation. Conversely, many primarily gay or lesbian adults have had heterosexual experience during adolescence or adulthood. Adolescent homosexual sexuality is common among various cultures. Before becoming eligible to marry, young men of the East Bay Melanesians are forbidden to have contact with girls, but are expected to be sexually active with older males.[40]

Accepting and affirming a homosexual identity and deciding to be open about it is known as "coming out." This includes admitting it to oneself, identifying and getting to know other homosexual people, revealing it to friends and family, and acknowledging it publicly. Much effort has been made to establish freedom from job discrimination on the basis of sexual orientation. Yet, such bias still exists in some places, and when it does, some homosexual people choose to remain "in the closet." Where homosexual people have chosen to be open about their orientation, they give their family, friends, and associates a greater chance to see them more realistically.

Lesbian Coupling

A **lesbian** is a female who is primarily homosexual. Lesbians, like other women, prize companionship. They seek affirmation and open communication in their relationships. Many lesbians make

homosexuality sexual attraction primarily to people of one's own sex.

lesbian a female who is primarily homosexual.

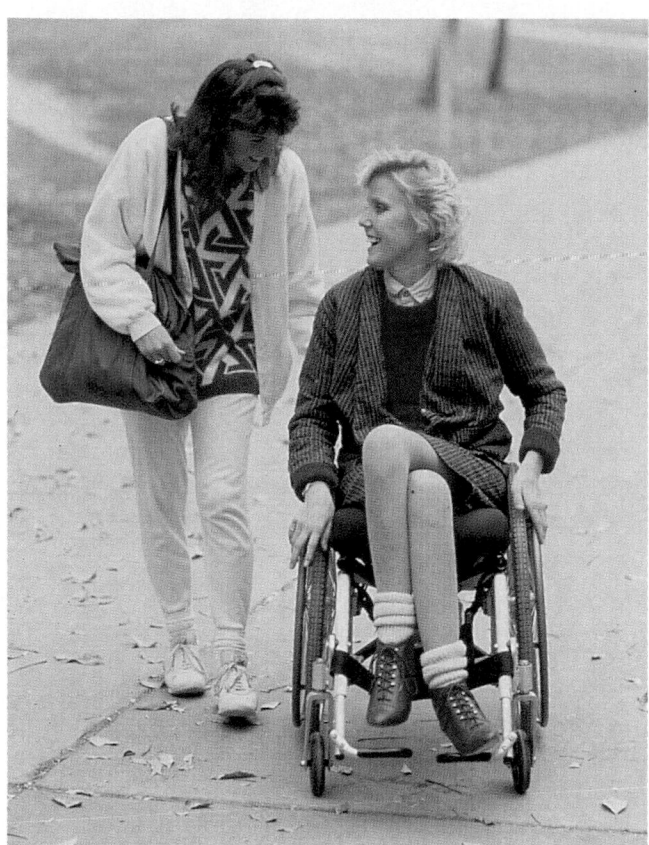

Friendships between people of the same gender often occur more readily than those between males and females.

long-term commitments to their partners; some of these relationships last a lifetime. Other lesbians, however, engage in short-term relationships.

Lesbian couples use many of the same general sexual techniques as heterosexual couples. In their relations with each other, lesbians commonly express themselves as equals, rather than adopting stereotypic dominant and submissive roles. They are likely to engage in full-body contact, including holding, kissing, and general caressing. They may also engage in oral and manual stimulation of the breasts and genitals.

Male Homosexual Coupling

Gays are males who are primarily homosexual. As with other groups of people, many gay males place an emphasis on freedom of personal expression. Many younger gay men tend to engage in sexual activity with many partners; gay partnerships

among older men, however, tend to be longer-lasting and monogamous.

Since the emergence of HIV as a serious health threat, more attention has been given to male homosexual behavior. Carried in body fluids, the virus, which is responsible for AIDS, is almost invariably transmitted in blood, semen, breast milk, and by vaginal or cervical secretions. The most effective mode of sexual transmission appears to be by anal intercourse. The impact of AIDS on the gay community has been monumental, dramatically influencing the multipartner practices of many men. As a result, many gay men now restrict their sexual practices to monogamous relationships or practice "safer sex" techniques, using condoms and avoiding the exchange of body fluids.

Gay men often affirm their commitment to a relationship by entering into a gay "marriage." While these marriages are not legally binding, they may be confirmed with marriage rituals such as the exchange of rings or the purchase of a shared home.

Homosexual males sometimes marry heterosexual women. Although this may represent a compromise for the gay male, he may marry for a variety of reasons. Pressure from family or friends, a desire to conceal his sexual orientation, or a wish to have children may encourage a gay man to enter a marriage relationship with a woman. Living in both the gay and heterosexual worlds is a concession that some gay men make in order to have economic and social security, as well as a family life.

Like lesbian couples, male homosexuals often express themselves as equals, rather than assuming dominant or submissive sexual roles. Sexually, gay men may engage in generalized hugging and kissing, may stimulate the genitals orally or manually, and may engage in anal intercourse.

BISEXUALITY

A person who forms sexual relationships with people of either gender is known as a **bisexual.** A bisexual may prefer people of one gender, and may have one or more partners of either sex. Some bisexuals are in transition between homosexual and heterosexual practices, while others may be

gay a male who is primarily homosexual.

bisexual a person who forms sexual relationships with people of either gender.

reluctant to admit primarily homosexual orientation.[41] Bisexual females tend to be happier with their sexual orientation than bisexual males.[42] Lesbians and gays may criticize bisexual men and women because they are not completely homosexual in their orientation, while heterosexuals may condemn them for not being fully heterosexual.

C H E C K P O I N T

1. Explain why divorce is often emotionally devastating to people.

2. Give some characteristics of lesbian coupling.

3. List some characteristics of homosexual coupling.

4. Define the term *bisexuality*.

SEX FOR SALE

Many people are willing to pay money for sex, whether the sex is represented through imagery, actual sexual contact, or through goods. There is a thriving market for sexual merchandise and services. Sex for money fulfills a variety of needs for some people. It can provide sexual variety, the thrill of illicit sex, and compensation for being rejected by a sexual partner, for example.

PROSTITUTION

Prostitution is the act of engaging in sexual activity in exchange for money or gifts. It is the only sex offense that is more often charged against women than men. Because prostitution is illegal in most places, a prostitute's life is often controlled by his or her criminal status and by the people who control the trade. The prostitute's support system consists of his or her clients, as well as people who live off his or her earnings, including the **panderer,** who recruits prostitutes, and the **pimp,** who "manages" the prostitute's time and money.

....

prostitution engaging in sexual activity in exchange for money or gifts.

panderer one who recruits prostitutes.

pimp one who "manages" the prostitute's time and money.

People who become prostitutes may seek emotional and financial affirmation of their worth. Some must support expensive drug addictions, and others are runaways from intolerable home situations. Once individuals become involved in prostitution, they may become trapped in the lifestyle.

One of the most serious risks associated with prostitution is the transmission of sexually transmitted diseases, including HIV. Some people advocate the legalization of prostitution, arguing that states could then exert control over the trade and thus reduce the incidence of sexually transmitted diseases among prostitutes and the transmission to their clientele.

Female Prostitutes

Prostitutes are known for their versatility in accommodating their clients. Call girls, the most highly paid prostitutes, make appointments to meet with and escort their clients. Streetwalkers solicit their customers on the streets. Because this is dangerous, streetwalkers must protect themselves from violence and avoid arrest. Other prostitutes may work in brothels, in massage parlors, or as supported mistresses. Many prostitutes in large cities were recruited as runaway minors.

Male Prostitutes

The male heterosexual prostitute, or gigolo, often provides escort and sexual services to well-to-do female clients. Hustlers, or homosexual male prostitutes, often are hired by older homosexual men. In large cities, runaway boys may be recruited to become prostitutes. As with female prostitution, health risks to male prostitutes include contracting HIV, as well as other sexually transmitted diseases, and violence.

PORNOGRAPHY

Pornography is the depiction of erotic behavior with the intent of stimulating sexual arousal. Most pornography is available in magazines, movies, and on cable television. Some is available in "adult only" stores, but much pornography is also sold at neigh-

....

pornography the graphic depiction of erotic behavior with the intent of stimulating sexual arousal.

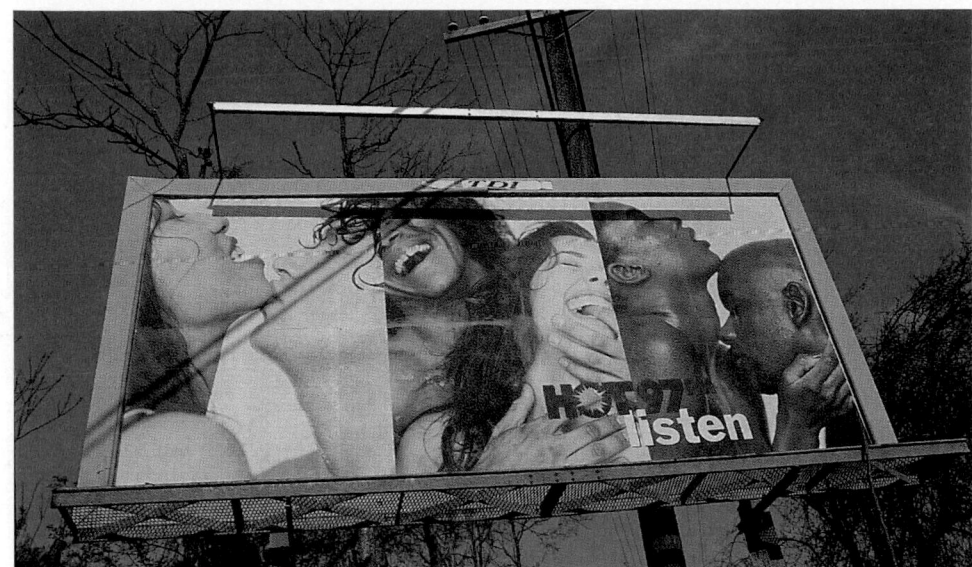

The desire for sexual excitement (fulfillment) is often used to sell commercial products.

borhood newsstands. Sexually explicit videocassettes are popular, as is adult cable television. To be ruled legally offensive, pornography must be obscene, or not fit to be displayed. Since this relies on a subjective value judgment, the courts allow local communities to determine what constitutes obscenity.

An industry larger than the record and film industries combined, pornography exaggerates and distorts reality. Those who oppose pornography are concerned about its promotion of violent, aggressive behavior by men toward women. A form of sadism, pornography often portrays the degradation of women and children as being sexually pleasurable to them and may show acts of brutality. Of special concern is the illegal publication of child pornography ("kiddie porn"), in which prepubertal children are featured. Exposure to this material may encourage people to act in response to what they see.[43]

SEX IN ADVERTISING

The advertising industry has contributed to a massive proliferation of sexually suggestive material on television, in print, and on billboards. Sexual suggestion in ad copy is used to sell everything from cosmetics to machine parts. One method of using sex to sell products is known as **subliminal seduction.** The intent of subliminal seduction is to

....

subliminal seduction a method of using sexual suggestions below the threshold of consciousness to sell products.

send subtle sexual messages to the viewer, which are received subconsciously. While the success of this particular advertising ploy is questioned, there is no doubt that appealing to consumers' sexuality helps to sell products.

Some advertisers have resorted to such sexually explicit material that some executives are concerned that they exceed the limits of acceptability. They fear that such advertisements will have the reverse of their desired effects, turning consumers off to the products. Merchandise can be sold effectively without the use of sexual messages.

CHECKPOINT

1. Define the terms *prostitution, pandering,* and *pimping.*

2. What are some of the reasons people become prostitutes?

3. Why do people view pornography with concern?

4. Describe subliminal seduction and why some advertisers attempt to use it.

COERCIVE SEX

Violence against an individual may be physical or mental. Sexual violence is especially damaging because it violates a person both physically and mentally. Ordinarily, sex is associated with intimacy and pleasure. After a sexual assault, a victim may associate sex with fear and pain, rather than

If you receive unsolicited and unwanted touching or closeness from someone else it may create feelings of helplessness and anger.

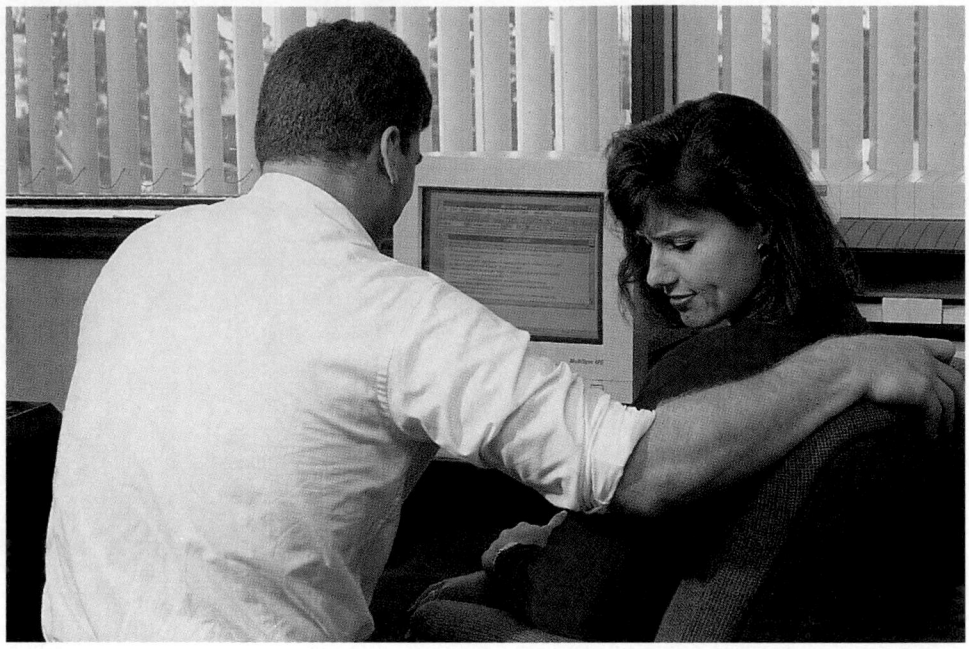

with gratification. **Coercive sex** occurs when one or more individuals victimize another in order to exert power and maintain control. Unfortunately, in some areas of our culture sexual violence has become eroticized by distorting it as sexual pleasure. Sex becomes coercive in sexual harassment, child sexual abuse, forcible rape, date (acquaintance) rape, and sometimes statutory rape (see Chapter 6).

SEXUAL HARASSMENT

Unwelcome sexual advances, requests for sexual favors, or other visual, verbal, or physical conduct of a sexual nature is **sexual harassment.** Sexual harassment can take many forms: It may be verbal or nonverbal, and may include actions such as unwanted touching, use of profanity, pressure to go out on a date, or pressure to engage in unwanted sexual activity. In situations involving sexual harassment, one person exerts power over another.

....

coercive sex use of sex to exert power and maintain control.

sexual harassment unwelcome sexual advances, requests for sexual favors, or other visual, verbal, or physical conduct of a sexual nature.

Sexual harassment, although unlawful, often occurs in the workplace. According to surveys, 90 percent of Fortune 500 companies have had to deal with sexual harassment complaints, and almost 25 percent have been sued. More than 50 percent of women executives in the United States report that they have been victims of sexual harassment.[44] Under Title VII of the 1964 Civil Rights Act, job-related harassment is defined as sexual discrimination.

In 1980, a ruling by the Equal Employment Opportunity Commission (EEOC) expanded the definition of sexual harassment to include unwanted verbal and nonverbal sexual behavior as being illegal. These revised guidelines were based on the 1964 Civil Rights Act that holds a company liable for sexual harassment by supervisors unless the company takes immediate and appropriate action. Revised again in 1986, these guidelines clarify that unwanted verbal and nonverbal sexual behavior is illegal, and that there is legal recourse for other employees if a co-worker uses sex to obtain job advancement. Due, perhaps in part, to an increasing number of court decisions awarding monetary judgments to victims, an increasing number of large corporations and companies are establishing programs for management and employees that identify what sexual harassment is and under what conditions the company can be held liable.

Sexual harassment also occurs in schools, between faculty and students. A reported 20–30

DEALING WITH SEXUAL HARASSMENT IN THE WORKPLACE

If and when you face sexual harassment at work, there are various steps you can take. Some of these points can also be used by students who are being sexually harassed by faculty members.

1. If you believe you have been sexually harassed on the job, report it to your supervisor, or if your supervisor is doing the harassing, report it to the harasser's boss.

2. You should keep a diary, listing the time, date, and place of each incident of harassment, when and how you responded, and whether or not there were any witnesses. Physical or emotional stresses caused by the incident should be noted. You should also list any professional person (psychologist, physician, counselor) whom you have consulted.

3. You should ask the offender to stop the harassment in as polite, unemotional, and clear a way as possible. If the harasser is head of the company, it is still important to ask that the harassment stop. You should not give the aggressor any information or emotional response that could be used against you later.

4. If the harassment continues, you should complain to the union, a grievance committee, the personnel department, or members of higher management who are sympathetic and willing to listen.

5. Also, if the harassment continues, you should write a low-key, polite, short letter to the aggressor: Experts recommend that the letter be divided into the following three parts:

• Part 1: A detailed statement of the facts as you see them.

• Part 2: Your feelings and what personal damage the harassment has caused you.

• Part 3: A short statement of what actions you would like the offender to take. You should ask that the harassment end, that you be reinstated in your former position if the harassment resulted in a termination or demotion, or that the objection to your advancement be withdrawn if the harasser is blocking a promotion.

You should hand deliver the letter to the offender, accompanied by a witness. You should keep a copy of the letter since this will be valuable legal evidence if you have to go to court.

Usually, the offender simply accepts the letter, says nothing, and the harassment stops. Once in a while, there is an apology, a discussion of perception of sexual harassment, or a denial. At any rate, a letter is a peaceable attempt to settle the problem. If it does not, you should keep the following additional points in mind.

6. Talk to other people on the job or at school. Often, these people have been victims of sexual harassment by the same person. Collaborative testimony will help you in pursuing the charge should you choose to take legal action, and will also make you feel better about complaining. Talking with other people about the harassment also puts your concern on record with someone else.

7. If you quit because of the situation, you should send a letter to the head of the personnel department. The letter should be a very detailed account of the sexual harassment and should be compiled from your diary.

8. If you are fired because you turned down sexual advances, you should talk to an attorney who is familiar with harassment cases. You may have to prove your complaint just to collect unemployment benefits.

9. To sue under the sexual discrimination act, Title VII, you must file a complaint with the local office of the Equal Employment Opportunity Commission within 180 days of leaving the company. To collect damages, you will need to sue the company, the offender, or both.

percent of female college students have been harassed by professors, administrators, teachers, staff, or fellow students.[45] This problem is recognized by most colleges, and policies have been established to deal with harassment-related complaints.

Victims of sexual harassment should seek recourse. It is important for the victim of sexual harassment to keep records so she or he can counter past and future incidents. Complaints may be in the form of a letter, a face-to-face confrontation with the offender, a complaint to management, testimony of others, or by retaining an attorney (see Feature 5.3). Some cases even go to court.

RAPE

Forcing a person to have unwanted sex is known as **rape.** Rape may include oral, anal, or vaginal penetration, and includes penetration by objects. Rape is often an act of violence, not sex, although in some forms, such as date rape, it may be both. It is often motivated by an individual's need for dominance and power, or anger and hatred of the other sex.

rape forcing a person to have unwanted sex.

Supportive counseling is needed to help a rape victim sort through her feelings of loss, hurt, and bewilderment.

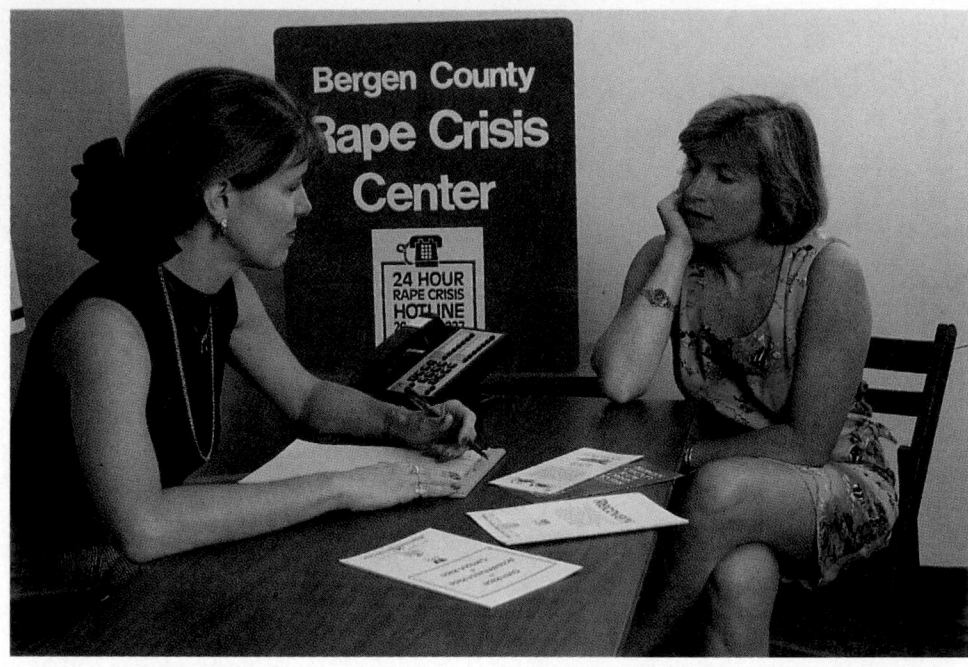

In 1991, there were almost 125,000 rapes *reported* in the United States; since 1987 the rate of reported forcible rape of women has risen 13 percent,[46] yet rape is one of the most underreported crimes. The National Victim Center estimates that there are more than three times the number of rapes each year than are reported by the Justice Department.[47] One in eight women now living in the United States has been raped, and it is estimated that one in four women will be raped in her lifetime.[48] Although women of all ages are raped, the average victim is 16–19 years old; the average assailant is 21–29 years old. Rape may be committed by strangers or by acquaintances of the victim.

Stranger Rape

Most people imagine rape as a sexual attack committed by an unknown assailant in a dark alleyway. Stranger rape often *does* occur after dark in a parking lot or on the street, but one-third of these rapes occur in the victim's home. About 53 percent of the assailants are white, while 46 percent are black.[49]

Women can reduce the chance of rape by learning self-defense techniques and avoiding situations in which they might be attacked. The best defenses against rape may fail, however, and it is important to remember that the victim is never responsible for the crime.

If a woman is raped, she should immediately go to a hospital emergency room. She should not bathe or change clothing, as doing so could destroy important evidence. Hospital treatment of the rape victim includes attending to any injuries received during the assault, as well as therapeutic treatment for sexually transmitted diseases and pregnancy. Many hospitals and mental health agencies offer the services of rape counselors. These individuals can be invaluable in aiding the victim to recover emotionally.

Acquaintance Rape

Acquaintance rape is a sexual assault in which the victim knows the assailant. Acquaintance rapes often occur on dates, and thus are sometimes referred to as **date rapes.** This category of rape includes group rapes in which fraternities, athletic teams, or other groups of men attack a woman of their acquaintance.

According to the National Victim Center, about 75 percent of all rapes are acquaintance rapes.[50]

acquaintance rape a sexual assault in which the victim knows the assailant.

date rape a sexual assault that occurs on a date.

FEATURE 5.4

AVOIDING DATE RAPE

To reduce the chance of becoming a victim of date rape, consider using these precautions:

- Know something about the men you date.

- If you do not know your date well, select a public place for your date, insist upon getting home by a specific time, or recruit a friend with whom to double date.

- If you do not know your date well, meet him at your destination rather than at your home to reduce the risk of having him in your apartment or room.

- Do not drink alcoholic beverages or use recreational drugs while on a date with someone you do not know well.

- If your date wants to come to your apartment or room, ask a friend to call you after 15–30 minutes to make sure that you are safe.

Source: Adapted from Byer, C., and Shainberg, L. *Dimensions of Human Sexuality,* 4th ed. Dubuque, IA: Brown and Benchmark, 1994.

Twenty to 25 percent of all college women have experienced forceful attempts at sexual intercourse by their dates.[51] Since victims of acquaintance rape are more hesitant than other rape victims to report the crime, it is believed to be the most underreported type of sexual assault.[52]

Acquaintance rape may be extremely difficult for the victim to discuss, even with her closest friends. The victim is violated both physically and mentally, and may feel shame, guilt, and fear of reprisal. A date rape victim may also wrongly feel responsible for the attack because she trusted the assailant, and she may feel betrayed by someone considered to be a friend. Some victims report feeling that they failed at being assertive or "holding the line," and many report problems in reestablishing trust in their own judgment. See Feature 5.4 for some tips on how to protect yourself from date rape.

In a Kent State University study, more than one-half of women students surveyed had at some time experienced sexual aggression, and one in eight had been raped. Of the men in the study, 4.3 percent admitted to the use of violence to obtain sex, with an additional 27 percent admitting to a lesser degree of physical or emotional coercion.[53] Such men commonly see themselves as "victims" of adolescent confusion. For some, the examples seen at home or in the media legitimize violence. According to the National Coalition on Television Violence, one out of eight Hollywood movies includes a rape theme.[54] Other men feel justified in their actions because their dates arouse them sexually, engage in petting, or use drugs with them.[55] Many young men—and some young women—believe that forced sexual intercourse is permissible under such circumstances.

Further muddying the waters of social interaction are what some see as confusing social signals. People often learn about sexuality without developing emotional understanding. Some people do not understand nuances of social behavior, and do not understand consent or the lack of it. Some women only want love, although the man expects sex. He may feel aggressive, while she feels the need to be coy. Both partners may ask for independence, yet may not be adept at communicating their real wants in the area of sexual interaction, an area in which innuendo and implied communication may not be sufficient. In an age when sexual experimentation is accepted, sexual misunderstandings are apt to occur. Unfortunately, such misunderstandings do damage to both the man and the woman, both of whom need reliable and caring intimacy.

Learning self-defense techniques can help prevent sexual assault by increasing a woman's awareness and preparing her to act when confronted with a potential assault (Feature 5.5, p. 136). As with stranger rape, a victim of acquaintance rape should seek medical attention as soon as possible. Hospital emergency rooms cannot legally deny treatment to a rape victim even if the victim is unable to pay for treatment. A victim should also contact a rape-crisis hotline or rape counselor for help in dealing with health care professionals, police, and family.

statutory rape sexual intercourse between an adult and a minor who are not married to each other.

FEATURE 5.5

REDUCING THE CHANCES OF STRANGER RAPE

To avoid becoming the victim of any crime, especially rape, consider following these guidelines:

- *Home Security* Use secure locks on doors and windows. Have dead-bolt locks installed on all exterior doors and windows on the ground floor, and install screens on all windows. Be certain to have your locks changed if you lose a key.

- *Lights* Leave lights on in your home if you plan on returning after dark. Keep lights on in all entrances.

- *Visitors* Identify all visitors before opening your door. Install a peephole to allow you to check before allowing someone to enter your home. If a visitor claims to be a representative of a service or company, request identification and verify its legitimacy by telephone before allowing him to enter.

- *Phone Book* If you wish to list your phone number in the directory, use only your first initial rather than your full first name. Do not list your address.

- *Walking* When walking alone, plan your route to avoid dark streets, high shrubbery, and isolated areas. Be cautious when approaching alleyways, recessed doorways, and open fields. Walk with authority, and be aware of what is going on around you. You might carry a whistle around your wrist. Dress so that you can move and run easily if in danger. If you are assaulted, shout "Fire!" rather than "Help!" or "Rape!"

- *Automobile* Keep your car in good repair to avoid highway trouble, and always keep at least a quarter-

tank of gas in it. Be certain to lock your car whenever it is parked, and check the back seat before you reenter it. When returning to your car, always carry your keys in your hand so that you are ready to unlock your car quickly. (Keys also make a good weapon if attacked.) When driving, keep all of the doors locked, and roll up the windows as far as possible. Avoid personalized license plates, and do not respond to someone who calls you by name if you do have personalized plates.

- *Hitchhiking* The best advice is to avoid hitchhiking. If you must take a ride with someone you do not know, check the door handle and keep your window open. Never accept a ride with more than one man.

- *Public Transportation* When using public transportation, know your route. If you are unfamiliar with your route, ask the driver and sit near the front of the car. Avoid standing among a group of men.

- *Hotel/Motel Room* Use the peephole and door chain before opening the door to a stranger. Open the door to a stranger only after confirming by telephone with the front desk the purpose of the caller.

- *Alertness* Remember to plan ahead, take precautions, and use common sense.

Source: Adapted from Byer, C., and Shainberg, L. *Dimensions of Human Sexuality*, 4th ed. Dubuque, IA: Brown and Benchmark, 1994.

STATUTORY RAPE

Statutory rape is sexual intercourse between an adult and a minor who are not married to one another. Generally, statutory rape, which is also known as *unlawful sex*, occurs between adult males and minor females. The basis of statutory rape laws is the contention that minors, being under the age of consent, may only have sexual intercourse if given permission by a parent or legal guardian. Some states have replaced statutory rape laws with laws regarding contributing to the delinquency of a minor. In some states only the actions of an adult male with a minor female are subject to statutory rape laws, whereas the actions of an adult female with a minor male are handled as contributing to the delinquency of a minor.

CHECKPOINT

1. What is coercive sex?

2. How are women now protected from sexual harassment?

3. Give statistics on the incidence of rape in the United States.

4. Distinguish stranger rape from acquaintance rape.

5. Why is acquaintance rape so difficult for a woman to deal with after the assault?

6. Contrast statutory rape with stranger and acquaintance rape.

SUMMARY

In learning how sexual values, intimacy, and love contribute to healthy relationships, you are better prepared to make sound decisions about your sexual life-style.

Humans are sexual beings, and may express this sexuality in a variety of ways. Because most sexual behavior is neither inherently right nor inherently wrong, you must make your own decisions regarding sexuality and relationships. Society helps to guide behavior by defining what is immoral and what is moral, but you must form your own sexual values. These values, based on what is important to you, help guide your sexual behavior.

The sexual climate in America has been affected by many factors. Behavior that was once condemned by society may now have greater acceptance. Currently, our society encompasses a wide variety of sexual life-styles. People may be married or single, heterosexual or homosexual. Divorce and cohabitation are common, as is single parenthood. Each life-style has unique rewards and liabilities, so you must determine how to best fulfill your needs.

Although most sexual relations are two-way affairs in which both partners desire intimacy and pleasurable relations, some people pay others to obtain sexual pleasure. This may be done through prostitution, pornography, or by using sex in advertising to sell a product.

A person's needs for intimacy and pleasure can be violated through coercive sexual relationships. Such violation occurs when people, against their will, are coerced into participating with another person sexually. Such coercion is a way of exerting and maintaining control over another person. Sexual coercion occurs in sexual harassment, child sexual abuse, forcible rape, and sometimes, statutory rape.

In making life-style decisions, it is important for you to determine what is important and to fulfill your needs without compromising your values.

REFERENCES

1. Hatfield, E., and Wolster, G. *A New Look at Love.* Lanham, PA: University Press of America, 1985.
2. Gregor, T. *Anxious Pleasures: The Sexual Lives of an Amazonian People.* Chicago: University of Chicago Press, 1985.
3. Briggs, D. "Teens Are Saying Give Chastity a Chance." *Los Angeles Times* (24 September 1993), E-6.
4. Sternberg, R. *The Triangle of Love.* New York: Basic Books, 1988.
5. Sternberg, R. "Triangulating Love." In R. Sternberg and M. Barnes (eds.), *The Psychology of Love.* New Haven, CT: Yale University Press, 1988.
6. Shapiro, J. "Teenage Sex: Just Say 'Wait'." *U.S. News & World Report* (26 July 1993), 56–59.
7. Ibid.
8. National Center for Health Statistics. "Cohabitation, Marriage, Marital Dissolution, and Remarriage: United States, 1988." *Advance Data* No. 194, DHHS Pub. No. (PHS) 91-1250 (4 January 1991).
9. Krier, B. "Why So Many Singles." *Los Angeles Times* (26 June 1988) Part IV, pp. 1, 8.
10. McGrath, A., et al. "Living Alone and Loving It." *U.S. News & World Report* (3 August 1987), 52–55.
11. Shapiro, op. cit.
12. Allgeier, E., and Allgeier, A. *Sexual Interactions,* 3rd ed. Lexington, MA: Heath, 1991.
13. McGrath, op. cit.
14. U.S. Bureau of the Census. *Statistical Abstracts of the United States, 1992,* 112th ed. Washington, DC: U.S. Government Printing Office, 1992.
15. National Center for Health Statistics, op. cit.
16. McGrath, op. cit.
17. Ibid.
18. U.S. Census Bureau, op. cit.
19. Sanoff, A. "19 Million Singles." *U.S. News & World Report* (21 February 1983), 53–56.
20. McGrath, op. cit.
21. Rempel, J., and Holmes, J. "How Do I Trust Thee?" *Psychology Today* (February 1986), 28–34.
22. Kantrowitz, B. "How to Stay Married." *Newsweek,* (24 August 1987), 52–57.
23. National Center for Health Statistics. "Births, Marriages, Divorces, and Deaths for 1992." *Monthly Vital Statistics Report,* U.S. Department of Health and Human Services, Vol. 41, No. 12, DHHS Pub. No. (PHS) 93–1120 (19 May 1993).
24. Kantrowitz, op. cit.
25. Booth, W. "WHO Seeks Global Data on Sexual Practices." *Science* 244 (1989), 418–419.
26. Greeley, A., Michael, A., and Smith T. "A Most Monogamous People: Americans and Their Sexual Partners." *GSS Topical Report No. 17.* Chicago: NORC, 1989.
27. Allgeier, op. cit.
28. Fulwood, S. "Out-of-Wedlock Births Rise Sharply Among Most Groups." *Los Angeles Times* (14 July 1993), A-1, 16.

29. Newcomb, M. "Sexual Behavior of Cohabitors: A Comparison of Three Independent Samples." *The Journal of Sex Research* 22 (1986), 492–513.

30. Thornton, A. "Cohabitation and Marriage in the 1980s." *Demography* 25 (1988), 497.

31. Marbella, J. "Heartbreak of Cohabitation Ends in Divorce." *Los Angeles Times* (16 November 1989), E-12.

32. Krier, op. cit.

33. Sanoff, op. cit.

34. National Center for Health Statistics, op. cit.

35. Wallerstein, J. *Surviving the Break Up: How Parents and Children Cope with Divorce*. New York: Basic Books, 1980.

36. Rosenfeld, M. "Study Tracks the Children of Divorce Into Adulthood." *Los Angeles Times* (12 November 1987), Sec. 5, 34, 35.

37. Wallerstein, op. cit.

38. Sanoff, op. cit.

39. Sanoff, op. cit.

40. Francoeur, R. "Sexual Archeotypes in Eastern Cultures Can Be Helpful in Creating Sex-Positive Views." *Contemporary Sexuality* 22 (1990), 6.

41. MacDonald, A. "Research in Sexual Orientation: A Bridge That Touches Both Shores but Doesn't Meet in the Middle." *Journal of Sex Education and Therapy* 8 (1982), 9–13.

42. Cook, K., et al. "The Playboy Readers' Sex Survey, Part 3." *Playboy* (May 1983), 126–128.

43. *Attorney General's Commission on Pornography, Final Report, July, 1986*. Washington, DC: U.S. Department of Justice, 1986.

44. Webb, S. *Step Forward*. New York: Master Media, 1992.

45. Hughes, J., and Sandler, B. *In Case of Sexual Harassment, A Guide for Women Students*. A publication of the Status and Education of Women. Washington, DC: Association of American Colleges, 1986.

46. U.S. Department of Justice Statistics. *Criminal Victimization in the United States 1990*. National Crime Survey Report NCJ-134126. Washington, DC: U.S. Department of Justice, 1992.

47. National Victim Center. *Rape in America*. Ft. Worth, TX: National Victim Center, 1992.

48. Gibbs, N. "When Is It Rape?" *Time* (3 June 1991), 48–54.

49. U.S. Department of Justice, Bureau of Justice Statistics. *Sourcebook of Criminal Justice Statistics, 1991*. Tim Flanagan and Katherine Maquire (eds.). NCJ-137-369. Washington, DC: Government Printing Office, 1991.

50. National Victim Center, op. cit.

51. Yegidis, B. "Date Rape and Other Forced Sexual Encounters Among College Students." *Journal of Sex Education and Therapy* Vol. 12, No. 2 (Fall–Winter 1986), 51–54.

52. Barret, K. "Date Rape—Campus Epidemic?" *Ms* (September 1982), 50.

53. Ibid.

54. Gelman, D., et al. "The Mind of the Rapist," *Newsweek* (23 July 1990), 46–52.

55. Yegidis, op. cit.

SUGGESTED READINGS

Blumfield, W., and Raymond, D. *Looking at Gay and Lesbian Life*. Boston: Beacon, 1993.

Buchwald, E., et al. *Transforming a Rape Culture*. New York: Milkweed, 1993.

Deitz, S. *Single File: How to Live Happily Forever After With or Without Prince Charming*. New York: St. Martin's Press, 1989.

Eisendrath, D. *You're Not What I Expected*. New York: Morrow, 1993.

Godek, G. *1001 Ways to Be Romantic*. Boston: Casablanca, 1993.

Kasl, C. *Women, Sex, and Addiction: A Search for Love and Power*. New York: Ticknor and Fields, 1989.

Langelay, M. *Back Off, How to Confront and Stop Sexual Harassment and Harassers*. New York: Simon & Schuster, 1993.

Lansky, V. *Divorce Book for Parents*. New York: New American Library, 1989.

Notarius, C., and Markham, H. *We Can Work It Out*. New York: Putnam, 1993.

Rich, H. *Get Married Now*. Holbrook, MA: Adams, 1993.

Simon, S. *In Search of Values*. New York: Warner, 1993.

Simring, S., and Simring, S. *The Compatability Quotient*. New York: Fawcett, 1990.

Smedes, L. *Shame and Grace*. New York: HarperCollins, 1993.

Stanway, A. *The Art of Sexual Intimacy*. New York: Carroll and Graf, 1993.

Thompson, C. *Single Solutions*. New York: Ballantine, 1990.

Vaughn, D. *Uncoupling*. New York: Vintage, 1990.

Wallerstein, G., and Blakeslee, S. *Second Chances*. New York: Ticknor and Fields, 1990.

Williamson, M. *A Return to Love*. New York: HarperCollins, 1992.

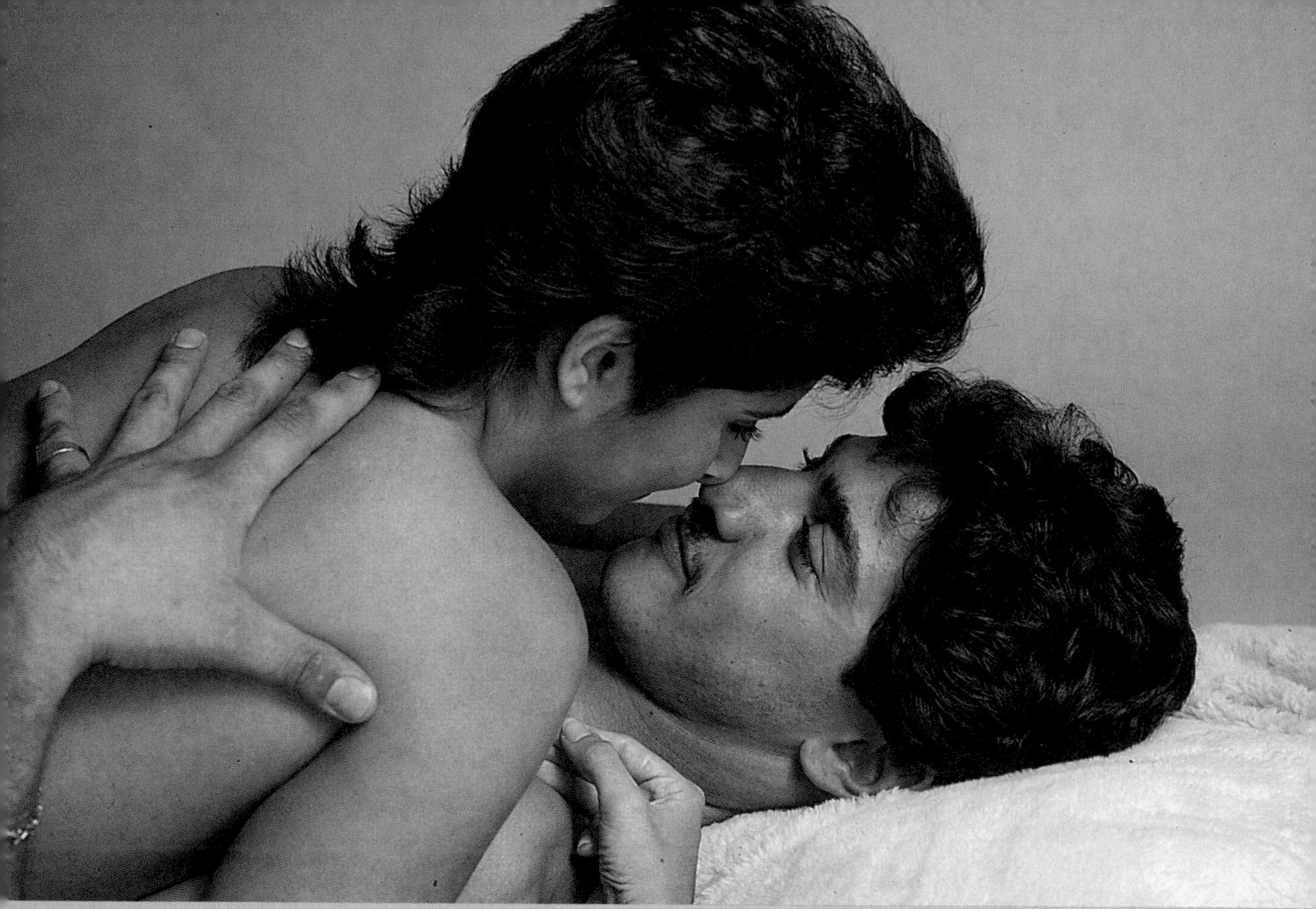

6
SEXUAL BIOLOGY AND BEHAVIOR

Upon completing this chapter, you will be able to:

KNOWLEDGE

- Distinguish between gender roles and gender identity.
- List the gonadotropins that govern sexual reproduction.
- Compare the reasons a woman might strive or might not strive to experience G-spot arousal.
- Explain the role of testosterone in libido.
- Name the four phases of sexual response.
- Define the term *erogenous zones*.
- List reasons why a person may choose to be celibate.
- Distinguish between sexual dysfunctions and sexual paraphilias.
- List the steps a woman who is not experiencing orgasm during sexual intercourse might take.
- List the characteristics of a sexually mature person.

INSIGHT

- Identify those factors that have contributed to your own sexual identity.
- Explain why it is as important for a man to understand a woman's menstrual cycle as it is for the woman herself.
- Examine your reasons for practicing or for not practicing masturbation.
- Explain whether you consider yourself to be sexually mature. Why or why not?

DECISION MAKING

- Determine your sexual role identification.
- Form a personal opinion on the practice of male circumcision.
- Identify some steps you plan to take to avoid developing a sexual performance disorder.
- Decide what steps you might take in the event your child was victimized by a child molester.

Gender is determined at conception by whether the sperm supplies the ovum with an X chromosome or a Y chromosome. Several weeks after conception, the embryo begins to develop sex organs. After birth, gender identity results from biological, social, and cultural events. Sometimes, people feel trapped in a body of the wrong sex. This happened to Ray Capwill (now April Capwill), who 18 years ago had an operation that changed him hormonally and physically into a female. Having a sex change operation is hardly newsworthy, yet April has been in the center of a controversy related to her sex change. A former runner, she has returned to that sport with significant success. She is regularly winning, or placing among the top finishers in her age class. This has sparked controversy about whether or not she should be allowed to race as a woman. While this question may seem simple, it is actually quite complex.

According to April's physical characteristics and hormones, she is female. However, by chromosome she is male. Twenty years of her life were spent as a male, the past 18 as a female. In certain sports, such as running, the basic physiology of males gives them a general advantage over females. There are claims *that since April was a male for 20 years, she has a physiological advantage over females who have female chromosomes.*

Gender verification tests, like those used in certain cases in the Olympics, recently have been debated by medical experts who are concerned about their validity and appropriate use. Most proponents of gender verification testing recommend that it be used only as a screening device prior to a physical exam. By physical examination, April Capwill is female. Is it then fair to use the physical exam as the gender verification test when some evidence points out that April may have certain athletic advantages over other females?

Most would agree that this is more than a legal question. A person could legally be a female, but have male characteristics that provide an unfair advantage. This issue may be one that will be debated for some time.

■ ■ ■

For some people, sexuality is seen as something that becomes evident when you realize a sexual attraction to someone else. Actually, humans are inherently sexual beings; from birth, ours is a sexual life cycle.

An understanding of your sexuality throughout your life helps bypass many of the obstacles you may face in seeking sexual satisfaction. A lack of learning about sexual processes and behaviors may lead you to not know what to expect and cause you to experience considerable self-doubt. At this point you are urged to complete In Your Hands: Assessing Your Level of Sexual Understanding.

From as early as infancy, a child has sexual feelings and experiences. His or her sexual expressions, however, may not be recognized as such because, as adults, we define sexuality with adult terms and standards. As we pass through the various stages of life, our sexual interests and activities change in nature and intensity.

A child may engage in sexual activity more out of curiosity than arousal. As his or her sexual development continues and the child passes through **puberty,** that period when a person becomes functionally capable of reproducing, and into adoles-

cence, hormonal activity leads to significant physical change. As the adolescent becomes a young adult, he or she is faced with many sexual choices, which may include decisions about sexual intimacy, relationships, marriage, and parenthood.

A person's reproductive capacity wanes as he or she ages, yet the sexual interests can remain very much alive; the older adult usually retains the ability to respond to sexual stimuli. Sexual interest and activity among older men and women is directly related to their sexual urges when younger. Older people who describe their sexual urges as being strong in youth tend to retain greater sexual interest than those whose describe sexual activity when young as weak.[1]

DEVELOPING SEXUALLY

All humans are born as sexual beings. Our **gender,** whether we are male or female, develops and defines a part of our sexuality. Most people perceive gender as an either/or matter; we are either male or female. While our sex may be categorized as male or female, a number of factors affect gender traits and behaviors. Some of these factors are biological and affect us genetically before birth, or *prenatally*. Other factors are social and psychological and affect us *postnatally,* or after birth.

BIOLOGICAL FACTORS

Biological factors play a major role in determining our gender identities. Some of these factors include our genetic, gonadal, hormonal, and genital make-up. All of these characteristics begin to form before birth.

Genetic Determinants

Each cell in the human body contains 46 **chromosomes** (*krō'mō-sōmz*), structures that contain genes. Of these chromosomes, two are called sex chromosomes. The two sex chromosomes in a female are identical and are known as XX; the two sex chromosomes in a male differ from each other and are known as XY. X chromosomes are consid-

puberty the period of time during which a person becomes functionally capable of reproduction.

gender the biological state of being male or female.

chromosomes structures in cells which contain genes.

IN YOUR HANDS

ASSESSING YOUR LEVEL OF SEXUAL UNDERSTANDING

Listed here are topics relating to human sexuality. Using the rating categories shown, indicate your level of understanding of each topic by checking the appropriate spaces.

	I know very little about this, and could use further information.	I understand this reasonably well, but could use more information.	I feel comfortable with this and do not need further information.
1. Psychosexual development of children and adolescents	____	____	____
2. Gender identity, masculinity, and femininity	____	____	____
3. Sex hormones of a male and female	____	____	____
4. Male genital anatomy and physiology	____	____	____
5. Female genital anatomy and physiology	____	____	____
6. Human sexual response	____	____	____
7. Sexual performance concerns	____	____	____
8. Sex counseling	____	____	____
9. Homosexuality and bisexuality	____	____	____
10. Erogenous zones	____	____	____
11. Masturbation	____	____	____
12. Sexual intercourse	____	____	____
13. Sexual variations	____	____	____

In reexamining your check marks, notice those areas where you feel you may need more information. For each of these, answer the following questions:

1. What are the personal implications in my wanting to understand this topic better?

2. Do I intend to seek more information on the topic?

3. Where will I look for more information on this topic?

You will learn more about all of these areas as you read this chapter.

erably longer than Y chromosomes and carry more **genes** (*jēnz*), the basic units of heredity.

The female's sex cells, or **ova (eggs),** each carry a single X chromosome. The male's sex cells, or **sperm,** carry either an X chromosome or a Y chromosome. If a sperm cell fertilizing an egg carries an X chromosome, the offspring will be female (XX). If the sperm cell carries a Y chromosome, the

offspring will be male (XY). The sex of the offspring is thus determined by which type of chromosome (X or Y) the male supplies.

Both XX and XY offspring develop identically for about the first seven weeks. At that point, a gene carried on the Y chromosome becomes active, which leads to the development of **testes** (*tes´tēs*), the male sex glands, and the embryo differentiates into a male. In the absence of this particular gene, **ovaries** (*ō´va-rēz*), the female sex

genes basic units of heredity located on chromosomes.

ova (eggs) female sex cells; ova is the plural of ovum.

sperm male sex cell.

testes male sex glands.

ovaries female sex glands.

EFFECT OF SEX CHROMOSOMES ON GONAD DEVELOPMENT AND SEX DIFFERENTIATION

Humans cannot survive without any X chromosomes; however, they can survive with only one X chromosome. Since the female has no Y chromosome, humans can obviously survive without a Y chromosome.

Errors occasionally occur during cell division, creating sex cells that have either more or less than one chromosome.

An embryo having anywhere from one to three X chromosomes, but no Y, will develop as a female. When an embryo develops with any number of Y chromosomes present, it will develop some male characteristics. Some persons may have one Y chromosome and more than one X, giving combinations such as XXY, XXXY, and XXXXY.

Total Chromosomes	Chromosomes	Gonad Produced	Gender of Individual	Condition	Effects on Genitals
45	X	ovary	female	Turner's Syndrome	Defective ovary
46	XX	ovary	female	normal	—
46	XY	testis	male	normal	—
47	XXX	ovary	female	Triple X Syndrome	No sex abnormality
47	XXY	testis	male	Klinefelter's Syndrome	Genitals are small and do not produce sperm
47	XYY	testis	male	XYY Syndrome	Sperm production reduced; may be sterile
48 and 49	XXXY XXXXY	testis	male	Variations of Klinefelter's Syndrome	Genitals are small and do not produce sperm

glands, develop. Sometimes cells divide improperly, resulting in the presence of an extra sex chromosome. This occurs in chromosomal abnormalities such as XXY or XXX (see Feature 6.1).

Gonadal (Sex Gland) Determinants

From conception to the fourth week of development, an embryo develops no sex organs. From the fourth to the sixth week of development, tissue that will become **gonads** (*gō'nadz*), either testes or ovaries, begins to form. If a Y chromosome is present, testes begin to develop during the sixth week. If, on the other hand, the embryo carries two X chromosomes, ovaries begin to develop several weeks later. If a female possesses only a single X chromosome and no Y chromosome, ovaries will not develop normally; the offspring may be mentally impaired and will be unable to reproduce as an adult.

Hormonal and Genital Determinants

The presence of specific hormones in the embryo also influences gender development. The testes begin to produce a hormone called **testosterone** (*tes-tos'ter-ōn*) early in their development. A masculinizing hormone, testosterone promotes the development of male genitals and reproductive structures and inhibits female development. Sexual development in a female does not rely on the presence of hormones. If testosterone is absent, female genitals and reproductive structures develop. Thus, testosterone is the critical factor in determining gender development.

SOCIAL AND PSYCHOLOGICAL FACTORS

At the time of birth, a newborn is assigned a sex based on the appearance of his or her genitals. This identification usually corresponds with the

gonads male and female sex glands.

testosterone a male sex hormone produced primarily in the testes.

child's genetic gender, though certain infrequent chromosomal abnormalities are exceptions. While a child's sex is determined prenatally, postnatal factors can have a profound effect on his or her gender development.

Gender Identity

A person's sense of being a male or a female is his or her **gender identity.** Gender identity is the result of a series of developmental events that may or may not correspond with his or her biological sex, although it ordinarily does. In some cases people feel uncertain about their gender identity; others become quite convinced they are of the other sex from that of their bodies. Confusion over gender identity is known as **gender dysphoria** (*dis-fō′ri-a*). An individual who is convinced that his or her true gender is the opposite of his or her anatomical sex is known as a **transsexual.** Transsexuality is not to be confused with homosexuality, bisexuality, or **transvestism** (*trans-vest′izm*) (sexual pleasure derived from cross-dressing). Transsexuals often feel that they are "trapped" in the body of the wrong sex; many seek surgical reassignment, or "sex changes," so that their bodies correspond with their sexual identities.

Although no one knows exactly how gender identity develops, it is accepted that the way a child is raised plays a dominant role in its formation. Gender identity is well developed by the age of four, and is not easily changed once it is established.[2]

Gender Roles

The way in which you behave as a male or a female is your **gender role.** The way in which you

....

gender identity an individual's sense of being male or female.

gender dysphoria confusion over one's gender identity.

transsexual an individual with a persistent sense of discomfort with his or her biological gender.

transvestism deriving sexual pleasure from dressing in the clothing of the other sex.

gender role a person's masculine or feminine behavior and appearance, as viewed in context of cultural classification.

perceive your gender role affects every aspect of your life. Our perceptions of others' gender roles are initially based on actions, mannerisms, and appearances; we judge how the behavior of others corresponds with our expectations. We judge the masculinity and femininity of people by how closely they correspond to our behavioral anticipations for each gender. Such anticipations affect how we relate to others in the home environment and the workplace.

Gender Role Identification

To varying degrees, people conform to cultural expectations of their gender. For example, some people may expect males to be assertive, competitive, and controlling, with little display of emotions; we may expect females to be sympathetic, caring, compassionate, beautiful in appearance, and sexually appealing. How an individual incorporates these cultural expectations into his or her personality is known as his or her **gender role identification.** A male or female may conform to these expectations or may reject them, preferring to adopt certain behaviors usually associated with the other sex. Males may be both aggressive and tender, and females may be both active and nurturing. Flexibility in gender roles by an individual is known as **androgyny** (*an-droj′i-nē*). In North America, it is currently accepted that behaviors and traits traditionally viewed as either masculine or feminine may be integrated into the personalities of people of both sexes, helping to produce well-rounded, fully functioning individuals. Androgyny permits an individual to choose behaviors from the complete range of human behaviors rather than limiting behavior to that traditionally associated with his or her assigned gender.

In her classic work, *Sex and Temperament in Three Primitive Societies,* Margaret Mead found wide cultural differences among three societies in New Guinea. Among the Mundugumor people, both males and females exhibited aggressive, nonnurturing behavior. Contrarily, both sexes among

....

gender role identification how a person incorporates expected gender roles into his or her personality.

androgyny an openness to and acceptance of one's own feminine and masculine nature.

There are few jobs/professional roles today that can be classified: "For women only." or "For men only." There is little to prevent either sex from participating in the full range of opportunities.

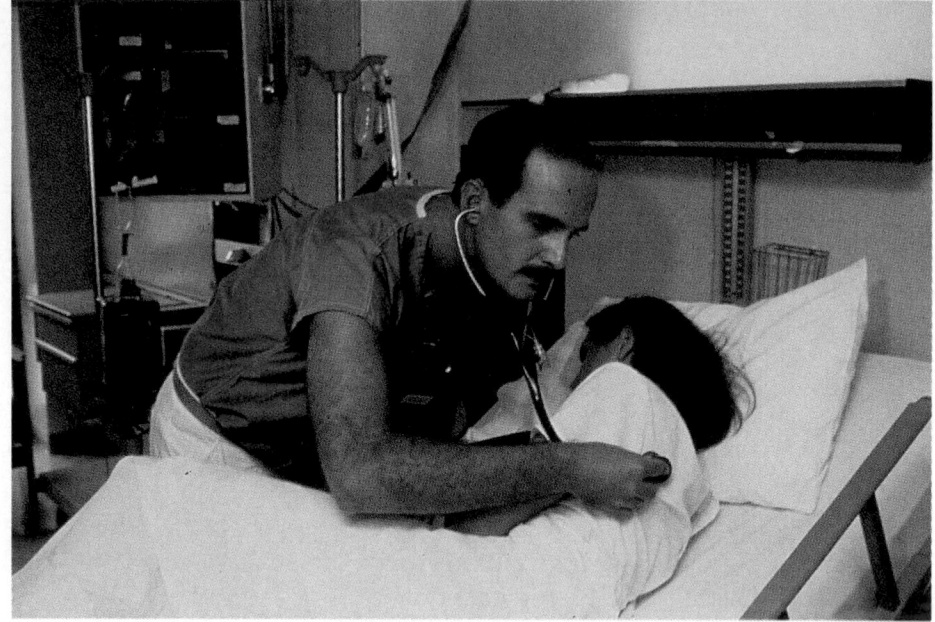

the Arapesh were gentle, nurturing, and nonaggressive. The Tchambuli culture exhibited yet a third pattern, in which traditional male and female behavioral patterns were a reversal of the typical American society.[3]

Gender Stereotypes

Gender stereotypes are oversimplified generalizations about male and female behaviors. These stereotypes are based on a person's values, behavior, and personality. Parents begin molding their children according to these stereotypes at an early age. Parents may be dismayed if their daughter is a tomboy or their son prefers quiet play to traditional "little boy" activities. The sexual revolution of the 1960s and 1970s fostered increased flexibility regarding sex and gender, but some gender role expectations are still ingrained in people, perpetuating gender stereotyping.[4]

CHECKPOINT

1. Describe the difference between the X and Y sex chromosomes, and state the kinds of sex chromosomes carried by male and female sex cells.

2. Distinguish among gonadal, hormonal, and genital determinants in the development of an embryo and fetus.

3. Define the term *gender identity*.

4. Discuss gender roles and gender role identification. Explain the difference between the two terms.

5. Explain how gender stereotyping differs from gender role identification.

SEXUAL ORIENTATION

As sexual beings, it is natural that humans are sexually attracted to others. An individual's sexual attraction to others of the same sex, other sex, or both sexes is known as his or her **sexual orientation,** as described in Chapter 5. To review, sexual orientation toward those of the other sex is known as heterosexuality, while attraction to members of the same sex is called homosexuality; orientation toward members of both sexes is known as bisexuality.

Until the beginning of this century, it was thought that people were clearly either homosexual or heterosexual.[5] Sexual orientation is now commonly viewed as a continuum, a wide range of

....

sexual orientation an individual's attraction to persons of the same, opposite, or both sexes.

behaviors between the two extremes of exclusive heterosexuality (0 on the scale) and exclusive homosexuality (6 on the scale),[6] with varying degrees of bisexuality being rated as 1–5 (see Figure 6.1).

Determining a person's place along the continuum of sexual behavior depends, in part, on his or her attraction to or sexual activities with members of both sexes. These behaviors may vary over a person's life span. Some people may shift their sexual orientation, such as from exclusive heterosexuality to some degree of bisexuality.[7] Another determinant of a person's placement on the continuum of sexual behavior is how others perceive him or her. Perceptions of others are based on mannerisms (masculine or feminine), choice of sex partners, and occupation, among other considerations. Another element used to determine a person's placement on the continuum is his or her self-perceptions. A person may engage in homosexual activities, yet not see him- or herself as homosexual. Others, however, may categorize such an individual as homosexual. Fear of publicly acknowledging homosexuality may cause some individuals to attempt to replace their homosexual urges with heterosexual marriage and parenting. Conversely, a person who is regarded as homosexual may wish for heterosexual contact, yet fear the rejection of his or her homosexual friends. Lastly, sexual orientation may change with time. Accordingly, any positioning of a person on the continuum is not firmly fixed.

DEVELOPMENT OF SEXUAL ORIENTATION

At what point does a person become aware of his or her sexual orientation? How does it develop? For some people, sexual orientation is determined by age 4 or 5; others, however, do not fully define their sexual orientation until adolescence, early adulthood, or even later. Some people who experiment with homosexual activity as adolescents may become confirmed heterosexuals. Conversely, men and women may marry and have children, and later confirm their homosexual orientations.

Theories regarding the development of sexual orientation vary and fall into several categories. One theory contends that sexual orientation is biological. During the last decade, the belief that biology plays some role in a person's sexual orientation has gained some acceptance. Evidence of such influence comes from studies linking the differences in the size of the brain to sexual orientation, and from studies showing that identical twins, who are genetically alike, have a greater similarity in their sexual orientation than do fraternal twins, who are not genetically alike. However, there is no evidence of differences of chromosomes or genes between people of various sexual orientations, whether heterosexual, bisexual, or homosexual. While the influence of some yet-to-be identified gene cannot be unequivocally ruled out, available evidence points to a nongenetic basis for sexual orientation. The role of sex hormones also has been researched, but conflicting information makes it difficult to draw valid conclusions.

Figure 6.1

A Continuum of Sexual Orientation

An individual's sexual attraction to persons of the opposite or same sex can be described as a scale, or continuum, between 0 (exclusively heterosexual) and 6 (exclusively homosexual).

Source: Adapted from Kinsey, A., et al. Sexual Behavior in the Human Male. Philadelphia: Saunders, 1948.

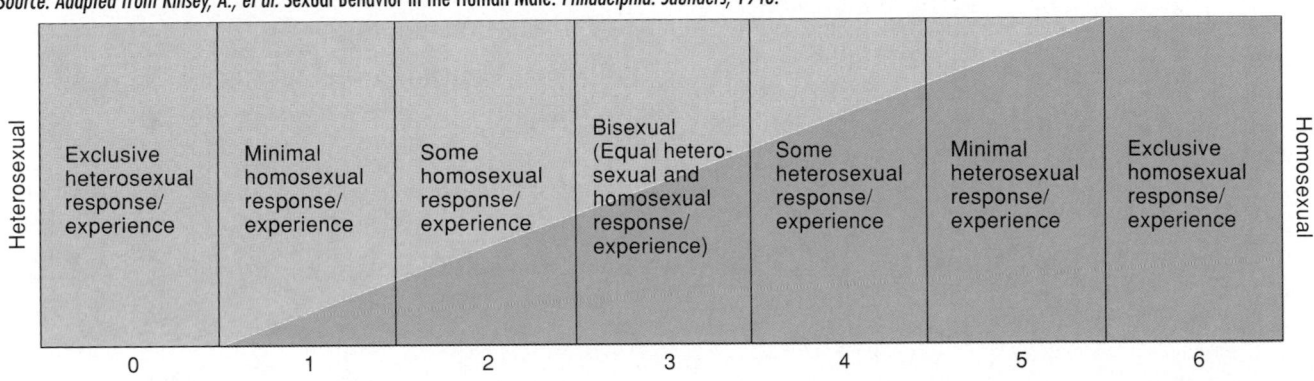

Another theory suggests that sexual orientation is psychologically based. Some contend that unresolved sexual attraction to a parent of the opposite sex, known as an Oedipus complex in males and an Electra complex in females, can create such fear in a child that he or she is unable to develop and maintain heterosexual relationships later in life.

The percentage of males in a given society who engage in homosexual activity at some time in their lives varies widely among cultures. In the Melanesian island society of East Bay, the percentage of males who engage in homosexual activity is almost 100 percent;[8] among the Mangaia islanders of Polynesia, virtually no males participate in it.[9] The So people of Uganda do not practice homosexual activity,[10] although homosexual relations among Sambia people of New Guinea is a normal activity of young males before they marry, after which they give it up for exclusively heterosexual behavior.[11, 12]

Because sexual expectations for males and females differ from culture to culture, another theory speculates that cultural factors influence sexual orientation. Although all cultures share the expectation that males and females will live together and produce children, most cultures also have elements of homosexual behavior. In North America, for example, **fellatio,** or oral stimulation of the male's genitals, between males is viewed as a homosexual act, while in New Guinea, it is viewed as a rite of passage for adolescent boys into male adulthood.[13]

There is no conclusive evidence to support any one of these theories over another. It is possible that biological, psychological, and cultural factors all play a part in the development of sexual orientation and homosexuality.

CHECKPOINT

1. Discuss the concept of the continuum of sexual orientation.

2. Describe the various theories regarding the development of sexual orientation.

3. Compare homosexual behavior among different cultures.

fellatio oral stimulation of the male's genitals.

SEXUAL ANATOMY AND PHYSIOLOGY

The entire body is involved in eliciting a sexual response. When a person's sexual organs are stimulated, all parts of the body—including the mind, glands, and skin—become involved in producing a pleasurable response. Central to the sexual experience are the brain, the body's sex hormones, the reproductive organs, and the genitals.

GONADOTROPINS

The hypothalamus is a portion of the brain that interacts with the pituitary gland, thereby controlling the body's reproductive system and sexual processes. The pituitary is a small gland, located at the base of the brain, which produces a number of hormones that regulate various processes and other glands, including the testes and ovaries. The hypothalamus initiates activity by releasing a hormone called **gonadotropin-releasing hormone** (GnRH) (*gon'a-dō-trō'pin*). When released, GnRH stimulates the pituitary gland to secrete two **gonadotropins,** hormones that affect the gonads. Females produce the gonadotropins **follicle-stimulating hormone (FSH)** and **luteinizing hormone (LH)** (*lū'tē-in-ī-zing*); males produce FSH and **interstitial-cell-stimulating hormone (ICSH)** (*in'ter-stish'al*). Under the influence of these gonadotropins, the testes and ovaries produce hormones that control the sex organs and influence the activity of the brain.

gonadotropin-releasing hormone (GnRH) hypothalamic hormone that acts on the pituitary gland.

gonadotropins hormones secreted by the pituitary gland that act on the gonads.

follicle-stimulating hormone (FSH) a gonadotropin that stimulates the ovary to produce a follicle in the female and sperm in the male.

luteinizing hormone (LH) a gonadotropin that stimulates the ovary to release an ovum.

interstitial-cell-stimulating hormone (ICSH) a gonadotropin that stimulates the testes to secrete testosterone.

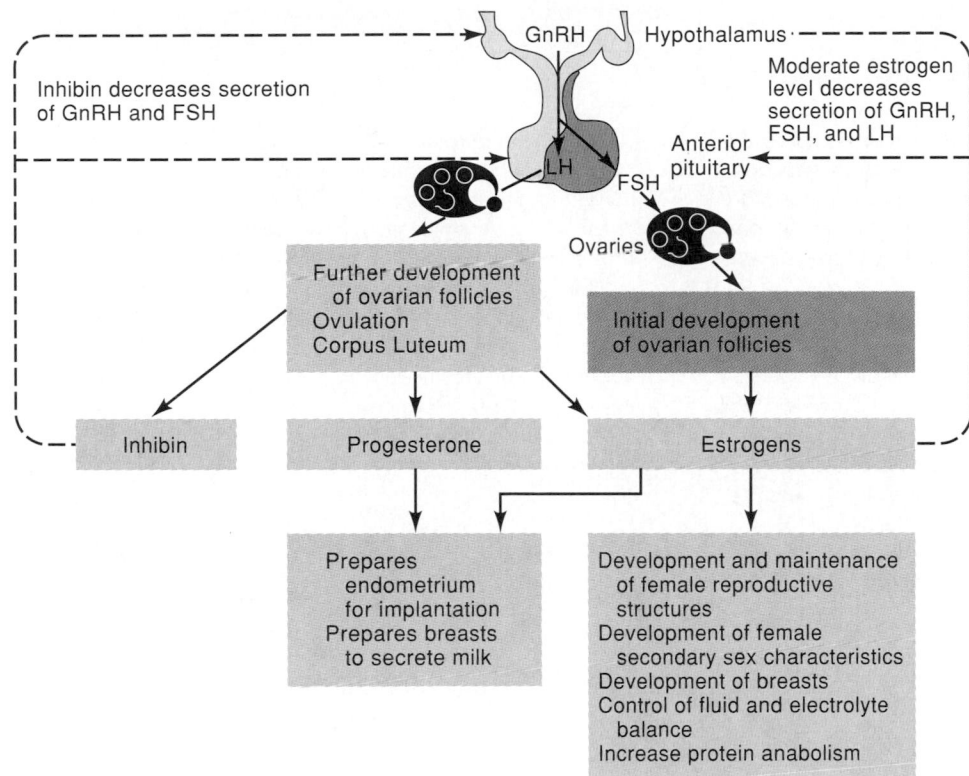

Figure 6.2

Hormonal Control of the Reproductive System in the Female

The human reproductive system functions under the control of a sequence of hormones.

Follicle-Stimulating Hormone

When the hypothalamus secretes GnRH, the pituitary is signaled to release FSH (see Figure 6.2). In the female, FSH stimulates the ovaries, leading to the maturation of ovum-containing follicles which secrete estrogens; in the male, FSH stimulates the testes to produce sperm.

Luteinizing Hormone

Upon the release of GnRH by the female's hypothalamus, the pituitary gland releases LH. LH causes the ovary to release an ovum from the ovary, a process known as **ovulation** (*ov-ū-lā'shun*). Once the egg is released, the empty follicle becomes a yellow mass known as the **corpus luteum** (*kor'-pus lū'tē-um*).

FSH and LH stimulate the ovaries to produce the hormones **estrogen** (*es'trō-jen*) and **progesterone** (*prō-jes'ter-ōn*). Estrogen is responsible at puberty for the development of female body characteristics such as breasts and fat deposits on the hips and abdomen. It also stimulates the development of the reproductive organs and the restoration of the uterine lining following menstrual discharge. Progesterone prepares the uterus for pregnancy and causes the breasts to enlarge in preparation for breastfeeding. The levels of both estrogen and progesterone provide feedback to the pituitary gland, helping control the release of FSH and LH. The corpus luteum secretes the hormone **inhibin** (*in-hib'in*). This hormone inhibits

ovulation the periodic release of an ovum (egg) from the ovary.

corpus luteum a yellow mass formed from an empty ovarian follicle after ovulation.

estrogen a hormone that stimulates development of the female reproductive tract and body characteristics.

progesterone a hormone that prepares the uterus for pregnancy and causes the breasts to enlarge in preparation for breastfeeding.

inhibin a hormone secreted by the gonads that inhibits FSH by the pituitary and GnRH release by the hypothalamus.

FEATURE 6.2

IS CIRCUMCISION NECESSARY?

The surgical removal of the foreskin of the penis is called *circumcision.* This minor surgical procedure is usually done within a day or two of the male baby's birth; the procedure exposes the glans of the penis. Circumcision is usually performed for health reasons or as a religious ritual by followers of Islam and of the Jewish faith.

Circumcision performed for hygienic reasons is based on the belief that *smegma,* an odorous cheesy-like substance secreted beneath the foreskin, collects beneath the foreskin and causes infections. Circumcision makes the penile glans easier to clean and as a result, smegma does not collect and inflammation and infections of the glans are less likely to occur. Also, with circumcision, cancer of the penis is less likely to occur.

In recent years, there have been a flurry of reports critical of routine circumcision. Arguments range from psycho-

logical trauma to reduced sensitivity to touch. These criticisms led the American Academy of Pediatrics to conclude, in 1975, that there was no absolute medical need for routine circumcision. As a consequence, the percentage of male babies being circumcised dropped.

Recently, a growing body of evidence has caused the Academy to revise its position. Studies show a link between noncircumcised boys and dangerous urinary tract infections. Not only do uncircumcised boys develop infections 10 times more often than circumcised boys, but one-third of those infected develop complications. Conversely, only 1 in 1000 boys have circumcision complications.

Source: "Report of Task Force on Circumcision." *Pediatrics* Vol. 4 (August 1989), 388–391.

secretion of FSH and GnRH, and, to a lesser degree, LH.

Interstitial Hormone

When GnRH is released in the male, it signals the pituitary gland to secrete ICSH, which then stimulates the interstitial cells of the testes to produce testosterone, the primary male sex hormone. Testosterone is essential for pubertal development of the male physique, male genitals, the larynx and vocal cords, and pubic and body hair. Testosterone, which is also produced in lesser amounts by the adrenal glands, in both males and females, is also responsible for the sexual drive of both males and females.

MALE SEXUAL SYSTEM

The male sexual system is composed of the penis, scrotum, testes, ducts, and fluid-producing glands (see Figure 6.3). For their own sexual wellness and pleasuring, it is important that men understand and feel comfortable with their sex organs.

Penis

The most conspicuous external organ of the male genitals is the **penis** (*pē'nis*). The penis is three to

four inches long when flaccid, and consists of three cylinders of spongy **erectile tissue.** When filled with blood, the erectile tissue causes the penis to enlarge to five to six inches in length and to become erect. The cone-shaped end of the penis is known as the **glans** or head. A loose flap of **foreskin** covers the glans. This flap of skin is often surgically removed during a procedure known as **circumcision** (see Feature 6.2). A small slit-like opening at the end of the penis, called the external urethral orifice, allows for urine and semen to pass out of the body.

Scrotum

Behind the penis is the **scrotum** (*skrō'tum*), or scrotal sac, which contains two testes. This thin-walled pouch is lightly covered with hair in adults and its skin contains many sweat glands. To pro-

....

erectile tissue tissue that becomes firm when it fills with blood.

glans the head of the penis (in the male), and of the clitoris (in the female).

foreskin a loose fold of skin covering the glans.

circumcision the surgical removal of part or all of the foreskin.

penis an external male genital organ through which urine and semen pass.

scrotum thin, loose pouch of skin that contains the testes.

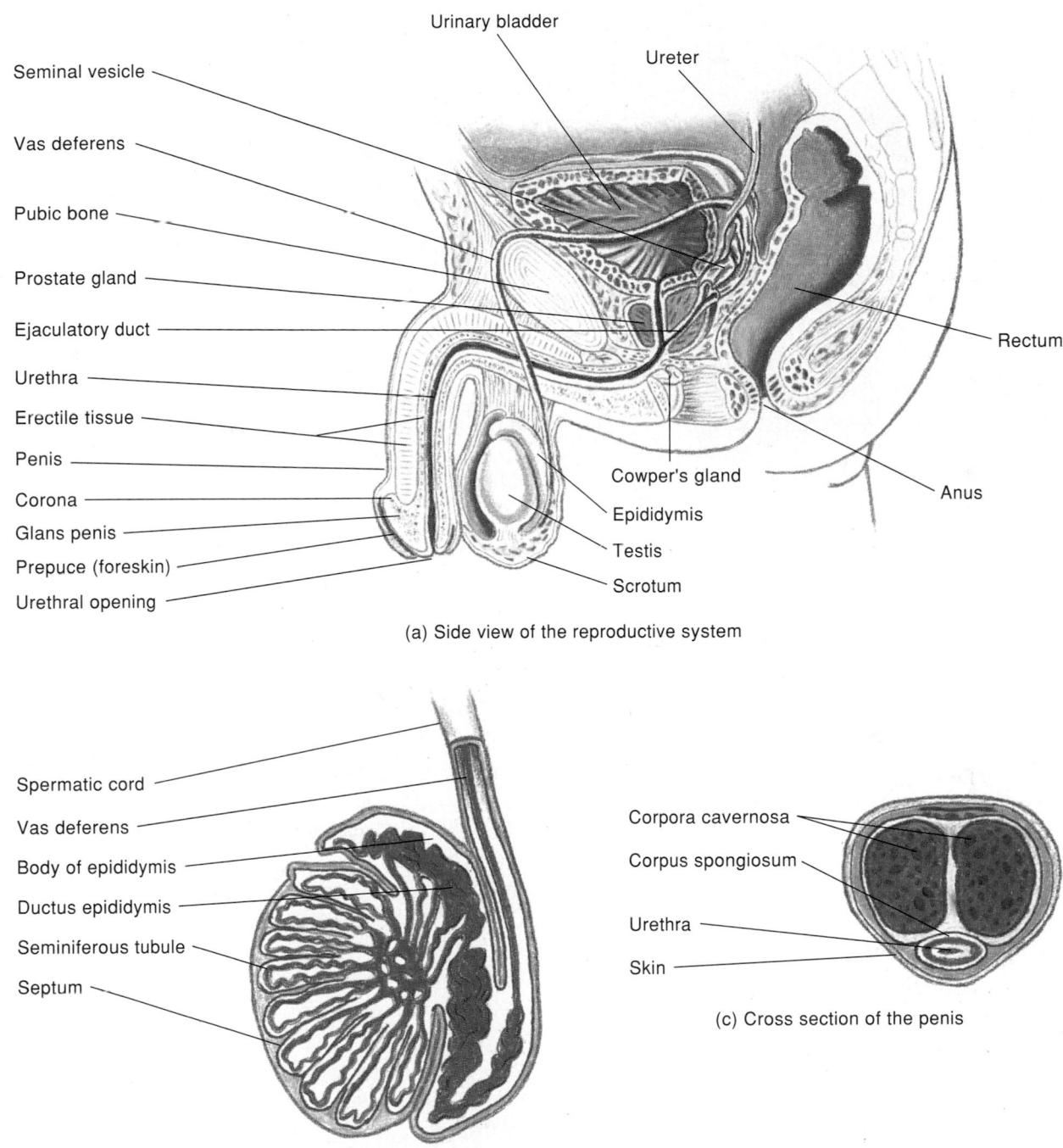

Urinary bladder

Ureter

Seminal vesicle

Vas deferens

Pubic bone

Prostate gland

Ejaculatory duct

Urethra

Erectile tissue

Penis

Corona

Glans penis

Prepuce (foreskin)

Urethral opening

Rectum

Cowper's gland

Epididymis

Testis

Scrotum

Anus

(a) Side view of the reproductive system

Spermatic cord

Vas deferens

Body of epididymis

Ductus epididymis

Seminiferous tubule

Septum

(b) Cutaway view of the testes

Corpora cavernosa

Corpus spongiosum

Urethra

Skin

(c) Cross section of the penis

Figure 6.3
Male Reproductive System and Surrounding Structures

(a) Side view of the male reproductive system. (b) Cutaway view of the testes. (c) Cross section of the penis.

Sources: Masters, W., Johnson, V., and Kolodny, R. Human Sexuality, 4th ed. New York: HarperCollins, 1992; Tortora, G., and Grabowsky, S. Principles of Anatomy and Physiology, 7th ed. New York: HarperCollins, 1993.

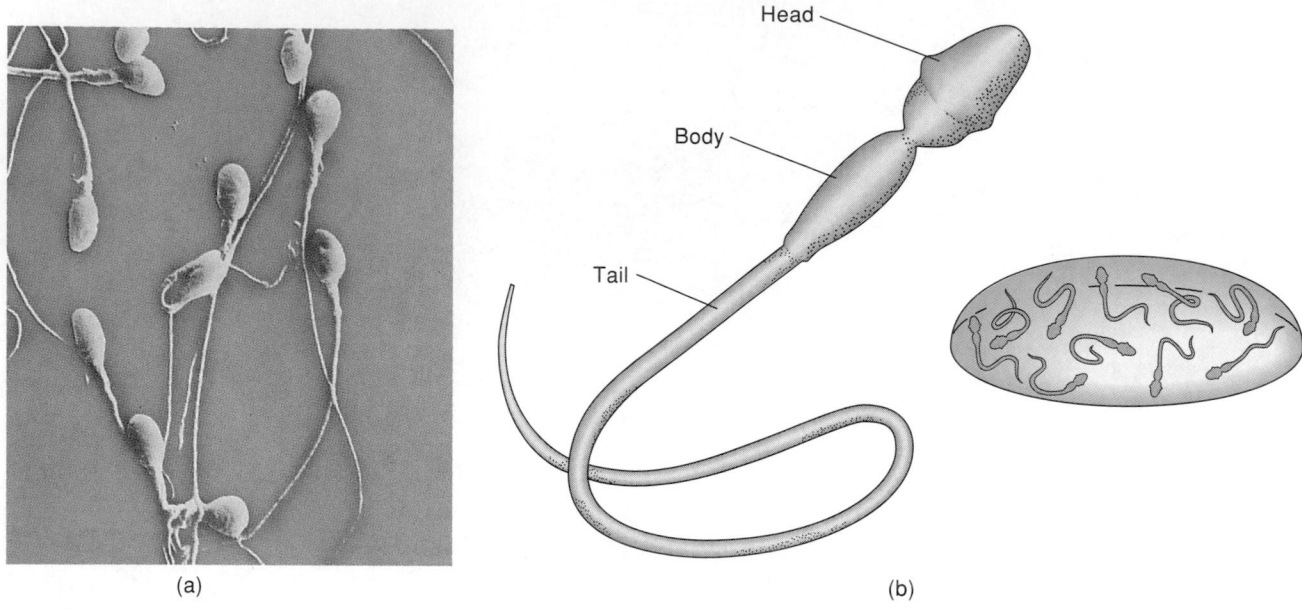

(a)

(b)

Figure 6.4
The Human Sperm

(a) An electromicrophotograph of a human sperm. (b) A rendering of the human sperm as seen in a drop of fluid and in detail.

duce viable sperm, the testes must maintain a temperature that is three to four degrees (Fahrenheit) cooler than body temperature. To aid in maintaining the proper temperature, the scrotum is suspended from the body; it hangs limply when warm, and draws closer to the body when cool.

Testes

The two testes produce sperm (see Figure 6.4) within a network of many threadlike **seminiferous tubules,** as well as the hormone testosterone. Sperm production begins early in puberty and continues until a man reaches his seventies and eighties. The hormone FSH stimulates the production of about 240 million sperm daily.

Duct Structures

Several ducts in the male sexual system store and transport sperm. These are the **epididymis** (*ep'i-did'i-mis*), the **vas deferens** (*vas def'er-enz*), the

seminiferous tubules highly coiled tubules in the testes that produce sperm.

epididymis a tightly coiled tube alongside the testis that stores sperm.

vas deferens a tube that carries sperm upward from each epididymis to the ejaculatory duct.

ejaculatory duct, and the **urethra** (*ū-rē'thra*). The epididymis is a tightly coiled tube that lies along the back of each testis. It is the site where sperm are stored and mature. The epididymis also forms a connection between the testis and the vas deferens. Each vas deferens is a tube about 18 inches in length. The vas deferens carries sperm from the epididymis through the body wall into the abdominal cavity. Near the termination of the vas deferens, it joins with the duct from the seminal vesicle to become the ejaculatory duct. In each ejaculatory duct, sperm mix with fluid from the seminal vesicles to form semen. The urethra runs from the urinary bladder through the **prostate gland** to the tip of the penis. In the prostate gland, the two ejaculatory ducts join the urethra. Since the urethra carries, at different times, both urine and semen, there are valves that prevent the two from mixing.

ejaculatory duct the near end of the vas deferens that joins with the urethra, where sperm mixes with seminal vesicle fluid.

urethra duct for the discharge of urine from the bladder and the carrying of semen.

prostate gland a gland that surrounds the neck of the bladder and urethra, and that secretes a fluid portion of semen.

Fluid-Producing Glands

The **seminal vesicles** (*sem'in-al*), the prostate gland, and the **Cowper's glands** (*kow'perz*) all produce fluid that becomes a part of semen. The paired seminal vesicles produce a fluid that activates sperm, increasing their capacity to swim. The prostate gland is a doughnut-shaped structure that surrounds the urethra and produces fluid that also enhances the movement of sperm. The paired Cowper's glands are located directly below the prostate gland. When a male is sexually aroused, the Cowper's glands secrete a small amount of clear, sticky preejaculatory fluid, which appears at the tip of the penis prior to ejaculation. Cowper's fluid neutralizes any urine that might remain in the urethra prior to ejaculation. Cowper's fluid may also carry sperm cells, making it possible for a female to be impregnated even if her partner withdraws his penis from the vagina before he ejaculates (see Chapter 7).

Semen

Semen (*sē'men*) is a grayish-white fluid that is ejaculated during orgasm. The number of sperm in semen is highly variable. At a volume of two to five milliliters of semen per ejaculate, the number of sperm in a single ejaculation may range from 140 to 350 million cells.

Ejaculation

Ejaculation (*ē-jak-ū-lā'shun*), the ejection of semen from the urethra, occurs in two stages. During the first stage, called *emission,* the ducts contract and the fluid-producing glands move semen into the urethra; this occurs when a male is about to climax. In the second stage, called *expulsion,* semen spurts from the penis. The rhythmic con-

tractions that cause the ejaculation are accompanied by the sudden release of neuromuscular tension perceived as intensely pleasurable sensations called **orgasm** (*or'gazm*), or the climax. Once the sperm is deposited into the vagina, its cells can survive for 48–72 hours. Sometimes, in the young adolescent, ejaculation occurs during sleep. Known as a **nocturnal emission,** or "wet dream," such an ejaculation is a normal process.

CHECKPOINT

1. Describe the types of gonadotropins, their sites of production, and their target sites in both males and females.

2. Name and describe the external organs of the male genitals.

3. How many sperm may a male produce daily?

4. List the three ducts in the male sexual system, and the three fluid-producing glands that help produce semen.

5. Describe what semen is. How many milliliters of semen might each ejaculate contain, and how many sperm cells might be contained in each ejaculate?

FEMALE SEXUAL SYSTEM

The female sexual system is more complex than that of the male because of the female's capacity for childbirth. The reproductive events in a woman's body follow a monthly cycle known as the **menstrual cycle.** Whereas the male can produce **viable** sex cells (those capable of living) daily, the female produces viable ova only one or two days per month.

---

seminal vesicles glands that produce fluid that activates sperm and increases their capacity to swim.

Cowper's glands paired glands located beneath the prostate gland on either side of the urethra which secrete preejaculatory fluid.

semen a grayish-white, sticky mixture of sperm and seminal fluid discharged from the urethra of the male during ejaculation.

ejaculation the sudden ejection of semen from the penis that occurs at the peak of sexual arousal; occurs in two stages, emission and expulsion.

orgasm the highly pleasurable body response that occurs at the climax of sexual arousal as the result of the sudden release of neuromuscular tension.

nocturnal emission an involuntary orgasm that occurs during sleep, usually associated with an erotic dream; also called a "wet dream."

menstrual cycle the monthly reproductive cycle in women that begins with the menstruation.

viable capable of living.

Figure 6.5
Side View of the Female Reproductive System

Source: Masters, W., Johnson, V., and Kolodny, R. Human Sexuality, 4th ed. New York: HarperCollins, 1992; Tortora, G., and Grabowsky, S. Principles of Anatomy and Physiology, 7th ed. New York: Harper-Collins, 1993.

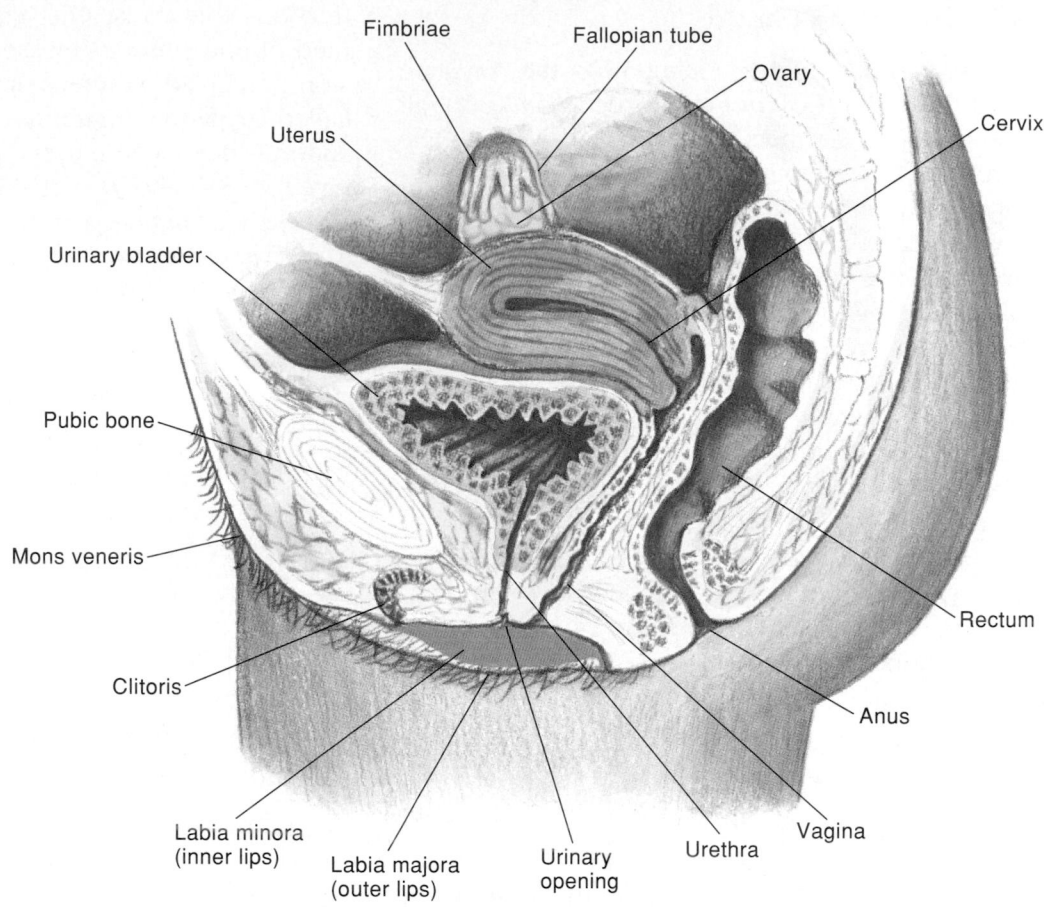

The female's sex organs, or genitals, include the following structures: the *mons veneris* and *labia,* the *vestibular structures,* the *uterus,* the *fallopian tubes,* and the *ovaries* (see Figure 6.5). For their sexual wellness and pleasuring, women need to understand their sex organs and feel comfortable with them.

Mons Veneris and Labia

The **mons veneris** (*monz ve-nē'ris*), also called the mons pubis, is the fatty pad that lies beneath a woman's pubic hair. The mons veneris divides and extends back to form the two **labia majora** (*lā'bi-a ma-jor'a*), or outer lips of the **vagina** (*va-jī'na*), the tubular passageway leading to the uterus.

These two thick, fleshy folds may be sparsely covered with pubic hair. Between the two outer lips is the slit-like *pudendal cleft* (*pū-den'dal*). Lining the inside of the cleft are two folds of erectile tissue known as the **labia minora** (*mi-nor'a*), or inner lips of the vagina. Recessed between these inner lips is a shallow cavity, or **vestibule,** in which the small, sensitive **clitoris** (*klīt'ō-ris*), urethral opening, and vaginal opening are located.

Vestibular Structures

The clitoris is a highly sensitive mass of erectile tissue and nerves. Resembling a tiny penis, this organ lies in the front of the vestibule, an area between the labia minora. Only the head, or glans, of the

----

mons veneris fatty, hair-covered pad over the female's pubic bone.

labia majora the outer lips covering the vaginal opening.

vagina a tubular organ that forms a passageway between the vestibule and the uterus.

labia minora the inner lips covering the vaginal opening.

vestibule an area between the labia minora.

clitoris a small, sensitive structure near the front end of the vestibule.

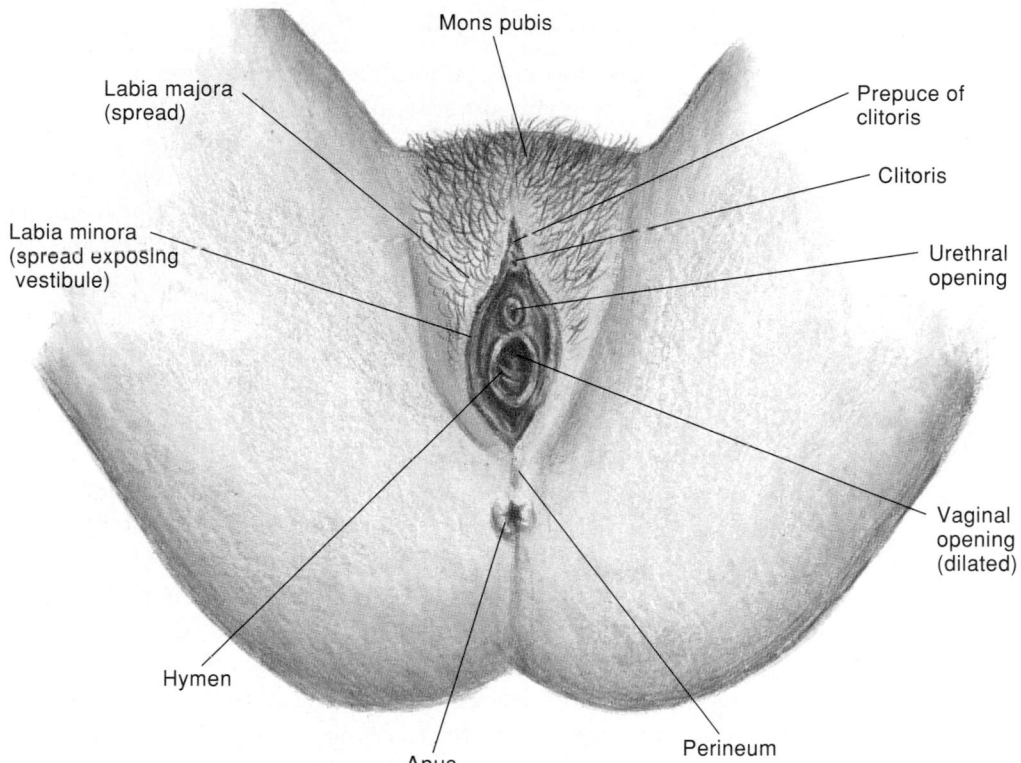

Mons pubis

Labia majora
(spread)

Prepuce of
clitoris

Clitoris

Labia minora
(spread exposing
vestibule)

Urethral
opening

Vaginal
opening
(dilated)

Hymen

Anus

Perineum

Figure 6.6
**External View of the
Female Genitals**

*Source: Masters, W., Johnson, V., and
Kolodny, R. Human Sexuality, 4th ed.
New York: HarperCollins, 1992; Torto-
ra, G., and Grabowsky, S. Principles of
Anatomy and Physiology, 7th ed. New
York: HarperCollins, 1993.*

clitoris is visible. When the female is sexually
aroused, the clitoris, like the penis, becomes erect
and hard. Stimulation of the clitoris generally leads
to female orgasm, which is the sudden release of
neuromuscular tensions and is perceived as
intensely pleasurable by the female. Below the clitoris is the tiny urethral opening, through which
urine is excreted.

The opening to the vagina is located at the
back of the vestibule. Located just behind the urinary bladder and urethra, the vagina serves as a
birth canal during childbirth and as a canal for the
monthly menstrual discharge. When the female is
sexually aroused, the vagina expands and its walls
secrete a lubricating fluid. This enables an erect
penis to enter. The vaginal opening in some
females is partially covered by a thin membrane
called the **hymen** (*hī'men*). The hymen usually
stretches easily when tampons are inserted or during masturbation, physical exercise, and sexual
intercourse.

Behind the vaginal opening is a flat section of
skin, the *perineum* (*per'i-nē'um*), which extends to

the anus. The perineum is sometimes surgically cut
to prevent tearing during childbirth in a procedure
known as an **episiotomy** (*e-pis'i-ot'ō-mē*). The
external genital structures of the female—the mons
veneris, the labia, and the vestibular structures—
are collectively known as the **vulva** (*vul'va*) (see
Figure 6.6).

Uterus

At the upper end of the vagina is an opening to the
uterus (*ū'ter-us*), also called the *womb*. The uterus
is a muscular, pear-shaped organ that is tipped forward over the top of the urinary bladder. The nonpregnant uterus is about the size of a fist; during
pregnancy, however, it expands to many times its
normal size to accommodate a growing fetus. During childbirth, the uterus contracts to expel the

episiotomy a surgical procedure in which the perineum is cut to facilitate childbirth.

vulva the external genitals of the female.

uterus a muscular, pear-shaped reproductive organ in
which the embryo and fetus develop.

hymen a thin membrane that partially covers the vagina.

fetus through the uterine neck, or **cervix** (*ser'viks*), and into the vagina.

The cervix is usually filled with mucus to prevent organisms from entering into the uterus. For conception to occur, this mucus must be dissolved by enzymes carried by sperm in order to allow them to penetrate it and enter the uterus.

Fallopian Tubes

Curving out from either side of the uterus are two 4-inch ducts, or **fallopian** (*fa-lō'pi-an*) **tubes.** The outer portion of each of these tubes is funnel-shaped and lies close to an ovary. The rim of each funnel is fringed with fingerlike projections.

Once every month, an ovum, or egg, is released from one of the two ovaries of a sexually mature female. The ovum is drawn into one of the two fallopian tubes, and muscular contractions of the walls of the tubes push the ovum toward the uterus. The process of moving the ovum through the fallopian tube takes approximately 3–4 days. During this time, sperm that may be in the fallopian tube may fertilize the ovum.

Ovaries

In sexually mature women, the two almond-shaped ovaries produce ova or eggs, as well as estrogen and progesterone. The ovaries are located in the female's pelvic cavity, and contain a lifetime's supply of immature ova; at birth, the ovaries contain about 2 million potential ova.

Each ovum is surrounded by a thin tissue, or **follicle** (*fo'lik-al*). During puberty, the first of the immature ova begin to develop. Once every month, one or more mature follicles, known as a *graafian* (*grā'fē-an*) *follicle,* rupture on the surface of the ovary and release their ova. During ovulation, a woman may experience transient abdominal pain, called *mittelschmerz* (*mit'el-shmārts*), as the follicle ruptures.

....

cervix the neck of the uterus.

fallopian tubes a pair of ducts that connect the ovary to the uterus.

follicle a small cavity in the ovary in which the ovum is located.

Menstrual Cycle

The monthly sequence of reproductive events in a sexually mature woman is collectively known as the menstrual cycle. The timing and sequence of events in the menstrual cycle are governed by hormones released from three sites: the hypothalamus, the pituitary gland, and the ovaries. Each month, the inner lining of the uterus prepares for a pregnancy. If pregnancy does not occur, the lining is shed and later replaced. The breakdown and loss of the inner uterine lining, or **endometrial tissue** (*en'dō-mē'tri-al*), and blood is called **menstruation** ("the period").

A woman typically experiences her first menstrual cycle between the ages of 12 and 13 years, though menstruation may begin as early as 10 years or as late as 16 years. This first menstrual cycle is known as **menarche** (*men-ar'kē*). After menarche, some girls may be *anovulatory* (*an-ov'ū-la-tō'rē*) (without ovulation) for a year or longer until their hormonal cycles become regular. A female's menstrual cycle ceases, usually between the ages of 45 and 50; this cessation of menstruation is known as **menopause** (*men'ō-pawz*), or "the change of life." Menopause is characterized by the loss of reproductive capacity, a thinning of the vaginal walls, and atrophy of the ovaries and uterus. Some women also experience unpleasant symptoms such as "hot flashes," irritability, and weight gain; these symptoms often disappear when the woman's body becomes accustomed to its new hormonal balance.

The length of the average menstrual cycle is approximately 28 days. While a few women consistently experience regular 28-day cycles, most women experience fluctuations of 2–8 days between their longest and shortest cycles. Other women's cycles vary even more widely.

The menstrual cycle consists of three phases (Figure 6.7), with the first day of menstrual bleeding

....

endometrial tissue the tissue located in the inner lining of the uterus.

menstruation the monthly shedding and discharge of endometrial tissue and blood from the uterus.

menarche the first menstrual period of a female during puberty.

menopause the period that marks the permanent cessation of menstrual activity.

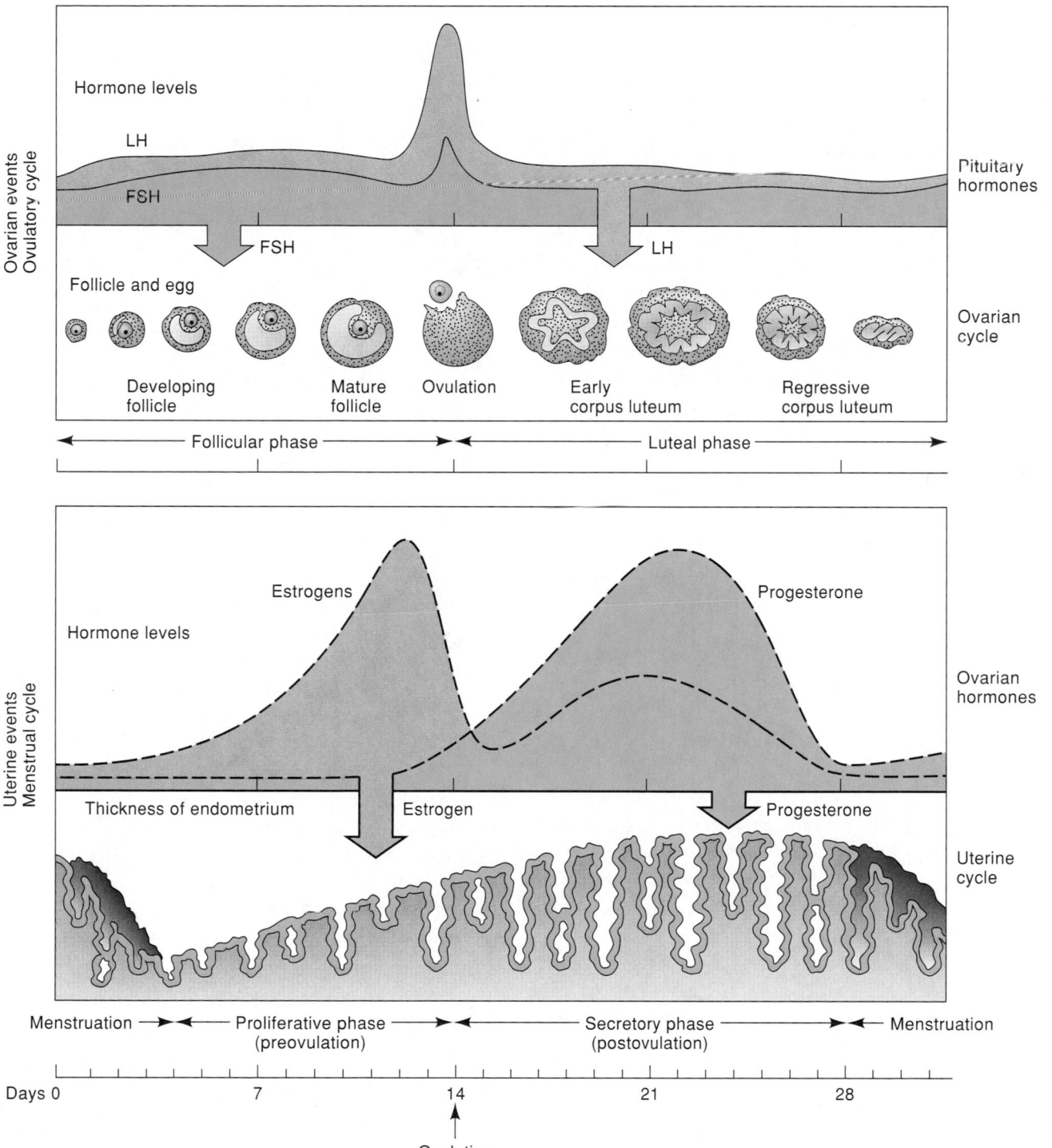

Figure 6.7
Monthly Reproductive Events in the Adult Female

The ovary and uterus go through monthly changes in response to hormonal secretions. Top: the pituitary gland releases the hormones FSH and LH, which stimulate the ovarian follicle to develop and release a mature egg (ovum). The follicle develops during the follicular phase and degenerates during the luteal phase. Bottom: the ovarian follicle produces and releases the hormones estrogen and progesterone, which prepare the endometrium to receive the fertilized egg. The endometrium builds up during the proliferative phase, secretes fluids during the secretory phase, and then degenerates during menstruation (the menstrual phase).

Source: Tortora, G., and Grabowsky, S. Principles of Anatomy and Physiology, 7th ed. New York: HarperCollins, 1993.

considered the first day of the cycle. The first phase is the *menstrual phase,* lasting 4 to 6 days; the second is the *proliferative phase* (preovulatory), lasting a week or longer; and the third is the *secretory phase* (postovulatory) lasting about 2 weeks. Each phase is characterized by different hormonal secretions.

The menstrual phase occurs when the uterine lining is shed. During menstruation, a woman loses a total of approximately one-fourth to one-half cup of blood and uterine tissue. Most of this is lost during the days of heaviest menstrual flow, usually the first few days of the menstrual phase.

When FSH is released from the pituitary gland, the body enters the second stage of the menstrual cycle, the proliferative phase. When menstrual discharge stops, FSH stimulates the ovaries to begin maturing 10–20 egg follicles. These follicles release estrogen, which in turn stimulates the endometrium to grow thick, spongy, and rich in blood vessels and mucus. As estrogen levels increase, the FSH production decreases, and estrogen stimulates the hypothalamus to release GnRH. GnRH, in turn, stimulates the pituitary gland to secrete luteinizing hormone (LH). As LH production surges, one graafian follicle undergoes ovulation, after which all other maturing follicles disintegrate.

In the third phase of the menstrual cycle, the secretory phase, the remains of the graafian follicle become the corpus luteum. Remaining inside the ovary, the corpus luteum produces estrogen and progesterone. Progesterone continues to stimulate the buildup of the endometrium, which becomes increasingly glandular in preparation for a potential pregnancy.

High levels of progesterone signal the pituitary to halt the release of LH, which causes the corpus luteum to stop its hormone production. Between days 24 and 28 of the menstrual cycle, the estrogen and progesterone levels drop significantly. As progesterone levels decline, the uterine lining disintegrates and menstrual bleeding begins. As estrogen levels decline, the hypothalamus releases GnRH, which signals the pituitary to release FSH. The menstrual cycle then repeats. If pregnancy occurs, however, the developing embryo produces a hormone called **human chorionic gonadotropin (HCG)**

....

human chorionic gonadotropin (HCG) gonadotropic hormone produced by the tissues of the embryo and fetus.

(*kō-ri-on'ik*), which is chemically similar to LH. HCG stimulates the corpus luteum to secrete the increased amounts of progesterone and estrogen needed to maintain the pregnant state.

Menstrual Concerns

For some women, menstruation carries significant discomfort. If this discomfort begins before the onset of menstruation, it is called **premenstrual syndrome (PMS),** if it occurs during menstruation, it is called **dysmenorrhea** (*dis-men-ō-rē'a*). Some women do not menstruate at all, a condition known as **amenorrhea** (*a-men-ō-rē'a*).

PMS is a group of symptoms experienced by as many as 70 to 80 percent of women late in their menstrual cycles, often postovulatory (after ovulation), but sometimes overlapping into menstruation. In 20–40 percent of women the symptoms are fairly severe; 3–10 percent of women experience such severe PMS symptoms that their routines are disrupted from one to two weeks each month.[14] PMS symptoms commonly increase in severity until the onset of menstruation, then disappear dramatically. Although some dispute the existence of PMS, those who are affected by it have little question that it exists.

PMS symptoms can be physical, emotional, and/or behavoral (see Table 6.1). PMS is related to the cyclic production of ovarian hormones, although the symptoms are not directly linked to changes in the levels of these hormones.[15] The basic cause of PMS remains unknown.

Effective treatment of PMS differs with the individual. Treatment depends on the type and severity of the symptoms. Common remedies are given in Feature 6.3 (p. 160). The management of PMS can include medical treatment, psychological treatment, and social education of the family, so that fears and myths regarding the menstrual cycle can be eliminated.

....

premenstrual syndrome (PMS) the physical discomfort and emotional mood swings that some women experience before menstruation.

dysmenorrhea painful menstrual flow.

amenorrhea absence of menstrual periods.

Table 6.1
Possible Symptoms of PMS

Physical Symptoms

Headache	Fatigue
Abdominal bloating	Swelling (water retention)
Constipation	Breast tenderness

Emotional Symptoms

Anxiety	Depression
Confusion	Irritability
Hostility	Mood swings
Paranoia	

Behavioral Symptoms

Increased alcohol consumption	Violence toward self and others
Binge eating	Crying spells

The term *dysmenorrhea,* or painful menstruation, is applied to the condition of severe discomfort accompanying menstruation. About one-half of all women who menstruate experience some degree of dysmenorrhea. Symptoms include painful abdominal cramps, diarrhea, and nausea. It is now believed that women who suffer from these symptoms produce high levels of **prostaglandins** (*pros'ta-gland-ins*).[16] The production of these potent substances causes uterine muscle contractions to increase, leading to more severe menstrual cramping. The severity of menstrual cramps can be mitigated by medications that inhibit prostaglandins, such as ibuprofen (*Motrin, Advil, Mediprin*) and aspirin. Increased sleep, exercise, relaxation techniques, orgasm (to relieve vasocongestion), and a diet low in sodium and caffeine also can provide relief from dysmenorrhea.

Amenorrhea, or the absence of menstruation, may be a transient or a chronic condition. During pregnancy and breastfeeding, missed periods are expected; other causes, however, are less well known. Eating disorders, malnutrition, anxiety, and stress may interfere with menstruation. Hormonal imbalances and certain diseases, such as diabetes, may also cause amenorrhea. Some athletes experience amenorrhea; experts attribute this to an

prostaglandins a group of substances produced by the body that affects the contraction of the uterus.

unusually low percentage of body fat in those who exercise strenuously. During amenorrhea, ovulation is irregular; it occurs less frequently, but may not stop completely.[17] Prolonged amenorrhea can have significant health consequences, including a loss of bone mass that can lead to early osteoporosis, discussed further in Chapter 8.

Toxic shock syndrome (TSS) is a rare but serious illness that occurs almost exclusively in menstruating women. It can cause fever, dangerously low blood pressure, a red rash on the palms of the hands and soles of the feet, redness of the lining of the throat and vagina, vomiting, severe diarrhea, and impaired kidney and liver function. In severe cases, TSS can cause death.

TSS is caused by a toxin (poison) released by the bacterium *Staphylococcus aureus,* a microorganism normally present in small amounts in the body. Most reported cases of toxic shock syndrome are associated with the improper use of menstrual tampons and contraceptive sponges. When left in the vagina for too long, these devices provide an environment for an unusual proliferation of *Staphylococcus aureus,* which spreads into the uterus and fallopian tubes. The toxins released by the larger bacterial population are quickly absorbed by the bloodstream and affect the body, causing the symptoms characteristic of the syndrome. Women who use tampons, contraceptive sponges, or diaphragms should be aware of the potential risks of TSS and should consult their physician for appropriate guidelines for use. These women should be aware of the symptoms of TSS and immediately report the occurrence of such symptoms to their physicians.

CHECKPOINT

1. Name and describe each of the organs of the external female genitals.

2. Describe the appearance of the uterus and the fallopian tubes. What are the parts of each?

3. List the functions of the ovaries.

4. Describe the three phases of the menstrual cycle. At what ages does the menstrual cycle characteristically begin and end?

5. Describe the following by giving symptoms, possible causes, and treatments: PMS, dysmenorrhea, amenorrhea, and toxic shock syndrome.

FEATURE 6.3

COMMON REMEDIES FOR PMS[a]

Remedy	Comments
Reduced sugar intake	Dietary sugar can cause moodiness through sudden swings in blood glucose levels.
Vitamins	Vitamins B₆, C, and E may help combat PMS. B₆ is often needed by women on oral contraceptives.
Over-the-counter medications	Midol (contains aspirin and caffeine) Pamprin (contains acetaminophen).
Low sodium	Reducing sodium (table salt and salt in foods) reduces bloating and weight gain due to water retention.
Caffeine	A diuretic that reduces body water, thus reducing bloating and weight gain, but can increase irritability. Found in coffee, tea, chocolate, and some soft drinks.

Remedy	Comments
Potassium	Replaces potassium lost through loss of body water. Needed for healthy nerves and muscles; helps reduce cramps. Found in bananas and dairy products.
Exercise	Increases blood flow and oxygen to muscles—thus reduces cramps and pains. Perspiration reduces excess water.
Sleep	Reduces fatigue. Fatigue makes pain seem worse.
Refraining from the use of alcohol	Drink no more than one ounce per day.

[a]It is appropriate that, if affected by PMS, you consult a physician before trying any of these remedies.

HUMAN SEXUAL RESPONSE

Human **sexual arousal** and response are highly pleasurable sensations that begin in the mind and then involve every part of the body. While physiologists measure sexual response in terms of vaginal lubrication and penile erection, these reactions result from conscious and unconscious processes that begin in the brain (see Feature 6.4).

Sexual arousal often begins in your mind, triggered by cues that you see, hear, smell, or think about, such as **sexual fantasies.** If given the proper opportunity, a receptive partner, and an allowable setting, you may decide to take advantage of these cues by beginning an exploratory process of touching. A caress, massage, hug, or kiss may set in motion the complex body response that may involve you in some sort of sexual activity that may range anywhere from a mere playful exchange to engaging in sexual intercourse. Along the way your entire body becomes engaged in a physical, emotional, and hormonal sexual response characterized by conspicuous bodily reactions.

Masters and Johnson, two well-known sex researchers, determined that the human sexual response generally occurs in a cycle of four phases

(stages): **excitement, plateau, orgasmic,** and **resolution** (Figure 6.8, p. 162). In the first phase of sexual response, or excitement, your sex organs fill with blood and the body muscles tense. In plateau, the second phase of response, there is an increased congesting of blood in your sex organs and an increase of your muscle tension. In the third phase, the orgasm or climax, there is a rhythmic contraction in your pelvic muscles and sex organs. After all of this, your body goes through the fourth phase, the resolution, during which your body returns to its unaroused condition.

Some researchers consider sexual desire to be the first stage of your sexual response cycle. Sexual desire, or **libido** (li-bē'dō), is an appetite or drive for sexual activity. When the libido is stimulated, testosterone levels in both males and females increase. When activated, libido may cause you to feel restless and more receptive to sex; when libido is inactive, you lose your drive, though not necessarily your ability to respond.

EXCITEMENT PHASE

Excitement marks the beginning of sexual arousal. The first physiological responses in both sexes are

sexual arousal the activation of reflexes involving the sex organs and the nervous system.

sexual fantasy any daydream of a sexual nature.

excitement, plateau, orgasmic, and **resolution** the cycle of four phases (stages) of the human sexual response.

libido the sexual desire; also called the sex drive.

FEATURE 6.4

THE G-SPOT

The G-Spot (Gräfenberg Spot) is a sensitive area located beneath the front wall of the vagina between the pubic bone and the cervix. Two researchers, John Perry, a psychologist, and Beverly Whipple, a sex counselor, contend that the stimulation of this spot during vagina penetration causes some women to orgasm with an ejaculate-like gush of fluid from the urethra. Varying percentages of women report this reaction. The initial researchers reported that 40 percent of sexually active women reported this response[a]; other researchers have found the figure to be considerably lower[b]. Some sex researchers contend that the fluid that is released is actually urine.

There has been no anatomical confirmation of a G-spot. Yet, it is observed that women can identify erotically sensitive areas in their vagina that contribute to the pleasure of orgasm.

One concern about placing so much emphasis on the G-spot is that women who are unable to find their G-spots may fear they are abnormal. Another concern is that a G-spot should not be seen as the expectation of a sexually liberated female. Although the possibility of a G-spot may be an important discovery, it is important that this issue not become an unnecessary concern for a woman.[c]

[a]Ladas, A., et al. *The G Spot and Other Recent Discoveries About Human Sexuality.* New York: Holt, Rinehart and Winston, 1982.

[b]Masters, W., and Johnson, V. *Human Sexuality,* 4th ed. New York: HarperCollins, 1992.

[c]Boston Women's Health Book Collective. *The New Our Bodies, Ourselves.* New York: Simon and Schuster, 1992.

---

pelvic **vasocongestion** and general **myotonia** (*mī'ō-tō'nēa*). Vasocongestion, or increased blood flow into the penis, labia, vagina, and breasts, causes swelling and sensations of warmth and fullness. During this stage, the penis becomes partially erect and the walls of the vagina begin to secrete a slippery lubricating fluid. The nipples and **areolae** (*a-rē'ō-lē*), the darkened rings surrounding the nipples, may swell. Both sexes may show a "sex flush," or reddening of the skin of the chest, neck, and head. Myotonia, or increased muscle tension, occurs throughout the body.

PLATEAU PHASE

During the plateau phase, sexual excitement intensifies. Muscle tension increases, vasocongestion continues, and the sex flush spreads. In the female, vasocongestion forms the **orgasmic platform,** a narrowing of the outer third of the vagina that intensifies when the erect penis comes in contact with it. With penetration, the upper part of the vagina elongates and opens to accommodate the

erect penis more easily. As the penis continues to harden, several drops of sticky, clear **preejaculatory fluid** may escape from its tip.

ORGASMIC PHASE

Orgasm, or climax of sexual arousal, is the highly pleasurable total body sensation that marks the peak of vasocongestion and myotonic buildup, with the sudden release of neuromuscular tensions. In the female, rhythmic contractions of the orgasmic platform, uterus, and anal sphincter occur. In the male, orgasm occurs in two stages: First, the seminal vesicles and prostate gland begin to contract, causing a feeling that orgasm is inevitable and imminent; secondly, contractions along the urethra and in the pelvic region cause ejaculation. In both males and females, orgasm is accompanied by increased pulse rate, faster and deeper breathing, and contractions of arm, leg, and lower abdominal muscles.

RESOLUTION PHASE

During the resolution phase, muscle tension and vasocongestion subside and the genital organs return to their unaroused state. The orgasmic response elicits deep body relaxation and a feeling of peace. Immediately after orgasm, males enter a

---

vasocongestion the filling of the genitals and breasts with blood during sexual arousal.

myotonia tensing of muscles.

areolae the pigmented rings surrounding the nipples; areolae is the plural of areola.

orgasmic platform the narrowing of the vagina entrance during sexual excitement.

preejaculatory fluid sticky fluid secreted prior to ejaculation, and which may contain sperm.

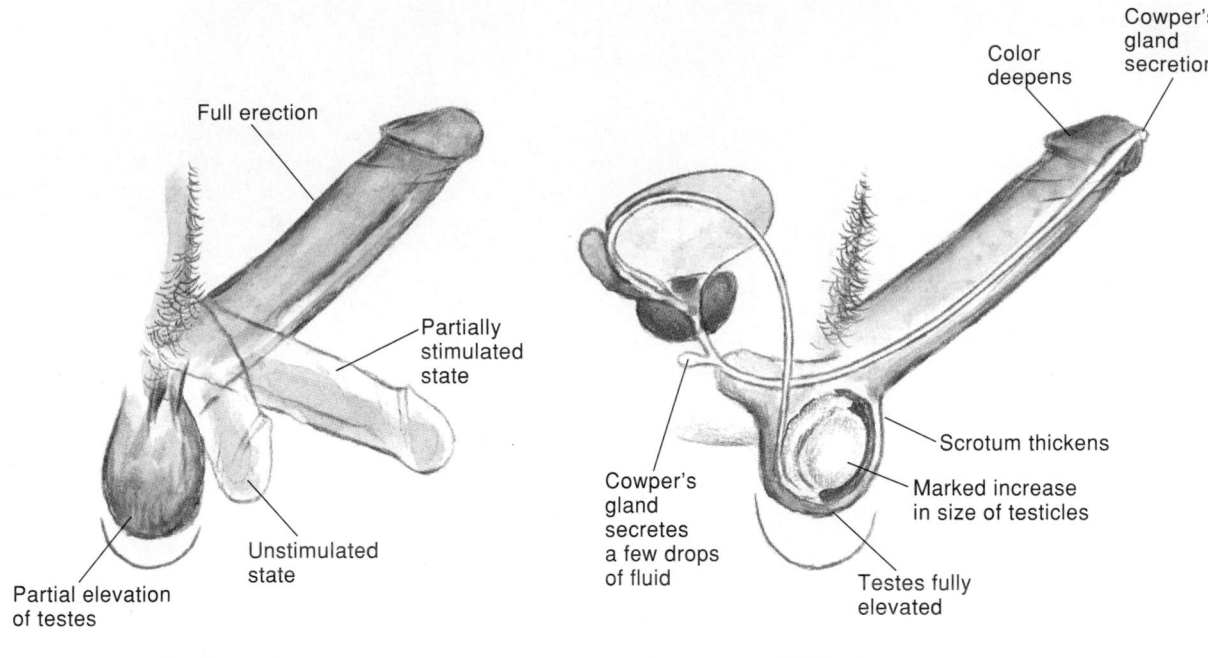

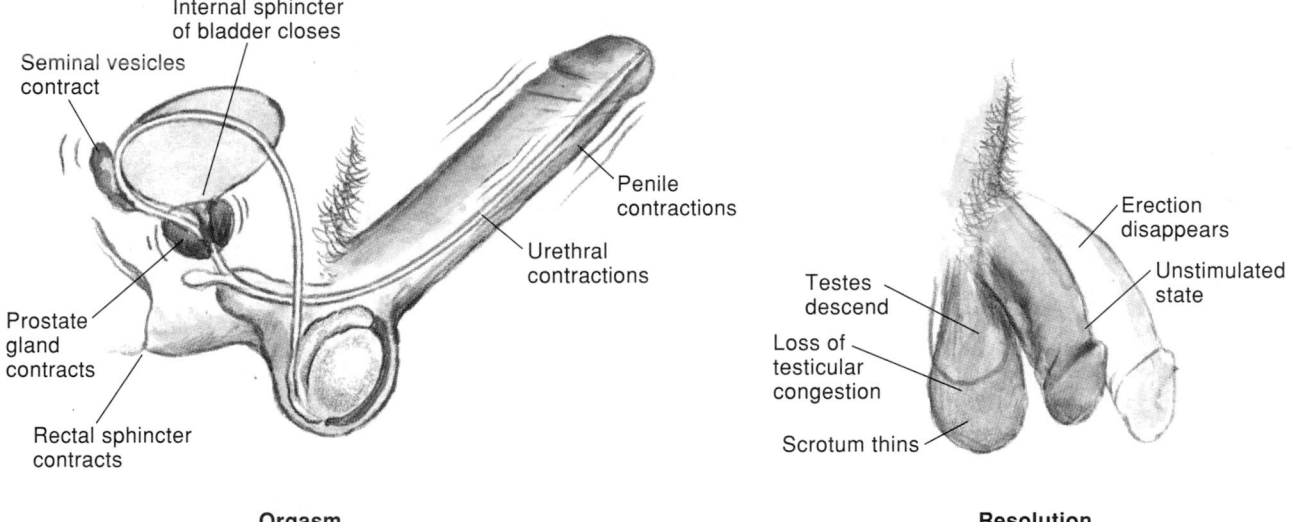

(a)

Figure 6.8
Changes in Sexual Response in:

(a) the male

Source: Masters, W., Johnson, V., and Kolodny, R. Human Sexuality, *4th ed. New York: HarperCollins, 1992; Byer, C., and Shainberg, L.* Dimensions of Human Sexuality, *4th ed. Dubuque, IA: Brown and Benchmark, 1994.*

(b) the female

Source: Masters, W., Johnson, V., and Kolodny, R. Human Sexuality, *4th ed. New York: HarperCollins, 1992; Byer, C., and Shainberg, L.* Dimensions of Human Sexuality, *4th ed. Dubuque, IA: Brown and Benchmark, 1994.*

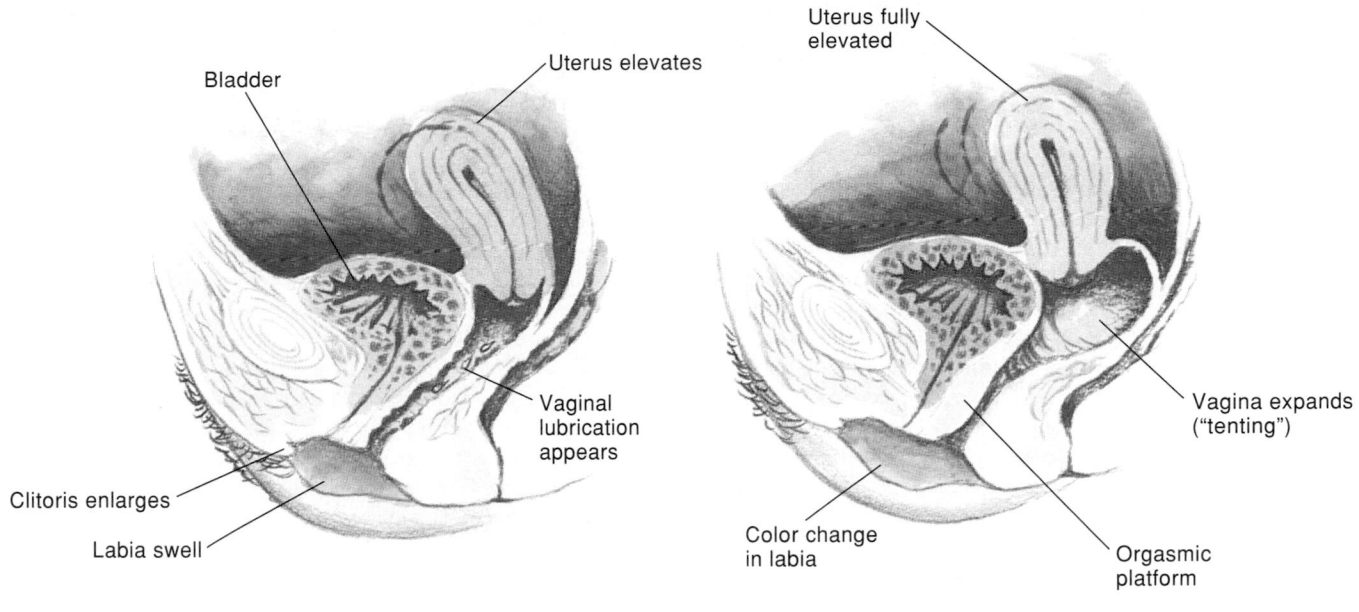

Bladder

Uterus elevates

Clitoris enlarges

Labia swell

Vaginal lubrication appears

Excitement

Uterus fully elevated

Vagina expands ("tenting")

Color change in labia

Orgasmic platform

Plateau

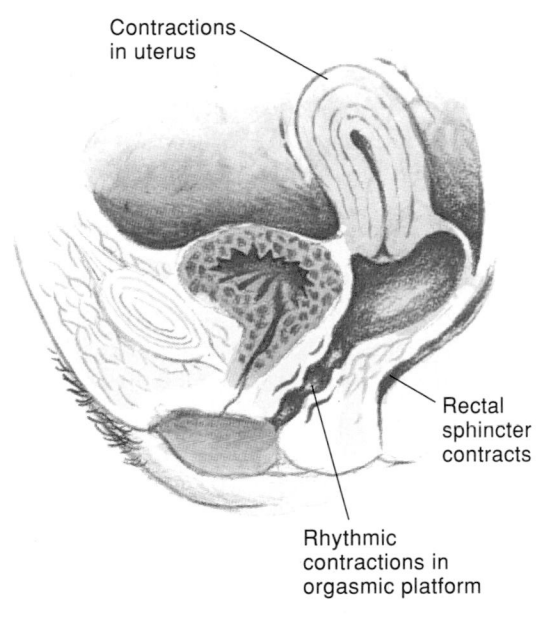

Contractions in uterus

Rectal sphincter contracts

Rhythmic contractions in orgasmic platform

Orgasm

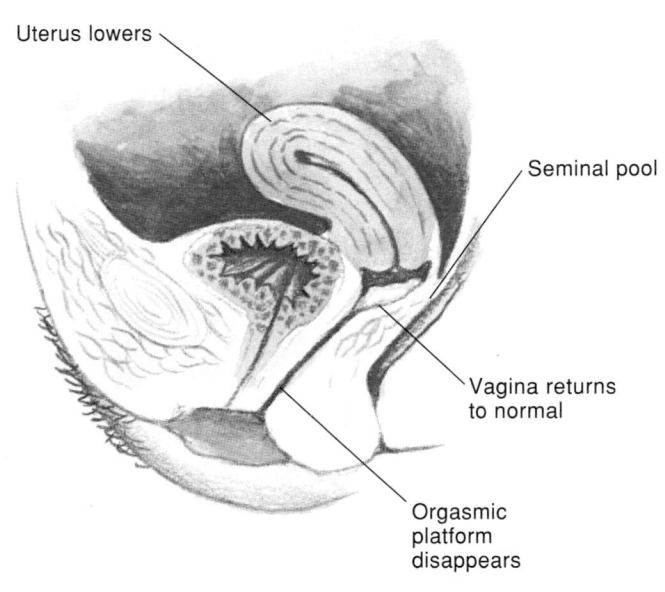

Uterus lowers

Seminal pool

Vagina returns to normal

Orgasmic platform disappears

Resolution

(b)

refractory period, during which the nerves will not respond to further stimulation. During the refractory period, a male cannot achieve another

....

refractory period the period immediately following ejaculation, during which males are unable to experience further orgasms.

orgasm; he remains unable to do so until his sexual tension returns to the level found during early sexual excitement. The refractory period can last from minutes to hours, lasting longer with age. Because females do not experience a refractory period, they may experience repeated orgasms within minutes.

Of course, any model of sexual response describes an average, in terms of degree and length

LEARNING TO SHARE YOUR SEXUAL DESIRES

Even in this supposedly enlightened era, many people do not communicate well on sexual topics, especially when it involves their own sexual interests and responses. Too many people apparently expect their partners to be clairvoyant, to somehow "just know" what to do sexually. Even the most sexually experienced and sophisticated person can not know exactly what his or her partner would enjoy because we are all different. Something that is a powerful turn-on for one person can be an equally powerful turn-off for another.

Yet, there are some givens for you to follow. Don't hesitate to tell your partner what you do and don't like sexually. Very few people will be offended by this and most will greatly appreciate knowing how to increase your pleasure. Further, most people will reciprocate. By talking about your sex-

ual likes and dislikes, you give your partner permission to do the same. Yet, be prepared for your partner not wanting to do what you would like him or her to do, especially if it would make him or her feel uncomfortable. It is also acceptable for you to reserve the right to not do something your partner requests if it would make *you* feel uncomfortable.

Someone who has never talked much about his or her sexual desires may at first feel uncomfortable about trying this. But after a few successes in expressing yourself, it seems quite natural to do so. Beyond the sexual benefits of this communication, the sharing of such personal feelings may lead you and your partner to a greater degree of emotional intimacy than you have previously experienced and thereby strengthens your total relationship.

of time, of how people respond sexually. It is important to realize that sexual response differs from person to person and from experience to experience. To enjoy a rich sexual life, then, a person should not compare him- or herself with any sexual standard or preconceived notion of how sex "should" be. No two orgasms are exactly alike, nor is there an "ideal" orgasm for which a person should strive. Contrary to popular beliefs, couples rarely experience simultaneous orgasms.

During sexual intercourse, one partner often responds more easily to sexual stimulation than the other. One partner may be extremely responsive and reach orgasm easily, while the other partner may not reach orgasm at all. In these cases, it may be necessary to use another form of stimulation, such as manual caressing or oral stimulation, to assist the nonorgasmic partner to climax. While women are able to achieve multiple orgasms more easily than men, sexual satisfaction should not be measured in terms of numbers; orgasms are profoundly satisfying whenever they occur, but are not the key to a satisfying sex life.

CHECKPOINT

1. Define the term *sexual desire* and enumerate the factors that lead to the beginning of sexual arousal.

2. Describe the events that occur during each of the four phases of sexual response.

3. List the major differences between male and female sexual response.

EXPRESSIONS OF SEXUAL BEHAVIOR

People engage in sexual behavior either with others or by themselves. Sexual pleasure can be experienced in a number of ways. The following activities represent some of the more common sexual behaviors.

TALKING

Sexual communication can greatly enhance an intimate relationship. Talking about sex is a special kind of communication that makes partners aware of each other's needs and desires. Verbal dialogue is one of the most effective ways to express caring, openness, and warmth, and is often the basis for improved satisfaction in sexual relationships. Any extra effort to express caring is usually rewarded with a reciprocal empathy from the partner (see Communication for Wellness: Learning to Share Your Sexual Desires).

TOUCHING

Humans are tactile beings, requiring touch from infancy. Of all the senses, touch is most often associated with sexual stimulation because it is often used in a sexual context. Touch applied to a person's **erogenous zones,** or body parts especially

erogenous zones areas of the body that are especially sensitive to sexual stimulation.

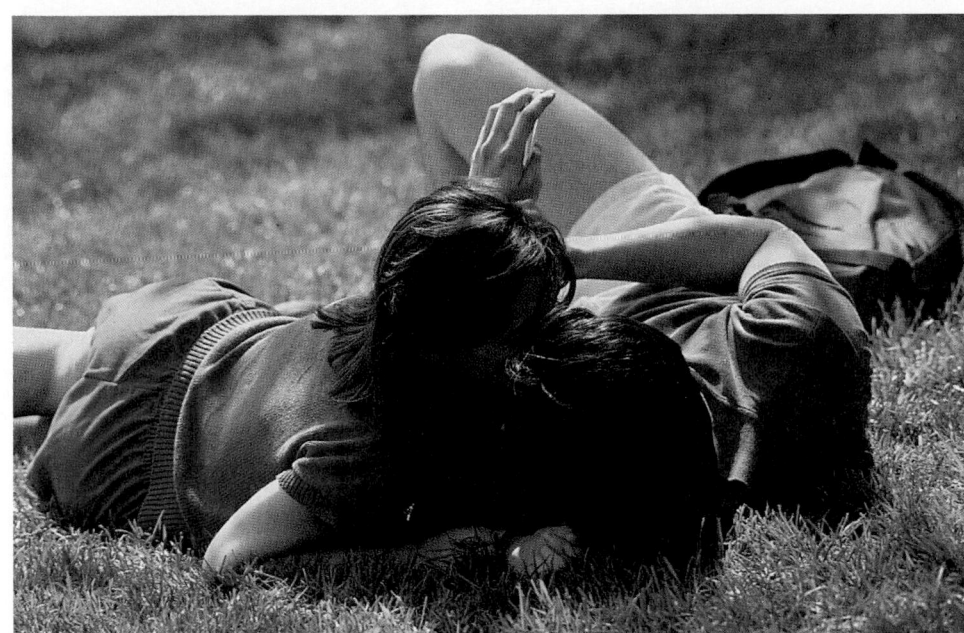

Of all the senses, touching (tactility) is the most significant in communicating sexual pleasure, especially when applied to an erogenous zone.

sensitive to sexual arousal, is particularly pleasurable. Especially erogenous are the genitals (clitoris, vaginal lips, penis, scrotum), the breasts, the lower body and thighs, and around the mouth. The use of a light touch is always preferred for early arousal. As arousal mounts, however, caresses can be more pressured and firm. A common form of erotic touch is the use of the tongue and lips in kissing. Kissing serves both to express feelings and arouse the partners.

ORAL SEX

A usual first step in sexual interaction in our culture is mouth-to-mouth kissing. Although we take romantic kissing for granted, one survey found it mentioned in only 21 cultures and a part of sexual intercourse in only 13.[18] In some cultures, it is as, or more, common to kiss or lick other body parts, including the genitals.

An erotic form of arousal is oral-genital sex. Fellatio consists of licking and sucking the male genitals, while **cunnilingus** (*kun-i-lin'gus*) is similar stimulation of the female genitals. Oral sex is a practice of many heterosexual and homosexual couples.

Oral sex has become more widely practiced in recent decades.[19–21] For women, cunnilingus provides more direct stimulation to the clitoris than

does intercourse. Many men enjoy oral stimulation as well. The person providing the stimulation can become as aroused as the person receiving it.

Anal stimulation for arousal is another practice used by some partners during sex play. Oral licking of the skin around the anus, or **anilingus** (*ā-ni-lin'gus*), is enjoyed by some as a pleasurable stimulation.

Oral sex should only be practiced if both partners enjoy it. In a loving relationship, a person should never force a reluctant partner to participate. Before engaging in oral sex, partners must insist that the genitals or anus be clean and disease-free. This is especially true in light of the prevalence of STDs, including AIDS (see Chapter 19). Small breaks in the skin of the genitals or anus, or around the gums in the mouth, can allow the transmission of HIV from an infected person to the bloodstream of a noninfected person. If practiced, it is wise to restrict oral genital/anal sex to monogamous relationships.

MASTURBATION

Masturbation (*mas-tur-bā'shun*) is the stimulation of one's own genitals to derive sexual gratification.

cunnilingus oral stimulation of the female's genitals.

anilingus oral stimulation of the anal area.

masturbation stimulation of one's own genitals to derive sexual pleasure.

(Although some texts refer to the caressing by each partner of the other's genitals as mutual masturbation, these authors restrict the use of the term to *self-stimulation*.) Masturbation often involves orgasm, though this does not need to be the case. Masturbation is an almost universal practice among people in the United States. Many teenagers, especially males, begin genital exploration early. By the time they are 18, as many as 80 percent of males and 59 percent of females have masturbated.[22] Eventually, as many as 94 percent of males and 63 percent of females have masturbated.[23] The majority of women who masturbate begin *after* they have had first intercourse, while the majority of men who masturbate begin *before* having had first intercourse. While many adults practice masturbation, they do so less often when frequent intercourse is available.

Masturbation can play an important role in sexual self-discovery. It can help both males and females discover their sexual preferences, which, in turn, allows them to help their partners please them sexually. Masturbation also helps relieve sexual tension when a partner is not available or when sexual intercourse is not appropriate. In a sexual climate of increasing caution and "safer sex," masturbation does not carry the risk of causing pregnancy or spreading sexually transmitted diseases.

Some people feel guilty when they masturbate. This is usually the result of cultural or religious teachings. As a rule, masturbation is not a harmful activity and can, in fact, be a part of a healthy sexual experience. It can become psychologically harmful, however, if it produces unresolved guilt or anxiety, if it is used as a preferred substitute for sexual relations with a marital partner, or if it is a compulsion chosen as a replacement for more rewarding interpersonal encounters.

SEXUAL INTERCOURSE

Sexual intercourse, or **coitus** *(kō'i-tus),* usually refers to insertion of the penis into the vagina. The term is applied by some, however, to other forms of sexual play, such as anal intercourse (insertion of the penis into the anus). Sexual intercourse is the natural culmination of intimate feelings between partners (see Chapter 5).

There is no "normal" way for a couple to engage in sexual intercourse, nor is there a "normal" position, time, or place. As with any sexual activity, couples should choose the time, place, and position for intercourse that are the most enjoyable for them. Factors affecting enjoyment include privacy, freedom from interruptions and distractions, caring and communication between partners, absence of negative feelings such as fear and guilt, and the willingness to experiment. Common positions for intercourse include the male on top with the partners facing each other (the "missionary position"), the female on top and partners facing each other, side by side with the partners facing each other, and rear entry with penetration of the vagina from behind. Two of these positions are illustrated in Figure 6.9. Many couples move into several different positions during a single lovemaking session. There is no standard dictating how often a couple "should" have intercourse; this will vary widely among couples.

Among societies where women are assigned low social status, the male-above position is more commonly practiced, but where females enjoy high status, such as among groups in the South Pacific, the woman-above position is the most popular.[24]

Some couples practice anal-penile insertion. The anus is a constricted circular muscle designed to normally keep the anus tightly shut and it usually tightens more when stimulated. Not designed for penile insertion, the anal canal is lined with sensitive internal tissues, and lacks natural lubrication. For penile penetration of the anus, it is essential that you use a lubricated condom. The canal is easily damaged by dry and abrasive objects. It is important that the anal tissues not be irritated or injured. Anal intercourse is one of the riskiest techniques for the transmission of HIV. It is important that infected ejaculate not be deposited into the anal canal.

CELIBACY

Celibacy *(sel'i-ba-sē)* is the avoidance of, or abstinence from, sexual intercourse. Some people choose to never have intercourse, while others are celibate for limited periods.

---

coitus heterosexual intercourse referring to insertion of the penis into the vagina.

celibacy abstinence or avoidance of sexual intercourse.

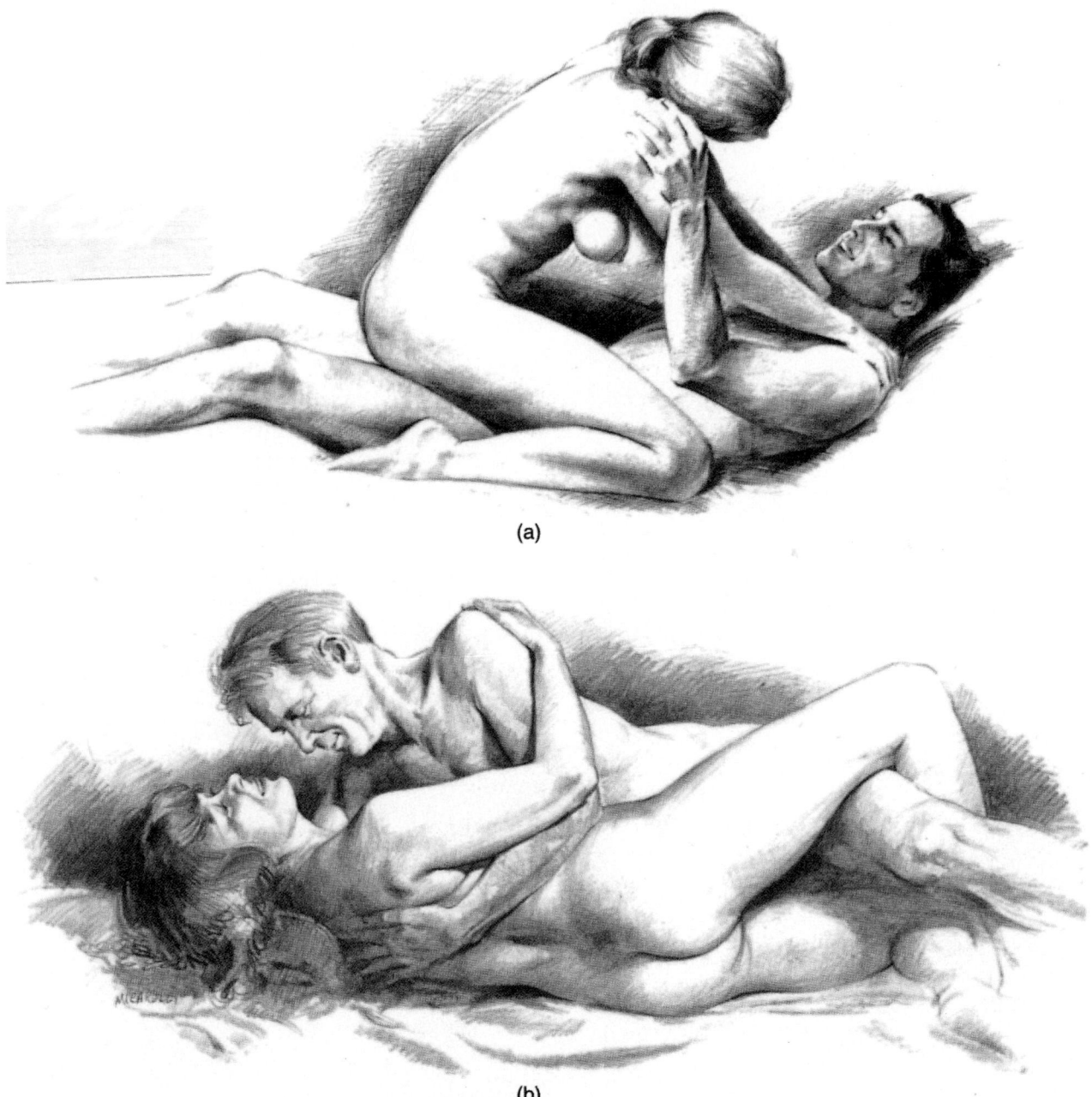

(a)

(b)

Figure 6.9
Two Intercourse Positions

(a) Female on top with the partners facing each other. (b) Side by side with the partners facing each other.

Sources: Masters, W., Johnson, V., and Kolodny, R. Human Sexuality, 4th ed. New York: HarperCollins, 1992; Byer, C., and Shainberg, L. Dimensions of Human Sexuality, 4th ed. Dubuque, IA: Brown and Benchmark, 1994.

A person may choose to be celibate for a variety of reasons. For example, celibacy is a requirement for some religious groups. Others remain celibate because they are opposed to intercourse outside of marriage or because their partners are absent or ill. Some couples find that through planned, time-limited celibacy, they are able to increase their desire for each other and thus intensify their pleasure when intercourse is resumed.[25] Celibacy can mean loneliness if an intimate relationship is preferred. On the other hand, individuals can be involved in sexually intimate relationships without engaging in sexual intercourse. Couples may choose to express their sexuality with oral sex or manual stimulation, achieving both sexual arousal and orgasm. They may choose to meet their needs for companionship by caressing and holding each other, or merely by being close to each other in social settings.

CHECKPOINT

1. Discuss the role of touching in sexual expression.

2. Distinguish between fellatio and cunnilingus.

3. Discuss masturbation as a sexual option. Include information concerning incidence, role in sexual expression, and potential benefits and problems.

4. Discuss sexual intercourse. What are the most common coital positions?

5. Define the term *celibacy* and explain the reasons people may choose to be celibate.

SEXUAL PERFORMANCE DISORDERS

Almost everyone experiences a sexual performance disorder sometime in his or her life. Sexual disorders fall into two categories: **sexual dysfunctions** (*dis-funk'shunz*) and **sexual paraphilias** (*par-a-fil'i-az*). A sexual dysfunction is a type of sexual disorder that interferes with a full or complete sexual response cycle. Such a disorder makes it difficult for a person to have or to enjoy sexual intercourse. A sexual paraphilia is a type of sexual disorder in which variations in sexual behavior occur, and in which a person's sexual arousal and gratification is based on a fanciful or unusual sexual experience.

SEXUAL DYSFUNCTIONS

Sexual dysfunctions are disorders in which a person is unable to experience a complete sexual

---

sexual dysfunction a sexual disorder that interferes with a full or complete sexual response cycle.

sexual paraphilia a sexual disorder in which sexual arousal and response is pleasurable, yet whose object and/or aim deviates from the norm.

response cycle and finds it difficult or impossible to have or enjoy sexual intercourse. Sexual dysfunctions may result from a variety of causes, including disease, damaged sexual organs, side effects of drugs, communication problems between partners, or previous negative or traumatic sexual experiences, such as rape or sexual abuse during childhood. Sexual dysfunctions may affect any phase of the sexual response cycle.

Lack of Interest

Sexual inhibitions may cause a lack of interest in sex for some people. These individuals, once aroused, have no difficulty responding sexually; however, they do not initiate sexual activity. A person may lack a normal sexual appetite for a number of reasons. He or she may be an incest or rape victim with a strong aversion to sex, or be from a home in which normal sexual expression was treated as "dirty" or "sinful." Some legitimate medications, such as antidepressants and drugs used to treat high blood pressure, diminish sexual desire. Users of recreational and illicit drugs also may have little or no interest in sex. Anxiety, stress, illness, fatigue, pregnancy, and childbirth may all temporarily reduce interest in sex.

To treat a lack of sexual interest, a physician or therapist must first identify the physical or emotional basis for the loss of libido. Then, he or she may be able to help remedy the problem. If, for example, a male has an abnormally low level of testosterone, a physician may administer the hormone, causing the male to show sexual interest and resume sexual activity.[26]

Premature Ejaculation

Premature, or involuntary, **ejaculation** is when ejaculation occurs quickly with such frequency that the enjoyment of the man, his partner, or both is adversely affected. Yet, applying a strict definition is difficult because there are so many variables in speed of response between two partners. It's impossible to quantify it in terms of minutes spent in penetration or the number of penile thrusts. The

---

premature ejaculation early, or involuntary, ejaculation with such frequency that a couple's sexual enjoyment is adversely affected.

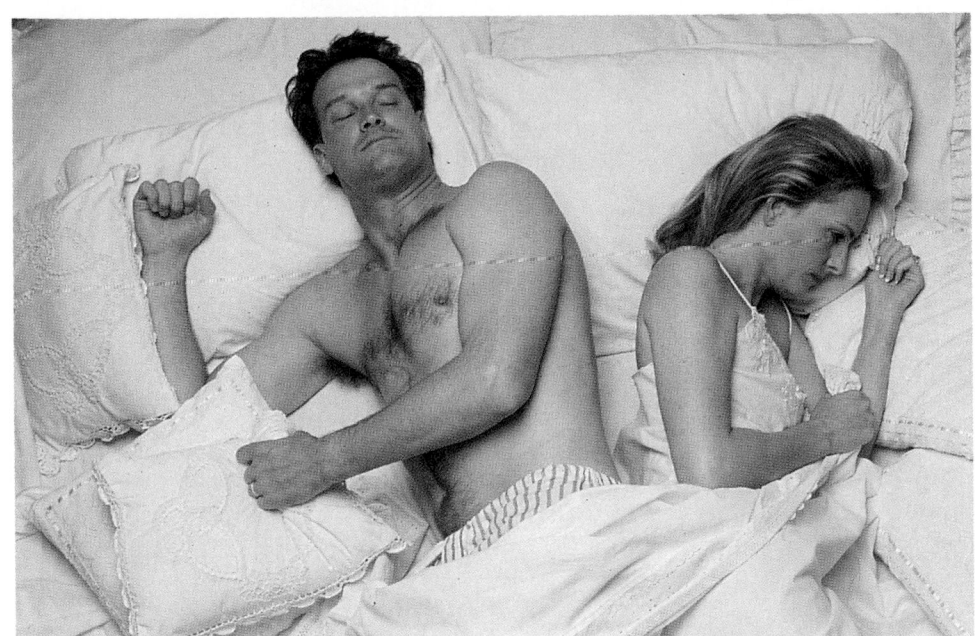

Inhibited sexual desire frequently reflects relationship problems. Early efforts at resolving differences can often improve the chances of saving the marriage.

female partner may experience orgasm rapidly or slowly; she may not climax at all, even though the man has learned to control his ejaculatory response. Nor should it be assumed that the speed of one person's response need match that of the partner. Although simultaneous orgasm may be enjoyable on occasion, it is not necessary for satisfying sexual activity. Nor is rapid ejaculation to be considered a problem if neither partner sees it as such.

Beyond certain variables, however, premature ejaculation may become regular and unwanted. Among young adults, about 50 percent complain of early ejaculation.[27]

The ability to delay ejaculation may depend on a man's increasing age, the position the couple uses in intercourse, how recently it has been since he last had intercourse, and his level of emotional comfort with his partner. For some men their masturbatory experience may have been marked by rapid ejaculation, without attempt to practice delay. Speed of ejaculation may also relate to the nature of the fantasies the man is experiencing, as well as his own arousability.

Therapy is available to treat premature ejaculation. The goal of such therapy is to recondition the man to anticipate orgasm and to gain control over the timing of ejaculation. Two such techniques are recommended to help a man gain control: the *stop-go* method, which is a starting-stopping sequence of caressing to stimulate the penis, but delay ejaculation, and the *basilar squeeze* method, in which

the base of the penis is squeezed to delay ejaculation whenever the man feels it is going to occur. Other methods to treat premature ejaculation might include using condoms to reduce sensory perception in the penis, using a coital position that is less exciting to the man, such as the woman atop the man, and trying to achieve orgasm a second time.

Erectile Dysfunction

The inability to achieve or maintain an erection that is sufficiently firm to penetrate the vagina is known as an **erectile dysfunction.** Also known as impotence, this condition affects millions of men. Impotence is not the same condition as infertility, the inability to conceive. A man with erectile dysfunction, though unable to maintain an erection, may be fully fertile. Common causes of erectile problems include diabetes, low testosterone levels, drug abuse, stress, and fatigue. Some men may experience anxiety that they will not be able to meet their partner's expectations; some men are frightened by the increased sexual assertiveness of many women and react to this fear by becoming unable to achieve or maintain an erection.

....

erectile dysfunction (impotence) the inability to achieve or maintain an erection of sufficient firmness for coitus.

Therapy for erectile problems necessitates determining the cause of the dysfunction. In about half of all cases of erectile dysfunction, the basis is psychological. Since erection must occur involuntarily ("determination" alone cannot cause an erection to occur), therapy for these cases includes **sensate focus exercises.** With these exercises, the man focuses on the pleasure of touching and being touched rather than on his ability to achieve an erection. By relaxing or disregarding the pressure to have an erection, many men find that they are able to respond to sexual stimulation. When the cause of erectile dysfunction is physical, the first step in therapy is to treat the physical cause, if possible. For example, administering testosterone to a man with low levels of the hormone will often restore normal erectile function. If the basis of the erectile dysfunction cannot be treated, as with permanent vascular damage from diabetes for example, the only available treatment consists of surgical insertion of a **penile implant.** This penile **prosthesis** (*prōs-the'sis*) mechanically induces erection.

Female Orgasmic Concerns

Some women are unable to experience complete sexual arousal. Obstacles to attaining satisfaction include insufficient vaginal lubrication, inability of the vagina to open or enlarge properly, and the inability to reach an orgasmic platform. Other women are unable to reach orgasm; these women may experience erotic feelings and produce enough lubrication, but are unable to become aroused beyond the plateau phase. In one survey, 40 percent of women reported that they achieve orgasm nearly every time they have intercourse; another 38 percent reported that they achieve orgasm sometimes.[28] In another study, 10 percent of sexually active women reported that they never experience orgasm.[29] In yet another survey of 745 nurses, it was found that 59 percent of the women had occasionally pretended to achieve orgasm.[30] While a male who does not reach orgasm may consider himself to have a performance problem, a woman who does not reach orgasm may not see it as unusual. If physical problems are ruled out, then therapy is similar to that for erectile dysfunctions. The woman is encouraged to concentrate on body sensations rather than on distractions, such as what her partner might think or whether she will achieve orgasm.[31] She is encouraged to enjoy the delightful sensations she is feeling. Women who are most likely to experience orgasm during intercourse are those who are most willing to surrender conscious control to their bodily sensations and behavior and who accept the feeling of getting "carried away" during arousal.[32] Many therapy programs also encourage women to become more familiar with the nature of their arousal by stimulating themselves. Once a woman learns to respond to stimulation and reach orgasm with masturbation,[33] she is encouraged to share her feelings and preferences with her partner so that he is better able to elicit a sexual response. She can also help him by instructing him in the types of clitoral and genital caressings that are most exciting to her.

Other sexual problems affect women. Some women experience **dyspareunia** (*dis-pa-rū'ni-a),* or pain during intercourse. This difficulty may occur during insertion, thrusting, orgasm, or even after intercourse. Other women may experience a spastic contraction of the vagina, a condition known as **vaginismus** (*vaj-in-iz'mus).* Vaginismus closes the vaginal opening so tightly that intercourse becomes difficult or impossible. Both of these problems require medical treatment and/or psychotherapy, which are often successful.

SEXUAL PARAPHILIAS

Most adults have affectionate sexual relationships with partners who are consenting adults. There are others, however, who engage in unusual sexual practices, either occasionally or exclusively. Sexual paraphilias, or variations, are sexual disorders in

---

sensate focus exercises a series of touching exercises designed to teach nonverbal communication and to reduce anxiety about achieving an erection.

penile implant a mechanical device inserted within the penis in order to aid in erection.

prosthesis an artificial organ or body part.

dyspareunia painful intercourse.

vaginismus involuntary spasm of the lower vaginal muscles when penetration by the penis is attempted.

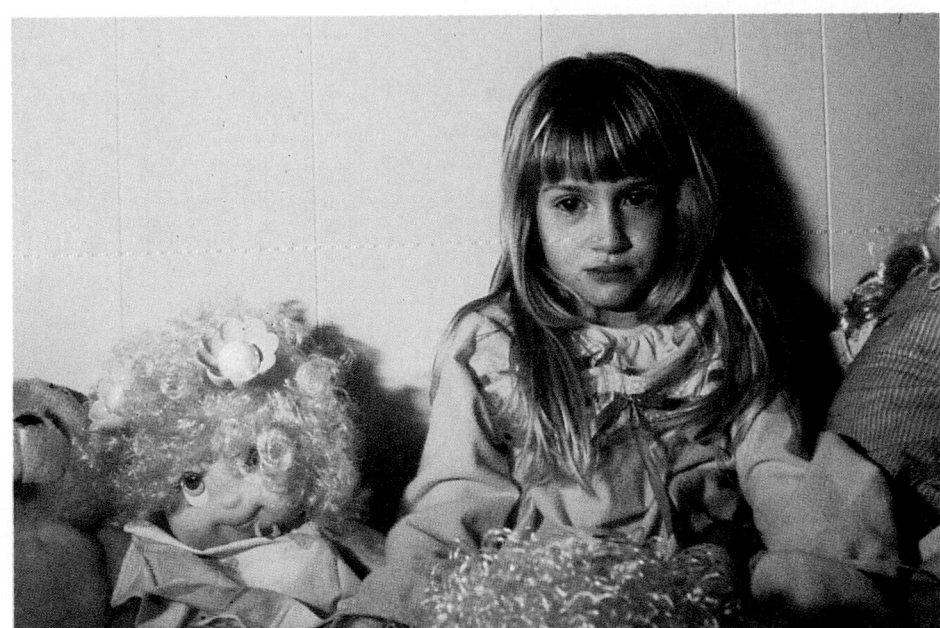

Therapy for the victim of child sexual abuse is essential so the victim can recover some sense of trust and stability.

which a person finds sexual activity pleasurable, but requires an extraordinary or bizarre experience as stimulus for sexual arousal.[34] The sexual experience may be performed with a consenting adult (who may or may not share the gratification), and thus be harmless; more often, however, the experience may be performed with a nonconsenting partner who finds the activity offensive, as with obscene phone calls. Those who practice illegal sexual paraphilias, such as child molestation, are known as *sex offenders*.

Child Sexual Abuse

Child abuse has been of increasing concern in recent years. Especially troubling is the sexual abuse of minors, which is defined as sexual involvement with dependent and developmentally immature children and adolescents. The prevalence of sexual abuse of minors is of such concern that addressing the problem has become a national priority. An estimated 20 percent of all female children and 9 percent of male children are victims of sexual abuse; only a fraction of these cases are reported to authorities. The effects of child sexual abuse are devastating, increasing the victim's vulnerability to further exploitation; victims of child sexual abuse often tend toward behaviors such as promiscuity, prostitution, abuse of their own children, and sexual dysfunctions.

Pedophilia

Pedophilia *(pē'dō-fil'i-a)*, or sexual contact between an adult and a child, is often known as child molestation, and is a common form of child sexual abuse. Most pedophilic acts involve touching or fondling of the victim's genitals; some cases also involve physical violence. About two-thirds of the victims of pedophilia are girls; most offenders are adult males, and usually are family friends, relatives, or acquaintances of the victim.

Incest

Incest is sexual abuse that occurs within a family. The most common form of incest occurs between siblings of the opposite sex, although the most reported form occurs between fathers and daughters. Most incest victims are females between the ages of 9 and 12; most offenders are males. Incest is an indicator of severe emotional instability within the family and of a possible breakdown in the marital relationship in the home. Incest carries a near-universal taboo; it causes the breakdown of

....

pedophilia a type of child sexual abuse in which there is sexual contact between an adult and a child.

incest sexual activity between persons too closely related to be allowed by law to marry.

familial stability and carries the risk of producing defective offspring.

Fetishism

Fetishism (*fet'ish-ism*) is a sexual paraphilia that involves using inanimate objects or the image of a body part to initiate sexual arousal. The object of fetishism varies, but is commonly an article of clothing, such as a shoe, a hat, or lingerie or a body part, such as hair, breasts, eyes, or feet. A person with a fetish may achieve sexual arousal and reach orgasm by masturbating while fondling, kissing, or smelling the object of desire. It is important to recognize that, for the fetishist, a body part is dissociated from the person; that is, while many men find women's breasts arousing, to the fetishist, they are an object of desire that takes the place of a human sexual partner.

Zoophilia

Zoophilia (*zo-o-fil'i-a*), or *bestiality* (*bēs-ti-al'i-tē*), is an uncommon sexual variance in which sexual arousal results from contact with animals. While zoophilia was once more common in farming areas when the country's population was mostly rural, it now occurs with equal frequency in rural and urban settings. While it is not uncommon for males to experiment with zoophilia, only those with deep psychological problems continue these sexual practices.

Exhibitionism

Exhibitionism is a paraphilia in which sexual arousal is achieved by exposing one's genitals or buttocks to unsuspecting and unconsenting strangers. Exhibitionists are usually men, who derive sexual pleasure from exposing themselves to women or children; however, exhibitionists can

be female. Because the victim's reaction to exposure enhances the offender's gratification, it is recommended that a victim of exhibitionism remain calm and attempt to ignore the act. While exhibitionists are a nuisance, they rarely become involved in more serious sexual offenses.

Sadomasochism

Sexual sadomasochism (*sā-dō-mas'e-kizm*) is deriving sexual arousal giving (sadism) or receiving (masochism) physical and/or psychological pain. Sadists inflict pain, while masochists receive it. Sadomasochistic acts range from fantasy, when the pain is imagined, to life-threatening criminal acts.

Some people believe that the orientation to sadomasochism can be traced to childhood experiences. Sadomasochism may provide sexual variety or a means of breaking sexual taboos. It may also be an expression of anger and resentment in the guise of a sexual game.

Voyeurism

Voyeurism (*voy'yer-ism*) is a form of sexual variance in which the offender secretly watches unsuspecting people as they disrobe, are nude, or engage in sexual activity. Voyeurs, often referred to as "peeping Toms," are usually young males, though some offenders are women. While it is normal to find nudity sexually arousing, voyeurs are compulsive in their need to view others in sexual situations.

Obscene Telephone Calling

Obscene telephone calling refers to the use of lewd language during anonymous telephone communication in order to achieve sexual arousal. It is important to make the distinction between the compulsive obscene telephone caller and the adolescent prankster who is trying to be a bother. As

fetishism the use of inanimate objects or body parts for sexual arousal.

zoophilia obtaining sexual arousal through sexual contact with animals; also known as bestiality.

exhibitionism deriving sexual gratification from exposing the genitals or buttocks to unsuspecting and unconsenting strangers.

sexual sadomasochism variant sexual behavior in which inflicting pain (sadism) and submitting to pain (masochism) occur simultaneously.

voyeurism deriving sexual gratification from secretly viewing people disrobing, nude, or engaging in sexual activity.

with exhibitionism, obscene telephone calls cause the victim to feel shock and embarrassment. Obscene telephone callers are most often males. They may masturbate during their phone calls, enhancing the victim's discomfort and disgust. Women who receive harassing obscene telephone calls may fear for their safety; there are, however, various strategies that can be used to protect one's privacy. It is recommended that a victim of an obscene caller blow a high-pitched whistle into the telephone receiver, or defuse the situation by allowing the receiver to remain off the hook. If a victim receives repeated calls from the same person, it may be necessary for him or her to have the telephone company assign a new, unlisted telephone number.

CHECKPOINT

1. Distinguish between the sexual performance disorders and sexual paraphilias.

2. List some of the causes of sexual dysfunctions.

3. List the sexual dysfunctions that affect males.

4. Discuss female orgasmic concerns.

5. Discuss the sexual abuse of minors, including its incidence and common ways in which it is expressed.

6. Compare and contrast the following paraphilias: fetishism, zoophilia, exhibitionism, sadomasochism, voyeurism, and obscene telephone calling.

SEXUAL MATURITY

Sexual maturity involves choices and requires understanding and responsibility. Sexuality is a very individual and personal part of development for which there is no specific timetable.

What is sexual maturity, and how can a person tell if he or she has achieved it? A sexually mature person displays the following characteristics:

- Accepts him- or herself as a sexual being, is able to choose a satisfying way of expressing his or her sexuality, and is able to integrate that choice into his or her life.

- Enjoys sexual activity to its fullest and brings joy to a partner by ensuring that he or she is sexually satisfied.

- Develops sexual values that increase the esteem of the partner as well as him- or herself.

- Demonstrates independence and capacity for self-direction.

- Accepts responsibility for sexual acts, both personally and for his or her sexual partner.

- Communicates needs, feelings, and preferences to a partner, and listens to the partner's needs.

- Makes compromises to ensure that the partner's needs are fulfilled.

- Admits the need for professional help when sexual problems that have no apparent solution arise.

A measure of your developing sexual maturity is your willingness to take an honest look at your sexual and reproductive preferences. Your answers to In Your Hands: Reproductive Life Plan (p. 174) are important to both you and your partner. After you have completed your answering, ask your partner to take the same test and then compare your answers.

CHECKPOINT

1. Define the term *sexual maturity*.

2. List the characteristics of a sexually mature individual.

SUMMARY

You are a sexual being from birth to death. Your gender is identified at birth, but other factors affect your sexual behavior throughout life. Some factors are present before birth; others, such as social and psychological influences, affect you after birth and help you to form a gender identity and a gender role.

Your sexual orientation is defined by the sex of the person to whom you are sexually attracted. The degree to which you are heterosexual, homosexual, or bisexual can be expressed on a continuum ranging from exclusive heterosexuality to exclusive

IN YOUR HANDS

REPRODUCTIVE LIFE PLAN

Intimate sexual relationships can have a great impact on your life, so make sure your sexual practices fit into your overall life plan. Ask yourself the following questions. Ask your partner the questions, too.

1. Of all the things I could do in my life, probably the most important thing would be _____ .

2. When I get older and reflect upon my life, what would make me most proud? Most regretful?

3. Do I want children one day? How many?

4. Do I want to get married one day?

5. What would make my marriage stronger?

6. How many years of schooling do I want to complete?

7. When do I want to start having intercourse?

8. Have I had or will I have intercourse with several partners?

9. When would I want to have my first child or my next child?

10. Would I be emotionally and financially ready to have this child?

11. How would I feel if I became pregnant before I got married?

12. How would I feel if I became pregnant before I wanted to?

13. If I became pregnant when I didn't want to, what would I do? Raise the child? Put the child up for adoption? Have an abortion?

14. Will I use birth control?

15. How would I feel if I couldn't have children? What would I do?

16. Will I work after I have children? When?

17. How do I expect my partner to help with child-rearing?

18. What would I do if my marriage were to end in divorce?

19. What if my spouse and I were to have intercourse outside of marriage?

20. What is my risk of AIDS? Do I or does my partner engage in behaviors that put me at some risk?

21. What do I believe in? Do my answers to these questions fit in with my religious and spiritual beliefs?

Source: Hatcher, R., et al. Contraceptive Technology, 1990–1992, 15th rev. ed. New York: Irvington, 1990, p. 7.

homosexuality. Your placement on this scale is determined by various factors, and may shift during your lifetime. Sexual anatomy and physiology relate to the nature of the human sexual response. Central to this response is the action of a person's sex hormones. These hormones direct the development and functioning of the male and female sexual systems. The female system provides an environment for nurturing an unborn child; the uterine events in the female occur on a monthly cycle.

Human sexual response is the result of the body reacting to sexual arousal. The sexual response cycle involves four phases: excitement,

plateau, orgasmic, and resolution. While sexual climax is highly pleasurable, sexually mature couples value the ability to communicate their feelings more than the ability to reach orgasm.

People express their sexuality by touching and engaging in oral sex, masturbation, and sexual intercourse. Some people are celibate, refraining from expressing their sexual feelings with a partner.

Sexual performance disorders include dysfunctions, which are problems with sexual arousal, and paraphilias, which are problems related to how a person expresses his or her sexuality.

Sexual maturity involves a variety of choices and requires understanding and responsibility.

REFERENCES

1. Dressel, P., and Avant, W. "Range of Alternatives." In R. Weg (ed.). *Sexuality in the Later Years: Roles and Behavior.* New York: Academic Press, 1983.
2. Doyle, J. *Sex and Gender.* Dubuque, IA: Brown, 1985.
3. Mead, M. *Sex and Temperament in Three Primitive Societies.* New York: Morrow, 1963.
4. Deau, K. "Structure of Gender Stereotypes: Interrelationships Between Components and Gender Label." *Journal of Personality and Social Psychology* 5 (1984), 991–1004.
5. Gordon, S., and Snyder, C. *Personal Issues in Human Sexuality.* Boston: Allyn and Bacon, 1986.
6. Kinsey, A., et al. *Sexual Behavior in the Human Male.* Philadelphia: Saunders, 1948.
7. Dixon, J. "The Commencement of Bisexual Activity in Swinging Married Women Over Age Thirty." *Journal of Sex Research* 1 (1984), 71–90.
8. Davenport, W. "Sexual Patterns and Their Regulation in a Society of the Southwest Pacific." In F. Beach (ed.). *Sex and Behavior.* New York: Wiley, 1965.
9. Marshall, D. "Sexual Behavior in Mangaia." In D. Marshall and R. Suggs (eds.). *Human Sexual Behavior: Variations in the Ethnographic Spectrum.* Englewood Cliffs, NJ: Prentice-Hall, 1971.
10. Laughlin, C., and Allgeier, E. *Ethnography of the So of Northeastern Uganda.* New Haven, CT: Human Relations Area Files, Inc., 1979.
11. Herdt, G. (ed.). *Ritualized Homosexuality in Melanesia.* Berkeley: University of California Press, 1984.
12. Herdt, G. *Guardian of the Flutes: Idioms of Masculinity.* New York: McGraw-Hill, 1981.
13. Carrier, J. M. "Homosexual Behavior in Cross-Cultural Perspective." In J. Marmor (ed.). *Homosexual Behavior.* New York: Basic Books, 1980.
14. Sara, M., and Camden-Main, B. "PMS Diagnosis and Management." *Medical Aspects of Human Sexuality* (October 1987), 73–79.
15. Tortora, G., and Grabowski, S. *Principles of Anatomy and Physiology,* 7th ed. New York: HarperCollins, 1993.
16. Boston Women's Health Book Collective. *The New Our Bodies, Ourselves.* New York: Simon and Schuster, 1992.
17. Cunningham, F., et al. *Williams Obstetrics,* 19th ed. Norwalk, CT: Appleton and Lange, 1993.
18. Ford, C., and Beach, F. *Patterns of Sexual Behavior.* New York: HarperCollins 1951.
19. Kinsey, A., et al. *Sexual Behavior in the Human Female.* Philadelphia: Saunders, 1953.
20. Petersen, J., et al. "The Playboy Readers' Sex Survey, Part 1." *Playboy* (January 1983), 241–250.
21. Whitley, B. "Correlates of Oral Genital Experience Among College Students." *Journal of Psychology and Human Sexuality* 2 (1989), 151–163.
22. Hass, A. *Teenage Sexuality.* New York: Macmillan, 1979.
23. Hunt, M. *Sexual Behavior in the 1970s.* Chicago: Playboy Press, 1974.
24. Ibid.
25. Aquilar, N. "Post-pill Couples Discover the Joy of Abstinence." *Los Angeles Times* (16 November 1980), Sec. 9, 28.
26. Rosellini, L. "Sexual Desire." *U.S. News & World Report* (6 July 1992), 61–66.
27. McCarthy, B. "Cognitive Behavioral Strategies and Techniques in the Treatment of Early Ejaculation." In S. Leiblum and R. Rosen (eds.). *Principles and Practices of Sex Therapy,* 2nd ed. New York: Guilford Press, 1989, pp. 141–167.
28. Petersen, J., et al. "The Playboy Readers' Sex Survey, Part 2." *Playboy* (March 1983), 90–92, 178–184.
29. Hite, S. *The Hite Report.* New York: Macmillan, 1976.
30. Darling, C., and Davidson, K. "Enhancing Relationships: Understanding the Feminine Mystique of Pretending Orgasm." *Journal of Sex and Marital Therapy* 3 (1986), 182–196.
31. Boston Women's Health Book Collective, op. cit.
32. Bridges, C., et al. "Hypnotic Susceptibility, Inhibitory Control, and Orgasmic Consistency." *Archives of Sexual Behavior* 4 (1985), 373–376.
33. Wakefield, J. "Female Primary Orgasmic Dysfunction: Masters and Johnson Versus DSM-IIIR on Diagnosis and Incidence." *Journal of Sex Research* 24 (1988), 363–377.
34. American Psychiatric Association. *Diagnostic and Statistical Manual (DSM-IIIR),* 3rd ed. rev. Washington, DC: American Psychiatric Association, 1987.

SUGGESTED READINGS

Boston Women's Health Book Collective. *The New Our Bodies, Ourselves.* New York: Simon & Schuster, 1992.
Buxton, A. *The Other Side of the Closet.* Santa Monica, CA: IBS, 1991.
Calderone, M., and Johnson, E. *The Family Book About Sexuality.* New York: HarperCollins, 1989.
Comfort, A. *The New Joy of Sex.* New York: Crown, 1991.
Covington, S. *Awakening Your Sexuality.* New York: HarperCollins, 1991.
Haug, F. *Beyond Female Masochism.* New York: Verso, 1992.
Johnson, J. *Mothers of Incest Survivors.* Bloomington, Indiana: University Press, 1992.
Kaplan, H. *How to Overcome Premature Ejaculation.* New York: Brunner-Mazel, 1989.

Lark, S. *Menstrual Cramps*. Los Altos, CA: Westchester, 1993.

Likosky, S., ed. *Coming Out*. New York: Pantheon, 1992.

McCarthy, B. *Male Sexual Awareness: Increasing Sexual Satisfaction*. New York: Carroll and Graf, 1988.

McCarthy, B., and McCarthy, E. *Female Sexual Awareness*. New York: Carroll and Graf, 1989.

Reinisch, J. *The Kinsey Institute New Report on Sex*. New York: St. Martin's, 1990.

Sedgwick, S. *The Good Sex Book*. Minneapolis: Comp-Care, 1992.

Sheehey, G. *Menopause, The Silent Passage*. New York: Pocketbook, 1993.

Smalley, G., and Trent, J. *The Language of Love*. Colorado Springs, CO: Focus on the Family, 1991.

Wade, B. *Love Lessons*. New York: Amistad, 1993.

Yaffee, M., and Fenwick, E. *Sexual Happiness for Women, A Practical Approach*. New York: Holt, 1992.

Young, E. *Romancing the Home*. Nashville, TN: Broadman and Holman, 1993.

Zilbergeld, B. *The New Male Sexuality*. New York: Bantam, 1992.

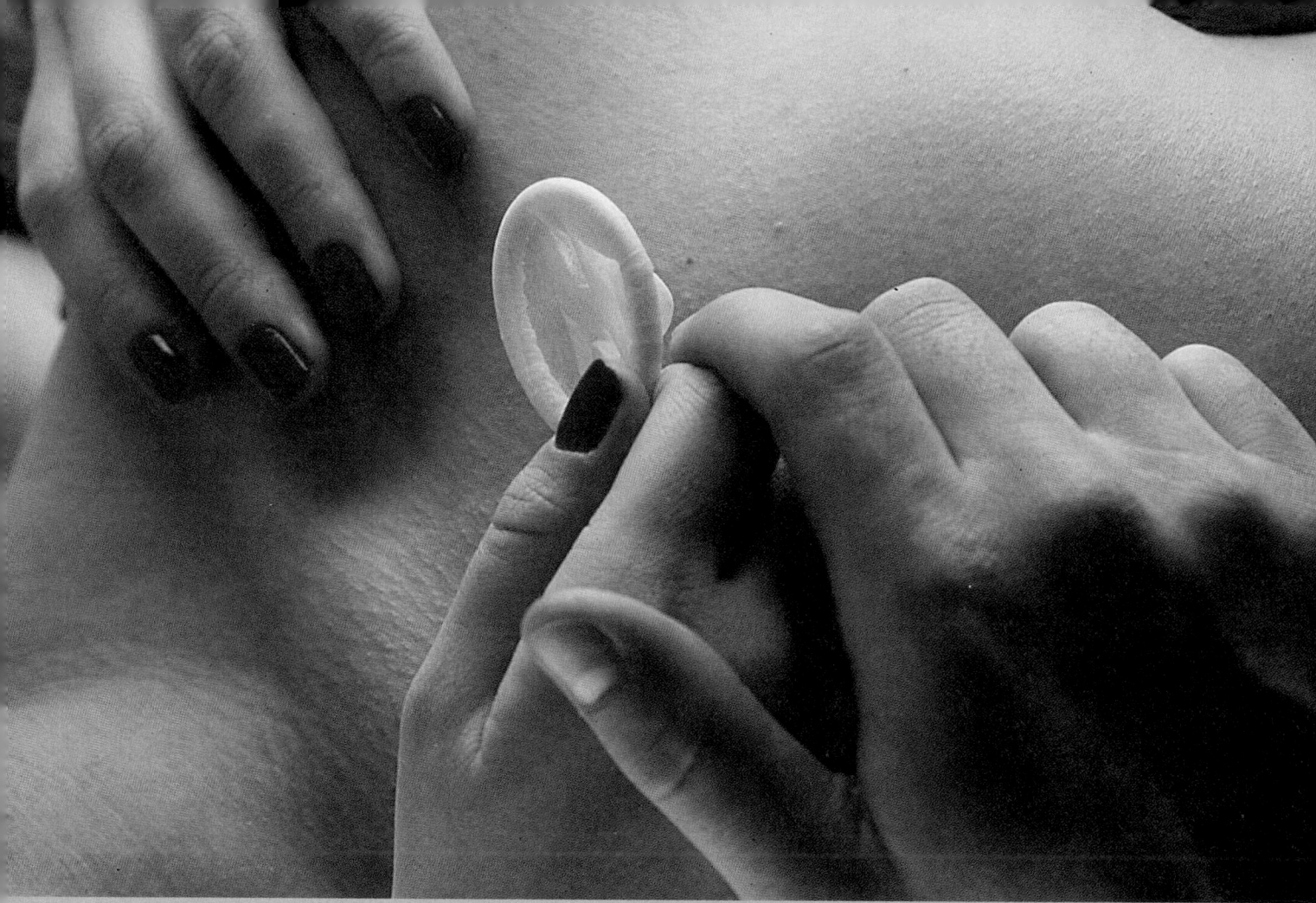

7
CONTRACEPTION

KNOWLEDGE

- List the various categories of temporary contraceptive devices.
- Define the terms lowest expected failure rate and typical failure rate.
- Identify the synthetic hormones contained in oral contraceptives.
- Define the acronym IUD.
- Name the most effective type of spermicide.
- Name the various materials of which male and female condoms are made.
- List the various vaginal barrier devices.
- Explain the meaning of natural family planning.
- Define the term vasectomy.

INSIGHT

- Identify what are for you the most important criteria favoring a given method of contraception.
- Discuss how a breastfeeding mother, in protecting herself from an unwanted pregnancy, decides what contraceptive she may or may not choose to use.
- Explain the reasons a woman would consider having Norplant embedded in her arm.
- Explain the significance of being certain that the chemical agent nonoxynol-9 is present in any spermicide you choose to use.

DECISION MAKING

- Explain how you plan to demonstrate responsible behavior if you are engaging in or plan to engage in sexual intercourse.
- Identify the contraceptive methods preferred by yourself and your partner. Explain the basis for your choice.
- Decide whether menstrual cycle charting and periodic abstinence as a contraceptive method hold any promise for you and/or your partner.
- Decide whether you would or would not consider having a sterilization performed on yourself.

A 1991 meeting of the United States National Academy of Sciences concluded with recommendations for new and improved contraceptives so that couples can be offered a wider variety of safer, more effective methods of contraception. This recommendation comes in light of the fact that the United States has one of the highest rates of unintended pregnancy in the Western world. Each year in the United States, over three million women have unwanted pregnancies and about half have abortions.

Some experts indicate that fear of lawsuits has kept American drug companies from aggressively pursuing better methods of contraceptive technology. Until 1980, 17 major U.S. drug companies were actively engaged in contraceptive development. In 1991, only one was doing so. As a result, many believe that the United States is far behind its European counterparts in contraceptive technology research and development.

The moral issues surrounding contraception and abortion also affect contraceptive development in the United States. Some lawmakers are strongly opposed to sexuality education in the schools, school-

based clinics, and young people's access to birth control devices. However, former Surgeon General Joycelyn Elders has been outspoken in her support of such programs to reduce the number of unwanted pregnancies and abortions among teens.

Worldwide, and among some Americans, price is a factor in the decision to use contraceptives. For example, an average woman in the country of Chad would have to pay nearly 75 percent of a year's income to afford an intrauterine device. For people in many countries, even condoms are not affordable. The price of the contraceptive implant, Norplant, has created a great deal of debate. The cost of Norplant is much less in some other countries than it is in the United States. Thus, some women who would choose to use Norplant, and who could significantly benefit from its use, do not because they cannot afford it.

Given these barriers to contraceptive research, development, and use there are some new trends in birth control research. These include the use of implant and injectables for women, vaginal delivery of hormones, new barrier methods (such as the female condom), and pills, implants, and injectables for men. It is hoped that advances in contraceptive technology will promote more effective and efficient methods of birth control and will reduce the number of unwanted pregnancies and abortions.

Source: Special Delivery, *Summer 1991, p 1(3).*

■   ■   ■

Almost everyone at some point in life enters a relationship that involves sexual intercourse. Whenever that occurs, consideration of contraceptive options becomes important. By presenting this information to you at this time, we are not assuming that you are having intercourse or that you should be, however you deserve this information so that whenever you need it you can make the choice that is best for you.

Sexual intercourse is one of the most satisfying expressions of love and sexuality. Engaging in sexual intercourse can be a statement of the need for intimacy, love, and belonging. At the same time, it can reveal how we see ourselves and how we regard our partner. While emotionally gratifying, sexual intercourse usually is also the way we initiate the biological process of human reproduction.

Humans have a unique choice not found among other animals; we have the option of minimizing the risk of conception as the result of sexual intercourse. Sexual intercourse without the risk of **conception,** the fertilization of the ovum by the sperm, has been an elusive dream for centuries. Yet, the reality is that most acts of sexual intercourse carry the possibility of conception; therefore, heterosexual sex partners must take measures to avoid an unwanted pregnancy. This responsibility involves not only each partner, but also the child that could result from their union.

Partners who engage in sexual intercourse may seek to avoid conception through the use of a **contraceptive;** however, there is no contraceptive that completely eliminates the risk of pregnancy. Yet, without using contraceptives sexually active partners stand an 85 percent chance of conceiving within a year.

The use of contraceptives, then, allows a couple greater control over their lives. By taking control of their own fertility, couples can tailor their sexual relations to their own needs and desires. In essence, birth control gives both men and women the freedom to enjoy sexual intercourse and to avoid parenthood.

CHOOSING TO USE CONTRACEPTION

Choosing whether or not to use contraceptives is a personal decision based on individual circumstances and beliefs. Many couples choose to use them because they are not prepared for the responsibilities and demands of parenting.

Many couples use contraception to protect their own interests as well as those of a potential child. Some need time to adjust to living together. Many want to feel confident that their union is stable before testing it further with the demands of pregnancy and a child. Other adults wish to complete their education or reach other personal and

conception the moment of fertilization of an ovum by a sperm.

contraceptive any technique, drug, or device that prevents conception.

professional goals before committing themselves to the responsibilities of parenting.

Some couples prefer not to have children, and find sufficient fulfillment in their interpersonal relationships and professional lives. Unfortunately, some individuals are carriers of genetic conditions, such as sickle-cell anemia or Tay-Sachs disease, or are HIV-positive, and must use contraception to avoid risking the transmission of such conditions to their partners or potential offspring. Some couples have children, but limit their family size to a preplanned number; some need time, before a second pregnancy, to adjust emotionally and financially to having a first child.

Not all couples view the use of contraceptives favorably. Some fear side effects of certain methods. Other couples view the use of them as being against God's divine order. Others see the advocacy of birth control as a sinister attempt by the "establishment" to adversely limit the population of a particular racial or ethnic group. As with adults, the use of contraceptives by sexually active teenagers depends on their self-perceptions and on their knowledge of contraception. Teenagers who use them tend to be older, more mature, and better informed; they also know more about their own bodies, have a positive attitude about themselves, and believe that what happens to them is a result of their own actions.[1]

Few teenagers who are engaging in sexual intercourse intend to become pregnant—even though many sexually active teenagers do not use birth control.[2] Teenagers avoid using contraceptives for various reasons. Some have little knowledge of the reproductive structures and processes, and don't know when the chances are best for "making a baby." They may believe the risk of pregnancy is small. Some are overcome by their sexual passions and have unplanned intercourse; others may be under the influence of alcohol and other drugs and not in full control of their actions. Some young people believe that by planning ahead (deciding to use a contraceptive and having it available) they are more "immoral" than if they get "helplessly carried away" and are unprepared. Many are driven by sexual feelings and desires, but have not developed skills in verbalizing their feelings or exploring the feelings or desires of their partner, or have been taught that talking about sexual matters is "dirty."[3]

To address the epidemic of teenage pregnancies in the United States, some high schools and colleges now provide information on and the dispensing of contraceptives as a part of their professional health services. Some public high schools have initiated school-based clinics, which provide students with birth control information and contraceptives.[4] Many college and university health services provide contraceptive counseling and devices at low cost.

All of the issues raised so far regarding the use of birth control deserve to be discussed frankly and openly between sexual partners as pointed out in Communication for Wellness: Talking About Birth Control.

CHECKPOINT

1. List some of the reasons couples choose to use contraception to avoid pregnancy.

2. What might be some reasons couples object to the use of contraceptives?

3. Give some of the reasons why sexually active teenagers do not use contraceptives.

COMMUNICATION FOR WELLNESS

TALKING ABOUT BIRTH CONTROL

"I thought *you* were taking care of that." Sad but true, this is a very common statement, made upon the discovery that *no one* was taking care of the birth control.

Failure to communicate about birth control is usually part of a larger failure to communicate about sexual issues in general. The same people who don't talk about birth control tend also not to talk about disease prevention, commitment, and other issues revolving about a sexual relationship.

So why don't people talk about birth control, disease prevention, commitment, and similar issues? Simply because confronting these issues makes them uncomfortable. Someone who is uncomfortable talking about sexual issues may not have come to terms with his or her own sexuality and/or the advisability of entering into the particular sexual relationship at hand. If you don't feel at ease with discussing birth control, disease prevention and other issues, perhaps you really aren't yet ready for the relationship to become sexual at this time.

CONTRACEPTION CATEGORIES

Various terms are used, correctly or incorrectly, to refer to the prevention of conception. **Contraception** is the prevention of conception. The term **birth control** defines the regulation of conception, pregnancy, or birth by preventive devices or methods. Sometimes the terms birth control and contraception are used interchangeably. **Family planning** refers to the spacing of conception of children according to the wishes of the couple, rather than leaving it to chance. This is accomplished by practicing some form of birth control.

Contraceptives are any processes, devices, or methods that prevent conception. Some methods are temporary, others permanent. Temporary contraceptive devices include *hormones,* taken by pill, injection, or by implantation, that inhibit ovulation; *intrauterine devices* that alter the movement of sperm and ova in the female and block implantation of the egg in the uterus; *spermicides* that immobilize or kill sperm; *barriers* that block the movement of the sperm toward the egg; *menstrual cycle chartings* that calculate the day of ovulation; *withdrawal* that attempts to keep the semen out of the vagina, and *complete abstinence,* or the total avoidance of intercourse. *Sterilization,* the surgical alteration of the reproductive tract, should always be considered permanent.

SELECTING AN APPROPRIATE METHOD

There is no one contraceptive method that will suit everyone. The "right" method of contraception is a choice made by couples based on personalized criteria. Some key considerations follow:

1. *Safety.* The most important consideration when deciding on a contraceptive method is safety. The method should pose minimal risk and minimal side effects to the health of yourself and your partner.

....

contraception the prevention of conception.

birth control the regulation of conception, pregnancy, or birth by preventive devices or methods.

family planning the spacing, or the timing, of conception according to the wishes of the couple.

2. *Effectiveness.* Effectiveness should be maximal, thereby preventing pregnancy. As discussed in Feature 7.1, there may be two reasons why a method does not work: defects in the method itself, or incorrect use of the method. The most realistic idea of the effectiveness of a particular method is expressed by the *typical failure rate,* the percentage of failure per 100 people who have used one method for a period of a year. While a 10 percent failure rate may seem high, consider that women engaging in intercourse and using no method at all have an 85 percent pregnancy rate.[5, 6]

3. *Ease of use.* Spontaneity and ease of use are of concern for couples who use devices that are *self*-administered, such as the pill, diaphragm, cervical cap, sponge, and spermicides. Some of these devices are inserted or placed at the site of use by the user before each act of intercourse. Others, such as the pill, alter the reproductive system chemically and must be taken orally. If the device depends on the action of the user, ease of use is important. Figure 7.1 shows the sites of effectiveness for the various methods.

4. *Acceptability.* Certain methods depend upon a person's medical history, susceptibility to side effects, religious beliefs, and personal preferences. The method ultimately chosen should not interfere with a person's enjoyment of intercourse.

5. *Reversibility.* Reversibility is essential if the user wishes, at some future time, to become a parent. Surgical methods of preventing conception (such as sterilization) are largely irreversible and should be used *only* if a person is reasonably certain he or she does not want children.

6. *Affordability* and *availability.* Some costs occur once every several years (intrauterine device), while others are ongoing (pills). The device should be easily accessible from a pharmacy.

C H E C K P O I N T

1. Define the terms *birth control, contraception,* and *family planning.*

2. List the various types of contraceptives.

3. List and describe the important criteria in selecting a contraceptive method.

4. Which criteria are viewed as the most important and why?

EFFECTIVENESS OF CONTRACEPTIVE METHODS

The effectiveness of contraceptive methods is best expressed as failure rates during the first year a given method is used. Based on 100 women who start and continue to use a method, it tells how many have become pregnant in the first year. This is essentially expressed as a failure percentage rate. For instance, it is estimated that if no contraceptive method is used, about 85 percent of women who engage in intercourse will become pregnant within one year.[7] This represents a 15 percent effectiveness rate of avoiding pregnancy.

The *lowest expected failure* rate is the percentage of those women who have experienced pregnancy during the first year of using a given method when it is used consistently and correctly (see Table 7.1). The *typical failure rate* is based on a random sampling of those who experience pregnancy during the first year for a given method, whether it was used correctly and consistently or not (see Table 7.1). The typical failure rate is most representative overall of the effectiveness of any given contraceptive device.

5. Why is the typical failure rate viewed as most representative of the effectiveness of a given device?

HORMONAL CONTRACEPTIVES

Hormonal contraceptives were introduced to the U.S. market in 1960. Today over 14 million women in the United States, or approximately 30 percent, and 60 million women worldwide use the pill or some other hormonal contraceptive.[8] Hormonal contraceptives are available in two forms:

- a *combination of estrogen and progestin* pills, and
- *progestin-only* pills, implants, and injectables.

ORAL CONTRACEPTIVES

Oral contraceptives (OCs), or contraceptive hormones taken by mouth, are also known as birth control pills, the pill, or combination pills. (These terms are not applied to progestin-only minipills.) Next to surgical sterilization, the pill is the most widely used form of contraception in the United States.

Birth control pills contain a combination of a synthetic *estrogen* and *progestin,* a synthetic progesterone. The two hormones in the combination pill perform specific functions. The synthetic estrogens inhibit ovulation, ovum transport, **implanta-**

tion (the embedding of the blastocyst into the uterine lining), and the degeneration of the corpus luteum (the remains of the ruptured ovarian follicle). Progestin causes the thickening of the cervical mucus (which hampers the movement of sperm into the uterus), and inhibits ovum transport.[9]

Figure 7.1

Location of Contraceptive Effects

This drawing indicates where male and female contraceptives affect the body.

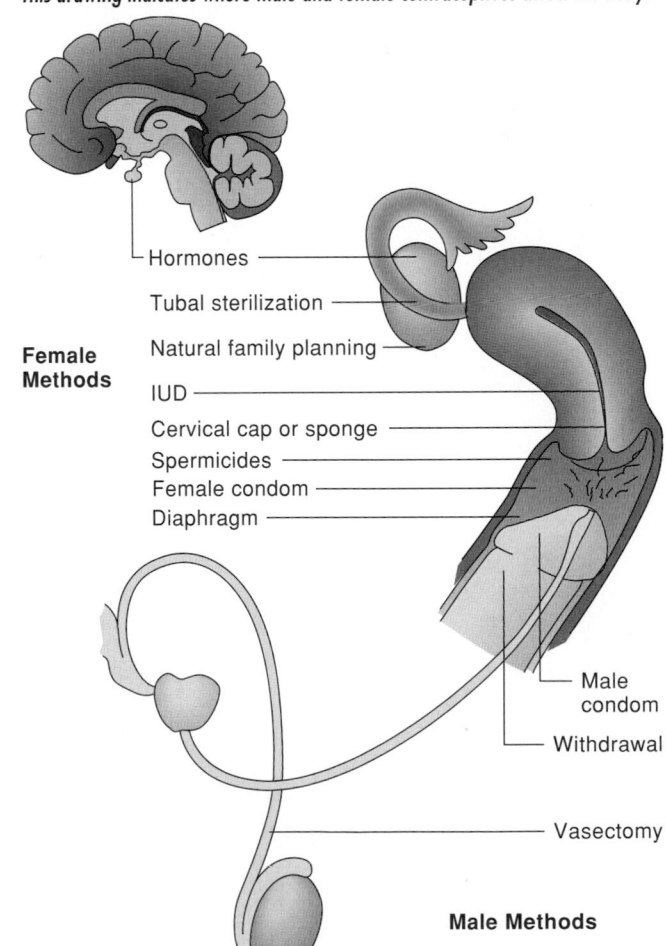

Female Methods

- Hormones
- Tubal sterilization
- Natural family planning
- IUD
- Cervical cap or sponge
- Spermicides
- Female condom
- Diaphragm
- Male condom
- Withdrawal
- Vasectomy

Male Methods

---

oral contraceptive a contraceptive hormone taken orally.

implantation embedding of the blastocyst into the uterine lining.

Table 7.1
Failure Rates, Costs, and Selected Advantages/Disadvantages of Contraceptive Methods During First Year

Method	Lowest Expected Failure Rate (%)	Typical Failure Rate (%)	Cost (approximation)	Advantages	Disadvantages
Chance (no protection)	85.0	85.0	0	No preparation; no hormones/chemicals	High risk of pregnancy; provides little peace of mind
Spermicides (aerosol foams, creams, jellies, and vaginal suppositories)	6.0	21.0	$5–$10/ container	Easy to obtain and use; no prescription required; completely reversible; no hormones; contain drugs that provide partial protection against some STDs	Continuing expense; requires high motivation to use correctly and consistently with each intercourse; may not be highly effective when used alone
Periodic abstinence or Natural Family Planning (calendar, ovulation, cervical mucus, symptothermal methods)	1.0–9.0	20.0	0	No cost; no hormones or chemicals	May be frustrating to full enjoyment of spontaneous intercourse; higher risk of pregnancy
Withdrawal (coitus interruptus)	4.0	19.0	0	No hormones or chemicals; acceptable to those who object to devices or hormones/chemicals	Requires much motivation and cooperation between partners; high risk of pregnancy may distract from full enjoyment of intercourse
Cervical cap (with spermicide)			$72	Can be left in place for several days; uses no hormones; no side effects	Continuous expense (spermicide); may be dislodged by intercourse; requires skill in insertion; may cause vaginal or cervical trauma
previous childbirth	26	36			
no previous childbirth	9	18			
Sponge (with spermicide)			$1.50/sponge	Easy to obtain and use; uses no hormones; no side effects	Continuing expense; may be inadvertently expelled; requires skill for removal; absorption of vaginal secretions may create dry vagina
previous childbirth	20.0	36.0			
no previous childbirth	9.0	18.0			
Diaphragm (with spermicide)	6.0	18.0	$40	Can be inserted up to six hours before intercourse; uses no hormones; no side effects; helps prevent disease; requires fitting by a physician or nurse-practitioner	Must be sized and fitted; continuing expense (spermicide) requires high motivation to use correctly and consistently with each intercourse; must be left in place six to eight hours after intercourse
Male condom (without spermicide)	3.0	12.0	$.50–$1.50/ condom	No side effects; easy to use; easy to obtain, helps prevent STDs	Continuing expense; must use every time; risk of tearing; may interrupt continuity of lovemaking; some loss of sensitivity
Female condom	5.0	21.0	$1/condom	No side effects; easy to use; easy to obtain; helps prevent transmission of disease	Continuing expense; must use every time; risk of tearing; may interrupt continuity
IUD			$225[a]	Needs little attention; no expense between insertion and removal	Side effects; possible expulsion; may perforate uterine wall; some incidence of pelvic inflammatory disease
Progestasert	1.5	2.0			
Copper T 380A	0.6	0.8			
Combined birth control pills	0.1	3.0	$25/month	Highly effective; easy to use	Daily use required; continuing expense; slight medical risk; side effects
Progestin-only (minipill)	0.5	3.0	$21/month	Highly effective; easy to use	May cause irregular menses; daily use required; continuing expense
Injectable progestin (Depo-Provera)	0.3	0.3	$140[b]	No day-to-day attention required; long-lasting protection	Some risk of regaining fertility; side effects; continuing expense

Method	Lowest Expected Failure Rate (%)	Typical Failure Rate (%)	Cost (approximation)	Advantages	Disadvantages
Implants (Norplant)	0.09	0.09	$500ᵃ	No day-to-day attention; low hormone levels for high protection; may protect against pelvic inflammatory disease	Tenderness at site; menstrual irregularities; expense involved in both implantation and removal
Female sterilization	0.4	0.4	$940ᵇ	Permanent relief from pregnancy worries	Low success of surgical reversal; possible postoperative and psychological complications
Male sterilization	0.10	0.15	$300ᵇ	Permanent relief from pregnancy worries	Low success of surgical reversal; possible postoperative and psychological complications
Abstinence	0.0	0.0	0	No chance of pregnancy	May require much motivation

ᵃExpense only for insertion and removal
ᵇExpense one time only

The available brands of birth control pills vary both in the specific forms and amounts of hormones present. Today, combination pills commonly contain 35–50 micrograms (mcg) of an estrogen and 1 milligram (mg) or less of a progestin. The estrogen component of the pill may range from a high of 80–100 mcg per pill down to a low of 20 mcg. Pills with an estrogen dosage of 30 mcg or less are known as low-dosage estrogen pills. The *biphasic pill* is a low-dose combination pill that contains a constant dose of estrogen (35 mcg), but provides less progestin during the first half of the cycle and more during the last half. The *triphasic pill* is a low-dose combination pill in which the amount of estrogen and progestin varies during each third of the menstrual cycle. Estrogen increases at the middle of the cycle, and progestin slowly increases throughout the cycle. The triphasic pill has a lower dose of estrogen than other combination pills and less progestin than the progestin-only pills.

The estrogen component of the pill is responsible for most of the major pill-associated complications that lead to discontinuation of use of the pill. The higher estrogen dosages are more effective in preventing contraceptive failure and bleeding irregularities, but may cause more pill-associated complications such as nausea, breast tenderness, water retention, and leg pains. Too low an estrogen content leads to breakthrough bleeding, spotting, and missed menstrual periods. If estrogen-related complications continue with the lowest estrogen dosage, the physician may prescribe a progestin-only pill (minipill).

Packaging of Oral Contraceptives

Different brands of combination pills are packaged with 21 and 28 pills, and may include different forms and dosages of hormones. With 21-pill packs, one active (hormone-containing) pill is

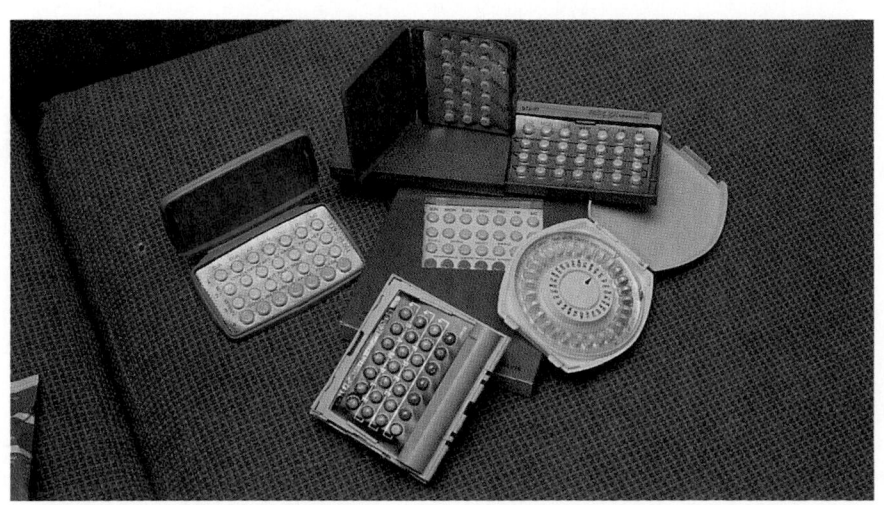

Some typical brands of birth control pills, showing 21- and 28-pill packs.

FEATURE 7.2

BEFORE STARTING TO TAKE THE PILL

Before a woman begins using the pill, her physician must know her medical history. An examination that includes a pelvic exam, breast exam, Pap smear, blood pressure check, and blood and urine tests should be conducted. Based on the information obtained from the exam, the physician will select the brand or dosage of pill best suited to the individual. The woman should only take the brand of pill prescribed, since another type of pill may affect her differently. Pills should not be accepted from a physician if an examination has not been done, nor should a woman ever give her pills to another woman.

Since the pill is given only by prescription, periodic visits to a physician are necessary for prescription renewal. Most physicians require that their patients who are on the pill return for a complete checkup at least once a year.

taken daily, starting on the fifth day after the beginning of menstruation. To maintain a uniform level of hormones in the body, a woman is advised to take a pill at the same time each day for the three weeks. During the fourth week, pill-taking is discontinued and menstruation is allowed to occur. After 7 days, a new pack is started.

In brands packaged with 28 pills, the first 21 pills are active, while the last 7 pills are inactive pills that often contain replacement iron for that lost during the menstrual period which occurs during this time. After 28 days, the woman immediately begins a new pack. By using the 28-pill pack, the woman does not have to remember the correct number of days before starting a new pack.

Using Oral Contraceptives

Oral contraceptives can only be prescribed by a physician, because a medical examination of the woman and knowledge of her medical history are necessary to make sure the pill is safe for her to use (see Feature 7.2). When first starting to take the pill, a woman is not protected from pregnancy until she has taken 14 pills over a period of 14 days. In the meantime, some other method of birth control should be used if sexual intercourse is desired.

If a pill is missed, nothing serious will happen. The woman may wish to double the next dose to minimize **breakthrough bleeding** (light vaginal bleeding between periods) and stay on schedule. If several pills are missed, another form of birth control should be used during intercourse. After menstruation, the pill can be resumed on schedule. If

menstruation does not occur, a pregnancy test may be necessary. If no pills have been missed, however, and a period is missed, and if there are no other signs of pregnancy, it is unlikely the woman is pregnant because the pill is 97 percent effective.

Although the use of the pill may not make a woman's periods regular, it often does. Even while on the pill, a period may be missed now and then. If a woman who is on the pill has irregular periods, she should continue to take the pill on schedule.

When a woman wants to become pregnant, she should finish her pill pack and not start another. Most women soon become fertile again. It's wise for the woman to use another method of contraception for 6 to 12 months after stopping use of the pill to allow her body to return to normal.[10]

Effectiveness of Oral Contraceptives

The oral contraceptive is the most effective nonsurgical, reversible form of contraception available. The combination pill has a typical failure rate of 3.0 percent and a lowest expected failure rate of 0.1 percent (see Table 7.1).

Examining the Pros and Cons of Oral Contraceptives

In deciding whether or not the pill is a viable form of birth control, individuals and couples should examine the following advantages and disadvantages:

Advantages

- is highly effective
- is easily administered
- reduces the amount of menstrual blood lost (thus conserving iron), menstrual cramps, and premenstrual complaints

breakthrough bleeding light vaginal bleeding between periods which may occur during use of progestin-containing pills.

- may decrease risk of rheumatoid arthritis, ovarian cysts, benign breast diseases, and endometrial and ovarian cancer

- protects against pelvic inflammatory disease (PID), which is a significant cause of infertility in women[11]

- causes fewer health risks than pregnancy.[12]

Disadvantages

- daily use required

- increased risk of blood clot disorders, which can lead to heart attacks, strokes, and pulmonary emboli (obstructions carried by the blood); this risk increases the longer a woman has been taking the pill, if she is a smoker, and if she is 35 years or older; overall, if you are a smoker and on the pill, your chance of death due to a circulatory disease is ten times that of nonsmokers who have never used the pill

- increased risk of hypertension (high blood pressure)

- increased frequency and intensity of migraine attacks

- increased risk of gallstones and gallbladder disease

- intensified bouts of preexisting diabetes

- reduction in milk production of nursing mothers with use of combined pill; should not be used until milk flow is well established; small amounts of hormones that appear in the milk have little effect on infant[13, 14]

- bothersome side effects (especially for first several cycles while adjusting to the pill) which resemble pregnancy, such as nausea, headaches, breast fullness and tenderness, fluid retention, breakthrough bleeding (vaginal spotting) between periods

- does not protect user against HIV infection, gonorrhea, syphilis, herpes, STDs, or cervical cancer

- ongoing costs of up to $30 or more per month (less if obtained through a college student health clinic or through a local Planned Parenthood office or affiliate).

CHECKPOINT

1. Describe the kinds of hormones contained in the combination pill and how these hormones function in preventing pregnancy.

2. Indicate the advantages of using the 28-pill pack versus using the 21-pill pack.

3. What should a woman who forgets to take one of her oral contraceptive pills do? If she forgets to take two or more of her pills?

4. List the pros and cons of using oral contraceptives.

PROGESTIN-ONLY CONTRACEPTIVES

Some of the most exciting new choices in birth control are progestin-only methods. These devices contain progestin only, rather than an estrogen-progestin combination. As indicated earlier, progestin inhibits ovulation, thickens the cervical mucus (thus impeding the entry of the sperm into the uterus), and causes the formation of a thin, less receptive uterine lining. In addition, sperm capacitation (ability to fertilize an ovum) may be inhibited, and ovum transport may be slowed.

Progestin-only contraceptives may be administered orally as a pill, through implants (Norplants), Progestasert, and by injection.

Minipills

The minipill is a low-dose progestin pill available in packets of 35–42 pills. One pill is taken daily without break for as many days as conception control is desired. Since progestin-only pills are most effective if ovulation is blocked consistently, as indicated by the absence of menstruation or prolonged intervals between menstruation, the pill must be taken at the same or nearly the same time daily. Due to the consistent blocking of ovulation for extended periods of time, one of the side effects of use of the minipill and other progestin-only agents is prolonged intervals without a menstrual discharge. Thus, the progestin-only pills are most effective when the normal menstrual patterns are most disturbed.

The significant advantage of a progestin-only pill over the combination pill is that a woman is saved from the potential adverse side effects of estrogen. Use of estrogen is known to increase the risks of high blood pressure, cardiovascular complications, and liver ailments.

The effectiveness of the progestin-only pills is slightly less than the oral contraceptive, with a typical failure rate of 3.0 percent (see Table 7.1). Older women and women who are nursing their children show a lower failure rate than other women.

Examining the Pros and Cons of Minipill Use

The pros and cons of minipill use are as follows:

Advantages

- no estrogen-related side effects
- fewer PMS symptoms than with an estrogen-containing pill
- lower levels of progestin than in combination pill
- blocks ovulation consistently
- woman may not have menstrual periods
- easy to use
- highly effective

Disadvantages

- requires a personal motivation to take the pill daily
- increased risk of ectopic pregnancy and ovarian cysts
- slightly greater risk of pregnancy than with oral contraceptives
- more difficult to find stocked in local pharmacy
- does not protect against STDs
- irregular menses
- continuing expense

Norplant

Norplant is a newly approved long-lasting contraceptive that is surgically implanted beneath the skin. The device consists of six matchstick-sized progestin-filled silicone tubes. Once implanted, these cylinders supply a slowly declining, low-level release of progestin into the bloodstream over the next 60 months. After 5 years it is recommended that the implants be replaced if continued contraception is desired. If the woman desires to become pregnant during the period of hormone release, the cylinders can be removed and the contraceptive effects soon end.

Norplant has a typical failure rate of 0.09 percent (see Table 7.1). Once implanted, the supply of hormone is constantly maintained and not subject to user error, as might be true with the pill, which must be taken daily. Norplant is being viewed by some as an answer to consistent pregnancy prevention, and as such to being used by some school-based clinics in programs to reduce the incidence of teenage pregnancies.[15] A high level of satisfaction is reported by users.[16]

Examining the Pros and Cons of Norplant Use

The pros and cons of Norplant use include:

Advantages

- no estrogen-related effects
- no day-to-day attention required
- long-term protection against pregnancy without periodic attention
- requires no preparation prior to intercourse
- little or no menstrual discharge during use
- reversible when discontinued; removable if pregnancy desired
- low hormone levels for high protection
- may protect against pelvic inflammatory disease

Disadvantages

- does not protect against STDs
- an expense involved for both the implantation and removal
- to initiate pregnancy the tubes must first be removed
- menstrual cycle irregularities range from an increase in duration of menstrual bleeding to no menstrual discharge
- tenderness at implant site on arm.
- increased risk of ovarian cysts
- enlargement of the ovaries and/or fallopian tubes
- headaches may occur; if severe, may prompt removal
- weight gain
- breast tenderness may occur; if so, treatable

Depo-Provera

Already in use in more than 90 countries, Depo-Provera was approved by the Food and Drug

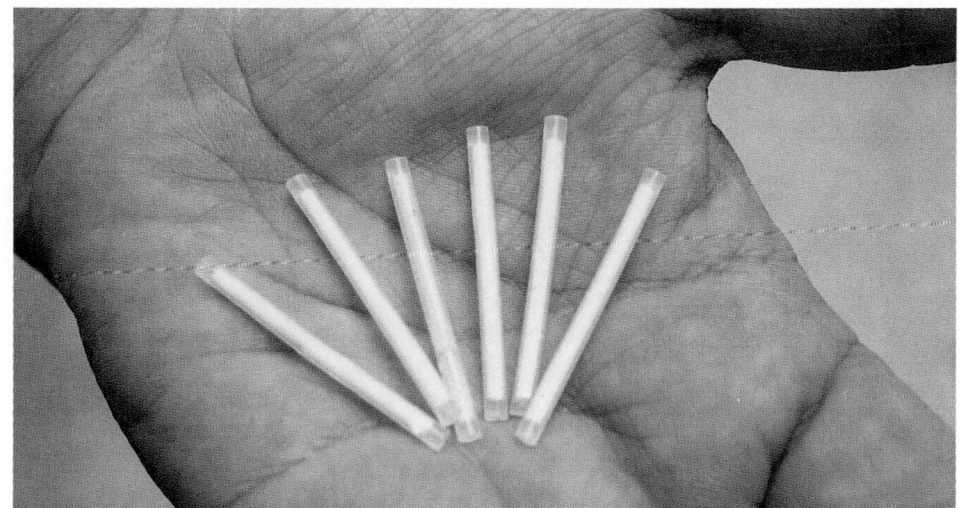

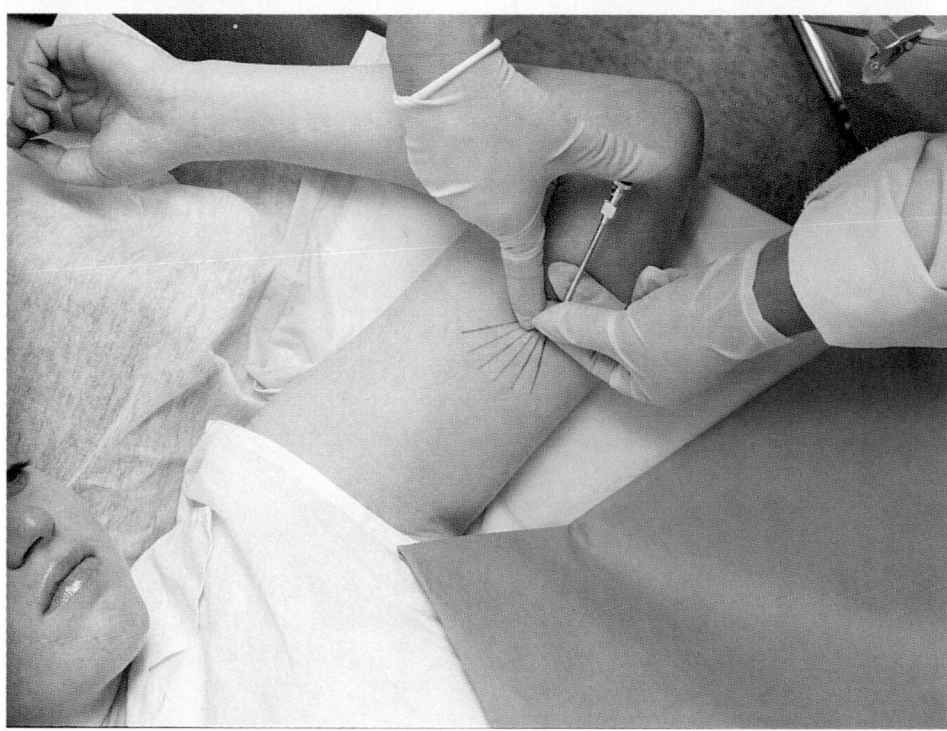

Norplant, the contraceptive implant: (top) the six implants; (bottom) implants beneath the skin of the upper arm.

Administration in 1992 for use in the United States. It is a progestin-only contraceptive which is injected into a woman two to four times per year. The popularity of Depo-Provera has been its convenience and reliability, and the belief by some societies that injections are preferable to oral medications.[17] Nor does its use require a surgical implantation, as with Norplant.

A given injection actually provides for more than three months of protection, giving four to six weeks of "grace period" in case the woman is late in coming in for her next injection. Highly effective, the typical failure rate is 0.3 percent (see Table 7.1).

Examining the Pros and Cons of Depo-Provera The pros and cons of Depo-Provera injection include:

Advantages
- no need for surgical implants
- no day-to-day attention required
- gives extended protection against pregnancy
- highly effective.

Disadvantages
- does not protect against STDs
- some users experience weight gain, headaches, and nausea

- possible delay in return of fertility following discontinued use
- menstrual irregularities (some women desire menstruation as indication of absence of pregnancy)
- some women are hesitant to take injections
- continuing expense.

Other Progestin-only Contraceptives

The progestin-containing IUD will be discussed in the next section. The following progestin-only devices are still undergoing development.

Capronor is a biodegradable capsule implant. Inserted under the skin in the hip or upper arm through a small incision, the implant is expected to provide contraceptive protection for 18 months or longer. Once implanted, the capsule cannot be removed. This device is still in development.[18]

Norethindrone is a biodegradable pellet about the size of a grain of rice. Implanted in the upper arm, the pellet, which may be effective for at least 12 months, cannot be removed. This device is still in development.[19]

Vaginal rings are plastic rings implanted with progestin. Placed around the cervix, the ring can be inserted by the woman for periods of time and left in place during the time between the menses. The hormone supply, which diffuses into the bloodstream through the vaginal wall, lasts one to six months.[20]

CHECKPOINT

1. How are Norplant and Depo-Provera administered?
2. For how long a period of days can minipills be taken without a break?
3. Compare the typical failure rate of Norplant with that of the combined oral contraceptives.

BREASTFEEDING AND HORMONAL CONTRACEPTIVES

Breastfeeding confers a brief period of infertility on the mother. Yet she can regain her fertility before she can detect signs that her menstrual cycle will resume. In other words, her first ovulation following delivery may precede her first menstruation.

Thus, breastfeeding is not a reliable method of controlling conception. In waiting for her first menses, the sexually active mother faces the risk of pregnancy.

Taking the combination pill during nursing decreases the volume and the protein content of the milk, although the progestins have minimal affect. Small amounts of the pill's hormones may be found in breast milk, although they have no bearing on the infant's nutrition and weight gain. It is recommended that a new mother avoid resuming the use of pill until she has established a good flow of breast milk.[21]

At the same time, it may also be important for a woman to avoid the risk of pregnancy during nursing. Thus, the new mother may be initially placed on a barrier device such as the diaphragm. If choosing an oral contraceptive during this time, the progestin-only contraceptives are seen as a better choice than the combination ones.[22, 23]

CHECKPOINT

1. Why is breastfeeding not a reliable method of controlling conception?
2. Why might a woman wish to avoid oral contraceptives during lactation?

INTRAUTERINE DEVICES

The **intrauterine device (IUD),** a device placed inside the uterus to interfere with the implantation of the fertilized ovum, was first used experimentally in Europe in the 1930s. During the 1950s and 1960s in the United States, the design and effectiveness were dramatically improved and the IUD became a viable method of birth control. Various forms of the IUD have been developed.

The IUD is a modern refinement of the centuries old practice of placing a foreign object into the uterus to avert pregnancy. Today, the IUD is a small (1 × 1½ inch) plastic device (some with a copper coil) that fits inside the uterus (see Figure 7.2). Once inserted through the cervical canal and posi-

intrauterine device (IUD) a device placed inside the uterus and left there to interfere with the implantation of the fertilized egg.

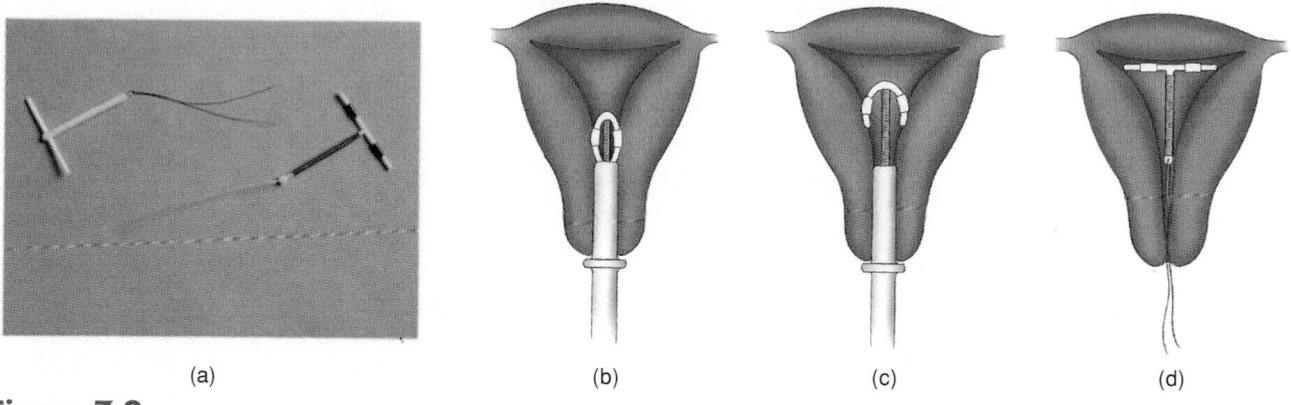

(a)   (b)   (c)   (d)

Figure 7.2
FDA Approved IUDs

(a) Several types of IUDs currently in use. Insertion of an IUD: (b) An applicator carrying an IUD is inserted past the cervix of the uterus. (c) The IUD is inserted into the cavity of the uterus. (d) The applicator is withdrawn.

tioned in the uterus, it remains in place until removed or accidentally expelled.

The IUD prevents pregnancy by affecting sperm, ova, fertilization, implantation, or the endometrial lining of the uterus. Its primary effects are that sperm mobility is reduced, ova transport through the fallopian tubes is speeded up, and fertilization is inhibited. In the event fertilization does occur, implantation is impeded due to the endometrium being adversely affected by copper or progesterone. Unfortunately, the IUD provides no chemical or physical protection against the passage of sexually transmitted diseases.

TYPES OF IUDS

IUDs are categorized according to their shape and the materials from which they are made. By the early 1990s, the only types of IUDs marketed in the United States were the progesterone T (Progestasert) and the Copper T 380A (ParaGard). In addition to these, types still available in other countries include the Lippes Loop and the Copper 7.

- The progesterone T contains a supply of progestin in the stem of the T, which is gradually released into the uterus. This concentration of progestin interferes with the endometrial cells and inhibits implantation of a fertilized egg. Due to the dissipation of the progestin within a year, this device is approved for one year of contraceptive protection, after which it must be replaced.

- The Copper T is a soft plastic T-shaped device around which a fine copper wire is coiled. The copper slowly dissolves into the uterine fluids, where it interferes with estrogen uptake by the endometrium. The most predominantly used IUD in the United States, the Copper T has the lowest failure rate of any IUD developed to date. This device is approved for four years of use.

- The Copper 7 is a plastic device, shaped like the numeral 7, around which a fine copper wire is coiled. Its action is similar to that of the Copper T. Its U.S. distribution was curtailed during the mid-1980s due to concerns over liability by its manufacturer.

- The Lippes Loop is an uncovered plastic device shaped into an open configuration which, once inserted into the uterus, can be left in place for an extended time. Its U.S. distribution was also stopped during the 1980s over liability concerns.

The use of IUDs became controversial in the United States during the 1980s because, in some cases, they were marketed before sufficient research was done to demonstrate their safety over a long period of time. Some of them were implicated in a number of cases of miscarriage and pelvic diseases, and were allegedly responsible for some deaths. As a consequence, certain IUDs became the focus for massive product liability suits. Manufacturers' decisions were based on their not being able to obtain liability insurance and on the fear of the high costs of defending themselves in the event of potential lawsuits being filed against them. Worldwide, IUDs are widely marketed and remain highly popular. They are the leading contraceptive in use in China, Egypt, Norway, and England.[24]

INSERTION

A physician or nurse-practitioner places an IUD into a woman's uterus. While insertion may be easier near the end of the menstrual period when the cervical canal is more dilated, it can be done at any time during the cycle. After insertion, the silk threads are clipped so that they are visible high inside the vagina. The device can then be left in place from one to several years, during which time no other contraceptive protection is required. Recommended replacement time depends on the specific device being used.

When the woman wishes to become pregnant, she should return to her physician or nurse-practitioner to have the IUD removed.

EFFECTIVENESS

The typical failure rate of IUDs is 0.8–2.0 percent. The lowest expected failure rate for the Copper T 380A is 0.6 percent and for the Progestasert is 1.5 percent (see Table 7.1).

EXAMINING THE PROS AND CONS OF IUDs

In deciding whether or not to use the IUD, it is important to examine the following advantages and disadvantages:

Advantages

- instantly reversible upon removal
- once inserted, it needs little attention
- no preintercourse planning or preparation; nothing to remove afterward
- no effect on the body's progesterone level
- failure is less common among users over 30 years of age and for those who have previously given birth
- no expense between insertion and removal.

Disadvantages

- initial cost to purchase the device and have it inserted
- periodic replacement of the device
- need to check for presence of silk thread before each act of intercourse
- small increase in blood loss during menstruation
- 10–15 percent of women have the IUD removed due to bleeding, spotting, or cramping; such removal is most common shortly after insertion
- possibility of perforating or embedding in uterine wall
- risk of pelvic inflammatory disease (PID), which may lead to sterility
- possibility of expulsion; about 5–20 percent of users spontaneously expel their IUDs within the first year of use
- possibility of ectopic (tubal) pregnancy within several months after the removal of an IUD
- possibility of miscarriage if pregnancy occurs with the IUD in place
- no protection against STDs

VAGINAL SPERMICIDES

Placing substances such as honey and lemon juice into the vagina to form a barrier to sperm is an ancient practice. Today, this practice has been refined in the form of **vaginal spermicides.** These products contain a combination of chemical contraceptives in an inert (inactive) chemical base. The active agent in most spermicide products in this country is *nonoxynol-9,* a drug that destroys or immobilizes sperm and provides at least partial protection against some STDs, including HIV, the virus that causes AIDS. Spermicides usually come in the form of a cream, jelly, foam, or **suppository.** The suppository is made of a semisolid sub-

vaginal spermicide a chemical agent applied in the vagina that kills or immobilizes sperm.

suppository a semisolid substance containing spermicide that is introduced into the vagina, where it dissolves.

stance containing spermicide, and is placed inside the vagina to dissolve.

USE

To effectively use the spermicide, it should be inserted into the vagina before intercourse. It works in two ways. First, the foam, jelly, or cream serves as a mechanical barrier to block sperm from moving into the cervical canal. Second, the spermicide kills sperm within the vagina.

Aerosol foam is inserted using an applicator (Figure 7.3). Aerosol foam is the most effective spermicide. Once the foam is dispensed, it forms a dense and even distribution over the cervical opening. Creams and gels, also widely available, are introduced into the vagina by means of an applicator. Tablet forms are also available.

EFFECTIVENESS

As contraceptives, the spermicides have a typical failure rate of 21 percent and a lowest expected rate of 6 percent (see Table 7.1). As with any contraceptive device applied or put in place by the user, wider disparity in failure rates is observed with the use of spermicides, condoms, diaphragms, sponges, and cervical caps. If your concern is with the transmis-sion of STDs, the Centers for Disease Control states that a spermicide containing nonoxynol-9 used in conjunction with a condom provides the most effective protection against HIV.[25]

EXAMINING THE PROS AND CONS OF VAGINAL SPERMICIDES

In deciding whether or not to use vaginal spermicides, consider the following advantages and disadvantages:

Advantages

- easy to obtain and use
- inexpensive and available over-the-counter; requires no pelvic examination or prescription
- fully reversible
- provides some protection against sexually transmitted diseases, thus may help prevent transmission of the virus that causes AIDS
- decreases chances of developing pelvic inflammatory disease (PID)
- increases the effectiveness of the condom, diaphragm, or IUD; it can be used as a lubricant with the condom

Figure 7.3
Vaginal Spermicides

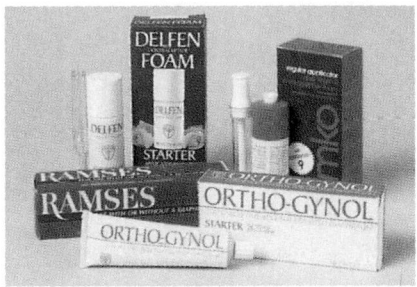

(a)

(a) Properly used, vaginal foams can be an effective method for averting pregnancy, as the spermicides immobilize or kill sperm on contact. In using an aerosol foam: (b) the applicator is filled with foam, and (c) the foam-filled applicator is inserted deep into the vagina. In (d) a vaginal suppository is inserted deep into the vagina.

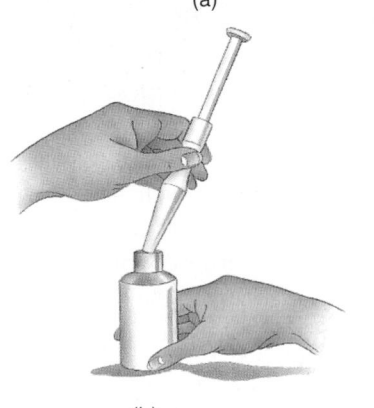

(b)

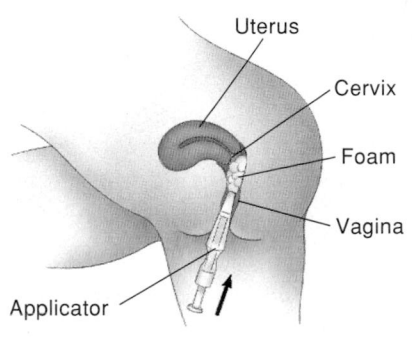

(c)

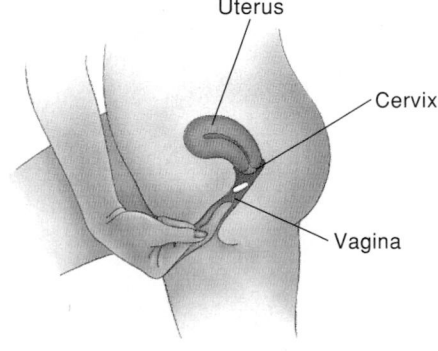

(d)

- can be used when no other method is available, as a backup method when pill use is beginning or terminating, or during menopause
- useful for persons who are sexually active on an infrequent basis.

Disadvantages

- not highly effective when used alone
- some require a 10- to 30-minute waiting period between insertion and intercourse
- requires preplanning and high motivation; must be used before *each* intercourse
- some women or their partners are allergic to, or irritated by, certain brands
- some spermicide suppositories may fail to liquefy completely; others tend to leak from the vagina
- continuing expense

CHECKPOINT

1. What is an IUD and how does its use affect pregnancy?

2. List the pros and cons of IUD use.

3. How does a spermicide protect a woman against pregnancy?

BARRIER METHODS

Barrier methods are contraceptives that are designed to serve as physical barriers to prevent sperm from meeting the egg. One, the male condom, is worn by the man; the others, the female condom, diaphragm, sponge, and cervical cap are worn by the female. Historically, the barrier contraceptives and spermicides were some of the most important and widely used forms of contraception until the arrival of the oral contraceptives in 1960 when they declined in popularity. In the last few years, with the great concern over STDs, especially HIV, the barrier devices are presently the only con-

traceptive devices which, when used with a spermicide containing nonoxynol-9, are effective in giving some measure of protection against the STDs.[26]

MALE CONDOM

Commonly referred to as "rubbers," "safes," and "prophylactics," the **male condom** is a sheath worn over the erect penis to catch the ejaculate and keep it from entering the vagina (Figure 7.4). Condoms are the second most widely used contraceptive device in the United States after the pill.

All condoms are approximately the same length and width, and are fitted with a ring at the open end to keep them from slipping off the penis. Condoms differ in shape and in the presence or absence of a reservoir end (nipplelike extension at the tip to hold ejaculate). Other differences include the presence or absence of lubricants (wet jellies or dry powders) and the presence or absence of spermicide on the inside and outside. While some condoms are tinted, most are a neutral color.

Most condoms available today are made of thin rubber latex; some are made of young lamb intestines, and are called "skins." Skin condoms used for disease prevention are of special concern. They contain tiny pores not found in latex condoms which allow the passage of viruses such as HIV and hepatitis B. The Food and Drug Administration does not allow skin condom packages to carry the "disease prevention" labeling found on packages of latex condoms.[27]

Use

The spermicidal condom, available since the early 1980s, is very effective in killing sperm within the condom. The active agent in the spermicide, nonoxynol-9, quickly inactivates sperm ejaculated into the condom.[28] Spermicidal condoms, along with spermicides and vaginal barriers, are the only available contraceptive products that help reduce the risk of sexually transmitted diseases. The use of condoms in combination with other methods can improve contraceptive effectiveness, encourage a

barrier methods contraceptive methods that use a physical barrier to block the sperm from meeting the egg.

male condom a thin sheath worn over the erect penis to stop sperm from entering the vagina.

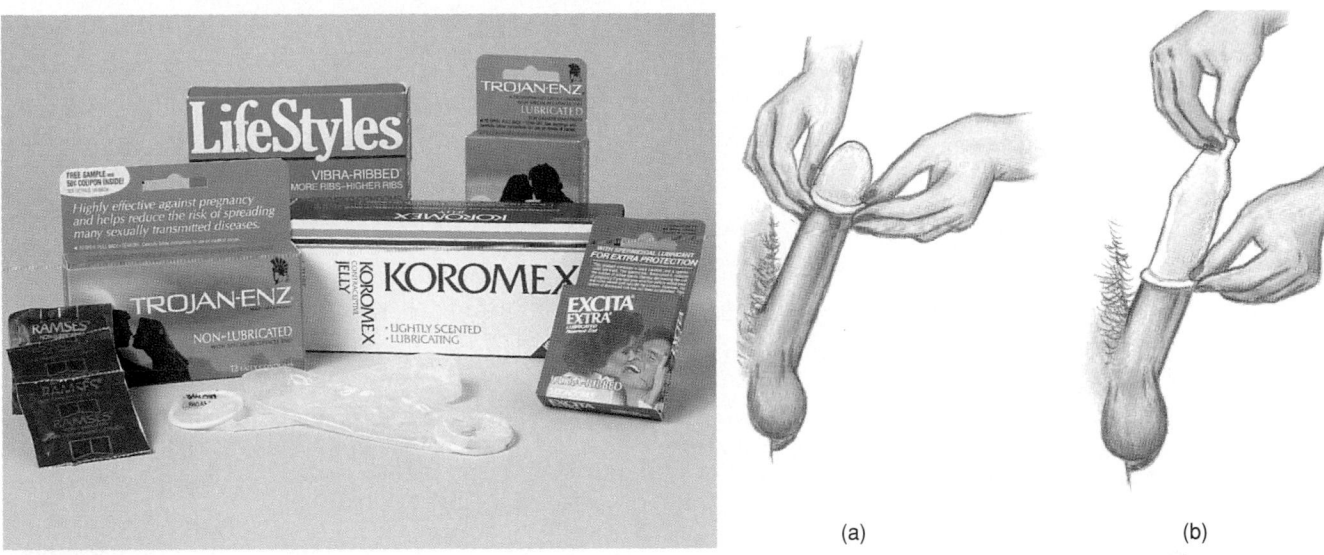

(a)   (b)

Figure 7.4
The Male Condom

Male condoms are one of the most accessible and affordable forms of birth control. Most condoms come packaged in foil and rolled, ready for convenient use. Using a condom: (a) Squeeze the air out of the tip of the condom and place it over the head of the penis, with space left at the tip to hold the semen when ejaculated. (b) Unroll the condom down over the glans and shaft of the penis to the scrotum. The condom should be placed on the penis before any vaginal contact and should be removed promptly after ejaculation.

shared responsibility for contraception, and reduce the risk of contracting HIV and other sexually transmitted diseases (see Feature 7.3, p. 196).

Effectiveness

The lowest expected failure rate of the condom is 3.0 percent, while the typical failure rate is 12 percent (see Table 7.1). The use of a foam inside and outside the condom significantly improves the condom's effectiveness.

Examining the Pros and Cons of Male Condoms

In deciding whether or not to use a condom, it is important to be aware of the following advantages and disadvantages:

People who are mature enough to engage in sexual intercourse are able to take accountability together for their sexual activities.

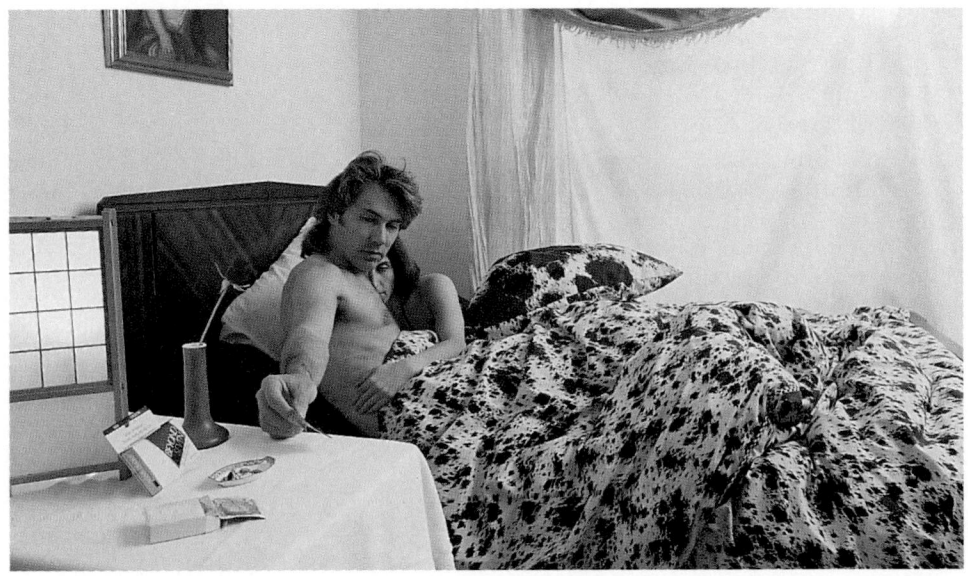

FEATURE 7.3

USING THE MALE CONDOM

To use the male condom successfully, remember to:

1. Use a condom every time you have intercourse.

2. Handle the condom carefully to prevent tearing by fingernails or rings.

3. Put the condom on the penis *before* the penis first touches the partner's genitals. (See Figure 7.4 for the proper method of applying a condom.)

4. Unroll the condom all the way to the base of the penis. Leave about one-half inch of empty space at the tip of the condom or use condoms with reservoir ends to hold the semen.

5. Lubricate the condom with K-Y Jelly, a spermicide, or saliva, if necessary. Do *not* use oil-based lubricating products, such as petroleum jelly (Vaseline), baby oil, vegetable oil, butter, mineral oil, and suntan oil; they adversely affect the condom.

6. Withdraw the penis soon after ejaculation and before erection is lost. Pinch the ring against the penis to prevent spilling the semen near the vagina to reduce the risks of pregnancy and of sexually transmitted diseases.

7. Check the condom for tears before throwing it away. In case semen is accidentally spilled into the vagina, apply some spermicide into the vagina immediately to minimize the risk of pregnancy.

8. Dispose of the condom after use. *Never* reuse a condom.

9. Store condoms in a cool, dry place. Avoid keeping them in your wallet for long periods of time, since body heat can cause rubber to deteriorate.

Advantages

- no side effects
- completely reversible; prior fertility is restored after use is discontinued
- inexpensive
- easily available over-the-counter; requires no examination or prescription; no prior fitting required
- can be purchased by either males or females
- there are no health hazards associated with use; contains no hormones
- if used for sexual intercourse (from start to finish), and for oral and anal sex, will reduce the risk of transmission of sexually transmitted diseases such as HIV[29]
- may prevent the occurrence of precancerous cervical growths. The growth of new abnormal tissue has been closely linked to STDs[30]

Disadvantages

- use requires motivation; it must be used consistently; there must be no contact between the genitals of the partners without the condom in place; no seminal fluids may be allowed to touch the female's genitals
- some users or partners are allergic to latex and may need to use a natural condom, which is ineffective in preventing the transmission of STDs
- placing the condom on the erect penis may interfere with the continuity of lovemaking
- the condom may reduce the sensitivity of the head of the penis
- some men are psychologically affected by the condom and are unable to maintain erection with it on
- continuing expense

CHECKPOINT

1. Describe how a male condom works. How effective is it in preventing pregnancy?

2. List the pros and cons of male condom use.

FEMALE CONDOM

The **female condom** is a vaginal pouch designed to offer contraception and STD protection. Several devices have been variously designed and made of latex or polyurethane. The Reality condom, approved by the Food and Drug Administration for sale in the United States in 1992, is made of polyurethane (a clear plastic similar to the material used in food storage bags).

female condom a pouch worn inside the vagina to serve as a barrier to sperm and to protect the woman against sexually transmitted disease transmission.

Use

Resembling a male condom, the "one size fits all" device consists of flexible rings connected by a polyurethane sheath (Figure 7.5). One ring is at the closed end of the sheath and fits loosely over the cervix in a manner similar to the diaphragm. The second ring, at the open end of the sheath, remains outside the vagina and covers the vulva, thus protecting the labia from exposure to microorganisms carrying sexually transmitted diseases. The design of the condom allows the penis to move freely inside the sheath during intercourse. The female condom is disposable after a single act of intercourse.[31]

Effectiveness

According to preliminary data available, the lowest expected failure rate of the female condom is 5.0 percent, whereas the typical failure rate is 21 percent.[32] The effectiveness of the device in blocking the passage of microorganisms, including HIV, appears to be about the same as for the male condom.

Figure 7.5
Female Condom

Insertion and positioning: (a) the inner ring is squeezed for insertion; (b) the sheath is inserted, similarly to a tampon; (c) inner ring is pushed up as far as it can go with index finger; (d) in place.

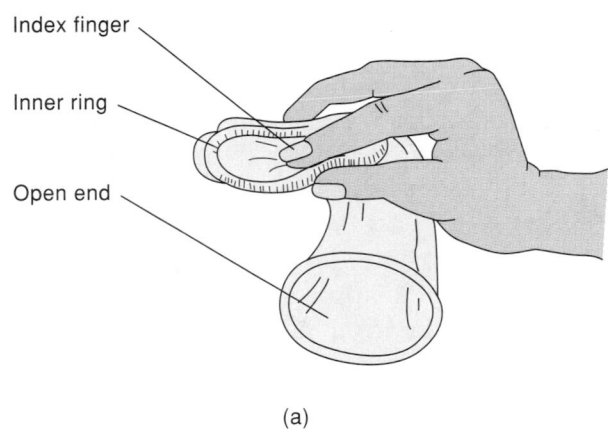

(a)

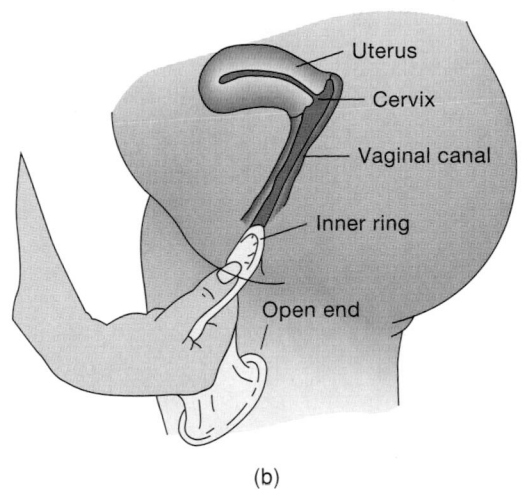

(b)

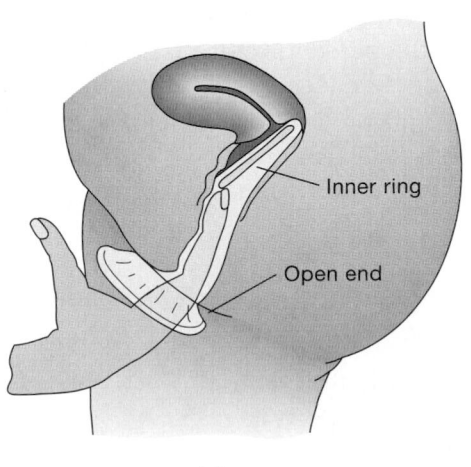

(c)

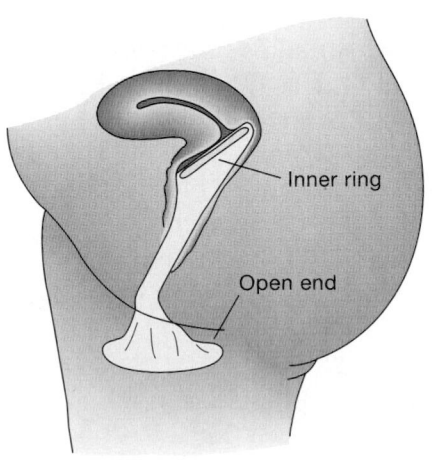

(d)

Examining the Pros and Cons of the Female Condom

Before deciding to use the female condom, consider the following pros and cons:

Advantages

- no side effects
- completely reversible
- can be purchased by either males or females
- no fitting required by a health professional
- one size fits all
- available over-the-counter

Disadvantages

- some loss of sensitivity
- use requires motivation; it must be used consistently
- must be no contact between the genitals of the partners without the condom being in place; no seminal fluids may be allowed to touch the female genitals

DIAPHRAGM

The **vaginal diaphragm** was the most commonly used contraceptive until the pill and IUD became the more popular forms of birth control. While the diaphragm has lost much of its earlier popularity, many women are rediscovering that when used with a spermicide it is a safe alternative to the pill and IUD.

The diaphragm is a shallow, round dome, 2–4 inches in diameter, made of soft latex rubber. Its rim covers a flexible metal spring or coil with rubber, which helps hold it in place when inserting it in the vagina. When placed in the vagina, it completely covers the cervix of the uterus (see Figure 7.6).

The diaphragm blocks sperm from entering the cervix and holds spermicide against the cervix to kill sperm that may have moved across the rim of the diaphragm. Along with male condoms, and

----

vaginal diaphragm a shallow, dome-shaped device that is positioned inside the vagina over the cervix to serve as a barrier to sperm.

spermicides, vaginal barriers such as the diaphragm are the only available contraceptive products that help reduce sexually transmitted disease rates.

Use

Women must be measured and fitted for a diaphragm by a physician or nurse-practitioner. Women are urged to practice inserting and removing the fitted diaphragm before leaving the physician's office. Size and fit should be checked again every year or two, and immediately after childbirth, miscarriage, abortion, or after any significant weight change.

Before each insertion, the diaphragm should be checked for holes or cracks. The inside dome and rim should then be covered with about a teaspoon of spermicide.

To insert the diaphragm, the woman squeezes the cup together and inserts it deep into the vagina so that it completely covers the cervix. After intercourse, it must be left in place for 6–8 hours to ensure that any sperm that have moved across the rim are killed. If intercourse is repeated before the 6–8 hours, spermicide should be applied with an applicator (leaving the diaphragm in place). The diaphragm should not be left in place more than 24 hours after intercourse.

To remove the diaphragm, the woman hooks a finger around the ring and pulls it out. After removal, the diaphragm should be washed with warm water and mild soap, rinsed, dried, and stored in a container away from heat and light.

Effectiveness

When used with a nonoxynol-9–containing spermicide, the diaphragm has a lowest expected failure rate of 6 percent, and a typical failure rate of about 18 percent (see Table 7.1). Failures are mainly due to inaccurate fittings, inaccurate insertion, or dislodging during intercourse. To be effective, the diaphragm must be used with each act of intercourse.

Examining the Pros and Cons of the Diaphragm

In deciding whether or not to use the diaphragm, the following advantages and disadvantages should be examined:

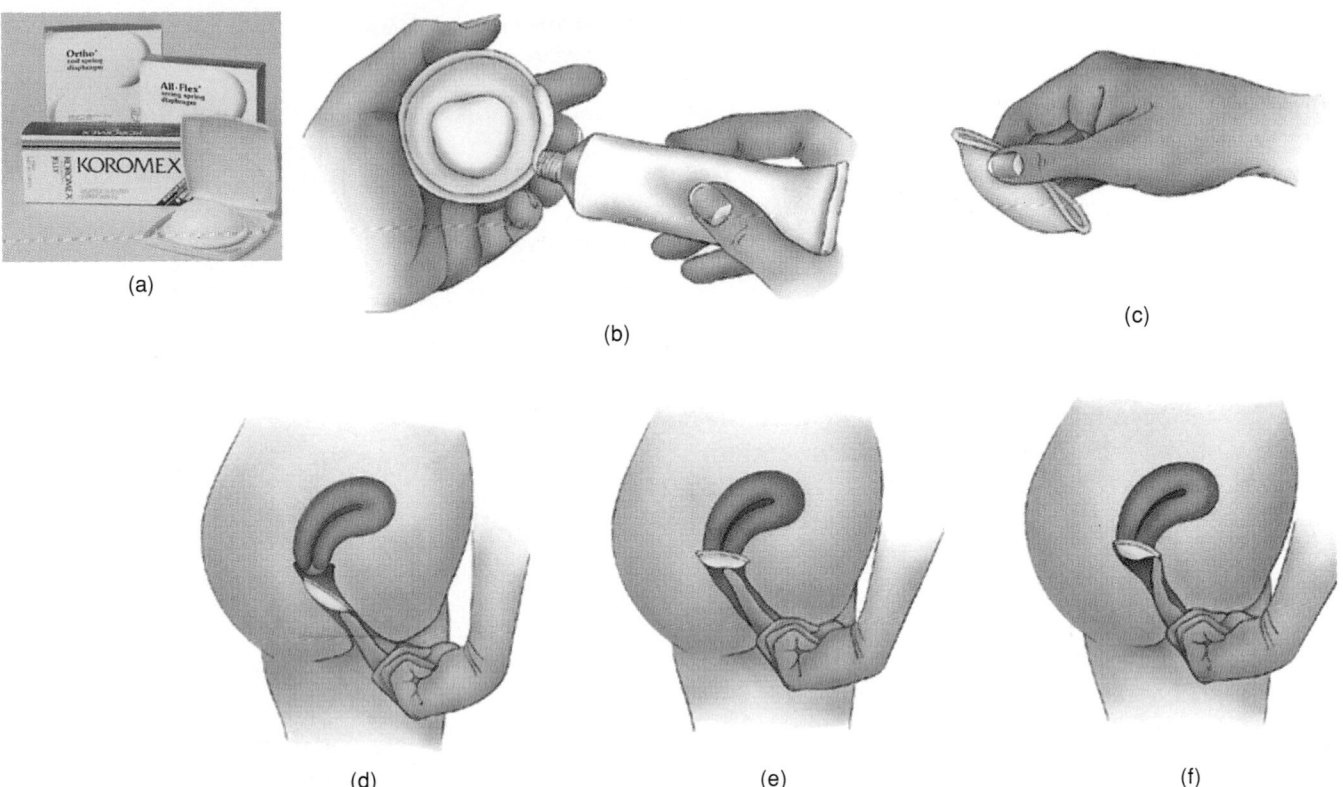

(a)

(b)

(c)

(d)

(e)

(f)

Figure 7.6
The Diaphragm

(a) Various types of diaphragms and spermicidal jellies and creams. Use of the vaginal diaphragm: (b) A spermicide is applied around the rim and in the dome. (c) The diaphragm is pinched between the fingers and the thumb. (d) The pinched diaphragm is inserted into the vagina and pushed in as deeply as it will go. (e) Proper positioning is checked by feeling the cervix through the soft rubber dome of the diaphragm. (f) To remove the diaphragm, hook a finger under the forward rim and pull.

Advantages

- can be inserted up to 6 hours before intercourse begins
- completely reversible; prior fertility is restored after use is discontinued
- no health hazards are associated with its use; uses no hormones
- can be used for one to two years after being properly fitted
- safer than the oral contraceptive or IUD when fitted properly and used consistently
- reduces the risk of contracting sexually transmitted diseases, pelvic inflammatory disease, and cervical cancer when used with spermicide

Disadvantages

- must be sized and fitted by a physician or nurse-practitioner
- requires some skill in its insertion
- requires motivation to use with each act of intercourse
- some users and partners are allergic to latex and/or spermicide
- taste of spermicide may make oral sex objectionable (user may wish to insert diaphragm after oral sex, but before intercourse)
- must be left in place for 6–8 hours after intercourse
- continuing expense (of spermicide)

CONTRACEPTIVE SPONGE

Natural sea sponges have been used since ancient times to prevent conception; however, it was not until the early 1980s that the Food and Drug Administration approved a contraceptive sponge in the United States. This device is a small (2½ inch × ¾ inch) pillow-shaped polyurethane pad or sponge containing spermicide.

Use

To use the sponge, it must be moistened with tap water, compressed, and inserted deep into the vagina by hand. Once in place, it expands to fill the space around the cervix, thereby blocking the cervical opening.

The sponge provides immediate and continuous protection for up to 24 hours, after which it is removed. After intercourse it must be left in place for at least 6 hours. It is removed by pulling on the loop and is then discarded.

Effectiveness

The sponge has a lowest expected failure rate of 9–18 percent and a typical failure rate of 18–28 percent. The failure rates are significantly higher, in contrast to the diaphragm and cervical cap, for women who have already had children.[33]

Examining the Pros and Cons of the Sponge

Before deciding to use the sponge, it is important to compare the following advantages and disadvantages to see if this method is right for you:

Advantages

- easy to obtain; available over-the-counter
- easy to use; comes in a single size (no fitting required)
- reversible
- effective for up to 24 hours after insertion; allows for repeated intercourse without interruption
- sponge absorbs the ejaculate
- uses no hormones; no side effects
- spermicide reduces transmission of sexually transmitted diseases
- a simple backup option when other methods of contraception are unavailable; its use increases the effectiveness of some other methods

Disadvantages

- some women have difficulty inserting and/ or removing it

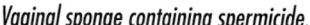
Vaginal sponge containing spermicide.

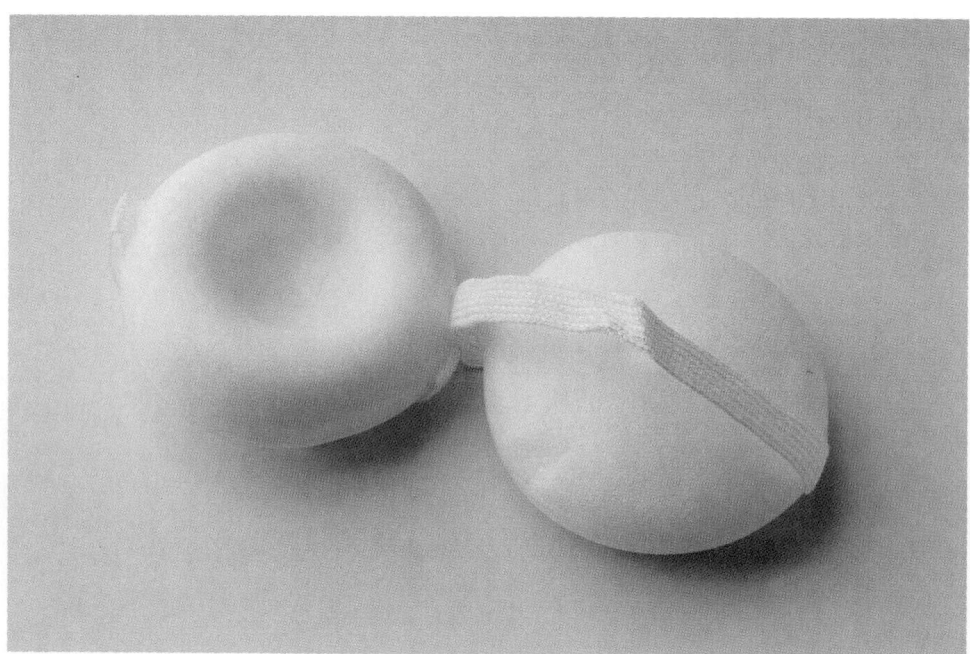

- anatomic abnormalities of the vagina, uterus, or rectum may interfere with its proper placement or retention in the vagina
- some users are allergic to polyurethane and/or spermicide
- the sponge may absorb excessive amounts of vaginal secretions, leading to vaginal dryness
- should not be used during menses
- may create unpleasant odor if left in place for more than 18 hours
- the sponge may be expelled involuntarily, such as during bowel movements
- use increases the risk of toxic shock syndrome (see Chapter 6)
- continuing expense

CERVICAL CAP

The **cervical cap** is a thimble-shaped soft rubber device with a rim that fits snugly over the cervix. The device is about 1½ inches long and comes in several different diameters. After being inserted, the cap is held in place by suction created by the near air-tight seal around the cervical opening. A small amount of spermicide is applied inside the cap prior to insertion to kill any sperm that might break through the seal. The cap resembles a miniature diaphragm, except the tighter seal around the cervix allows fewer sperm to pass around the edge of the rim.

Early forms of the cervical cap, which were made of metal, were common in Europe. Newer forms of the cap, which are used today, are made of soft rubber. In 1988 the Food and Drug Administration approved the cervical cap for nationwide use in the United States.[34]

Use

In many ways, using the cervical cap is similar to using the diaphragm. The cap must be sized and

....

cervical cap a small plastic or rubber contraceptive device that fits snugly over the cervix to serve as a barrier to sperm.

fitted by a physician. As with the diaphragm, the woman should practice inserting and removing the cap before leaving the physician's office.

The cap should be one-third to two-thirds full of spermicide before it is inserted. The cap is pushed deep into the vagina until the rim forms a seal around the cervix.

Once inserted, no more spermicide is needed for several days regardless of sexual activity. After intercourse, the cap must be left in place for at least 8–12 hours.

Strong odors may develop in the vagina if the cap is left in place longer than 36–48 hours; some women remove the cap daily or every other day to let cervical secretions pass. Prolonged wear may also increase the risk of toxic shock syndrome.[35] During a woman's period, the cap should not be used. If it is used, it should be removed at least daily to let secretions flow. The seal of the cup may be broken by the menstrual flow.

Effectiveness

The cap, used by the woman with no previous childbirth, has a lowest expected failure rate of 9 percent and a typical failure rate of 18 percent, or about equal to that of the diaphragm (see Table 7.1).

Examining the Pros and Cons of the Cervical Cap

The following advantages and disadvantages should be considered before deciding whether or not to use the cervical cap:

Advantages

- relatively inexpensive
- completely reversible
- no hormones; no side effects
- less spermicide is used with the cap, thus it is less messy than the diaphragm
- can be inserted as long as one to two days before intercourse, thus insertion need not interfere with lovemaking; once inserted, it can be left in place for three to four days
- may reduce the incidence of cervical cancer.

Disadvantages

- must be sized and fitted

- more difficult to insert and remove than the diaphragm
- may be dislodged by intercourse
- may irritate the cervix after prolonged use
- strong odors tend to develop if cap is in the vagina for more than 36–48 hours
- must be removed during menses or secretions may break seal around the cap
- may not protect against sexually transmitted diseases, including HIV
- may need replacement (resizing and refitting) after birth of a child or after more than 20 pounds of weight gain or loss
- continuing expense (spermicide)

C H E C K P O I N T

1. List the kinds of barrier devices.

2. What are the advantages and disadvantages of using a diaphragm to prevent pregnancy?

3. Where is the contraceptive sponge placed in order to prevent conception?

4. What is a cervical cap and how is it used?

5. Describe the differences between the construction of the female condom and male condom.

MENSTRUAL CYCLE CHARTING AND PERIODIC ABSTINENCE

Charting of the menstrual cycle is based on observations of the menstrual changes during a cycle. Documenting any changes allows for preventing or planning for pregnancy by pinpointing the day on which a woman ovulates and identifying her fertile days, those days on which an ovum is present to be fertilized. The success of this method in preventing pregnancy depends on abstinence from intercourse during a woman's fertile days. As such, this is not a method of contraception since there is the use of no device or chemical to prevent conception on the days a woman might be fertile.

Using these natural rhythms for preventing, or planning for, pregnancy is identified by various

terms. **Natural family planning (NFP)** is using menstrual cycle charting and the postponing of intercourse during the fertile days to avoid conception. **Fertility awareness** is the use of charting combined with barrier methods during the fertile days to avoid conception.

The NFP methods take into account that sperm inseminated into the woman's body and kept at normal temperature during the fertile, or unsafe, period remain alive from two to seven days, and that the ovum is estimated to remain viable for up to 72 hours. Thus, conception can occur only if intercourse takes place from seven days before ovulation to three days afterward. This period is called the fertile, or unsafe, period.

CHARTING METHODS

Several charting methods are used to pinpoint the day of ovulation. Some refer to these as the rhythm methods. They include: (1) the *calendar method*, (2) the *basal body temperature method*, (3) the *cervical mucus method*, and (4) the *symptothermal method*. Each of these methods is based on three assumptions: (1) that ovulation occurs 14 days (plus or minus 2 days) *before* the beginning of menstruation; (2) that sperm deposited into the vagina remains viable for 2–3 days; and (3) that unless fertilized by sperm within 12–24 hours after ovulation, the egg degenerates.

Calendar (Rhythm) Method

The **calendar method** is a way of calculating the onset and duration of the fertile period each month. This method requires that the woman record the length of her menstrual cycles for a period of eight months. The first day of menstruation is day one of

....

natural family planning (NFP) use of menstrual cycle charting and the postponing of intercourse during the fertile days to avoid conception.

fertility awareness use of menstrual cycle charting with the use of barrier methods during the fertile days to avoid conception.

calendar method use of the calendar to calculate the onset and duration of the fertile, or unsafe, period each month in a woman.

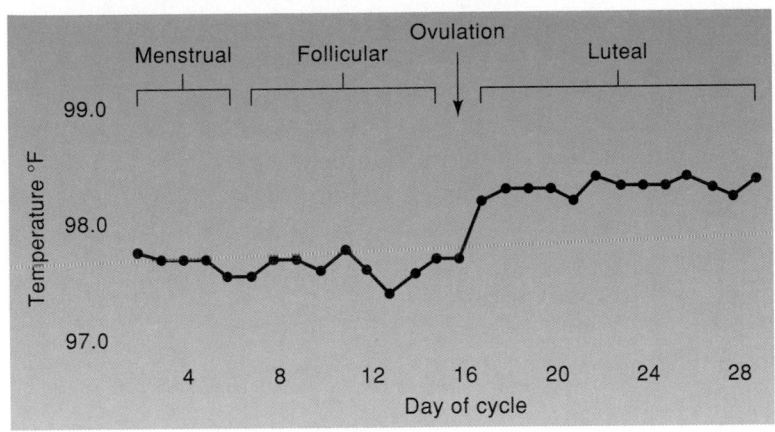

Figure 7.7
Basal Body Temperature (BBT) Chart

Note that the temperature pattern for this average woman includes a sharp rise in BBT on day 17, indicating the point of ovulation as day 16.

the new cycle. She can then calculate the fertile period of the new cycle by subtracting 18 days from the length of the shortest recorded cycle to find the *first* fertile (unsafe) day, and 11 days from the length of the longest cycle to find the *last* fertile (unsafe) day. For example, if all the cycles are 28 days long, the first unsafe day is the tenth day and the last unsafe day is the seventeenth day. If the shortest cycle is 26 days and the longest cycle is 30 days, the first unsafe day each month is the eighth day, and the last unsafe day each month is the nineteenth day. To be safe, there must be no intercourse between the first and last fertile day *every* month.

Basal Body Temperature Method

This method is based on the theory that a correlation exists between body temperature and ovulation. The **basal body temperature (BBT)** is defined as the lowest body temperature of a healthy person during the time he or she is awake.

A woman using the BBT method should take her temperature daily, immediately upon waking and *before* getting out of bed or engaging in any physical exercise. The temperature should be taken orally or rectally with a basal temperature thermometer (with 0.1 degree intervals from 96 to 100 degrees Fahrenheit). The BBT is recorded on a chart. Generally low two weeks prior to ovulation, a woman's BBT usually dips slightly a day before ovulation, *then rises sharply*. The temperature stays

....

basal body temperature use of the lowest body temperature of a healthy person during the time he or she is awake.

high the rest of the cycle, then falls at the start of the next period and stays low until the next ovulation (Figure 7.7).

Cervical Mucus Method

The cervical mucus method, also known as the Billings or ovulation method, depends on the woman's awareness of "dryness" and "wetness" in her vagina. She must be aware of changes in the amount and kind of cervical mucus secreted at different times in her menstrual cycle.

A yellow, viscous (sticky), cloudy mucus is normally present during most of the cycle. Near the time of ovulation, the secretion becomes clear and slippery (like a raw egg white). The last day of this clear, slippery mucus is called the peak day. Ovulation usually occurs on the day *after* the peak day. A woman may be fertile from the time the clear mucus appears until the fourth day *after* the peak day. Infertile, safe days are likely to occur during the relatively dry days just before and after menstruation.

Symptothermal Method (STM)

The STM combines the BBT with the cervical mucus method. With it, a woman uses mucus observations *before* ovulation, and changes in cervical mucus and BBT to confirm ovulation. The fertile period ends either at the end of the third day, when her temperature is elevated or on the fourth day after peak mucus, whichever occurs later. The temperature method, when used alone, is of little value in determining the infertile or fertile days *before* ovulation.

EFFECTIVENESS

Overall, the lowest expected failure rate is between 1 and 9 percent and the typical failure rate of NFP is 20 percent (see Table 7.1). The wide margin between the lowest expected and typical failure rates is due in part to the fact that some women and men find it difficult to follow procedures carefully. Yet, for couples who avoid all intercourse contact on fertile days, the effectiveness is much better. Of the four charting methods, the symptothermal method has the lowest expected failure rate.[36]

Examining the Pros and Cons of Natural Family Planning

Before deciding to use NFP, the following advantages and disadvantages should be examined:

Advantages

- no cost
- no health risks to the partners; no drugs or hormones
- completely reversible
- helpful for those who object (religiously or otherwise) to mechanical or chemical methods of contraception
- helps a woman know her own body

Disadvantages

- requires motivation by both partners, with careful record keeping and observation of the woman's body
- intercourse must be avoided on fertile days (and in some or many cases, preovulatory days) or else some other device must be used
- may be frustrating if there are no other sexual outlets during the days of abstinence
- failure rate is higher than many other methods

ABSTINENCE

Sexual abstinence is the voluntary avoidance of sexual intercourse. Also known as celibacy, it may be a temporary or long-standing practice.

Abstinence is practiced by some persons to avoid the possibility of pregnancy; as such, it is the most effective form of birth control (see Table 7.1). Some individuals abstain from intercourse to avoid contracting or transmitting sexually transmitted diseases. Others avoid sexual intimacy until they find a person with whom they think they may want a long-term relationship. (For more about celibacy, see Chapter 6.)

EXAMINING THE PROS AND CONS OF SEXUAL ABSTINENCE

There is good reason to reflect on the advantages and disadvantages of sexual abstinence:

Advantages

- no chance of pregnancy
- avoids sexually transmitted diseases, such as the HIV (although if the couple engages in oral sex while practicing abstinence, diseases can be transmitted)
- may intensify sexual desire
- may fulfill a religious commitment

Disadvantages

- may create feelings of loneliness
- denies the person the satisfaction he or she could get from a sexual relationship
- it may lead to frustration if a person is sexually aroused and is unable to find ways of releasing his or her sexual tensions

WITHDRAWAL

Withdrawal (*coitus interruptus,* "taking care," "pulling out") is perhaps the oldest of all contraceptive methods. This practice involves withdrawing the erect penis from the vagina just before ejaculation of semen. The partners' expectation is that sperm will not be deposited within the vagina or on the genital lips.

·······································

withdrawal the removal of the penis from the vagina prior to ejaculation as a method of controlling conception; also called coitus interruptus.

Very few couples successfully use withdrawal to control conception as this method requires both timing and considerable discipline. The man must be alert to the first signs of ejaculation and be prepared to terminate intercourse at the first sign of climaxing. Sperm can move on their own and, if deposited on *any part* of the woman's genitals, may continue moving up into the fallopian tubes.

Withdrawing the penis before climax runs counter to the sexual instincts of both partners. Women often prefer continued thrusting movements so they can attain orgasm, and some men prefer deep penetration at the moment of ejaculation. Withdrawal tends to curtail complete sexual pleasure for both partners.

The woman may be unable to fully enjoy intercourse due to worry the man may not pull out in time. Some couples find little disruption in early withdrawal, others find it unfulfilling.

Even if the man withdraws before climaxing, this method is not foolproof. Evidence shows that the preejaculatory (Cowper's) fluid that leaves the penis early in the erection may carry millions of sperm. This fluid may be deposited deep in the vagina before the man has any feelings of ejaculation.

EFFECTIVENESS

The typical failure rate of 19 percent, and the lowest expected failure rate of 4 percent (see Table 7.1), does not make withdrawal a highly promising method of preventing pregnancy.

EXAMINING THE PROS AND CONS OF WITHDRAWAL

In assessing the advantages and disadvantages of withdrawal, consider the following:

Advantages

- it requires no preparation or devices
- it costs nothing
- it involves no chemicals or hormones
- the man takes the primary responsibility (yet the woman's cooperation is necessary)

Disadvantages

- impossible for the man to avoid preejaculatory seepage into the vagina

- difficult for man to judge the timing of actual ejaculation; emission of semen may occur both before and after climax
- some couples have trouble controlling themselves at height of sexual excitement and tend to suspend good judgment
- high failure rates for withdrawal makes this the method of last resort

CHECKPOINT

1. What is meant by natural family planning? What are the four methods of natural family planning described in this chapter?

2. Discuss the pros and cons of sexual abstinence.

3. Explain the principle of withdrawal and clarify how this technique might help prevent pregnancy.

4. Give some reasons why withdrawal is not the most reliable method of birth control.

STERILIZATION

Since 1982, **sterilization** has been the predominant method of birth control in the United States. Today in the United States better than 39 percent of all users of contraception have undergone surgical sterilization.[37] Also known as surgical contraception, sterilization is the voluntary surgical interruption of the reproductive tracts of either the male or female to prevent the passage of sperm and egg cells, and thus prevent fertilization. Because sterilization is generally permanent and provides complete protection, it has great appeal to couples who do not desire children, or to those who already have children and do not want to have more. Other than abstinence, sterilization is the most effective method of contraception.

Surgical alteration of the reproductive tract must be considered cautiously before it is chosen

....

sterilization the surgical interruption of the male or female reproductive tracts, preventing the passage of sex cells, and thus fertilization.

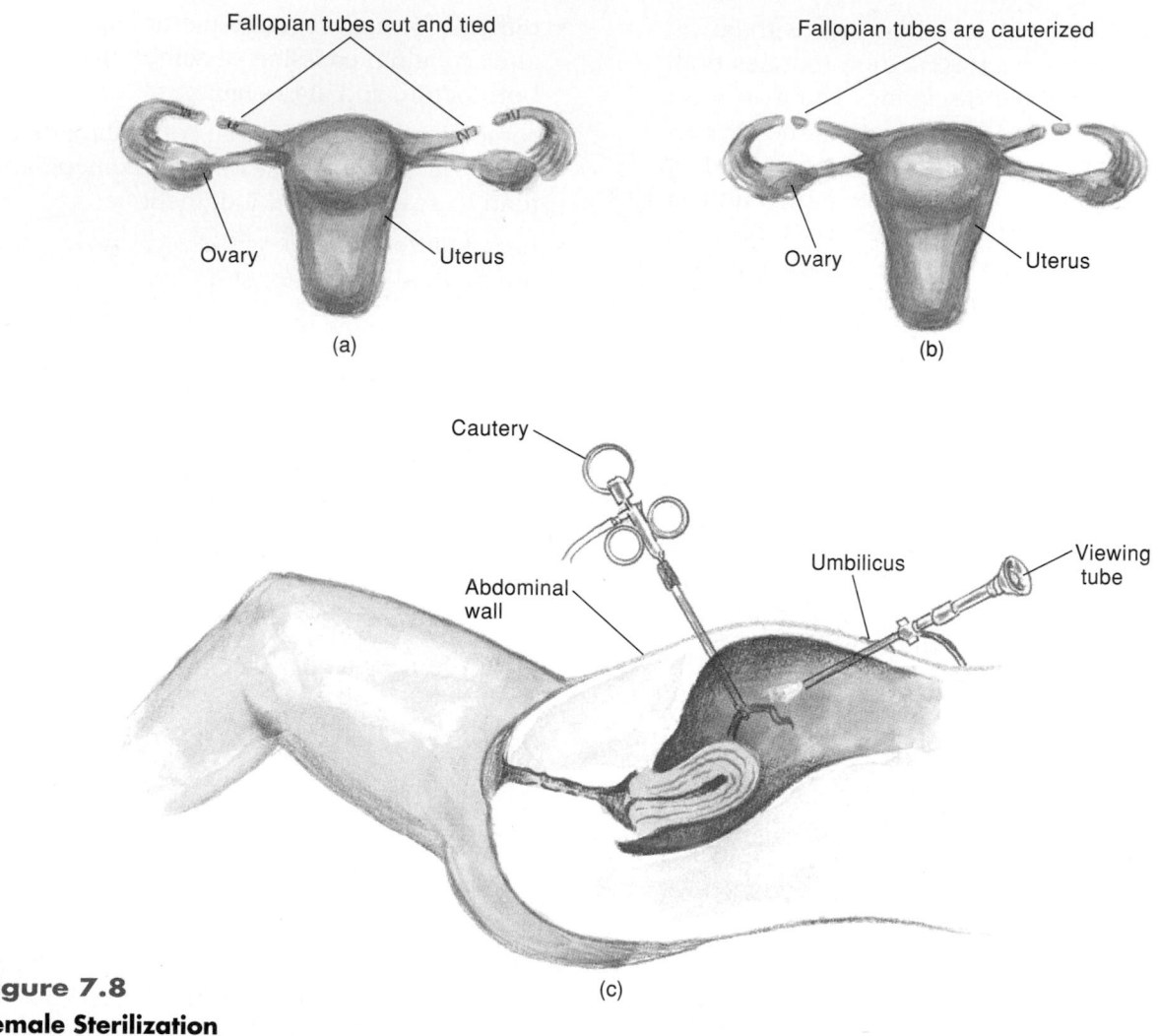

Fallopian tubes cut and tied

Ovary   Uterus

(a)

Fallopian tubes are cauterized

Ovary   Uterus

(b)

Cautery

Abdominal wall

Umbilicus

Viewing tube

(c)

Figure 7.8

Female Sterilization

The fallopian tubes may be interrupted by: (a) cutting and ligating (tying) them, or (b) by cauterizing (heat-sealing) them. (c) Sterilization is commonly performed by means of a laparoscope, a lighted optical instrument which a physician inserts through a small incision in the abdominal wall.

as an option. Once sterilization has been performed, it is generally irreversible. Some sterilized persons have, for various reasons, later wished to regain their reproductive capacity. While such procedures are sometimes successful, restoration of fertility is far from assured.

FEMALE STERILIZATION

The usual method of female sterilization is by a tubal blocking, or sterilization, of the fallopian tubes so that sperm and the egg cannot meet. Tubal sterilization is usually performed by way of the abdominal wall (minilaparotomy or laparoscopy), but may also be approached by way of the vagina, entering the end, or dome, of the vagina

(Figure 7.8). Female sterilization can also be accomplished by a partial or complete **hysterectomy** (*his-ter-ek'tō-mē*), or removal of the uterus.

In a **minilaparotomy** (*min-i-lap-ar-ot'ō-mē*) a tiny incision is made in the lower abdomen and each fallopian tube is lifted from the abdomen and surgically interrupted by one of several techniques. A **laparoscopy** (*lap-ar-os'kō-pē*) may be per-

....

hysterectomy surgical removal of part or all of the uterus.

minilaparotomy a tiny surgical opening of the abdomen.

laparoscopy the use of an endoscope for abdominal exploration.

formed by making one or two tiny openings in the abdominal wall. A lighted tubal optical instrument called an **endoscope** (*en'dō-skōp*) is inserted and the fallopian tubes are located and surgically interrupted inside the abdomen. This is performed by **ligation** (*lī-ga'shun*) (tying), mechanical closure, or **occlusion** (*ō-kloo'zhun*) by means of clips or rings, or by **electrocoagulation** (*ē-lek-trō-kō-ag-ū-la'shun*), in which electric current is used to cause a thickening and closure of the tube.

Effectiveness

Considering the various techniques used, overall female sterilization has a lowest expected failure rate of 0.2 percent and a typical failure rate of 0.4 percent (see Table 7.1). Some sterilizations have failed, however, due to regrowth or reconnection of the severed tubes.

Examining the Pros and Cons of Tubal Sterilization

Due to the general irreversibility of sterilization, any woman considering it should weigh its advantages and disadvantages very carefully:

Advantages

- highly effective, permanent method of birth control
- it is immediately effective
- some women have heightened interest in sexual activity due to allayed fear of pregnancy
- one-time procedure
- no long-term side effects
- no effect on a woman's ability to enjoy intercourse and experience orgasm
- tubal sterilization poses far less of a threat to life and health of a woman over 35 than does oral contraception or term pregnancy

---

endoscope a long tubular device with an optical system inserted through a small body opening for observing internal body parts or cavities.

ligation tying off.

occlusion closure of a passage.

electrocoagulation thickening and closure of a tube by use of electric current.

Disadvantages

- some women face unexpected psychological adjustment over knowing they can no longer reproduce
- attempts to reverse the sterilization are costly, difficult, and uncertain (overall, 50 percent or less are successful; the risk of subsequent tubal pregnancy is higher)
- postoperative complications are possible

MALE STERILIZATION

Males are sterilized through **vasectomy,** which is minor surgery that consists of cutting and tying the two vas deferens, the tubules that carry sperm from each testis to the penis (see Figure 7.9, p. 208). This procedure can be performed under local anesthesia in a physician's office.

After the procedure is done, the man must have two consecutive sperm counts of zero before he is considered sterile. Since many sperm are stored in the vas deferens *above* the site of surgery, and only some of these sperm leave the vas deferens after each ejaculation, some contraceptive method must be used for six to eight weeks after a vasectomy.

Some men feel anxiety about having a vasectomy because they believe it may affect their ability to have an erection, produce ejaculate, or enjoy orgasm. Such fears are unfounded because the vasectomy leaves the man's genital system and hormones operative. Vasectomy does not affect erection or feelings of orgasm, and the volume of ejaculate remains relatively unchanged. The bulk of semen comes from the prostate gland and seminal vesicles (neither of which is affected by the surgery); sperm cells make up only about 3 percent of a man's semen. After vasectomy, the sperm cells remain in the epididymis and vas deferens, where they disintegrate and are absorbed by blood vessels.

Some men face psychological adjustment over losing their ability to impregnate. They may view their genitals as central to their anatomy and equate fertility with virility and masculinity. Men who are subject to the fear of becoming impotent may not be good candidates for vasectomy; they

---

vasectomy the surgical closing of the vas deferens to prevent conception.

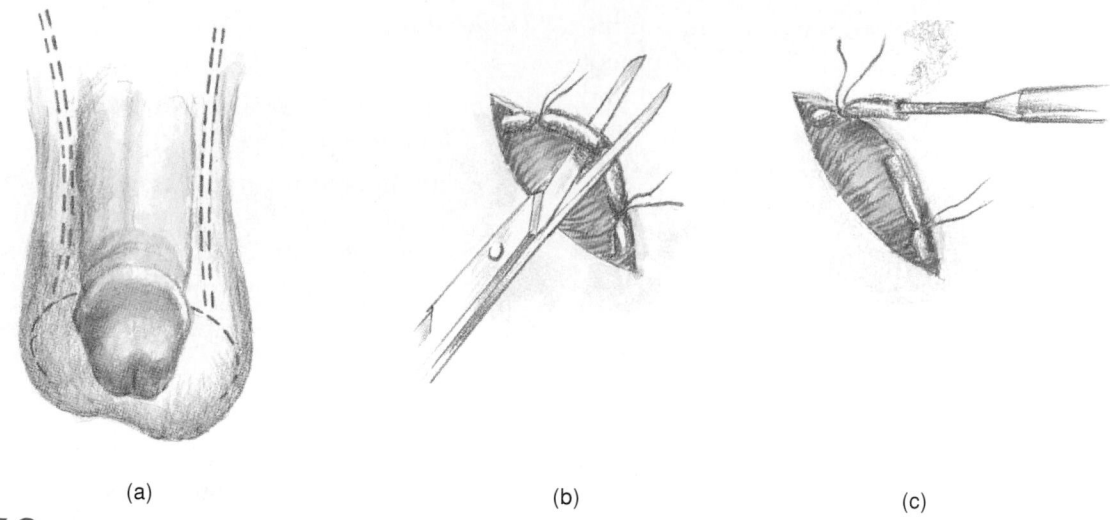

(a)   (b)   (c)

Figure 7.9

Male Sterilization by Vasectomy

To prevent sperm from (a) traveling from the testes up into the reproductive trace, (b) each vas deferens is ligated (tied) and cut, and (c) cauterized (heat-sealed) to block the passage of sperm.

Source: Masters, W., Johnson, V., and Kolodny, R. Human Sexuality, 4th ed. New York: HarperCollins, 1992.

may risk sexual dysfunction after surgery. (For more on sexual dysfunctions, see Chapter 6.)

Effectiveness

The failure rates of vasectomy are 0.2 and 0.15 percent (see Table 7.1). Mistakes in performing the surgery, regrowth of the cut ends of the vas deferens, or unprotected intercourse before the sperm count is negative account for these failures.

Examining the Pros and Cons of Vasectomy

Due to the general irreversibility of vasectomy, a man considering it should carefully compare its advantages and disadvantages.

Advantages

- a highly effective, permanent method of birth control
- it is much less expensive than tubal sterilization
- it is a one-time procedure
- complication rates are low; no long-term clinical side effects

Disadvantages

- male may have feelings of lost masculinity due to his lost fertility

- male is not immediately sterile
- attempts to restore fertility do not always succeed (the longer the period of time since the sterilization, the lower the rate of success; overall no higher than a 50 percent success rate)

CHECKPOINT

1. Why should a couple consider the pros and cons of sterilization carefully before agreeing to have it performed on either partner?

2. How is female sterilization performed?

3. What common name is given to male sterilization and how is such sterilization performed?

4. Explain the effectiveness of female and male sterilization in avoiding pregnancy.

CONTRACEPTION RESEARCH

Following much activity in contraception research, ongoing development slowed dramatically in the 1980s. Largely a casualty of the product-liability crisis involving contraceptive devices, many companies halted research or abandoned the market. Still, some research has continued. Some of the new products in various stages of investigation or testing include the following:

Male pills (gossypol). Currently undergoing testing by the Food and Drug Administration, this non-hormonal pill is derived from cottonseed meal. Developed and used by the Chinese, the pill alters sperm production, structure, and motility without causing a reduction in levels of testosterone, the hormone critical to the male sex drive. After discontinuing use of the pill, the man's sperm count usually returns to normal, although in some cases infertility is prolonged after use has been discontinued. Some toxic effects have also been reported in the use of the pill.

Filshie Clip. The clip is a female sterilization device that closes off the fallopian tubes. Upon removal reversal is far easier than with other sterilization techniques.

Antisperm vaccine. Research is going on for a vaccine that attacks sperm. An enzyme called lactic dehydrogenase is extracted from sperm and injected into the woman, whose body develops antibodies that attack sperm and reduce their motility and ability to fertilize eggs.

Male injectables. One such blocks GnRH, the hormone that regulates sperm production and which may be paired with another hormone that maintains libido.[38] A synthetic form of testosterone is being researched, which when injected, reduces sperm counts to safe levels by inhibiting sperm production.

Plug sterilization. In a reversible male sterilization procedure, two tiny puncture holes are made in each vas deferens, through which two silicone plugs are inserted into each vas. Upon removal of the plugs, a small stitch closes the hole, which heals almost immediately.[49]

DECISIONS REGARDING CONTRACEPTION

In this chapter you have been given information on kinds of contraceptive devices, their costs, rates of effectiveness, how to use them, and the pros and cons of their use.

Yet, having information about contraceptive devices and having access to them is often not sufficient motivation for persons to want to protect themselves against unintended pregnancy. Beyond this, and in a personal way, you need to examine questions and give answers to your own feelings and fears regarding the use of contraceptive devices. In Your Hands: Contraceptive Comfort and Confidence Scale presents a list of questions

---

IN YOUR HANDS
CONTRACEPTIVE COMFORT AND CONFIDENCE SCALE

It is important to choose a method of contraception that is effective and that is comfortable for you. Answering the following questions will help you assess the method you are using or thinking of using, and will help you decide which method is best for you. Interpretations to your answers are found at the end of these questions.

Method of contraception you are considering using: .

1. Am I afraid of using this method?   yes   no
2. Would I really rather not use this method?   yes   no
3. Will I have trouble remembering to use this method?   yes   no
4. Have I or my partner ever become pregnant while using this method?   yes   no
5. Will I have trouble using this method correctly?   yes   no
6. Do I still have unanswered questions about this method?   yes   no
7. Does this method make menstrual periods longer or more painful?   yes   no
8. Does this method cost more than I can afford?   yes   no
9. Could this method cause me or my partner to have serious health complications?   yes   no
10. Am I opposed to this method because of any religious beliefs?   yes   no
11. Is my partner opposed to this method?   yes   no
12. Am I using this method without my partner's knowledge?   yes   no
13. Will using this method embarrass my partner?   yes   no
14. Will using this method embarrass me?   yes   no

(continues)

15. Will I or my partner enjoy intercourse less because of this method?   yes   no
16. If this method interrupts lovemaking, will I avoid using it?   yes   no
17. Has a nurse or physician ever told me *not* to use this method?   yes   no
18. Is there anything about my personality that could lead me to use
    this method incorrectly?   yes   no
19. Am I at risk of being exposed to HIV (the AIDS virus) or other sexually
    transmitted infections?   yes   no

Total number of "yes" answers: _____.

INTERPRETATION

Most individuals will have a few "yes" answers. "Yes" answers mean that potential problems may lie in store. If you have more than a few "yes" responses, you may want to talk to your physician, a counselor, partner, or a friend. Talking it over can help you to decide whether to use this method, or how to use it so it will really be effective for you. In general, the more "yes" answers you have, the less likely you are to use this method consistently and correctly.

Source: Hatcher, R., et al. *Contraceptive Technology, 1990–1992,* 15th ed. New York: Irvington, 1990.

you should ponder and answer at this point. Evaluate your results and follow the directions at the end.

SUMMARY

Sexual intercourse can provide one of the most satisfying expressions of your sexuality. Yet, sexual intercourse often carries with it the threat of an unwanted pregnancy.

Conception may be controlled by using contraceptives, the various types of which include: combination estrogen and progestin oral pills; progestin-only pills, implantations, and injections; IUDs containing copper and progesterone; spermicides in cream, jelly, foam, and suppository form; male condoms; vaginal barriers, such as diaphragms, cervical caps, sponges, and female condoms; periodic abstinence; withdrawal; celibacy; and sterilization. Research continues into other contraceptive devices. The selection of a method of contraception is a very personal decision that you and your partner must agree upon to ensure mutual satisfaction and to minimize the risk of an unwanted pregnancy.

REFERENCES

1. Stark, E. "Young, Innocent and Pregnant." *Psychology Today* (October 1986), 28–35.
2. Wallis, C. "Children Having Children." *Time* (9 December 1985), 78–90.
3. Stark, op. cit.
4. Wallis, op. cit.
5. Hatcher, R., et al. *Contraceptive Technology, 1990–1992,* 15th rev. ed. New York: Irvington, 1990.
6. Boston Women's Health Book Collective. *The New Our Bodies, Ourselves.* New York: Simon and Schuster, 1992.
7. Hatcher, R., et. al. *Contraceptive Technology, 1994–1996,* 16th rev. ed. New York: Irvington, 1994.
8. Haub, C. "Survey Report, United States Contraception Prevalence." *Population Today,* Vol. 19, No. 3 (March 1991).
9. Hatcher, 1990 op. cit.
10. Ibid.
11. Boston Women's Health Book Collective, op. cit.
12. Hatcher, 1990 op. cit.
13. Ibid.
14. Cunningham, F., et al. *Williams Obstetrics,* 19th ed. Norwalk, CT: Appleton-Lange, 1993.
15. Hatcher, 1990 op. cit.
16. Kantrowitz, B. "The Norplant Debate." *Newsweek* (15 February 1993) 37–41.
17. Kantrowitz, B. "A 'Silver Bullet' Against Teen Pregnancies." *Newsweek* (14 December 1992) 4.
18. Hatcher, 1990 op. cit.
19. Ibid.
20. Ibid.
21. Ibid.
22. Ibid.
23. Stewart, F., et al. *Understanding Your Body.* New York: Bantam, 1987.
24. Roan, S. "The Quiet Rebirth of the IUD." *Los Angeles Times* (22 July 1993), A-1, 20, 21.

25. Centers for Disease Control. "Condoms for the Protection of Sexually Transmitted Diseases." *Morbidity and Mortality Weekly Report* 9 (1988), 133–137.
26. Cunningham, op. cit.
27. Consumers Union. "Can You Rely on Condoms?" *Consumers Reports* (March 1989), 135–141.
28. Hatcher, 1990 op. cit.
29. Ibid.
30. Ibid.
31. Segal, M. "Cervical Cap: Newest Birth Control Choice." *FDA Consumer* (September 1988) 32–35.
32. Hatcher, 1994 op. cit.
33. Hatcher, op. cit.
34. Hatcher, 1990, op. cit.
35. Ibid.
36. Ibid.
37. Haub, 1990, op. cit.
38. Begley, S. "If You Don't Like Implants." *Newsweek* (15 February 1993), 42.
39. Hatcher, 1990 op. cit.

SUGGESTED READINGS

Boston Women's Health Book Collective. *The New Our Bodies, Ourselves*. New York: Simon & Schuster, 1992.

Cassell, C. *Straight Talk from the Heart: How to Talk to Your Teenagers About Sex and Love*. St. Paul, MN: S and S, 1987.

Chesler, E. *Woman of Valor: Margaret Sanger*. New York: Anchor, 1992.

Hatcher, R., et al. *Contraceptive Technology*, 16th rev. ed. New York: Irvington, 1994.

McCoy, K., and Wibbelsman, C. *The New Teenage Body Book*. Los Angeles: The Body Press, 1987.

Reinisch, J. *The Kinsey Institute New Report on Sex*. New York: St. Martin's, 1990.

Sedgwick, S. *The Good Sex Book*. Minneapolis: CompCare, 1992.

Stewart, F., et al. *Understanding Your Body: Every Woman's Guide to Gynecology and Health*. New York: Bantam, 1987.

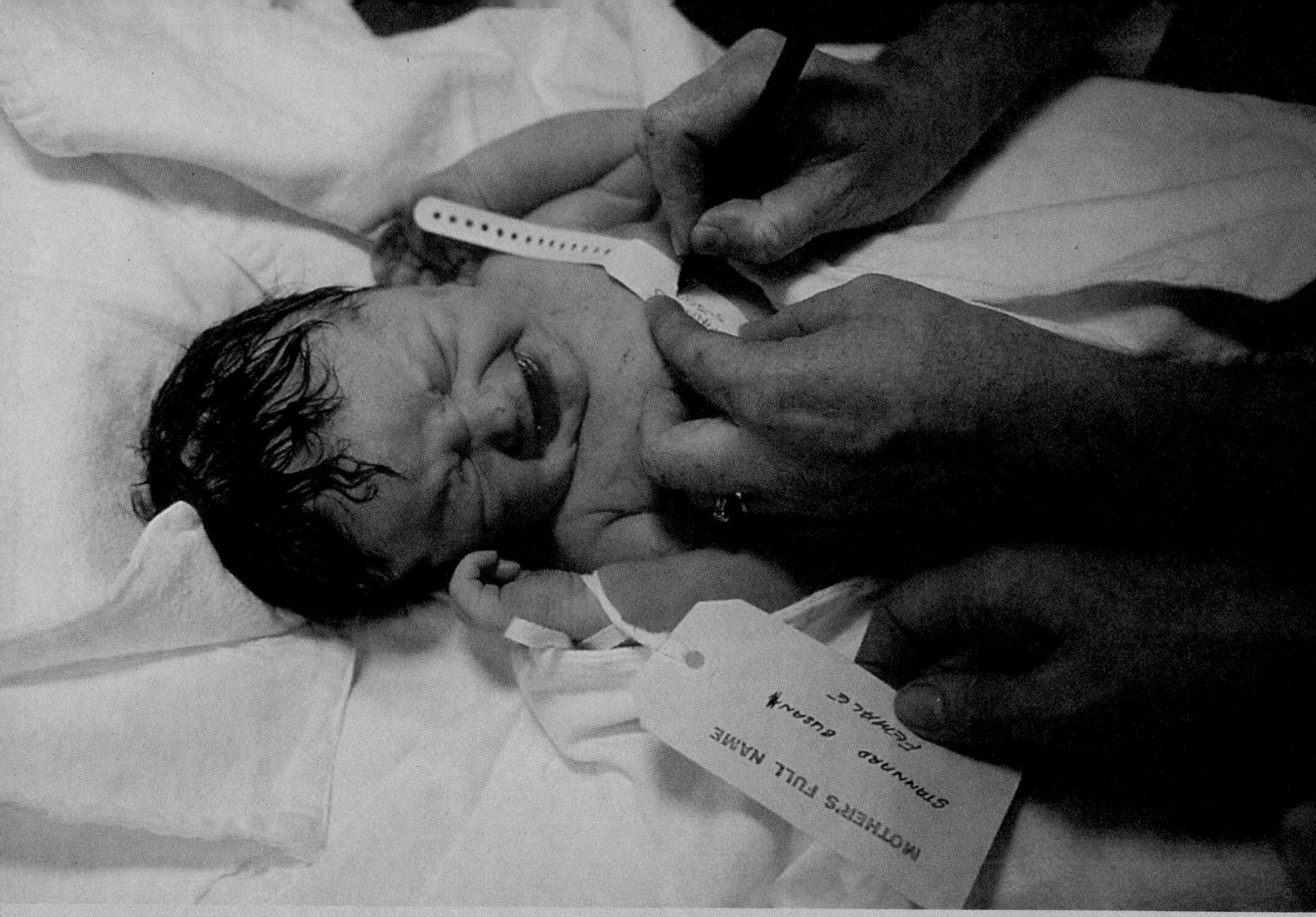

8
PREGNANCY AND PARENTING DECISIONS

Upon completing this chapter, you will be able to:

KNOWLEDGE

- Describe the trend in the percentage of couples who become parents.
- Contrast the processes of conception and implantation.
- Define the term fetus.
- Outline the main events that take place each month in the life of the embryo/fetus.
- Define the term teratogen.
- Define the term miscarriage.
- Identify when a birth can be called a premature birth.
- Define the term infertility.
- Distinguish an induced abortion from a miscarriage.

INSIGHT

- Explain how you feel about learning the gender of your unborn child before birth.
- Describe how you might respond when, seeing your newborn for the first time, you realize it is carrying a recognizable birth defect.
- Identify your current position on abortion.
- Explain your opinion on women using RU 486 to abort an embryo.

DECISION MAKING

- Discuss your willingness to make the immense emotional, physical, and monetary investment needed to produce and raise a child.
- Explain how, as an expectant parent, you plan to curtail or stop any smoking, alcohol or drug use of yours that could adversely affect a fetus or infant.
- Form an opinion on abortion if you did not have one before reading this chapter, and explain the reasons for your opinion.
- Describe the steps you might take in the event you or your partner are unable to reproduce any or as many children as you might wish for.

A baby girl was born to Cara Clausen in February 1991. Cara gave her child up for adoption because she was single and did not feel she was able to care for the baby by herself. The elated adoptive parents named the infant Jessica and took her to her new home in Ann Arbor, Michigan. In March of that year, however, Cara revealed that the man who signed the adoption consent was not Jessica's biological father (Cara had apparently lied), and now the real father, Dan Schmidt, wanted custody. Cara and Dan eventually married, settling in Blairstown, Iowa, and the legal battle began in full force.

Difficult questions abounded. Whose rights are more important: those of the biological parents or those of the adoptive parents? What rights does little 2-year-old Jessica have? Eventually, the case made it all the way to the United States Supreme Court. The 6-to-1 custody decision awarded little Jessica to her biological parents.

Jessica, 2½ years old by the time of the decision, had to leave the only parents she had ever known, as well as her familiar surroundings. Her name was changed to Anna once she arrived in Iowa to live with her "new" parents. Her adoptive parents were grief-stricken, losing a daughter they had reared since *infancy. On the other hand, her new parents were relieved about the verdict and happy to be reunited with their biological child, Anna.*

This case indicates the strong commitment that our judicial system has made to protecting the rights of biological parents. Should those rights be preserved in cases such as this one? Parenthood is a huge responsibility that should come only after serious thought and consideration. As in the case of Jessica, there are many people, especially the innocent young child, who can be affected by the decision to become a parent.

Source: People, *July 19, 1993, pp. 47-51, 53-54.*

■   ■   ■

Deciding to become a parent will perhaps be the most important decision you will make during your lifetime. Parenthood requires enormous amounts of time, energy, and financial commitment; but most of all, it requires love and the willingness to take full responsibility for a child's development. Because it is such an enormous decision, couples or individuals considering parenthood need to assess whether or not they are ready to make this lifelong commitment.

Experiencing the pregnancy and nourishing the developing embryo and fetus is physically demanding for the woman. Once pregnant, she will reflect many times on why she made the decision to become pregnant, how it will change her appearance and life, what being a mother will be like, and who the child will resemble and what she or he will be like. She will experience a mixture of fear, joy, exhilaration, and reflection. Her relationship with her partner becomes more important. Will he continue to accept her, and help her when she needs it? She needs his unqualified reassurances on all of these points during this exciting and stressful time.

For the man, sensing the responsibility of creating and providing for the needs of a new person may create both apprehension and elation. He must now share his partner's attentions with another person; he wants her to become a caring mother, yet may fear the loss of her exclusive attention as a lover. He needs her reassurances also. He is concerned with both her health and that of the developing child. The father should want, and deserves, to become as much a part of the pregnancy and birthing process as possible. His atten-dance at birthing classes, presence during labor and delivery, and actual interaction with the newborn will help him become a nurturing caregiver. Both partners need to work together to lay the groundwork for a strong family.

The purpose of this chapter is to bring to light the many factors involved in preparing for pregnancy, childbirth, and child rearing. The information conveyed here may help you decide whether you are prepared to take on the many responsibilities of parenthood.

THE DECISION TO BECOME A PARENT

Couples today generally have different views on child rearing than parents did in past generations. Today only 66 percent of married couples are becoming parents, compared to 80 percent in 1950. Couples are having fewer children than their parents, and are having them later. Forty-five percent of today's children are living or will live with only one parent.[1] Sometimes this is the result of the divorce or death of a parent, while other times it is the result of single individuals choosing to become parents.

Parenthood is not always the result of a planned pregnancy. Teenage pregnancies comprise a high percentage of unplanned children. Eighty percent of pregnancies among women under 20 years of age are conceived out of marriage, and only 12 percent of these parents are married by the time the child is born.[2] There are many consequences of having a child before being properly prepared. Studies in the United States show that teenage women who have early first births have more closely spaced subsequent births, more unwanted children, face greater marital instability, are less educated, and have fewer assets and lower income later in life.[3]

The decision to have a child is strictly between both potential parents; it is not a decision that anyone's relatives or friends can make for them. Couples who are considering having a child should educate themselves and become prepared to make many adjustments and accommodations to guarantee the best future for their child. At the same time, couples who decide not to have a child owe no one a rationale for that choice.

IN YOUR HANDS

TO BE OR NOT TO BE PARENTS

Deciding to have a child should be a joint decision, and the result of a candid discussion in which a couple assesses the effect that pregnancy and childbirth will have on their lives.

DIRECTIONS:

You and your partner should separately write a sentence or two in response to each of the following questions. Next, read through what you have written and indicate, by a check in the proper column, whether each response amounts to a "yes," a "no," or a "not sure" response.

	Yes	No	Not sure
Do we really want to have a child?	_____	_____	_____
Are we ready to accept the responsibility of having a child?	_____	_____	_____
Are we willing to give up much of the freedom we now have and some of the things we enjoy doing for the sake of a child?	_____	_____	_____
Are we prepared to alter our monthly budget so that we can accommodate the needs of a child?	_____	_____	_____
Can we handle the emotional obligations of taking care of a child for the next 18 years?	_____	_____	_____
Are we willing to accept the responsibility of making decisions affecting someone else's life?	_____	_____	_____
Do we feel uncomfortable bringing a child into our current social and economic situation?	_____	_____	_____
Are we prepared to live with a child who challenges (and perhaps rejects) our social values, view of life, religious outlook, and political philosophy?	_____	_____	_____

SCORING:

Compare your answers with those of your partner. A discussion about the realistic expectations of parenthood can quiet some fears and be a starting point for a decision.

Source: "To Be or Not to Be Parents" adapted from *Your Sexuality, A Personal Inventory* by R. Valois and S. Kammerman. Copyright © 1984 McGraw-Hill, Inc. Reprinted by permission of McGraw-Hill, Inc.

CHECKPOINT

1. What percentage of married couples become parents today as compared with the percentage that became parents in 1950?

2. What percentage of children are presently living or will live with only one parent?

3. What are some of the liabilities of being a teenage mother?

PREPARING FOR PREGNANCY

Once a couple decides to have a child, they need to prepare for the birthing process from conception to birth. There are many stages in this process, and anticipating what is to come during each stage will help both partners to understand and support each other's needs. Most importantly, it will also ensure healthy fetal development.

It is important that a pregnancy be planned. A top priority is to ensure the mother-to-be's and fetus's health during the pregnancy. A woman can even begin preparing before conception by visiting a physician who will counsel her on proper nutrition, advise her on how to curtail her particular birth control method, discuss any medications she is taking, and develop a fitness program that will promote a healthy pregnancy. She should be certain to tell her physician *all* drugs she is taking, including over-the-counter drugs (Feature 8.1, p. 216).

It is very important for a pregnant woman to understand her body, and regular visits to a physi-

FEATURE 8.1

CHOOSING A PHYSICIAN

If you suspect you are pregnant, see your physician to confirm the pregnancy. In case you need to select a physician, first choose the type of care you may need—private physician, medical group, clinic, or hospital. Do you want an obstetrician, family practitioner, or a midwife?

Your final selection should be someone you are comfortable talking to about all health matters. You should also be comfortable with his or her philosophy and delivery practices. Does he or she advocate the Lamaze method or induce delivery? Does he or she practice in a traditional hospital or in a birthing center?

Consider the following factors when choosing a physician:

1. Be satisfied with your physician's sex, age, location, hospital, and delivery practices.

2. Talk to your family, friends, or call the local medical society to ask them to recommend a physician.

3. Set up a visit to discuss philosophy and fees.

4. Select a physician who appears the most competent, not merely popular.

5. Be open and frank with your physician, and expect him or her to be open with you. If relations with your physician become unsatisfactory, even midpregnancy, consider choosing another physician.

6. Be prepared for the possibility that you may need to have your baby delivered by another physician if your own physician is ill, on vacation, or tied up in a medical emergency.

---

cian for **prenatal** checkups will help her to learn about the changes she is experiencing. Her physician will monitor any condition, such as diabetes, that might complicate the pregnancy, as well as help her learn how to avoid infectious diseases. Because traces of some drugs can remain in the body for weeks and months, a physician will also monitor the woman's blood to ensure that any contaminants are gone when the woman is ready to conceive. The father must also be monitored to ensure that he is free from drugs or harmful chemicals that could harm the fetus at the time of conception.

Both parents need emotional support to endure the stresses of pregnancy. For the woman, this support can help her accept the changes in her body. The love and support of the people around her is essential in helping her to develop confidence in her ability to give birth successfully. For the male, the support can help him to understand and support the changes his partner is going through.

EGG AND SPERM FORMATION

As was discussed in Chapter 6, once every month during a woman's childbearing years, at about the middle of the interval between her menstrual periods, ovulation occurs. After ovulation, an unfertil-

ized egg lives for about 24 hours before it disintegrates. The remains are then expelled during menstruation along with the uterine discharge.

Beginning around 12 years of age, these eggs are released at the rate of one every 28 days. At most, only 400–500 of the eggs will ripen and be released during the female's lifetime.[4]

Sperm cells are much smaller and more numerous than egg cells. There may be 140 to 350 million sperm in a single ejaculation.[5] Produced in the testicles, the sperm pass into the epididymis, where they mature. Upon ejaculation the sperm cells travel through the vas deferens into the urethra, which ends at the tip of the penis. Along the way the sperm cells mix with fluid secretions from the seminal vesicles, prostate gland, and Cowper's glands to become seminal fluid (semen). During the ejaculation phase of sexual intercourse, seminal fluid is expelled into the vagina with some force. The sperm cells must then be transported upward into and through the uterus and fallopian tubes. Although sperm may live from 48 to 72 hours in the female's body, many are killed by the acidic environment of the vagina, or swim into the one of the two fallopian tubes not containing an ovum. It is estimated that fewer than 200 sperm get close to the egg[6] (Figure 8.1).

CONCEPTION

Once ejaculated into the vagina, some of the sperm reach the ovum within an hour, then secrete an

---

prenatal before birth.

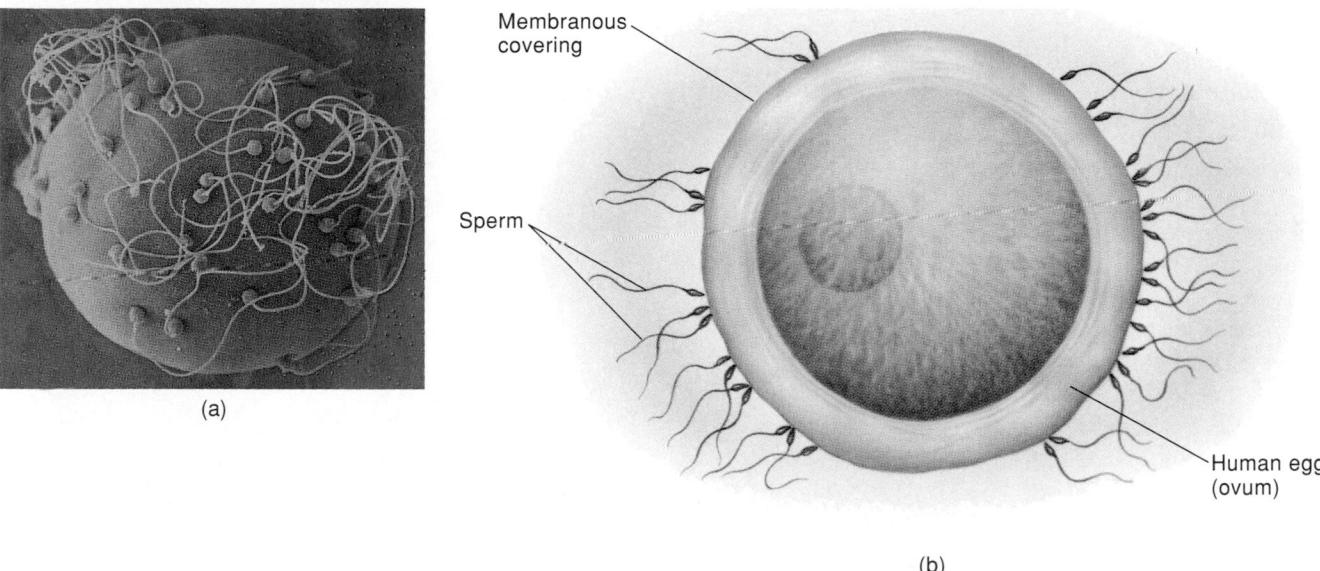

Figure 8.1

Human Ovum (egg) Surrounded by Sperm

(a) Photomicrograph of a human egg surrounded by sperm. (b) One sperm will break through to fertilize the egg.

enzyme that dissolves the protective coating around the ovum. Only one sperm actually enters the ovum, after which the coating around it becomes impenetrable to any other sperm. At the moment the sperm unites with the nucleus of the ovum, **fertilization,** or conception, occurs.

Fertilization produces a single cell called the **zygote** *(zī'gōt)*. The sex of the developing baby is determined at the moment of conception, based on whether a sperm bearing an X chromosome or a Y chromosome has united with the ovum. Within about 30 hours after fertilization, the single-celled zygote begins to divide. As division proceeds, it splits into two cells, then four cells, eight cells, and so on as it continues moving through the fallopian tube (see Figure 8.2, p. 218). Within three or four days, it has become a mass of cells that resembles a tiny raspberry and is called a **morula** *(mor-ū'la)*; it now enters the cavity of the uterus.

IMPLANTATION

At this stage, the lining of the uterus, or endometrium, has become thick and profuse with blood vessels due to the supply of hormones in the woman's body. Within a few days after entering the uterus, the young **embryo,** now called a **blastocyst** *(blas'tō-sist)*, attaches itself to the lining of the uterus in a process called implantation. By five to nine days after fertilization, implantation is complete. On occasion an implantation takes place outside of the uterus (see Feature 8.2, p. 218).

An indentation marking the beginnings of the embryo's nervous system forms on one side of the blastocyst as cell division accelerates. By the twelfth day, the beginnings of the head, heart, and limbs are evident.

HORMONE SECRETION

Shortly after conception, the embryo begins producing the human chorionic gonadotropin (HCG)

fertilization the union of the sperm cell nucleus with the ovum cell nucleus; also called conception.

zygote the fertilized ovum.

morula the young embryo, which consists of a solid mass of cells.

embryo the unborn child during the first eight weeks after conception.

blastocyst the young embryo when it consists of a fluid-filled ball of cells.

Figure 8.2

Stages in the Development of the Early Embryo

The unfertilized egg is released from the ovary and moves into the fallopian tube where it is fertilized by a sperm cell. As the fertilized egg is moved by the cilia through the tube toward the uterus, the egg divides to form a two-cell stage, a four-cell stage, and an eight-cell stage. As cell divisions continue, the embryo becomes a hollow blastocyst which becomes implanted into the endometrium lining the inside of the uterus.

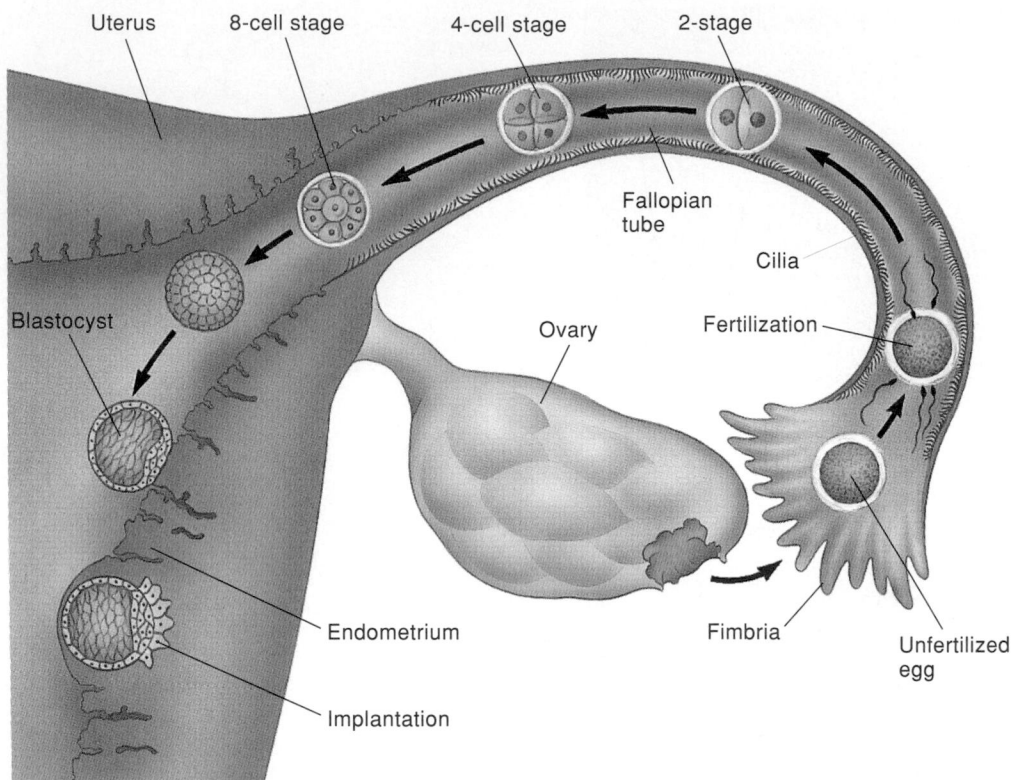

Uterus   8-cell stage   4-cell stage   2-stage

Fallopian tube

Cilia

Blastocyst   Ovary   Fertilization

Endometrium   Fimbria   Unfertilized egg

Implantation

 FEATURE 8.2

ECTOPIC PREGNANCY

When a fertilized egg is implanted anywhere other than in the uterus, it is called an **ectopic,** or misplaced, **pregnancy.** More than 90 percent of all ectopic pregnancies occur in the fallopian tube. Such ectopic pregnancies are called *tubal* pregnancies.

Tubal pregnancies may occur due to scarring of the fallopian tubes from infections, such as gonorrhea or pelvic inflammatory disease, tumors, appendicitis, or a failed sterilization attempt on the tubes. Unfortunately, ectopic pregnancies are on the increase. This increase is greater for nonwhite women than for white, and greater for older women (35–44 years) than for younger ones. The incidence of ectopic pregnancies has more than tripled in recent years. Causes for this increase include the following:

- more cases of sexually transmitted diseases

- use of some intrauterine contraceptive devices

- use of low-progestin contraceptives

- use of drugs to induce pregnancy

- unsuccessful tubal sterilizations

- tendency of women to delay childbearing until later in life

- induced abortion followed by infection

Ectopic pregnancy may produce many of the same symptoms as a normal pregnancy, but with severe pain. Tubal pregnancies usually result in rupture of the fallopian tubes during the first two months, with death of the embryo and severe hemorrhaging. If such is the case, the affected tube and embryo must be removed. As long as the other fallopian tube is intact, removal of one tube does not preclude pregnancy.

Although the incidence of ectopic pregnancies has increased since 1970, the death rate for such pregnancies has been reduced from 35 to 3.4 per 10,000. Yet, ectopic pregnancy remains the second leading cause of maternal mortality in the United States, with nonwhite women having a 1.8 times greater chance of dying from an ectopic pregnancy than white women.

Source: Moore, K. *Before We Are Born,* 3rd ed. Philadelphia: Saunders, 1989; Centers for Disease Control. "Ectopic Pregnancy in United States, 1984–1985." *Morbidity and Mortality Weekly Report,* 21 October 1988, 637–639; Cunningham, F., et al. *Williams Obstetrics,* 19th ed. Norwalk, CT: Appleton-Lange, 1993.

---

ectopic pregnancy a fertilized egg implanted outside of the uterus.

FEATURE 8.3

"DO-IT-YOURSELF" PREGNANCY TESTS

A number of types of relatively inexpensive over-the-counter home pregnancy test kits are available today. Some of these tests use *antibodies* (chemical substances) that will react with any HCG hormone present in the woman's urine.

To date, women using home tests have a relatively low false positive rate (about 5 percent), but a high false negative rate (about 20 to 25 percent). Investigators who analyzed home pregnancy test results found that only one-third of women using the test kits complied with the instructions.

Some physicians advise against women using the kits because they are afraid that women who obtain false nega-

tive results may delay seeing a physician, thereby delaying these women from starting appropriate prenatal care. Another reason against using these kits is that they may be almost as expensive as a physician's pregnancy test. Women who use home pregnancy testing kits are strongly advised to follow the kits' instructions *exactly* and to follow up any negative test with a physician's visit.

Source: Cunningham, F., et al. *Williams Obstetrics,* 19th ed. Norwalk, CT: Appleton-Lange, 1993.

hormone (see Chapter 5), and releases it into the bloodstream. This hormone is responsible for sustaining the corpus luteum during the early stages of pregnancy. The presence of the corpus luteum, which produces the hormone progesterone, helps keep the endometrium inside the uterus intact. Since HCG is secreted into the urine, its presence or absence is a common indicator used in pregnancy tests (see Feature 8.3).

PLACENTA AND FETAL MEMBRANE FORMATION

The embryo continues to develop through the embryonic stages, or the first eight weeks. From this time until the end of pregnancy, the developing child is referred to as a **fetus.** During the embryonic stage a complex, spongy structure called the **placenta,** or afterbirth, begins to form (see Figure 8.3, p. 220). The placenta is responsible for exchanging nutrients and wastes between the mother and fetus through the tubelike **umbilical cord.** Nutrients pass from the mother to the fetus and fetal wastes are returned to the mother's system through a reverse sequence. The blood of the mother and fetus do not mix, but remain separated

by a thin membrane through which these other materials diffuse.

Other parts of the blastocyst develop into the fetal membranes, an innermost **amnion** (*am'ni-on*) and an outermost **chorion** (*kō'ri-on*). The membranes are thin sacks of tissue that enclose the developing embryo and fetus. The amniotic sac is filled with a liquid called **amniotic fluid,** which keeps the temperature constant and serves as a shock absorber to protect the fetus from physical injury.

CHECKPOINT

1. Discuss the various considerations a woman should review with her physician when planning a pregnancy.

2. Describe the process of production of egg cells by a woman and of sperm cells by a man. Compare the number of egg cells produced with the number of sperm cells produced.

3. Once an egg is fertilized by a sperm cell it goes through a developmental process. Detail these developmental steps prior to implantation.

4. Following conception, how soon does implantation of the fertilized egg occur?

5. Describe the source and function of the hormone, human chorionic gonadotropin (HCG).

fetus the developing child from the eighth week after conception until birth.

placenta a spongy structure in the uterus through which the fetus obtains nourishment.

umbilical cord a cordlike attachment containing blood vessels which connects the fetus with the placenta.

amnion the innermost of the fetal membranes.

chorion the outermost of the fetal membranes.

amniotic fluid the fluid contained in the amnion that protects the fetus from injury.

Figure 8.3
The Placenta

The enlargement shows how only a thin membrane keeps the fetal and maternal blood separate.

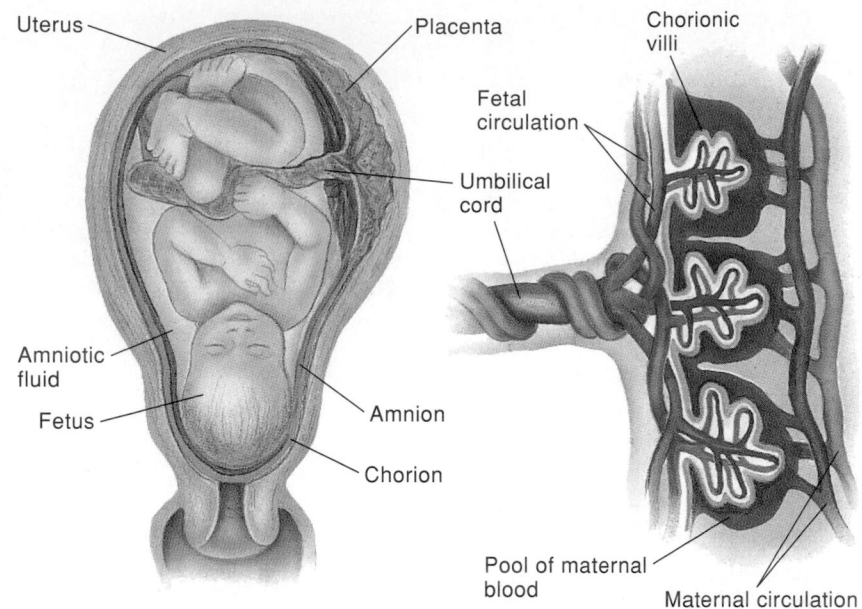

DURING PREGNANCY

An actual pregnancy lasts approximately 266 days. Since ovulation usually occurs about midway between periods of menstrual flow, conception usually commences about the middle of the menstrual month *after* a woman's last flow, or *last menstrual period* (LMP). Using the LMP as a starting point, delivery can be expected in approximately 280 days (266 days plus 14 days). Using 280 days, pregnancy can be divided into 10 *lunar* (moon) months of 28 days each, or 40 weeks. The 9 calendar months of pregnancy can be divided into 3 *trimesters* of almost 13 weeks each (see Figure 8.4).

ESTABLISHING THE DUE DATE

The names for the periods during the pregnancy depend upon the point at which the physician starts counting toward a woman's due date. If the counting began two weeks before ovulation, the periods during the pregnancy are referred to as

Figure 8.4
A Calendar of Pregnancy

Birth occurs at the end of 10 lunar months, each of which are 28 days (4 weeks) in duration. Calculations begin with the beginning of the last menstrual period before conception. Conception occurs about 2 weeks later. An embryo develops during the 8 weeks following conception, then continues development as a fetus. The events of pregnancy can be divided into three trimesters.

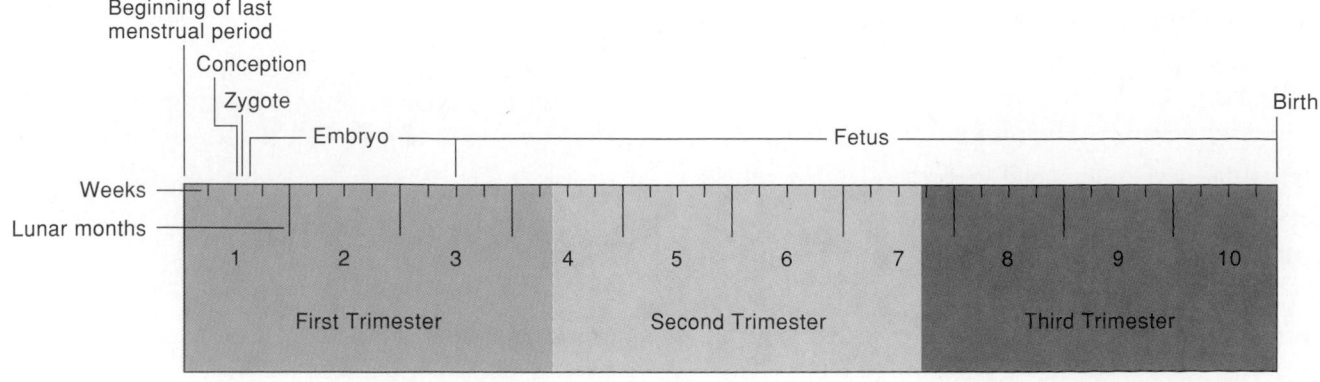

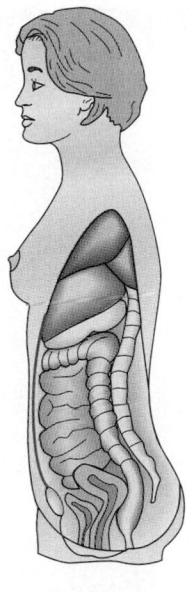

First trimester

(a)

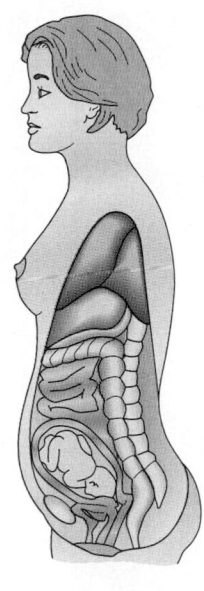

Second trimester

(b)

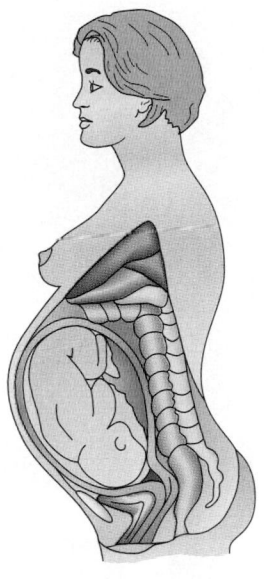

Third trimester

(c)

Figure 8.5

Changes in a Woman's Body During Pregnancy

(a) First trimester. (b) Second trimester. (c) Third trimester. Pregnancy leads to dramatic changes in a woman's body.

either the **gestational age** or *menstrual age.* If the counting began from the time of ovulation (about two weeks later), these events are described as the *ovulatory age* or the *fertilization age.* Physicians frequently prefer to use the term gestational age.

The expected day of delivery can be estimated by adding 7 days to the date of the first day of the last normal menstrual period and counting back 3 months. For instance:

LMP	March 20, 1994
add 7 days	March 27, 1994
subtract 3 months	
add 1 year	December 27, 1994

The majority of women deliver within 10 to 14 days, either before or after, their due date.

FIRST TRIMESTER

The Mother

Each woman reacts to pregnancy differently. Some have a new sense of well-being and energy, while others experience fatigue, emotional letdown, and appetite loss. Approximately half of all women feel nauseated around the end of the first month. Although this is commonly known as "morning sickness," it can occur at any time of the day. While

some women are hospitalized to control the dehydration that results from excessive vomiting, symptoms usually disappear a month or two after they begin. For many women, symptoms are relatively mild or do not occur at all.

Other signs of early pregnancy are fatigue, irritability, and apprehensiveness. Some women become anxious over the changes they know will be occurring in their bodies. Although women are unable to detect any changes inside their uterus (Figure 8.5), other physical changes occur, such as increased frequency of urination, irregular bowel movements, swollen and tender breasts, and increased vaginal secretions.

The Embryo/Fetus

The embryo's growth and development begins at the moment of fertilization. By the end of the fourth week, the embryo is about one-quarter inch long (Figure 8.6, *First Month*). It has an incomplete heart muscle that has started to beat. The brain, spinal cord, nervous system, throat, and face have all begun to develop. The eyes also start to form on a head that is large relative to the rest of the body. The embryo's body is elongated, and tapers off into a small, pointed tail.

During the second month, the embryo grows to about 1½ inches long (Figure 8.6, p. 222 *Second Month*). The face develops more fully—but eyes are far apart, eyelids are fused, and nose is flat. The neck becomes apparent. Limbs become distinct—

---

gestational age the estimated age of a fetus as calculated from the first day of the last normal menstrual period; also called the menstrual age.

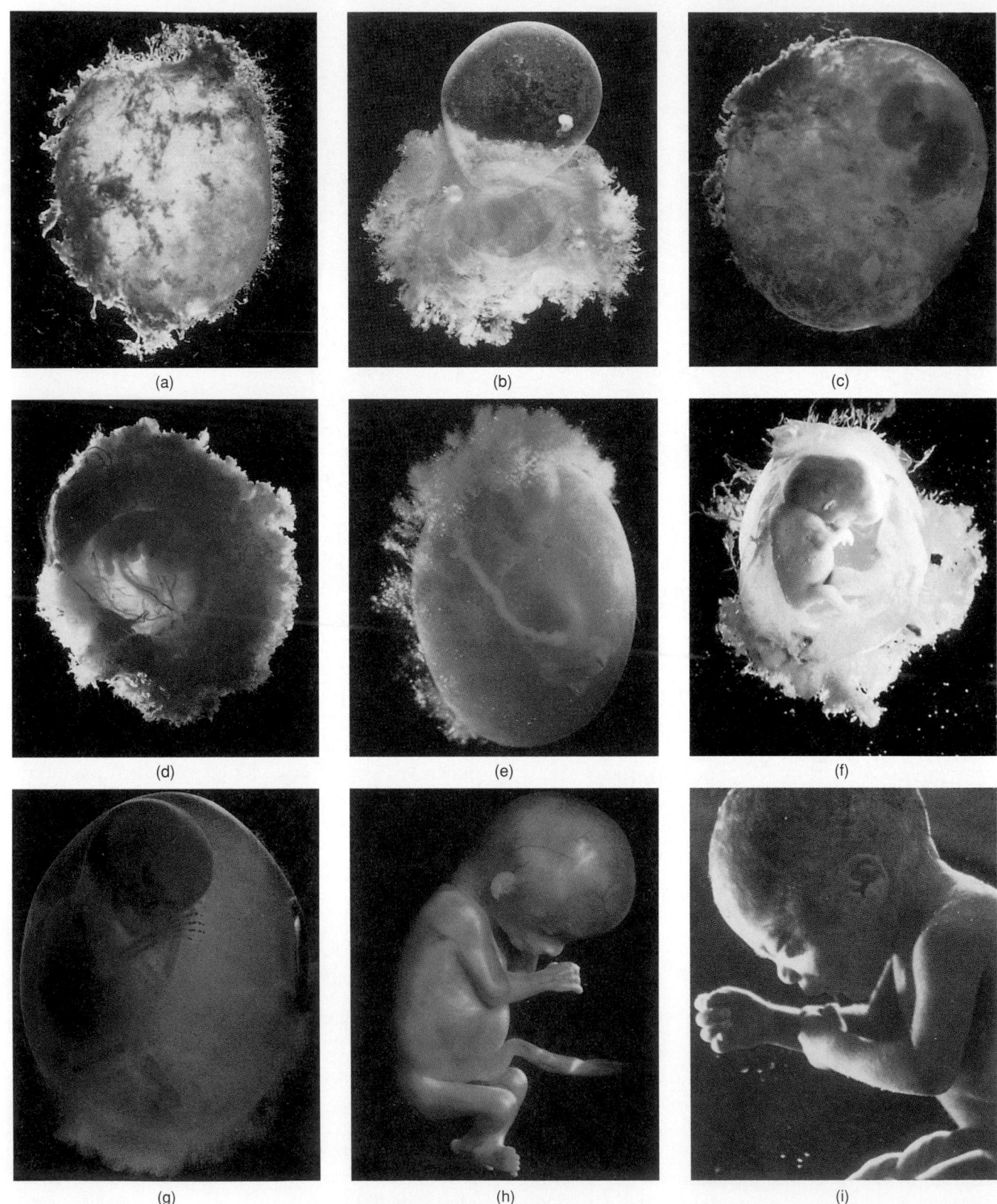

(a)   (b)   (c)

(d)   (e)   (f)

(g)   (h)   (i)

Embryo and fetal development by weeks: (a) two weeks; (b) three weeks; (c) four weeks; (d) six weeks; (e) eight weeks; (f) nine weeks; (g) ten weeks; (h) fourteen weeks; and (i) an eight-month-old fetus.

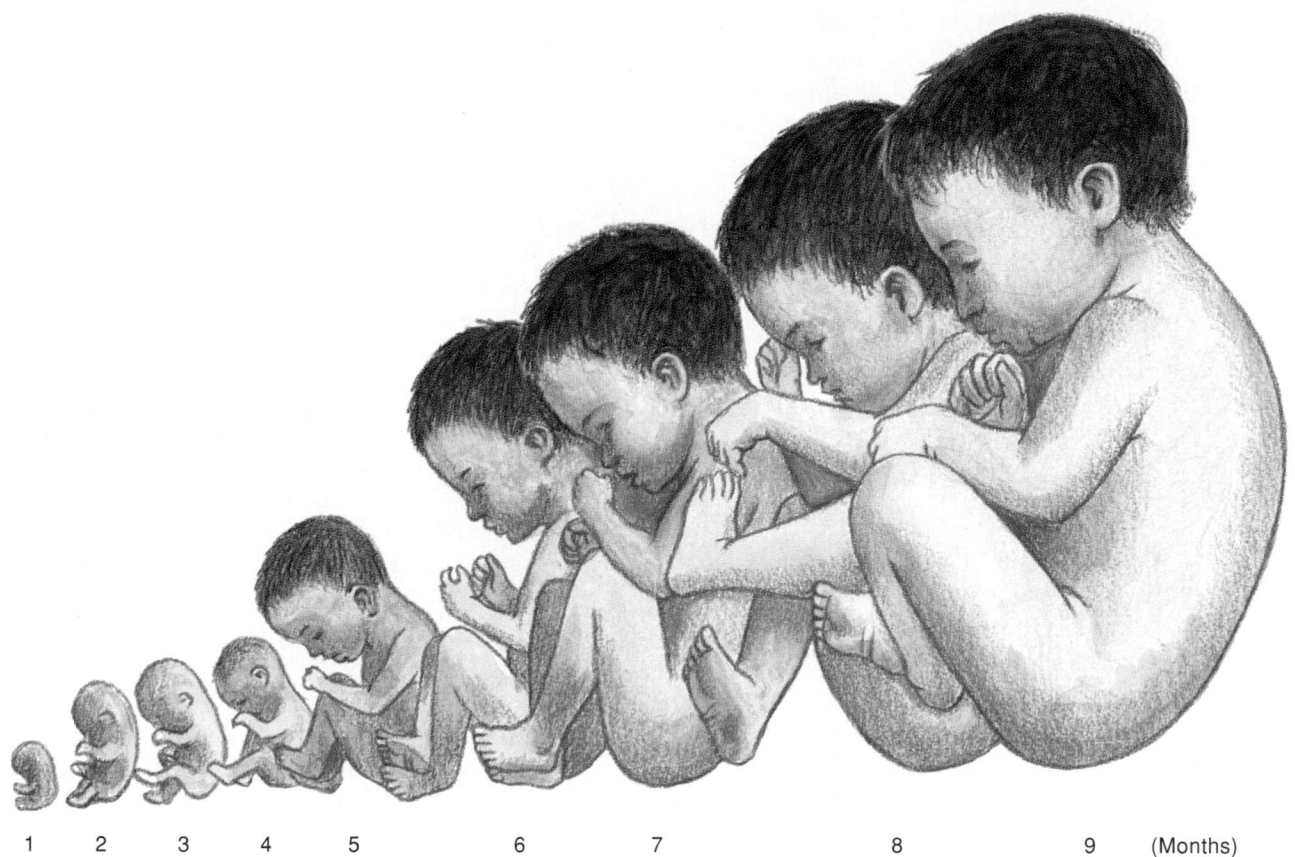

1   2   3   4   5   6   7   8   9   (Months)

Figure 8.6
Changes Occurring with Embryonic and Fetal Growth

arms with hands and fingers, legs with feet and toes. The blood vessels and muscles begin to form. Skin begins to envelop the developing organs and features. Testicles also begin to form in the male, although ovary formation occurs a bit later in the female. The eighth week marks the end of the embryo stage; for the remainder of the pregnancy, the developing child is known as a fetus.

By the end of the third month (Figure 8.6, *Third Month*) fingernails, toenails, and eyelids are forming. Teeth are apparent under the gums. The limbs are properly proportioned in relation to the rest of the body. The genitals in both the male and female are apparent, and the sex of the fetus is distinguishable. All the major organs have formed and have limited functioning. At the end of the first trimester, the fetus is about three inches long.

SECOND TRIMESTER

The Mother

During the second trimester, many women have a feeling of well-being and pleasure. Symptoms of morning sickness, sleepiness, and frequent urination may lessen or disappear entirely.

In the fourth month, the woman may feel the fetus move (the "quickening") for the first time. At about the same time, the skin over the abdomen stretches and the abdomen itself begins to protrude to accommodate the growing fetus (see Figure 8.5). The breasts and nipples increase in size, and the nipples and areolar rings around her nipples become darker. Fluids may begin seeping from the nipple. At this point in the pregnancy, visits to the physician for prenatal checkups should increase to once a month.

The Fetus

In the fourth month, the fetus's entire body structure is formed and the head is large in proportion to the rest of the body. As physical features are refined, fingernails, eyebrows, and eyelashes become clearly visible. The skin is covered by a fine downlike hair. Sucking motions begin. The fetus is about 4½ inches long and weighs 3½–4 ounces (Figure 8.6, *Fourth Month*).

By the fifth month (Figure 8.6, *Fifth Month*) the fetus moves freely inside the uterus and its heartbeat is audible. The skin is a bright pink and covered by a cheeselike substance, which will remain until after birth.

During the sixth month (Figure 8.6, *Sixth Month*) the eyelids separate and eyelashes form. The fetus opens its eyes and fine hair is on its head. There is a substantial weight gain, and by the end of the second trimester the fetus is about 12 inches long and weighs 1¼–1½ pounds.

THIRD TRIMESTER

The Mother

The size and firmness of the uterus increase significantly by the third trimester. As the uterus pushes forward, the mother may begin walking with her head and shoulders back to maintain her sense of balance; this posture often leads to backaches. While the fetus averages a total weight of up to 6½–7½ pounds, the mother's total weight gain during her pregnancy may average 20–27 pounds due to fetus, fat stores, body fluids, breast size increase, uterus, placenta, and amniotic fluid[7] (see Feature 8.4). The enlarged uterus and fetus put pressure on the blood vessels in the lower body, which may cause leg cramps and **varicose** veins in the legs and **hemorrhoids** in the rectum.

The fetal movements, which earlier may have been a source of fascination may become bothersome, especially when the mother is trying to relax or sleep. Because of the pressure the growing fetus places on the bladder, frequent urination may recur as a symptom. Heartburn is also common due to compression of the stomach by the displaced uterus.

Late in pregnancy, contractions of the uterus may become frequent; many women mistake this for labor. During the last few weeks, the head of the fetus lowers into the pelvis, until it is positioned against the pelvic bones (see Figure 8.5). The "dropping" may not occur until labor, especially in the case of women who have had previous births.

The Fetus

By the end of the seventh month (Figure 8.6, *Seventh Month*) the head and body are more proportionate. The brain and nervous system are completely developed. The downlike hair disappears over most of the fetus's body. As fat deposits beneath the skin, the fetus's skin becomes smoother. The eyelids, which may have fused closed earlier, reopen. The testes of the male descend into the scrotum. The lungs of the full term fetus secrete **surfactant** (*sur-fak'tant*), a secretion produced inside the lungs that reduces surface tension within the air sacs, making breathing easier.

In the eighth month the fetus becomes larger (Figure 8.6, *Eighth Month*), and the space around it in the uterus becomes smaller, so the mother and fetus feel each other's movements. The fetus falls asleep when rocked and may be startled by loud noises, but usually calms down when the mother speaks softly.

In the ninth and final month, the fetus reaches 18–20 inches in length and 6½–7½ pounds in weight (Figure 8.6, *Ninth Month*) Because of its cramped quarters this late in the pregnancy, it may be less active than it was earlier (see Figure 8.6). Until delivery, the fetal skin is light, even in dark-skinned parents, and the fetus's eyes are blue.

CHECKPOINT

1. Describe the duration of a pregnancy, in terms of days, weeks, and trimesters, from the last menstrual period (LMP).

2. List the changes that take place within a woman as a result of pregnancy.

3. List the changes that occur in the embryo/fetus during the first, second, and third trimesters of development.

4. Explain the difference between an embryo and a fetus.

5. By the time of birth, what is the approximate length and weight of the fetus?

---

varicose distended, swollen veins.

hemorrhoids enlarged varicose veins in the rectal lining.

surfactant a secretion produced inside the fetal lungs that makes breathing by the newborn easier.

PRENATAL CARE

Many pregnancies progress without incident for both the fetus and the mother, yet, for others, problems may occur. The ultimate welfare of the developing fetus and of the mother depends on her role in *preventing* problems. Prenatal care protects the mother's and the developing fetus's health. Medical supervision by a physician or nurse is part of prenatal care, which helps to detect potential problems. Following are some of the most important aspects of prenatal care.

NUTRITION

A pregnant woman's diet has lifelong importance for her unborn baby. Proper nutrition is needed for the developing fetal brain, bones, and teeth during the pregnancy and for as long as the mother nurses her infant. A healthy diet for the mother during her pregnancy may be especially critical for women who are under 16 years of age, pregnant for the third time in two years, carrying more than one fetus, strict vegetarians, smokers, users of alcohol or drugs, underweight before pregnancy, or anemic.[8, 9]

The best source of vitamins and minerals is a well-balanced diet. A pregnant woman's diet should provide sufficient amounts of the four basic food groups, and extra amounts of protein, calcium, iron, and vitamins A, B, C, and D. Milk or milk products (fresh low-fat milk, buttermilk, yogurt, or cottage cheese) provide a wide range of nutrients. Poultry, fish, eggs, low-fat cuts of red meat, and fresh fruits and vegetables are the best sources of vitamins and minerals for a well-balanced diet.

The National Academy of Sciences advises that pregnant women should avoid multivitamins and mineral supplements except iron, and get the extra nutrients they need from a balanced diet. Nutrient supplements should be used only under medical supervision.

Maternal weight gain during pregnancy is an important factor in determining fetal growth and birthweight. In the past, the medical community has recommended a weight gain of 22–27 pounds for a full-term pregnancy. In 1990, the National Academy of Sciences recommended that weight gain be geared to the mother's weight and height, and that for an optimal fetal development, an average-sized mother should gain 25–35 pounds during normal pregnancy[10] (see Feature 8.4).

EXERCISE

Exercise is important to overall fitness during pregnancy. Well-conditioned women who engage in aerobics or run regularly have shorter active labors and fewer cesarean deliveries, although such exercise does result in reduced birthweight, due to less fat mass.[11]

The American College of Obstetricians and Gynecologists recommends that women who are accustomed to aerobic exercise before pregnancy be allowed to continue during pregnancy, but without starting new exercise programs or intensifying existing ones. For women who are sedentary before pregnancy, activity no more strenuous than walking is recommended.[12] Exercise during pregnancy can condition the body's muscle tone so that the woman's body will return to its original shape soon after delivery.

The American College of Obstetricians and Gynecologists has given safety guidelines for women who wish to continue exercising during pregnancy:

FEATURE 8.4

IDEAL WEIGHT GAIN DURING PREGNANCY

The National Academy of Sciences recommends that healthy pregnant women gain more weight. The ideal weight for pregnant women varies. Women who are near their ideal weight before pregnancy should gain 25–35 pounds, and follow their physician's advice. Underweight women should gain 28–40 pounds. Overweight women should try to limit their weight gain, and gain no more than 15–25 pounds.

Women with special health circumstances need specific weight-gain recommendations from their physician.

Source: Institute of Medicine. Subcommittee on Nutritional Status and Weight Gain During Pregnancy. *Nutrition During Pregnancy.* Washington, DC: National Academy Press, 1990.

1. Consult your physician. She or he may recommend against exercise, depending upon whether your condition is special.

2. Limit aerobic exercise to 15-minute sessions and check your heart rate regularly; keep it below 140 beats per minute.

3. Avoid generating too much body heat. Avoid exercising in hot humid weather. Stay out of saunas, steam rooms, and hot whirlpools.

4. Avoid jumping and running, as done in aerobic classes. Avoid jerky stretchings and exercises. During pregnancy a woman is more susceptible to joint injury due to hormonal changes that affect soft tissue in the joints. Walking is usually excellent exercise.

5. Protect the abdomen from injury, especially in games of baseball or basketball in which accidents are likely.

6. Drink fluids before and after exercise. If you become thirsty, stop and drink immediately. Dehydration occurs more rapidly in pregnant women than in nonpregnant women.

7. After the fourth month of pregnancy, avoid any exercises performed while lying on your back. The enlarged uterus can affect blood flow to the woman's heart and to the fetus.

8. Eat enough food to support the additional needs of pregnancy plus exercise.[13]

Specific kinds of exercise routines are of particular help in preparing women for childbirth. One of these, Kegel exercises, is also recommended for use by women following childbirth (see Feature 8.5).

Plenty of rest and sleep are as important as exercise. While women vary in the amount of rest and sleep they need, it is important to make enough time for both.

SEX DURING PREGNANCY

For a healthy pregnant woman, sexual intercourse is a perfectly safe option. In fact, unprotected intercourse, free from worry about contraception, can be one of the enjoyable bonuses of pregnancy for women in monogamous relationships. A question in the mind of some women, however, is how far along during pregnancy intercourse is safe. Feature 8.6 (p. 228) helps answer this and other questions relating to intercourse during pregnancy.

TERATOGENS

Environmental agents or factors that cause congenital malformations by affecting the embryo or fetus

Walking is recommended during pregnancy.

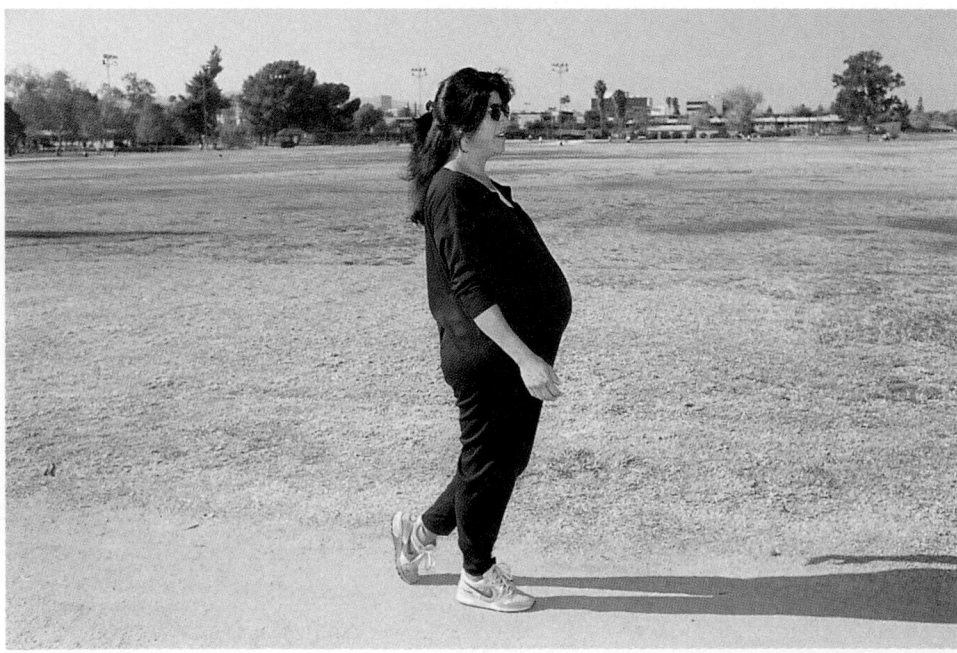

FEATURE 8.5

KEGEL EXERCISES

Kegel exercises, named after the physician who developed them, strengthen the pelvic floor muscles of the female (see figure below). These exercises not only help you prepare for childbirth, but help restore tone in the muscles lost during childbirth, as well as enhancing sexual enjoyment. Loss of tone in these muscles makes it more difficult to control urination; urine may also be lost when coughing or sneezing.

You can locate these muscles by voluntarily stopping and starting the flow of urine. The muscles that stop the flow of urine also tighten the vagina around an inserted object, such as a finger or penis. These are the muscles to be strengthened by the Kegel exercises. These muscles can be exercised by contracting these muscles hard for several seconds, and then releasing completely.

Once you have learned which muscles to concentrate on, you should contract those muscles, hold the contraction for two to three seconds, and then release. Perform this exercise for ten repetitions, five to six times a day, gradually working up to more. You can do this exercise at any time, while sitting in class, watching a movie, riding in a car, or lying in bed.

Women who have followed the Kegel routine notice improved muscle tone. Some also notice an increased sensitivity in the vaginal area, and an increased ability to stimulate their sexual partner by applying vaginal pressure against the inserted penis.

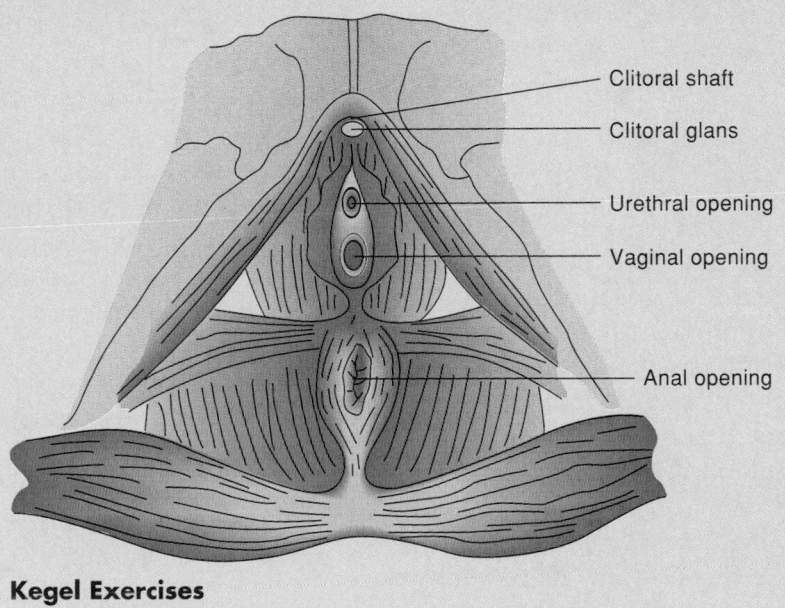

Clitoral shaft

Clitoral glans

Urethral opening

Vaginal opening

Anal opening

Kegel Exercises

The underlying muscles of the vulva can be strengthened by the Kegel exercises.

during its rapid growth and development are called **teratogens** (from the Greek *terato* meaning monster, and *gennan,* to produce). Various drugs and microorganisms are such agents.

The placenta is a porous barrier between the mother and embryo or fetus. The molecules of many drugs are able to pass freely from the maternal blood to the fetal blood. Any drug or chemical

dangerous to an infant may be considered potentially dangerous to the fetus when taken by the mother.

Virtually every drug a pregnant woman uses, and some infectious agents, can pass into the placenta and enter the fetus. Our culture has become accustomed to relying on drugs to alter life situations. Many prescription, nonprescription, and street drugs can damage the fetus. Examples include alcohol, tobacco, cocaine, marijuana, LSD, numerous prescription drugs, antibiotics, some hormones, industrial chemicals, and pesticides. Irradiation can also affect the fetus, as can viruses.[14, 15]

····················

teratogens environmental agents that cause congenital malformations by affecting the embryo or fetus.

FEATURE 8.6

SEX DURING PREGNANCY

All couples do not respond the same to pregnancy and sexual expression. For some, there is a steady decline in sexual activity during each trimester. For others, there is a decline during the first trimester because of morning sickness, with heightened sexuality during the second trimester, then a sharp decrease or stopping of sexual intercourse during the third trimester. The reasons for this drop may be due to the woman's physical discomfort, fear of hurting the fetus, physical awkwardness, or advice from her physician.

Until recent years, women were advised to avoid intercourse during the final six weeks of pregnancy. Today, many physicians advise couples to engage in sexual activities that are comfortable for the woman, unless certain problems arise.

When vaginal or uterine bleeding occurs, couples should avoid intercourse until the physician approves. Rupture of the amniotic sac, dilation of the cervix, or indications of premature labor are further reasons to avoid intercourse. Blowing air into the vagina, as during cunnilingus, may lead to maternal death from *air embolisms* (air bubbles in a blood vessel).

Intercourse with a partner who has a sexually transmitted disease is hazardous at any time, but especially during pregnancy, since such infections can be transmitted to a fetus during pregnancy or in vaginal delivery. If there is any cause to question whether the male partner of a pregnant woman may be infected with a sexually transmitted disease, the male should use a condom for all acts of intercourse.

Women should consult their physician regarding when the couple should abstain from intercourse. For those couples who need to abstain from intercourse, other forms of sexual pleasure, such as genital caressing, are still possible.

Alcohol

The number one fetal teratogen by far is alcohol.[16] Long suspected to be a teratogen, only in recent years has the relationship between maternal alcohol intake and characteristic fetal malformations been shown. Intrauterine exposure to alcohol causes **fetal alcohol syndrome (FAS),** which is characterized by growth retardation, facial malformations, and dysfunction of the central nervous system, including mental retardation and behavioral disorders. In addition to FAS, alcohol use can cause low birthweight.[17]

In a recent study, the average IQ of FAS adolescents and adults averaged from 20 (severely retarded) to 105 (normal), with an average of 68. Yet none of the persons studied was capable of living alone or earning a living because of accompanying behavioral disorders such as high anxiety, excessive impulsiveness, and poor attention spans. Such findings confirm that FAS is not just a childhood disorder, but that there is a long-term progression of the disorder into adulthood.[18]

Although the risks of a maternal drinking problem have been well documented, even the effects of light-to-moderate drinking during pregnancy may be damaging. As little as one drink a day may have measurable effects[19] (see Feature 8.7). The use of prescription or nonprescription drugs along with drinking may increase the effects of even light drinking. Even beyond this, pregnancies are not always planned. A woman may not realize for several weeks that she is pregnant, and may not stop drinking in time to prevent harm to the fetus.

FAS and related effects are entirely preventable. The U.S. Surgeon General and the National Institute on Alcohol Abuse and Alcoholism advise pregnant women or women about to become pregnant to abstain completely from alcohol. No level of alcohol consumption by the pregnant woman has been shown to be safe.[20]

Cigarette Smoking

Cigarette smoking during pregnancy is extremely dangerous for the fetus. The carbon monoxide in tobacco smoke reduces the oxygen carried in the blood, and the nicotine constricts blood vessels leading to the uterus and placenta, thus reducing blood and nutrient flow. Women who smoke eat less and thus may gain an inadequate amount of weight during pregnancy. Mothers who smoke have higher chances of premature birth, spontaneous abortion, complications during pregnancy and labor, and giving birth to a low-birthweight baby. The rate of ectopic pregnancy is higher. Smoking during pregnancy is an important cause of hyperactive behavior, as well as physical and mental retardation in children.[21]

fetal alcohol syndrome (FAS) physical malformations to the embryo and fetus caused by intrauterine exposure to alcohol.

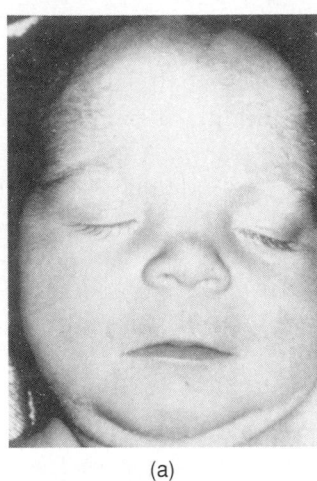
(a)

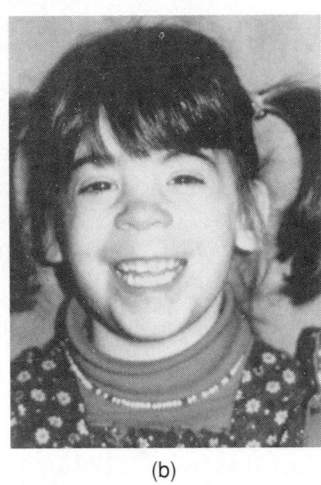
(b)

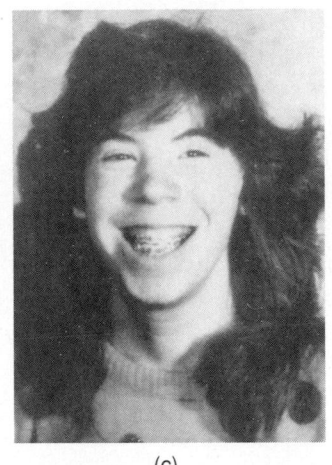
(c)

Child suffering from fetal alcohol syndrome. (a) At birth. (b) 5 years. (c) 14 years. Note the characteristic facial features of the sunken nose, smooth space between the nose and upper lip, and the small upper lip. These features are characteristic at birth.

Smoking during pregnancy is especially common among white mothers. White mothers are not only more likely than black mothers to smoke during pregnancy, but those who are smokers smoke much more. Hispanic women are much less likely to smoke than non-Hispanic women. Maternal smoking is relatively rare among Asian women.[22]

Cigarette smoke may be teratogenic, causing cardiac abnormalities and *anencephaly* (absence of a cerebrum). Smoking by the mother may also be a significant factor in the occurrence of cleft lip and palate and *sudden infant death syndrome* (SIDS). Gastrointestinal disturbances are higher in infants nursing from a smoking mother. Exposure to secondhand cigarette smoke (in the air we breathe) increases the incidence of respiratory problems during the first year of life, including bronchitis and pneumonia.[23] It is best that women who smoke before pregnancy find a way to curtail the habit *before* becoming pregnant.

Cocaine

A woman who uses cocaine, or "crack," in her childbearing years greatly reduces her chances of producing a healthy baby. (*Crack* is the more dangerous, smokable form of cocaine, since it is cheap and plentiful and enters the body more quickly.) This is crucial, since a reported 17 percent of inner city women use cocaine.[24] Cocaine use by the mother affects her heart action, and causes aortic rupture, strokes, seizures, and sudden death. The fetus of a cocaine-using mother may be affected with birth defects affecting the heart, brain, limbs, blood vessels, and fetal death.[25]

One dose of cocaine, or crack, taken by a pregnant woman may be enough to cause a defect or even kill the fetus. And if the mother is a cocaine or crack abuser, she can produce a baby with low birthweight, small head, kidney malformation, and neurological injury. Even if the drug-using mother

FEATURE 8.7

WHO DRINKS DURING PREGNANCY?

Alcohol use during pregnancy, reported as 3.7 percent, appears to be substantially underreported. Evidence from other studies suggests alcohol use of perhaps 20 percent or more during pregnancy.

Alcohol use is associated with maternal age and race. The rate of use by mothers aged 30 years and older is twice that reported by teenage mothers. African-American women are not only more likely than white women to report alcohol use, but they report a substantially larger number of drinks per week. By comparison, white and Hispanic women are half as likely to use alcohol. The impact of alcohol use on

birthweights is particularly severe for black babies. For example, nearly one-third of births of black women who use alcohol are babies of low birthweight, compared with 13–14 percent of nondrinkers of the same age. The proportions of low-birthweight babies born to white women in their thirties is 7–8 percent for drinkers and 5–6 percent for nondrinkers.

Source: National Center for Health Statistics. "Advance Report of Maternal and Infant Health Data from the Birth Certificate, 1990." *Monthly Vital Statistics Report* Vol. 42, No. 2, Suppl. Hyattsville, MD: Public Health Service, 1993.

stops cocaine use during pregnancy, her fetus will go through withdrawal inside the uterus. The fetal exposure to the drug will be longer than for the mother, because traces of cocaine remain in the body longer. This can be especially crucial if exposure occurs early in pregnancy during organ formation (kidneys, brain, heart, and lungs). Exposure later in pregnancy can have a negative effect on the development of speech and motor skills in the young child.[26]

Other Drugs

There are other legal drugs, both prescription and over-the-counter, that are safe for the mother, but may adversely affect the unborn child. Some drugs can produce malformations in an unborn child. Drug use during the first half of pregnancy, when fetal organs are forming, is particularly harmful. Examples of such drugs include the sulfonamides (sulfa drugs) which during the third trimester cause increased bilirubin and may cause encephalopathy, and combination oral contraceptives, which can cause limb defects, cardiovascular abnormalities, and skeletal malformation.[27] Due to the long list of commonly used drugs that may adversely affect the pregnant mother and/or the fetus, the American Pharmaceutical Association advises women to "avoid the use of drugs, in general, at any stage of pregnancy."[28]

Exposure to Radiation

Exposure to the radiation produced by x-rays during pregnancy can do irreversible damage to fetal tissues. Ionizing radiations are potent teratogens. The dangers include *microcephaly* (small head in relationship to the rest of the body), mental retardation, and skeletal malformations. Dangers also include *mutations* (chromosomal accidents) and increased incidence of cancer later in life for the unborn child. Actually, radiation poses a risk to the developing ovum *prior* to ovulation, as well as afterward. There is, in fact, no time when it is safe for a potential mother to be exposed to radiation.

This is not to imply that all pelvic x-rays should be avoided. There are times when pelvic x-rays are justified, but the benefits must always be weighed against the risks.

Exposure to Heat

Women exposed to heat sources, such as hot tubs and spas, during the first month of pregnancy, have two to three times the normal risk of bearing a child with central nervous system defects as those who are not exposed to such sources. Most common are neural tube defects, such as spina bifida.[29] If, in addition to exposure to such heat sources, the mother runs a fever due to infection, her total risk can be as much as six times greater than normal. Animal studies indicate that increased body temperature induced by overly vigorous exercise can adversely affect the fetus. No significant increase in risk has been found from the use of electric blankets.[30]

Diseases

One of the diseases most devastating to the fetus is rubella, commonly known as the German measles. Pregnant women infected with the virus are in danger of having children with serious birth defects, especially when infection occurs during the first third of the pregnancy. The degree of risk drops later in pregnancy. Results of this viral infection include babies born deaf, or with cataracts, heart defects, mental retardation, and retarded growth. Exposure to rubella during later stages of development may cause functional defects in the central nervous system.

Some states require proof of rubella immunization before they will issue a marriage license. The problem with this requirement is that the rubella vaccine uses a live virus, and receiving the vaccine may pose the same problem as contracting the disease. Because live virus is used, women receiving it are cautioned against conceiving for six months. The safest time for the young female to receive a rubella vaccination is before she becomes sexually active.

A disease which may be carried by cats is *toxoplasmosis.* Caused by a microscopic parasite that cats ingest by eating raw meat (birds and mice), it can be passed by food, water, or dust contaminated by cat droppings. It is carried in the mother's blood and crosses the placenta into the fetal blood, where it can damage the eyes or brain, or cause fetal death. The mother's symptoms may be mild or absent. Pregnant women should avoid cleaning cat litter pans, prevent cats from hunting rodents, and avoid contact with cats of unknown eating habits.

PROBLEMS DURING PREGNANCY

While many women have uneventful pregnancies, others encounter many problems. Following are several of the more common afflictions.

TOXEMIA

Toxemia (*toks-ē'mi-a*) is a condition marked by the retention of toxic body wastes, high blood pressure, protein in the urine, severe swelling, and fluid retention. The cause of toxemia is unknown, yet it occurs in about 6 percent of all pregnancies. It generally occurs during the third trimester, and is more common during a woman's first pregnancy, especially in very young women, or in women over age 35. This disease is also more common in women who have gained excessive weight during pregnancy. If toxemia goes untreated, it can cause maternal and fetal death; however, toxemia can be controlled if treated. If the symptoms of toxemia reach dangerous levels, early termination of pregnancy is often recommended.

BIRTH DEFECTS

Children born with **birth,** or **congenital, defects** account for approximately 3 percent of all live births. About 2 percent of these defects are inherited; others result from chromosomal abnormalities, infections, drugs the mother took during pregnancy, or exposure to environmental chemicals.

Chromosomal disorders may occur when the union of the sperm and egg does not result in the usual 46 chromosomes. The infant may be born with a missing chromosome or with an extra one. These disorders occur in about 1 in every 170 live births.[31] As the female ages, the eggs in her ovaries get older and less fertile.[32] The age of the mother at conception relates to the incidence of the defect known as Down's syndrome. *Down's syndrome* (mongolism, trisomy 21), which results in severe mental retardation and defects of the heart, kidneys, and intestines, usually occurs in infants with an extra number 21 chromosome. At maternal age 30 the risk of an affected newborn is less than 1 in 900, but the risk increases to 1 in 100 by age 40, and to 1 in 32 by age 45. The father's age at conception does not appear to relate to the incidence of this disorder.[33]

Genetic disorders occur when there is a flaw in genetic instructions (see Feature 8.8, p. 232). Different kinds of genetic disorders may express themselves at different ages in the life of an individual—before birth, during infancy or childhood, or in later years. It is estimated that these disorders are responsible for one-third to one-half of all congenital abnormalities.

In a society that places a premium on perfection and beauty, parents of a child with a birth defect may question whether the defect was caused by a deficiency within themselves or whether they are being punished for their own shortcomings. While some parents are able to accept and love a child with a birth defect, others may have more trouble coping with the condition.

Early Detection of Birth Defects

Parents with a history of genetic or chromosomal disorders, women who have already given birth to

---

toxemia a condition during pregnancy in which poisonous body wastes are retained by the body.

birth or **congenital defect** a defect present at the time of the birth of an individual.

FEATURE 8.8

GENETIC DISORDERS

Sickle-cell anemia is a condition caused by a defective gene that causes the formation of misshapen (sickled) red blood cells. About 8 percent of the U.S. population, predominantly persons with Central African ancestry, carry this gene. When persons with sickle-cell anemia lack tissue oxygen, there is a blockage of capillaries by sickled red blood cells. There is a high death rate among infants with this condition.

Another defective gene condition called *phenylketonuria (PKU)* involves the inability to produce specific enzymes. In normal enzyme functioning, the amino acid phenylalanine is bro-

ken down. The defective gene results in only a partial breakdown of this amino acid; the accumulation of the resulting toxic products interferes with the normal activity of the child's nervous system. Untreated, the condition usually results in severe retardation. The condition can be treated by monitoring the child's diet to restrict or eliminate the intake of phenylalanine.

Tay-Sachs disease is a genetic defect found among Jews of Eastern European origin. People inheriting this condition experience early blindness, deterioration of mental and physical abilities, and death.

children with birth defects, and pregnant women over the age of 35 may wish to confirm the absence of birth defects in the unborn child. There are several ways to detect certain birth defects in a developing fetus.

One method used to detect birth defects is **amniocentesis** (*am ni-ō-sen-tē'sis*). Around the sixteenth to eighteenth week of pregnancy, the physician maps the position of the fetus inside the uterus. Then amniotic fluid is withdrawn with a needle inserted into the uterus through the abdominal wall. The fluid is analyzed and a number of disorders can be identified.

In **chorionic villus sampling (CVS),** a thin **catheter** (tube) is inserted through the vagina and cervix into the uterus so that a tissue sample can be taken from the **chorionic villus,** the vascular projections from the chorion. CVS can be done by the eighth week of pregnancy, shortly after the woman knows she is pregnant. Thus, CVS allows for a much earlier detection of birth defects, and a safer decision regarding any possible abortion.

Alpha-fetoprotein (AFP) screening is a blood test that measures a substance produced by the fetal kidneys in the mother's blood, between the thirteenth and twentieth weeks of pregnancy. Down's syndrome can be indicated by levels that are too low, and neural tube defect by levels that are too high. Further testing is done to confirm an abnormal level.

Ultrasound examination, or sonography, is the producing of high-frequency ultrasound waves which are beamed into the body and reflected off fetal tissue. The reflection of these waves is used to form a picture of the fetus (Figure 8.7).

Performed in more than one-half of all pregnancies, ultrasound is used both to check the sex of the fetus and for diagnostic purposes. The procedure is simple and painless, poses no risk to the fetus, and can be used between 20 and 24 weeks of pregnancy.

MISCARRIAGES AND STILLBIRTHS

A **miscarriage,** also called a spontaneous or natural abortion, occurs when the body spontaneously terminates the pregnancy by expelling the

amniocentesis obtaining amniotic fluid through surgical penetration of the abdomen to assist in the detection of birth defects.

chorionic villus sampling (CVS) the use of a catheter for removing a small sample of chorionic villi of the fetal membranes.

catheter a tube passed through the body and used to remove from or inject fluids into body cavities.

chorionic villi vascular projections from the chorion, or outermost fetal membrane.

alpha-fetoprotein (AFP) screening a test measuring a substance produced by the fetal kidneys in the mother's blood.

ultrasound examination taking a picture of a developing fetus using sound waves.

miscarriage a natural termination of the embryo or fetus before it is capable of living outside the uterus; a spontaneous abortion.

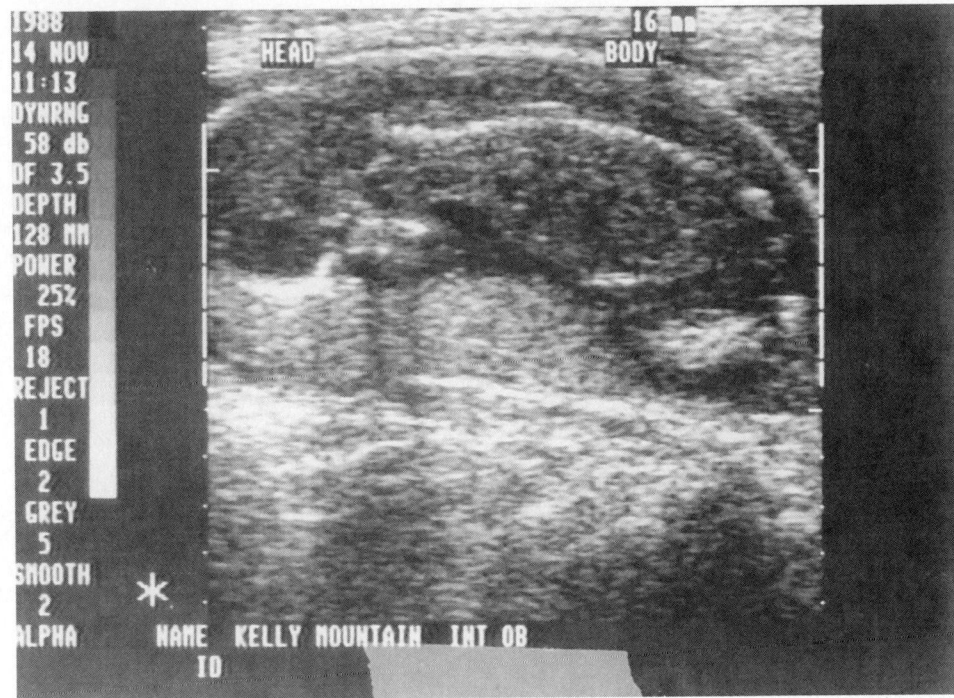

Figure 8.7
Ultrasound Imaging

In ultrasound imaging, sound waves are used to form a visual image of the fetus.

Source: Masters, W., Johnson, W., and Kolodny, R. Human Sexuality, 4th ed. New York: Harper-Collins, 1992.

embryo or fetus, which is too young to live outside the uterus. A **stillbirth** is the birth of a dead fetus at a stage where, if born alive, the fetus would have been capable of living outside the uterus. The birth of any dead fetus 20 weeks or after is viewed today as being a stillbirth. Approximately 15 percent of all recognized pregnancies end in miscarriage.[34]

Many miscarriages and stillbirths are the result of chromosomal abnormalities in the fetus. Others may be due to maternal infections. In many of these cases, had the fetus lasted the full term, it would have been born with birth defects.

PREMATURE BIRTH

It is to the fetus's advantage to remain in the uterus for the full term of pregnancy. Generally, birth anywhere between 38 and 42 weeks of gestation is seen as an optimal development, or **term birth.**[35] A birth earlier than 37 weeks is called a *preterm* birth, and more than 42 weeks is a *postterm* birth.

....

stillbirth birth of a dead fetus which, if born alive, would have been capable of living outside the uterus.

term birth the duration of a normal pregnancy.

A newborn weighing 5½ pounds or less is considered to have a *low birthweight*. Low-birthweight infants comprise about 8 percent of all children born in the United States. Generally, the lower the birthweight, the riskier the delivery becomes. A newborn weighing 1⅓ pounds or less (23 weeks of development) has virtually no chance of survival (see Feature 8.9, p. 234). Survivability gradually increases with birthweight. A newborn weighing 2⅛ pounds or more (27 weeks of development) and who is given **neonatal** intensive care, or intensive care during the first 6 weeks, has a good to excellent chance of survival, depending on birthweight.

The proportion of low-birthweight infants is different among various ethnic groups, ranging in incidence from about 60 per 1000 for white mothers to about 120 per 1000 for African-American mothers. It is believed that these are mainly a result of lack of access to medical care.

The development of neonatal intensive care has significantly reduced the death rate of low-birthweight infants in the United States over the past several decades. This kind of care involves controlling oxygen, temperature, and humidity levels, and intravenous feeding. The lower the birthweight, the

....

neonatal the first six weeks after birth.

FEATURE 8.9

LOW BIRTHWEIGHT

A newborn infant is considered to have low birthweight when the first weight is 5½ pounds, or 2500 grams (g), or less. Birthweight has significant effects on survival at birth, the frequency of severe handicap, and the average length of hospital stay, as you can see in the accompanying table.

Depending on birthweight, a low-birthweight infant is further classified as:

an *abortus:*	0–1⅛ lbs (0–499 g)
extremely low birthweight	1⅛–2⅛ lbs (500–999 g)
very low birthweight	2⅛–5½ lbs (1000–2499 g)

Source: Pritchard, J., et al. *Williams Obstetrics,* 17th ed. Norwalk, CT: Appleton-Century-Crofts, 1985; Cunningham, G., et al. *Williams Obstetrics,* 19th ed. Norwalk, CT: Appleton-Lange, 1993.

Weight	Newborn Mortality (%)	Frequency of Severe Handicap (%)	Average Length of Hospital Stay	Total Cost of Hospital-ization
1.1–1.3 lb (500–599 g)	100			
1.3–1.5 lb (600–699 g)	97	100	125 days	$443,618[a]
1.5–1.7 lb (700–799 g)	76	26		
1.7–1.9 lb (800–899 g)	62	29		
1.9–2.2 lb (900–999 g)	40	33	76 days	$63,442[a]

[a]Costs are from 1984.

longer the period of intensive care required. The cost of care for surviving infants may be extremely expensive. Even with proper care, the lower the birthweight the higher the frequency of severe handicaps.

The reasons for many low-weight births are unknown, although some factors have been found to affect the developing fetus, as has been indicated earlier in this chapter. A mother's health is important to the fetus's development; therefore, when a pregnant woman has an infection, it may affect the development of the fetus, and could result in a low-birthweight baby. A pregnant woman's nutritional habits and other behaviors, such as smoking, may also affect the fetus. A woman who is carrying multiple fetuses (see Feature 8.10), such as twins and triplets, may end up with low-birthweight babies as well. Teenage mothers often have low-birthweight babies because they are not physically mature enough to carry their pregnancy to term.

CHECKPOINT

1. Describe the causes, effects, and symptoms of toxemia during pregnancy.

2. What are the various techniques used in detecting early birth defects?

3. Distinguish between a miscarriage and stillbirth.

4. Explain the significance of low birthweight to the survivability of a newborn.

BIRTH

If a couple has prepared themselves for the birth of their child, much of the uncertainty and fear of delivery is reduced. To prepare for childbirth, both parents should learn as much as they can about the birthing process and how they can each be active participants. As a part of the process, the parents should explore their options with their physician. Considerations that need to be addressed involve deciding which birthing site and birthing alternative they will want for the delivery. As is increasingly the case when the mother is without a partner, these preparations and decisions may need to be made by the mother alone.

LABOR

The whole process of childbirth is called **labor,** or parturition (*par-tū-rish'un*). Late in the third trimester, the fetus usually positions itself deeper in the pelvic cavity, in a process known as **lightening,** or engagement. The fetal body rotates and the head engages more deeply into the mother's pelvic girdle. When this happens, the baby is said to have "dropped."

....

labor the act of giving birth; also called parturition.

lightening fetal descent into the pelvis; also called engagement.

FEATURE 8.10

MULTIPLE PREGNANCIES

When mothers learn that their physician can detect two fetal heartbeats rather than one, many react with elation, but others react with distress. A multiple pregnancy is one in which two or more embryos develop. While incidence varies among studies, overall the incidence of twins is believed to be about 1 in every 89 births, and triplets, about 1 in every 7921 births. Twins are more common among women who have already had children; among blacks than among whites; and among older mothers.

Twins develop from the fertilization of either two separate eggs or from a single one. Twins from two separate eggs are known as *fraternal twins*. Fertilized by different sperm, they develop as two separate embryos. They are no more alike than any two separate pregnancies of the same mother. They may not be the same sex and may or may not share the same placenta.

In about 1 out of every 3 sets of twins, one mature ovum fertilized by a single sperm separates into two embryos during development. These two embryos, containing the same genetic material, develop into *identical twins*. In 1 in every 60,000 cases, the two embryos do not separate from each other completely before birth, forming conjoined twins (popularly known as *Siamese twins*).

Triplets may come from one, two, or three eggs. There could be three embryos, or two (with one dividing into two during development), or one (with one dividing into three during development). This is also the case for quadruplets, quintuplets, and all other types of multiple births. In the case of the famous Canadian Dionne quintuplets, it is believed that all five girls were identical, or developed from a single egg fertilized by a single sperm.

Source: Cunningham, G., et al. Williams Obstetrics, 19th ed. Norwalk, CT: Appleton-Lange, 1993.

Another indication that delivery may be imminent is the increased reportings of **Braxton Hicks contractions.** While these painless uterine contractions occur with mild intensity and at irregular intervals throughout pregnancy, they become more frequent during the last weeks of pregnancy.

As the uterine pressures intensify, force is exerted against the cervix, shortening it from a short necklike canal to a narrow ring (Figure 8.8, p. 236). This funneling of the cervix is known as **cervical effacement.** Cervical effacement may take place prior to the onset of labor or as a part of the first stage of labor.

When uterine contractions become more intense and occur at regular intervals, actual labor has begun. Labor can be divided into three stages (see Figure 8.8).

First Stage (Opening of the Cervix)

The first stage of labor is by far the longest of the three stages, averaging 13 hours for first pregnancies and 8 hours for later ones. This stage often begins with the dislodging of the cervical mucus plug. When this happens, it results in a "bloody show," consisting of the mucus plug and a small amount of blood in the cervical canal. This show indicates that dilation of the cervix has begun.

Around this time, the amniotic sac around the fetus may burst. The breaking of the "water" usually happens near the beginning of labor and results in the release of a variable amount of amniotic fluid.

The first stage continues until the cervix dilates to about 10 centimeters (4 inches). Early in this stage, the contractions last from 15 to 60 seconds and occur 20 minutes apart. As the cervix dilates, these contractions become more forceful and occur closer together.

During the late phase of the first stage, known as *transition,* the cervix has dilated to a full 10 centimeters to allow the fetus to move into the vaginal (birth) canal. During transition, labor contractions last 60–90 seconds each, with brief intervals of 30–60 seconds between. Although this is the most intense part of labor, it is the shortest phase for most women. Until the cervix has fully dilated, the woman is instructed not to "push" the fetus. Concentrating, using breathing techniques, and the support of her partner help a woman through the first stage.

....

Braxton Hicks contractions intermittent painless uterine contractions that do not represent true labor pains.

cervical effacement the shortening of the cervical canal.

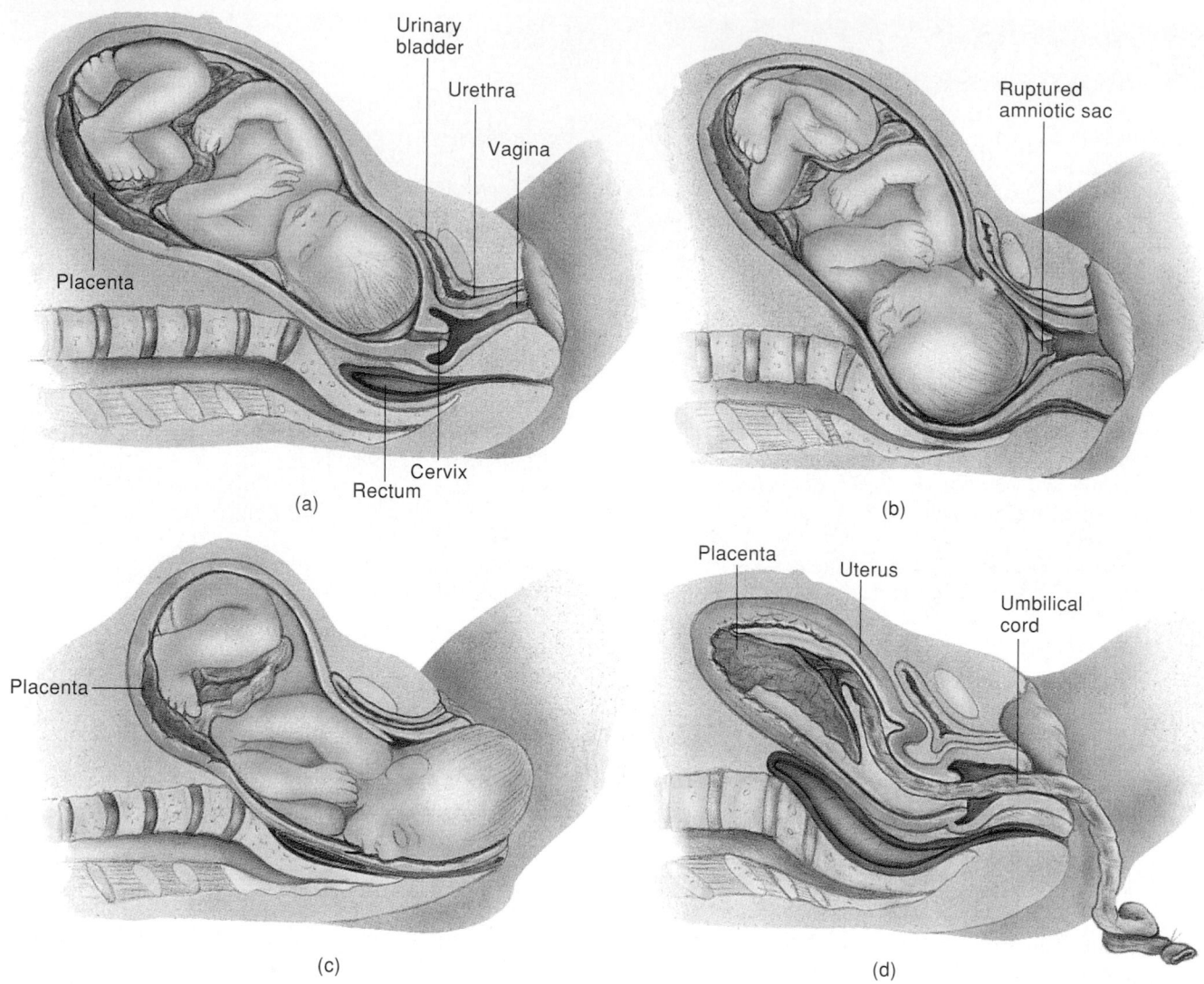

Figure 8.8
The Stages of Labor

(a) Early first-stage labor. (b) Later first-stage: the transition stage. (c) Early second-stage labor. (d) Third-stage labor: delivery of afterbirth.

Second Stage (Expulsion of the Fetus)

When the cervix is fully open, the baby begins the descent through the uterus, usually head first. With the mother now pushing with her abdominal muscles, the uterine contractions become less forceful, are of shorter duration, and occur farther apart.

The first sight of the baby's head is known as **crowning.** Before crowning, the physician or midwife may perform an episiotomy, which is an incision at the lower end of the vagina toward the anus, to reduce tearing of tissue. This cut enlarges the vaginal opening and allows the baby's head more room to emerge. Once the baby's head is delivered, its body rotates and, with the next few contractions, its shoulders emerge. When the baby is delivered in a more difficult position, such as its feet or buttocks emerging first, this is referred to as a **breech birth.**

....

crowning the first appearance of the fetal head in childbirth.

breech birth when the fetal buttocks emerge first rather than the head.

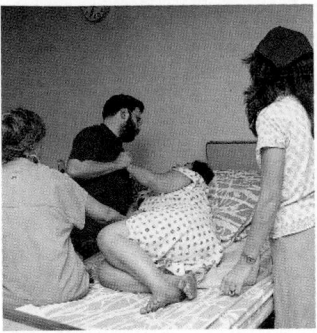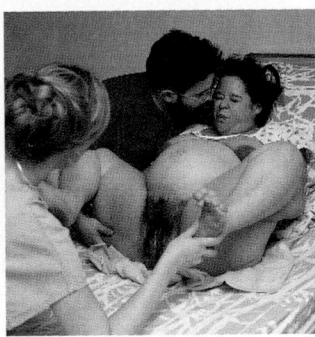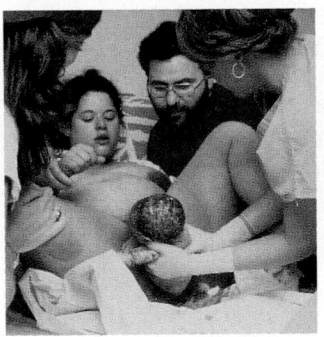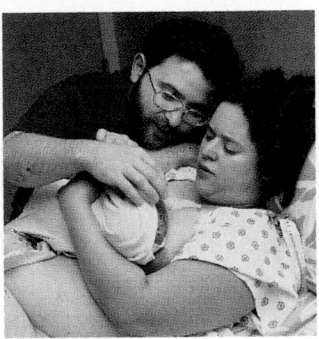

The process of childbirth.

The baby is cleaned and his or her breathing is monitored. The baby's color changes from bluish to pinkish as regular breathing begins. The umbilical cord is clamped and cut about 1¼ inches from the baby's body; this stump dries and drops off within several days, leaving a "navel." Within several days, the baby's head will have lost the misshapen appearance caused by the passage through the vagina.

Third Stage (Expulsion of the Placenta)

The uterus again begins contractions to deliver the placenta, or afterbirth. Within 10–12 minutes the placenta is separated from the uterus and expelled. It is important that the physician ensures a clean removal of any placental remnants to avoid later hemorrhaging. The physician next repairs the episiotomy and any damage that may have occurred to the vagina and uterus.

Once all of the placental tissue has been removed, uterine contractions slowly diminish and the uterus begins its return to its original size. This period, called **postpartum,** is a time of both physical and psychological adjustments as the mother makes the transition from pregnancy to motherhood.

CESAREAN DELIVERY

About 24 percent of all deliveries in the United States are **cesarean** (*sē-sār'i-an*) **deliveries** (also

postpartum the days and weeks following childbirth.

cesarean delivery delivery of a child through a surgical incision in the abdominal and uterine walls; also called cesarean section or C-section.

called cesarean section or C-section).[36] A cesarean delivery is a procedure in which a baby is delivered through an incision in the abdominal and uterine wall. C-sections are generally performed when vaginal delivery is unsafe for the fetus, the mother, or both. Cesarean deliveries are recommended when one or more of the following conditions exists[37]:

- the fetus is improperly aligned
- the pelvis of the mother is too small
- the fetus is larger than usual
- fetal cardiac or respiratory distress is apparent
- the umbilical cord is compressed
- delivery of the placenta would occur before the fetus
- maternal diabetes or herpes infection are present

Although a cesarean delivery is considered to be major surgery, the mother's hospital stay is only prolonged by a few days. Cesarean deliveries need not interfere with the mother nursing her baby, although the pain of the surgery may be uncomfortable, or the baby may have been affected by painkilling drugs given to the mother during delivery. Some mothers who have cesarean deliveries may feel a sense of failure over not being able to deliver vaginally; a C-section is no less an accomplishment than a vaginal delivery. Also, giving birth via a C-section does not preclude the mother from delivering vaginally in the future.

From 1965 to 1988 the rate of cesarean sections increased from 4.5 per 100 births to 24.7. Since then the rate increase has leveled off. A part of this shift is a significant recent increase in the rate of vaginal births by women who have had previous cesarean sections.[38]

PAIN RELIEF

In spite of the popularity of various methods of prepared delivery, such as the Lamaze method, many women receive medication during labor. Before delivering, a woman will want to become familiar with the various types of pain relief available and to discuss her options with her physician.

Analgesics are drugs that reduce pain. The milder analgesics, which may be taken orally (Percodan, Vicodin) or be injectable (Demerol, Nubain), can reduce the mother's pain and cause relaxation without slowing labor or affecting the fetus. Anesthetics are drugs that block all sensations. These may be general anesthetics, such as inhaled gases, which can also depress the fetal nervous system. More commonly, the anesthetics used are regional or local (Marcaine, Lidocaine), and are used to block pain in specific areas such as the uterus, cervix, or vulval areas as the fetus moves through the birth canal.

BIRTHING ALTERNATIVES

There are a variety of methods that couples can use to prepare for their baby's delivery. Known as *prepared delivery,* these methods involve prebirth classes, which facilitate the birthing process. Several popular approaches are the Read, Lamaze, and Leboyer methods.

In 1944, Dr. Grantly Dick Read emphasized that the fear of pain, rather than the pain itself, was largely responsible for the discomfort of childbirth. He urged expectant mothers to become educated about the birthing process and tension-relieving exercises. He believed that with training in breathing and muscle control, women could give birth much more easily, often with fewer pain-relieving drugs or no drugs at all.

In 1970, Dr. Fernand Lamaze expanded on these techniques by including methods of controlled breathing, birthing posture, and mental concentration. He included the father or a friend as a coach in preparation classes, as well as in the actual exercises. Lamaze method enthusiasts feel that this method is beneficial during delivery, has a more positive influence on the couple's relationship, and contributes to the positive bonding with the child.

In 1975, French physician Frederick Leboyer introduced a method for reducing the trauma that newborn infants experience. He believed that the ideal birth occurs in a quiet, dimly lit room where people speak softly. With the Leboyer method, the child is placed in a warm bath for a few minutes immediately after delivery, then placed on the mother's abdomen; cutting the umbilical cord is delayed. Parents who find success with this method report improved bonding with their infant.

In Lamaze classes expectant mothers and expectant fathers are given excellent information about normal labor and birth, relaxation techniques, and the importance of having someone present at the birth, other than the hospital staff, trained in coaching.

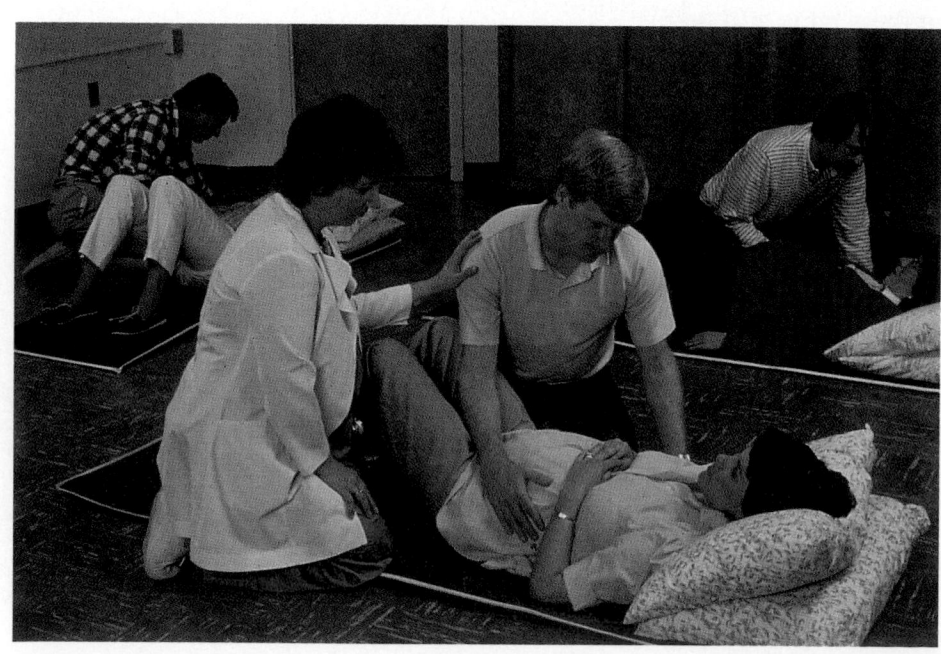

They also report that their infant appears calmer and more alert.

BIRTHING PLACES

There is no ideal location for labor and delivery. The choice of the *where* and *how* to deliver usually depends on the practitioner and clinic a woman chooses. We will discuss the most popular choices.

Many women prefer to give birth at hospitals or clinics. After admission, the woman usually must give a brief medical history, undergo a vaginal examination, and have blood tests done. In the traditional labor room, the staff monitors the progress of the mother and fetus. The mother is then prepared for delivery. Labor either is allowed to occur naturally or is stimulated with medications. When ready, the mother is transported to a delivery room to give birth, often with a family member present.

Delivery rooms are often sterile. In fact, for many people, the emotional detachment of that kind of environment is one of the primary disadvantages of a hospital delivery. The advantage, however, is in the hospital's preparedness in case of emergency complications such as premature labor, mother-fetus blood incompatibility, multiple birth, or illness.

An increasing number of parents are opting for *birthing rooms* or *birthing centers*. Birthing rooms are located in hospitals, and provide a homey, private setting in which the woman goes through labor and delivery in one room with her husband, a friend, or a family member present. Delivery may take place in a comfortable bed or in a birthing chair. After delivery, mother and family may be allowed to "room in" with the newborn. In case of an emergency, staff and facilities are close at hand.

Birthing centers are freestanding (nonhospital) and are generally located near a fully equipped hospital. These facilities are staffed with registered midwives and birthing assistants. Birthing center deliveries are made without drugs, monitoring, or surgical procedures. With the increasing demand for such centers, many states are establishing licensing rules.

BREASTFEEDING

Mothers have the choice of either breastfeeding or bottlefeeding their newborn babies. Although some mothers feel that breastfeeding creates a

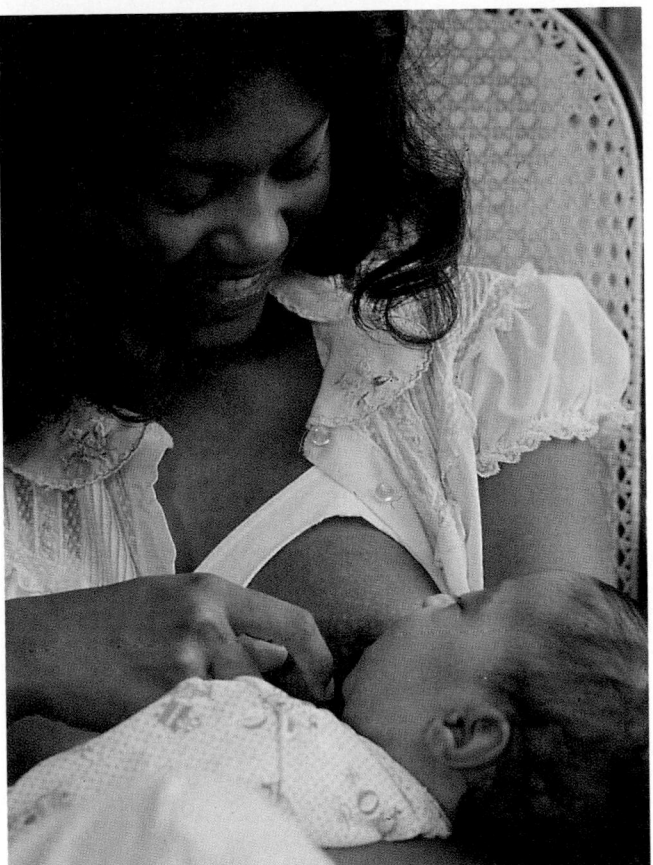

Breastfeeding provides superior nutrition for an infant and helps build a strong emotional bond between mother and baby.

unique bond between mother and baby that bottlefed babies do not establish, studies have found that the way a baby is fed is not a factor in a baby's emotional development.[39] In fact, the quality of the relationship is more important than the feeding method. For instance, a woman who breastfeeds her child while harboring resentment is more harmful to the baby than the mother who bottlefeeds her baby in a relaxed and loving manner. For those mothers choosing not to nurse their babies, medications can be taken to stop milk production by suppressing the milk-producing hormones.

Today more than half of all babies in the United States are breastfed. After being out of fashion in the 1960s and 1970s, breastfeeding is once again widely promoted. Because of the numerous benefits to the baby, the American Academy of Pediatrics urges every mother who can nurse to do so.

During the last weeks of pregnancy and for the first few days after delivery the breasts secrete

colostrum (*kō-los'trum*), a thin yellowy, milky fluid rich in vitamins A and E with twice the breast milk protein that is produced later. Within several days after delivery, the breasts stop producing colostrum and become engorged with milk. After some initial adjustment, milk production accommodates the needs of the baby.

Breast milk is the perfect food for infants and provides all the nutritional needs of an infant during its first six months. Its content of fatty acids, protein, and calories is superior to cow's milk. The enzymes in breast milk also help the infant absorb nutrients. Breast milk contains antibodies that passively protect against disease and stimulate the child's own defenses against disease.

Breastfeeding has other advantages. It is convenient; there are no bottles to warm and sterilize and no formula to warm. Breast milk is always readily available and is economical. Breastfeeding provides a special visual, tactile, and olfactory contact between the mother and child that some mothers feel is not found with bottlefed babies.

When a woman breastfeeds her baby, her menstrual periods may not return for 7–15 months after birth, because the hormone prolactin that stimulates milk production also suppresses menstruation (see Chapter 7, p. 190). Although breastfeeding does delay ovulation, it should not be considered a reliable form of contraception. Some women ovulate and conceive before resuming their menstrual periods following delivery.

Breastfeeding also has some disadvantages. Some mother's breasts and nipples may become tender and sore, or may seep milk at times other than during feeding. For as long as the mother is breastfeeding, she may need to restrict her routine somewhat to accommodate her baby's schedule, although a working mother can express (squeeze out) milk for baby's feedings and leave it with the caregiver while the mother returns to work. The mother may also endanger her infant if she consumes any toxic substances (alcohol, nicotine, or other drugs) because these substances will pass to the baby through the mother's milk. Babies whose mothers have had the equivalent of one beer consumed 23 percent less milk than usual. Such milk smells, and probably tastes, distinctly different.

This challenges the old adage that anxious nursing mothers should have a drink to relax.[40] Any alcohol the baby ingests may also impede her or his motor development.[41]

AFTER CHILDBIRTH

Immediately after childbirth the mother, child, and father must make many adjustments, both physically and emotionally. A special emotional process called **bonding** begins immediately between the mother and child (as explained in Communication for Wellness: Bonding with the Newborn). During the first day or two after delivery there is an immense sense of accomplishment. Family and friends offer support and share in the parents' joy. However, when the excitement dies down and everyone settles into their daily routines, the new parents are confronted with a new set of responsibilities and demands.

Psychological Effects

Not long after her child's birth, the mother's high from all the excitement may lead to a low called **postpartum depression.** She may feel irritable, anxious, tearful, or explosive. This emotional letdown is a normal consequence of delivery and comes from her fatigue and stress, hormonal changes, and mixed feelings over being a new mother.

After leaving the hospital, there is an immediate set of new adjustments—the baby's welfare, diaper changes, nighttime feedings—in addition to all the other daily demands. Everyone wants attention and time. The mother may feel vulnerable, confused, and exhausted. The postpartum period is an appropriate time for friends and family to give the mother help and time to adjust to her new baby's needs. Fathers also may suffer postpartum blues and need time to adjust.

Physical Effects

After delivery, the uterus begins to shrink back gradually to its normal size and returns to a

bonding the special emotional attachment that occurs between mother and newborn following birth.

postpartum depression an emotional low that may follow the birth of a child.

colostrum a thin, yellow, milky fluid secreted by the breasts soon after delivery.

COMMUNICATION FOR WELLNESS

BONDING WITH THE NEWBORN

Within the several hours following childbirth, it is believed, a special emotional attachment between mother and child, called bonding, occurs. Professionals in human development believe that this special period of bonding not be unnecessarily interfered with by medical personnel or procedures.

The elements of this bonding include:

1. *Odor* Upon the birth of the infant there is a unique odor emanating from the lining of the placenta, an odor which seems to stimulate in the mother the desire to communicate with her child—to hold, to cradle, and to embrace. This odor has been observed to stimulate a similar response in other women helping in the delivery. In addition, the child recognizes unique odors in the parents that trigger "at home" perceptions, which may last a lifetime.

2. *Voice* New mothers are observed to vocalize at the sight of their newborn, and to elevate their voices and speak directly to them. Some believe the mother is programmed to speak in this higher pitched voice, a sound to which the newborn seems unusually attentive.

3. *Eyes* The visual bonding of the extended stare is seen as an involuntary fixation between mothers and newborn, similar to the visual fixation between lovers. It's observed that for a short time immediately after birth, newborn infants can follow objects with their eyes, even turning their head to follow.

4. *Warmth* The first embraces of the infant by the mother provide a kind of warmth for the infant, who, until now, has enjoyed the continual warmth of the mother's body.

5. *Touch* The contact between the nude skin of the mother and child starts a type of contact that creates lifetime yearnings. This first touching between between them helps to seal their special relationship with each other. Even fathers are sometimes coached to expose the skin of their chests to the bare body of the newborn in order to create the special touch bonding between them.

Source: Joy, D. *Bonding, Relationships in the Image of God.* Waco, TX: Word, 1985.

---

prepregnant state in about six weeks. Breastfeeding hastens the process. The mother's body must adjust to an abrupt decline in estrogen and progesterone once the placenta has been removed. The cervix regains much of its tone within the first week. During the first several weeks the lining inside the uterus grows back, and a bloody discharge, called **lochia** (*lō'-ki-a*), is produced from the placental attachment to the uterine lining. The very stretched vagina shrinks, but may not return completely to its original size. Following delivery, the pelvic floor and abdominal walls of many women are slack. Kegel exercises (see Feature 8.5, p. 227) started soon after birth, followed by mild abdominal exercises and leg lifts, may help in restoring the abdomen to its prior tone, shape, and size.

RESUMING SEXUAL INTERCOURSE

Physicians often recommend that women refrain from intercourse for four to six weeks after delivery. This allows the uterus and vagina to return to the prepregnancy size, and also allows the episiotomy to heal. The woman's physician can let her know when it is safe for her to resume intercourse.

....

lochia a bloody uterine discharge following delivery.

CHECKPOINT

1. Discuss the expected due date of a birth, both in terms of gestational (menstrual) age and of ovulatory (fertilization) age of the fetus.

2. Compare the three stages of labor in terms both of duration of time and of changes that occur in the mother and the fetus.

3. Describe a cesarean delivery and give reasons why it may or may not be recommended.

4. What are some advantages to the mother of giving birth in birthing rooms and birthing centers over giving birth in a traditional hospital delivery room?

5. List the advantages of breastfeeding a newborn baby over bottlefeeding.

INFERTILITY

Couples who are unable to conceive after a year or more of sexual intercourse are said to be **infertile.**

....

infertile inability or diminished ability to produce children.

Ten to 15 percent of couples are not able to conceive within one year if they are using no contraception and attempting to achieve a pregnancy.[42] In 40 percent of these cases the difficulty lies with the woman, in another 40 percent it lies with the man, and in about 20 percent the problem is a combination of both.[43]

Some reasons for the rise in infertility include: the high incidence of sexually transmitted diseases; the tendency of American women to postpone marriage and childbearing into their 30s; the increase in environmental and industrial toxins; and the widespread use of the pill (which may lead to ovulatory problems).[44]

When a couple decides to have a child, it is a decision they have thought about carefully. The prospect of infertility, therefore, is extremely painful. The inability to conceive, or if conception has occurred, the inability to maintain a pregnancy, becomes a life crisis. The desire to reproduce is a strong inborn need with many couples. To be denied this fulfillment may produce feelings of anger, guilt, envy, and depression.

CAUSES

Male infertility may be due to any of the following:

1. Too few sperm that mature. This may be the result of infectious diseases after puberty, such as mumps, undescended testes, exposure of the scrotum to high temperatures, drugs, or varicose veins in the scrotum (see Feature 8.11).

2. Reduced sperm motility due to abnormal seminal fluids, which could be caused by drugs the person may be taking.

3. Blockage of the sperm ducts by scar tissue, which may have resulted from infections or untreated sexually transmitted diseases.

4. Inability to ejaculate sperm deeply into the vagina due to erectile problems or other sexual dysfunctions.

5. Poor health or malnutrition.

Female infertility may be due to any of the following:

1. Damage to the fallopian tubes caused by infections or intrauterine devices.

2. **Endometriosis** (*en-dō-mē-tri-ō'sis*), a condition in which endometrial tissue grows outside the uterus, which can lead to bleeding, inflammation, and tubal blockage.

3. A hormonal imbalance, so the endometrium is not adequately prepared to receive the fertilized ovum.

4. Failure to ovulate regularly due to insufficient hormone production or release.

5. Improper formation of reproductive organs, such as the uterus or cervix, which results in a failure to ovulate or receive the egg.

6. Cervical mucus of an incorrect consistency or pH, which prevents sperm from entering the uterus.

7. Extreme weight loss or gain, malnutrition, environmental toxins, or excessive exercise.

Some shared causes may include the following:

1. Immobilization and destruction of sperm by the woman's antibodies.

2. Lack of knowledge about how to time intercourse to increase the possibility of conception.

3. Infrequent coitus.

EVALUATING INFERTILITY

The infertility evaluation process includes educating the patients on fertility awareness and the timing of intercourse. A medical history is taken and physical examination given, which includes blood tests and semen analysis, and may include a laparoscopy, examination for sexually transmitted infections, and determining whether, by checking BBT and cervical mucus, ovulation takes place.

HOPE FOR THE INFERTILE

In the past, couples either resigned themselves to infertility or decided to adopt a child. Now all of

....

endometriosis growth of endometrial tissue outside the uterus.

SPERM COUNTS: INDICATORS OF INFERTILITY

Infertility is often detected by testing a man's sperm count. While estimates vary, for semen to be considered normal the ejaculate should contain:

- a minimum volume of 3–5 milliliters of semen per ejaculate (5 milliliters = 1 teaspoonful),

- at least 40 million sperm per milliliter of ejaculated semen,

- at least 60 percent of motile (moving) sperm two hours after ejaculation, and

- at least 60 percent of normally formed sperm.

Males are considered to be functionally infertile if their sperm counts are less than 10 million per milliliter of semen, or if the percentage of normal sperm falls below 60 percent.

---

this is changing. In 1990, more than a million new patients sought treatment for fertility problems.[45] Fortunately for those who seek assistance with their infertility, medical science is opening up new doors in fertilization. Physicians today can manipulate almost every aspect of the reproductive cycle (see Feature 8.12, p. 244).

DECIDING WHETHER TO TERMINATE PREGNANCY

COUNSELING THE PARTNERS

Once an unwanted pregnancy has been confirmed, the woman needs support and counseling to help her explore feelings and options. Abortion is not the *only* option; the pregnancy can be carried to term and the child placed for adoption. The woman or couple might also carefully explore, with professional counsel, whether she or they may wish to keep and raise the child. Issues that need to be discussed include values about life, religious beliefs, whether there is pressure for an abortion, the nature of the couple's relationship, and the support the woman feels from the man who impregnated her, and from family and friends.

Another serious consideration is the medical risks involved. Complications of an abortion may include infection, intrauterine blood clotting, incomplete removal of tissue, or continuing pregnancy after an attempted abortion. Abortions can also lead to injury to the uterine wall (perforation), to the cervix by reducing its competence (ability in a subsequent pregnancy to retain the fetus in the uterus until term), and hemorrhaging.

A woman may feel confused and frightened. She may need to deal with fears of her partner abandoning her, another unwanted pregnancy, or of the inability to have a later pregnancy. She may feel anger toward the partner who impregnated her. She may also experience sadness, loneliness, and guilt.

The male partner may share some of the same feelings. He may want the child and may not have been consulted about the decision to have an abortion. He may also feel guilty about the burden placed on the woman and about abandoning her once he found out about her pregnancy.

Both partners should receive counseling. There should be opportunity for open communication between them. This may help the decision-making process and, if she or they wish to proceed, may serve to provide added support to the couple during and following the abortion.

CHECKPOINT

1. Describe the considerations that need to be looked into by a woman with an unwanted pregnancy before she decides on any course of action.

2. Identify some of the medical concerns related with having an abortion.

TERMINATING PREGNANCY

The decision to terminate a pregnancy is an extremely personal one, and should be undertaken by both partners with great care and consideration of all of the implications. Women in the United States currently have the option of terminating a pregnancy. To carry out this decision, there are several choices available which may include the following.

FEATURE 8.12

ADVANCES IN FERTILITY

Today, new techniques are creating a revolution in reproductive technology. The advances in reproductive technology include the following:

1. **Artificial insemination.** When the husband's sperm count is low, his sperm is collected and then inserted (inseminated) artificially, by syringe, into the vagina at the mouth of the cervix near the expected time of ovulation. If the husband's sperm does not successfully result in conception, an anonymous donor may be used. **Artificial insemination** is successful in about 75 percent of cases where fresh semen is used, and in about 60 percent of cases where it is frozen.

2. **In vitro fertilization (IVF),** or "test-tube baby" procedure. When the woman's fallopian tubes are blocked, she is given hormones to stimulate the release of eggs. These are then retrieved by an endoscope and the eggs are united with the husband's sperm outside the body in a laboratory dish. The ova are allowed to develop into embryos and then inserted into the uterus. The insertion can be disruptive to the uterus and the embryo may fail to implant. In vitro fertilization fails 75–85 percent of the time.

3. *Gamete intra-fallopian tube transfer (GIFT).* A variation on IVF, sperm and unfertilized ripe eggs are inserted into the fallopian tube with a catheter, where fertilization occurs. The fertilized egg drifts into the uterus, as it would naturally. The fertilized egg is more likely to be successfully received than with IVF.

4. *Zygote intra-fallopian transfer (ZIFT).* A variation of GIFT, ZIFT allows the sperm to fertilize ripe eggs in a laboratory dish. The resulting fertilized eggs (zygotes) are placed in the fallopian tube. The advantage is that only those eggs successfully fertilized are transferred. Success rates of GIFT and ZIFT now approach 50 percent.

5. *Opening blocked fallopian tubes.* A balloon catheter is inflated to clear a passageway for the egg. This technique benefits women whose tubes are clogged with scar tissue or other obstructions and who cannot conceive by natural means because their eggs have no way of getting to the uterus. Microsurgery is also used to open obstructed tubes.

6. *Microinjection.* Using a thin needle, a single sperm is inserted through the egg's outer membrane. This is useful for men with extremely low sperm counts. This is a variation of artificial insemination which places sperm directly into the cervix.

7. *Zona drilling.* This fertilization technique removes part of the outer layer (*zone pellucida*) of an unfertilized egg before mixing it with sperm. A variation of this is sperm washing, in which sperm of couples with sperm allergy problems is cleaned of chemical antigens that trigger the allergic reaction.

8. *Surrogate mother.* A woman agrees, for a fee, to bear a child that another woman will raise as her own. The surrogate is fertilized artificially with sperm from the husband of the infertile woman. The surrogate bears the child and then gives it to the infertile couple according to their agreement. Such agreements are sometimes challenged by mothers who renege on their agreements.

9. *Pregnancy after menopause.* Eggs are collected from a younger woman, are combined with sperm, and fertilization occurs. After two days multicelled embryos are removed. An embryo is transferred into the uterus of the postmenopausal woman. Such a woman, able now to bear children into her late 40s and 50s, is infertile not because her uterus is too old, but because her ovaries have stopped functioning. The problem—children of such pregnancies carry the genes of the younger egg donor, not of the mother who bears them.

10. *Other techniques. Frozen embryos*—drugs are used to induce the ovary to produce a dozen or more ripe eggs, which may then be used or frozen for later thawing and use. *Selective reduction of pregnancy*—when more than one egg has been fertilized and are developing, a lethal substance is injected into one or more of the developing embryos to improve the chances of only one embryo surviving.

Source: Elmer-Dewitt, P. "A Revolution in Making Babies." *Time,* 5 November 1990, pp. 76–77; Blackman, A., et al. "Making Babies." *Time,* 30 September 1991, pp. 56–63; Roan, S. "Ethics and the Science of Birth." *Los Angeles Times* 8 December 1990, pp. A-1, 38, 39.

EARLY METHODS

Morning After Pill

The morning-after pill is a postcoital drug that women can take after unprotected intercourse to

artificial insemination introducing sperm into the vagina or uterus by means other than intercourse.

in vitro fertilization (IVF) fertilization of the egg by sperm outside of the body.

ensure that pregnancy has not occurred. Only about 4 out of 100 women who have an unprotected act of intercourse during a given cycle get pregnant, whereas the rate of pregnancy is 15–25 percent if the act occurs midcycle.[46]

Consisting of a high dose of synthetic estrogen, or progesterone, or a combination of both, the pills must be started within 72 hours of unprotected intercourse. The most common pill used to be DES (diethylstilbestrol), a synthetic estrogen that had serious side effects. A newer regimen is the use of

Ovral, a combination pill approved by the Food and Drug Administration (FDA) as an oral contraceptive. Not intended for use as morning-after pills, neither of these pills was approved by the FDA for this purpose.[47]

Before using Ovral as a morning-after pill, a woman should be examined by a physician. Used only for one-time protection against pregnancy in emergency situations, such as in cases of rape or incest, the pill when used for morning-after purposes may pose risks to the user not found with its use as a contraceptive.

Taken within 72 hours after unprotected intercourse, the pill affects the transport of the fertilized ovum in the fallopian tube and the ability of the uterus to support it, ensuring that no pregnancy has resulted. The failure rate of this method is about 1 percent.[48]

Oral Abortion Pill

A pill has been developed which, when taken orally, interrupts pregnancy in its early stages. Known by the drug manufacturer's shorthand RU 486, the drug was developed in France, where it is approved for use.

RU 486 blocks the effects of progesterone, the hormone that supports pregnancy. Without progesterone, the lining of the uterus, in which the embryo must become implanted, breaks down. When administered late in the menstrual cycle (within ten days of the next usual period) it leads to menstrual discharge and loss of the fertilized egg in 85 percent of the women given the pill.[49]

Opponents to the public use of RU 486 claim that the use of the drug as an **abortifacient** (any substance or device used to cause an abortion) is not acceptable, and that the use of the drug can lead to prolonged uterine bleeding and incomplete or failed abortion. Proponents argue that RU 486 is an effective and noninvasive method of terminating early pregnancy, that it is less expensive than other methods, and that it is generally safe. Supporters point to research on other possible medical uses for the pill. While approved for public use in France, Britain, and various other European countries, the Food and Drug Administration has currently approved the use of RU 486 in the United States only for testing and research purposes.

Menstrual Extraction

Menstrual extraction (menstrual aspiration) may be performed before pregnancy is confirmed. Some women prefer not to know whether they are actually pregnant, even though a missed period does not always indicate a pregnancy. Menstrual extraction is a procedure that involves the application of light suction through the use of a small tube that is inserted into the cavity of the uterus. The tube is moved around the inside of the uterus and through it, endometrial lining and other uterine contents are withdrawn. This is done without dilating the cervical canal, as is done in an abortion.

Menstrual extraction is performed in a physician's office and may occur between the fourth and sixth week after the last menstrual period (LMP), which is up to two weeks after a missed menstrual period, yet before a pregnancy has been confirmed. This procedure is relatively safe. Blood loss is minimal and complications are uncommon. The use of this method may not guarantee that all of the endometrial tissue has been removed. Remaining tissue could still result in pregnancy.[50] Failure to locate and remove the implanted blastocyst could result in the continuation of the pregnancy.[51]

CHECKPOINT

1. Explain the action of the morning-after pill.
2. Describe the technique of menstrual extraction.

ABORTION

Abortion is the termination of pregnancy before the fetus is viable, or sufficiently developed to survive. A fetus may be viable as early as the twentieth week of development or as late as the twenty-eighth week. In the following sections we will

menstrual extraction suctioned removal of the uterine lining just before the next menstrual period.

abortion the termination of pregnancy before the fetus is viable.

abortifacient any substance or device used to cause an abortion.

FEATURE 8.13

CHANGES IN ABORTION DECISIONS

In the summer of 1989, the United States Supreme Court handed down a decision that began to modify *Roe* v. *Wade,* the landmark 1973 decision that established a woman's right to terminate a pregnancy by abortion. In the case of *Webster* v. *Reproductive Health Services,* a 5–4 majority of the Court upheld a Missouri law that sharply restricted the availability of publicly funded abortion services and required physicians to test whether a 20-week-old fetus could survive outside the womb. While stopping short of reversing *Roe* v. *Wade,* the so-called Missouri case not only narrowed its meaning, but invited state legislatures to experiment with new laws designed to limit access to abortion.

In 1992, the U.S. Supreme Court heard *Planned Parenthood* v. *Casey.* This case pertained to a Pennsylvania law restricting access to abortion. The Court, in a 5–4 vote, held that Pennsylvania could require a 24-hour waiting period, mandate that physicians inform women about other options ("informed consent"), demand parental notification for minors seeking an abortion, and require that physicians provide statistical information about their abortions. Pennsylvania was forbidden from requiring a woman to notify her husband before an abortion (an "undue burden" on the woman).

The public debate over abortion covers a wide spectrum of personal positions. It ranges from those who feel that a woman has the right to control her own body, including the right to have the embryo or fetus she is carrying aborted (*pro-choice*) to those who feel that from the moment a sperm cell fertilizes an egg a new life has been created that is a separate growing organism that has the right to life (*right-to-life; pro-life*).

Pro-choice persons hold that a woman considering an abortion should not be subject to interference from the state or church, that she is entitled to the support and advice of trusted friends and professionals, and that she has the right to easy access to a qualified physician trained in performing an abortion. They hold that a "quality of life" ethic gives her the right of deciding the quality of her life over the quality of any other life. Pro-life persons hold that an embryo or fetus is a human life that is not an integral part of the woman's body, that the embryo or fetus has legal rights including the right to life regardless of the woman's condition or wishes, and that abortion poses both emotional and physical hazards to the woman. They hold that an "absolute value of life" take precedence over the woman's wishes.

In its recent decisions the Supreme Court has been backing away from a federal policy based on judicial decision. In effect, the Court is saying that decisions on abortion belong to the people rather than to the courts. The language of the decisions clearly invites state legislatures to experiment with new laws structured to limit access to abortion and to call for parental consent, informed consent of the mother, and new standards for abortion clinics.

By moving the debate from the judiciary to the state legislatures, the effect may be to pull the various extreme positions into the middle where, it is believed, the majority of Americans are positioned. Such center ground may be found if both extremes can hear each other's concerns and find tolerance for each other's apprehensions.

Source: Salholz, E. "Abortion Angst." *Newsweek,* 13 July 1992, pp. 16–19.

---

discuss various methods used for aborting an embryo or fetus.

A pregnancy that terminates involuntarily before the fetus is viable is known as a spontaneous (natural) abortion, or miscarriage (as discussed earlier in this chapter). Miscarriages are unintended and often unwanted, and cause grief for the couple anticipating the birth. Miscarriages occur in 10–15 percent of all pregnancies. About 75 percent of all miscarriages terminate before the twelfth week.

An **induced abortion** is an intentional ending of a pregnancy before the fetus is viable. Abortions may be induced to protect the mother's health, or to respond to the mother's request, which need not

be health related. Almost 25 percent of all pregnancies in the United States are now terminated by induced abortion[52] (see Feature 8.13). In 1973, the United States Supreme Court (in *Roe* v. *Wade*), by a 7–2 vote, ruled that the fetus is "potential life" and not a "person," and that, as such, the fetus does not have a "right to life." The Court states that an elective, voluntary abortion may be legal within the following guidelines:

1. During the first three months of pregnancy (first **trimester of pregnancy**), the decision to abort a fetus lies with the woman and her physician.

---

induced abortion an abortion brought on intentionally.

trimester of pregnancy a third of pregnancy, or approximately 13 weeks.

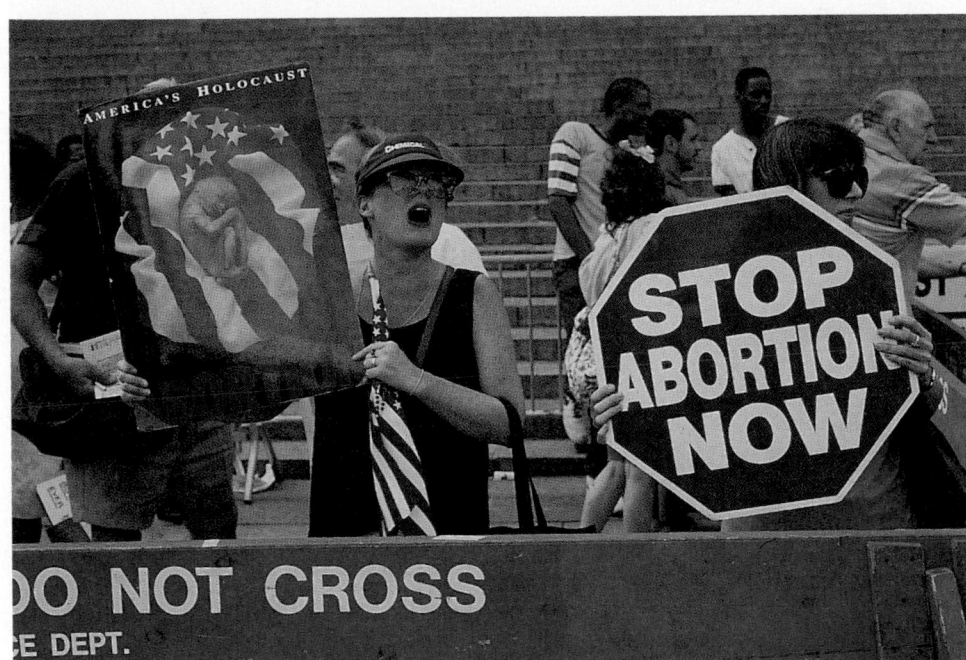

The public debate on abortion has been intense and sometimes bitter. Many believe that people in this country will need to find a balance between the concern for the pregnant mother and for fetal life.

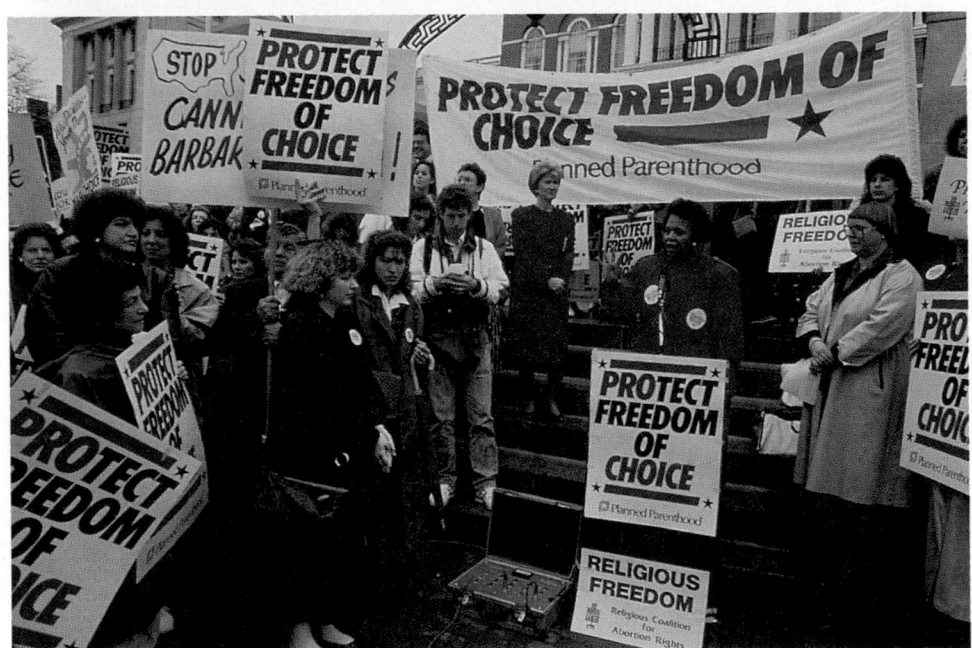

2. During the next six months (second and third trimesters), the state may regulate abortion procedures in ways that protect the health of the mother.

3. During the last three months of pregnancy (third trimester), when the fetus is viable, the state may regulate or prohibit abortion except in those cases in which the mothers' life or health is endangered.

The Court also stated in its 1973 decision that a woman's right to privacy overrides any state interest in using abortion statutes to regulate sexual conduct.

First Trimester Methods

First trimester abortion is performed within the first 12 weeks of pregnancy. The methods used are vacuum aspiration and dilation and curettage.

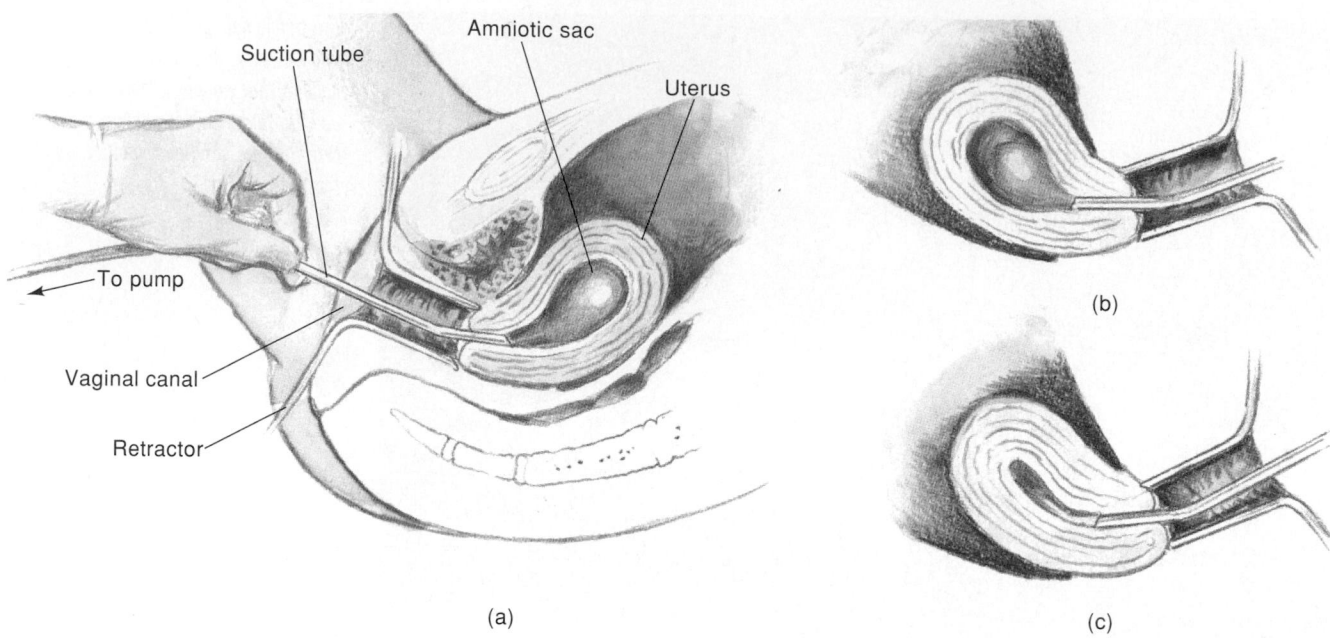

Figure 8.9
Vacuum Aspiration

(a) Removal of fetal material. (b) and (c) As fetal material is removed, the uterus contracts to its original size.

Source: Masters, W., Johnson, W., and Kolodny, R. Human Sexuality, 4th ed. New York: HarperCollins, 1992.

Vacuum Aspiration **Vacuum aspiration** is used until the twelfth week of pregnancy. Approximately 97 percent of all abortions in the United States are performed using this method.[53]

This is one of the safest surgical procedures. It involves dilating the cervical canal and inserting into the uterine cavity a **cannula** (a small tube) attached to an aspirator. The uterine contents are then sucked out (see Figure 8.9). Side effects of this procedure may include bleeding and menstrual-like cramps.

Dilation and Curettage **Dilation and curettage** (D and C) may be used between the sixth and twelfth weeks of pregnancy. While the patient is under general anesthesia, the physician dilates the cervical canal and inserts a small, spoon-shaped metal curette into the uterine cavity. The curette is used to scrape and remove the fetal and endometrial tissue.

Hospitalization is usually required since there is increased risk of uterine perforation, bleeding, and infection. The D and C procedure is routinely used to scrape the inside of the uterus in cases of spontaneous abortion and suspected uterine malignancies.

Second Trimester Methods

Second trimester methods may be used after the thirteenth week of pregnancy. These include instillation and dilation and evacuation.

Instillation (Induced Contraction) After the thirteenth week of pregnancy, the fetus is too large to be removed using first trimester methods. During the second trimester, the safest way to perform an abortion is for the physician to induce uterine contractions that stimulate the uterus to expel the fetus and placenta in a process similar to that of childbirth.

Contractions may be induced by withdrawing a measured amount of amniotic fluid, the uterine fluid surrounding the fetus, and injecting (instilling) a *hypertonic saline* solution through the

....

vacuum aspiration the removal of a fetus by suction.

cannula a small tube used to withdraw the uterine lining.

dilation and curettage a first trimester abortion procedure in which the inner lining of the uterus is scraped.

abdominal wall into the amniotic sac surrounding the uterus, or by injecting (instilling) *prostaglandins* intramuscularly. The induced contractions lead to the expulsion by the mother of the embryo or fetus in the same manner as a childbirth. The entire instillation-expulsion may require 12–48 hours of hospitalization.

Dilation and Evacuation **Dilation and evacuation** (D and E) is used for abortions during the second trimester (between the thirteenth and eighteenth week of pregnancy). This procedure is performed while the patient is under general anesthesia in a hospital.

The D and E first involves dilation of the cervix. Then, the fetus is removed using a combination of vacuum aspiration and forceps. The aspirator removes the fetal tissue the forceps has been unable to extract. After the fetus and fetal tissue is removed, the physician uses a metal curette to scrape the uterine wall.

Safety of Abortions

Abortions are relatively safe. Induced abortions performed during the second month of pregnancy are responsible for a mortality rate of less than 0.6 per 100,000 abortions, compared with a mortality rate from natural childbirth of 7.8 per 100,000.[54] The least risky procedure is the vacuum aspiration at less than eight weeks of pregnancy; the risk factor rises noticeably when the abortion is delayed until the second trimester.

Incidence of Induced Abortion

The incidence of induced abortion in the United States is about one abortion for every three live births. For African American women there are more than twice as many induced abortions per 1000 women as there are for white women. African American women seeking abortions tend to be slightly older than white women. Among married women, less than 10 percent of pregnancies end in induced abortion, but among those married women, the abortion ratio for African American women is more than three times greater than that

dilation and evacuation a second trimester abortion procedure.

for white women. Among unmarried women there are more than nine induced abortions for every ten live births, but among those unmarried women the abortion ratio is almost one-and-a-half times greater for white women than for African American women. Over all, women having abortions are typically young, white, unmarried, and have had no prior live births. A little more than half of these women have had no prior abortions. More than 90 percent of abortions are performed during the first trimester.[55]

CHECKPOINT

1. What is an abortion?
2. Distinguish between spontaneous and induced abortions.
3. Explain the guidelines under which the U.S. Supreme Court legalized abortion in 1973.
4. Describe the methods used to perform a first trimester abortion.
5. How may a second trimester abortion be performed?

SUMMARY

Deciding to become a parent is one of the most important decisions you will make during your lifetime. Careful assessment of many issues is required. Parents need both physical and emotional preparation for pregnancy.

The female matures 400–500 eggs during her lifetime; the male produces several hundred million sperms with each ejaculation. Conception occurs when the sperm unites with the egg. The fertilized egg moves through the fallopian tube and implants in the uterus as it is dividing. Upon implanting into the uterine wall, it forms a placenta to connect the embryo and uterine blood supply.

A pregnancy lasts approximately 266 days, but is often calculated as 280 days from the last menstrual period. Pregnancy is divided into 10 lunar months, 40 weeks, or 3 trimesters. During the first trimester, major embryo/fetal organs and structures are formed. During the second trimester, the mother first feels fetal movements and her abdomen begins to protrude. During the third trimester, most fetal weight gain occurs.

Proper prenatal care includes good nutrition, exercise, no smoking, no alcoholic drinks or other drugs, rubella immunization, and avoidance of unnecessary radiation. Problems that occur during pregnancy may include birth defects, toxemia, miscarriage, stillbirth, and premature delivery.

Birth occurs close to nine calendar months after conception. The process of childbirth is called labor, and occurs in three stages. Childbirth may involve cesarean delivery, pain relief with drugs, prepared delivery techniques, and use of special birthing facilities.

As many as 10–15 percent of American couples are infertile. Some of these couples resort to test-tube pregnancy, artificial insemination, hormone treatment, microsurgery, or surrogate motherhood.

Abortion is the termination of a pregnancy before the fetus is viable. Abortion may be induced using different methods, and may be recommended for medical reasons or because the mother is unable to carry the fetus to term. Abortion is least risky if performed during the first trimester of pregnancy. Induced abortion is less risky to the mother than natural childbirth. A woman contemplating abortion ought to seek counseling to help her to examine the pros and cons. It is best to counsel both the male and female partners during this process.

REFERENCES

1. U.S. Bureau of the Census. *Statistical Abstract of the United States: 1993,* 113th ed. Washington, DC: U.S. Department of Commerce, 1993.
2. Hatcher, R., et al. *Contraceptive Technology, 1990–1992,* 15th rev. ed. New York: Irvington, 1990.
3. Wallis, C. "Children Having Children." *Time* (9 December 1985), 88–90.
4. Cunningham, G., et al. *Williams Obstetrics,* 19th ed. Norwalk, CT: Appleton-Lange, 1993.
5. Ibid.
6. Ibid.
7. Ibid.
8. Ibid.
9. Institute of Medicine, Subcommittee on Nutritional Status and Weight Gain During Pregnancy. "Nutrition During Pregnancy." Washington, DC: National Academy Press, 1990.
10. Ibid.
11. Cunningham, op. cit.
12. Ibid.
13. Whitney, E., and Rolfes, S. *Understanding Nutrition,* 6th ed. Minneapolis: West, 1993.
14. Tortora, G., and Grabowski, S. *Principles of Anatomy and Physiology,* 7th ed. New York: HarperCollins, 1993.
15. Hole, J. *Human Anatomy and Physiology,* 6th ed. Dubuque, IA: Brown, 1993.
16. Tortora, op. cit.
17. National Center for Health Statistics. "Advance Report of Maternal and Infant Health Data from the Birth Certificate, 1990." *Monthly Vital Statistics Report,* Vol. 42, No. 2, Supplement. Hyattsville, MD: Public Health Service, 1993.
18. Streissguth, A., et al. "Fetal Alcohol Syndrome in Adolescents and Adults." *Journal of the American Medical Association,* Vol. 265, No. 15 (17 April 1991), 1961–1967.
19. U.S. Department of Health and Human Services. *Sixth Special Report to the U.S. Congress on Alcohol and Health* (DHHS Publ. No. (ADM) 87-1519). Washington, DC: U.S. Government Printing Office, 1987.
20. Ibid.
21. Cunningham, op. cit.
22. National Center for Health Statistics, op. cit.
23. Tortora, op. cit.
24. Miller, S. "Moms: No 'Safe' Time for Cocaine." *Los Angeles Times* (28 November 1989), E-1, 2.
22. Ibid.
23. U.S. Department of Health and Human Services, op. cit.
24. Milunsky, A., et al. "Maternal Heat Exposure and Neural Tube Defects." *Journal of the American Medical Association,* Vol. 268, No. 7 (12 August 1992), 882–885.
25. Cunningham, op. cit.
26. Ibid.
27. Ibid.
28. Cunningham, op. cit.
29. Milunsky, et al., op. cit.
30. Ibid.
31. Cunningham, op. cit.
32. Elmer-Dewitt, P. "Making Babies." *Time* (30 September 1991), 56–63.
33. Cunningham, op. cit.
34. Moore, K. *Before We Were Born: Basic Embryology and Birth Defects.* Philadelphia: Saunders, 1989.
35. Cunningham, op. cit.
36. Scott, J. "25-Year Rise in Cesarean Births Levels Off." *Los Angeles Times* (11 July 1991), A-28.
37. Cunningham, op. cit.
38. Scott, op. cit.
39. Papalia, D., and Olds, S. *A Child's World: Infancy Through Adolescence,* 4th ed. New York: McGraw-Hill, 1987.
40. Mennella, J., and Beauchamp, G. "The Transfer of Alcohol to Human Milk." *The New England Journal of Medicine* Vol. 325, No. 14 (30 October 1991), 981–985.

41. Little, R., et al. "Maternal Alcohol Use During Breast-feeding and Infant Mental and Motor Development at One Year." *The New England Journal of Medicine* Vol. 321, No. 7 (17 August 1989), 425–430.

42. Hatcher, op. cit.

43. Boston Women's Health Book Collective. *The New Our Bodies, Ourselves.* New York: Simon & Schuster, 1992.

44. Ibid.

45. Elmer-Dewitt, P. "A Revolution in Making Babies." *Time* (5 November 1990), 76–77.

46. Boston Women's Health Book Collective, op. cit.

47. Hatcher, op. cit.

48. Ibid.

49. Cunningham, op. cit.

50. Hatcher, op. cit.

51. Cunningham, op. cit.

52. National Center for Health Statistics. "Induced Terminations of Pregnancy: Reporting Rates, 1988." *Monthly Vital Statistics Report,* Vol. 39, No. 12, Suppl. 7. Hyattsville, MD: National Center for Health Statistics, 1991.

53. Ibid.

54. Cunningham, op. cit.

55. National Center for Health Statistics. "Induced Terminations of Pregnancy: Reporting Rates, 1988," op. cit.

SUGGESTED READINGS

Borg, S., and Lasker, J. *When Pregnancy Fails,* rev. ed. New York: Bantam, 1989.

Boston Women's Health Book Collective. *The New Our Bodies, Ourselves.* New York: Simon & Schuster, 1992.

Gillespie, C. *Your Pregnancy Month by Month.* New York: HarperCollins, 1992.

Hausknecht, R., and Heilman, J. *Having a Cesarean Baby.* 2nd rev. ed. New York: Plume, 1991.

LaLeche International. *The Womanly Art of Breastfeeding,* 4th ed. New York: Plume, 1987.

Nilsson, L. *A Child Is Born,* completely revised. New York: Delacourte, 1977.

Novak, J. *Enhancing Lamaze Techniques.* Los Angeles: The Body Press, 1988.

Odent, M. *The Nature of Birth and Breast-feeding.* Westport, CT: Bergin and Garvey, 1992.

Queenan, J., and Queenan, C. *A New Life: Pregnancy, Birth, and Your Child's First Year—A Comprehensive Guide,* 2nd rev. ed. Boston: Little, Brown, 1992.

Rosenberg, H., and Epstein, Y. *Getting Pregnant When You Thought You Couldn't.* New York: Warner, 1993.

Shapiro, H. *The Pregnancy Book for Today's Woman,* 2nd ed. New York: HarperPerennial, 1993.

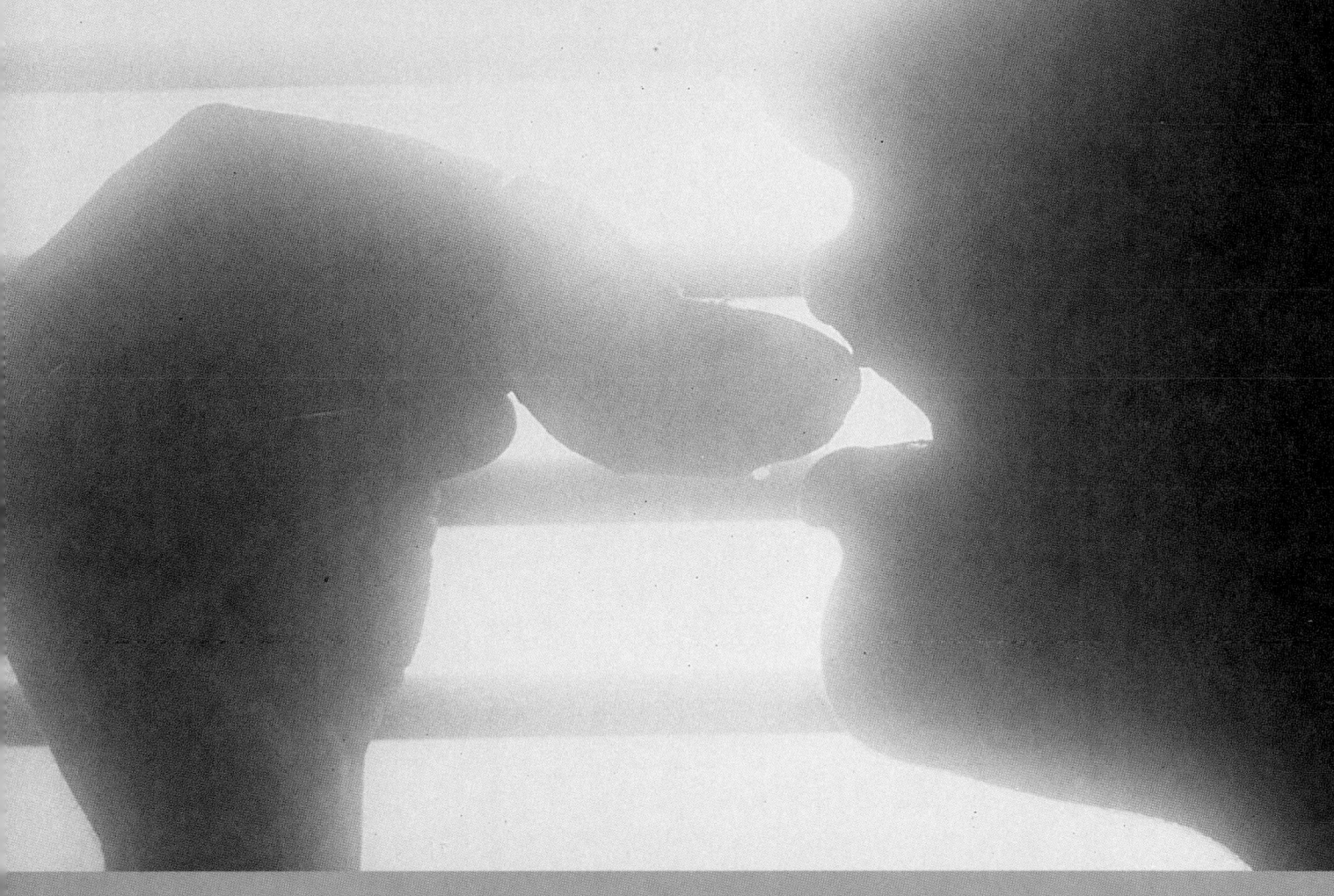

FOUR
FOOD AND FITNESS

Whether we wear the latest fashions or drive the latest model of import, our bodies are essentially the same model used by our pioneer ancestors. While we sit in front of our computers synthesizing new languages, our bodies process food and energy in exactly the same way as our forefathers' bodies did centuries ago.

Over the years, immense technological changes have occurred in our ability to grow and process foods. New farming techniques ensure greater yields of certain crops while new processing breakthroughs allow for easy transport of foods across town and across the world. We not only have the greatest selection of foods ever, but more leisure time to spend indulging (and overindulging) in them.

With these dramatic changes has come a greater freedom of choice. Accompanying this freedom, however, are risks and responsibilities; do we overindulge our bodies with too many calories and too little exercise, or do we eat well, manage our weight, and stay physically fit? This unit deals with how we can develop and maintain high levels of nutritional and physical fitness.

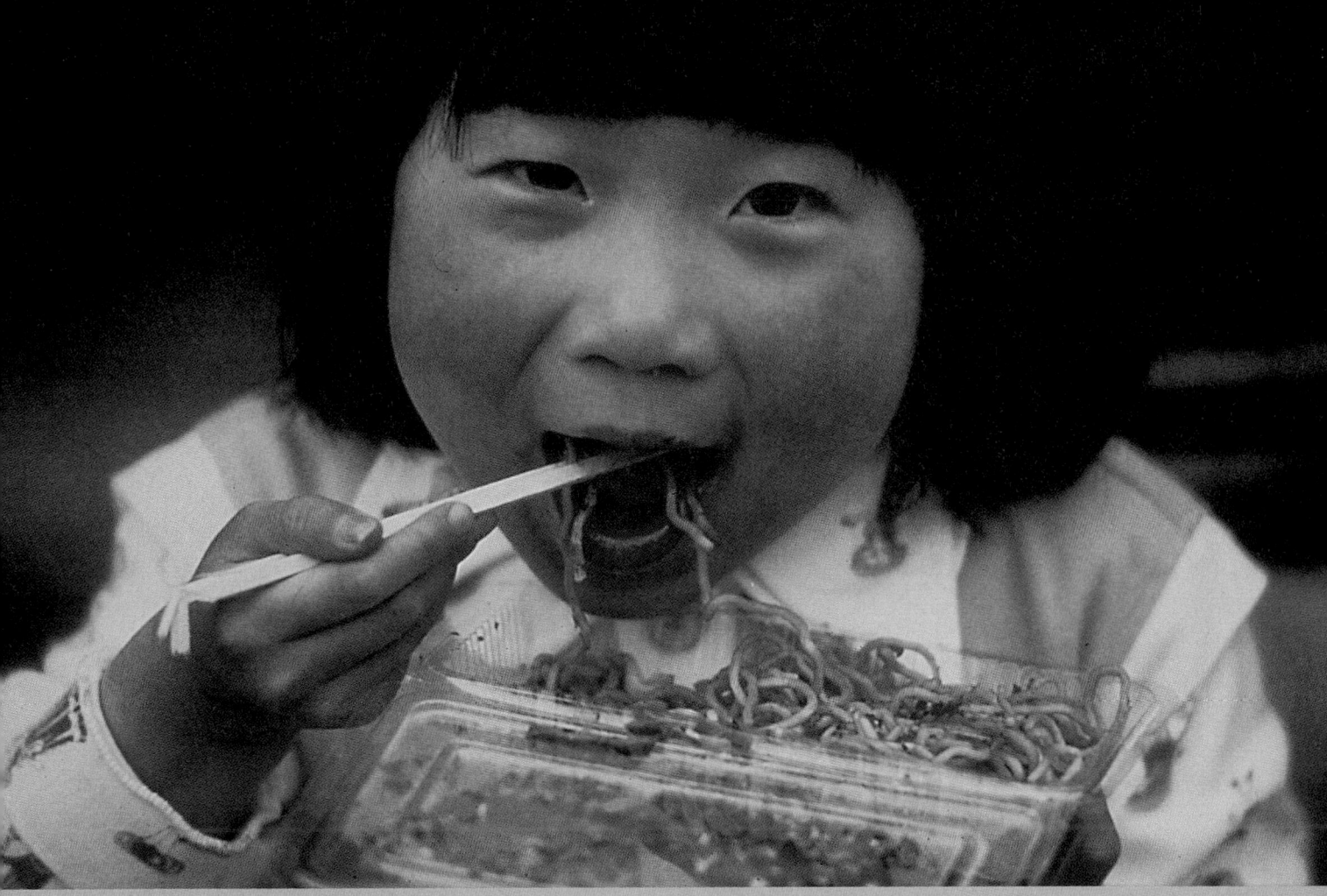

9
NUTRITION

KNOWLEDGE

- List the six major types of nutrients needed by the body.
- Explain the consequences of a person taking in more calories than expended.
- Classify the kinds of fatty acids.
- Name the four common chemical elements in an amino acid.
- Describe how a vitamin differs from carbohydrates, fats, and proteins.
- Name the five food groups.
- Explain the meaning of the term *Daily Values*.
- Explain the Food Guide Pyramid.
- List some rules to follow in improving your dietary balance when eating in restaurants.
- Explain why food additives may be seen as beneficial.

INSIGHT

- Determine your nutrition quotient.
- Discuss the reasons you might consider using an artificial sweetener in place of sugar as a food sweetener.
- Distinguish organic foods from natural foods.
- If you were an athlete, how would you go about "carbohydrate loading"?

DECISION MAKING

- Describe the steps you might take to avoid developing osteoporosis.
- Make an informed decision about the use of vitamin supplements.
- In comparing your typical diet with the Daily Food Guide, what changes do you see that you need to make to match the Guide?
- Explain how you expect the new food labeling Nutritive Facts to help you improve your nutritional intake.

Actress Angela Lansbury, star of the popular television series "Murder, She Wrote," knew she needed to address her nutrition habits when she saw herself at 165 pounds on a home video. While she had no desire for the superthin, Madison Avenue look, she did want to get rid of some excess weight and start feeling better again. Not only had she noticed that she looked overweight, but she also had begun to feel sluggish, and have more headaches and stomach problems.

Weight watching was not new to Ms. Lansbury, but she had never been a compulsive dieter like many in her business. Rather than go on some diet that would be unhealthy and unsuccessful, her solution was to change her eating habits and begin observing some simple, basic nutritional principles. Her old idea of a good meal—large portions of a meat and two vegetables followed by a dessert—would not work. She and her husband began a low fat, high-fiber eating plan with lots of fruits, vegetables, and grains. Protein was limited to only about 6 ounces per day. Whenever she feels that she needs to lose a pound or two, she simply limits the size of the servings to reduce her caloric intake. Ms. Lansbury tries to keep her caloric intake at around 2000 per day, without overdoing the calorie counting. However, she does recognize that a big slab of cheesecake may contain about 1000 calories, mostly from fat, so she just takes a *bite or two instead of eating the entire piece. Also, Ms. Lansbury recognizes the importance of exercise in combination with a healthful diet in achieving a healthful life-style. In fact, she recently made her own fitness video, which emphasizes these principles.*

Everyone should find their own healthful way of eating; Ms. Lansbury recommends the American Heart Association and American Cancer Society as good starting points for nutritional information. Not only does she look and feel better since adopting her improved eating habits, but she also acknowledges the impact it has had on her self-esteem. Now, she feels good about herself, eliminating the guilty feelings she used to have when she overate. She doesn't awaken in the morning feeling sluggish from a huge meal the night before. From these positive experiences with good nutrition, Angela Lansbury has come to realize that it really is worth it to eat right.

Source: Saturday Evening Post, *March 1991, pp. 42 (5).*

■ ■ ■

In the last ten years, nutrition has been emphasized more than ever before. The trend toward a healthful life-style calls for healthful eating and exercise. But what is nutrition? How can you determine the best eating patterns and foods? These issues will be discussed further throughout this chapter so that you will be able to make informed choices.

Food is part of everyday life, whether we are socializing with friends over meals, gathering with family for the holidays, or discussing a business proposition over lunch. Certain foods may even trigger memories, good or bad, of certain events from our childhood. Whatever the association, food is essential to life, and establishing a healthful life-style will improve your quality of life.

Nutrition is the process of taking in and using food for growth, repair, and maintenance of the body. The science of nutrition is the study of foods and how the body uses them. Many North Americans define nutrition as eating a healthful diet. But what is healthful? Our food choices may be influ-

enced by fads, advertising, or convenience. We may reflect on the meaning of nutrition while pushing a cart down a supermarket aisle, or while making a selection from a restaurant menu.

People are becoming more health conscious in their food choices. We are increasingly aware of **nutrients,** those substances needed by the body to maintain life, and the pros and cons of kinds of sugars and sweeteners, dairy products, eggs, and meat. *Cholesterol, fiber, saturated fats, polyunsaturates,* and *carbohydrates* are part of our daily conversations. Mark Twain once stated that, "Part of the secret of success in life is to eat what you like and let the food fight it out inside." We are finding that this philosophy may lead to health risks not addressed in Mark Twain's lifetime.

COMMONSENSE NUTRITION

In the effort to eat nutritiously, many people wonder if they are truly eating a balanced diet or if they have been duped by fads and best-selling diet books. Who are the experts? Whom should you believe? Better yet, how much good information do you already have on foods and diet? As a beginning exercise to determine your own understanding of nutrition at this time you should complete the assessment, In Your Hands: What Is Your Nutrition Quotient?

While some foods are more nutritious than others, no food is by itself good or bad; all foods have some nutritional value. Conversely, there is no such thing as a perfect food. Some foods are a fine source of some nutrients and a poor source of others. For example, most fruits are an excellent source of carbohydrates, but a poor source of protein. High fiber diets, "natural foods," or high carbohydrate diets are all good in some ways and not good in others.

Some of the nutrients the body needs can come only from the foods we eat. These are known as the **essential nutrients.** There are approximately

....

nutrition the process of absorbing and using food substances for growth, repair, and maintenance of the body.

nutrients substances needed by the body to maintain life.

essential nutrients those nutrients a person *must* obtain from food, because the body cannot make them or make enough of them to satisfy its needs.

IN YOUR HANDS

WHAT IS YOUR NUTRITION QUOTIENT?

Your understanding of nutrition, or your nutrition quotient, can serve as a basis for you to improve your knowledge of nutrition. To evaluate your knowledge of nutrition, complete the following self-test:

1. If your carbohydrate intake is greater than your energy needs, the excess is
   a. eliminated
   b. converted to fat and stored
   c. used to build muscle
   d. converted to protein

2. Which of the following food groups contains the greatest amounts of cellulose and other food fiber?
   a. meat and dairy products
   b. whole grain cereals
   c. fruit juices
   d. refined sugars

3. The normal functioning of fiber in the diet
   a. promotes normal operation of the lower intestine
   b. raises the body's calcium levels
   c. increases caloric reserve
   d. lowers blood glucose levels

4. The greatest array of amino acids is found in
   a. animal products
   b. vegetable products
   c. nuts
   d. cereal grains

5. Amino acids that cannot be manufactured by the body are called
   a. essential
   b. nonessential
   c. complete
   d. incomplete

6. Proteins are synthesized from
   a. simple sugars
   b. fatty acids and glycerol
   c. starches
   d. amino acids

7. B complex vitamins
   a. are water soluble
   b. help the clotting of blood
   c. are fat soluble
   d. promote absorption of calcium

8. Niacin
   a. is also known as vitamin C
   b. is found in abundance in meats, poultry, and fish
   c. is fat soluble
   d. is none of the above

9. The vitamin most closely related to calcium utilization is
   a. Vitamin A
   b. Vitamin D
   c. Vitamin K
   d. phosphorus

10. The most reliable food source of chloride is
    a. meats and whole grain cereals
    b. salt
    c. dark green vegetables
    d. public water

Correct Answers: 1-b, 2-b, 3-a, 4-a, 5-a, 6-d, 7-a, 8-b, 9-b, 10-b.

INTERPRETATION

8–10 correct: *excellent*—you have a good understanding of nutrition. 6–7 correct: *good*—you have some incorrect concepts of nutrition, but have good awareness. 5 or less correct: *improvement needed*—you need to increase your nutritional knowledge by studying this chapter carefully.

40 such nutrients known.[1] Other nutrients either come from the foods we eat or can be made by the body itself. Since it's not crucial that we obtain them in our diets, they speak of these as the **nonessential nutrients.** This is not to say that these nutrients are unimportant, just that supplementation in the diet is nonessential.

···

nonessential nutrients nutrients that may come from the foods a person eats, or be made by the body, in sufficient amounts to satisfy its needs.

Some of our nutritional needs are influenced by our genetic makeup. Therefore, what is a healthy diet for one person may not be so healthy for another. For example, persons with high blood pressure might need to cut down on salt consumption; for someone with low or normal blood pressure, high salt consumption does not carry the same risk. High blood pressure is often hereditary; therefore, if your relatives have high blood pressure you may want to stay away from salt as an added precaution.[2]

Following oversimplified dos and don'ts in the foods you eat without understanding them may

In commonsense eating a combination of foods is needed. No food is by itself good or bad. All foods have some nutritional value, yet no one food is nutritionally perfect.

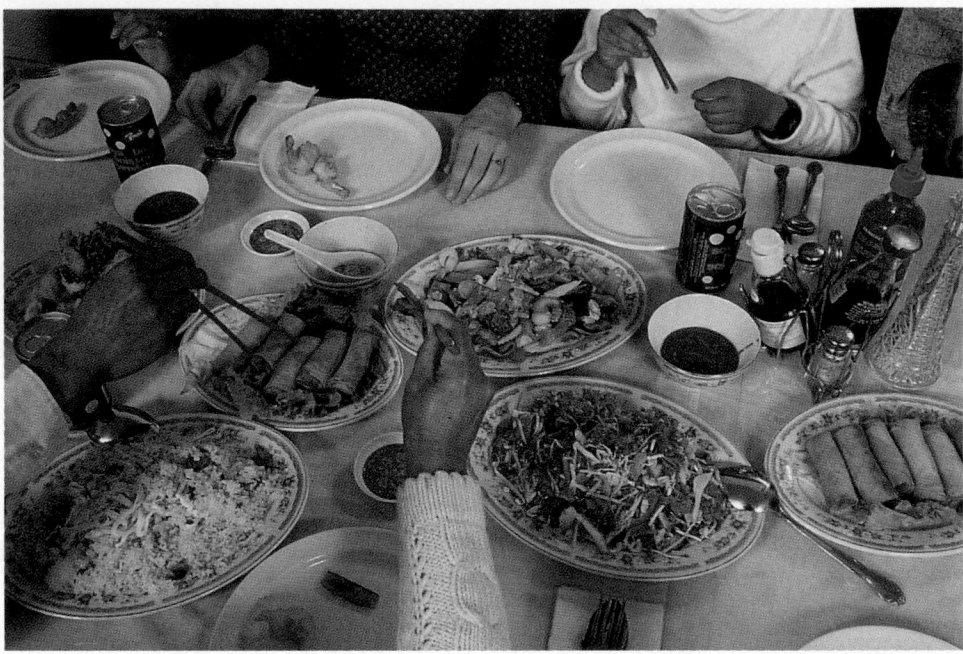

lead to unnecessary fears or dietary abuses. For example, many people believe that "natural," or unprocessed, foods are not harmful, even if consumed in large amounts. The truth is that natural foods may contain potentially harmful substances.[3] By following unproven food practices, you are experimenting on your body.

Proper nutrition allows the body to reach its maximum genetic potential; however, the body can't exceed that potential. Eating well cannot make you bigger, stronger, or healthier than you are genetically capable of being. Proper nutrition can help prevent diseases, but may not be able to cure diseases (except those caused by nutritional deficiency). Nutrition is only one factor that contributes to health and fitness. Other factors include accidents, toxic waste, infectious diseases, and emotional stress. You have limited control over many of these factors, but you have significant control over diet and exercise. Thus, within the limits of your genetic heritage, diet and exercise are the most effective ways to influence your health and fitness.

NUTRITIONAL NEEDS

Food supplies essential nutrients that your body needs for energy and for building and maintaining body tissues. The energy found in carbohydrates, fats, and proteins is measured in **calories,** or units of heat. Calories are such small units and common foods contain so many of them that in order to use smaller numbers, amounts of energy are expressed in 1000-calorie units called **kilocalories** (abbreviated **kcalories,** or **kcal**). But in order to keep terms as simple as possible in this text, the term *calorie* will be used. Whenever the term *calorie* is used it will be referring to a kilocalorie.

The calories in food represent stored energy. To produce energy the body uses ("burns") these calories in a manner similar to the way burning firewood produces light and heat. The body breaks apart complex chemical molecules and puts together new ones. All of these chemical processes in the body are collectively known as **metabolism** (*me-tab'ō-lizm*). Depending on wide differences in life-style and metabolism, adult males use an average of 2000–3000 calories a day and adult females an average of 1400–3000 calories a day.[4] If a person takes in more energy than is expended, regardless

....

calorie a unit of heat; a unit by which energy is measured.

kilocalorie a unit of heat that is the equivalent of 1000 calories.

metabolism the sum of all the chemical reactions that occur in the body.

of the nutrient source of that energy, the result is a weight gain of body fat.

CHECKPOINT

1. What is the risk of following unproven food practices?
2. What are the advantages of proper nutrition?
3. How is energy that is found in carbohydrates, fats, and proteins measured?
4. What term defines all of the chemical processes in the body?
5. Give the range of calories used per day by the adult male and the adult female.

TYPES AND SOURCES OF NUTRIENTS

When we eat food we are impressed by its appearance, taste, and smell. Often we fail to stop and think of its nutrient composition, although people are increasingly interested in the health consequences of what they eat.

There are six major types of nutrients needed by the body:

- carbohydrates
- fats
- proteins
- vitamins
- minerals
- water

Carbohydrates and fats are both the richest energy sources and the ones preferred by the body. One gram of fat yields 9 calories and carbohydrates yield 4 calories per gram. Protein, which yields 4 calories per gram, may serve as an energy source when the other energy sources are limited. A gram is a unit of weight in the metric system.

CARBOHYDRATES

Carbohydrates (*car-bō-hī'drāts*) have a questionable reputation in the minds of some people who

carbohydrate a group of chemical substances, including sugars and starches, that can be used efficiently as an energy source.

mistakenly think they are the "fattening" agent in foods. The basis for such a notion might be that high carbohydrate foods are often eaten with fat, such as the addition of butter to potatoes or bread. Carbohydrate can be used efficiently as an energy source; it is readily available and inexpensive. It is also recommended as a source of more than half of the energy the body needs.[5]

Carbohydrates are found in all foods, but are especially abundant in grains, fruits, and vegetables. These foods may be processed into products such as breads, pastries, pasta, jams, and jellies. Chemically, carbohydrates in food are made up of atoms of the elements carbon, hydrogen, and oxygen, and may vary in combinations from a few to hundreds. Carbohydrates may be classified according to complexity and are divided into two categories: simple and complex. Chemical compounds that contain carbon are referred to as **organic** compounds.

Simple Carbohydrates

The basic unit of all carbohydrates is the sugar called **glucose** (*gloo'kōs*). Often called "blood sugar," glucose is the predominant carbohydrate in the blood. The atoms of glucose may be rearranged to form *fructose* (*fruk'tōs*), which is common in fruits, berries, and honey, or *galactose* (*ga-lak'tōs*), which is not found free in nature. Fructose and galactose are usually converted into glucose by the liver, and glucose is the carbohydrate most commonly used by cells as fuel. Glucose, fructose, and galactose are known collectively as **monosaccharides** (*mon-ō-sak'a-rīdz*), or simple (one-unit) sugars (*mono* means one).

Glucose and fructose together form **sucrose** (*sū'krōs*), which is a **disaccharide** (*dī-sak'a-rīd*), or double (two-unit) sugar (see Figure 9.1, p. 260). Sucrose, also known as table sugar, is found natu-

organic carbon-containing compounds.

glucose a simple sugar sometimes known as blood sugar.

monosaccharide a descriptive term for a single-unit sugar.

sucrose a double sugar known as table sugar.

disaccharide descriptive term for a double sugar.

Figure 9.1
Simple and Complex Carbohydrates

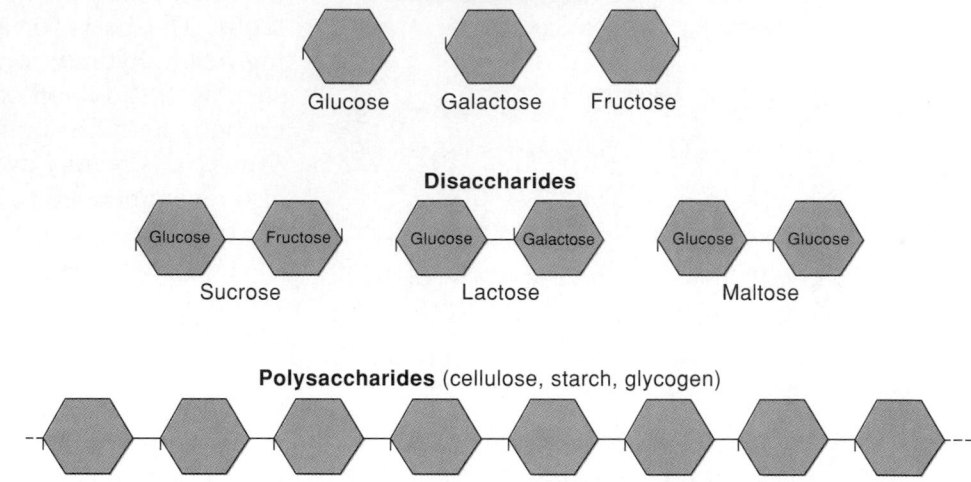

Monosaccharides

Glucose Galactose Fructose

Disaccharides

Glucose—Fructose   Glucose—Galactose   Glucose—Glucose
Sucrose   Lactose   Maltose

Polysaccharides (cellulose, starch, glycogen)

rally in sugar cane, sugar beets, and many fruits and vegetables. Other disaccharides, such as lactose and maltose, are formed from other combinations of simple sugars. Disaccharides must be broken down into monosaccharides before they can be absorbed by the blood. Sucrose can be found in candy, honey, jams, jellies, syrups; lactose in milk and milk products; and maltose in malt and sprouting seeds. Some people are lactose intolerant and must avoid milk and milk products (see Feature 9.1).

Complex Carbohydrates

Known as **polysaccharides** (*pol'ē-sak'a-rīdz*), complex carbohydrates consist of three or more saccharide units and are often long chains. The three most common forms of complex carbohydrates are *starch, glycogen* (*glī-kō-jen*), and *cellulose* (*sel'ū-lōs*).

Starch is the principal form in which plants store energy. Although foods containing starch are not as large a part of the U.S. diet as they once were, they are the most important source of carbohydrates and they supply nutrients such as vitamins and minerals. Starches are abundant in potato tubers, although the largest food sources for starches are grains, such as rice, wheat, corn, millet, rye, barley, and oats. Starch can be found in bread, biscuits, crackers, rolls, dry cereal, pancakes, and pasta.

....

polysaccharide many monosaccharides linked together.

starch a plant polysaccharide composed of many units of saccharide.

Since glucose is the basic carbohydrate unit used by each cell of the body, the body systems must disassemble the disaccharides and polysaccharides and convert them to glucose for absorption by the blood for transport to the cells. Cells may use glucose immediately or convert and store it for future use. If more glucose is delivered than a cell needs, muscles and the liver take up the excess. Some of it is stored as **glycogen,** a so-called animal starch. Muscles claim two-thirds of the stored glycogen, which they use during times of intense exercise. The liver stores one-third of the glycogen and slowly releases it as glucose into the blood, always maintaining a blood glucose concentration near 0.1 percent. Excess glucose beyond what the body is able to store as glycogen is stored as fat.

Cellulose and **pectin** are complex carbohydrates that cannot be broken down (digested) by body enzymes. Cellulose and pectin occur in abundance in fruits, vegetables, and the outer coverings (bran layers) of grain seeds. They both supply **dietary fibers,** which play a major role in provid-

....

glycogen a polysaccharide composed of glucose, made in the body and stored in the liver and in muscles.

cellulose a plant polysaccharide composed of glucose, indigestible by humans.

pectin a plant polysaccharide composed of glucose, indigestible by humans.

dietary fiber a food component that resists chemical digestion and provides bulk to keep material in the digestive tract moving.

FEATURE 9.1

LACTOSE INTOLERANCE

The enzyme lactase, normally present in the body, breaks down the lactose of milk into simple sugars so they can be absorbed by the body. Lactase levels are highest in infants, which is appropriate for their early milk-only diet. Although some infants are born without lactase, many people lose lactase activity to some degree with age. For those with little or no lactase, lactose molecules remain in the intestine undigested, creating diarrhea, bloating, and abdominal discomfort, all symptoms of lactose intolerance. Among North American adults, lactose intolerance occurs among 80 percent of Native Americans, 75 percent of blacks, 50 percent of Hispanics, and 20 percent of Caucasians. The rate of lactose intolerance drops among children from interracial marriages, indicating a genetic basis for the condition.

Although there are people with only a partial lactose intolerance, some affected persons must follow lactose-free diets. This becomes difficult because of the presence of milk in many food and pharmaceutical products. Excluding milk products from the diet can also mean risking deficiencies of calcium and the vitamin riboflavin.

Some affected people can tolerate yogurt, hard cheeses, cottage cheese, and acidophilus milk. Many can use commercially prepared milk products that contain a lactose-destroying enzyme, and some take enzyme tablets.

Lactose intolerance should be diagnosed by a physician in order to rule out any other serious disorder. Lactose intolerance, which is treatable although not curable, should not be treated by a person on his or her own.

Source: Whitney, E., and Rolfes, S. *Understanding Nutrition,* 6th ed. St. Paul, MN: West, 1993.

---

ing bulk to keep material moving in the digestive tract. Some of the fibers are insoluble in water and others soluble. Insoluble fibers absorb water, swell up, and help in the elimination of intestinal wastes. In so doing they help reduce the incidence of constipation, colon cancers, and other colon disorders. Water-soluble fibers tend to be digested by bacteria in the digestive tract that release intestinal gases, which is a side effect of a high fiber diet. While the average U.S. citizen consumes about 11 grams of fiber daily, the National Cancer Institute recommends that adults eat 20–30 grams of fiber per day.[6] Fiber intake can be increased by eating more whole grain breads and cereals, fruits, vegetables, and dried beans and peas.

Artificial Sweeteners

We have been conditioned to expect a degree of sweetness in our foods. The time-honored source for this is sugar. Yet, too high a sugar consumption carries certain risks, and many people seek to avoid sugar or cut down on the amount they use.

There are two kinds of alternative sweeteners people can choose. One kind are the *nutritive sweeteners,* the other, the *artificial sweeteners.*

The nutritive sweeteners are sugar alcohols, and are known by the names of mannitol, sorbital, xylitol, and maltitol. Energy-yielding, the nutritive sweeteners provide as much energy as sugars, but are absorbed by the body more slowly or converted to glucose more slowly. This is especially true in the mouth, where bacteria metabolize them more slowly, leading to fewer dental caries. For these reasons nutritive sweeteners are used in "sugar-free" chewing gums and in some carbonated beverages and canned fruits.

Artificial sweeteners, although providing a sweet taste, provide virtually no energy. These nonnutritive sweeteners carry the names *cyclamate, saccharin,* and *aspartame.* By comparison with sugar, weight for weight, their sweetness far exceeds that of sugar or the sugar alcohols (Table 9.1).[7]

Public acceptance of artificial sweeteners, especially saccharin and cyclamate, in soft drinks and as a tabletop sweetener has been clouded by

Table 9.1
Relative Sweetness of Sugar Alternates

Sweetener	Relative Sweetness[a]
Sorbitol	½
Mannitol	¾
Maltitol	¾
Xylitol	1 (equivalent)
Aspartame	180–200
Acesulfame-K	150–200
Saccharin	300–400

[a] The relative sweetness, compared with sucrose (table sugar), is the standard by which the approximate sweetness of sugar substitutes is compared.

Source: Schlicker S., and Regan C. "Innovations in Reduced-caloric Foods: A Review of Fat and Sugar Replacement Technologies." Topics in Clinical Nutrition 6, 1990, 50–60; Bertorelli, A., and Czarnowski, J. "Review of Present and Future Use of Nonnutritive Sweeteners." The Diabetes Educator 16, 1990, 415–420.

questions about their safety. Lab experiments have suggested that they cause cancerous tumors in humans. In the United States, products containing saccharin are now required to carry the warning label that "use of this product may be hazardous to your health. This product contains saccharin, which has been determined to cause cancer in laboratory animals." Cyclamate use has been banned in the United States since 1970. Aspartame, approved by the FDA in 1981 for use in the United States is known by the brand name NutraSweet in diet drinks, chewing gum, presweetened cereal, gelatines, and puddings, and as the sugar substitute Equal.[8, 9]

FATS

Everyone these days seems to have some awareness of the terms **triglycerides** (*trī-glis'er-īdz*), **cholesterol** (*kō-les'ter-ol*), **fats,** and **oils.** Your physician can advise about fats in your diet. Whether found in butter, salad oil, or cream for your coffee, all of these fats and oils fall under the umbrella term **lipids** (*lip'idz*).

From all the attention fats receive, you might get the idea that they are bad or that we are better off eliminating them from the diet. Like all nutrients, fat is useful in appropriate quantities. It is harmful to eat too much or too little of it. Yet, in the United States people tend to ingest too much fat.

Fats benefit the body in a number of ways. First, fats are a richer source of energy than carbohydrates; fats yield more than twice the number of calories per gram than do carbohydrates.[10] Second, fats are the body's chief way of storing energy; the body can store much more fat than glycogen. When more fat is ingested than the body needs it is stored in *adipose,* or fat cells. If this occurs to excess an individual becomes obese; obesity is one

of the major nutritional problems in the United States today. Stored fat also provides insulation for the body against cold temperatures and provides protective padding.

A third benefit is that fats carry fat-soluble vitamins—A, D, E, and K. Fourth, fats move slowly through the stomach, so they reduce hunger by making us feel full. This explains why we stay satisfied longer after a meal of fried chicken and buttered biscuits than after salad and melba toast. Finally, fat makes food more flavorful and tender; it gives ice cream its smoothness, potato chips their aroma, and butter and cheeses their flavor and texture.

Fats are composed of atoms of carbon, hydrogen, and oxygen, the same elements found in carbohydrates. A fat molecule is known as a triglyceride. A triglyceride consists of a *glycerol* backbone to which three *fatty acids* are attached (Figure 9.2). A fat is identified by the types of fatty acids it contains. Glycerol molecules are all alike, but fatty acids vary in two ways: length of chain and degree of saturation (see the following).

Fatty acids consist of hydrogen (H), and carbon (C) atoms. When the fatty acid is fully loaded with hydrogen atoms, it is *saturated* (Figure 9.2). Saturated fats are more common in palm oil, beef tallow, palm kernel oil, and coconut oil. Look for them in animal sources such as dairy products, and fat from beef, chicken, and pork (Table 9.2). Saturated fats, such as lard, tend to be solid at room temperature.

When hydrogen atoms are removed from a fatty acid it is unsaturated (Figure 9.3, p. 264), and the carbon atoms in the chain form what is called a *double bond*. If only one double bond is present, the fatty acid is *monounsaturated* (Figure 9.3[a]). If two or more double bonds are present, the fatty acid is *polyunsaturated* (Figure 9.3[b]). Unsaturated fats are more commonly vegetable products. However, some plant oils, such as palm and coconut oil, which are common ingredients in processed foods, are more saturated than animal fats.

The more unsaturated a fat is, the more liquid it is at room temperatures. A food manufacturer may want to use an unsaturated oil to make a spreadable (solid) margarine. To do this, the manufacturer would **hydrogenate** an oil. Hydrogen is

---

triglyceride the major class of dietary lipids containing three fatty acids.

cholesterol a fat-derived sterol made in humans and animals and available in the diet.

fat a lipid that is solid at room temperature.

oil a lipid that is liquid at room temperature.

lipid a group of chemical substances, including fats and oils, that contain carbon, hydrogen, and oxygen.

hydrogenate to add hydrogen to an unsaturated fat to make it more solid.

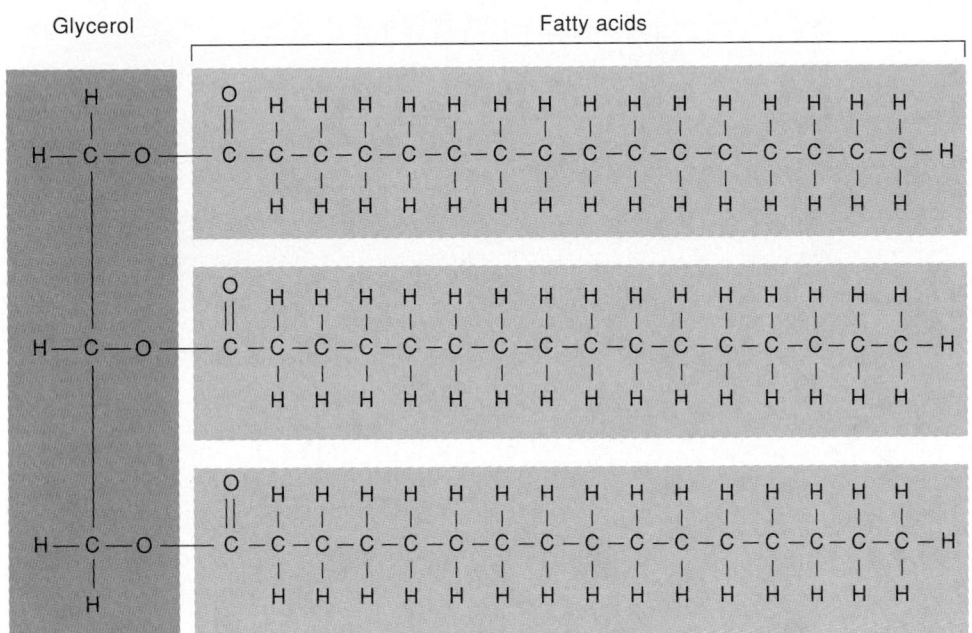

Glycerol   Fatty acids

Figure 9.2
Lipid Molecule

Recipe for a fat (triglyceride): one glycerol, three fatty acids.

forced into the oil and some of the unsaturated fatty acids accept the hydrogen and the oil becomes solid. This process alters the texture of foods. Hydrogenated fats help make puddings creamy and pie crusts flaky. It also reduces the health value of the polyunsaturated oil.

The degree of unsaturation among fatty acids has health implications. Although total fat intake is important, people threatened with heart disease are told to reduce their intake of saturated fats. There is evidence that monounsaturated fats and polyunsaturated fats, and low-fat diets, in general, are all effective in controlling blood lipid concentrations.[11] Yet, with cancers, the type of polyunsaturated fat may make a difference. The polyunsaturated fatty acids occur in two families: the omega-6 family and the omega-3 family (Table 9.2). Cancer patients are now being told to restrict the intake of omega-6 fatty acids, especially linoleic acid.[12, 13] (See Table 9.2.) It is believed that monounsaturated and omega-3 fatty acids do not promote cancer. Omega-3 fatty acids may help prevent cancer by delaying cancer development and reducing the rate of growth and the size and number of tumors. Omega-6 fatty acids are more likely to promote cancer development.[14]

Table 9.2
Lipids

Fatty Acid (kind)	Higher Amounts Found In	Common Food Sources
Triglycerides (e.g., fats and oils)		
Saturated (stearic)	Lard, coconut oil, palm	Meat and
	Oils: palm, coconut, palm kernel	dairy products
Unsaturated		
Monounsaturated (oleic)	*Oils:* olive, canola	Avocados, peanuts, nuts in general, olives
Polyunsaturated		
omega-3 (linoleic, arachadonic)	*Oils:* corn, safflower, soybean, cottonseed, sunflower, sesame	Vegetable oils
omega-6 (linolenic)	*Oils:* soybean, canola	Fish, seafoods
Phospholipids (e.g., lecithins)		
Sterols (e.g., cholesterol, testosterone)		

Source: Whitney, E., and Rolfes, S., Understanding Nutrition, 6th ed. Minneapolis: West, 1993.

Figure 9.3
Unsaturated Fatty Acids

(a) Monounsaturated Fatty Acid

Oleic Acid (an 18-carbon fatty acid)
Because it has one point of unsaturation, oleic acid is monounsaturated.

(b) Polyunsaturated Fatty Acid
Linoleic Acid (an 18-carbon fatty acid)
The two points of unsaturation in linoleic acid make it polyunsaturated. Linoleic acid is one of the essential fatty acids.

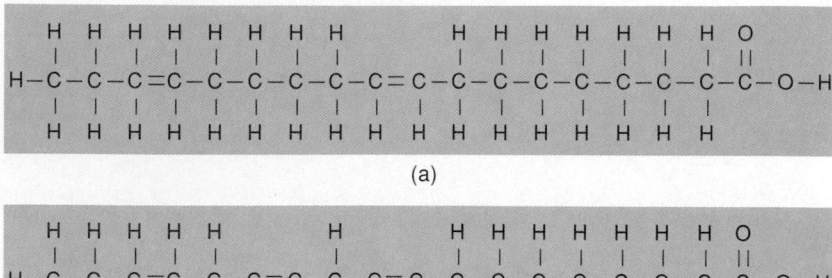

Phospholipids

Similar to the triglycerides, *phospholipids* have only two fatty acids in each fat molecule. In place of the third fatty acid is a phosphate group, which is why they are known as phospholipids. One of the best known phospholipids is lecithin. Made by the body, lecithins are a major constituent of cell membranes. Because they are produced naturally by the body (thus are nonessential), they are not needed as supplements to the diet.

Sterols

The *sterols,* unlike the triglycerides and phospholipids, have a large complex structure (with which we refuse to bore you). Yet the significance of one of the sterols, called cholesterol, is anything but boring.

Cholesterol

Cholesterol is a substance that comes from fat, but is more complex. An important compound in the body, cholesterol is a part of every cell. Cholesterol is the starting material from which sex hormones are made and is essential in the formation of liver bile (which helps in digestion), cell membranes, and nerve fiber coverings. Cholesterol can be made in the body as well as obtained through eating foods of animal origin, such as red meats, fish, milk, and eggs. Elevated blood cholesterol levels are known to be responsible for an increased incidence of coronary heart disease (CHD).[15] (See Feature 9.2.)

FEATURE 9.2

THE CHOLESTEROL RIDDLE

No other nutritional topic has received more attention in the media than the role of cholesterol and fats in causing disease. Cholesterol is important. Many health-conscious persons recognize high levels of cholesterol as the result of overeating and underexercising. It is known to be a primary risk factor for CHD, which causes 1.5 million heart attacks and 550,000 deaths in the United States each year.

Depending on level and type, cholesterol may be either friend or foe. Cholesterol is an essential substance that plays a central role in building cell membranes and sex hormones, and it aids in digestion. Cholesterol in the bloodstream comes from two sources: a person's diet and natural production of the body's cells. Dietary cholesterol comes from foods containing saturated fats and pure cholesterol, such as butter, cheese, liver, eggs, and animal fat. In the body, cholesterol is manufactured mainly in the liver.

Problems begin with the way cholesterol travels through the body. In the liver, cholesterol, along with dietary fats known as triglycerides, is loaded onto carrier particles called very low density lipoproteins (VLDLs) for transport through the bloodstream. Triglycerides are used for energy and stored for future use. As triglycerides are released into body tissues the VLDL carriers are transformed into low density lipoprotein (LDL) carriers. LDLs deliver the cholesterol to the cells. Another carrier particle, the high density lipoprotein (HDL), or "good" cholesterol, acts to pick up excess cholesterol in the bloodstream and carry it back to the liver where it is converted into bile acid and eliminated.

Dietary indulgence can upset this delicate balance. The problem is with excess LDLs, which circulate freely in the bloodstream. LDLs are called "bad" cholesterol because any excess of cholesterol carried by them can trigger the buildup of **plaque** on the interior walls of coronary arteries, a condition known as **atherosclerosis.** Eventually these plaques can narrow the artery, allowing a clot to form and block the blood flow; this blockage is one of the causes of heart attack.

The lower the amount of LDLs in the bloodstream, the lower the risk of coronary heart disease. But scientists also know that too little HDL may be as important a factor as too much LDL. The higher level of HDL the more it can counteract the effects of bad cholesterol. In fact, low levels of HDL can result in heart disease even if a person's total cholesterol is within the safe range below 200 milligrams per deciliter (mg/dl) of blood.[a]

The National Heart, Lung, and Blood Institute has concluded that those individuals with a total cholesterol count of between 200 and 239 mg/dl are borderline high risk, and anyone with a count of 240 or more may be at high risk. The Institute suggests that a person should not have an LDL count higher than 130. Levels of HDLs in the 70s and 80s are believed to be protective against heart disease; but HDL levels below 35 place a person at risk of CHD, even though total cholesterol readings are in the safe zone. The best indicator of coronary risk is the ratio of total cholesterol to HDL. For example, an overall reading of 200 and an HDL of 50 gives a ratio of 4. A ratio of 4.5 or higher is typical of people who develop CHD.[b]

Strategies for increasing HDLs and lowering overall cholesterol include diet and exercise. The recommendation is for less total fat, less saturated fat, and control of obesity. Most reports also recommend a lowering of dietary cholesterol and replacement of saturated fat with polyunsaturated fat. While polyunsaturates lower both HDL and LDL, those high in monounsaturates are better replacements for saturated fats such as bacon fat and lard than are the polyunsaturates such as corn and safflower oil. Bran is believed to draw LDLs out of blood circulation while sparing the HDLs. Excess weight, a sedentary life-style, and smoking are other risk factors that raise cholesterol levels in the body. For additional factors affecting vascular health, the American Heart Association has published the following guidelines for reducing heart disease.[c]

TO CONTROL THE AMOUNT AND KIND OF FAT YOU EAT

- Limit your intake of meat, seafood, and poultry to no more than 5–7 ounces per day.
- Eat chicken or turkey (without skin) or fish in most of your main meals.
- Choose lean cuts of meat, trim all the fat you can see, and throw away the fat that cooks out of the meat.
- Substitute meatless or "low-meat" main dishes for regular entrees.
- Eat no more than a total of 5–8 teaspoons of fats and oils per day for cooking, baking, and salads.
- Eat only low-fat dairy products.

TO CONTROL YOUR INTAKE OF CHOLESTEROL-RICH FOODS

- Use no more than two egg yolks a week, including those used in cooking.
- Limit your consumption of shrimp, lobster, sardines, and organ meats.

[a]Dolan, B., and Nash, M. "Searching for Life's Elixir." *Time,* 12 December 1988, 62–66.

[b]U.S. Department of Health and Human Services, *The Surgeon General's Report on Nutrition and Health, 1988.* DHHS (PHS), Publication No. 88-50210. Washington, DC: U.S. Government Printing Office.

[c]The American Heart Association Diet, *An Eating Plan for Healthy Americans.* Dallas, TX: The American Heart Association, 1985.

Lipoproteins

Lipoproteins (*lip'ō-prō'tenz*), as the name implies, are complexes of lipids and proteins. The more protein in the lipoprotein the higher its density. The several types of lipoproteins have different functions, but all are transport vehicles for the pick up and delivery of lipids to and from cells. The three classes of lipoproteins are the low-density lipoproteins (LDLs), high density lipoproteins (HDLs), and very low density lipoproteins (VLDLs). HDLs consist of about 50 percent lipids, LDLs are about 75 percent lipids, and VLDLs contain about 80 percent lipids. HDLs and LDLs carry most of the cholesterol in the blood. High LDL levels are associated with a high risk of heart attacks, and high HDL levels with a low risk.[16]

Fat Substitutes

Since 1960, food chemists have been working on artificial fats, or so-called *fat substitutes.* One such fat substitute is olestra, a synthetic combination of sucrose and fatty acids. Yet, unlike either substance by itself, olestra is indigestible. It passes through the intestine without being absorbed. In addition, olestra interferes with the body's absorption of

---

plaque a deposit of fatty substances in the inner lining of the artery wall.

atherosclerosis a blood vessel disease in which the inner layers of artery walls become thick and irregular due to deposits of fat and cholesterol.

lipoprotein a cluster of lipids associated with a protein.

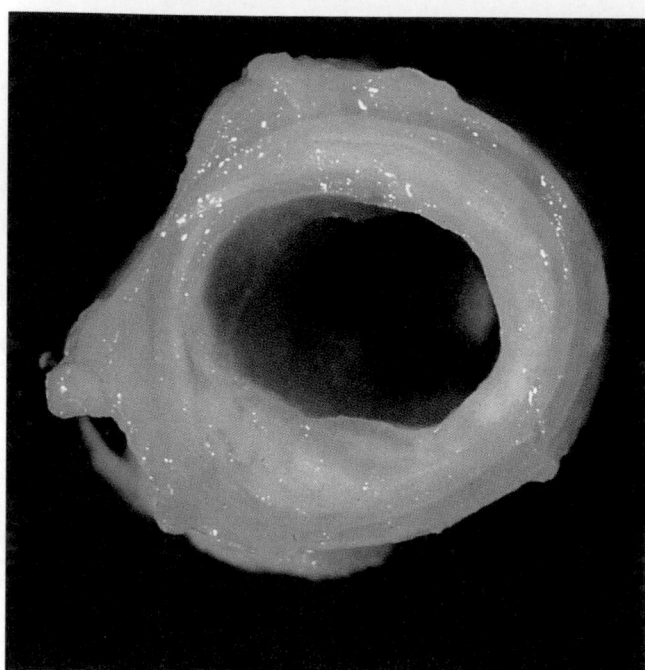

Plaque, which is a depositing of fatty substances and cholesterol, may build up in the inner lining of an artery. Affecting large and medium size arteries, plaque buildup may eventually partially or totally block the flow of blood. Known as atherosclerosis, such a slow and progressive buildup may lead to heart attack or stroke.

both dietary and natural cholesterol. Olestra resembles fats in taste and in cooking properties, yet it adds no energy and does not raise blood lipid concentrations. Vitamin E absorption may be interfered with by olestra, but Vitamin E can be supplemented when necessary.[17]

Another fat substitute is Simplesse. Unlike olestra, Simplesse is made of protein and is digested by the body and absorbed, adding to energy intake. Yet, its calorie content is far less than from a similar amount of fat.[18]

CHECKPOINT

1. Give the name of a simple sugar that is classified as a monosaccharide and one that is classified as a disaccharide.

2. Name the four most common forms of complex carbohydrates.

3. What is the difference between a saturated fatty acid and an unsaturated one?

4. Distinguish between a low-density lipoprotein and a high-density one.

PROTEINS

Proteins are extraordinary and versatile substances. The body uses them in more ways than it does any other nutrient. There are an estimated 50,000 different kinds of protein in the body. Protein is the most abundant substance in the body next to water.

All protein molecules have certain features in common. They contain atoms of the four common elements: carbon, hydrogen, oxygen, and nitrogen, and are put together to form a basic unit called an **amino** (*a-mēn'o*) **acid.** There are 20 different amino acids in the body important to human nutrition; the body produces 11 of them (nonessential) and receives 9 only from the protein in food (essential).

It takes hundreds of amino acid units strung together like beads to make a single protein molecule. Anywhere from several dozen to as many as 300 amino acid units assembled from the 20 different amino acids in the body allow an almost limitless number of combinations. Proteins take on dramatically different shapes, such as rods, spirals, and balls.

The proteins produced in the body get their amino acid building blocks principally from the digestion of dietary proteins. The *hydrolysis,* or breakdown, of dietary protein begins in the stomach and is completed in the intestine. The final products of protein digestion, the amino acids, are carried away from the intestine by the blood to the cells of the body where they are reformed into proteins.

Role of Amino Acids

Besides serving as units of proteins, amino acids have many individual roles in the body. They serve as a source of energy, especially when other energy sources are limited.

Role of Proteins

Proteins carry on important tasks. Proteins serve as **enzymes,** or organic catalysts, that facilitate the

···

protein a compound composed of carbon, hydrogen, oxygen, and nitrogen arranged as a strand of amino acids.

amino acid a building block of protein.

enzyme a protein catalyst that speeds up the rate of a reaction without becoming a part of the process.

breakdown of food substances in digestion, the building of new substances, and the transformation of one body substance into another. Proteins are especially important in building new tissue rapidly, such as during pregnancy and infancy. Beyond this, proteins in red blood cells transport materials and maintain fluid balance. They form clots that help to close wounds, mend damaged tissue, and reinforce tendons, ligaments, and blood vessel walls.

Those dietary proteins that contain all the essential amino acids, and in the same amounts the body requires, are defined as **complete proteins.** Most of the proteins derived from animal foods (meat, fish, poultry, eggs, and milk) are quite complete. Those derived from some plant foods (rice, potatoes) may be complete, however many are **incomplete proteins,** or lack one or more of the essential amino acids in sufficient amount.

Protein quality is measured not only in completeness of amino acids, but also in digestibility and absorbability. For a protein to be of the highest quality, sufficient numbers of a protein's amino acids must reach the body cells to allow the cells to make the proteins they need. **Biological value (BV)** is the measurement of such quality. One of the finest proteins available, by these standards, is egg protein. It has been assigned a top biological value by the Food and Agriculture Organization (FAO) of the United Nations, which sets world standards.[19]

People whose diets lack one or more essential amino acids may suffer one or more consequences. The highly publicized protein deficiency **kwashiorkor** (*kwash-i-or'kor*), often found in developing countries, develops when infants weaned from breastfeeding are not provided with a protein supply similar to that found in human milk. The child will fail to grow and put on weight, muscles waste away, and anemia, diarrhea, and vomiting occur.

The child becomes weak, apathetic, and vulnerable to all sorts of infections and diseases. When calories and protein are both inadequate in a diet, **marasmus** (*mar-az'mus*), an energy-protein malnutrition occurs. Since the protein eaten is not sufficient for both energy and protein needs of the body, death from malnutrition and infections is virtually certain.

A person whose carbohydrate and fat intake is inadequate to meet the body's energy needs will turn to dietary and body protein to supply energy. The body's need for energy takes priority over its need for amino acids to build protein. Over time, breakdown of protein to meet energy needs will lead to muscle wasting. If a person consumes more protein than needed for body nutrition, the amino acids are converted to fat and stored; thus, valuable, expensive, protein-rich foods can add to obesity.

Vegetarians and Protein

People who prefer plant food products to animal products—**vegetarians**—have the same nutritional needs as any one else. Some vegetarians omit only meat, fish, and poultry from their diets; some also exclude eggs, but use milk. Others, called **vegans,** exclude foods that come from animals in any form. Meats, milk, and eggs provide the highest quality protein available, and anyone eating them will not experience protein deficiency. Plants offer less protein per unit (by weight or measure) of food than animal protein. Those who eat an all-plant diet should give consideration to their protein intake.

Vegans need to learn how to combine plant proteins to make up for any missing proteins. Called *mutual supplementing,* the idea is to match two foods so as to provide for essential amino acids missing in either one. The two proteins chosen are called *complementary proteins.* Examples of such combinations would be black beans and rice, peanut butter and wheat bread, tofu and stir-

complete protein a protein containing all of the essential amino acids in proper balance.

incomplete protein a protein lacking one or more of the essential amino acids.

biological value (BV) the measurement of a protein's efficiency in supporting the body's needs.

kwashiorkor a disease, usually found in children, resulting from protein deficiency.

marasmus a disease resulting from a caloric-protein deficiency, most often in young children.

vegetarian a general term for a person who prefers plant food products to animal products.

vegan a person who excludes all animal-derived food from his or her diet; pure, or total, vegetarian.

fried vegetables. Vegetarians who eat some foods from animal sources can enrich protein quality by using combinations such as cereal with milk, vegetable omelettes, and eggplant Parmesan.

VITAMINS

Vitamins, like energy-yielding nutrients, are organic compounds. Vital to life, vitamins are available in foods. Vitamins differ from carbohydrates, fats, and proteins in that they are much smaller, they act singly rather than being strung together to make larger compounds, and do not provide energy when broken down. They help with energy production, help cells multiply for growth and healing, and are commonly available in foods in amounts ranging from a few micrograms to many milligrams per day. Dietary deficiency diseases result if vitamins are absent or inadequate in the diet. Only those chemical compounds shown to be necessary to the diet and whose absence will lead to a deficiency disease are called vitamins.

The first vitamins were discovered in 1912 and were identified by letters of the alphabet (A, B, C, D); the recent trend has been to name them according to their chemical identification. Vitamins are classified into two categories: *water soluble,* capable of being dissolved in water, and *fat soluble,* capable of being dissolved in fat (see Tables 9.3 and 9.4).

Water-soluble vitamins (B-complex, C, folacin, biotin, and pantothenic acid) are widely found in foods. They work together with enzymes, which we have already identified as proteins that govern metabolism. In this capacity they are called **coenzymes** (*kō-en´zīmz*). Because water-soluble vitamins are not stored by the body they need to be consumed daily. The body eliminates any excess vitamins through urine. Water-soluble vitamins are vulnerable to heat and are often broken down in cooking or processing. When fresh vegetables and fruit are overcooked or soaked for too long, many of their water-soluble vitamins may be lost.

vitamins organic compounds vital to body function.

water-soluble vitamins vitamins soluble in water.

coenzymes compounds that work with enzymes to promote the work of the enzyme; some vitamins are coenzymes.

The **fat-soluble vitamins** (A, D, E, K) are absorbed into the body with fats. Excessive amounts of these vitamins, especially vitamins A and D, can be stored in fat, or adipose, cells. Unlike water-soluble vitamins, fat-soluble vitamins are not coenzymes; they operate independently. Vitamin A can be obtained pre-formed in animal food; in plant sources it is available as beta-carotene, which produces vitamin A. Because fat-soluble vitamins are stored, it is possible to consume too much and reach toxic levels.

Vitamin Supplements

Vitamin supplements are those vitamins a person takes, often as pills, beyond those eaten in a normal balanced diet. In a recent survey of adults, two-thirds of those surveyed used some form of food supplement.[20] The most commonly taken are multivitamins and Vitamin C.

Some contend that recommendations for the taking of vitamin and mineral supplements are not warranted. They insist that vitamin supplements represent an unnecessary cost if you are eating a balanced diet. Taking supplements might, in fact, induce a person to eat carelessly on the excuse that in any event they are protected nutritionally. The use of vitamin supplements may even be dangerous. The **toxic,** or poisonous, risks of excessive use of fat-soluble vitamins, especially A and D, are widely known; even some of the water-soluble vitamins, such as Vitamin B$_6$, have a potential for toxicity.[21]

Some people do demonstrate marginal vitamin deficiencies, along with protein and mineral deficiencies. Although the incidence of such people is thought to be low, for them vitamin supplements are useful. Such people may include habitual dieters, ill people with little or no appetite, people with illnesses that impair nutrient absorption, vegetarians, women whose menstrual discharge is excessive, and women who are pregnant or lactating.[22] For most vitamin-deficient persons, a multivitamin-mineral supplement supplying the RDA would be adequate.

If a person needs vitamin-mineral supplements, the first step is to be certain the person's diet is

fat-soluble vitamins vitamins soluble in and absorbed into the body in fats.

toxic pertaining to or caused by a poison.

Table 9.3
Water-soluble Vitamins

Vitamin	Functions	Important Sources	Adult RDAs	Prolonged Deficiency Syndrome	Toxic Effects of Megadosages
Thiamin (B₁)	Helps convert carbohydrates, fats, and proteins to energy	Liver, pork, oysters; whole grain breads and cereals; enriched cereals and bread; peas, nuts	1.1–1.5 mg	Moderate: depression, fatigue, constipation, muscle cramps. Severe: beri-beri (nerve damage, paralysis, heart failure)	None presently known
Riboflavin (B₂)	Helps convert all fuel foods to energy; cell division; red blood cell formation	Liver, meat; dairy products; eggs; dark green vegetables; whole grain breads and cereals; nuts; produced in human intestines	1.3–1.7 mg	Sore mouth, tongue, throat; dry, cracking skin; anemia, depression; personality shifts	None presently known
Niacin (nicotinic acid)	Release of energy from all fuel foods; protein and fat synthesis	Liver, poultry, meat; eggs, whole grain bread, and cereals; nuts and legumes (peas, beans)	15–19 mg	Pellegra (seen as rash, diarrhea, sleeplessness, confusion, and death)	Irritated stomach lining, diabetes, loss of liver function, jaundice; flushing of face, neck, and hands
Pyridoxine (B₆)	Release of energy from fuel foods; regulates nervous system activity; regenerates red blood cells; produces antibodies	High protein foods in general; bananas; some vegetables; whole grain cereals and breads; liver; green vegetables; fish, meat, poultry, nuts	1.6–2.0 mg	Moderate: rash, mouth lesions Severe: nausea, vomiting, anemia, confusion, severe nervous disturbances	Nerve damage; depending on megadose, numbness, tingling in extremities, difficulty walking, poor coordination
Cobalamin (B₁₂)	Helps produce red blood cells; growth and function of nervous system	Liver, kidney, meat, fish; eggs, dairy products; yeast	2.0 mcg	Moderate: fatigue, weakness, weight loss, tingling in extremities; sore tongue. Severe: low immune response; paralysis; possibly fatal anemia	None presently known
Folacin (folic acid)	Helps produce nucleic acids; aids cell division; formation of red blood cells; fetal development	Liver; dark green vegetables; wheat germ; legumes; oranges, orange juice; fish; poultry, eggs	180–200 mcg	Anemia; mouth and throat sores; rheumatoid arthritis; infections; toxemia in pregnancy; often deficient in alcoholics	Convulsions in some epileptics
Biotin	Helps release energy from fuel foods	Eggs; liver; dark green vegetables; widely found in foods	30–100 mcg	Rash; sore tongue; muscular pain; sleeplessness; nausea; loss of appetite; fatigue; depression	None presently known
Pantothenic acid	Release of energy; helps form cholesterol	Liver; whole grain cereals and breads; widely found in plant and animal foods	4–7 mg	None known in humans on natural diet	Diarrhea and water retention
Ascorbic acid (C)	An antioxidant; promotes healing and fights infection; required for forming connective tissue; increases iron absorption	Citrus fruits; melons; tomatoes; strawberries; potatoes; dark green vegetables	60 mg	Moderate: restlessness; swollen or bleeding gums; bruises; painful joints; energy loss; anemia. Severe: scurvy (bleeding gums, poor wound healing, loose teeth, poor skin, irritability)	Diarrhea, bloating, abdominal pain, nausea, vomiting, kidney stones, loss of red blood cells, bone marrow changes

mcg = micrograms; mg = milligrams

Source: Adapted from the Food and Nutrition Board, National Academy of Sciences–National Research Council, Recommended Dietary Allowances, revised 1989.

Table 9.4
Fat-soluble Vitamins

Vitamins	Functions	Important Sources	Adult RDAs	Prolonged Deficiency Syndrome	Toxic Effects of Megadoses
A	Normal (especially night) vision; formation of cells, particularly skin; aids in resistance to infections	Fat-containing and fortified dairy products; liver; leafy dark green and yellow vegetables	800–1000 RE	Poor night vision, blindness; dry skin, eyes	Blurred vision; headaches; nausea; roughened skin; diarrhea; depression; spontaneous abortions and birth defects in pregnant women
D	Promotes absorption and use of calcium and phosphorus; bone growth; neuromuscular activity	Fortified milk; liver, cod liver; fish; egg yolk; formed in skin upon exposure to sunlight	5–10	Children: deformed bones (ricketts). Adults: softened (osteomalacia); brittle bones (osteoporosis)	Children: poor appetite; retarded growth; deformed bones. Adults: headaches; vomiting; diarrhea; weight loss; muscular weakness
E	Antioxidant to prevent cell membrane damage; helps form and protect red blood cells, muscles, and other tissue	Vegetables and fish oils; liver; whole grains breads and cereals; nuts and seeds	8–10 αTE	Rare in healthy children and adults; possible anemia; possible muscle loss	Reduced vitamin A storage; possible blood disorders in anemic children
K	Helps blood clot; promotes bone formation	Green leafy vegetables; other vegetables (peas, cabbage, cauliflower); produced in human intestine	65–80 mcg	Impaired blood clotting and bone formation, especially in some newborns; hemorrhaging; bruising	Rare, since not available in over-the-counter supplements; loss of red blood cells; jaundice; risk of brain damage

RE = retinal equivalents; mcg = micrograms; αTE = alpha tocopherol equivalents

Source: Adapted from the Food and Nutrition Board, National Academy of Sciences—National Research Council, Recommended Dietary Allowances, revised 1989

well balanced and adequate. Then, when purchasing a supplement, choose one that provides all the RDA nutrients in amounts below or very close to the RDA. Avoid taking concentrations above the RDA, called **megadosing,** unless recommended by a physician.[23] Also avoid products with high potency claims, preparations with items not needed in human nutrition, geriatric "tonics" that contain alcohol (unless prescribed by a physician), and "organic" or "natural" preparations that are no better or more effective than standard pharmacy preparations. The best counsel is to take vitamin supplements only on the recommendation of your physician.

megadosing taking concentrations above those recommended by the RDA.

MINERALS

Minerals are inorganic substances that make up nearly 5 percent of the body. Minerals function primarily as structural components of teeth, muscles, blood cells, and bones, but may also work together with enzymes in controlling metabolic reactions. They are essential to muscle contraction, blood clotting, protein synthesis, and cell membrane permeability. There are about 21 minerals that are seen as being critical to human health. Since the body is unable to produce any minerals on its own, it must obtain minerals from foods. Many minerals are water-soluble and are readily excreted in the urine.

mineral a naturally occurring inorganic substance.

Minerals are divided into two categories: **macrominerals** and **trace minerals.** The body needs macrominerals, which include calcium, phosphorus, potassium, sulfur, sodium, chlorine, and magnesium, in fairly large amounts (*macro* means large). Trace minerals, which include iron, manganese, copper, iodine, cobalt, zinc, and fluorine, are equally important but are needed in smaller, "trace" amounts. Tables 9.5 (p. 272) and 9.6 (p. 273) list these two categories of minerals and their functions, sources, and recommended dosages.

Several of the minerals combine chemically with other minerals to form salts, which when dissolved in fluids, have the capacity to carry electrical charges. Minerals with this capacity are called **electrolytes,** and include sodium, calcium, potassium, and chlorine. These substances are able to maintain the balance of fluids in the body, control acid-base balance in these fluids, and play an important role in transmitting nerve impulses and contracting muscles, especially the heart. The kidneys are able to excrete and reabsorb electrolytes as needed to maintain the proper level of these electrolytes in the body.

Sodium

Sodium is the major factor in maintaining proper blood–fluid balance in the body. Yet as important as sodium is, the body requires relatively little. The National Academy of Sciences recommends a daily intake of 500 milligrams (mg), but with a daily limit of less than 6 grams (the equivalent of 2400 mg sodium). One teaspoon (tsp) of salt contains nearly 2000 mg of sodium.[24]

Much of our sodium intake is consumed in the form of table salt (sodium chloride). About 40 percent of table salt is sodium. Its estimated that men in the United States consume an average of 3300 mg of sodium a day (1⅔ tsp of salt).[25] The bulk of the sodium in the U.S. diet comes from processed foods. About 75 percent of the sodium in the U.S.

....

macrominerals minerals needed by the body in fairly large amounts.

trace minerals minerals needed by the body in minute amounts.

electrolytes ionized salts in blood, tissue fluid, and cells.

diet comes from salt added in food processing; about 15 percent comes from salt added during cooking and while eating; and only 10 percent comes from the natural content of foods.[26] The level of salt concentration in the blood is maintained by the kidneys and other body organs. Most people excrete the excess sodium in urine. Some people, perhaps with a genetic predisposition, are salt sensitive and cannot handle the excess this way. Instead it is drawn into the circulation, causing the blood to retain liquids, adding to the volume of blood to be pumped. The result is **hypertension,** or sustained high blood pressure.[27] Hypertension is of wide concern due to its relationship to coronary heart disease, heart failure, and kidney disease.

Research is inconclusive regarding the overall effects of sodium. While we eat more salt than we need, little evidence exists that shows that the excess is bad for all of us. Except for those who already have high blood pressure, changes in salt intake may not result in changes in blood pressure. People are urged to monitor their blood pressure and, if it is high, seek help in lowering it. For those who want, or are medically advised to lower their sodium intake, the easiest route is through reduced table salt intake.

Calcium

Calcium is the most abundant mineral in the body and is essential in the formation of bones and teeth. Almost all of this calcium (about 99 percent) is in the bones and teeth. There is a continuing exchange of minerals and nutrients between bone tissues and body fluids all during life. When there is a dietary surplus of calcium, some is stored in bones. When supply is low, calcium is released from this storehouse.[28] The other 1 percent of the body's calcium is found in solutions in the blood and body fluids. Here calcium helps in the clotting of blood, nerve transmission, heartbeat, and muscle functions.

People of all ages need calcium and its companion mineral, phosphorus, in their diets. The demand is especially critical in children and pregnant women. But contrary to some opinion, the body's need for calcium does not lessen with age.

....

hypertension sustained high blood pressure.

Table 9.5
Macrominerals

Mineral	Functions	Important Sources	Adult RDAs	Prolonged Deficiency Symptoms	Toxic Effects of Megadosages
Calcium (Ca)	Bone and tooth formation; essential to blood clotting and membrane structure; fluid balance; nerve impulses; muscle contraction; enzyme activation	Dairy products; cheeses; liver; fish; egg yolk; green leafy vegetables; cereals; molasses; soybeans	800–1200 mg	Muscle cramps, pain, spasms; tingling sensations and stiffness in hands and feet; deformed bones in children; osteoporosis in adults	Loss of appetite; nausea; vomiting; constipation; loss of weight; fever; weakness
Phosphorus (P)	Bone and tooth formation; acid-base balance; energy release; fat transport; synthesis of enzymes, proteins, nucleic acids (DNA/RNA)	Liver; meats; dairy products; fish; egg yolk; legumes; dried fruit; nuts	800–1200 mg	Loss of appetite; weakness; demineralization of bone and loss of calcium; bone pain	Reduced levels of calcium in blood; reduced bone-building capacity
Potassium (K)	Works with sodium to regulate blood pressure, transmit nerve impulses, regulate heart function; protein and carbohydrate metabolism	Meats; fish, poultry; potatoes; bananas; apricots; legumes; peanut butter; nuts; cocoa; molasses; cereals	2000 mg	Vomiting and diarrhea; loss of appetite; irregular heartbeat; weakened pulse; lowered blood pressure	Weakened muscles; abnormal heart rhythm; kidney disorders
Sulfur (S)	Blood clotting; detoxification of body fluids; collagen synthesis	Protein foods (meat, dairy products, eggs, legumes)	Not established	Not clearly established	No toxic effects established
Sodium (Na)	Regulation of blood pressure; nerve impulse transmission; acid-base balance; formation of digestive secretions	Table salt; cured meats; cheese; sauerkraut; salted nuts	500 mg	Loss of appetite; thirst; vomiting; muscle cramps. Extreme cases: convulsions; coma	Dehydration; higher body temperature; vomiting; depression
Chloride (Cl)	With sodium and potassium, transmits nerve impulses; acid-base balance; helps blood cells transport carbon dioxide	Table salts; cured meats; cheese	750 mg	Vomiting; diarrhea; sweating; alkalinity of body fluids	No toxic effects established
Magnesium (Mg)	Energy production; regulates heart function; activates enzyme system; release of energy	Leafy green vegetables; whole grains; soybeans; nuts; molasses; animal proteins; milk	280–350 mg	Muscle pain, tremors, spasms; vertigo; convulsions; altered heart rhythm; apathy; depression	Depressed respiration and central nervous system function

Source: Adapted from the Food and Nutrition Board, National Academy of Sciences—National Research Council, Recommended Dietary Allowances, revised 1989.

Table 9.6
Trace Minerals

Mineral	Functions	Important Sources	Adult RDAs	Prolonged Deficiency Symptoms	Toxic Effects of Megadosages
Iron (Fe)	Oxygen and carbon dioxide transport; red blood cell formation	Liver; heart; shellfish; beans and peas; vegetables	10–15 mg	Iron-deficiency anemia	Liver damage
Manganese (Mn)	Nerve action, muscle action; bone and connective tissue formation	Meat; fruits; vegetables; whole grains and cereals	2.0–5.0 mg	No specific description	No specific description
Copper (Cu)	Hemoglobin synthesis; energy release of fats and carbohydrates; bone formation	Meat, liver; shellfish; whole grain cereals	1.5–3 mg	Occurs along with kwashiorkor and cystic fibrosis	Ingestion of large amounts toxic to humans
Iodine (I)	Thyroid regulation of metabolism; synthesis of Vitamin A	Iodized table salt; shellfish; green vegetables	150 mcg	Cretinism (stunted growth); goiter (thyroid gland enlargement)	Hypothyroidism (toxic goiter)
Cobalt (Co)	Part of Vitamin B$_{12}$ molecule	Shellfish; nuts	Not established	No specific description	No specific description
Zinc (Zn)	Promotes healing and growth; immune functions	Meat; shellfish; whole grain cereals; nuts	12–15 mg	Impaired wound healing; decreased sense of taste and smell	Ingestion of large amounts is toxic to humans
Fluorine (F)	Tooth and bone formation	Drinking water	1.5–4.0 mg	Tooth decay	Mottled stains on teeth

The recommended intake of calcium for adults is 800 mg daily. Unfortunately, the average American intake is only 450–550 mg daily.[29]

Body calcium is increased by eating more dairy products, bean and pea seeds, fish, dark leafy vegetables, dates, raisins, and grain products.

Osteoporosis Osteoporosis (*os'tē-ō-por-ō'sis*) is a condition in which bones become weakened due to calcium loss. Experienced almost universally with aging, it is more common in women, especially after menopause, since osteoporosis is known to be hormonally and genetically related. The bones of women are not as dense as those of men, and their drop in estrogen production following menopause leads to the formation of less

....

osteoporosis increased porosity of bone resulting from excessive calcium loss, seen most often in elderly women.

new bone. Osteoporosis affects whites more often than blacks, and can also occur in young female runners, ballet dancers, male marathoners whose calorie intake is inadequate, teenagers on junk food diets, and young women suffering from eating disorders.[30] Over 1 million fractures attributable to osteoporosis occur yearly in people over age 45. It is now recommended that postmenopausal women should increase their dietary calcium by taking calcium supplements, especially within the first few years after menopause when the bone loss is greatest.[31]

Bone loss in later life is a natural process, but it can be reduced by the building of maximally dense bones during the years of growth.[32] This depends upon factors such as adequate calcium and Vitamin D intake and sufficient exercise. Excessive dieting, smoking, and alcohol use may also promote bone loss.

A well-balanced diet, drinking milk, and regular exercise throughout life helps minimize bone loss. Regular exercise helps retain peak bone mass.[33]

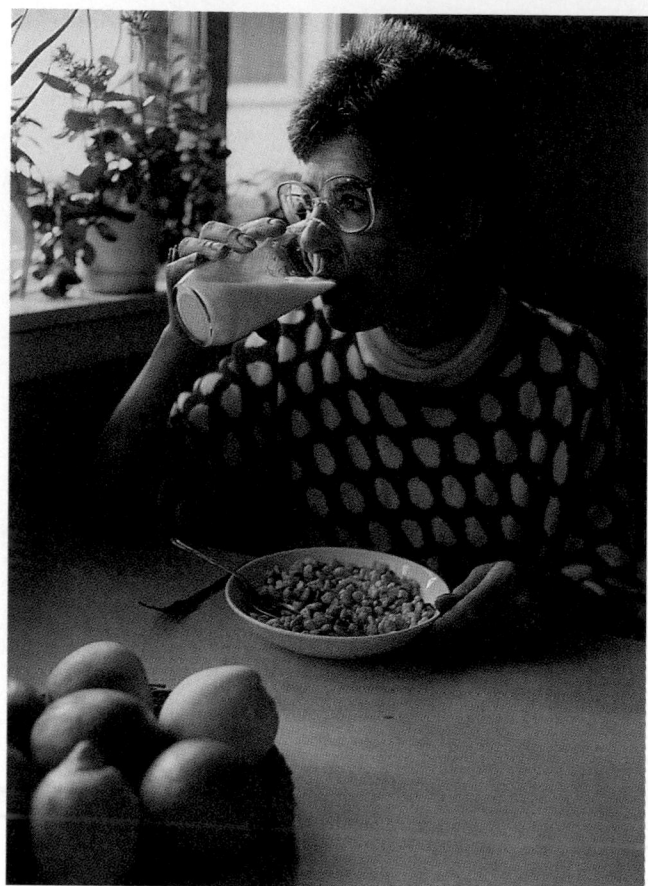

Calcium is essential in the formation of bones and teeth. It's important that people of all ages maintain an adequate calcium intake in their diet.

WATER

Water is one of the most essential nutrients in the body, and comprises about two-thirds of the body's weight. It is a major component of all body fluids, as well as a solvent that distributes nutrients throughout the body and eliminates waste products. Water also plays a major role in regulating body temperature, maintaining the body's acid-base balance, and taking part in every chemical reaction that occurs in the body.

Human beings can go without food for two weeks or more, but can survive only five to seven days without water. When the amount of water in the body is reduced by 1 percent of its weight, a person becomes thirsty. When 10 percent of water is missing, a person may experience kidney failure. Death from dehydration occurs when 20 percent of body water is lost.[34]

The body loses 2–3 quarts of water each day through breathing, perspiration, urination, and defecation. To replace this, adults should drink about six to eight glasses of water a day. The rest of the required water intake can be found in other beverages and foods. Many foods, especially fruits and vegetables, have a high water content. Lettuce and cucumbers are more than 95 percent water, cantaloupe, cauliflower, spinach, peppers, and watermelon are more than 90 percent water; and many fruits, such as pears, oranges, plums, and pineapples, are over 80 percent water. Fruit juices, milk, and other beverages also have a high water content.

CHECKPOINT

1. Compare a nonessential amino acid with an essential one, and a complete protein with an incomplete one.

2. As a source of energy, how do vitamins and minerals differ from carbohydrates, fats, and proteins?

3. List the water-soluble vitamins and the fat-soluble vitamins.

4. What are the functions of minerals in the body?

5. Discuss the importance of water to the body.

ACHIEVING NUTRITIONAL ADEQUACY

The National Academy of Sciences has selected two national committees of scientists to participate in a federally funded study to define the amounts of dietary factors that best support health. The *Committee on Dietary Allowances* is concerned with maintaining health and focuses on energy and nutrient needs. The *Committee on Diet and Health* deals with reducing the risk of chronic disease and focuses on dietary inadequacies and excesses. The Committee on Dietary Allowances produces a set of nutritional standards, which is periodically reviewed.

RECOMMENDED DIETARY ALLOWANCE

The standard used in the United States today to evaluate nutritional value of food and beverages is the **Recommended Dietary Allowance (RDA).**

....

Recommended Dietary Allowance (RDA) nutrient intakes suggested for the maintenance of health in people in the United States.

The recommended dietary allowance was established after World War II and is updated periodically by the Food and Nutrition Board of the National Research Council. Table 9.7 provides a solid basis for planning a balanced diet.

To arrive at these standards, nutritionists determined average requirements, over a period of time, for protein, vitamins, and minerals. The recommended dietary allowances are not minimal requirements, nor are they necessarily optimal for all persons, but with their margin of safety they cover nearly everyone in the population. No one receiving the recommended dietary allowances will suffer nutrient deficiency.[35]

DIETARY GUIDELINES

In the 1977 *Dietary Goals for the United States,* published by the Senate Select Committee on Nutrition and Human Needs, a major shift was rec-

ommended in caloric intake from fats to carbohydrates, with the following suggested goals of:

- reducing fat consumption from 42 percent to 30 percent of energy intake
- a recommended increase in consumption of complex carbohydrates from 22 percent to 45 percent of intake
- a reduction of sugars from 24 percent to 13 percent of energy intake (see Table 9.8, p. 277; Figure 9.4).

This recommendation was followed in 1980 by the issuance of *Dietary Guidelines for Americans* (Table 9.9, p. 277). Issued by the USDA and the U.S. Department of Health and Human Services (USDHHS), the dietary guidelines addressed dietary excesses and what we should *not* eat, as well as the need to maintain an ideal diet. Those two major recommendations reflected a growing understanding of the relationship of diet to the

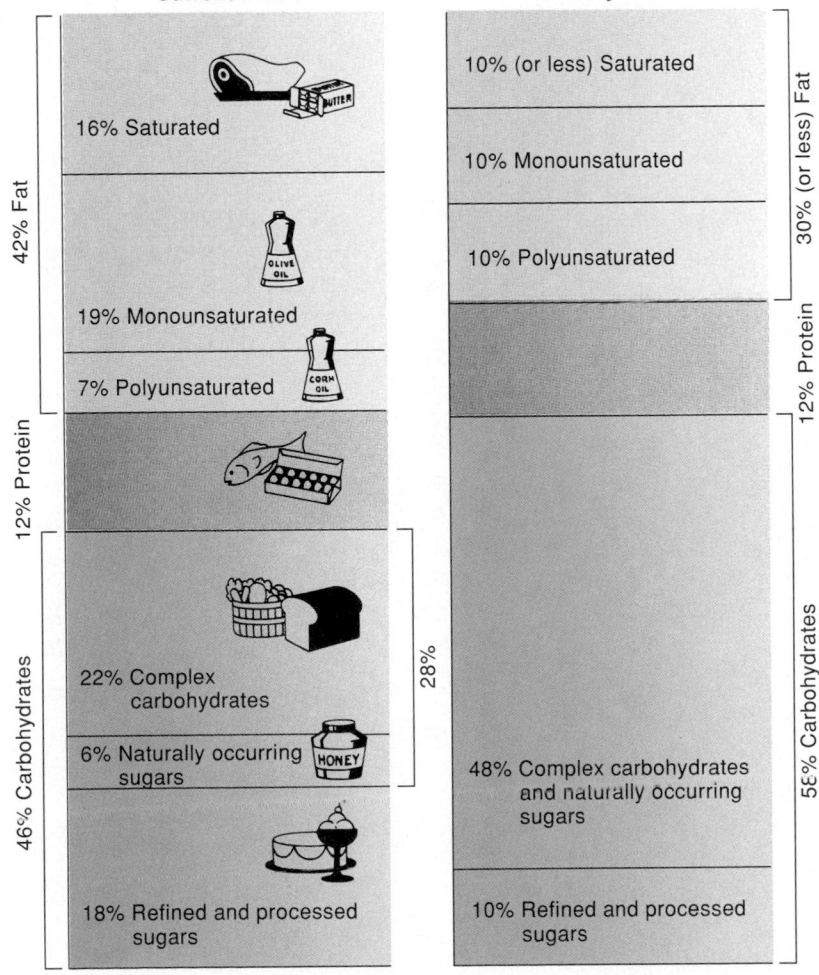

Figure 9.4
Sources of Calories—Current Sources vs. Dietary Goals

Percent of calories from different nutrients. Our present source of calories is compared with the sources that were recommended by the U.S. Senate Select Committee on Nutrition and Human Needs. Where are the changes?

Source: Adapted from the U.S. Senate Select Committee on Nutrition and Human Needs, Dietary Goals for the United States. Washington, DC: December, 1977.

Table 9.7
Recommended Dietary Allowances,[a] Revised 1989

Category or Condition	Age (years)	Weight[b] (kg)	Weight[b] (lb)	Height[b] (cm)	Height[b] (in)	Protein (g)	Fat-Soluble Vitamins Vitamin A (µg RE)[c]	Vitamin D (µg)[d]	Vitamin E (mg α-TE)[e]	Vitamin K (µg)
Infants	0.0–0.5	6	13	60	24	13	375	7.5	3	5
	0.5–1.0	9	20	71	28	14	375	10	4	10
Children	1–3	13	29	90	35	16	400	10	6	15
	4–6	20	44	112	44	24	500	10	7	20
	7–10	28	62	132	52	28	700	10	7	30
Males	11–14	45	99	157	62	45	1000	10	10	45
	15–18	66	145	176	69	59	1000	10	10	65
	19–24	72	160	177	70	58	1000	10	10	70
	25–50	79	174	176	70	63	1000	5	10	80
	51+	77	170	173	68	63	1000	5	10	80
Females	11–14	46	101	157	62	46	800	10	8	45
	15–18	55	120	163	64	44	800	10	8	55
	19–24	58	128	164	65	46	800	10	8	60
	25–50	63	138	163	64	50	800	5	8	65
	51+	65	143	160	63	50	800	5	8	65
Pregnant						60	800	10	10	65
Lactating	1st 6 months					65	1300	10	12	65
	2nd 6 months					62	1200	10	11	65

Water-soluble Vitamins							Minerals						
Vitamin C (mg)	Thiamin (mg)	Riboflavin (mg)	Niacin (mg NE)[f]	Vitamin B₆ (mg)	Folate (mcg)	Vitamin B₁₂ (mcg)	Calcium (mg)	Phosphorus (mg)	Magnesium (mg)	Iron (mg)	Zinc (mg)	Iodine (mcg)	Selenium (mcg)
30	0.3	0.4	5	0.3	25	0.3	400	300	40	6	5	40	10
35	0.4	0.5	6	0.6	35	0.5	600	500	60	10	5	50	15
40	0.7	0.8	9	1.0	50	0.7	800	800	80	10	10	70	20
45	0.9	1.1	12	1.1	75	1.0	800	800	120	10	10	90	20
45	1.0	1.2	13	1.4	100	1.4	800	800	170	10	10	120	30
50	1.3	1.5	17	1.7	150	2.0	1200	1200	270	12	15	150	40
60	1.5	1.8	20	2.0	200	2.0	1200	1200	400	12	15	150	50
60	1.5	1.7	19	2.0	200	2.0	1200	1200	350	10	15	150	70
60	1.5	1.7	19	2.0	200	2.0	800	800	350	10	15	150	70
60	1.2	1.4	15	2.0	200	2.0	800	800	350	10	15	150	70
50	1.1	1.3	15	1.4	150	2.0	1200	1200	280	15	12	150	45
60	1.1	1.3	15	1.5	180	2.0	1200	1200	300	15	12	150	50
60	1.1	1.3	15	1.6	180	2.0	1200	1200	280	15	12	150	55
60	1.1	1.3	15	1.6	180	2.0	800	800	280	15	12	150	55
60	1.0	1.2	13	1.6	180	2.0	800	800	280	10	12	150	55
70	1.5	1.6	17	2.2	400	2.2	1200	1200	320	30	15	175	65
95	1.6	1.8	20	2.1	280	2.6	1200	1200	355	15	19	200	75
90	1.6	1.7	20	2.1	260	2.6	1200	1200	340	15	16	200	75

[a]The allowances, expressed as average daily intakes over time, are intended to provide for individual variations among most normal persons as they live in the United States under usual environmental stresses. Diets should be based on a variety of common foods in order to provide other nutrients for which human requirements have been less well defined. . . .

[b]Weights and heights of Reference Adults are actual medians for the U.S. population of the designated age, as reported by NHANES II. The median weights and heights of those under 19 years of age were taken from Hamill et al. (1979). . . . The use of these figures does not imply that the height-to-weight ratios are ideal.

[c]Retinol equivalents. 1 retinol equivalent = 1 µg retinol or 6 µg β-carotene. . . .

[d]As cholecalciferol. 10 µg cholecalciferol = 400 IU of Vitamin D.

[e]α-Tocopherol equivalents. 1 mg- d-α tocopherol = 1 α-TE. . . .

[f]1 NE (niacin equivalent) is equal to 1 mg of niacin or 60 mg of dietary tryptophan.

Source: Subcommittee on the Tenth Edition of the RDAs Food and Nutrition Board, Commission on Life Sciences, National Research Council. Recommended Dietary Allowances, 10th ed. Washington, DC: National Academy Press, 1989.

Table 9.8
Dietary Goals for the United States

1. To avoid becoming overweight, consume only as much energy (calories) as is expended; if overweight, decrease calorie intake and increase calorie expenditure.

2. Increase the consumption of complex carbohydrates and "naturally occurring" sugars from about 28 percent of energy intake to about 48 percent of energy intake.

3. Reduce the consumption of refined and processed sugars by about 45 percent to account for about 10 percent of total energy intake.

4. Reduce overall fat consumption from approximately 40 percent to about 30 percent of energy intake.

5. Reduce saturated-fat consumption to account for about 10 percent of total energy intake; balance that with polyunsaturated and monounsaturated fats, which should account for about 10 percent of energy intake each.

6. Reduce cholesterol consumption to about 300 milligrams a day.

7. Limit the intake of sodium by reducing the intake of salt to about 5 grams a day.

Source: Select Committee on Nutrition and Human Needs, Dietary Goals for the United States, *2nd ed. Washington, DC: U.S. Senate Select Committee, 1977.*

Table 9.9
Dietary Guidelines for Americans

- Eat a variety of foods.
- Maintain healthy weight.
- Choose a diet low in fat, saturated fat, and cholesterol.
- Choose a diet with plenty of vegetables, fruits, and grain products.
- Use sugars only in moderation.
- Use salt and sodium in moderation.
- If you drink alcoholic beverages, do so in moderation.

Note: Dietary Guidelines for Americans *is a government document developed by the U.S. Department of Agriculture and the U.S. Department of Health and Human Services. These guidelines are based on* The Surgeon General's Report on Nutrition and Health, *DHHS (PHS) Publication No. 88-50211. Washington, DC: Government Printing Office, 1988;* Diet and Health: Implications for Reducing Chronic Disease Risk. *Washington, DC: National Academy Press, 1989; and the* Recommended Dietary Allowances, *10th ed. Washington, DC: National Academy Press, 1989.*

development of major health threats, such as coronary heart disease, hypertension, and liver disease.

THE FOOD GROUPS

The key behind a nutritious diet is to get adequate amounts of nutrients from a variety of foods. Two popular tools for diet planning are food group plans and exchange lists. To help people plan a proper diet, the U.S. Department of Agriculture (USDA) has organized foods into food groups. These are clusters of foods similar in origin and rich in the same key nutrients. They started with the "Basic Eleven," which were later reduced to the "Basic Seven," and later to the "Basic Four." These four food groups were variously displayed into easy-to-remember schematics and graphics. Many adults can still remember the "food wheel" hanging on classroom bulletin boards illustrating the basic four food groups in proportion that everyone was told to eat daily: two servings of meat and meat alternates, two servings of milk and milk products, four servings of bread and cereals, and four servings of vegetables and fruits.

The Four Food Group Plan was useful in laying a strong foundation for a healthy diet by teaching people about meal planning, and by helping children understand nutrition. A major shortcoming was that it failed to specify food energy intake.

Users of the plan could easily overconsume fat and energy foods. Among the foods in each of the four groups there were large fat and energy differences, such as between nonfat milk and ice cream, fish and hot dogs, and avocados and green beans. Following the plan, some people could grow overweight, while others would become undernourished. Worse yet, following this plan enhanced the development of diseases of the heart or cancers.[36] Today, many people are becoming informed on nutrition and want to eat properly.

Daily Food Guide

The Daily Food Guide replaces the old Four food groups. It splits vegetables and fruits into separate groups, and recommends more generous servings of carbohydrates, vegetables, and fruits in comparison to meats and dairy products. It clusters foods into five food groups and one miscellaneous group that makes little contribution to nutrient intake, for a total of six groups (Feature 9.3, p. 278). Within each group it subdivides foods in terms of **nutrient density,** which is a measure of the nutrients of a food relative to the calorie the food provides.[37] Within each group there is a listing of foods of

nutrient density a measure of the nutrients a food provides relative to the energy it provides. The more nutrients and the fewer the calories, the higher the nutrient density.

THE DAILY FOOD GUIDE

BREADS, CEREALS, AND OTHER GRAIN PRODUCTS

These foods are notable for their contributions of complex carbohydrates, riboflavin, thiamin, niacin, iron, protein, magnesium, and fiber.

- 6–11 servings per day.

- Serving = 1 slice bread; ½ c cooked cereal, rice, or pasta; 1 oz ready-to-eat cereal; ½ bun, bagel, or English muffin; 1 small roll, biscuit, or muffin; 3–4 small or 2 large crackers.

  *A Whole grains (wheat, oats, barley, millet, rye, bulgur), enriched breads, rolls, tortillas, cereals, bagels, rice, pastas (macaroni, spaghetti), air-popped corn.

  B Pancakes, muffins, cornbread, crackers, low-fat cookies, biscuits, presweetened cereals.

  C Croissants, fried rice, granola.

VEGETABLES

These foods are notable for their contributions of Vitamin A, Vitamin C, folate, potassium, magnesium, and fiber, and for their lack of fat and cholesterol.

- 3–5 servings per day (use dark green, leafy vegetables and legumes several times a week).

- Serving = ½ c cooked or raw vegetables; 1 c leafy raw vegetables; ½ c cooked legumes; ¾ c vegetable juice.

  A Bean sprouts, broccoli, brussels sprouts, cabbage, carrots, cauliflower, cucumbers, green beans, green peas, leafy greens (spinach, mustard, and collard greens), legumes, lettuce, mushrooms, tomatoes, winter squash.

  B Corn, potatoes, sweet potatoes.

  C Avocadoes, french fries, olives, tempura vegetables.

FRUITS

These foods are notable for their contributions of Vitamin A, Vitamin C, potassium, and fiber, and for their lack of sodium, fat, and cholesterol.

- 2–4 servings per day.

- Serving = typical portion (such as 1 medium apple, banana, or orange, ½ grapefruit, 1 melon wedge); ¾ c juice; ½ c berries; ½ c diced, cooked, or canned fruit; ½ c dried fruit.

  A Fresh apricots, cantaloupe, grapefruit, oranges, orange juice, peaches, strawberries, apples, bananas, pears.

  B Canned fruit.

  C Dried fruit, coconut.

MEAT, POULTRY, FISH, AND ALTERNATES

These foods are notable for their contributions of protein, phosphorus, Vitamin B_6, Vitamin B_{12}, zinc, magnesium, iron, niacin, and thiamin.

- 2–3 servings per day.

- Servings = 2–3 oz lean, cooked meat, poultry, or fish (total 5–7 oz per day); count 1 egg, ½ c cooked legumes, or 2 tbs peanut butter as 1 oz meat (or about ⅓ serving).

  A Poultry, fish, lean meat (beef, lamb, pork, veal), legumes, egg whites.

  B Fat-trimmed beef, lamb, pork; refried beans, egg yolks, tofu, tempeh.

  C Hot dogs, luncheon meats, peanut butter, nuts, sausage, bacon, fried fish or poultry, duck.

MILK, CHEESE, AND YOGURT

These foods are notable for their contributions of calcium, riboflavin, protein, vitamin B_{12}, and, when fortified, Vitamin D and Vitamin A.

- 2 servings per day.

- 3 servings per day for teenagers and young adults, pregnant/lactating women, women past menopause.

  4 servings per day for pregnant/lactating teenagers.

- Serving = 1 c milk or yogurt; 2 oz process cheese food; 1½ oz cheese.

  A Nonfat and 1 percent low-fat milk (and nonfat products such as buttermilk, cottage cheese, cheese, yogurt); fortified soy milk.

  B 2 percent low-fat milk (and low-fat products such as yogurt, cheese, cottage cheese), sherbet, ice milk.

  C Whole milk (and whole-milk products such as cheese, yogurt, cottage cheese), cream, sour cream, cream cheese, custard, milk shakes, pudding, ice cream.

MISCELLANEOUS GROUP

These foods are notable for their contributions of sugar, fat, salt, alcohol and food energy. These foods are not in the pattern because they provide few nutrients. Note that some of the following items could be placed in more than one group or in a combination group. For example, potato chips are high in both salt and fat; doughnuts are high in both sugar and fat.

A Miscellaneous foods, not high in calories, include spices, herbs, coffee, tea, and diet soft drinks.

C Foods high in fat include margarine, salad dressings, oils, mayonnaise, cream, cream cheese, butter, gravy, and sauces.

C Foods high in salt include potato chips, corn chips, pretzels, pickles, olives, bouillon, prepared mustard, soy sauce, steak sauce, salt, and seasoned salt.

C Foods high in sugar include cake, pie, cookies, donuts, sweet rolls, candy, soft drinks, fruit drinks, jelly, syrup, gelatin, desserts, sugar, and honey.

C Alcoholic beverages include wine, beer, and liquor.

*KEY

A Foods generally higher in nutrient density (good first choice).

B Foods moderate in nutrient density (reasonable second choice).

C Foods lowest in nutrient density (limit selections).

Note: Serve children at least the lower number of servings from each group, but in smaller amounts (for example, ¼–⅓ cup rice). Children should receive the equivalent of 2 cups of milk each day, but again in smaller quantities per serving (for example, four half-cup portions). Pregnant women may require additional servings of fruits, vegetables, meats, and breads to meet their higher needs for energy, vitamins, and minerals.

Source: Whitney, E., and Rolfes, S. *Understanding Nutrition*, 6th ed. St. Paul, MN: West, 1993.

highest, moderate, and lowest nutrition density. Foods highest in nutrient density give the greatest nutrition with the lowest calorie. Thus a person who is inactive should choose foods of highest nutrition density but of lowest calorie, whereas a physically active person could choose foods with the lowest nutrition density, but the highest calorie. High calorie foods are the perfect "ticket" for a young athlete, whereas an inactive person could easily grow fat on the same foods. The important thing is that every person get the needed nutrients, and focusing on nutrition density provides for this.

The Food Guide Pyramid

Although the mission in overall dietary goals remains the same, the USDA sought to promote a newly designed graphic. The result is the *Food Guide Pyramid* (Figure 9.5).

The pyramid makes it plain visually:

- that amount of intake of all food groups should *not* be equal
- and that there should be no confusion as to which foods are safe for larger percentage of intake (bread, cereal, rice, and pasta group) and which ones should be consumed in small quantities (fats, oils, and sweets).

It's important not to assume that groups higher in the pyramid are less important or bad for you. All foods in the pyramid are included because they are needed.

By placing preferred foods, which include bread, cereal, rice, and pasta, in larger-sized spaces toward the base of the pyramid, the message is that we should be moving toward more of these foods and away from those foods in the apex of the pyramid, which are high in fat, sodium, and sugar. Not only does the pyramid tell us the direction of our diet selections, but also reminds us of the number of servings of each group we should be getting daily. Each group covers a wide enough group of foods that it allows for substitutions. For example, milk products such as cheese, yogurt, and cottage cheese can be substituted for whole milk.

Exchange System

The premise of the **food exchange system** is different from the food group system in that it does not categorize food groups by their nutritional value, but by their caloric value.

These categories are organized into six food lists. In each list, portions are recommended so that all items in each list have the same amount of energy nutrients such as fats, carbohydrates, and proteins. This system was originally developed for people with diabetes, but has become a popular way to monitor the diets of participants in weight-control programs, such as Weight Watchers.

The food group plan is useful in ensuring that all classes of nutritive foods are included. The exchange system provides calorie and fat intake

food exchange system lists of foods having the same number of calories and the same amounts of energy nutrients.

Figure 9.5
Food Guide Pyramid

The breadth of the base shows that grains (breads, cereals, rice, and pasta) deserve the most emphasis in the diet. The top is smallest: use fats, oils, and sweets sparingly.

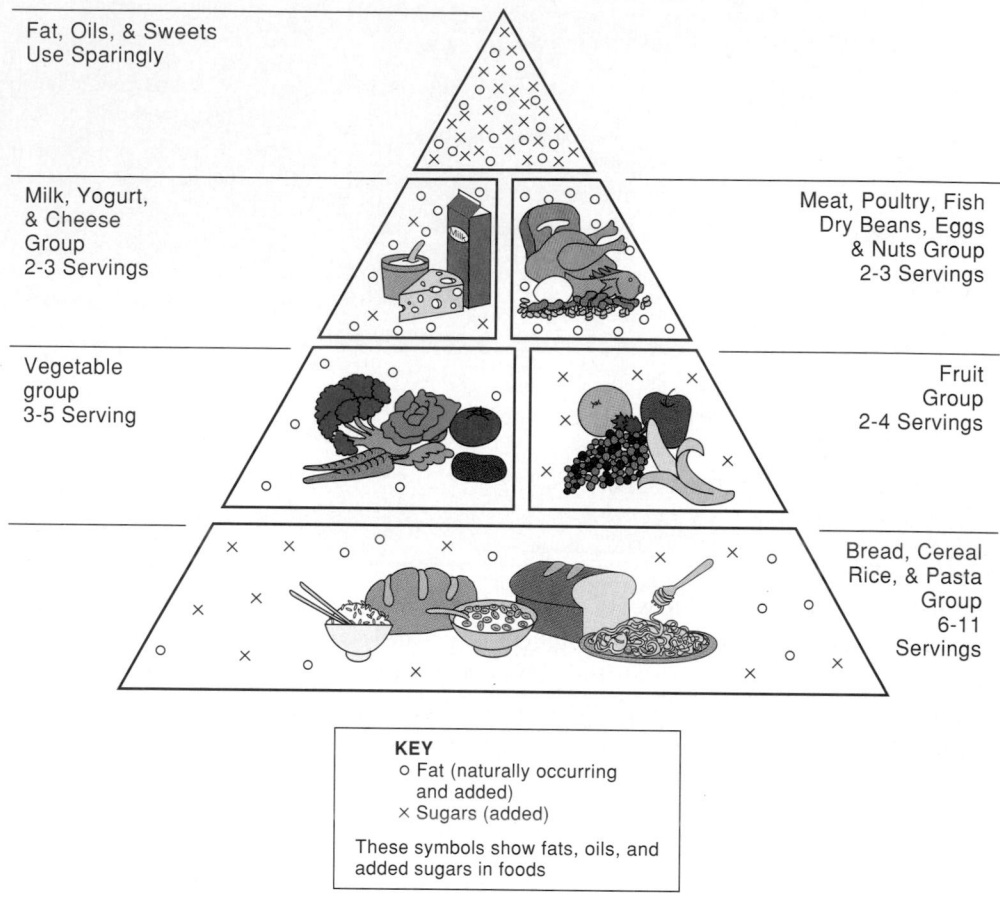

Fat, Oils, & Sweets
Use Sparingly

Milk, Yogurt,
& Cheese
Group
2-3 Servings

Meat, Poultry, Fish
Dry Beans, Eggs
& Nuts Group
2-3 Servings

Vegetable
group
3-5 Serving

Fruit
Group
2-4 Servings

Bread, Cereal
Rice, & Pasta
Group
6-11
Servings

KEY
o Fat (naturally occurring
and added)
× Sugars (added)

These symbols show fats, oils, and
added sugars in foods

controls. For example, the Food Guide suggests 6–11 servings of grains (breads and cereals) per day. The exchange system may allow 9 exchanges from the starch/bread list so calorie intake can fall within a target range. Food groups and exchange systems can work together to make a healthful, well-balanced diet.

THE U.S. RDA AND DAILY VALUES

For the past 25 years the Recommended Daily Allowance (U.S. RDA) has been used to express nutrient information on labels. The U.S. RDA is a set of standard values determined for the typical consumer, which the FDA designated for use on food labels. Based on the 1968 edition of the RDA, the U.S. RDA was useful for some individuals in determining a percentage expression of nutritional needs, but was not useful for others. Some persons have confused the U.S. RDA (U.S. Recommended Daily Allowance) with RDA (Recommended Dietary Allowance), a name that has been used for decades.

In an effort to improve on food product labeling, the FDA has replaced the U.S. RDA with the

Daily Values. The Daily Values are based on two sets of reference values, the *Reference Daily Intakes (RDI),* which are the average allowances for proteins, vitamins, and minerals as based on the RDA, and the *Daily Reference Values (DRV),* which are average allowances for food components, such as fat and fiber, which do not have an established RDA but have an important relationship to health.[38] All of the required nutrients are now listed as a *Percent (or %) of Daily Value.* Slightly lower than the U.S. RDA, the Percent of Daily Values is based on a 2000 calorie diet and is a percentage of the recommended intake for the "typical consumer."

CHECKPOINT

1. Name the standard used in America to evaluate the nutritional value of foods and beverages.

2. What were the shifts in fat and carbohydrate consumption that were contained in the 1977 *Dietary Goals for the United States?*

daily value standard nutrient value developed by the FDA for use on food labels.

3. What is the significance of the placement of foods in the Food Guide Pyramid?

4. Explain the Food Exchange system.

LABELING

About half of all consumers say they depend on food labels to determine which foods to buy. Yet, deception in food labeling is widespread.[39] Examples include: "light and healthy Salisbury steaks" labeled as "low fat" although deriving 45 percent of total calories from fat; "fresh choice orange juice" made from concentrate; and "fruit juice drinks" containing only 10 percent fruit juice.

In 1992 the federal government, under a mandate from Congress, adopted new regulations for the most sweeping revision ever of nutritional labeling of processed foods to help people choose their foods more wisely. By mid-1994, new revised labels appeared on over 257,000 food items.[40]

The prior food product labels provided *Nutrition Information* (Figure 9.6), and listed serving size, number of servings, breakdown of nutrients per serving, statement of percent of U.S. RDA for protein, vitamins, and minerals, and ingredients in descending order of amount in the package. The prior labeling regulations did not require food manufacturers to present complete and consistent information, which would allow the customer to compare the nutritional value of different products.

Titled *Nutrition Facts,* the new labeling panels are built around a new set of labeling components (Figure 9.7). Every food label must display:

- the common name of the product
- the name and address of the manufacturer, packer, or distributor
- the net contents in terms of weight, measure, or count, and the nutritional value of the product
- the ingredient list
- the serving size and number of servings per container

Figure 9.6
Old Format for Nutrition Labeling

The federal government required that this information be listed on the labels of all food packages.

NUTRITION INFORMATION PER SERVING			COMMENTS
SERVING SIZE: 1 OUNCE (ABOUT 1 CUP) CEREAL ALONE AND IN COMBINATION WITH 1/2 CUP VITAMIN D FORTIFIED WHOLE MILK.			Defines the size of a serving or portion.
SERVING PER CONTAINER: 8			Number of servings or portions in container.
	1 OZ.	CEREAL WITH 1/2 CUP WHOLE MILK	
CALORIES	110	180	Breakdown of calories, protein, carbohydrates, and fat. Total fat and cholesterol content is optional.
PROTEIN	2 g	6 g	
CARBOHYDRATES	25 g	31 g	
FAT	0 g	4 g	
PERCENTAGE OF U..S. RECOMMENDED DAILY ALLOWANCE (U.S. RDA)			
	1 OZ.	CEREAL WITH 1/2 CUP WHOLE MILK	
PROTEIN	4	15	Statement of protein, vitamin, and mineral content in percentages of the U.S. Recommended Daily Allowances for each.
VITAMIN A	25	30	
VITAMIN C	25	25	
THIAMIN	25	25	
RIBOFLAVIN	25	35	
NIACIN	25	25	
CALCIUM	*	15	
IRON	10	10	
VITAMIN D	10	25	
VITAMIN B6	25	25	
FOLIC ACID	25	25	
PHOSPHORUS	*	10	
MAGNESIUM	*	4	

*CONTAINS LESS THAN 2% OF THE U.S. RDA OF THESE NUTRIENTS.

INGREDIENTS: MILLED CORN, SUGAR, SALT, MALT FLAVORING, SODIUM ASCORBATE (C), VITAMIN A PALMITATE, NIACINAMIDE, ASCORBIC ACID (C), REDUCED IRON, PYRIDOXINE HYDROCHLORIDE (B6), THIAMINE, HYDROCHLORIDE (B1), RIBOFLAVIN (B2), FOLIC ACID AND VITAMIN D2. BHA AND BHT ADDED TO PRESERVE PRODUCT FRESHNESS.

Ingredients in descending order of predominance, except when blends of fats or oils are used. Fat and oil ingredients must be listed by common or usual names, such as lard, coconut oil, beef oil, or soybean oil shortening blend, instead of more generalized names such as animal fat, vegetable oil, or shortening.

Figure 9.7
Food Labeling

Nutrition Facts

Source: FDA Consumer, "Nutrition Facts to Help Consumers Eat Smart" by Paula Kurtzweil, May 1993, pp. 22–27. Actual figure used, p. 23.

New heading signals a new label. ⟶

More consistent serving sizes, in both household and metric measures, replace those that used to be set by manufacturers. ⟶

Nutrients required on nutrition panel are those most important to the health of today's consumers, most of whom need to worry about getting too much of certain items (fat, for example), rather than too few vitamins or minerals, as in the past. ⟶

Conversion guide helps consumers learn caloric value of the energy-producing nutrients. ⟶

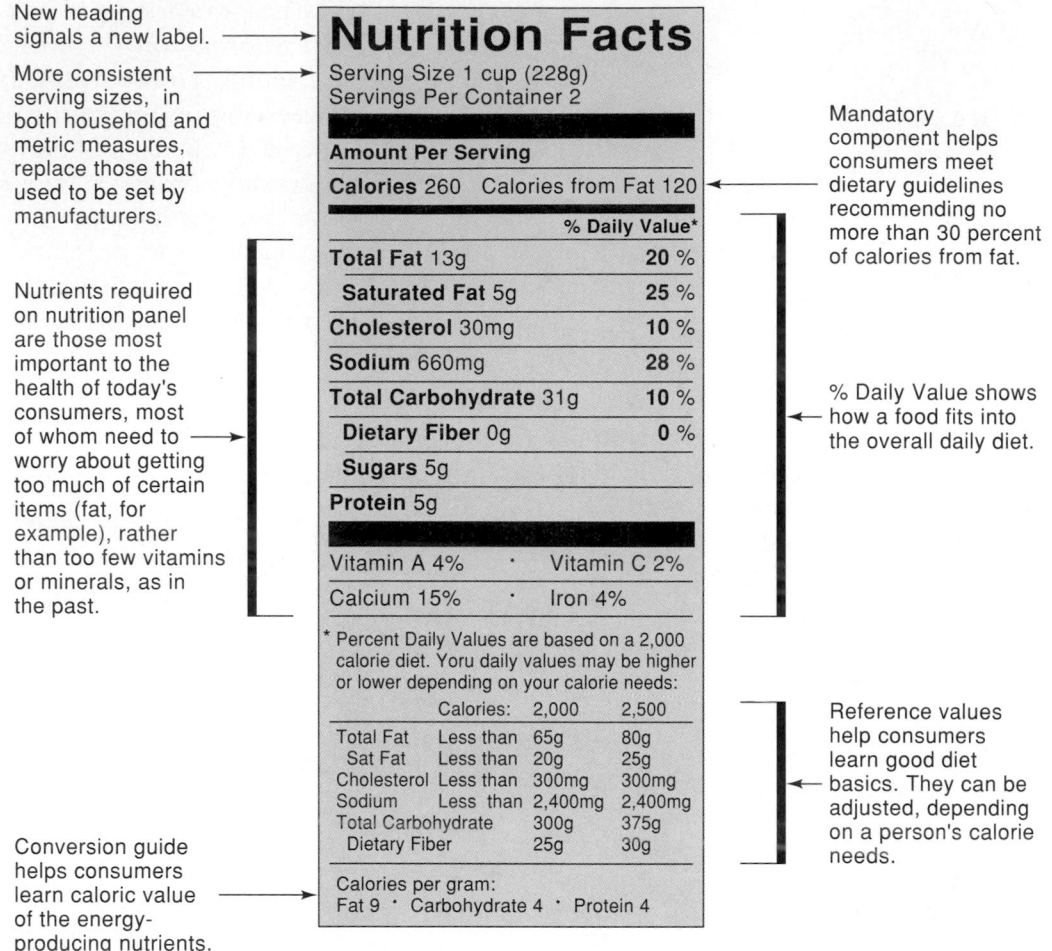

Mandatory component helps consumers meet dietary guidelines recommending no more than 30 percent of calories from fat.

% Daily Value shows how a food fits into the overall daily diet.

Reference values help consumers learn good diet basics. They can be adjusted, depending on a person's calorie needs.

- the quantities of specified nutrients and food constituents.

All ingredients must be listed in descending order of predominance by weight. Specific fats and oils used in manufacturing must be listed, as well as all additives. Serving sizes that people customarily consume must be given in both common household measures, such as cups, and in metric measures. Most importantly, the labels show the quantities of certain nutrients in a serving. **Macronutrients,** such as fat, cholesterol, sodium, carbohydrates, and protein, are declared as an amount in grams or milligrams per serving, and as a Percent of the Daily Values. The amounts by themselves may appear large or small, but as a Percent of Daily Value there is basis for accurate comparison of recommended

intakes for the "typical consumer." **Micronutrients,** such as vitamins and minerals, are expressed as a percentage. Only those vitamins whose deficiencies is viewed as a public health problem must be listed. Others may or may not be listed. Some larger labels will give reference values, or a Percent of Daily Values of selected nutrients for 2000 and 2500 calorie diets, as well as calorie conversion information for fats, carbohydrates, and proteins.[41] (See Figure 9.7.)

Significant changes from the old system include the following:

- listing of total calories *compared* with the calories from fat per serving (formerly unlisted)
- listing of percentage of Daily Value (daily maximal intake) for fats, carbohydrates,

macronutrients energy-producing and nonenergy-producing nutrients such as fats, carbohydrates, proteins, sodium, and cholesterol needed by the body in greater amounts.

micronutrients nonenergy-producing nutrients, such as vitamins and minerals, needed by the body in lesser amounts.

sodium, protein, and fiber for a 2000 calorie diet. A 2000 calorie intake is the approximate need of an average adult woman. For instance, if a product contains 13 grams (g) of fat, the label will list this amount as 20 percent of the Daily Value (a maximum intake of 65 g) (formerly unlisted).

- listing of Daily Value, or the daily maximum intake, for a 2000 calorie diet and for a 2500 calorie diet (formerly unlisted)

- a uniform definition for terms such as "light," "fat free," "low fat," "low calorie," "cholesterol free," and "high fiber." For example, the term "fat free" can be used only if there is less than 0.5 g of fat per serving (with no added fat or oil) (formerly unregulated)

- allowing products to print health claims on the food package *only* if supported by scientific evidence (formerly unregulated).

The new labeling applies only to foods regulated by the FDA. Exempted from the new rules are advertising and items on restaurant menus, which are under Federal Trade Commission regulation (yet, an increasing number of restaurants provide nutrition information upon request). Also exempted are low-fat milk and low-fat yogurt, products covered by existing federal regulations. The new labeling changes are expected to result in savings of billions of dollars in health care costs, according to the Department of Health and Human Services.[42]

CHECKPOINT

1. What is the significance of Percent of Daily Value on food product labels?

2. Why are some vitamins omitted from food labeling?

DIETARY CHANGES

Two approaches to dietary changes may be used, the preventive approach and the medical approach. The medical approach is to wait for a disease to show up and then have the affected person make dietary changes. The preventive approach is aimed at everyone and offers the same advice to all. The idea is to recommend changes that may delay or prevent any disease that may be related to diet. The message of this approach is that correct eating patterns are beneficial and attainable. Communication for Wellness: Right Eating (It Might Be Easier Than You Think!), p. 284, gives a number of easy-to-follow dietary tips for improving the quality of your diet and for preventing disease.

Dietary guidelines drawn up by government agencies and other organizations opt for the preventive approach. A decade of work and a series of dietary guidelines has brought about the practical and easy-to-follow *Dietary Guidelines for Americans* (see Table 9.9, p. 277). The message of this approach is that right eating patterns are both beneficial and attainable.

VEGETARIAN DIETS

As mentioned earlier in this chapter, vegetarian diets depend largely or entirely on plant products, and restrict intake of animal protein. The dietary practices of vegetarians vary, ranging from strict vegetarians, who eat no animal products of any kind, *vegans,* to those who eat certain types of animal products. The majority of vegetarians eat some animal products, and as a consequence consume more nutrients than strict vegetarians.

Vegetarian diets are advantageous for many reasons, one being that vegetarians have a lower risk of cardiovascular diseases than do nonvegetarians. Not only do vegetarians have lower blood cholesterol, but more of their cholesterol tends to be high density lipoprotein (HDL or "good cholesterol"). Vegetarians are less likely to be overweight or to have high blood pressure than are nonvegetarians.[43] They also face reduced risks of diabetes and cancer.[44]

One caution with a vegetarian diet is the potential for deficiencies of certain nutrients. Nutrient and energy needs are greater during pregnancy, lactation, infancy, childhood, and during times of illness. During pregnancy and lactation, dietary deficiencies can have significant consequences on the pre- and postnatal development of a child. A completely vegetarian diet during infancy and childhood can also have adverse consequences. Because of the small bulk of food a child can eat, it is difficult to provide the range of nutrients a child needs on a strict vegetarian diet.[45] A child is apt to be full of food before nutrient needs are met. As a result, vegan children tend to be smaller in height and lighter in weight than children who eat

COMMUNICATION FOR WELLNESS
RIGHT EATING (IT MIGHT BE EASIER THAN YOU THINK!)

Misunderstanding and fears over dietary change may be why some people delay taking steps to improve their diets. People fall in love with what they are used to doing. Nutritionists are telling us that with a little effort, we can change our "average diet" into an "ideal diet." Taken from "Are You Eating Right?" (*Consumer Reports,* October 1992), here are some tips for improving the quality of your diet:

- Try low fat products. If not available, use the real thing sparingly.
- Avoid deep-fried foods (and foods that are breaded and fried).
- Cut off visible fat from meat before cooking and remove the skin from poultry.
- When eating red meat, choose lean cuts.
- When using stews and soups, cook them a day early, chill, then skim off the fat.
- Choose flavorful ingredients so you can cut down on the portions of fatty foods.
- Select milk and yogurt, rather than other higher fat dairy foods.
- Limit sodium by going easy on soy sauce, steak sauce, catsup, pickles, olives, most cheeses, and canned soups. Cook with less salt.

- Eat fruits and vegetables with skins on, when possible, and cook them as little as possible.
- Snack on raw, refrigerated vegetables immersed in water.
- Add shredded carrots, tomatoes, or bean sprouts to sandwiches.
- Add vegetables to casseroles, soups, salads, and pastas.
- Add sliced fruit to cereals, frozen yogurt, plain yogurt, and other food.
- Select brown rice and whole grain breads, cereals, and pastas for extra vitamins, minerals, and fiber.

The foods you choose to eat should fit easily into your dietary plan. Don't count nutrients too closely. By eating recommended numbers of servings and a variety of foods (according to the Food Guide Pyramid), you should do well. Make room for favorites. Don't allow yourself to feel deprived. Just keep portions small if the food is high in fat. Adopt a new eating style gradually, perhaps over several years. Be easy on yourself. Don't expect to change overnight.

Source: Adapted from Consumers Union, "Are You Eating Right?" *Consumer Reports.* October 1992, pp. 644–653.

---

meat.[46] The most critical factor in vegan children is low food energy intake.[47]

Most animal proteins are complete, whereas no single plant protein is complete. This problem can be overcome by combining two incomplete but complementary proteins in the same meal to yield a complete protein.

Strict vegetarians may be deficient in Vitamin B_{12} since no plant food provides an ample amount of this vitamin; they may also be in danger of consuming insufficient amounts of Vitamin D, calcium, iron, and zinc. Strict vegetarians should consider a daily multivitamin containing these nutrients missing from their diets, in addition to a calcium supplement.

CHECKPOINT

1. What are the two approaches to dietary change?

2. List the precautions a person must take if eating a vegetarian diet.

ETHNIC DIETS

People of every country and of regions within countries, have their own favorite foods and ways of using them in meals. The United States is a great "melting pot" of ethnic peoples, and the menus popular in this country reflect many subcultures. American-style restaurants feature tacos (Mexican), french fried potatoes (French), spaghetti (Italian), hot dogs with sauerkraut (German), Yorkshire pudding (English), and wonton soup (Chinese). We accept these foods as an integral part of the American diet. The older and newer immigrant groups in the U.S. have made significant contributions to our national patterns of eating. The following sections include a selection of popular ethnic cuisines.

NORTHERN EUROPE

Many North Americans emigrated from Northern Europe. They brought with them their appetites for roast meat, mashed potatoes with gravy, cabbage, and desserts of fruit pies. Northern European diets are high in proteins and fats from meats, and more limited in the vitamins, fibers, and minerals that come from fruits and vegetables. The Food Guide Pyramid recommends *larger* servings of complex carbohydrate foods, vegetables, and fruits, and *smaller* servings of meat and meat products.

The English have given us tea as a beverage, breakfasts of bacon and eggs with biscuits, and beans, which we have largely replaced with hash browns or grits.

French descendants in the southern states have given us the distinctively flavored Cajun foods. These dishes include thick, spicy soups; sausages; Tabasco pepper sauce; red beans; rice; and seafood. High in carbohydrates and fibers, and low in fats, many Cajun dishes come close to meeting or meet the Daily Food Guide recommendations.[48]

SOUTHERN EUROPE

The Italians have given us pizza, spumoni (ice cream with fruits and nuts), and pastas. But Italy is known for its distinctive regional differences in food preferences. Northern Italians have given us animal-derived foods such as egg-based pastas, meat, butter, cheese, and eggs. Southern Italians have contributed wheat pastas made without eggs, along with vegetables such as eggplants, tomatoes, peppers, and artichokes, and beans, all seasoned with olive oil rather than butter.

Some Italian dishes represent healthful eating. With a spread of ingredients from three or four food groups, pizza gives eating nutritional balance, as do the pastas served with eggplant Parmesan, other vegetables, and beans. Yet, people who select from Italian dishes may need to reduce the intake of fats found in oils, high-fat cheeses, butter, and cream.[49]

WEST AFRICA

Peanuts and peanut products in our diets find their origins in Africa. Brought to the United States by slaves, peanuts, okra, and black-eyed peas have been absorbed into Southern cuisine of both blacks and whites. Southern cooking includes both benefits and cautions. Dishes commonly include corn, green leafy vegetables, and sweet potatoes, rich sources of vitamins and minerals. Yet, many of these foods are rich in fat and salt, such as spare ribs, fried chicken, pork cuts, along with biscuits rich in shortening and served with butter or fatty gravy. Southern cooking can be nutritious if you choose beans, rice, and cornbread dishes, along with plenty of vegetables prepared without extra salt, and if you go easy on fatty biscuits, gravy, and meats.[50]

MEXICO

Mexican eateries are famous for their tortillas, along with fried rice, refried beans, guacamole (avocado sauce), sour cream, and salsa (tomato sauce). At home, Mexican families typically eat a stew of beans, meat, and rice served with tortillas, and salsa, along with eggs for breakfast, and cooked vegetables and salads of lettuce and tomatoes for other meals.

Mexican fast food taco stands often sell beans, which are low in fat and high in nutrient density and fiber. These may be used in soft corn tortillas, along with lettuce and salsa for a nutritious meal. On the other hand, the tortilla can be fried and filled with ground beef, along with cheese and sour cream, and served with refried beans that may have been cooked in lard, making for a high fat meal. By using soft, nonfried tortillas filled with lean grilled meats topped with salsa, a dish called *fajita,* a nutritious meal can be prepared. As with other ethnic foods, Mexican foods can be nutritious or not depending on a person's ability to select.[51]

CHINA

Due to limited access to meat products, Chinese meals consist of large amounts of rice, vegetables and fruits, and small amounts of meat. Although Chinese consume 20 percent more calories per day than people in the United States, Chinese people have few obesity or malnutrition problems.[52] They eat three times as much fiber and take in half the amount of fat, and have half the blood cholesterol levels of people in the United States.[53]

The Chinese diet is ideal in many ways. Each person has his or her own cup of rice and then chooses from vegetable, meat, and noodle dishes, along with ample tea and soup. Flavoring is done largely with fat-free seasonings, and sauces, rather than with the typical butter, gravies, and sour cream. Wok cooking requires only a small amount of oil per dish. Meals tend to contain higher amounts of sodium, although they can be prepared without it.

Chinese cooking tends to preserve nutrients. Cooking rice in water, using bite-sized pieces of food that have not been overcooked, and using cooking water for food preparation, all help to avoid nutrient loss.[54]

RELIGIOUS FOOD TRADITIONS

Worldwide, religious groups practice dietary traditions. Immigrant religious traditions, as well as those originating in the United States, often have distinctive food requirements. Whether from Eastern Europe, the United States, or the Middle East, Orthodox Jews place a set of restrictions, known as keeping **kosher,** on the preparation of foods. Kosher rules govern the kinds of products allowed, as well as the method of slaughtering, butchering, and preparing such foods. Observance of these dietary laws is a religious commitment, although an ancillary health benefit has been attributed to their adherence. All forms of scavenger animals (those eating garbage and decaying matter), such as pig, shellfish, and catfish are prohibited. Dairy products and meats or poultry may not be consumed in the same meal. Thus, in food preparation, cooks may replace milk, which is high in fat, with soy "milk," which is not. As with any cultural eating patterns, dishes must be examined for nutrient content. Reducing fats, such as schmaltz (rendered chicken fat), used in cooking, can improve the nutrient balance. Bagels with lox (smoked salmon), along with other foods make a unique and nutritious breakfast, especially if served without the usual cream cheese.

Various other religions teach special food restrictions. During Lent, Christians may give up meat in favor of vegetable dishes. Eastern Orthodox Christians observe fast days on which no animal products are consumed. Mormons are taught to avoid all alcohol, coffee, and tea. Seventh Day Adventists are admonished to drink no alcohol, coffee, and tea, and to avoid meat, although they may allow for eggs and milk products.

Knowing a person's ethnic and religious backgrounds allows dieticians to respect those preferences and yet provide nutritious foods. Some ethnic and religious practices have sound nutritional bases, although others deliver too much fat and are short on vitamins and minerals associated with fruits and vegetables.[55]

....

kosher the ritual fitness of food according to Jewish law.

SPORTS AND NUTRITION

Athletes seek athletic prowess in their desire to become champions. Inherited abilities, physical training, and good nutrition also influence success. Some athletes insist that certain foods by themselves, eaten certain ways, can give them the winning edge or improve their performances. Many persons who do not consider themselves to be athletes, but who regularly engage in sports, share some of the same concerns. While there is no magic diet that by itself enhances performance, an incorrect diet may negate the effects of hard training.

The three major sources of energy are carbohydrates, protein, and fat, but carbohydrates are the primary source of energy during exercise. Carbohydrates furnish the fuel for anaerobic exercises (such as sprinting) in which muscles work faster than the heart and lungs can supply needed oxygen. During aerobic activities (such as running a marathon or cross-country skiing) muscles work slowly and permit the heart and lungs to meet immediate oxygen demands. During aerobic exercise the body burns both carbohydrates and fat. The longer the activity lasts the more energy is derived from fat.

Carbohydrates are available to the muscles as glucose, or sugar circulating in the blood, and glycogen, the form in which glucose is stored in muscle and the liver. Since the body stores only about 1800 calories worth of glycogen, an athlete must replenish this supply by eating carbohydrates. Fats, on the other hand, are easily stored by the body; it can store an average of 140,000 calories of fat. Any excess carbohydrate, protein, or fat a person takes in is stored as fat.[56]

The American Dietetic Association suggests that anyone engaging in a sport should get at least

55 percent of his or her calories from carbohydrates and no more than 35 percent of his or her calories from fat. When extra calories are needed they should be obtained from carbohydrates such as starches, rather than from fats. Protein needs of athletes are little different from those of nonathletes. Appropriate sources for these proteins include meat, eggs, and dairy products.

The water needs of athletes may be much greater than those of nonathletes. Exercise results in the production of considerable amounts of heat, which if not disposed of through the evaporation of sweat, can lead to a dangerous increase in body temperature. It is not unusual for athletes engaging in strenuous activities to lose 2 to 4 quarts of water (4 to 8 pounds) per hour. The loss of as little as 3 percent of body weight from sweating (5.4 pounds for a 180 pound person) leads to fatigue. Greater amounts of water loss can lead to lowered blood pressure and heat stroke. Because an athlete's thirst may not accurately indicate water loss, it is suggested that an extra pint of water be consumed for every pound of body weight lost during exercise. Those who lose more than 4 quarts of water as sweat (8 pounds of weight during an activity) may need to supplement sodium and potassium during competition. The supplementation should be done only under the direction of a physician.[57]

Some athletes believe they can enhance performance by using unique nutritional techniques. One such belief is *carbohydrate-loading,* a technique of packing muscles with higher than normal levels of glycogen. A regimen is followed in which the person exercises to exhaustion one week before an event in order to reduce glycogen in the muscles, then exercises moderately for three days while reducing carbohydrate intake, then exercises lightly for four days while "loading up" on carbohydrate to replenish the glycogen. Nutritionists raise questions about the safety of this technique. Both reducing carbohydrate intake and then "loading up" may be dangerous, but are especially risky for diabetics, heart patients, and adolescents.[58]

The best advice for people engaging in sports is to eat a well-balanced diet from a wide variety of foods in amounts great enough to meet energy needs. You should be alert to any nutritional inadequacies you may have and to seek qualified nutritional and medical advice to remedy specific nutritional deficiencies.

CHECKPOINT

1. Which type of food is the primary source of energy during exercise?

2. What are the recommendations of the American Dietary Association for athletes regarding percentages of carbohydrates and fats in their total food consumption?

3. What are the special needs of athletes regarding water intake?

4. What is "carbohydrate loading"? Describe how it is done by athletes.

WHERE TO GO TO EAT

Norman Rockwell's portrayal of the American family no longer exclusively typifies the American lifestyle; we are not a nation of three or more family members sitting around a table twice a day eating a nourishing, home-cooked meal. As life-style factors have evolved, emphasis has shifted from the family to the individual. This shift also represents a change in food styles, which is influenced by social fads, financial status, and advertising in a very competitive food industry.

HOME COOKING

There are many advantages to home cooking, even though it is not our only food style. For one, it is more economical than eating out. It also allows you to choose the kinds of foods you use, such as fresh fruits and vegetables as opposed to frozen varieties. But this preparation takes time and skill. Vitamin C and riboflavin can be lost if too much heat is applied for too long. Microwave cooking and stir frying are methods that can be used to prevent vitamin loss in the process of preparing food. There are, of course, many more methods of cooking for a healthful diet. Cooking by breaking down carbohydrates and proteins and by softening the cellulose walls of fruits and vegetables enables enzymes to work more effectively. As a result foods are more digestible.

Home cooking allows you more control over your fat intake. While saturated fatty acids help create the flaky texture of baked goods, it is better to replace them with polyunsaturated vegetable oils or monounsaturated olive oil. If a nonstick pan is used, less oil may be necessary. Fat intake at home can be further reduced by trimming the exterior fat from meat, by pouring off accumulated fats, and by choosing leaner cuts of beef. Substituting poultry or fish for beef with also reduce fat intake as 40–50 percent of the fatty acids in red meat are saturated, compared to about 30 percent in chicken fat.

FROZEN FOODS AND DINNERS

The frozen meals available in supermarkets are considerably more nutritious than in past years. While providing a good supply of proteins, manufacturers have sought to control the content of fat as well as calories. Despite efforts to add nutrients to these meals, people with high blood pressure should be careful in selecting frozen foods because *sodium levels* tend to be high in proportion to calories.

Frozen fruits and vegetables, unlike fresh produce, are available at any time of the year. The freezing process itself does not nutritionally damage produce, meat, fish, and poultry, but losses may occur during the steps taken in preparation for freezing. Even so, there may be less loss with frozen foods than with fresh fruits and vegetables that have been in the produce department too long. While the price may be higher for the convenience, these alternatives offer the same nutritional value as fresh foods.

SNACKING

Snacking patterns begin early in life. As babies, our parents quickly respond to our cries for food. Not only do babies dictate *when* they eat, but *what* they will eat. While parents may try to shape children's eating patterns, young children and adolescents do a good deal of snacking, and they may consume as much as one-fifth of their food from *grazing* (irregular snacking at home and elsewhere).[59]

Snacking may or may not be bad. Some snacks, like potato chips, carry not only excess calories but surplus fat and salt. While some snacks do not provide the best balance of nutrients, they may be fortified with various nutrients. Some snacks contain sucrose, which has the reputation of promoting tooth decay. Recent evidence indicates that the fac-

tor most responsible for tooth decay is not necessarily the amount of sugar in the diet, but *when* it is eaten, the type of sugar (sucrose or glucose), and its acidity. The worst offenders seem to be sticky, sugary foods eaten between meals.

DINING OUT

Dining out has become a convenient and pleasurable life-style alternative to home cooking. While eating in restaurants can be nutritious, it is not always easy to maintain a nutritional balance. Traditional restaurants may give large portions of high calorie foods. Restaurants often cook with a lot of oil and butter and may not offer alternatives to their usual menus, which would include more fruits and vegetables.

To improve your dietary balance when eating out, you should:

- eat at restaurants offering a variety of soups and salads;
- eat at restaurants that have a selection that includes vegetables, salads, and fruits;
- build your own salad with fresh green vegetables and fresh fruits, and avoid the sauces, egg, ham, croutons, and bacon bits;
- ask for your salad dry, or request salad dressing or oil and vinegar on the side;
- order fish or poultry rather than steak, and ask that it be dry broiled without butter;
- ask that gravy or other sauces be left off of your food;
- choose baked potatoes over french fries and ask for light sour cream or sour cream substitutes rather than margarine or butter;
- ask for a "doggy bag" for portions you can do without, or just leave the excess on your plate so you don't overeat simply to "get your money's worth."

FAST-FOOD RESTAURANTS

A favorite topic for food columnists, consumer advocates, and nutritionists is fast-food restaurants. They are also a favorite of the average U.S. family. People in this country spend over $47 billion a year in these restaurants and derive 10–15 percent of their total nutrition from them.

Fast-food restaurants, in general, have the reputation for serving food that is high in calories and low in nutritional value. While the food these restaurants serve does indeed contain nutrients, many items may, in fact, be *too* rich in certain nutrients, such as cholesterol, salt, and sugar.

The good news is that these meals may be more than adequate in protein, some of the B vitamins, and iron. Some of the fast-food chains are now responding to an increasingly nutrition conscious public. For instance:

- Some are switching from lard to vegetable oil for frying certain foods. The percentage of vegetable oil used is important, but the percentage of saturated fats in these oils is equally important.

- More fast-food establishments now feature salad bars, plain baked potatoes, grilled chicken sandwiches on whole grain buns, and leaner cuts of meat.

- Some restaurants make nutrition information available by putting ingredient information on their menus.

Fast foods tend to be short on fresh fruits and vegetables, and are low in calcium, although calcium can be obtained in shakes and milk. Pizza is a fast-food exception. It contains grains, meat, vegetables, and cheese, which represent four of the food groups. Pizza is often only about 25 percent fat, most of which comes from the crust. Overall, studies have shown pizza to be highly nutritious.

Fast-food restaurants can be economical while providing a healthy diet. If we select our food carefully and balance it with the rest of our daily intake such as snacks of fresh fruit and yogurt, a fast-food lunch or dinner may offer a reasonable alternative to home cooking or expensive restaurants (see Table 9.10).

CHECKPOINT

1. List some of the advantages of home cooking.

2. Why should people with high blood pressure be careful when eating frozen foods and dinners?

3. Give some pros and cons of snacking.

4. How can fast-food meals be nutritionally sound?

FOOD SAFETY

People are increasingly concerned about food safety, and matters such as food-borne illnesses, environmental contaminants, natural toxicants in foods, pesticides, and food additives. Moving the food from the field to processors, stores, and onto your table requires a vast network. Public agencies monitor this huge network. The Food and Drug Administration (FDA) works within the Public Health Service to ensure the safety and wholesomeness of foods sold in interstate commerce, except meat, poultry, and eggs, which is checked by the U.S. Department of Agriculture (USDA). The Environmental Protection Agency (EPA) monitors pesticides and water quality, and the Centers for Disease Control (CDC) looks for food-borne diseases. Beyond all of this, you as a food consumer can help by knowing about kinds of foods, food risks, and ways of avoiding them.

NATURAL AND ORGANIC FOODS

Terms used in referring to *natural* and *organic* foods are applied in various ways, since there are no federal guidelines as to what these terms mean. *Natural foods* may refer to unprocessed foods or it may mean that no synthetic fertilizers or pesticides were used while they were grown. If the product has been processed, natural food connotes that no artificial substances were added. *Organically* grown foods generally refers to foods grown without use of pesticides or synthetic fertilizers.

An increasing number of farmers are using organic farming methods for raising crops and livestock. Such farming uses only organic fertilizers such as animal manure, compost, and legumes, and also uses natural pest control. Pest control without use of pesticides may be successful through use of integrated pest management, which includes use of crop rotation, planting two or more different crops in alternate rows or strips, adjusting planting times, removing debris in which pests breed, and interfering with insect mating and life cycles by introducing insect predators, such as lady bugs. Organic farming as a practical option to conventional agriculture is more than a novel idea. Organic farming produces crop yields comparable to nonorganic farming, and the net financial returns are compatible; also organic farming

Table 9.10
Fast-food Facts

	Serving Size (wt in gms)	Calories (1 serving)	Carbohydrates (gm)	Protein (gm)	Fat (gm)	Sodium (mg)
Arby's						
Roast beef sandwich (regular)	147	353	32	22	15	588
Jr. Roast beef sandwich	86	218	22	12	8	345
Ham and cheese sandwich	156	292	19	23	14	1350
Beef 'n Cheddar	197	455	28	26	27	955
Jamocha milkshake	326	368	59	9	10	262
Kentucky Fried Chicken						
Original dinner (2 pcs, dark, mashed potatoes, gravy, cole slaw, buttermilk biscuit)	556	1157	110	41	60	2962
Extra crispy dinner (same combination)	615	1314	115	44	74	3093
Long John Silver's						
Fish/fries meal (3 pcs.)	350	853	64	43	48	2025
Seafood platter	410	976	85	29	58	2161
Shrimp dinner, batter fried	300	711	60	17	45	1297
Seafood salad	480	426	22	19	30	1086
McDonald's						
Big Mac	215	500	42	25	26	890
Quarter pounder (with cheese)	194	510	34	28	28	1110
Filet-o-fish	142	373	38	14	18	735
French fries, small	68	220	26	3	12	110
Egg McMuffin	138	286	29	18	11	726
Low-fat sundae, hot caramel	168	270	59	7	3	180
Pizza Hut						
Thin 'n crispy cheese pizza (2 pcs)	148	398	37	28	17	986
Pan pizza, pepperoni (2 pcs)	211	540	62	29	22	1127
Taco Bell						
Burrito (beef, beans, red sauce)	191	393	44	17	15	1095
Taco	78	183	11	10	11	276
Tostada (with red sauce)	156	243	27	9	11	596
Wendy's						
Big Classic hamburger	241	470	36	26	25	900
Cheeseburger, bacon	147	460	23	29	28	860

Source: Whitney, E., and Rolfes, S. Understanding Nutrition, 6th ed. St. Paul, MN: West, 1993.

requires about 40 percent less energy per unit of food produced than conventional agriculture. The U.S. Department of Agriculture indicates that a total shift to organic methods of farming in the United States could continue to meet our domestic food needs.[60]

Any hope for an early agreement on a complete shift to organic farming in this country is unrealistic. Food buying preferences change slowly, and people select organically or nonorganically grown food for varying personal and technical reasons.

FOOD ALLERGIES

Behavioral and physical problems, especially in children, are sometimes blamed on food allergies. A true **food allergy** (a hypersensitivity response) is a reaction that occurs shortly after a person has eaten a certain food. In such a response, the reaction commonly occurs within minutes, but may not show up for several hours. The person may break out in a rash, become nauseated, vomit, have trouble breathing, turn blue, become convulsive, or collapse. In severe cases, death may occur unless emergency treatment is received.

The reaction is created when some food protein or other large molecule enters the blood circulation, which leads to a reaction by the person's immune system. Normally, large molecules are broken down into smaller ones in the digestive tract and absorbed uneventfully. In an allergy reaction, the person's immune system responds the way it would to an antigen, such as bacteria, poisons, or foreign blood cells. The body responds by producing antibodies, histamines, or other defensive agents.

In a true food allergy the person will always produce antibodies, but may or may not display symptoms. If a person displays symptoms without producing antibodies, he or she is displaying a *food intolerance,* such as to the monosodium glutamate (MSG) often found in Chinese food. Only a physician can test for and identify a true food allergy.

Various foods can cause allergies. Foods that commonly cause allergic reactions include nuts, eggs, milk, and soy. Allergies to peanuts, chicken, fish, and shellfish are also widespread. Parents are advised to be alert to food dislikes in their children, especially with toddlers and when a new food is introduced into their diet. Food aversions may be whims, or they may indeed be a reaction to a substance the child cannot handle.

FOOD ADDITIVES

Natural or synthetic substances that are added to processed foods to retard spoilage, provide missing nutrients, or to enhance flavor, color, or texture are called **food additives.** The regulation of food additives is in the hands of the FDA. For a food manufacturer to receive approval from the FDA, the additive must be:

- effective (do what it is supposed to do),
- detectable and measurable in the final product, and
- safe when fed in large doses to animals.

Approval is given for additives specific to a particular food preparation, for a limited period of time, and is subject to periodic review.

When the FDA established regulations for food additives in 1958, those substances already in use, for which no hazards were known at the time, were put on a GRAS (Generally Regarded As Safe) list, and exempted from complying with the procedure. Any substance on the GRAS list is subject to evaluation at any time if there is scientific or public question about it.

Additives are allowed in foods if their benefits outweigh the risks, and make the risks worth taking. The manufacturer is responsible for adding only as much additive as is necessary to achieve the desired effect.

Intentional food additives are substances put into foods to give a desirable color, flavor, texture, stability, nutritional value, or resistance to spoilage. Some drawing public attention include the following:

- *artificial colors:* used to make foods look pretty, such as beta-carotenes added to color margarine or cheese[61];
- *artificial flavors and flavor enhancers:* the largest single group of food additives includes the well-known additive monosodium glutamate (MSG);
- *antimicrobial agents:* added to keep food from going bad through spoilage or loss of attractiveness, such as salt used with meat and fish, sugars with jellies and jams, or nitrites used to preserve the color of hot dogs;
- *antioxidants:* to keep food from oxidative discoloration or change in flavor, such as Vitamin E to bacon, or BHA and BHT to pre-

food allergy allergic reaction resulting from ingestion of foods to which a person has become sensitized.

food additives natural or synthetic substances that are added to processed foods to retard spoilage, provide missing nutrients, or to enhance flavor, color, or texture.

vent rancidity in baked goods and snack foods[62];

- *nutrient additives:* to improve or maintain the nutritional value of foods, such as iodine added to salt, vitamins A and D added to dairy products, and nutrients to breakfast cereals[63];

- *radiation:* used as an alternative to chemical additives to kill microorganisms and insect pests, extend refrigerated shelf life, and delay some fruit ripening, such as the radiation of pork to kill the parasitic trichinella worm. Although the irradiation of food never makes it radioactive, all food so treated must bear a label identifying it as being so treated.[64]

Incidental food additives are accidental additives found in food as a consequence of some phase of harvesting, processing, or packaging. Bits of papers, plastic, tin, or chemicals used in processing may find their way into foods. Incidents of such adverse effects in processed foods are rare.

NUTRITION AND AGING

While many nutrient needs of the elderly are the same as for the young, several aspects deserve special emphasis. Energy needs decrease with advancing years. This is because the number of active cells in each organ decreases, reducing the body's overall metabolic rate. In addition, older people tend to be less active physically.

Calorie intake may be a little less for an older person, yet must be adequate. Consuming too few calories can cause protein-calorie malnutrition, resulting in muscle wasting and weakness. At the same time, foods that provide calories only (empty calories) such as sugar, sweets, fats, oils, or alcohol should be carefully controlled.

To maintain good health in later years, regular exercise is necessary. The exercise should be intense enough to increase heartbeat and respiration rate, and to prevent muscle atrophy. Even modest exercise can improve cardiovascular and respiratory function and promote muscle tone, while controlling the accumulation of body fat.

Older adults have the same protein needs as younger adults. But as overall food intake is reduced, an older person must get this protein from less food. To avoid using protein for energy needs rather than for building and replacing tissue, ample complex carbohydrates must be included in the diet.

The fat in the older person's diet should be limited. Reduced fat intake helps cut calories and may curb the development of atherosclerosis, cancer, arthritis, and other degenerative diseases. About 20 percent of the calories eaten may come from fat, half of which should come from unsaturated fats.[65]

As already indicated, foods containing complex carbohydrates should be emphasized in the older person's diet. Complex carbohydrates contribute a wide array of vitamins, minerals, and fiber. Fiber intake should be emphasized through the increased intake of fruits, vegetables, and whole grain cereals. These foods help in preventing constipation and keeping cholesterol levels down.

At any age, adequate vitamin intake can be assured by eating foods from all of the food groups. Older adults, however, frequently bypass vegetables and fruit. Some do not drink milk (thus risking Vitamin D deficiency) or do not eat whole grain breads or cereals (thus losing a source of B vitamins). Many older people tend to eat processed or convenience foods, in which Vitamin E is destroyed by heat processing and oxidation.[66] Frequent laxative use may speed food movement through the digestive system, reducing the time during which vitamins can be absorbed by the body. And prescription and over-the-counter drugs regularly taken by older people may also cause vitamin deficiencies.

It is essential that older people consume enough minerals. Iron deficiency is common due to reduced intake and poor absorption. Iron may also be lost through hemorrhaging of ulcers and hemorrhoids, as well as through the use of antacids and arthritis medications. Zinc deficiency may slow wound healing. Calcium intake is necessary to offset bone deterioration, such as occurs in osteoporosis. The use of alcohol impairs calcium absorption, as does the use of some medications. The use of alcohol and medications at the same time may severely increase calcium deficiency.[67] To obtain the necessary variety and amount of minerals, food from each food group should be eaten daily.

And finally, water is very important. Older persons may need to be reminded to drink enough fluids. Six to eight glasses of liquid a day, be it water and/or fruit juices, is preferable.

CHECKPOINT

1. In what ways does a naturally grown food differ from an organically grown one?

2. What is a true food allergy?

3. List the intentional types of food additives.

4. What dietary changes should a person make as he or she grows older?

SUMMARY

No food by itself is good or bad. All foods have some nutritional value; yet none by itself is the perfect food. More important than the kind of food you eat is how much you eat, when you eat it, and the combinations of foods you eat. Proper nutrition allows the body to reach its maximum genetic potential.

The dietary standard in the United States is the Recommended Dietary Allowance. The RDA sets standards for males and females of different ages. A generalized recommendation used in nutrition labeling is the Daily Food Guide.

Food supplies essential nutrients your body needs for energy and for building and maintaining body tissues. Energy content in foods is measured in calories. Of the six major nutrients, three supply energy (carbohydrates, fats, protein), and three do not (vitamins, minerals, water). The primary energy foods are carbohydrates and fats (lipids).

The key to a nutritious diet is to get adequate amounts of nutrients from a variety of foods. The Daily Food Guide plan helps you organize your eating on a daily basis. The six food groups include grain products, vegetables, fruits, milk and milk products, meats and meat alternates, and a miscellaneous group (salad dressings, oils, cakes, etc.).

Your food styles reflect your life-style. Whether you prefer home cooking, frozen dinners, snacking, dining out, or fast-food restaurants, it is important that you be alert to food preparation excesses and lack of balance in nutrients so that you can maintain a healthful, balanced diet.

REFERENCES

1. Whitney, E., and Rolfes, S. *Understanding Nutrition,* 6th ed. Minneapolis: West, 1993.
2. Tortora, G., and Grabowski, S. *Principles of Anatomy and Physiology,* 7th ed. New York: HarperCollins, 1993.
3. Whitney, op. cit.
4. National Research Council. *Recommended Dietary Allowances,* 10th ed. Washington, DC: National Academy Press, 1989.
5. Yetiv, J. *Popular Nutritional Practices: A Scientific Appraisal.* Toledo, OH: Popular Medicine Press, 1986.
6. Ibid.
7. Drucker, D. "Sweetening Agents in Food, Drinks, and Medicine: Carcinogenic Potential and Adverse Effects." *Journal of Human Nutrition* 33 (1979), 114–124.
8. Lecos, C. "The Sweet and Sour History of Saccharin, Cyclamate, and Aspartame." *FDA Consumer* (September 1981), 8–11.
9. Council on Scientific Affairs, American Medical Association. "Saccharin: Review of Safety Issues." *JAMA* 254 (1985), 2622–2624.
10. Whitney, op. cit.
11. Mattson, F. "A Changing Role for Dietary Monounsaturated Fatty Acids." *Journal of the American Dietetic Association* 89 (1989), 387–391.
12. Bingham, S. "Meat, Starch, and Nonstarch Polysaccharides and Large Bowel Cancer." *American Journal of Clinical Nutrition* 48 (1988), 762–776.
13. Grosvenor, M. "Diet and Colon Cancer." *Nutrition and the M.D.* (April 1989).
14. Whitney, op. cit.
15. "NIH Consensus Development Conference Statement: Lowering Blood Cholesterol to Prevent HD." *JAMA* 253 (1985), 2080.
16. Whitney, op. cit.
17. Ibid.
18. Ibid.
19. Ibid.
20. Yetiv, op. cit.
21. Ibid.
22. Heber, D., et al. "Foods vs. Pills vs. Fortified Foods." *Dairy Council Digest* (March–April 1987).
23. Ibid.
24. Whitney, op. cit.
25. Wright, H., et al. "The 1987–88 Nationwide Food Consumption Survey: An Update on the Nutrient Intake of Respondents." *Nutrition Today* (May/June 1991), 21–27.
26. Matles, R. "Discretionary Salt Use." *American Journal of Clinical Nutrition* 51 (1990), 519.
27. Miller, R. "Diet, Exercise and Other Keys to a Healthy Heart." *FDA Consumer* (February 1986), 8–13.
28. Tortora, op. cit.
29. Miller, op. cit.
30. Tortora, op. cit.
31. Whitney, op. cit.
32. Avioli, L. "Calcium and Osteoporosis." *Annual Review of Nutrition* 4 (1984), 471–491.

33. Halioua, L., and Anderson, L. "Lifetime Calcium Intake and Physical Activity Habits: Independent and Combined Effects in the Radial Bone of Healthy Menopausal Caucasian Women." *American Journal of Clinical Nutrition* 49 (1989), 534–541.
34. Stare, F., and McWilliams, M. *Living Nutrition,* 4th ed. New York: Wiley, 1984.
35. Whitney, op. cit.
36. Grosvenor, op. cit.
37. Whitney, op. cit.
38. Ibid.
39. Gorman, C. "The Fight Over Food Labels." *Time* (15 July 1991), 52–55.
40. Cimons, M. "U.S. Boosts Nutrition Data on Food Labels." *Los Angeles Times* (3 December 1992), A-1, 28, 29.
41. Kurtzweil, P. "'Nutrition Facts' To Help Consumers Eat Smart." *FDA Consumer* (May 1993), 22–27.
42. Ibid.
43. Yetiv, op. cit.
44. American Dietetic Association. "Position of the American Dietetic Association: Vegetarian Diets." *Journal of the American Dietetic Association* 88 (1988), 351–355.
45. Whitney, op. cit.
46. Sanders, T. "Growth and Development of British Vegan Children." *American Journal of Clinical Nutrition* 48 (1988), 822–825.
47. Acosta, P. "Availability of Essential Amino Acids and Nitrogen in Vegan Diets." *American Journal of Clinical Nutrition* 48 (1988), 868–874.
48. Whitney, op. cit.
49. Ibid.
50. Ibid.
51. Ibid.
52. Roberts, L. "Diets and Health in China." *Science* 240 (1988), 27.
53. Ibid.
54. Whitney, op. cit.
55. Ibid.
56. Henderson, D. "Nutrition and the Athlete." *FDA Consumer* (May 1987), 18–21.
57. Ibid.
58. Ibid.
59. Dolan, B., and Nash, M. "Searching for Life's Elixir." *Time* (12 December 1988), 62–66.
60. Miller, G. Tyler. *Living in the Environment,* 7th ed. Belmont, CA: Wadsworth, 1992.
61. Whitney, op. cit.
62. Wilkens, W., and Gray J. "Reduce N-nitrosamine Formation in Bacon." *Food Engineering* 548 (1986), 68–69.
63. Shank, F., and Wilkening, V. "Considerations for Food Fortification Policy." *Cereal Food World* 31 (1986), 728–740.
64. Rogan, A., and Glaros, G. "Food Irradiation: the Process and Implications for Dietitians." *Journal of the American Dietetic Association* 887 (1988), 833–838.
65. Whitney, op. cit.
66. Ibid.
67. Ibid.

SUGGESTED READINGS

American Heart Association. *The American Heart Association Cookbook,* 5th ed. New York: Random House, 1991.
Gershoff, S. *The Tufts University Guide to Total Nutrition.* New York: HarperPerennial, 1990.
Grundy, S., and Winston, M. (eds.). *The American Heart Association Low-Fat, Low-Cholesterol Cookbook.* New York: Random House, 1989.
International Life Science Institute. *Present Knowledge on Nutrition,* 6th ed. Washington, DC: International Life Science Institute, Nutrition Foundation, 1990.
Kraus, B. *Calories and Carbohydrates,* 9th rev. ed. New York: Plume, 1991.
McDougal, J. *The McDougal Program.* New York: Plume, 1990.
Margen, S. *The Wellness Encyclopedia of Food and Nutrition.* New York: Random House, 1992.
Monk, A., and Franz, M. *Convenience Food Facts.* Wayzata, MN: Diabetes Center, 1987.
Pennington, J. *Food Values,* 15th ed. New York: HarperPerennial, 1989.
Saltman, P. et al. *The University of California San Diego Nutrition Book.* Boston: Little, Brown, 1993.
Shils, M., and Young, V. (eds.) *Modern Nutrition of Health and Disease,* 7th ed. Philadelphia: Lea and Febiger, 1988.
Somer, E. *Nutrition for Women, The Complete Guide.* New York: Holt, 1993.
Starke, R., and Winston, M. *The American Heart Association Low-Salt Cookbook.* New York: Random House, 1990.
Tanny, M. *Body Building Nutrition.* New York: HarperPerennial, 1991.
U.S. Department of Health and Human Services. *The Surgeon General's Report on Nutrition and Health.* New York: Warner, 1987.
Woteki, C., and Thomas, P. *Eat for Life.* New York: HarperPerennial, 1992.

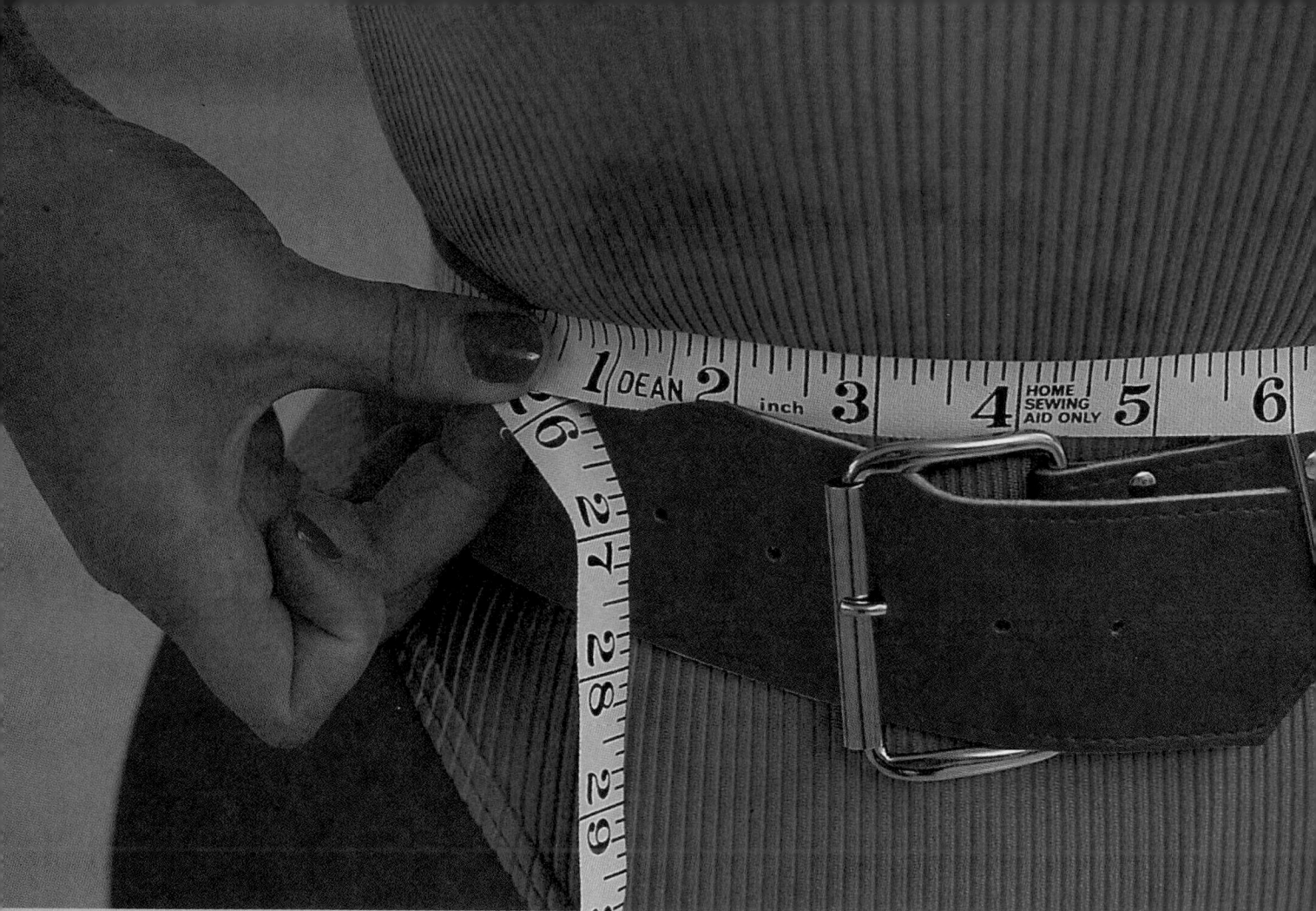

10

WEIGHT MANAGEMENT

CHAPTER OBJECTIVES

Upon completing this chapter, you will be able to:

KNOWLEDGE

- Explain why insurance company height/weight tables are viewed as being biased.
- Identify the percentage body composition of protein, fat, carbohydrate, water, and minerals for the average person.
- Contrast the terms *overweight* and *obesity*.
- Compare the ideal amount of body fat for the average man with that for the average woman.
- Identify some of the health risks of obesity.
- Know why diet fads are to be avoided in any weight-loss program.
- Define a very-low-calorie diet and identify the minimum number of calories needed in any diet plan.
- Determine the differences between an underweight person and an anorexic.
- Define the term *behavior modification*.
- Determine your current eating patterns.

INSIGHT

- From the information presented here, determine your acceptable weight based on the Body Mass Index.
- Discuss the tendency of your parents and relatives to be overweight or obese and determine how this family pattern might affect you.
- Identify the fad diets (if any) that you have used and explain why you could not recommend them.
- Describe your experiences of weight cycling (yo-yoing).

DECISION MAKING

- Determine how you will, as you become older, adjust your food intake to changes in your basal metabolic rate.
- Explain the steps you intend to take, if and when you have children of your own, to help them avoid becoming obese.
- Outline the ways in which exercise might help you in any weight-loss program you undertake.

Oprah Winfrey, actress and talk show host, allowed the world to watch as she learned (the hard way) about successful dieting and weight management. In 1988 she appeared before one of her largest audiences to reveal her new slender figure after losing 67 pounds. Just five months before the show she had begun a 400-calorie-per-day liquid diet administered and supervised by a physician. After the first 12 weeks, the dieter is allowed to begin eating small amounts of solid foods. This liquid diet is only recommended for those who are at least 30 percent heavier than their desirable weight, or at least 50 pounds overweight. She said then, "Every day for the rest of my life is going to be a struggle not to succumb once more to the old buffet table. I am by no means through."

It turns out that she was right. Soon after her acquiring her new look, she began to gain back her old one. She sank steadily into despair as the pounds crept back in the months and years that followed. Then Oprah, about to turn 40, decided to work toward the goal of "healthy-at-40." She gave up the liquid diet *and turned toward a more balanced approach to weight control. This new approach combined reducing calories from fat in her diet and making a habit of regular exercise. Five months into her new exercise and eating regime, she had dropped 60 pounds and was in good enough shape to run a half-marathon. She had learned more about herself, uncovering some of her own eating triggers, such as the fear of not being liked. Now she worries less about whether others like her, and focuses more on maintaining her healthful life-style.*

Many physicians and other experts point to Oprah Winfrey's experiences as evidence that reasonable eating accompanied by regular exercise is the only reliable way to manage weight. Diet plans that do not incorporate these basic principles will not be successful in the long run. These quick-fix diet plans often create a roller-coaster pattern of weight loss and weight gain that has been shown to increase the risk of health problems such as heart disease. Long-term weight control is an important step toward a healthful life-style.

■   ■   ■

For millions of people in the United States, the resolution to lose weight fluctuates somewhere between concern and obsession. After weekend partying, vacation cruises, holiday revelries, or any other event where food is one of the main attractions, we must face up to the bad news reported by the bathroom scale—we weigh too much.

Many of us have a degree of preoccupation with our weight. The results of a recent survey show that almost 90 percent of us perceive of ourselves as weighing too much, and more than one-third want to lose at least 15 pounds. At any one time it's estimated that one-third to one-half of U.S. women, and up to one-fourth of U.S. men, are dieting.[1] Polls indicate that almost one-third of U.S. women, ages 19–39, diet at least once a month, and 16 percent consider themselves as perpetual dieters.[2]

With such acute awareness of our tendency to overeat, we should be a country of thin, fit people, yet, obesity has become the number one nutrition problem in the United States. Approximately 34 million people in the United States are considered by the National Institutes of Health to be obese.[3] Close to one-fifth of American youth are overweight by the time they graduate from high school.

While the proportion of overweight adults increases with age, overweight people are found at all age levels.

People vary widely in size, height, and weight. Some of this variance is beyond our control and depends on our genetically determined structure. Yet, some of our body's size depends on how we treat and feed it, and how much fat it produces.

This chapter discusses the nature of body composition and the relationship of fat to body composition and weight. We will also discuss how we determine a healthy weight, and ways in which we can safely practice weight management.

BODY COMPOSITION

The exact degree of fatness of the body is not simply measured. It depends on the composition of the body, which includes both its fat and nonfat components. The fat component by itself is called the *fat mass* or *percent body fat,* the nonfat component is known as the *lean body mass.* The **body composition** is defined as the ratio of fat to fat-free mass (bone and muscle).

An ideal body composition is one in which there is enough fat to provide for the body's essential needs, yet not enough to create health risks. For the average person the body composition has been determined to be as follows (the weight in parentheses are those for a 150-pound person): *protein,* 18 percent (27 pounds); *fat,* 14 percent (21 pounds); *carbohydrate,* 1 percent (1.5 pounds); *water,* 61 percent (91.5 pounds); and *minerals,* 6 percent (9 pounds).[4]

It used to be thought that an easy and reliable way to determine whether a person was "fat" was to compare that person's weight to those listed on *ideal weight* tables. If the person's weight were 10–20 percent above the listed weight, the person was said to be overweight; if the weight was more than 20 percent above that on the table, the person was judged to be obese.

....

body composition a term used in reference to the fat and nonfat components of the body; the ratio of fat to fat-free (bone and muscle) body mass.

Actually, body weight alone says little about body fatness. When comparing two people whose body weight is the same, but whose activities are far different, there may be a significant difference in fatness. For example, a sedentary person who is physically inactive or an actively dieting person who fails to exercise may be too fat, while an athlete of the same weight might actually be the proper weight. Both physical inactivity and constant dieting lead to loss of lean body mass. Weight alone is a poor indicator of fatness and as a result, today the term *ideal weight* has become obsolete.

Obesity can be determined by using one of several methods for measuring body composition. These methods, from the least accurate to the most precise include: height/weight charts, body mass index, waist-hip ratio, skinfold measurement, hydrostatic weighing, and bioelectrical impedance.

HEIGHT AND WEIGHT

A refinement of weight tables was the development of height/weight tables. Height/weight tables are based on actuarial data collected by insurance companies. In the 1950s a number of insurance companies pooled the data they gained from noting at what age insurees purchased life insurance policies, their weight and height at the time of purchase, and their ages at the time of death. Using such data, the Metropolitan Insurance Company developed its 1983 tables of desirable body weights for each height for adults aged 25–29. These tables show how long people who purchased their life insurance lived, excluding those who had major diseases, such as diabetes, cancer, and heart disease. Because these tables are not based on a representative population for the country, some researchers reject insurance-based tables. A more acceptable table has been developed by the United States Department of Agriculture (USDA) and the Department of Health and Human Services (USDHHS) (Table 10.1).

The best weight tables can do is give a range of weights for a person, rather than one actual body composition. They tell you the quantity of the weight, not its quality. At best, height/weight tables are only gross estimates. Without more precise measurements, you are unable to determine whether you are an "ideal weight."

Table 10.1
Suggested Weights for Adults

Height[a]	Weight (lb)[b]			
	19–34 Years		35 Years and Over	
	Midpoint	Range	Midpoint	Range
5'0"	112	97–128	123	108–138
5'1"	116	101–132	127	111–143
5'2"	120	104–137	131	115–148
5'3"	124	107–141	135	119–152
5'4"	128	111–146	140	122–157
5'5"	132	114–150	144	126–162
5'6"	136	118–155	148	130–167
5'7"	140	121–160	153	134–172
5'8"	144	125–164	158	138–178
5'9"	149	129–169	162	142–183
5'10"	153	132–174	167	146–188
5'11"	157	136–179	172	151–194
6'0"	162	140–184	177	155–199
6'1"	166	144–189	182	159–205
6'2"	171	148–195	187	164–210
6'3"	176	152–200	192	168–216
6'4"	180	156–205	197	173–222
6'5"	185	160–211	202	177–228
6'6"	190	164–216	208	182–234

Note: The higher weights in the ranges generally apply to men, or women with larger frame sizes, who tend to have more muscle and bone; the lower weights more often apply to women, or men with smaller frame sizes, who have less muscle and bone. The higher weights for people aged 35 and older reflects recent research that seems to indicate that people can carry a little more weight as they grow older without added risk to health.
[a]Without shoes.
[b]Without clothes.

Source: U.S. Department of Agriculture and U.S. Department of Health and Human Services. Home and Garden Bulletin No. 232, Nutrition and Your Health: Dietary Guidelines for Americans, 3rd ed. Washington, DC: U.S. Government Printing Office, 1990.

BODY MASS INDEX

Recognizing that height/weight tables have limitations, other measurements of body weight have been devised. One such is the **body mass index (BMI).** The BMI indexes the person's weight to height by dividing the weight by the square of the

body mass index (BMI) indexing a person's weight to height by dividing the weight by the square of the height.

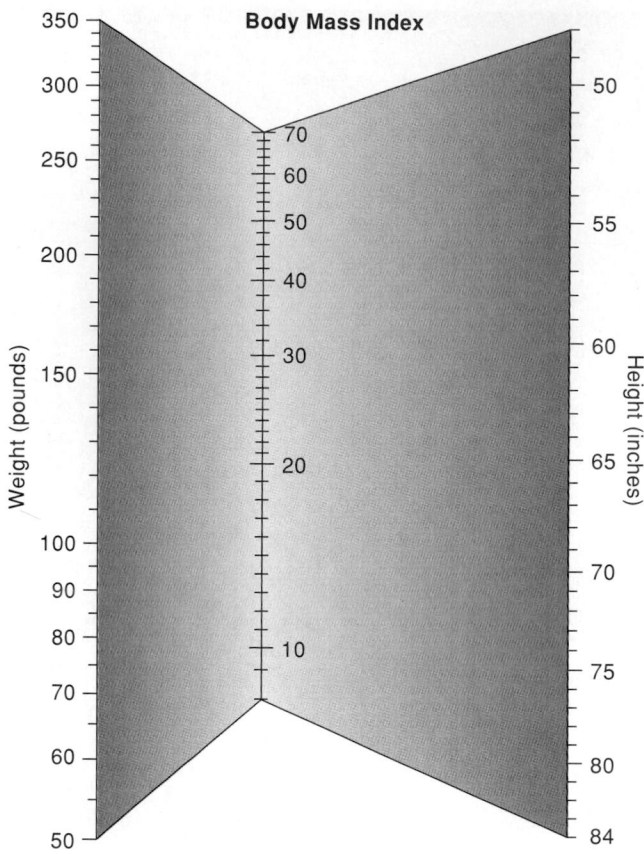

Figure 10.1
Body Mass Index (BMI)

Source: Adapted figure "Lifting Weight Myths" by D. Schardt from Nutrition Action Health Letter, October 1993, p. 819. Copyright © Center for Science in the Public Interest. Adapted from Nutrition Action Healthletter (1875 Connecticut Ave., N.W., Suite 300, Washington, D.C. 20009-5728. $24.00 for 10 issues). Reprinted by permission.

height. You can determine it mathematically by calculating:[5,6]

BMI = weight (lb) × 700 divided by height (in.) divided again by height (in.)

An easier way is to use the Body Mass Index Chart (Figure 10.1).

WAIST-TO-HIP RATIO

The location of body fat has become an important variable in body weight. The sites of fat on the body can be determined easily by measuring the circumference of the waist at its smallest point and the circumference of the hips at their widest point, and then calculating a ratio of the two. Your goal should be to have a waist-to-hip ratio below 0.95 (for women) or 0.85 (for men). The ratio distinguishes the "apples," or people who carry excess weight above the waist, or abdominal fat, from the "pears," or those who carry it around the hips and buttocks. The higher the waist-to-hip ratio, the more apple-shaped the figure.[7]

SKINFOLD THICKNESS

Measurement of body composition is most frequently done by the **skinfold thickness (fatfold) test.** The use of the skinfold as an assessment is based on the principle that about half of the fatty tissue of the body is located directly beneath the skin. The clinician lifts a fold of skin and measures its thickness with a **caliper,** an instrument for measuring the thickness of materials. Since skin fat is not uniformly thick in all body areas, measurements are taken at several body sites and then averaged.

The most common sites for the female are the back of the triceps (back of the upper arm), suprailium (just above the hipbone), and thigh (front outside, midway between the hip and knee). For the male, the most common sites are the chest (just in front of the armpit), the abdomen (an inch to the right of the navel), and the thigh. Readings from the three sites are added together, and this sum is marked on a nomogram. The **nomogram** (*nom'ō-gram*), a graph representing a relationship between numerical variables, converts the sum of the three skinfold measurements into the percent of body fat (see Table 10.2), which can then be used for classifying the degree of excess fat.

HYDROSTATIC WEIGHING

A more precise assessment of body composition is **hydrostatic weighing,** an underwater weighing technique in which the measure of body density, or weight, is compared with volume. Since lean tissue (muscle) is denser than fat tissue, the less

....

skinfold thickness test a method for determining the thickness of fat beneath the skin; also called the fatfold test.

caliper an instrument for measuring the thickness of materials.

nomogram a graph representing the relationship between numerical variables.

hydrostatic weighing underwater weighing technique in which the measure of body density, or weight, is compared with volume.

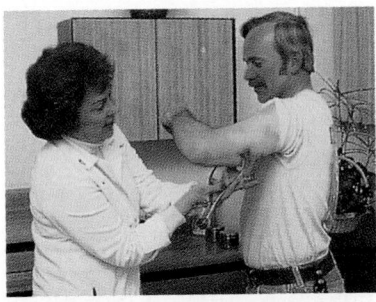

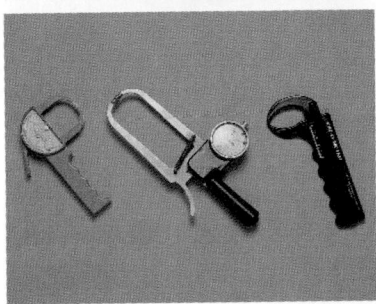

Obesity has become America's number one nutrition problem. Body fat needs to be assessed to determine overfatness. Since fat attached to the skin approximates body fat, the skin fold test is one measure of body fat. Using a caliper, this test measures the relative thickness of a fold of skin at specific locations on the body.

dense a person's body, the more fat it must contain. A person is weighed while being submerged in a tank of water. The amount of water displaced is measured. From the density, the percent of body fat can be calculated. This method requires special equipment and trained technicians and is not readily available except in research centers.

BIOELECTRICAL IMPEDANCE

Bioelectrical impedance is a technique that is fast to use, but requires costly equipment. The person being measured is hooked up to a machine that sends a weak, totally painless, electric current through the body to analyze composition (body fat, lean body mass, and water).

Fat tissue is not as good a conductor of an electric current as lean tissue, thus the leaner the person the easier the conductance. Because of cost, time, and complexity of the test procedure, some fitness centers do not use this method.[8]

A word of caution regarding using body composition assessments: Each of these laboratory assess-

....

bioelectrical impedance a technique in which a weak electric current is run through the body to measure body composition.

Table 10.2
Nomogram to Determine Percentage of Body Fat

Locate and mark your age (left), then locate and mark the sum of your three skin-fold measurements (right). With a ruler, connect these two marks. The point at which this line transects the male or female scale (center) expresses your percentage of body fat.

Percent Body Fat—Classification

	Male	Female
Lean	Less than 8%	Less than 15%
Healthy	8–15%	15–22%
Plump	16–19%	23–27%
Fat	20–24%	28–33%
Obese	Above 24%	Above 33%

Male ————
Chest, abdomen, thigh
Female ————
Triceps, thigh, suprailium

Source: Baun, W., et al. "A Nomogram for the Estimate of Percent Body Fat from Generalized Equations." The Research Quarterly for Exercise and Sport, **52,** *1981, pp. 380–384. Reprinted by permission of the American Alliance for Health, Physical Education, Recreation and Dance, 1900 Association Drive, Reston, VA 22091 and the author, W. Baun.*

ments has an error percentage, and even when administered by a skilled technician, the test results for a given procedure will vary when given and assessed at different times by different technicians. In addition, the test results can be interpreted improperly, such as by people with eating disorders. Most overweight people know they need to lose weight, without having to resort to these assessments.

HEALTHY WEIGHT

Many people continue to use weight as an indication of body fatness. Professional health care providers usually use weight/height tables, which factor in height, gender, and frame size.

Increasingly, however, researchers are speaking in terms of *healthy weight*. According to the *Dietary Guidelines for Americans*, guidelines prepared by the USDA and the USDHHS, a healthy weight can be defined by three criteria.[9]

- a weight within the suggested range for height and age (as seen in Table 10.1)
- a fat distribution pattern not associated with high-risk illness or death
- the absence of any medical condition for which weight loss would be indicated.

If a person meets these criteria, her or his weight can be considered appropriately healthy, and there is little reason to change it. Yet if a person whose weight falls within the listed range has a disease that would benefit from a weight loss, that person may not be at a healthy weight.

At this point you may be anxious to answer the question, "How much should I weigh?" Completing In Your Hands: Choosing a Weight Goal may help provide an answer.

CHECKPOINT

1. Determine your desirable weight according to Table 10.1: Suggested Weights for Adults.

2. Why are insurance company weight tables not viewed as appropriate guides for people to use in determining an approximate weight goal?

3. For what reasons might the desirable weights, as found on the weight chart, not be the exact desirable weight for everyone of a given age and height? ✔

OVERWEIGHT VS. OBESITY

There are varying degrees of being overweight. An **overweight** person may be defined technically as one who weighs more than the suggested weight, using the insurance tables. This is widely determined by comparing body weight with life insurance height/weight tables. Using these, a weight 10–20 percent above that listed in the tables is overweight, and obesity is a weight more than 20 percent above the one listed. Underweight is 10 percent below the weight listed.[10]

Being overweight, by itself, may not identify excess body fat. Weight that exceeds desirable weight may be primarily lean tissue, such as muscle and bone. A 240-pound weight lifter or football player would be considered overweight according to the weight tables, but his body fat is likely low. Yet, a sedentary executive secretary might be "just right" according to the tables and still be "overfat." At some point either too much extra muscle mass or too much extra body fat can be unhealthy.

THE BODY FAT "IDEAL"

A certain amount of body fat is essential. Fat serves as an integral part of cell membranes, nerve tissue, and bone; it helps protect and pad internal organs, such as the kidneys and liver; and makes it more comfortable for sitting, lying down, and keeping warm.

A person's ability to maintain **homeostasis** (*hō-mē-ō-stā'sis*), or equilibrium of the body's internal environment, is threatened if he or she loses too much of any of the body components. Loss of more than 10 percent water, 11 percent protein, 33 percent mineral content, 40 percent carbohydrate, or 90 percent body fat threatens the body's ability to maintain homeostasis.[11] Sports physicians recommend an absolute minimum of 3–7 percent body fat for adult males and a minimum of 10–20 percent for adult females. Any fat beyond this is seen as storage fat. The extra body fat allowed for females is considered "sex-specific" fat and relates to a female's functional and anatomical childbearing needs.[12, 13] For both males and females, some

overweight any weight above table weight, some specify 10–20 percent above.

homeostasis equilibrium of the internal environment of the body.

CHOOSING A WEIGHT GOAL

What is an appropriate weight for you? When physical health alone is considered, a wide range of weights is acceptable for a person of a given height. Within the safe range, the definition of appropriate weight is up to the individual, depending on factors such as family history, occupation, physical and recreational activities, and personal preferences.

1. Determine the safe range for a person your height and sex.
   a. Record your height: _____ ft. _____ inches.
   b. Look up the acceptable weight range for a person your height and age in Table 10.1. Record the entire range: _____ to _____ lb.

2. If your weight is below the bottom end of this safe range, you need to gain weight for your health's sake. If your weight is above the top end of the range, check your health history for further confirmation. A family or personal medical history of diabetes (non-insulin-dependent type), hypertension, or high blood cholesterol indicates the need for weight loss.

3. Choose a goal weight within the acceptable range. Answering the following questions should help you to determine where, within the safe range, your personal appropriate weight may be:
   a. Does your occupation demand that you have a certain body shape? If so, record the weight, within the safe range, that would most nearly approximate this body shape: _____ lb.
   b. Do you engage in a sport or other physical activity that requires a particular body weight for optimal performance? Consult your instructor or other expert in that sport or activity, and record the weight recommended on that basis: _____ lb.
   c. Do you hope to start a pregnancy soon? If so, consult your health care provider about the healthy weight with which to begin a pregnancy: _____ lb.

4. Based on all of these considerations, choose a final goal weight. No formula exists for this estimate, but don't choose a weight outside the acceptable range without a professional assessment.

   Your goal weight:_____ lb.

5. Diets can be planned using the exchange system to gain weight, lose weight, or stay the same. For practice in the use of this convenient system, try planning two diets, one for weight maintenance or gain, the other for weight loss.

storage fat is recommended. The optimal body fat (minimum plus storage) is 12–18 percent for adult males and 18–24 percent for adult females.[14]

OBESITY

A male who has 23 percent body fat has at least 5 percent excess fat. If he weighs 150 pounds, this would amount to 7½ pounds of excess fat. Some males would consider a lower percentage of body fat or a higher percentage as ideal depending on whether they were sprinters or offensive linemen. Using 18 percent body fat as an allowable limit for males and 24 percent for females, excess storage fat beyond these limits is **obesity.**[15] (See Table 10.3, p. 304.)

....

obesity excess storage fat.

OBESITY AND HEALTH

As stated earlier, the most important basis for an acceptable weight is the condition of your health. The ideal is to have enough fat to meet your body's basic needs without developing health risks. Health problems have been found to develop when body fat exceeds 22 percent in younger men, 25 percent in older men, 32 percent in younger women, and 35 percent in older women. In terms of a health definition, these values also help define obesity.[16]

   The health risk indicators that can rise and fall with body fatness include blood glucose, blood cholesterol, and blood pressure. Heart attack, stroke, and complications of Type II diabetes are responsible for earlier deaths among obese people. The location of the fat around the body may indicate greater risk (see Figure 10.2, p. 308). Abdomi-

Table 10.3
Body Fat and Classification

This table is based on 18 percent allowable body fat for males and 24 percent for females. Body fat beyond these percentages is considered excessive.

Males	Females	Classification
21–23%	27–29%	Slightly obese
24–29%	30–34%	Moderately obese
30–34%	35–39%	Obese
35%	40%	Very obese

Source: Johnson, P. and Mallon, T. Fitness and You. New York. Copyright © 1988 by Saunders College Publishing. Reprinted by permission of the publisher.

nal (belly) fat can increase five- to tenfold the risks of heart disease, stroke, diabetes, and premature death. Abdominal fat, which is more common in males, is more easily broken down and carried to the liver, where it may lead to dangerous elevations in blood fat and insulin levels.[17] Fat around the hips and thighs (more common in women) does not carry the same risks. In fact, a comparison of the waist-to-hip measurements is becoming a standard part of body fatness assessments.[18]

Related to problems of obesity are the risks of improper dieting. Fad dieting is frequently not only poorly advised, but may actually be hazardous (see Fad Diets, p. 311). The prevention of obesity is the ideal. Where prevention has failed, treatment should be started. Obesity carries identifiable physical hazards, yet it can be corrected. With medical supervision dieting can be both safe and effective.

CHECKPOINT

1. What functions does fat serve in the body?

2. How does obesity differ from overweight?

3. Describe two methods for assessing excess fat. Which method is considered to be the most accurate?

4. What is homeostasis?

5. Which nutrient can you lose the most of before upsetting your homeostasis: protein, fat, carbohydrate, water, or minerals?

CAUSES OF OBESITY

Researchers have tried to identify factors that will explain why people become obese, yet many questions remain unanswered. Why can some people seem to eat and never gain weight, while others perpetually diet and retain their fat? Factors considered when explaining these differences can be broken down into two categories: the physiological reaction to food, which is controlled by metabolism and genetic makeup; and environmental pressure, which includes psychological, social, and cultural factors.

GENETIC FACTORS

A genetic predisposition is now believed to play the most important part in determining a person's body weight and body composition. It is observed, for example, that adopted children's distribution of fat and the size of their fat cells is more similar to that of their biological parents than to that of their adoptive parents.[19] It is also found that if both of your parents are obese your risk of becoming obese is about 80 percent. If both parents are lean, the risk of becoming obese is less than 10 percent.[20]

To separate the effects of genetic and environmental factors on body weight and body composition, researchers have studied identical twins. In one study, 600 pairs of identical and fraternal twins were studied (identical twins are alike genetically; fraternal twins are alike genetically only in the same way as brothers and sisters). Whether reared together or apart, identical twins were twice as likely to have similar weights than were fraternal twins, supporting the conclusion that genetics is the most important factor in determining a person's weight.[21]

In another study of identical twins, there was evidence some people have a genetic tendency to gain more weight than others with the same amount of food intake. When fed 1000 extra calories daily for 100 days, some twins gained more than three times as many extra pounds as others. Further, the amount of weight gain was similar between each pair of twins, suggesting a genetic basis for the amount of weight gain.[22]

Set-point Theory

Within the body are a number of internal physiological variables, such as blood glucose, blood pH, and body temperature, which are maintained within certain limits. It is proposed that these factors have an effect on body weight. According to the **set-point** theory, the body has a certain amount of fat that it is "biologically set," or programmed, to carry. This is the weight the body *wants* to weigh. This set-point may be a weight different from some "ideal" weight. If so, the person who seeks to *lose* or *gain* more or less weight than the body *wants* may not succeed in his or her effort.

The body may *defend* its set-point by increasing or decreasing appetite by speeding up or slowing down its metabolic rate. This way the body expends more or fewer calories, depending on how much energy from food it receives.

Initially, the level of the set-point may be determined largely by genes. Exercise may lower the set-point, which makes it possible for the body to settle on a lower level of fatness. Dieting seems to have little effect on adjusting the set-point.[23] When dieting displaces someone from a set-point, a whole series of physical forces fight that displacement, which makes it possible to regain (or lose) that weight more efficiently.

The concept of a set-point is theoretical. No one has yet been able to determine the biological mechanisms that may make it work; yet there is a belief among researchers that fatness may be regulated by the body in this way.

Fat as a Fattening Agent

Some people have a tendency to store fat. In fact, some people grow more obese even while reducing their total energy food intake. A major factor in the determination of body weight is the intake and expenditure of fats and carbohydrates, whereas proteins play only a minor role. It may not be surprising that people who get more of their calories from a higher-fat diet gain more weight than people who get fewer of their calories from fat. For instance, drinking whole milk versus nonfat milk leads to greater weight gain. Of particular interest is the part played by dietary carbohydrate. In one study, it was found that regardless of the amount of fat in the diet, the determining factor in dietary satisfaction was the intake of carbohydrate. If fed a

higher-fat, lower-carbohydrate diet, persons ate more food (and calories) than on a lower-fat, higher-carbohydrate diet. In either case, reaching a satisfying level of carbohydrate intake appeared to be the critical issue.[24]

As to why high-fat diets lead to more fatness in body composition, the body appears to either store fat more efficiently than it does carbohydrates, or use the fat less efficiently. It costs the body only 3 percent of ingested energy to store dietary fat, whereas it costs the body 23 percent of ingested energy to store the same amount of carbohydrate. It is also known that the body stores less carbohydrate than fat. The body's fat reserves exceed the body's carbohydrate reserves by about 100-fold.[25]

Fat-cell Metabolism

Another cause of obesity may relate to the enzyme lipoprotein lipase (LPL). Both fat cells and muscle cells produce LPL to assist them in storing energy as fat. Obese people have more LPL activity in their fat cells than do lean people.[26] LPL activity appears to be regulated to some degree by gender-specific hormones, such as testosterone in men and estrogen in women. In men, fat cells in the abdomen produce more LPL, explaining why men often develop "pot bellies." In women, abundant LPL is produced in the breasts, hips, and thighs, causing fat to accumulate in those body locations.

Weight loss in a person affects LPL activity, and may explain why weight is regained so easily.[27] In a study it was found that people who are fatter before weight loss regain more LPL afterward, perhaps explaining why it's easy for a previously fat person to regain weight after having successfully lost it, and why repeated attempts at weight loss are so difficult and often futile. The activity of LPL levels may suggest that people have a predetermined weight level, and that even after a weight loss, the body resets its set-point.

Metabolic Rate and Exercise

There are two major components of energy output: metabolic processes and voluntary activities. The total energy a person spends is the total of these two processes.

Metabolism is the sum of all chemical reactions that occur in the body. Those functions that sustain life, such as heartbeat, breathing, body tempera-

....

set-point the concept that there is a point at which the body's weight is set.

ture, and kidney action constitute **basal metabolism.** The **basal metabolic rate (BMR)** is the measure of the number of calories your body uses each day to take care of these needs. The energy needs for basal metabolism must be met before energy is expended for any voluntary physical activities, such as exercising. At least two-thirds of the calories a person ingests are used for these basic functions.[28] The BMR is higher in people with more lean body mass (growing children, pregnant women, and males), people who are tall for their weight, and people under stress or with a fever. The BMR is lowered by less lean body mass, inactivity, fasting, and malnutrition.

The second factor in energy expenditure is voluntary physical activity involving skeletal muscles. The greater the number of muscles involved, the intensity of use, and the length of time they are used all determine the total amount of energy expenditure. The heavier a person, the more effort it takes to move and the more energy is used up by moving. The energy expenditure is also higher for a person undertaking a physical conditioning program. Regular vigorous physical activity leads to the development of more lean tissue, and lean body tissue is more metabolically active than fat tissue. Yet even on a given day, basal metabolism remains elevated for several hours following intense and prolonged exercise.[29] Basal metabolism is influenced by a person's age, sex, height, and muscle mass. As a person gets older, his or her basal metabolism drops about 2 percent per decade.

Some glandular secretions, such as the adrenal hormone epinephrine, cause the body to increase its metabolic rate. This hormone is often secreted in response to stress, which can explain why some people lose weight during stressful periods in their lives.

EXTERNAL FACTORS

The **external cue** theory holds that environmental cues prompt us to eat. This means that rather than

basal metabolism the basic body functions that maintain life.

basal metabolic rate (BMR) the measure of the number of calories the body needs for basal metabolism.

external cue an environmental factor that prompts us to eat.

relying on internal physical hunger cues, we respond to the sight, color, and availability of food or to the time of day when we are programmed to eat. This is further complicated by the fact that food is available around the clock—at home, at work, in restaurants and grocery stores (some restaurants even offer home delivery!).

Other factors that may contribute to people's attitudes toward food are the way in which individual families perceive food. Some families are "food-centered," which means they tend to overeat at mealtime, eat rapidly, snack excessively, eat for reasons other than hunger, or eat until all their dishes are empty. Unwittingly, family members may become involved as *codependents* in the exercise of overeating, and serve as *enablers* for a person whose eating habits are out of control (see Chapter 14 for a discussion of codependency). Overeating by children may be an imitation of overeating by parents. Obese children, over a given time interval, tend to take more bites of food and chew their food less thoroughly than nonobese children.[30] Some parents preach the "clean plate ethic" by which they praise their children for eating all the food on their plates as a token of thanks for having enough food to eat.

Some people eat in response to stress, boredom, insecurity, anxiety, loneliness, or as reward for being good. Parents who console a child with food may be initiating a life-long behavior pattern. Some people use food as an inappropriate response to psychological stimuli. As you experience pain, anxiety, insecurity, stress, arousal, or excitement, the brain responds by producing substances that soothe pain and lessen arousal. Another effect of these substances is that they enhance appetite for food and reduce activity.[31] If, in addition, you are unusually sensitive to stress, you are likely to eat to compensate for stress, whether negative or positive. Eating may be an appropriate response to all of these stimuli on occasion, but the person who uses them to overeat creates a whole new set of emotional problems relating to his or her overeating. They may get caught in a vicious cycle—depression causing overeating and vice versa.

Exacerbating the effect of external factors on eating habits is the tendency of many people to underexercise. In this age of automation, everything can be done with the press of a button—opening the garage door, turning the television on and off, and riding elevators. With such conveniences available, the temptation to remain sedentary may be overpowering, leading to underactivity. With reduced physical activity and with sustained or increased amounts of food intake, weight gain is bound to occur.

CHECKPOINT

1. List several reasons why people become obese.

2. Why might an adopted child be more like his or her biological parents than adoptive parents in a predisposition to become obese?

3. Explain what is meant by the set-point theory.

4. Define the term *basal metabolism.*

5. What are the external cues that may prompt a person to eat?

FAT CELLS AND THE ONSET OF OBESITY

The body is composed of many kinds of cells, such as muscle, bone, nerve, and fat. Most of the space inside a fat or adipose cell is filled with triglycerides; its nucleus and other cell components are squeezed into a small area. Active in storing unused fat in the body, fat cells are able to expand considerably as they store triglycerides. The fat cells in an obese person may be 100 times as large as those in a thin person.[32]

The total amount of fat in the body depends on two factors: the *number* and the *size* of fat cells (Figure 10.2). The degree of a person's fatness depends on how many of these cells a person has and how full the cells are. When we eat more energy foods than we use, we accumulate fat, which fills and expands the individual cells. When we use up more energy than we take in, these cells shrink, although their number remains the same. Every calorie eaten must be either burned or stored.

There are two forms of obesity: **juvenile-onset obesity** and **adult-onset obesity.**

......

juvenile-onset obesity obesity arising in childhood and/or adolescence.

adult-onset obesity obesity arising after adolescence.

JUVENILE-ONSET OBESITY

Growth in the body occurs mainly during the period from before birth through adolescence. Growth is especially rapid during the last three months of fetal development, the first three years of childhood, and adolescence. During growth the body has the potential for an excess accumulation of fat cells. Obesity that starts during childhood and adolescence results in a significantly greater number of fat cells than in a nonobese person.[33] The increased number of fat cells makes it difficult to lose weight as an adult and thus maintain a proper weight, and easier to later regain excessive weight previously lost. Diet and exercise help reduce the *size* of fat cells, but once established, do not change the *number* of fat cells.

ADULT-ONSET OBESITY

Obesity that occurs in adults is mainly the result of an increase in the size of fat cells. People who show adult-onset obesity may find it easier to lose weight and to maintain a proper weight, since the adult-onset person may have fewer fat cells than a juvenile-onset person.

Yet, even fat gain during adulthood may be hard to lose. When fat cells enlarge, they respond more slowly to insulin, even though insulin levels may be high. As a result, excess glucose stays in the bloodstream longer, which in turn stimulates the pancreas to produce even more insulin.[34] These elevated insulin levels finally get the fat cells to respond, but the fat cells then store more than the normal fat levels. Weight loss can reverse insulin levels to normal, but it requires great effort.

CHECKPOINT

1. On what two factors does the total amount of fat in the body depend?

2. Explain the difference between juvenile-onset and adult-onset obesity.

HAZARDS OF OBESITY

Of the ten leading causes of death in the United States, four of them (including the top three), are related to diet.[35] These four conditions, which

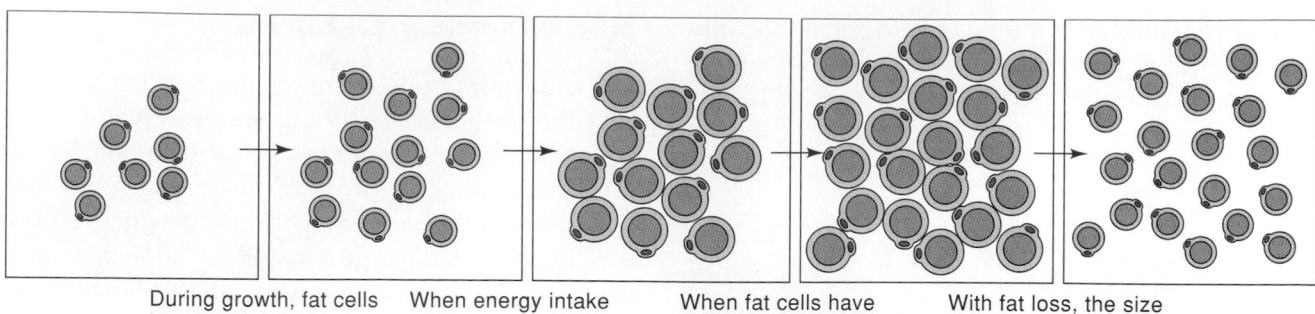

During growth, fat cells increase in number.

When energy intake exceeds expenditure, fat cells increase in size.

When fat cells have reached their maximum size and energy intake continues to exceed energy expenditure, fat cells increase in number again.

With fat loss, the size of the fat cells shrinks, but not the number.

Figure 10.2
The Number and Sizes of Fat Cells

include (in order of incidence) heart disease, cancer, stroke, and diabetes mellitus, together account for two-thirds of the 2 million deaths each year in the United States.

Obesity can be linked to many major health threats (see Figure 10.3). These health threats include diabetes, cardiovascular diseases, and certain cancers, among others. In fact, the evidence is now overwhelming that obesity has adverse effects on health and longevity.[36] A panel of nutritionists with the National Institutes of Health concluded that being 20 percent above recommended body weight constitutes an established health hazard. In the United States, for persons between the ages of 20 and 74, more than 15.4 million men (24.2 percent) and 15.6 million women (27.1 percent) are clinically obese.[37]

Diseases of the heart and blood vessels, known as cardiovascular diseases (CVDs), have been a major cause of death in many countries. CVDs increase with obesity. Of especial risk is abdominal, or central, obesity. Independent of total body fat, abdominal obesity may increase the risk of heart disease as much as the three leading CVD risk features (smoking, hypertension, and high blood cholesterol) combined.[38, 39] Excess body fat can lead to hypertension, which then can lead to stroke and heart attack. Weight loss of as little as 10 pounds in an overweight person often lowers blood pressure significantly.[40] The heart of an obese person must work harder to pump blood to

the lungs and to excess fat tissue. Obesity affects heart size; an enlarged heart can result in high blood pressure and an erratic heartbeat. High blood cholesterol levels and subsequent atherosclerosis is more common in obese people. This can result in high blood pressure, which increases the risk of stroke, kidney failure, and heart attack (Figure 10.4, p. 310). About one-fourth of all heart and blood vessel problems are related to obesity.[41]

Obesity also contributes to other major risk factors, such as diabetes and high blood lipids. The prevalence of reported diabetes is 2.9 times higher in overweight people than in those who are not overweight.[42] Studies show a direct relationship between non-insulin-dependent diabetes mellitus (NIDDM) and obesity. NIDDM is also sometimes referred to as Type II diabetes, or adult-onset diabetes. About 90 percent of adults with NIDDM are obese. When diabetic, obese people require much more insulin than normal-weight people to maintain normal blood glucose. With increase in body fat, there is insulin resistance, and adipose and muscle cells are less able to take up needed glucose.[43] All of this is especially true among older people.[44]

Obesity puts more stress on the muscles and joints and reduces their functional capacity. This is especially evident in the knees, hips, and lower back. Low back pain is more common in people who are obese. The muscles supporting the belly may give way, leading to abdominal hernias. Abnormally fatty leg muscles contract less efficient-

Lungs
Overweight people experience difficulty in breathing due both to their excess weight and to the buildup of carbon dioxide in their blood resulting from lowered respiratory capacity. Abdominal fat, in particular, restricts breathing.

Blood Pressure
High blood pressure (hypertension) is more common among overweight persons. Blood pressure is increased both by the increased blood volume and the need for the heart to pump harder. Hypertension can result in heart disease, stroke, and kidney disease.

Gallbladder
Gallbladder diseases are more common in overweight persons. The majority of those undergoing surgery for gallstones are overweight.

Pregnancy
Being overweight during pregnancy can be a hazard to both mother and fetus. Labor may be longer and more difficult, which may affect fetal well-being. Infant and maternal mortality is higher among overweight mothers.

Joint diseases
Burden of extra fat places strain on the skeletal system. Arthritis is more common, especially in the knees, hips, and lower spine. The more weight an individual carries, the greater the wear will be on the joints, which will in turn cause pain. Increased pain leads to less physical activity and risk of yet greater weight gain.

Atherosclerosis
Atherosclerosis, or hardening of the arteries due to deposits of fatty material in the arterial wall lining, may lead to rupture or closure of vessels. It is most life-threatening when it affects the coronary arteries (vessels on the surface of the heart) and cerebral arteries (vessels in the brain). Coronary heart disease and stroke are more common in overweight persons.

Heart
Because the heart must work harder to circulate the blood as a person's weight increases, the more overweight a person is, the more strain is put on the heart. Heart disease is more common among overweight persons.

Diabetes
90 percent of non-insulin dependent (adult-onset) diabetics are significantly overweight. Weight control is a primary means of treatment.

Muscles
Muscles supporting the belly may weaken, leading to abdominal hernias. A weakened diaphragm muscle may lead to displacement of the stomach into the chest cavity. Leg muscles, which are abnormally fatty, may fail to contact effectively enough to help return blood from the leg veins to the heart.

Surgery
Overweight patients have a thick layer of fat that may make surgery dangerous. Anesthetic risk is increased with overweight patients. Postsurgical complications are also increased.

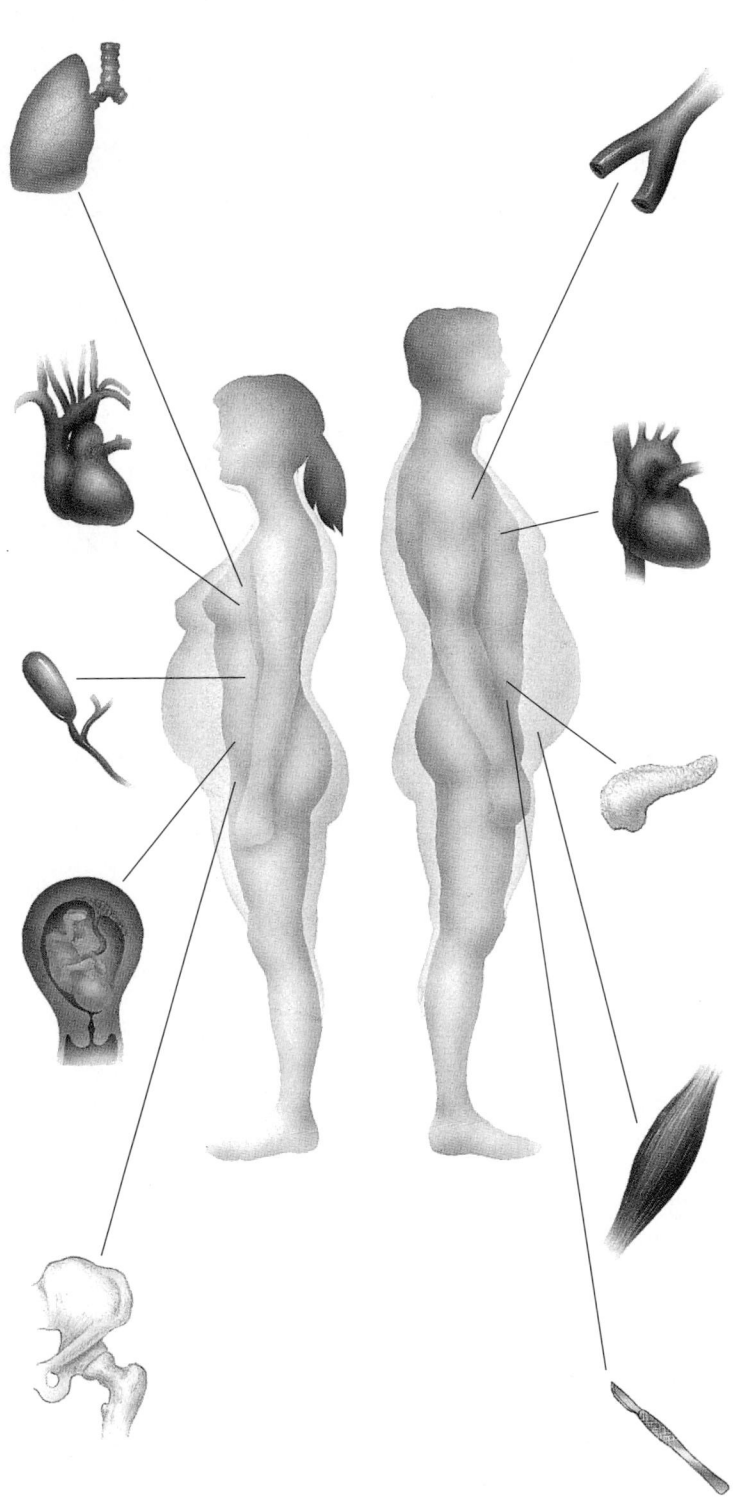

Figure 10.3
Fat Sites in the Body and Accompanying Health Risks

Figure 10.4
Obesity and Related Risk Factors

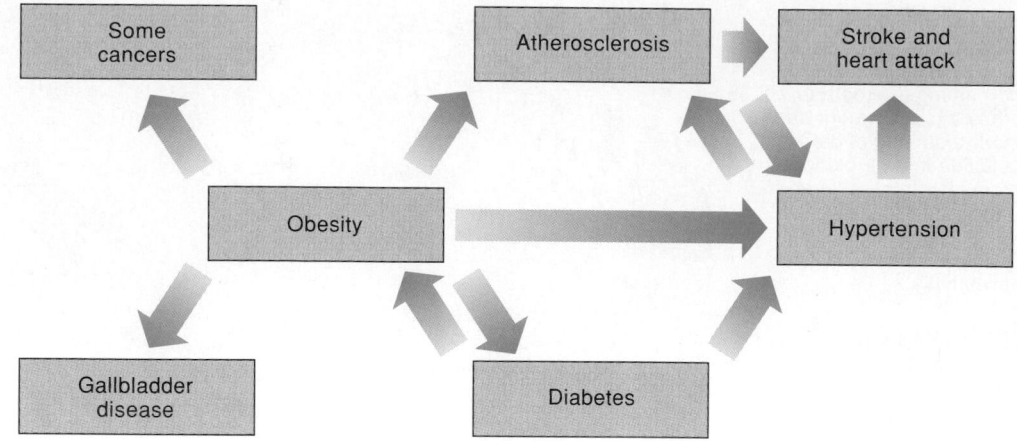

ly, causing the blood in the leg veins to return to the heart more slowly.

Sterility is more common in obese women. Excess fat tissue leads to the production of too much estrogen and too little progesterone. This imbalance may disrupt the menstrual cycle and release of the egg from the ovaries. Pregnant women who are obese tend to have more gallstones, blood clots, and toxemia during pregnancy; childbirth difficulties are also more common.[45]

Of all dietary components, fat is uniquely related to cancer. Although fat is not the cause of cancer, it appears to be a cancer promoter; certain forms of cancer are more prevalent in obese persons. Men who are obese have a higher incidence of cancers of the colon, rectum, and prostate; women who are obese have a higher incidence of cancers of the gallbladder, ovaries, uterine lining, and after menopause, the breasts.[46] Body fat is believed to be a storehouse for cancer-producing chemicals in both men and women.[47]

Because of the aforementioned problems, obesity tends to shorten an individual's life span. Studies examining the relationship between obesity and mortality have shown that obese persons are twice as likely as persons of normal weight to die prematurely.[48] The greater the degree of overweight, the higher the mortality ratio. In people whose weight is twice normal, the death rate soars to 12 times normal.[49]

An obese person has a reduced ratio of skin to body mass. This produces excessive sweating, with sweat becoming trapped in the fatty folds of skin where disease-producing organisms grow more readily. Fatty folds of skin tend to be more subject to rubbing and bruising. In men, fatty folds of tissue around the scrotum increase temperature and can cause male infertility. Skin irritation often occurs around the abdomen and, in women, below the breasts.

SOCIETY'S REACTION TO OBESITY

Aside from the physical consequences of being obese, people may react to obesity in negative ways. For example, obese people are less sought after socially and romantically. They may be the subject of cruel jokes or referred to in disparaging terms. They may be viewed as lacking willpower and social skills. Obese children may develop negative self-images due to being ridiculed or ostracized by slimmer peers; or they may be ignored when choosing up sides in competitive sports or may be unable to keep up with other children athletically.

Obese persons often face discrimination when seeking employment. Very heavy people may move more slowly, which may give the impression of apathy or even illness. They may have difficulty in getting accepted into police academies, competing for positions as firefighters, being selected as airline attendants, or acquiring other positions for which fitness, athletic ability, and size are of importance to job performance.

Obese persons may be limited to a smaller selection of clothing styles and often need to locate specialty shops that carry clothing for stout people or stores that carry a selection of colors or styles in their sizes.

TREATING OBESITY: POOR CHOICES

Millions of people in the United States want to lose weight without sacrificing their favorite foods, without pain, and without great effort. If only we could be thin and firm by waving a magic wand!

It's very popular to resort to well-publicized weight-loss programs that involve special food requirements such as high-fat, high-protein, low-carbohydrate, or liquid protein. There are hundreds of such programs that continue to come and go; many of them are reported as "breakthroughs," but if this were the case, even newer breakthroughs would not be needed. The problem is that most diet plans focus on short-term (and often futile) weight loss which results in weight cycling, or "yo-yo" dieting and psychological problems that result from repeated failures to keep weight off. Only 5 percent of people who try are able to maintain their weight losses.[50] Much better is a program of lifetime weight management, which involves learning new eating and exercise habits as discussed in the Successful Weight Management section later in this chapter.

Unwilling or unable to lose weight through diet and exercise, many people in the United States pour over $5 billion each year into diet pills, water pills, diet drugs, hormones, health spas, surgery, and fad diets.[51] Many of these products and procedures, if they work at all, may commit a person to a cycle of quick weight loss, rebound weight gain when normal eating is resumed, then greater difficulty with weight loss in the next diet attempt.

Weight loss has become a fertile field for quick-fix methods, gimmicks, and quackery. We will discuss fad diets, chemical strategies, and surgical procedures in the following sections.

FAD DIETS

There is usually at least one fad diet book on the best-seller list in any given week. Some fad diets are simple variations of a basic 1000–1200 calorie balanced diet. Others may be dangerous because they emphasize one food or food group and the elimination of others, and advise people to follow diets low in energy and nutrients. Some fad diets are more hazardous to a person's health than the obesity they propose to cure, creating adverse reactions ranging from headaches to death. Of 29,000 claims, treatments, and therapies for losing weight, fewer than 6 percent are effective, and 13 percent are downright dangerous.[52] Feature 10.1 (p. 312) provides some guidelines for recognizing unsound weight-loss promotions.

Diet Books

Fad diet books are long on advertising and packaging and short on unique approaches. Many of them are products of advertising specialists, not of scientists who are experts in dietetics. Although they list "degrees" after their names, the writers/practitioners sometimes have no training in nutrition or food science, or have credentials from unaccredited schools. "Doctor" Robert Hass, author of *Eat to Win,* was awarded a Ph.D. by Columbia Pacific University, in San Rafael, California, from which students could earn degrees in one year or less. "Doctor" Harry Diamond, author of *Fit for Life,* was a graduate of the former American College of Health Science in Austin, Texas, which stopped awarding degrees after the State of Texas said it was not qualified to operate as a college. Even a legitimate degree may not prevent a person from authoring scientifically inaccurate advice. Such was the case with Robert Atkins, a medical doctor, who authored *Diet Revolution,* which advised meals rich in animal fats and cholesterol and almost devoid of carbohydrates. Fad diets may be neither dangerous nor beneficial to a person's health, although this is not always the case.[53]

FEATURE 10.1

RECOGNIZING UNSOUND WEIGHT-LOSS PROMOTIONS

1. They promise dramatic, rapid weight loss (i.e., substantially more than 1 percent of total body weight per week).

2. They promote diets that are extremely low in calories (i.e., below 800 calories per day) without competent, close medical supervision.

3. They apply strong pressure to buy and consume only the program's foods, rather than teaching how to make good choices from the conventional food supply.

4. They fail to encourage permanent, realistic life-style changes, including regular exercise and behavior modification.

5. They misrepresent salespeople as "counselors" supposedly qualified to give guidance in nutrition and/or general health. Even if adequately trained, such "counselors" would still be of questionable value because of the obvious conflict of interest that exists when providers profit directly from products they recommend and sell.

6. They collect large sums of money at the start or require that clients sign contracts for expensive, long-term programs. Programs should be on a pay-as-you-go basis.

7. They fail to inform clients of the risks associated with weight loss in general or the specific program being promoted.

8. They promote unproven or spurious weight-loss aids such as human chorionic gonadotropin hormone (HCG), starch blockers, diuretics, sauna belts, body wraps, passive exercise, ear stapling, acupuncture, electric muscle-stimulating (EMS) devices, spirulina, amino acid supplements (e.g., arginine, ornithine), glucomannan, or methylcellulose (a "bulking" agent).

Source: Whitney, E., and Rolfes, S. *Understanding Nutrition*, 6th ed. St. Paul, MN: West, 1993.

Very-Low-Calorie Diets

One class of weight-loss diets, the **very-low-calorie diets (VLCDs),** are diet plans that provide from 400 to 800 calories a day, along with a protein intake about two times the RDA, little or no fat, and a little carbohydrate. These diet plans gained popularity in the 1980s, and were especially spotlighted by the weight loss of Tommy Lasorda, manager of the Los Angeles Dodgers, and Ed Koch, former mayor of New York City. The VLCDs have popular appeal. All a person does is drink a formula, which may come in a powdered form. VLCDs provide short-term relief from having to deal with foods. Unfortunately, VLCDs do not allow a person to break with their defective eating habits, and become monotonous. Some people tire of them and abandon their plans before they are finished; others lose the weight then regain it when they return to "normal" eating patterns.

The current VLCDs are safer than the early low-protein diets, whose use has led to the unfortunate deaths of many users.[54] Yet, VLCDs need to be carefully administered. Because they effect changes in electrolyte balance, organ functions, and metabolic activities, VLCDs are useful for only short periods of time. They should be limited to carefully selected patients who are a minimum of 30 percent overweight, and should be administered only by physicians trained in their use. Hazards can occur when the physician is untrained in clinical nutrition.[55] A critical element in the use of such diets is the retention of lean body mass. Mildly obese persons lose more lean mass when using these diets than people who are severely obese. Large losses of lean mass can have unanticipated, even fatal, results.[56]

Unfortunately, many patients who use VLCDs alone regain weight almost as fast as they lose it, especially if not taught how to modify their former faulty eating habits (see Feature 10.2). Even with such instruction, few such dieters may be able to maintain the lower weight.[57] The American Medical Association insists that a long-term weight control program is the only effective treatment for obesity.[58]

CHEMICAL STRATEGIES

The majority of proposals for losing weight include chemical strategies. Each of them includes some drug that the dieter must take. Although widely

very-low-calorie diet diet plans that provide from 400 to 800 calories a day, a protein intake about two times the RDA, with no fat and little carbohydrate.

publicized, none of them are both safe and effective and many are hazardous.

Diet Pills

Amphetamines (*am-fet'a-mēnz*), such as Dexedrine and Benzedrine, were the first diet pills. Amphetamines ("speed") and related drugs are thought to suppress the appetite by affecting the appetite centers in the brain. It is now known that while they raise a person's metabolic rates, hunger is reduced only temporarily. The dependency-creating properties of these drugs makes their long-term use undesirable; when use is terminated, depression is common.[59] The effectiveness of amphetamines is limited to short-term use.

Common appetite suppressant drugs include the active agent phenylpropanolamine. This agent can be found in brand name products such as Dexatrim, Anorexin, Appendrine, and Ordinex, and are available over-the-counter. Chemically similar to amphetamines, these drugs may increase the risk of stroke when taken at over-the-counter doses.[60] Other adverse side effects are nervousness, insomnia, headaches, nausea, and excessive increase in blood pressure.[61]

Water Pills

Water pills are **diuretics** (*dī-ū-ret'ikz*), drugs that speed up body water loss through urination. While some obese people would like to believe that their excess weight is due to water accumulation, the fact is that excess weight is due to stored fat. While users of water pills may lose a few pounds of water while taking the pills, as soon as use of the pill is stopped the lost water is regained. No fat is lost with the use of diuretics. Obese people have a smaller percentage of body water than people of normal weight. Any water loss through the use of diuretics is done at the risk of dehydration.

Diet Gums

Diet gums and candies are available over-the-counter. Some of them may contain *benzocaine* as

....

amphetamine a group of synthetically-produced drugs that serve as nervous system stimulants.

diuretic a drug that speeds up body water loss through increasing the production of urine.

an active ingredient. Benzocaine is supposed to work as a local anesthetic by numbing the taste buds on the tongue, thus reducing the sense of taste. No sound evidence has been found that it works as a long-term diet aid.[62]

Glucomannan

Glucomannan (*glū-kō-man'nan*), a derivative of a vegetable used in Japanese cuisine, was reportedly used by the Japanese for weight control for over 1500 years. In 1982, the FDA reported that it is ineffective in weight loss. Although glucomannan adds bulk in the stomach, thus producing a feeling of fullness, it is useless in effecting weight loss.[63]

Hormones

Hormones have been used by some clinicians as weight-loss drugs. *Thyroid* hormone, for example, may speed up the body's metabolic rate, causing the body to burn more lean mass (muscle) than fat. It has been found to be useless in fat control, however, and is potentially dangerous. *Human chorionic gonadotropin* (*kō-ri-on'ik gon-a-dō-trō'pin; HCG*), another hormone that has been examined, is extracted from the urine of pregnant women. Both the FDA and the American Medical Association have stated that this hormone is also useless for weight loss.[64] *Cholecystokinin* (*ko-le-sis'to-kī-nin; CCK*) is a hormone involved in secretion of bile by the gallbladder. Advertised as effective in decreasing hunger and causing sudden and dramatic weight loss, CCK may create adverse side effects. Further, the FDA has not found any data to support claims of weight loss for this hormone.[65] No hormones have yet been shown to be effective in promoting weight loss.

OTHER QUESTIONABLE METHODS

Surgical Procedures

Although surgery may appear justified, it is potentially a hazardous approach to weight correction. There are a number of health considerations that should be looked into before deciding to have it done.[66]

Stapling the stomach (gastroplasty) and shortening the small intestine (gastroresection) are the most common surgical steps for obesity. Gastrointestinal surgery reduces the amount of food a person can eat. The long-term success of such surgery depends on how successfully a person can comply with dietary directions. Short-term risks include infection, nausea, vomiting, and dehydration; long-term risks are vitamin and mineral deficiencies and psychiatric disorders.[67]

To force themselves to use a liquid diet, some patients request having their jaws wired shut; although there is little question that this technique can bring about weight loss, the issue is the ability to resist food once the wires are removed.

Suction lipectomy (*li-pek'tō-mē*), or liposuction, is a surgical method of selectively removing localized fat deposits, such as "saddlebags" on the thighs or "fat-roll" above the belt. By inserting a small tube under the skin, tunnels of fat are suctioned off. The procedure is used to remove the evidence rather than to treat obesity. Most weight control specialists regard it as unsafe and ineffective. It is also expensive and may lead to cosmetic complications such as sagging of the skin and temporary numbness.[68]

Spas and Salons

Some people resort to trips to spas or salons for weight loss results. Machines that jiggle parts of the body may make a person feel good, but they do not provide a form of exercise. Steam and sauna baths cause dehydration and temporarily reduce total body weight *without* any fat loss. Hot baths do not speed up the basal metabolic rate. Any device designed to break down cellulite fails because the existence of cellulite (*sel'ūlīt*) is a myth. The lumpy appearance in fatty areas of the body is from strands of connective tissue that attaches skin to underlying muscles. If the fat is thick at these points of attachment, lumps appear between them. When the fat in these areas disappears, so do the lumps. This fat is no different from fat elsewhere in the body.[69]

WEIGHT CYCLING

Weight-loss schemes can be dangerous because persons using them may be unable to maintain weight losses. Repeatedly losing weight, then regaining it (the "yo-yo" effect), leads to very effi-

....

suction lipectomy removal of fatty tissues.

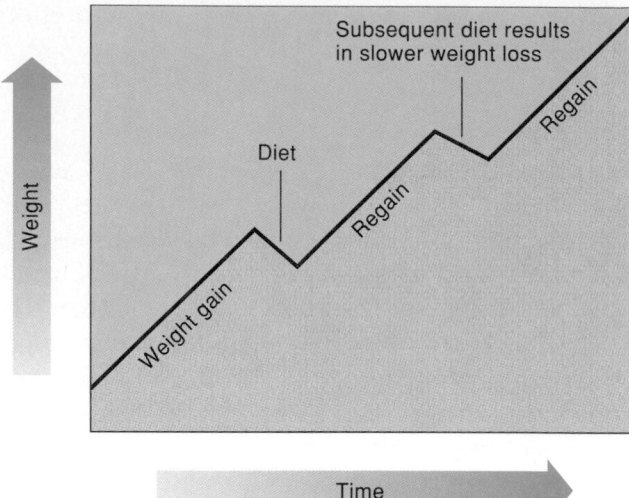

Figure 10.5

The Weight-Cycling ("Yo-Yo") Effect of Repeated Dieting

Each round of dieting is followed by a rebound of weight to a higher level than before. Each time the dieter tries to lose weight, it becomes harder and takes longer, and the lost weight returns more quickly.

cient making and storing of fat. In fact, chronic dieting may permanently change metabolism to favor weight *gain*.[70] Some describe this as a "dieting-induced obesity," or getting fatter because of dieting. Each time the dieter tries to lose weight, it becomes harder, and takes longer, and the weight returns more easily and quickly (Figure 10.5). Fluctuations in body weight increase the risks of diabetes, hypertension, high blood lipids, and even death.[71] In addition, such failure creates the psychological burden of being a failure in this important life aspect.

CHECKPOINT

1. How much money do Americans spend per year on weight-loss programs other than diet and exercise?

2. Identify the hazards that are associated with chemical strategies, such as diet pills, water pills, diet gums, glucomannan, and hormones.

3. Describe stomach stapling and suction lipectomy.

4. If you wanted to lose weight, which method would appeal to you most? Which the least? Why?

BEING UNDERWEIGHT

With so much concern over losing weight, it is hard for many people to conceive of people who have a hard time gaining weight. Using the life insurance tables, as done earlier in the chapter, a body weight 10 percent below the body weight can be defined as **underweight.** In other words, a person whose weight is less than 90 percent of his or her desirable weight, as shown in Table 10.1, would be underweight. No serious health problems accompany mild degrees of underweight. It does not pose hazards unless it is accompanied by undernutrition. The reasons people become underweight are similar to those why people become overweight; they include psychological, metabolic, and genetic factors.

Underfeeding during childhood may lead to fewer fat cells in the same way overfeeding increases their number. An extremely active child may need as many as 3000–4000 calories a day to maintain weight. If this child has an aversion to food or is too busy to eat, it may be just as difficult for him or her to gain weight as it is for an overweight person to lose it.[72]

To gain weight, underweight people need to adopt behavioral and dietary patterns conducive to weight gain. A continuing program of effective physical exercise must be included to build up muscle tissue so that the weight gain is not all fat. The person should increase food intake by using foods that pack a high number of calories into a small volume in order to avoid feelings of being too full. Bread with peanut butter, starchy vegetables with butter, meat with gravy, and high-calorie desserts such as diary products and pastries are recommended. The strategy is just the reverse of that of the overweight person. Eating large meals, eating more times per day, eating faster, and eating high-calorie snacks systematically between meals, may accomplish the desired weight gain.

Weight gain cannot be accomplished by any quick-fix strategies, such as pills, hormones, shots, or surgeries. It is essential that a balanced program of physical activity be maintained, unless it is recommended against because of some other overriding health reason.

---

underweight any weight more than 10 percent below desirable weight.

EATING DISORDERS

Our society has a preoccupation with food; eating is one of our most popular activities. At the same time, we are extremely image conscious and are pressured to match an "ideal" of thinness as portrayed by models in magazines and on television. This is further perpetuated by adult authority figures such as team coaches, cheerleader advisors, and dance instructors. Yet, the perception of thinness may become an obsession and therefore lead to eating disorders. Two such disorders common in today's society are *bulimia* and *anorexia nervosa.*

BULIMIA

Patricia is a single woman in her early twenties. Intelligent and well-trained, she was a high achiever in school. Of normal body weight, she has experienced more than her share of social anxiety and finds it difficult to develop personal relationships. This leaves her depressed and she has compensated by displaying impulsive behavior. Trying not to let it interfere with her work, she periodically goes through eating binges, usually after having deprived herself of food. At night, when no one else is around, she badly overeats and then induces vomiting. Patricia knows she shouldn't do it, is ashamed of what she does and feels guilty after it's all over.

Binge eating followed by purging is a serious psychological and medical problem known as **bulimia** (*bū-lim'i-a*) or **bulimarexia** (*bū-lim'a-reks'i-a*). Both mean to "eat like an ox." A related term, **bulimia nervosa** (*ner-vō'sa*), applies to recurring cycles of binge eating followed by vomiting.[73]

---

bulimia recurring binge eating; also called **bulimarexia.**

bulimia nervosa recurring binge eating followed by purging.

People who have bulimia, or bulimics, are typically overcome with a powerful urge to eat, especially "forbidden" sweets or starches, most often in secret. This is a compulsive behavior; the food is not consumed for its nutritional value.

Bulimia usually begins in conjunction with a diet that gets out of control and may follow a period of rigid dieting. A binge may be set off by the taste or even the perception of food and may be accelerated by hunger. The first bite triggers the loss of control and the person goes into a compulsive eating frenzy. During the binge the person consumes massive quantities of food—ice cream, cakes, pastries, croissants—stopping only when the stomach pain is unbearable. In the case of bulimia nervosa, the bulimic then vomits everything that has just been eaten. Using the well-trained reflex, he or she may then return and begin the binge process all over again.[74] Some victims binge as often as ten times a day, others only a few times a week. The binge may be ended by self-induced vomiting through gagging or use of a chemical to induce vomiting, or by taking laxatives, diuretics, or enemas. Some end their binges only when the pain is too intense, when interrupted, or by falling asleep.[75] Repeated use of **emetics** (*e-met'ikz*) can cause poisoning and lead to heart failure. The binge eater often goes through stages: "anticipation and planning, anxiety, urgency to begin, rapid and uncontrolled consumption of food, relief and relaxation, disappointment, and finally shame or disgust."[76]

Overall, bulimics tend to maintain a near normal weight. Yet the female menstrual cycle often becomes irregular, sexual interest is reduced, and the bulimic may evidence impulsive behavior such as alcohol, cigarette, or drug abuse and shoplifting.[77]

Purging can upset the body's balance of electrolytes (mineral tissue fluids) and lead to abnormal heart rhythms and injury to the kidneys. Kidney and bladder infections can lead to kidney failure. Repeated vomiting may damage the esophagus and stomach and induce bleeding; it may cause receding gums and damage to tooth enamel from the wash of gastric acid.

Bulimia often begins when individuals are between 17 and 25 years of age, and may follow a

long series of failures with weight-reduction programs. Bulimics commonly intersperse restrictive dieting with bulimic behaviors and may experience weight fluctuations of 10 pounds up and down over short periods of time. Most often females, victims are typically of higher than average intelligence and are close to their recommended weight.[78] They may appear healthy, successful, and competent. In the January 1985 issue of *Cosmopolitan*, Jane Fonda told her story of having been a secret bulimic from age 12 to 35, bingeing and purging up to 20 times a day. For individuals obsessed with food, the binges are often associated with great distress and marked by feelings of loss of self-control, self-disgust, anger, and depression. The vomiting may be a **catharsis** (*kath-ar'-sis*), or release from guilt feelings as well as from the food itself.

ANOREXIA NERVOSA

Marie is in her first year of college and a fine dancer. Living at home, she eats very carefully and works out daily at the fitness center. Although slender, she still feels her weight is too high. Unaware that she is actually undernourished, she says she feels fine, although she stopped menstruating some months ago. The concern of her family bothers her. Marie has worked hard to please her parents, who she feels have set her goals for her. Unable to gain control of her life from her parents the way she wants, she insists on severely controlling her weight, even though she is usually hungry. Even though she looks physically exhausted, she still contends that she is fat. Her friends and family are becoming concerned. Marie has anorexia nervosa.

Anorexia nervosa (*an-ō-reks'i-a ner-vō'sa*), meaning "nervous lack of appetite," is a condition in which a person, usually a female teenager, takes dieting to the point of self-starvation and loses 25 percent or more of his or her body weight.[79] The condition is estimated to occur in 1 of every 200

emetics substances that produce vomiting.

catharsis release from guilt feelings.

anorexia nervosa a disorder, seen usually in teenage girls, involving self-starvation.

females, usually aged 12–18; about 5–10 percent of anorexics are males.[80] The victim of this disorder is most commonly an adolescent or young adult who has an intense fear of fat and is plagued with a distorted body image. The victim of anorexia nervosa is so obsessed with losing weight that he or she sees even normal body contours as fat.[81] Refusing to maintain a minimum normal weight, the anorectic individual maintains a body weight below the weight expected for his or her age and height.

Anorexia, like bulimia, may begin as a diet that has gotten out of control. It may occur suddenly and for a limited time, or it may develop gradually and over many years. The behavior and body changes of an anorexic are typical of a starving person. An anorexic's behavior toward food may be atypical; for instance, he or she may crumble food, minutely dissecting it before eating it, or may not eat when others eat.[82] As weight is lost, the absence of fat tissue padding the body makes sitting or lying down uncomfortable. The body tries to protect its two main organs—the brain and the heart—by slowing down or stopping other less vital functions. Menstruation stops, blood pressure and body temperature both drop, and respiratory rate slows down. Constipation, intolerance of the cold, and light-headedness follow. Due to severe electrolyte imbalance, irregular heartbeat, heart failure, and bone loss may occur.[83] The anorexic may not sleep well and may withdraw from friends. *Lanugo* (*la-nū'gō*), or soft hair, forms over the skin.

In addition to starvation, some anorexics purge the little bit of food they do eat, further risking their health. Recording artist Karen Carpenter was an anorexic who died when the effects of induced vomiting irreversibly damaged her heart.[84]

Anorexics are often from educated, successful, middle-class families, and are usually competitive perfectionists who have lost control, or fear losing control, of their lives. The anorexia may be induced by a life situation with which the person is unable to cope—puberty, death of a loved one, first sexual contact, ridicule over weight, or over-controlling parents. The anorexic may feel the media/culture imposed "body concept" of being thin is the "ideal." Victims of this disorder become skilled in manipulating their appetites, which gives them a sense of control (even though self-destructive) over their emotions, family, and friends.[85]

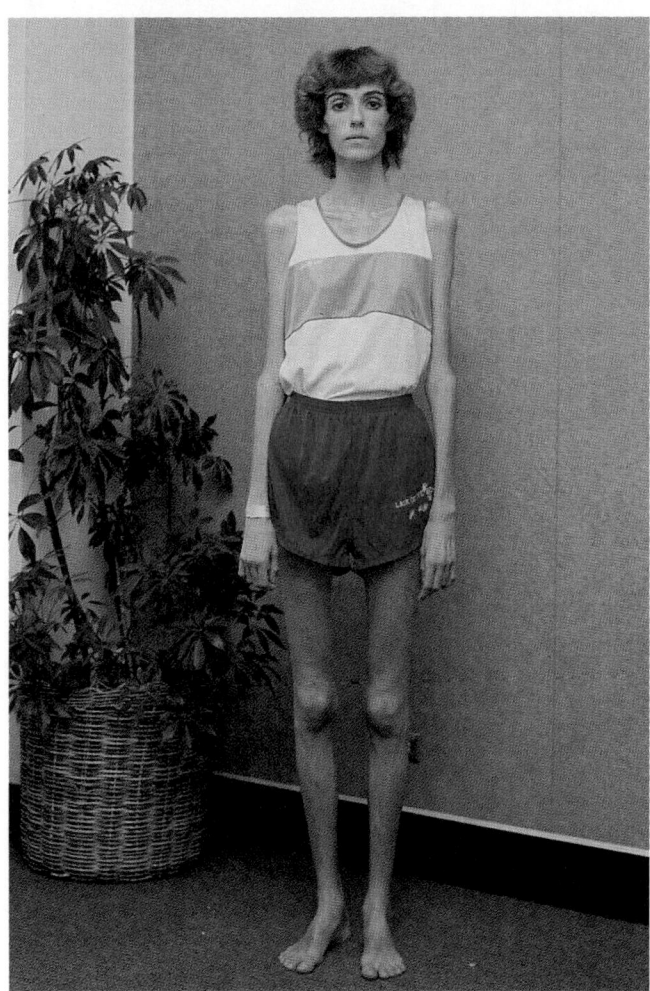

Anorexia nervosa is a condition brought on by a voluntary weight loss carried to the extreme. Obsessed with losing weight, such a person views even normal body contours as fat. Early treatment of the condition to avoid irreparable damage is imperative.

TREATMENT

Early treatment of eating disorders is imperative; however, there is no quick cure for either anorexia or bulimia. Due to their denial of being too thin and not eating enough, it may be hard to convince anorexics to gain weight. Bulimics tend to cooperate with treatment more easily and may actually seek treatment. The longer bulimia and anorexia persist, the more the damage to the body becomes irreversible. A realistic body image is necessary for recovery, especially with anorexia. Since family dynamics are a common cause of eating disorders, treatment programs need to involve the family. Medical care by a physician is necessary, as is psychotherapy, so that victims can deal with their low self-esteem, depression, and helplessness. Behavior modification may be used as another method of treatment for eating disorders. Some people with eating disorders find effective help by joining self-help groups such as Bulimic and Anorexic Self-Help (BASH). Tables 10.4 and 10.5 give some nutritional recommendations for the treatment for each condition.

CHECKPOINT

- What is bulimia? Why do people practice binge-eating, and what are the hazards of bulimia?

- Define the term *anorexia nervosa*. Who tends to practice it? What are the effects of that practice?

- Describe some of the approaches taken in treating eating disorders.

✓

Table 10.4
Nutrition Recommendations for Bulimia

- Avoid finger foods; eat foods that require the use of utensils.

- Enhance satiety by eating warm foods.

- Include vegetables, salad, and/or fruit at meals to prolong eating time.

- Choose whole-grain and high-fiber breads and cereals to maximize bulk.

- Eat a well-balanced diet and meals consisting of a variety of foods.

- Use foods that are naturally divided into portions, such as potatoes (rather than rice or pasta); 4- and 8-ounce containers of yogurt, ice cream, or cottage cheese; precut steak or chicken parts; and frozen dinners and entrees.

- Include foods containing adequate amounts of complex carbohydrates (for satiety) and fat (to slow gastric emptying).

- Eat meals and snacks sitting down.

- Plan meals and snacks, and record plans in a diary prior to eating.

*Source: Adapted from Rock, C., and Yager, J. "Nutrition and Eating Disorders" International Journal of Eating Disorders **6**, p. 276, New York: Wiley, 1987.*

Table 10.5
Nutrition Recommendations for Anorexia Nervosa

- Increase food energy intake slowly, beginning with 800–1200 cal/day.

- Eat well-balanced diets, with *some* individual variations according to your preferences (e.g., vegetarian).

- Take multiple vitamin-mineral supplements at RDA levels.

- Enhance elimination with dietary fiber from grain sources.

- Reduce sensations of bloating with small, frequent feedings.

- In behavioral programs, link rewards to food energy intake, not weight gain.

- Use liquid supplements when you cannot achieve desired intake with solid food.

- Reduce satiety sensations by eating cold or room-temperature foods and finger foods (e.g., snacks).

- Seek interactive nutrition counseling as an ongoing process.

- Reduce excessive caffeine intake.

- Take intravenous nutritional support only in severe states of ill health, malnutrition, and wasting.

*Source: Adapted from Rock, C., and Yager, J. "Nutrition and Eating Disorders" International Journal of Eating Disorders **6**, p. 276, New York: Wiley, 1987.*

SUCCESSFUL WEIGHT MANAGEMENT

The *only* workable means of reducing body fat is to shift the energy balance so that energy input is less than energy outgo. This is a simple principle to understand. The task of putting it into practice is more difficult. For example, less than 10 percent of obese patients who lose weight are able to maintain the weight loss for more than seven years.[86] One reason for this lack of success is that many of these obese patients do not learn coping skills to alter the habits that led to obesity in the first place.

Successful weight-control techniques do exist. Basic to any effective treatment are three approaches: a low-calorie diet, aerobic exercise, and behavior modification. To be most effective, all three strategies must be integrated into any weight management plan and must become part of a long-term change in life-style.

How each individual manages his or her weight is very personal. There is no one method that will suit everyone's needs. As you read the next few pages, reflect on healthy alternatives you can find to counteract any potentially unhealthy habits you may display.

ADOPTING AN EATING PLAN

There is no "surefire" diet you can buy into that's going to guarantee results. The only measure of success of any reducing diet is whether the pounds come off and stay off. The most successful kind of diet is a plan you adopt for life. Because you are the one who must live with the diet you choose, you must be involved in planning it. It should, therefore, consist of appealing foods that are available to you and that you can afford.

Two sets of behavior must be practiced: first weight loss, then maintaining the weight loss. These are two separate tasks; of the two, maintenance is the more difficult to manage. Dieters often have difficulty transferring successfully from a "diet" to an "eating plan." While a diet may be necessary for rapid weight loss, it must be replaced by an eating plan for long-term weight maintenance. It is best to adopt an eating plan from the start. That way, when you arrive at your ideal weight or the goal you have for yourself, you will have already laid the groundwork for long-term success in maintaining that reduced weight (see Feature 10.2).

DEVISING THE RIGHT EATING PLAN FOR YOU

First off, whatever your diet plan, it's important that you give yourself adequate nutrition. This is very difficult to achieve on fewer than 1000–1200 calories a day. It's easier and safer to lose weight on a plan that allows more calories per day and provides you with adequate nutrition, than to launch into a plan with a larger calorie deficit that leaves you feeling starved. Facing feelings of being deprived can help create the temptation for you to break the plan and "pig out."

This means that you need to choose an energy level. Remember that a calorie deficit of 500 calories a day for 7 days equals 3500 calories a week, which equals one pound of body fat. A workable rule is that your diet plan should give you ten calories per day per pound of current weight.

Your first priority is to provide for nutritional adequacy. Choose foods that appeal to you. Select low-calorie foods with a variety of nutrients, such as appealing vegetables and fruits, whole grain breads and cereals, a limited supply of lean, protein-rich foods, such as poultry, fish, eggs, nut alternates such as dried beans and peas, and low-fat milk products such as nonfat milk and yogurt. Plan to include a certain number of daily servings of food that you like from each of these food categories. This way it will be easier to eliminate high-calorie foods from your daily intake.

Of the carbohydrate foods you select, choose from the unrefined complex-carbohydrate foods that provide fewer calories. These are the starch foods—grains (rice, corn, barley, oats, wheat) and legumes (beans, and peas). These provide lower energy levels than concentrated simple carbohydrates, such as sugars, and sugar products such as candies.[87] It takes about 20 minutes from the time you start eating until the signal indicating your sense of fullness reaches the brain. Since you tend to eat complex carbohydrate grain products more slowly than simple carbohydrate concentrated sweets, you tend to "put away" more calories in 20

FEATURE 10.2

CRITERIA FOR A SUCCESSFUL WEIGHT MANAGEMENT PLAN

Before spending any money in a weight-loss plan, ask yourself whether it meets all of the following five criteria for successful weight management:

1. Does it work (does a person lose weight)?

2. Can the diet be easily followed?

3. Can the diet be followed for a long period of time?

4. Is it safe and relatively free from side effects?

5. Can weight loss be maintained after the diet period is over?

Source: Yetiv, J. *Popular Nutritional Practices.* Toledo, OH: Popular Medicine Press, 1986.

minutes of eating sweets than in 20 minutes worth of eating complex carbohydrate grain products.

Equally important is watching dietary fats. A knifeful of butter can add more calories than a spoonful of sugar. Dietary fat correlates more directly to body fat than do dietary carbohydrates.[88] People who eat low-fat foods consume fewer calories. Reducing fat in the diet has multiple health advantages.[89]

Drink plenty of water. Food should not take the place of water. Drinking water fills your stomach, it moistens the mouth, and it is a useful activity. It also dilutes metabolic wastes. Remember, water contains *no* calories.

Eat on a regular schedule and, if possible, before you become very hungry. When you do, eat all that you have planned to eat. After that, do not eat again until the next meal. Eat slowly and chew each mouthful thoroughly.

Weigh yourself at least once a week. Better yet, every seven days, weigh yourself for three consecutive days and determine the average. Daily weighing is not recommended because of the normal ups and downs in body weight. Weigh yourself in the morning, after eliminating. By weighing yourself regularly you can determine how your food intake is affecting your weight-loss program. You may notice plateaus after several weeks of weight loss. This may be due to temporary water gain as your body adjusts to reduced stored fat. If you follow your eating plan, however, your eventual weight loss will reflect it.

Avoid those situations that prompt you to eat. Shop at the grocery store only when you are *not* hungry, and buy only those foods you have planned for. Do not keep any foods around the house that you are trying to avoid. If you must have snack foods, keep a supply of low-calorie foods on hand.

If you slip and exceed your daily caloric intake, don't punish yourself by overcompensating the following day. In other words, if you overeat 1000 unnecessary calories, don't deprive yourself of 1000 calories the next day. Pick up the diet plan and go back to it. On the other hand, if there's an event coming up with foods not included in your plan, such as cakes, pastries, and chocolate, you might ease up on your calorie intake several days in advance.

If you lose your long-term resolve and begin to gain weight, realize that losing the excess weight is something that is within your control. You may need to go back and review your original weight-loss goals. You may decide to go into a holding pattern and plateau at a certain weight before losing more. This is *your* decision. Don't let yourself suffer from feelings of guilt or failure; your goal will always be within your reach.

EXERCISE

Your body is a complex machine, and its level of activity affects what your body does with its nutrients. The amount of energy you spend and how it is spent has an impact on your health and fitness. Although it is possible to lose weight without exercising, weight loss without exercise denies an understanding of how the body functions (see Feature 10.3). Part of the popularity of certain fad diets is that they appeal to those who want to lose weight without moving their bodies.

The amount of energy used (calories burned up) increases as physical activity increases. The number of calories used up in a given exercise varies depending on the type of exercise and how long it takes. For instance, a 150-pound person running a 6-minute mile burns off about 102 calories. The same person walking the same mile in 15 minutes, burns off about 93 calories, or close to the same amount. Caloric expenditure also varies with the weight of the person exercising. A 200-pound person running the same 6-minute mile as the 150-pound person burns off about 136 calories, and uses 124 calories when walking a mile in 15 minutes. To use up energy, a person does not need to work quickly. The same number of calories can be used up by walking as by running, although it will take you longer to "walk it off."[90]

Exercise leads to an increased metabolic rate. This occurs both during the exercise and afterward. Basal metabolism remains elevated for several hours after intense and prolonged exercise.[91] Another bonus is that as excess fat is eliminated, the overall body composition has a higher percentage of lean tissue. Since lean tissue is more metabolically active than fat tissue, even more calories end up being expended. With sufficient exercise, you can eat more food and still maintain a given weight. Exercise also helps control appetite. People are not automatically hungry after exercising. The basis for this is that the body responds to the stress of physical exertion by releasing stored glu-

FEATURE 10.3

DIET WITH OR WITHOUT EXERCISE

Exercise is very effective in weight control. In a study by Stanford University researchers, 71 moderately overweight men and women were given a low-fat diet for a year, while another 71 similar persons were placed on the same foods, along with a three-day-a-week program of aerobic exercise. At the end of the year, the diet-plus-exercise group has lost more weight overall, and more pounds of fat, although they had actually consumed more calories per day than the diet-only group.

This result happened because of the activity of basal metabolism. More than half of the calories we take in are spent on basal metabolism, that energy expended while the body is at rest. But something else occurred. Exercise, even of the moderate kind, increases the basal metabolic rate, so the body burns *more* calories while at rest. It is now known that the more muscle (lean tissue) in the body, the higher the metabolic rate. As exercise builds up muscle, the metabolic rate

rises with it. In fact, even if exercise does not result in weight loss, you build up muscle and lose fat. You also lose inches, since a pound of fat takes up more space than a pound of muscle.

Weight loss can take place without exercising; when on a weight loss program you lose weight whether you exercise or not. There is one important qualification, however. The person who exercises while dieting loses more fat than lean tissue, whereas the person who diets without exercising loses more lean tissue. In addition, those who diet and exercise are less likely to regain weight than are those who diet without exercise.

Source: Consumer Reports. "Losing Weight: What Works, What Doesn't." *Consumer Reports,* June 1993, pp. 347–352; Wood, P., et al. "Changes in Plasma Lipids and Lipoproteins in Overweight Men During Weight Loss Through Dieting as Compared with Exercise." *New England Journal of Medicine,* 319, 1988, pp. 1173–1179.

cose and fatty acids into the blood. At the same time, digestive functions are suppressed. The person is not hungry again until there is a drop in levels of glucose and fatty acids in the blood. Exercise also provides an interesting activity that replaces boredom and anxiety, feelings that, as we have discussed, may cause a person to eat.[92]

The exercise activity you choose should be something you want to do and enjoy doing regularly. You can also build more activity into things you must do every day. Take the stairs rather than using the elevator; park farther away from where you usually park so you must walk longer distances; get off the bus one stop early and walk the rest of the way; use an old-fashioned push-type lawn mower instead of a gasoline-powered one; do jobs in ways that require more exertion. Also consider getting out and walking rather than sitting and watching that next TV program!

MODIFYING BEHAVIOR

Many people engage in behaviors each day involving overeating and underexercising. These eating patterns are a learned behavior. Behavior follows environmental cues, or stimuli. The cues determine the likelihood of the behavior occurring. The more intense the cues, the greater the chance of the behavior occurring. The behavior in turn leads to consequences. The more intense the consequences the more or less likely the behavior is to occur.

In order to encourage desirable eating and exercising behaviors and to eliminate undesirable ones, **behavior modification** is necessary. Modifying behavior requires that you understand why you overeat, analyze your eating patterns, set up new patterns of what and how you eat, reward yourself for proper eating, and establish an exercise program.[93]

Understand Why You Overeat

To begin with, you must understand *why* you became overweight in the first place. What causes you to overeat? Are there unresolved emotional problems—loneliness, anxiety, or personal conflicts? Is there encouragement to overeat from your parents or your friends? If your social needs are not being met in other ways, are you trying to meet them with food? Analyzing your eating habits will be necessary to arrive at answers to these and other questions. Completing In Your Hands: Why Do You Eat? (p. 323) will help you do this.

Analyze Your Eating Patterns   Start by keeping a food log (diary) for five to seven consecutive days. The log should include what you eat, the circumstances (when, where, and with whom), asso-

behavior modification the systematic replacement of one set of behaviors for another.

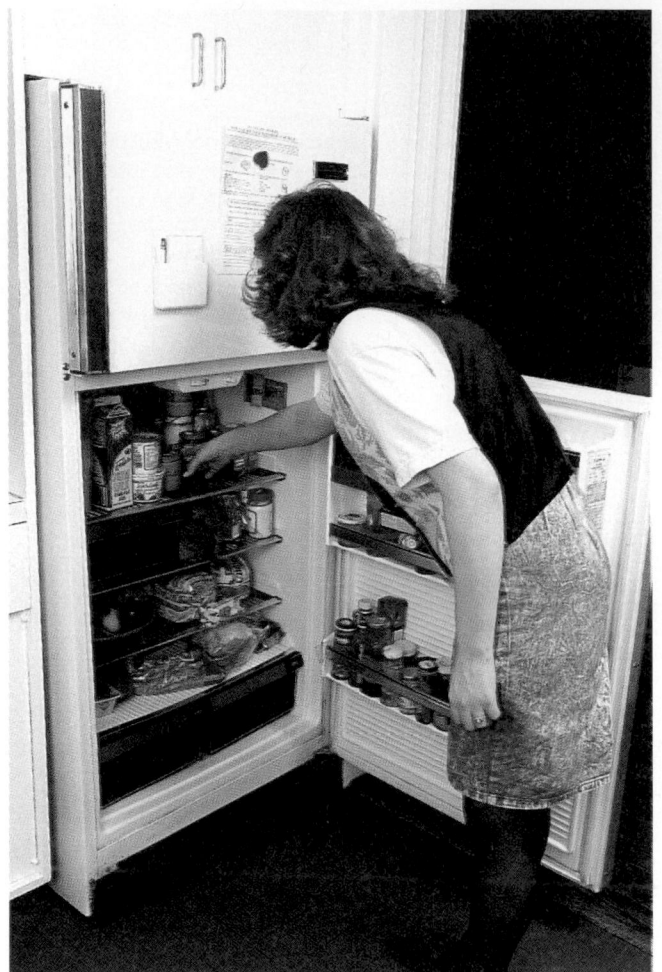

To control weight some basic rules need to be followed including: choosing easily available foods that are nutritious yet low in calories, including foods you like, eating regularly, and eating only as much as you plan on.

ciated activities (sitting, standing, driving, watching TV, reading, talking), and why you eat (hunger, mealtime, something to do).

In analyzing your food log, look for behavior patterns. Do you eat when you're with another person? When you're alone? When you're studying? How do you feel when you eat? Are you lonely? Fatigued? Angry? Bored? Do you overeat at certain times, such as after a frustrating experience? After an argument? When you're tired? Your analysis of your food log will reveal cues that will shed new light on your behavior.

Taking Charge of Your Thinking

A significant element in successful weight management is breaking faulty patterns of thinking. Some of the success in weight management depends on what occurs in your mind. You have the choice of

rationalizing faulty eating behavior and denying the consequences. Communication for Wellness: Keeping Weight Off After It's Been Lost (p. 326) provides some strategies for developing new patterns of thinking.

Setting Up New Patterns of* What *and* How *You Eat Once you have documented and analyzed your behavior, you are ready to break negative habits and replace them with new, acceptable ones.

You will need new patterns of *what* you eat:

- If you eat a bowl of ice cream each night while watching the late news, replace it with slices of carrots and celery.
- Rather than eating or sucking candy while studying, place the candy out of reach or in another room.
- If you select high-calorie food from a snack bar for lunch, pack your own lunch of half a sandwich and some fruit.
- If you eat candy in your car as you are driving to and from work or school, keep food out of your car, chew on a toothpick, eat an apple, or listen to the radio.

You will also need to develop new patterns of *how* you eat:

- If you are used to eating one 12-inch plate full of food each night for dinner, reduce the plate size down to 10 or 8 inches.
- If you are accustomed to second helpings, limit yourself to one plateful.
- When eating ice cream, if you're used to a soup bowl full, cut it down to a cup.
- If you give yourself only 15 minutes to eat increase the time to 30 minutes for the same amount of food.
- If you're used to eating a full evening meal followed by a late-night snack, either cut down the amount of food eaten at dinner or eliminate the late-night snack.

Rewarding Yourself When you succeed in developing a new behavior, reward yourself. Don't minimize the gains. Treat yourself to something that is not associated with eating, such as a haircut or a manicure. You deserve to be pampered for good behavior.

IN YOUR HANDS

WHY DO YOU EAT?

The following inventory will help you to answer the question, "Why do you eat?" The answers you provide may help you understand your reasons for eating and whether any of these reasons need to be modified. The answers may also give you clues on how such modification can be made.

DIRECTION

Here are some statements describing reasons for eating. How often do you feel this way about eating? Circle one number for each statement.

IMPORTANT

Answer every question.

	Always 5	Frequently 4	Occasionally 3	Seldom 2	Never 1
A. I eat to keep myself from slowing down.	5	4	3	2	1
B. Handling food is part of the enjoyment of eating.	5	4	3	2	1
C. Eating is pleasant and relaxing.	5	4	3	2	1
D. When I feel angry about something, I eat.	5	4	3	2	1
E. When I run out of my favorite foods I find it almost unbearable until I can get more.	5	4	3	2	1
F. I eat automatically without even being aware of it.	5	4	3	2	1
G. I eat to stimulate me, perk myself up.	5	4	3	2	1
H. Part of the enjoyment of eating comes from the steps I take to prepare the food.	5	4	3	2	1
I. I find eating pleasurable.	5	4	3	2	1
J. When I feel uncomfortable or upset about something, I eat.	5	4	3	2	1
K. I am very much aware of the fact when I am not eating.	5	4	3	2	1
L. I eat without realizing what I am doing.	5	4	3	2	1
M. I eat to give myself a "lift."	5	4	3	2	1
N. When I eat, part of the enjoyment is seeing, smelling, and tasting food.	5	4	3	2	1
O. I want food most when I am comfortable and relaxed.	5	4	3	2	1
P. When I feel "blue" or want to take my mind off cares and worries, I eat.	5	4	3	2	1

Q. I get a real gnawing
hunger for food when I
haven't eaten for a while.   ___5___   ___4___   ___3___   ___2___   ___1___

R. I've found food in my
mouth and didn't
remember putting it there.   ___5___   ___4___   ___3___   ___2___   ___1___

This inventory and interpretation is adapted from *Smoker's Self-testing Kit,* PHS Publication No. 1904, 1969, developed by Daniel Horn, Director of the National Clearinghouse for Smoking and Health of the Public Health Service and members of the Clearinghouse staff.

SCORING

1. Enter the numbers you have circled in the following spaces, putting the number you circled to question A over line A, to question B over line B, and so on.

2. Total the three scores on each line to get your totals. For example, the sum of your scores over lines A, G, and M gives you your score on "Stimulation"; lines B, H, and N give you the score on "Handling," and so on.

___ + ___ + _____ = _____
A   G   M   Stimulation

___ + ___ + _____ = _____
B   H   N   Handling

___ + ___ + _____ = _____
C   I   O   Pleasurable relaxation

___ + ___ + _____ = _____
D   J   P   Crutch: tension reduction

___ + ___ + _____ = _____
E   K   Q   Craving: psychological addiction

___ + ___ + _____ = _____
F   L   R   Habit

Scores can vary from 3 to 15. Any score of 11 and above is high; any score of 7 and below is low.

INTERPRETATION

What kind of eater are you? What do you get out of eating? What does it do for you? This instrument is designed to provide you with a score on each of six factors that describe many people's eating patterns. Your eating may be well characterized by only one, or by a combination of factors. In any event, this inventory will help you identify why you eat other than to satisfy your hunger, and what kind of satisfaction you think you get from eating.

The six factors measured by this instrument describe one or another way of experiencing or managing certain kinds of feelings. Three of these feeling states represent the positive feelings people get from eating: (1) a sense of increased energy or *stimulation;* (2) the satisfaction of *handling* or manipulating things; and (3) the enhancement of *pleasurable feelings* by reducing the state of tension in feelings such as anxiety, anger, and shame. The fourth is "crutching" that eating plays a part in reducing *negative feelings.* The fifth is a complex pattern of increasing and decreasing "craving" for eating that represents a *psychological addiction* to food. The sixth, *habit,* is eating that occurs in an absence of feeling—purely automatic eating.

A score of 11 or above on any factor indicates that this factor is an important source of satisfaction for you. The higher your score (15 is the highest), the more important a particular factor is in your eating and the more useful the discussion of that factor can be in your attempt to cut down on eating.

A few words of warning: If you cut down on eating, you may have to learn to get along without the extra satisfactions that food gives you. Either that, or you will have to find other acceptable ways of getting these satisfactions. In either case, you need to know just what you get out of eating before you can decide whether to forego the satisfactions or find another way to achieve them.

1. *Stimulation.* If you score high or fairly high on this factor, it means that you are stimulated by food—you feel that it helps wake you up, organize your energies, and keep you going. If you try to give up eating, you may want a safe substitute: a brisk walk or modest exercise, for example, whenever you feel the urge to eat. Try chewing gum or eating celery or carrot sticks.

2. *Handling.* Handling things can be satisfying, but there are many ways to keep your hands busy without placing food into your mouth. Why not toy with a pen or pencil? Or try doodling. Or play with a coin, a piece of jewelry, or some activity other than eating, such as knitting, crocheting, painting, or other handicraft.

3. *Accentuation of pleasure—pleasurable relaxation.* It is not always easy to find out whether you use food to feel good—that is, get honest pleasure out of eating (Factor 3) or to keep from feeling bad (Factor 4). Those who get pleasure out of eating often find that an honest consideration of the harmful effects of their habit is enough to help them quit. They substitute chewing gum, drinking fluids, or participating in social and physical activities. With these methods, they find they do not miss the excess food they are not eating.

4. *Reduction of negative feelings or "crutch."* You may be using eating as a kind of crutch in moments of stress or discomfort, and, on occasion, it may work; food sometimes is used as a tranquilizer. But if you are an excessive eater who tries to handle severe personal problems by snacking many times a day, sooner or later you will discover that foods do not help you deal with these problems effectively.

    When it comes to cutting down, you may find it easy to do so when everything is going well, but you may be tempted to start excessive eating again in a time of crisis. Again, physical exertion, chewing gum, drinking fluids, or engaging in social activity may serve as useful substitutes for eating, even in times of tension. Your choice of a substitute depends on whether the activity will achieve the same effect.

5. *"Craving" or psychological addiction.* Stopping excessive eating will be difficult for you if you score high on the "psychological addiction" factor. Probably, for you, the craving for food will continue to build up as your plate begins to empty. To be successful in changing your desire for excess food, you must go "cold turkey"—that is, cut off extra helpings completely.

    You will have to isolate yourself from your favorite rich foods, second helpings, and snacks until the craving is gone. Giving up excess food intake may be so difficult and cause such discomfort that once you do cut down, you will find it easy to resist the temptation to go back to excessive eating.

6. *Habit.* If you are a habitual eater, you probably are not getting much satisfaction from your food. You probably just eat without realizing you are doing so. You may find it easy to control caloric intake if you can break the habit patterns you have built up. Cutting down gradually may be quite effective if there is a change in the way the food is served and the conditions under which you eat. An example of this might be serving the food from the pots on the stove rather than from bowls on the table. This will make piling on "seconds" a conscious effort. The key to success is becoming aware of all the calories you eat. This can be done by asking yourself, "Do I really want this food?" You may be surprised at how often you do not really want the extra calories.

SUMMARY

If you do not score high on any of the six factors, chances are that you are not an excessive eater. If so, cutting down calories should be easy.

If you score high on several categories, you apparently get several kinds of satisfaction from eating and will have to find several solutions. Certain combinations of score may indicate that reducing food intake will be especially difficult. If you score high on both factor 4 and 5, "reduction of negative feelings and craving," you may have a hard time cutting down caloric intake. However, there are ways to do it; many excessive eaters represented by this combination have been able to cut down on caloric intake.

Others who score high on factors 4 and 5 may find it useful to change patterns of eating and cut down at the same time. You can try to eat foods that are lower in calories, such as carrots, fresh fruits, or crackers, or to substitute exercise and other physical activities for eating. After several months of trying this solution, you may find it easier to develop a habit pattern of low-calorie intake.

You must make a decision to cut down caloric intake either by (1) substituting appropriate volumes of less-fattening foods for the high-calorie foods currently in your diet; or (2) reducing or eliminating excess calorie food (such as junk foods) from your diet without the substitution of low-calorie foods.

Source: Sorochan, W. *Promoting Your Health,* New York: Wiley, 1981, pp. 175–179. Adapted from *Smoker's Self-Testing Kit,* PHS Publication No. 1904, 1969, developed by Daniel Horn, Director of the National Clearinghouse for Smoking and Health of the Public Health Service and members of the Clearinghouse staff.

KEEPING WEIGHT OFF AFTER IT'S BEEN LOST

The well-known consultant in weight management, Dr. Joyce Nash, says weight-loss failure need not happen. Writing in *Healthline*, Dr. Nash states that we are prone to "addictive thinking" which, after we have lost weight, allows us to rationalize dangerous behavior and seduces us into believing that we can eat the way we want to without regaining weight. Such thinking uses denial, which helps us ignore the returning pounds. We use excuses such as, "I think I can handle this treat." Such addictive thinking weakens motivation, and leads to guilt, blame, anger, and self-doubt, all of which makes things worse.

One way to counter addictive thinking is to learn positive "self-talk." Such self-talk reminds us of our achievements, in weight loss and other areas, and helps increase self-esteem. (Conversely, negative self-talk that reminds us of our failures erodes motivation and self-esteem.)

Kinds of positive self-talk include:

• *instructional self-talk,* which uses a problem-solving approach to reach goals, such as telling yourself to delay before eating a certain food, or letting yourself think about something else to avoid temptation.

• *statements about negative consequences* of regaining weight. Health problems, such as high blood pressure, economic consequences such as having to buy a new wardrobe, and psychological consequences, such as depression, low self-worth, frustration, and self-abuse.

Above all, avoid critical self-talk, such as "I don't deserve any better," or "I guess I was just meant to be fat." Like the alcoholic troubled with addictive thinking ("One drink—one drunk"), you need to tell yourself, "Beware of being a fat-thinking person in a thin body." Positive self-support comes from learning to think, and talk, in a supportive way.

Source: Nash, J. "Keeping Weight Off Once You've Taken It Off," *Healthline*, June 1991, pp. 2–4; Whitney, E. and Rolfe, S. *Understanding Nutrition,* 6th ed. St. Paul, MN: West, 1993.

Establish New Exercise Programs

Modifying your exercise behavior is as important as modifying eating behavior, and the same rules apply. Many health club memberships entitle you to an exercise program tailored specifically to your needs. The same results can be obtained independently at little or no cost by constructing and following a program of jogging, walking, bicycling, or swimming. A related incentive is to enlist a "buddy" with whom you share your exercise routine. Having a friend with whom you exercise may serve to stimulate you to maintain exercise habits when you might otherwise lighten up or drop out from lack of drive.

CHECKPOINT

1. State the principle behind successful weight management.

2. Discuss the steps a person might take in developing a program for losing weight.

3. List some things a person who is attempting to lose weight should *not* do and explain why.

4. Explain why exercise is so essential to a weight-loss program.

5. What is behavior modification? What are some of the behaviors that need to be modified by a person who is attempting to lose weight?

SUMMARY

Obesity in the United States has become the number one nutrition problem. Approximately 34 million people in the United States are considered obese. An estimated one-third to one-half of all American women and up to one-fourth of all American men are dieting at any one time.

Height/weight tables of desirable weights have been established for insured persons for a given sex and height. The most accurate weight table has been developed by the USDA and USDHHS. This table gives a range of recommended weights rather than an ideal weight. The preferable assessment of weight is a *healthy* weight based on this weight table and on the absence of any high-risk illness to which weight would be related. There is no ideal amount of body fat for a person. Yet, there is an average range that is recommended for a person, depending on gender and activity level.

An overweight person is one who weighs more than his or her recommended weight. Obesity is an excess of more than 18 percent stored fat in a male, and 24 percent in a female. Factors responsible for obesity may be physiological, and be controlled by a person's genetic makeup and by their rates of metabolism. External, or environmental, factors may provide cues that tell us when and when not to eat.

The onset of obesity may occur during childhood or adolescence, as with juvenile-onset obesity, or during adulthood, as with adult-onset obesity.

People often resort to fad diets, take chemical substances, or turn to surgical procedures to control their weight. Some people develop eating disorders such as *bulimia nervosa,* or binge-eating with purging, and *anorexia nervosa,* which is intentional starvation.

Successful weight management requires a lifetime maintenance of a recommended weight, a continuing exercise program, and behavior modification that changes faulty eating habits. Taking charge of this very important area can increase your self-esteem as well as providing lifelong health benefits.

REFERENCES

1. Toufexis, A. "Dieting: The Losing Game." *Time* (20 January 1986), 54–60.
2. Ibid.
3. National Institutes of Health, 1985 National Institutes of Health Consensus Development Panel on the Health Implications of Obesity, *Annals of Internal Medicine* 103, 1073–1077.
4. Johnson, P. *Fitness and You.* New York: Saunders, 1988.
5. Consumer Reports. "Losing Weight: What Works, What Doesn't." *Consumer Reports* (June 1993), 347–352.
6. Committee on Diet and Health, Food and Nutrition Board, National Academy of Sciences, *Diet and Health Implications for Reducing Chronic Disease Risk.* Washington, DC: National Academy Press, 1989.
7. Schardt, D. "Lifting Weight Myths." *Nutrition Action Health Letter* (October 1993), 8–9.
8. Neiman, D. *Fitness and Sports Medicine, An Introduction.* Palo Alto, CA: Bull, 1990.
9. USDA and USDHHS, Home and Garden Bulletin No. 232. *Nutrition and Your Health: Dietary Guidelines for Americans,* 3rd ed. Washington, DC: U.S. Government Printing Office, 1990.
10. Whitney, E., and Rolfes, S. *Understanding Nutrition,* 6th ed. Minneapolis: West, 1993.
11. Johnson, op. cit.
12. Lehman, T. "Body Composition Methodology in Sports Medicine." *The Physician and Sports Medicine* 10 (1982), 47–58.
13. Johnson, op. cit.
14. Ibid.
15. Ibid.
16. Whitney, op. cit.
17. Grady, D. "Bad News Bellies." *American Health* (May 1989), 20.
18. Whitney, op. cit.
19. Saltman, P., et al. *The California Nutrition Book.* Boston: Little, Brown, 1987.
20. Whitney, op. cit.
21. Stunkard, A., et al. "The Body-Mass Index of Twins Who Have Been Reared Apart." *New England Journal of Medicine* 322 (1990), 1483–1487.
22. Bouchard, C. "The Response of Long-Term Overfeeding in Individual Twins." *New England Journal of Medicine* 322 (1990), 1477–1482.
23. Saltman, op. cit.
24. Dreon, D., et al. "Dietary Fat: Carbohydrate Ratio and Obesity in Middle-aged Men." *American Journal of Clinical Nutrition* 47 (1988), 995–1000.
25. Flatt, J. "Effect of Carbohydrate Intake on Postprandial Substrate Oxidation and Storage." *Topics in Clinical Nutrition* 2 (1987), 15–27.
26. Whitney, op. cit.
27. Kern, P. "The Effects of Weight Loss on the Activity and Expression of Adipose-Tissue Lipoprotein Lipase in Very Obese Humans." *New England Journal of Medicine* 322 (1990), 1053–1059.
28. Saltman, op. cit.
29. Whitney, op. cit.
30. Ibid.
31. Mandenoff, A., et al. "Endogenous Opiates and Energy Balance." *Science* 215 (1982), 1536–1538.
32. Whitney, op. cit.
33. Saltman, op. cit.
34. Krieger, D., et al. "Role of Hormones in the Etiology and Pathogenesis of Obesity." In Frankle, R., and Yang, M. (eds.), *Obesity and Weight Control: The Health Professional's Guide to Understanding and Treatment,* Rockville, MD: Aspen Publishers, 1988, 35–52.
35. Centers for Disease Control, "Mortality Patterns— United States, 1989." *Morbidity and Mortality Weekly Report* 41 (1992), 121–125.
36. National Institutes of Health, op. cit.
37. Ibid.
38. Pi-Sunyer, F. "Health Implications of Obesity." *American Journal of Clinical Nutrition* 53 (1991), 15955–16035.
39. Bouchard, op. cit.
40. Corrigan, S., et al. "Weight Reduction in the Prevention and Treatment of Hypertension: A Review of Representative Clinical Trials." *American Journal of Health Promotion* 5 (1991), 208–214.

41. Weck, E. "The Dangerous Burden of Obesity." *FDA Consumer* (December 1986), 16–19.
42. National Institutes of Health, op. cit.
43. Whitney, op. cit.
45. Ibid.
46. National Institutes of Health, op. cit.
47. Weck, op. cit.
48. Yetiv, J. *Popular Nutritional Practices: A Scientific Appraisal.* Toledo, OH: Popular Medicine Press, 1986.
49. Weck, op. cit.
50. Whitney, op. cit.
51. Toufexis, op. cit.
52. Whitney, op. cit.
53. Yetiv, op. cit.
54. Wadden, T., et al. "Responsible and Irresponsible Use of Very-Low-Calorie-Diets in the Treatment of Obesity." *JAMA* 1 (1990), 83–85.
55. Ibid.
56. Van Itallie, op. cit.
57. Wadden, op. cit.
58. Council on Scientific Affairs. "Treatment of Obesity in Adults." *JAMA* 17 (1988), 2547–2551.
59. American Pharmaceutical Association. *Handbook of Nonprescription Drugs,* 9th ed. Washington, DC: American Pharmaceutical Association, 1990.
60. Papazian, R. "Should You Go on a Diet?" *FDA Consumer* (September 1993), 31–33.
61. American Pharmaceutical Association, op. cit.
62. Ibid.
63. Willis, J. "The Fad-Free Diet: How to Take Weight Off Without Getting Ripped Off." *FDA Consumer* (July/August 1985), 26–29.
64. Ibid.
65. Ibid.
66. National Institutes of Health, op. cit.
67. Whitney, op. cit.
68. Ibid.
69. Fenner, L. *Cellulite: Hard to Budge Pudge.* USDHHS Publ. No. 80–1078. Washington, DC: U.S. Government Printing Office, 1982.
70. Blackburn, G., et al. "Weight Cycling: The Experience of Human Dieters." *American Journal of Clinical Nutrition* 49 (1989), 1105–1109.
71. Lissner, L., et al. "Dietary Fat and the Regulation of Energy Intake in Human Subjects." *American Journal of Clinical Nutrition* 46 (1987), 886–892.
72. Whitney, op. cit.
73. Ibid.
74. Ibid.
75. Ibid.
76. Whitney, op. cit.
77. Farley, D. "Eating Disorders: When Thinness Becomes an Obsession." *FDA Consumer* (May 1986), 20–23.
78. Ibid.
79. Whitney, op. cit.
80. Yetiv, op. cit.
81. Farley, op. cit.
82. Farley, op. cit.
83. Ibid.
84. Ibid.
85. Whitney, op. cit.
86. Yetiv, op. cit.
87. Hammer, R., et al. "Calorie-Restricted Low-Fat Diet and Exercise in Obese Women." *American Journal of Clinical Nutrition* 49 (1989), 77–85.
88. Dreon, op. cit.
89. Lissner, op. cit.
90. Whitney, op. cit.
91. Poehlman, E., and Horton, E. "The Impact of Food Intake and Exercise in Energy Expenditure." *Nutritional Reviews* 47 (1989), 129–137.
92. Whitney, op. cit.
93. Ibid.

SUGGESTED READINGS

American Heart Association. *The American Heart Association Cookbook,* 5th ed. New York: Random House, 1991.
Cooper, K. *Controlling Cholesterol.* New York: Bantam, 1988.
Eades, M. *Thin So Fat.* New York: Warner, 1989.
Freiden, M. *The Calorie Factor.* New York: Fireside, 1989.
Hirschman, J., and Munter, C. *Overcoming Overeating.* Reading, MA: Addison-Wesley, 1988.
Kraus, B. *Calories and Carbohydrates,* 8th ed. New York: Signet, 1989.
Magee, E. *Fight Fat and Win.* Minneapolis: Chronimed/DCI, 1990.
Piscatella, J. *Controlling Your Fat Tooth.* New York: Workman, 1991.
Rhoades, J. *Fat to Fit Without Dieting.* Chicago: Contemporary, 1990.
Saltman, P., et al. *The University of California San Diego Nutrition Book.* Boston: Little, Brown, 1993.
Sheats, C. *Cliff Sheats' Lean Bodies.* Ft. Worth: Summit Group, 1993.
Stark, R., and Winston, M. *The AHA Low-salt Cookbook.* New York: Random House, 1990.
U.S. Department of Health and Human Services. *The Surgeon General's Report on Nutrition and Health.* DHHS (PHS) Publ. No. 88-50210. Washington, DC: U.S. Government Printing Office, 1988.
Vargas, P. *50 Ways to Lose Your Blubber.* Deerfield Beach, FL: Health Communications, 1993.
Waterhouse, D. *Outsmarting the Female Fat Cell.* New York: Hyperion, 1993.

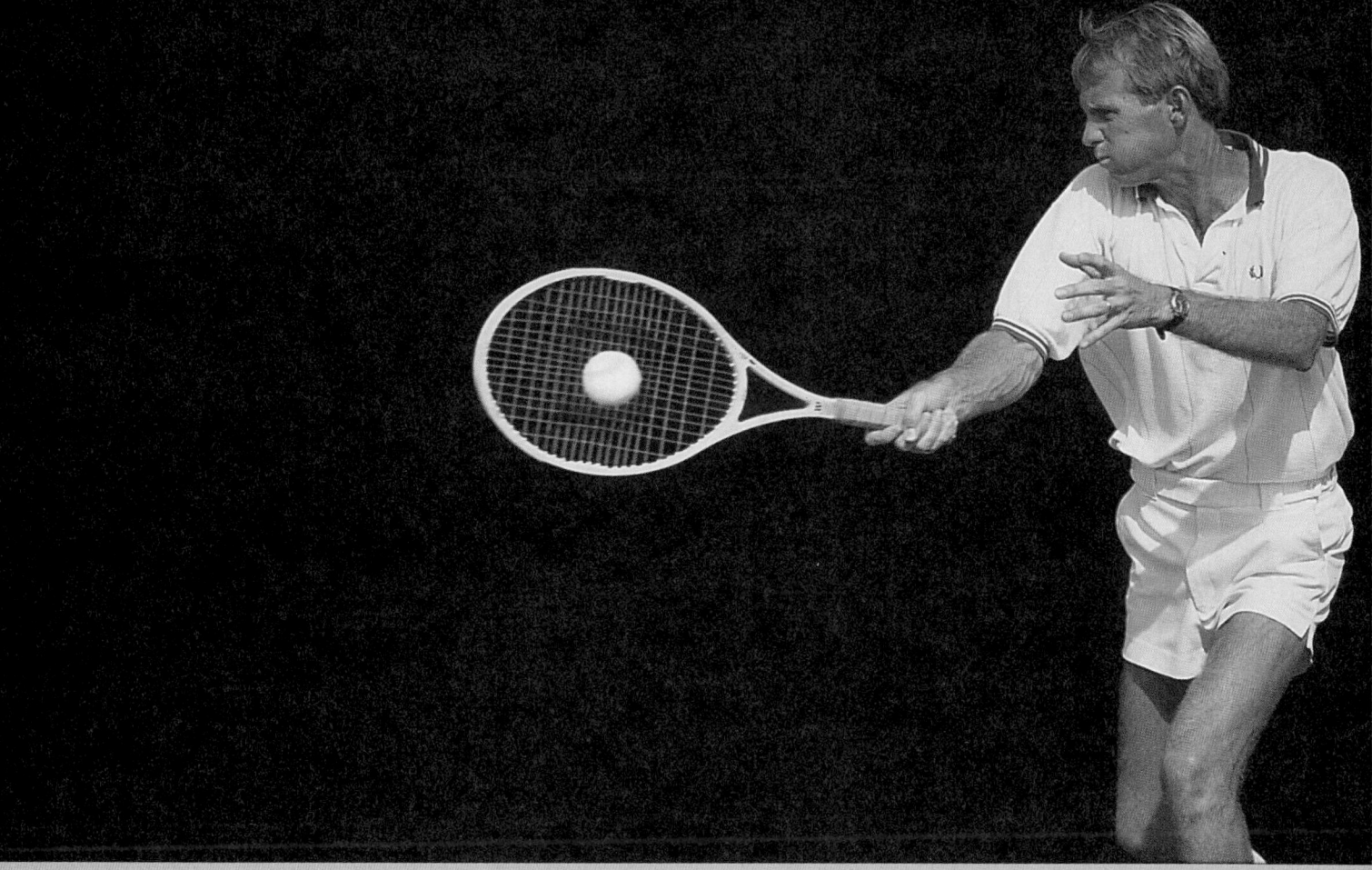

11
TURNING ON TO FITNESS

CHAPTER OBJECTIVES

Upon completing this chapter, you will be able to:

KNOWLEDGE

- List the significant physical advantages of exercise.
- Contrast anaerobic exercise with aerobic exercise.
- Identify the psychological benefits of exercise.
- Classify the components of physical exercise.
- Contrast muscular strength with muscular endurance.
- Discuss the significance of intensity, mode, duration, and frequency in developing cardiorespiratory endurance.
- Discuss the significance of the target training zone.
- Discuss the advantages of dressing in layers of clothing for cold weather exercise.
- Distinguish among heat cramps, heat exhaustion, and heat stroke.

INSIGHT

- Based on the self-test for fitness, describe your own level of fitness.
- Determine which fitness components might be best for improving your cardiovascular health.
- Determine your readiness to begin an exercise program.
- Calculate your heart rate reserve (HRR).

DECISION MAKING

- Determine which component of physical fitness you most need to improve.
- Develop a program to meet your specific fitness goals.
- Develop an effective schedule for you to develop maximum cardiovascular fitness.
- Develop a list of fitness activities that best fit your interests, age, and health.

How do celebrities such as Bruce Dern, Melissa Gilbert-Brinkman, and Joan Chen stay in shape? Many people probably believe that these folks rely on expensive personal trainers or go on elaborate diet regimens to maintain their superstar bodies. However, while many of the "rich and famous" do have personal trainers, others use very ordinary, inexpensive, and certainly not elaborate methods.

Film star Bruce Dern, known for his roles in Middle Age Crazy, Coming Home, and Silent Running, has made physical fitness a way of life. He has jogged roughly 160,000 miles over the past 40 years. His diet is simple—avoid the junk foods to keep down the cholesterol and weight. Melissa Gilbert-Brinkman, grown up since her days of running across the prairie in the television series "Little House on the Prairie," is the mother of a toddler. She uses fitness workouts as a way to bring her and her family together, through such activities as water aerobics. To maintain her weight, she simply chooses fruits, vegetables, and grains over fats and sweets. Joan Chen, costar of television's "Twin Peaks," relies on the foods of her native China, such as rice and fish, to help her keep trim. She chooses a rather unique way to exercise— her hobby, carpentry.

These celebrities realize the importance of regular physical exercise in the quest for fitness; it is clear that their workouts are not elaborate or expensive. Simple and inexpensive, running, aerobics, and even *carpentry, are excellent ways for virtually anyone to maintain or improve their level of physical fitness. The message is clear: Physical fitness does not require a big budget or a great deal of time. What it does require is a conscious decision to be active as a way to improve your looks, health, and overall quality of life.*

Source: American Fitness, *September/October 1991, p. 16.*

■   ■   ■

WELLNESS

Most of us are aware of the benefits of physical activity and a positive healthful life-style, and know that these help improve health. Yet many do not realize the benefits because they do not know how to go about a program that will give them results. Led on by persuasive advertising and by old habits, many follow practices that severely threaten health and lead to premature illness and death.

Wellness is something more than the absence of disease. Wellness is the constant and deliberate effort to stay healthy and achieve the highest potential for well-being. This concept of wellness brings together a healthy life-style and a level of physical fitness. It includes proper nutrition, stress management, disease prevention, not smoking, control or cessation of alcohol use, spiritual values, personal safety, and physical fitness.

WHY BE FIT?

Most people who exercise do it to improve their **fitness.** Fitness to them may mean anything from being able to fit into last year's clothes to working productively or sleeping soundly. For athletes, fitness is the ability to perform certain sports skills. The American Medical Association gives fitness a working definition by stating: *physical fitness is the general capacity to adapt and respond favorably to physical effort.* The meaning here is that persons are physically fit when they meet everyday, as well as unusual, demands of daily life, safely and effectively and still have enough energy left for leisure and recreational activities.

....

fitness the general capacity to adapt and respond favorably to physical effort.

EXCUSES FOR NOT STAYING FIT

Few personal physical activities are taken more seriously than exercising. People exercise in order to maintain youthfulness, to delay aging, to improve body image, to trim and keep off unwanted fat, and to increase their sense of vitality and well-being. The intensity and devotion with which people approach fitness programs makes them prime candidates for fitness myths. Such misconceptions find their way into the conversations of fitness enthusiasts and often become accepted as fact as they are passed from one person to another.

Before we proceed further with the positive aspects of fitness, here is a sampling of these physical fitness myths, along with the factual answers. How many of these myths have you heard and believed?

1. *Exercising makes you tired.* Although any physical activity produces temporary fatigue, as you become conditioned, you commonly have more energy than before. Regular vigorous exercise, in fact, helps you to resist fatigue and stress.

2. *You have to be an athlete to exercise.* Most aerobic exercise activities require no special athletic abilities. In fact, aerobic exercises are often found to be more enjoyable and manageable than participation in school sports.

3. *All kinds of exercise activities provide the same benefits.* All physical activity, vigorous or not, can be enjoyable. But only aerobic exercises, which are sustained and performed on a regular schedule, improve cardiorespiratory endurance (CRE) and burn off excess calories. Other less-demanding activities can help maintain flexibility and strength, but without excess calorie burnoff and CRE training (pp. 337, 353).

4. *Perspiration is a prime indicator of a workout's effectiveness.* Since some people naturally perspire more easily than others, sweat droplets are no measure of cardiovascular conditioning.

5. *Passive exercise is an easy, effective way to fitness.* Effective exercise requires that you increase your metabolic rate and calorie expenditure. If exercise is too easy and you aren't doing much work, you're not getting much fitness benefit. Toning tables and sauna belts are not recommended for fitness and general conditioning.

6. *Exercise makes women less feminine.* There is no evidence that exercise will increase growth

rates, muscle bulk, or body weight. Any person, regardless of sex, who maintains a healthful lifestyle will be more attractive.

7. *Men are superior to women in all types of exercise activities.* Women possess greater manual dexterity than men and have as great a skill-learning rate as men. Since women have more fatty tissue than men, they are more buoyant in water (an advantage in swimming). Since girls mature earlier, they are often superior to men in physical strength and endurance until ages 12–14, after which boys reach and surpass them in these capacities.

8. *Exercise takes too much time.* A regular program of aerobic exercises takes no more than 25–40 minutes, 3 times a week, which works easily into most schedules. If made a priority, exercising can become a natural, nonintrusive part of your life.

9. *If you stop exercising, your muscles will turn into fat.* Ceasing exercise will cause muscles to diminish in size, and being sedentary will increase fat stores. Yet, muscle tissue and fat tissue are two different kinds of tissue and are not interrelated.

10. *Eating before workouts isn't wise.* This depends on the kind of food and the amount. For example, eating a little fruit shortly before a workout is all right, but a full meal is not. Allow at least an hour between a full meal and exercising.

11. *Exercising through colds or the flu can lessen their severity.* Exercise is no foolproof way to working through colds. When a cold is coming on, especially with a fever, stay away from exercise and allow your body to fight the disease. When recovering from a cold, mild exercise may help circulation and body functioning.

These are just a few of the myths that exist about exercise. What other things do you believe about fitness? The material on the following pages will help you to determine your level of fitness and provide you with what you need to know to achieve your fitness goals.

CHECKPOINT

1. Define wellness.
2. Give the working definition of fitness.

BENEFITS OF EXERCISE

Exercise is any muscular activity that maintains fitness. Exercise, especially running, tends to increase muscle mass and bone density. When you ask people who exercise regularly how they have benefited, they usually say that it makes them feel better. Whether exercise is moderate or vigorous, feeling better and having an improved sense of satisfaction provides more drive and zest for life. Exercise has both psychological and physical benefits.

PHYSICAL BENEFITS

Statistics on early death are alarming. It's estimated that 83 percent of all deaths prior to age 65 are preventable.[1] More than 1.5 million people have heart attacks each year and over half of them die as a result. About half of those who die are men between the ages of 40 and 65—their most productive years.[2] For these reasons it's worth looking at the physical benefits of exercise. The following sections describe some of the significant physical advantages of exercise.

Body Composition

A person's body composition is affected by **aerobic exercises,** those continuous exercises involving major muscle groups and requiring oxygen, such as swimming, fast walking, jogging, and fast bicycling. Exercise alters a person's metabolism, causing increases in daily energy expenditures, even while resting. In fact, vigorous exercise speeds up the rate of metabolism by about 5 percent for as long as two days after the exercise has taken place.[3] An aerobic exercise program results in an increase in lean body mass and a decrease in body fat. The consequence is that an exercising person greatly improves overall body composition.

Muscle Conditioning

When a person exercises, hormones that signal the liver and fat cells to liberate their stored energy nutrients, such as glucose and fatty acids, are

....

exercise any muscular activity that maintains fitness.

aerobic exercise those continuous exercises involving major muscle groups and requiring oxygen.

released into the bloodstream. Muscle cells are thus exposed to more energy nutrients by the circulation of blood. The more fit a muscle is the more oxygen it draws from the blood to burn these food nutrients, which in turn means that more oxygen is drawn from the lungs. In response to this demand for oxygen the cardiovascular system increases its capacity to deliver oxygen to the body to produce the necessary energy to carry out the activity.

Stress Reduction

Physical activity is one of the easiest ways to control stress. Exercise not only reduces the intensity of the stress itself, but also reduces the amount of time needed to recover. Diverting the stress to working muscles causes the emotional strain to disappear and the mind to clear. Since a fatigued muscle is a relaxed muscle, exercise reduces muscular tension. Oxygen is needed in muscular exertion, and the physically fit person draws more oxygen from the lungs than the person who is not fit. In vigorous physical exercise, the pituitary gland releases morphinelike substances called *endorphins,* which not only serve as painkillers, but also create a soothing, calming effect associated with feelings of well-being. Exercise also stimulates alpha-wave activity in the brain. These are the same brain wave patterns seen during periods of relaxation and meditation.

Cardiovascular Conditioning

Regular aerobic exercise improves the condition of the whole cardiovascular system. As the cardiovascular system is conditioned, the total blood volume and number of red blood cells increases, raising the amount of oxygen the blood can carry. The heart muscle becomes larger and stronger, so that with each beat the heart chambers empty more completely, and thus pump more blood per beat. Since fewer heartbeats are necessary, the pulse rate drops. Along with an improved heart muscle, the muscles that inflate and deflate the lungs become stronger with the increased demand for oxygen, and breathing becomes more efficient.

Regulation of Levels of Cholesterol and Triglycerides

The term *blood lipids* is often used when referring to cholesterol and triglycerides. Their elevation in the blood is definitely linked to cardiovascular diseases, especially coronary heart disease (see Table 11.1). Cholesterol is carried in the blood by one of three proteins called lipoproteins: high density lipoproteins (HDL), low density lipoproteins (LDL), and very low density lipoproteins (VLDL) (see Chapter 9). The way in which cholesterol is carried in the blood and the total amount of cholesterol in the blood are both important. The levels of the three lipoproteins indicate the presence or absence

Exercise is any muscular activity that maintains fitness. Activities such as running tend to increase muscle mass and bone density.

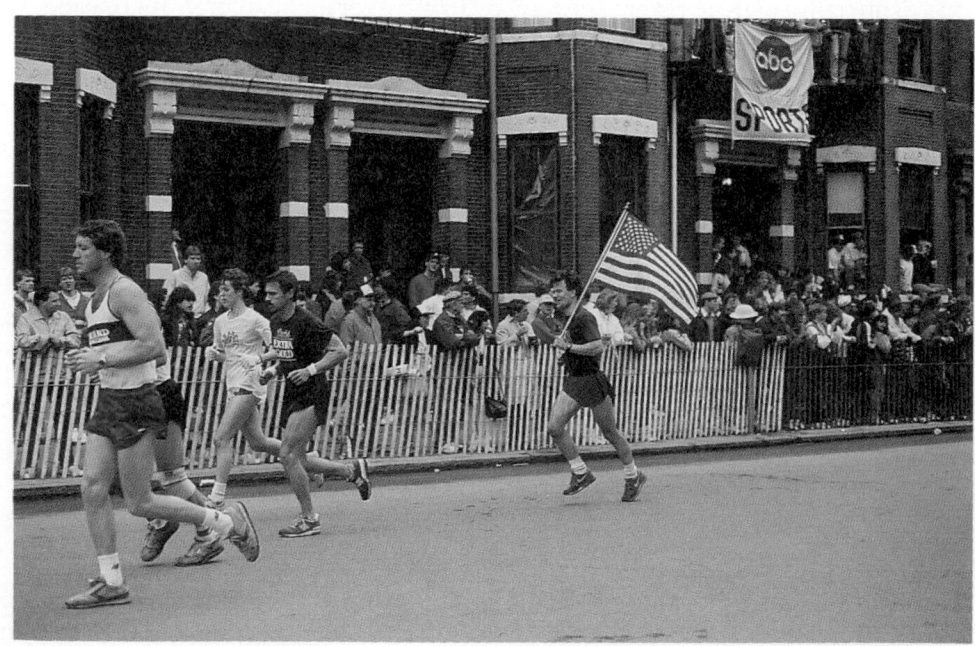

Table 11.1
Standards for Blood Lipids

	Level	Effect
Total Cholesterol[a]	≤200 mg/dl	Desirable
	200–239 mg/dl	Borderline high
	≥240 mg/dl	High risk
LDL-Cholesterol	≤130 mg/dl	Desirable
	130–160 mg/dl	Borderline high
	≥160 mg/dl	High risk
HDL-Cholesterol[a]	≥45 mg/dl	Desirable
	36–44 mg/dl	Moderate risk
	≤35 mg/dl	High risk
Triglycerides	≤250 mg/dl	Desirable
	251–499 mg/dl	Borderline high
	≥500 mg/dl	High risk

[a]The best indicator of coronary risk is the ratio of total cholesterol to HDL. For example, an overall reading of 200 and an HDL of 50 gives a ratio of 4. Ratios above 4 are viewed as being undesirable. The higher the ratio, the greater the risk of developing coronary heart disease.

Source: *"Standards for Blood Lipids,"* Annals of Internal Medicine. *December 1987.*

of cardiovascular disease risks. Of the three cholesterol-carrier lipoproteins, HDL is the most beneficial in handling cholesterol. The more HDL-cholesterol, the better. There is a clear effect between HDL-cholesterol and aerobic exercise; the greater the amount of exercise, the higher the level of HDL-cholesterol in the blood. The levels of blood lipids can be reduced by cutting back on foods containing lipids, by reducing excess body weight, and by engaging in aerobic exercise.

Reduced Incidence of Coronary Heart Disease

One of the major causes of unnecessary death in the United States is coronary heart disease (CHD). Risk factors for CHD include too little exercise, elevated blood cholesterol, cigarette smoking, high blood pressure, diabetes, and obesity. Of these, the most prevalent modifiable risk factor is too little exercise.[4]

Control of Diabetes

Diabetes is a disease characterized by insufficient production or utilization of insulin and by high blood glucose levels. Exercise can help reduce a

diabetic's insulin requirements. There is increased muscle sensitivity to insulin during exercise, so that muscle cells use more of the glucose in the blood. In fact, as with metabolic rate, this effect lasts after the exercise period has ended. Exercise not only helps prevent the onset of diabetes, but helps reduce the daily amount of insulin or insulin-producing drugs diabetics require. Another benefit is that people with diabetes who exercise experience weight loss, and excess body fatness is one of the significant risk factors in Type II diabetes.[5]

Reduction in Blood Pressure

There is increasing evidence of the importance of the role of aerobic exercise in managing high blood pressure (hypertension). Generally, people who are cardiovascularly fit have lower blood pressures than people who are unfit. In an 18-year study of exercising and nonexercising people, the exercising group had an average resting blood pressure of 120/79, compared to an average of 150/90 for the nonexercising group.[6] Aerobic exercise is often used in treating hypertensive patients, often with a significant effect after only a few weeks of training.

Reduced Incidence of Cancers

Some cancers, such as those caused by cigarette smoking and heavy use of alcohol, could be prevented completely, and other cancers, such as skin cancers, can be prevented by protection from the sun's rays, according to the American Cancer Society. Some cancer cases, such as these mentioned, are related to our physical surroundings, personal habits, or life-styles.[7] Many of these cancers are preventable through positive life-style habits. The American Cancer Society and the National Cancer Institute report that three most important general health habits in lowered cancer mortality rates are abstinence from smoking, adequate sleep, and regular physical activity.[8]

Slowing the Aging Process

Physical activity slows the aging process. People who maintain a high level of physical activity have a higher level of functional capacity. It is estimated that in a functional sense, the typical person in the United States is 30 years older than his or her chronological age. In other words, a person who is physically active at 60 years of age can have a work capacity similar to the sedentary 30-year-old.[9]

Reducing Death Rates

Cardiovascular fitness relates to levels of mortality (death), regardless of age and other risk factors. Studies show that among men, the least fit have a death rate 3.4 times higher than the most fit. Among women, the death rate is 4.6 times higher in the least fit than in the most fit. In fact, even a moderate level of fitness reduces the rate of premature death.[10]

PSYCHOLOGICAL BENEFITS

People who exercise regularly report a number of psychological benefits:

- *Reduction in negative emotion* Exercise has been shown to reduce feelings of frustration, aggression, anger, and hostility.
- *Development of discipline* A regular program of exercise helps a person prioritize significant activities.
- *Improved self-image* Exercise and its results promote self-confidence, alertness, and an improved body image. Persons who are fit have an increased feeling of well-being.
- *Improved motivation* An improved feeling of well-being helps motivate a person toward further positive life-style changes—better nutrition, stopping smoking, control or cessation of alcohol and other drug use, stress management, and disease prevention—and a desire to maintain wellness.

ARE YOU FIT?

The President's Council on Physical Fitness and Sports has proposed a scale of physical fitness ranging from an "abundant life" at one extreme to "death" at the other. According to this scale, anyone who is alive has at least some degree of physical fitness.

This spectrum of physical fitness can be thought of as a *continuum* (Figure 11.1). At the low end of the scale are impaired persons or those recovering from a severe illness who need help performing even daily routine tasks. At the other end are athletes who are trained and conditioned for competition. Each of us is at a point along the continuum of increasing physical fitness. *A person may be physically fit without reaching a high level of physical fitness.*

If you are fit enough to perform the daily activities your life-style requires, you may be content with where you fit along the continuum. To determine whether your level of physical fitness is adequate for your present life-style, check yourself using the test for adequate levels of fitness (see In Your Hands: Self-test for Fitness).

Simply being fit enough to fulfill your daily activities may seem sufficient, yet it leaves no extra energy should you decide to take on active leisure activities. Skiing, hiking, or getting back in shape after an illness for someone whose degree of fitness is less than average may lead to dropping the activity. It is important to build up your level of fitness gradually for such activities, to avoid both discouragement and injury. For the person in good condition, such activities are enjoyable.

Figure 11.1

A Physical Fitness Continuum

Source: Kusinitz, I., and Fine, M. *Your Guide to Getting Fit,* 2nd ed. Mountain View, CA: Mayfield, 1991.

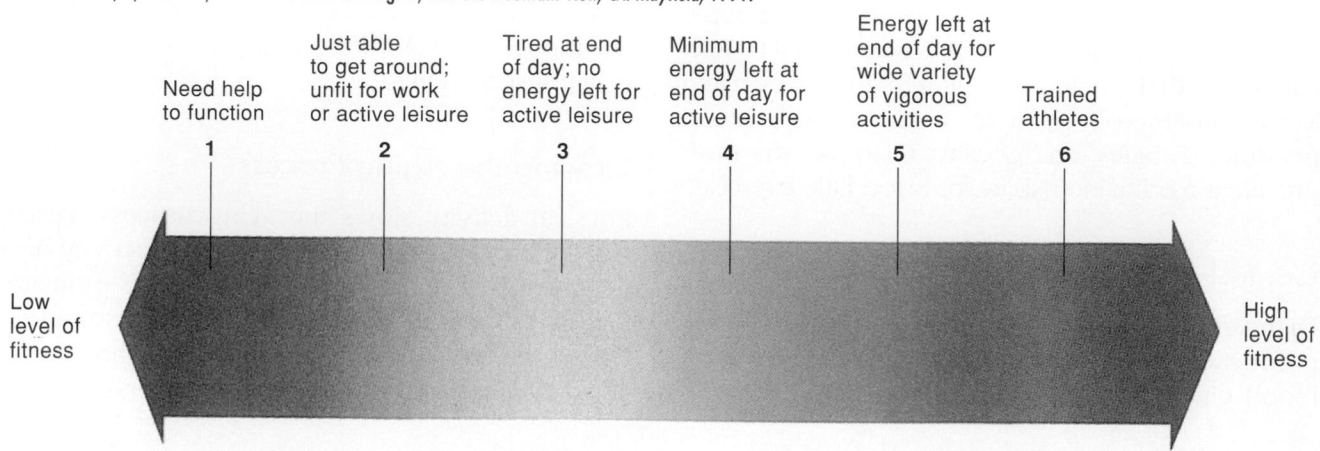

IN YOUR HANDS
SELF-TEST FOR FITNESS

This easy-to-take self-test can help you determine your level of fitness. Gaining an early understanding of your fitness level can provide you with information on what kind of fitness program you need to develop.

A person can be considered as having less than an adequate level of physical fitness if several of the following apply. Check the boxes that are applicable to you:

Yes   No

_____ _____ Do you yawn regularly throughout the day?

_____ _____ Do you feel tired when you wake up in the morning and often do not really want to get out of bed?

_____ _____ Do you become fatigued from tasks requiring minimal energy, such as climbing a flight of stairs or walking around a shopping mall?

_____ _____ Do you run out of energy by the middle of the day or early afternoon?

_____ _____ Do you experience a drowsy feeling for much of the day?

_____ _____ Do you look or feel flabby?

_____ _____ Do you fall asleep early in the evening while reading or while watching television?

_____ _____ Do you experience difficulty in coping with daily pressures?

_____ _____ Do you experience nagging aches and pains?

_____ _____ Do you find it difficult to relax?

_____ _____ Do you often have an irritable disposition toward others?

_____ _____ Are you often too tired to participate in active leisure activities?

_____ _____ Are you vulnerable to a variety of health problems, such as frequent colds and back pains?

_____ _____ Do you generally lack energy and vitality?

If you participate regularly in a well-designed exercise program you should have answered yes to very few, if any, of these and should develop and maintain an optimal level of health, performance, and appearance.

Source: Hockey, R. *Physical Fitness, the Pathway to Healthful Living,* 7th ed. St. Louis: Mosby, 1993.

CHECKPOINT

1. Explain the scale of physical fitness proposed by the President's Council on Physical Fitness and Sports.

2. Have you taken the Self-test for Fitness?

COMPONENTS OF PHYSICAL FITNESS

As our concepts of physical fitness have developed, it has become apparent that no single test is adequate in assessing overall fitness. Because several specific components are needed in order to determine an individual's overall level of fitness, a group of tests is needed. There are four specific health-related components of fitness: cardiorespiratory endurance, muscular strength and endurance, flexibility, and body composition.

CARDIORESPIRATORY ENDURANCE

Cardiorespiratory endurance (CRE) is the ability to perform moderately strenuous activity over an extended period of time. Also known as cardiovascular endurance, CRE is a measure of how well the heart and lungs supply the body with increased oxygen during sustained physical activity. As mus-

cardiorespiratory endurance (CRE) or **aerobic capacity** the ability of the body to perform moderately strenuous activity over an extended period of time; also called *cardiovascular endurance.*

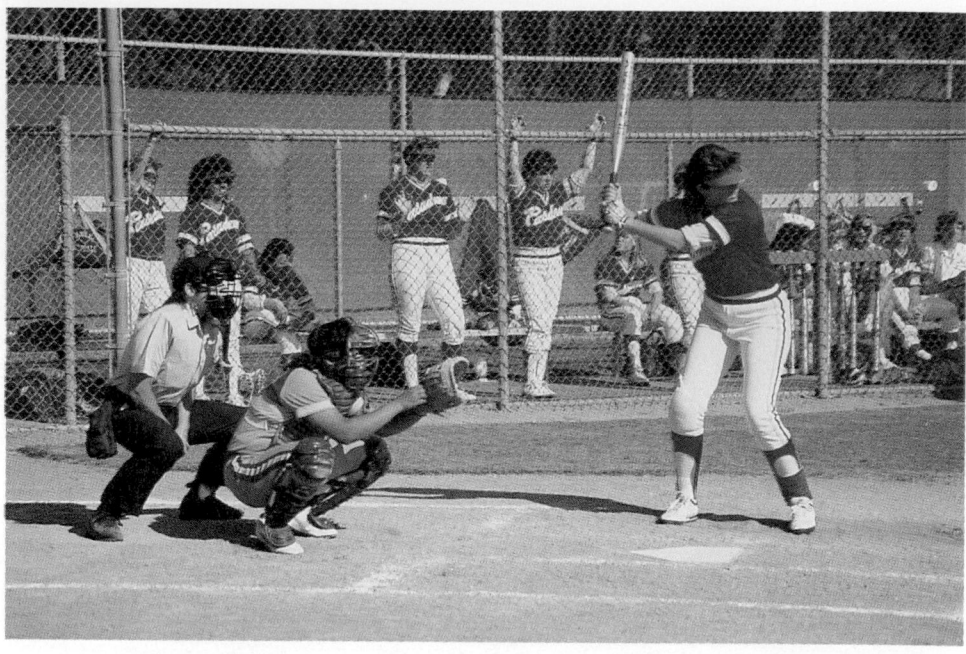

Exercise such as softball, that involves sudden bursts of muscle activity, is an anaerobic activity. In such activities the sudden vigorous activity may momentarily outstrip the ability of the body to maintain the needed supply of oxygen.

cles work they consume oxygen and give off carbon dioxide. Any activity, whether it is sleep or running, depends upon the cardiovascular and respiratory systems. Also referred to as **aerobic capacity,** this consumption of oxygen is the most important of the fitness components.[11]

Aerobic exercise is a method of conditioning the cardiorespiratory system by performing activities that increase the demand by muscles for oxygen over a period of time. This kind of exercise improves the cardiovascular and respiratory systems' capacity to deliver oxygen to and remove carbon dioxide from working muscles. As continuous exercise trains the heart, it is able to pump more blood per beat than the untrained heart. The more strenuous the exercise and the longer it is sustained over time, the higher the body's capacity. Assess your cardiorespiratory endurance by testing yourself according to the Modified Step Test in Feature 11.1.

Improving CRE Through Exercise

There are two types of exercise, aerobic and anaerobic. **Aerobic** (*a-rō'bik*), meaning "with oxygen," is exercise using energy that requires oxygen for continuous exertion. **Anaerobic** (*an-ā-er-ō'bik*),

meaning "without oxygen," is exercise that uses energy stored by the body for fast bursts of speed.

The energy that cells use is stored in a compound called **adenosine triphosphate (ATP)** (*a-den'ō-sēn trī'fos'fāt*). ATP is found in all cells, particularly muscle cells, and stores energy derived from carbohydrates, fats, and proteins. Cells have only a small reserve of ATP on hand; this is just enough to last for a few seconds of intense activity.[12] Muscle cells have an additional reserve material, which with ATP can supply energy without oxygen for 15–20 seconds. The release of further energy requires a supply of oxygen.

Continuous rigorous exercise lasting more than two minutes, such as jogging, long-distance swimming, bicycling, and cross-country skiing, brings about an aerobic training effect. Because aerobic exercise is rhythmic in nature, using large muscle groups and elevating heart rate for prolonged periods of time, the cardiovascular system is challenged to deliver oxygen to muscles.[13, 14] Muscles produce energy efficiently when oxygen is present. A small amount of ATP can be extracted from glucose stored within the muscle cells, without oxygen, during anaerobic exertion, but oxygen is needed to extract the maximum amount of ATP from glucose.

....

aerobic in the presence of oxygen; such exercise requires oxygen for continuous exertion.

anaerobic without oxygen; such exercise uses energy stored by the body for fast bursts of speed.

....

adenosine triphosphate (ATP) a substance found especially in muscle cells which, when split, releases stored energy.

FEATURE 11.1

MODIFIED STEP TEST

OBJECTIVE

To complete 3 minutes of stepping at 24 steps per minute.

DIRECTIONS

1. Step up (start with either foot) on a stair or bench that is 8 inches from ground level and then step down again. Continue stepping up and down, alternating feet, for three consecutive minutes at a rate of 24 steps per minute—about 2 steps every five seconds. (A metronome can help you maintain the rhythm.)

2. Stop at exactly three minutes, and immediately sit in a chair.

3. At exactly one minute after you complete the test, count your pulse for 30 seconds . . . and multiply by 2 to obtain your one-minute pulse recovery score.

4. Determine the rating for your score by consulting the Heart Beats per Minute table which follows. If you are unable to step for the full 3 minutes, consider yourself very low in cardiorespiratory endurance.

RATING

The scores in the table are for heartbeats per minute, measured one minute after completion of the modified step test.

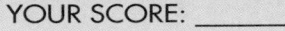

YOUR SCORE: _____

HEART BEATS PER MINUTE

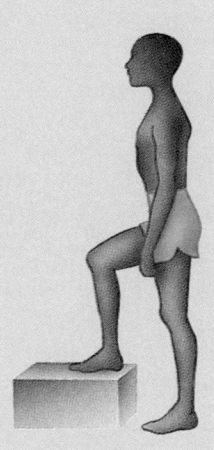

Age	Very high	High	Moderate	Low	Very low
Female					
10–19	Below 82	82–90	92–96	98–102	Above 102
20–29	Below 82	82–86	88–92	94–98	Above 98
30–39	Below 82	82–88	90–94	96–98	Above 98
40–49	Below 82	82–86	88–96	98–102	Above 102
Over 50	Below 86	86–92	94–98	100–104	Above 104
Male					
10–19	Below 72	72–76	78–82	84–88	Above 88
20–29	Below 72	72–78	80–84	86–92	Above 92
30–39	Below 76	76–80	82–86	88–92	Above 92
40–49	Below 78	78–82	84–88	90–94	Above 94
Over 50	Below 80	80–84	86–90	92–96	Above 96

Source: Kusinitz, I., and Fine, M. *Your Guide to Getting Fit,* 2nd ed. Mountain View, CA: Mayfield, 1991.

Exercise such as karate, weight lifting, sprinting, tennis, handball, squash, volleyball, and racquetball train the anaerobic system. Depending on the intensity and length of time the game is played, these exercises can also train the aerobic system. Anaerobic exercises are those that are performed in spurts and that do not effectively challenge the cardiovascular system due to the lack of sustained and vigorous exertion. When a person makes an all-out effort lasting one to two minutes, cells are able to make more ATP from the simple sugar glucose, which is stored in the cells. Such an intense burst of activity exceeds the ability of the heart and lungs to supply the necessary oxygen, thus leaving the person gasping for breath. To restore this oxygen, the heart and lungs work hard for the next several minutes to "repay" this oxygen debt. Although anaerobic activities may help develop strength, they do not provide aerobic benefit to the cardiovascular system.

Anaerobic sports require intense bursts of activity. These sports are usually safe for healthy young adults wishing to start a program. But for the sedentary older adult, they may be dangerous to the heart. The intensity of such sports also increases the risk of injury when compared with the more sustained and rhythmic forms of aerobic exercise. To avoid overexertion it is important not to engage in anaerobic activities until you are aerobically fit. This can be accomplished through participating in an aerobic program for several weeks. Unless you are

Anaerobic exercises, such as karate, call for sudden rigorous bursts of activity. Exercises performed in spurts do not effectively challenge the cardiovascular system. Because they exceed the ability of the heart and lungs to supply the necessary oxygen, such exercises may leave the person gasping for breath.

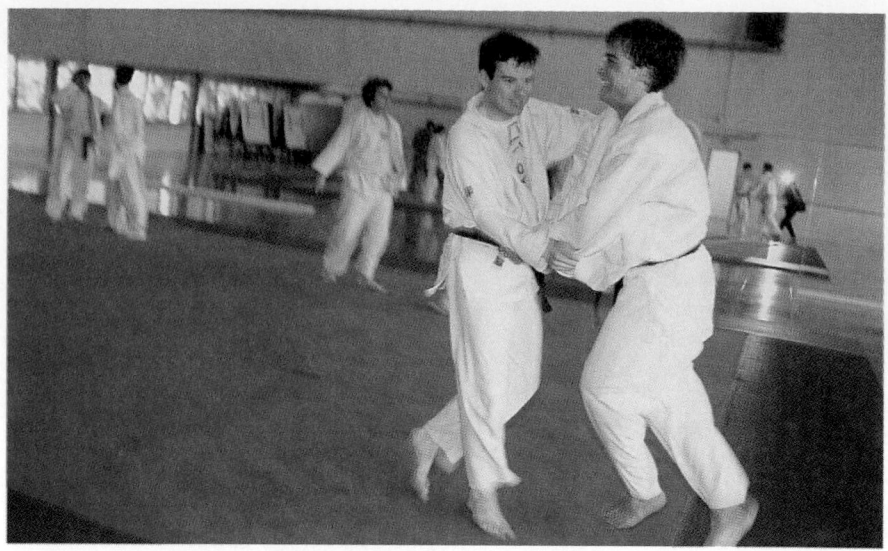

interested in competitive sports, anaerobic types of training can be eliminated from your program with little effect on cardiorespiratory endurance.

MUSCULAR STRENGTH AND ENDURANCE

Muscular strength is measured by the amount of force a muscle can exert when lifting, moving, or pushing an object.[15] A single muscle group can be tested using a hand dynamometer, which measures the strength of a hand's grip (see Feature 11.2).

Everyone needs some strength to carry out simple everyday tasks. Without maintaining strength, even the simplest activities, such as walking, become more difficult, and the risk of injury increases.

Muscular strength is needed to lift a suitcase off the floor and to hold it off the floor. **Muscular endurance** involves sustaining muscular contraction or repeatedly contracting a muscle group for a certain period of time.[16] Exercises such as sit-ups test the endurance of the abdominal muscles while push-ups measure the endurance of the shoulders, chest, and arm muscles. By following the instructions in Feature 11.3 (p. 342) you can test your muscular endurance.

Muscular endurance is important for performing everyday tasks. People who work at computer word processors, for example, need enough endurance in their fingers, forearms, shoulders, and back muscles to work at a keyboard hour after hour.

Improving Muscle Strength and Endurance

Muscles become stronger with use; they also become smaller and weaker if not used regularly. Your muscular strength and endurance determine your limits; increasing your limits makes your muscles more efficient.

Muscular strength and endurance can be improved in a program using any of three types of muscular contractions: isotonic, isometric, and isokinetic. Meaning "equal tensions," **isotonic contractions** occur, for example, when lifting a weight. The force exerted by the muscle is greater than the resistance, causing the joint to move and the muscle to shorten. As your arm muscles contract, the elbow bends, the forearm moves, and you lift the weight.

Isometric contractions occur when, for instance, you push against a wall with all your strength. The force exerted is equal to or less than the resistance and no movement occurs at the joint. Meaning "equal measure," isometric contractions cause the muscle to contract without shortening.

....

muscular strength the ability to exert maximum force, usually in a single exertion.

muscular endurance the ability to repeat a particular action or hold a particular position for an extended time.

isotonic contraction contraction in which the force exerted by the muscle is greater than the resistance; the object moves and the muscle shortens.

isometric contraction contraction in which the force exerted is equal to or less than the resistance; the object does not move and no shortening of the muscle occurs.

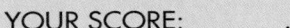

FEATURE 11.2
TAKING THE GRIP-STRENGTH DYNAMOMETER TEST

OBJECTIVE
To assess your grip strength by using a hand dynamometer.

DIRECTIONS
Hold the dynamometer in one hand (preferably the hand with which you write). Squeeze the device as hard as you can; then read your score in pounds (or kilograms) on the dial. Consult the Grip Strength table for an interpretation of your grip score. The scores are given in pounds.

YOUR SCORE: _____.

GRIP STRENGTH (IN POUNDS)

	Very high	High	Moderate	Low	Very low
Female	Above 89	83–89	56–82	49–55	Below 49
Male	Above 154	136–154	105–135	91–104	Below 91

Source: Kusinitz, I., and Fine, M. *Your Guide to Getting Fit,* 2nd ed. Mountain View, CA: Mayfield, 1991.

Meaning "equal motion," **isokinetic contractions** are like isotonic contractions in that the muscle shortens, yet are different in that the resistance matches the force. The force exerted is maximal throughout the full range of motion. Isokinetic exercises require mechanical devices that provide maximal resistance throughout the entire range of motion. This equipment is expensive and is usually found only in elaborately equipped fitness centers.[17]

Types of strength training include body building, weight training, and weight lifting. *Body building* emphasizes developing massive muscles which are well-proportioned and well-defined. Body builders use many repetitions involving specific body areas to enlarge and shape the appearance of the body. Although the effects are viewed by many as desirable, body building requires time, hard work, and self-discipline in terms of diet and consistency of training, and many body builders and other athletes take extreme measures to achieve the desired results (see Feature 11.4, p. 343).

Weight training is used to improve muscular strength and endurance, as well as flexibility and body composition. Weight-training programs require the use of free weights (barbells and dumb-

bells) or machines offering similar resistance, with weights and repetitions progressively increased. It involves taking the amount of weight or resistance through the full range of motion for 7–12 consecutive repetitions. While body building emphasizes developing well-defined muscles beyond what most weight trainers see as desirable, weight training is a means to reach a fitness goal.

Weight lifting is a sport in which a person attempts to lift his or her maximum amount of weight. Such an effort can only be done one time, followed by an interval for recovery. There are two categories of weight lifting: (1) *olympic lifts* include the snatch and the clean and jerk; (2) *power lifts* include the squat, the bench press, and the dead lift.

FLEXIBILITY

Flexibility is the ability to move a joint through its entire range of motion. Flexibility of our hips, knees, and ankles allows us to bend, stretch, and twist for routine activities such as walking, reaching, or turning to see who's behind us. Loss of flexibility may result in muscle tears or strains.[18] Overall flexibility is not assessed by a single test; one

isokinetic contraction contraction in which the resistance matches the force throughout the full range of motion resulting in the shortening of the muscle.

flexibility the ability to flex and extend each joint through its maximum range of motion.

FEATURE 11.3

TESTING YOUR MUSCULAR ENDURANCE

OBJECTIVE

To complete as many push-ups or modified push-ups as you possibly can.

DIRECTIONS

1. *Push-up:* Start in push-up position (a) with arms straight, fingers forward. Lower chest to floor with back straight; then return to starting position. (Note: Many people may have insufficient strength to perform even a single push-up when using the push-up technique described here. The modified push-up (b) allows such people to support themselves with their knees, thus reducing the need for upper-body strength in a test of muscular endurance.)

2. *Modified push-up:* Same as push-up, except that you support yourself with your knees and keep your back straight.

RATINGS

Your score is the maximum number of push-ups performed in succession. See the accompanying tables.

Your score for the push-up or modified push-up test: _____.

ASSESSING YOUR PUSH-UP TEST SCORE:

This test evaluates the muscular endurance of your shoulder, arm, and chest muscles. You can improve a low or very low score by weight training exercises for these muscles.

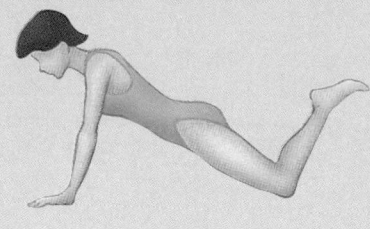

(a)

(b)

RATINGS FOR PUSH-UP AND MODIFIED PUSH-UP TESTS

Age	Very high	High	Moderate	Low	Very low
Push-up					
15–29	Above 54	45–54	35–44	20–34	Below 20
30–39	Above 44	35–44	25–34	15–24	Below 15
40–49	Above 39	30–39	20–29	12–19	Below 12
50 and over	Above 34	25–34	15–24	8–14	Below 8
Modified push-up					
15–29	Above 48	34–48	17–33	6–16	Below 6
30–39	Above 39	25–39	12–24	4–11	Below 4
40–49	Above 34	20–34	8–19	3–7	Below 3
50 and over	Above 29	15–29	6–14	2–5	Below 2

Source: Kusinitz, I., and Fine, M. *Your Guide to Getting Fit.* 2nd ed. Mountain View, CA: Mayfield, 1991.

measure of flexibility, however, is your ability to bend your body forward. You may evaluate your own flexibility by testing your trunk flexibility as described in Feature 11.5.

BODY COMPOSITION

Body composition is the proportion of body fat to lean body tissue (see Chapter 10, p. 298). In measuring fitness, the balance of these two components is a better standard than measuring body weight to height. For example, a professional athlete may have a healthier body composition than a college administrator even though both weigh the same and are the same height.

As discussed in Chapter 10, height/weight charts, despite their shortcomings, are of some use in assessing body composition. For someone whose weight exceeds the average for his or her height, the extra weight may be due to excessive fat. A more accurate assessment of body composition is the skinfold thickness test, as described in

FEATURE 11.4

STEROID USE BY ATHLETES

Fitness at any cost. In the past decade many believed this statement to be true and used whatever methods they could to improve their fitness, particularly for competitive sports. Many athletes felt they could gain a higher level of fitness and that competitive edge through the use of anabolic steroids, a synthetic version of the human hormone testosterone. The average male steroid abuser often takes 10–40 times per day more anabolic steroids than the amount of testosterone his body produces naturally. Although the use of steroids in competitive sports is banned and it is illegal to obtain them without a prescription, they are widely available. Steroid use among athletes has reached epidemic proportions, with an estimated $100 million spent on them annually in the United States alone. Do the benefits these athletes derive from steroids outweigh the consequences?

A case in point is Canada's world-class sprinter, Ben Johnson, who was stripped of a gold medal won in the 1988 Summer Olympics, after setting a world record in the 100-meter sprint. Johnson had traces of the anabolic steroid stanolozol in his system. The 1988 Olympics also had to disqualify many members of the Bulgarian weight-lifting team after it was discovered that they too had been using anabolic steroids. Why did these athletes decide to use steroids? What was the drug giving them that made them take the chance of being disqualified? Their reasoning no doubt included the facts that steroid use:

- builds the muscles that are key to athletics

- creates a sense of explosive power

- improves one's physique through muscular weight gain, giving that "muscular look"

- increases aggressiveness

- helps prove that "winning is the only thing"

- appeals to a basic tendency to go for quicker results without concern for the long-term adverse effects of drug abuse.

Losing a medal or being disqualified from competition is not the only price an athlete may pay for abuse of these drugs. Steroids fool the body into thinking that it is producing excess testosterone, and shuts down bodily functions involving testosterone, such as bone growth. Anabolic steroids have a host of side effects and adverse reactions in males, including liver cancer, heart disease, wasting away of the testicles, baldness, stunted growth, and death. Effects in females include unwanted facial hair, deepening of the voice, enlargement of the clitoris, male-pattern baldness, menstrual irregularities, and an increase in body hair. Steroids appear to be addictive, and withdrawal can bring on depression and encourage other drug use (see Chapter 15 for further discussion of the effects of steroid use).

Adding to the danger is how anabolic steroids are made and distributed. Many steroids are made outside the United States and smuggled into the country. Their potency, purity, and strength is neither known nor regulated. Steroid "alternative" drugs, such as gamma hydroxybutyrate (GHB) and clenbuterol are being illegally sold and used by athletes in order to avoid penalties for steroid use. These "alternatives" are potentially deadly drugs.

Steroids and steroid "alternatives" have been most abused by athletes in sports dependent on strength, such as weight lifting, body building, shot put, discus, javelin throwing, and by football linemen. Athletic organizations such as the U. S. Olympic Committee, the National Football League, and the National Collegiate Athletic Association maintain strict testing policies and discipline steroid users rigorously. Body-building authorities are now advising readers of muscle magazines that the best body-building gains come with serious training and good nutrition, rather than steroid use. The courts are handing down stiff sentences to people dealing in illegal steroids and similar drugs. Programs to educate high school and collegiate athletes about the dangers of steroid abuse are being put into practice.

Being fit is certainly part of a healthful life-style. Developing muscular strength for successful competition is certainly an acceptable goal. Does using steroids to reach that goal fit into the profile of long-term well-being? You decide.

Source: Mishra, R. "Steroids and Sports Are a Losing Proposition." *FDA Consumer,* September 1991, pp. 25–27.

Chapter 10 (p. 300). The layer of fat beneath the skin should be one-half to one inch thick. A skinfold total much greater than one inch indicates excessive body fat.[19]

CHECKPOINT

1. List the four categories by which physical fitness is measured.

2. Define the term *cardiorespiratory endurance.*

3. Explain the difference between aerobic and anaerobic exercise.

4. Contrast muscular strength with muscular endurance.

5. Distinguish among isotonic, isometric, and isokinetic muscular contractions.

6. Define the term *flexibility.*

7. What is the skinfold test used for? How would you fare?

FEATURE 11.5

TESTING YOUR TRUNK FLEXIBILITY

OBJECTIVE

To reach as far forward as possible while sitting with your knees straight.

DIRECTIONS

Before beginning this test, do some warm-up stretching exercises, such as bending sideways, forward, and backward several times, and rotating your trunk.

1. Place a box on the floor against a wall.

2. Tape a ruler on the box so that the 4-inch mark is on line with the near edge of the box and the 12-inch mark is farthest from you at the wall end of the box.

3. Sit on the floor with your legs extended so that your heels are about 5 inches apart and your feet are flat against the box.

4. Slowly reach with both hands as far forward as possible. Touch your fingertips to the yardstick and hold this position for about three seconds. Check the yardstick and note the distance you have reached.

5. Try this three times. (Do not attempt to add length by jerking forward.) Your flexibility score is the best of three trials.

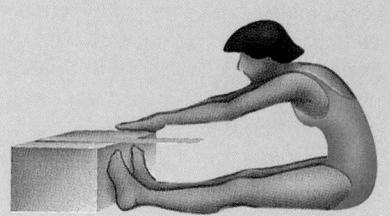

RATING

The scores in the Trunk Flexibility table are for the number of inches you reached.

YOUR SCORE: _____.

TRUNK FLEXIBILITY RATINGS (IN INCHES)

	Very high	High	Moderate	Low	Very low
Female	Above 11	10–11	6–9	2–5	Below 2
Male	Above 10	8–10	3–7	1–2	Below 1

Source: Kusinitz, I., and Fine, M. *Your Guide to Getting Fit,* 2nd ed. Mountain View, CA: Mayfield, 1991.

DETERMINING YOUR FITNESS

Once you've completed the tests outlined in Feature 11.1, Feature 11.2, Table 10.2, Feature 11.3, and Feature 11.5, record each result and rating in the feature In Your Hands: A Summary of Your Fitness. Use the Fitness Paradigm in the self-assessment to determine your fitness profile.[20] Mark your fitness rating for each of the four basic components with a small circle (for muscular endurance and muscular strength, use the ratings of muscular endurance unless you are specifically interested in muscular strength and have access to a hand dynamometer). Connect the four circles with straight lines. The smaller and more symmetrical the square you draw by connecting the four categories, the better your fitness level. If you begin a fitness program, repeat the paradigm every six to eight weeks to chart your progress.

CHOOSING AN EXERCISE PROGRAM

As part of starting an exercise program, you may wish to give yourself a self-test on your readiness to begin such a program. At this point complete In Your Hands: Self-test for Exercise Readiness (p. 346).

There are many exercise programs to choose from when setting a fitness goal. Of the full array of activities, no single one can meet everyone's needs. The exercise you choose should take into consideration your age, health, interests, as well as convenience and cost of the activity. If you're not a part of an organized aerobics class or health club, acquaint yourself with one of the many excellent books detailing training programs at the end of the chapter.

Your choice of an activity does not need to be permanent. Your first selection should be one that is most convenient and most enjoyable for you. After several weeks or longer, you may wish to switch to a different activity or to mix activities. Because you are experimenting, try to avoid spending too much money at the beginning of your program (Table 11.2).

What follows is a brief description of some of the more popular exercise activities according to fitness needs.

IN YOUR HANDS

A SUMMARY OF YOUR FITNESS

OBJECTIVE

To summarize the results of the physical fitness self-assessment tests in this chapter.

DIRECTIONS

After completing the tests, fill in this worksheet to get a rough estimate of how you rate in each of the five components of physical fitness.

COMPONENTS OF PHYSICAL FITNESS

Components and tests	Results	Rating	Components and tests	Results	Rating
Cardiorespiratory endurance			Muscular endurance		
Modified step test (Feature 11.1)	___	___	Push-ups (Feature 11.3)	___	___
Body composition			Flexibility		
Percentage body fat (Table 10.2)	___	___	Trunk flexibility (Feature 11.5)	___	___
Muscular strength					
Grip strength (Feature 11.2)	___	___			

The Fitness Paradigm

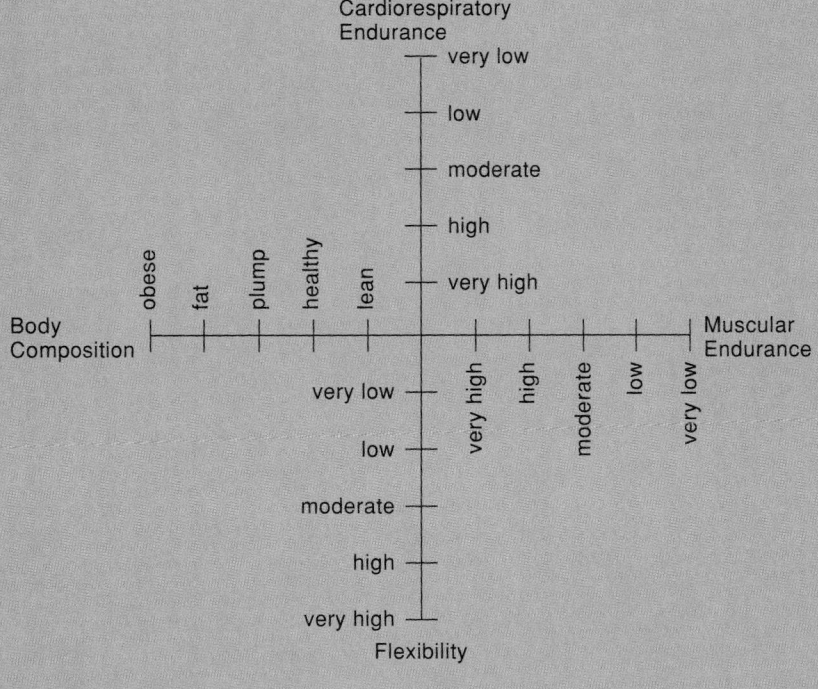

Source: Kusinitz, I., and Fine, M. *Your Guide to Getting Fit,* 2nd ed. Mountain View, CA: Mayfield, 1991.

WALKING

Walking is movement in which at least one foot is in contact with the ground at all times, as opposed to jogging or running. One of the best activities to use in beginning a conditioning program, walking is by far the most popular, particularly among older people.[21] Most people can walk, whether they are overweight, obese, or out of shape. A person who wishes to build up aerobic capacity will need to walk at a given speed for a set period of time. An example of a walking program is a 2-mile walk at a speed of 4 miles per

IN YOUR HANDS

SELF-TEST FOR EXERCISE READINESS

Exercise Readiness Questionnaire

Name: _____   Date: _____

Carefully read each statement and circle the number that best describes your agreement with each statement. Please be completely honest with your answers.

	Strongly Agree	Mildly Agree	Mildly Disagree	Strongly Disagree
1. I can walk, ride a bike (or a wheelchair), swim, or walk in a shallow pool.	4	3	2	1
2. I enjoy exercise.	4	3	2	1
3. I believe exercise can help decrease the risk for disease and premature mortality.	4	3	2	1
4. I believe exercise contributes to better health.	4	3	2	1
5. I have previously participated in an exercise program.	4	3	2	1
6. I have experienced the feeling of being physically fit.	4	3	2	1
7. I can envision myself exercising.	4	3	2	1
8. I am contemplating an exercise program.	4	3	2	1
9. I am willing to stop contemplating and give exercise a try for a few weeks.	4	3	2	1
10. I am willing to set aside time at least three times a week for exercise.	4	3	2	1
11. I can find a place to exercise (the streets, a park, a YMCA, a health club).	4	3	2	1
12. I can find other people who would like to exercise with me.	4	3	2	1
13. I will exercise when I am moody, fatigued, and even when the weather is bad.	4	3	2	1
14. I am willing to spend a small amount of money for adequate exercise clothing (shoes, shorts, leotards, or swimsuit).	4	3	2	1
15. If I have any doubts about my present state of health, I will see a physician before beginning an exercise program.	4	3	2	1
16. Exercise will make me feel better and improve my quality of life.	4	3	2	1

SCORING YOUR TEST

This questionnaire allows you to examine your readiness for exercise. You have been evaluated in four categories: mastery (self-control), attitude, health, and commitment. Mastery indicates that you can be in control of your exercise program. Attitude examines your mental disposition toward exercise. Health provides evidence of the wellness benefits of exercise. Commitment shows dedication and resolution to carry out the exercise program. Write the number you circled after each statement in the corresponding spaces below. Add the scores on each line to get your totals. Scores can vary from 4 to 16. A score of 12 and above is a strong indicator that particular factor is important to you, and 8 and below is low. If you score 12 or more points in each category, your chances of initiating and adhering to an exercise program are good. If you fail to score at least 12 points in three categories, your chances of succeeding at exercise may be slim. You need to be better informed about the benefits of exercise, and a retraining process may be required.

Mastery: 1. _____ + 5._____ + 6._____ + 9._____ = _____
Attitude: 2. _____ + 7._____ + 8._____ + 13. _____ = _____
Health: 3. _____ + 4._____ + 15. _____ + 16. _____ = _____
Commitment: 10. _____ + 11. _____ + 12. _____ + 14. _____ = _____

Source: Hoeger, W., and Hoeger, S. *Fitness and Wellness,* 2nd ed. Englewood, CO: Morton, 1993.

Table 11.2
Fitness Potential for Popular Sports

| Sport | Cardiorespiratory Endurance | Muscular Strength and Endurance | | Flexibility | Caloric Range | |
		Upper Body	Lower Body		Calories per Minute	Calories per Hour
Back packing[a]	2–3	2	3	2	5–10	300–600
Badminton	2–3	2	2	2	5–10	300–600
Baseball/Softball	1–2	2	2	2	4–7.5	240–450
Basketball	3	2	3	2	10–12.5	600–750
Bowling	1	2	1	1	2.5–4	150–240
Canoeing	2–3	3	1	1	4–10	240–600
Football (touch)	1–2	2	2	2	5–10	300–600
Golf	1	2	3	2	4–5	240–300
Handball	3	3	3	2	10–12.5	600–750
Karate	2	3	3	4	7.5–10	450–600
Racquetball	4	3	3	2	7.5–12.5	450–750
Scuba diving	1	2	2	2	5–7.5	300–450
Skating (ice)	4	1	2–3	2	5–10	300–600
Skating (roller)	2–3	1	2–3	2	5–10	300–600
Skiing (alpine)	2	3	3	3	6–10	360–600
Skiing (nordic)	4–5	3	4	3	7.5–15	450–900
Soccer	3–4	2	3–4	3	7.5–15	450–900
Surfing[b]	2	3	3	3	5–12.5	300–750
Tennis	2–3	2–3	3	2	5–10	300–600
Volleyball	2–3	2	2–3	2	5–10	300–600
Waterskiing	1	3	3	2	5–7.5	300–450

[a]Benefits depend on walking terrain and weight of pack.
[b]Paddling the board out beyond the breaking waves can be demanding.

1 = poor, 2 = fair, 3 = good, 4 = excellent.

Source: Getchell, B. The Fitness Book, Indianapolis: Cooper, 1987, p. 63.

hour, taken 5 times a week. Walking uses large muscle groups and is rhythmic, self-pacing, and safe.

JOGGING AND RUNNING

Jogging is a slow form of running at a comfortable pace. Jogging and running are popular and accessible methods of developing cardiorespiratory endurance. They give maximum benefits within a minimum amount of time and require few skills. In correct jogging and running the heel touches the ground first, as easily as possible, then the person rocks forward on the ball of the foot and pushes off on the toes. Wearing jogging shoes with padded heels reduces any jarring of the legs. Jogging and running are best done with a natural, relaxed movement, with minimal arm action. When possible avoid extended running on hard surfaces. High mileage runners should pay special attention both to their shoes (see Feature 11.6, p. 348) and running surface to ensure adequate cushioning. Jogging or running 3–5 times a week, 30 minutes at a time, for a maximum of 15 miles a week is sufficient to reach an acceptable level of cardiovascular

Walking is the most popular exercise program, especially for older people. Brisk walking can provide the same aerobic benefit as running, but it takes longer.

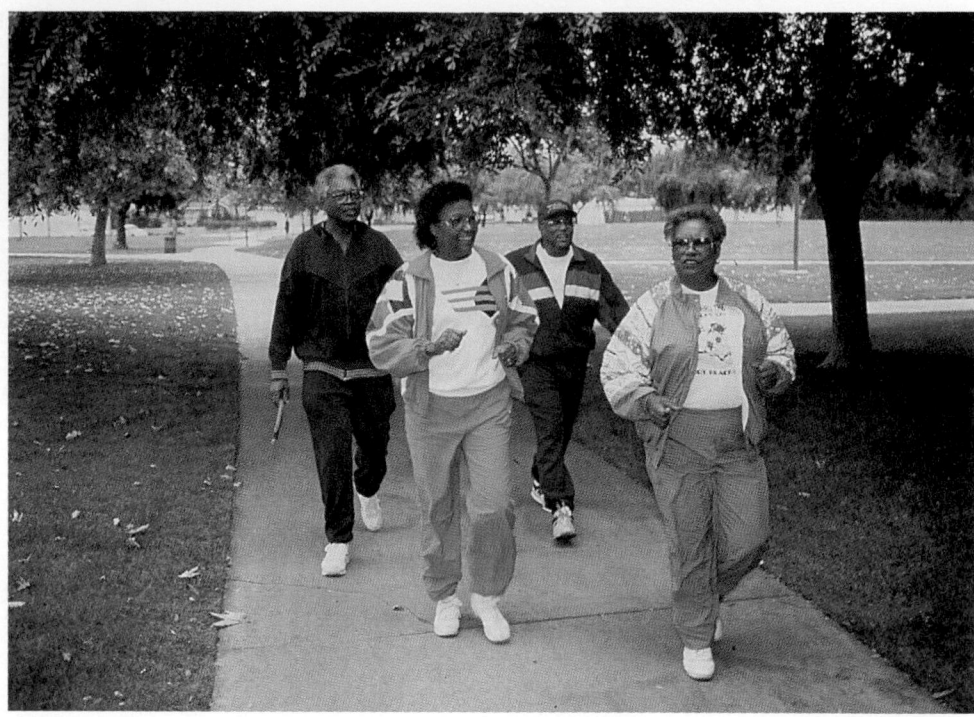

SELECTING AN ATHLETIC SHOE

When buying a new pair of athletic shoes, take a good look at your old pair before you discard them. Look for signs of wear. Athletic shoes begin to lose their shock absorbency after about 500 miles of use. In particular, look at:

- *Outer Sole* People with high arches tend to wear down the outer side of the heel, while those with flat feet tend to wear down the inner side. Such wear unduly reduces the shock absorbency of the shoe.

- *Midsole* This is the shock-absorbing layer between the outer sole and insole. Uneven compression may lead to a poor shock absorbency by the shoe, possibly leading to ankle strain or stress fractures.

- *Heel Counter* This rigid back of the shoe stabilizes the heel. If the counter leans or bulges to one side, this may destabilize the heel.

- *Upper Shoe* If the upper part of the shoe hangs over the sole on both sides, it may be too small; if it hangs over the sole on one side, the basic shape (or *last*) of the shoe may be wrong for your foot. People who roll their foot inward need a straight last, while those who roll it outward need a curved last. When you put all of your weight on one foot, there should be ½ inch of space between your longest toe and the tip of the shoe.

Shoe Construction

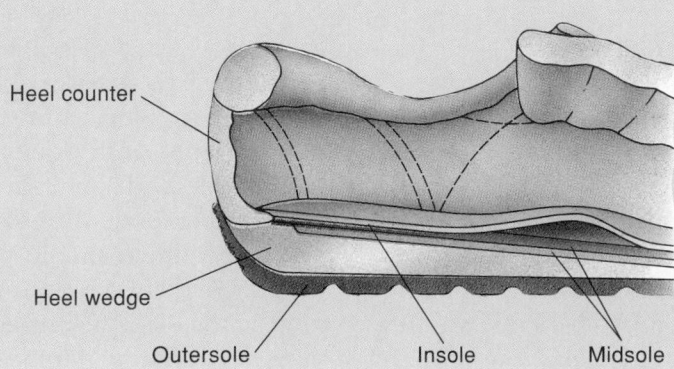

Heel counter

Heel wedge

Outersole   Insole   Midsole

When buying new shoes remember the following:

- Take an old pair of shoes with you so the salesperson can evaluate the wear pattern. Bring a (clean) pair of the socks you normally run in.

- The uppers should be perpendicular to the sole, rather than leaning to one side.

- Hold the front and back of the shoe and bend it. It should bend at the ball—where your foot bends. If it bends at midfoot it will offer little support. If it bends only slightly, it is too stiff; if it bends too easily, it will offer little support. Hold the heel and try to move the counter (see diagram)—it should not move from side to side.

- If your foot rolls outward when you exercise, you need a strong heel counter, a soft midsole, a curved last, and a more flexible sole. If your foot rolls inward, you need a good arch support, a strong last, and a less flexible sole.

In addition, there are criteria specific to particular sports.

A *walking shoe* should be lightweight and flexible, with a well-cushioned, curved sole, and enough room for your toes to move. Good heel support, and an upper made of material that allows air in and out are also important.

A *running shoe* should provide adequate cushioning under the ball of your foot, as well as a firm insole, a solid, but not snug, heel cup, a firm and well-padded heel counter, a slightly elevated heel, and room for your toes to move.

A *court shoe* should have plenty of toe reinforcement, some heel elevation, a long "throat" to ensure greater lace control, sturdy sides, and a toe box with ample room and some cushioning at the tips.

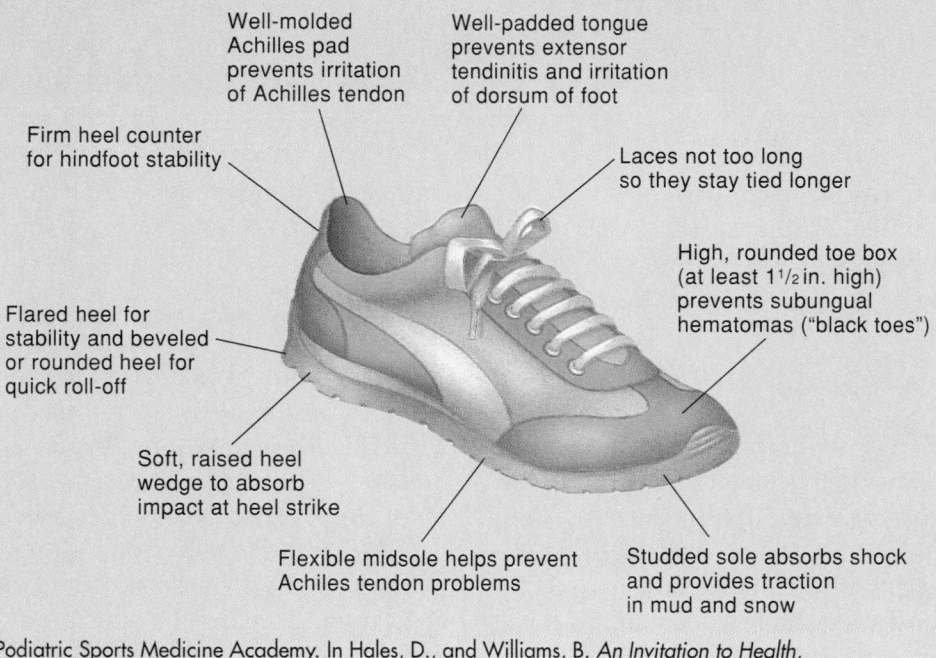

Well-molded Achilles pad prevents irritation of Achilles tendon

Well-padded tongue prevents extensor tendinitis and irritation of dorsum of foot

Firm heel counter for hindfoot stability

Laces not too long so they stay tied longer

High, rounded toe box (at least 1½ in. high) prevents subungual hematomas ("black toes")

Flared heel for stability and beveled or rounded heel for quick roll-off

Soft, raised heel wedge to absorb impact at heel strike

Flexible midsole helps prevent Achilles tendon problems

Studded sole absorbs shock and provides traction in mud and snow

Source: Canadian Podiatric Sports Medicine Academy. In Hales, D., and Williams, B. *An Invitation to Health,* 3rd ed. Menlo Park, CA: Benjamin/Cummings, 1986.

fitness. Jogging may be abused by running too fast for too long a period of time.

SWIMMING AND BICYCLING

Swimming is one of the best exercises for developing cardiorespiratory endurance and involves the entire muscular system with extensive use of the upper body. It also helps to develop flexibility. Since swimming is non-weight-bearing, there is less stress on the joints and fewer muscle prob-

lems. Swimming involves more skill than some other activities and requires access to a pool. Swimming results in fewer injuries than jogging due to the buoyant effect of the water. Overtraining can result in swimmer's shoulder, tendonitis, and arm pain.

Bicycling, whether done on a ten-speed bicycle or a stationary indoor model, builds muscle strength and endurance as well as cardiorespiratory endurance. As with swimming, cycling is a high-energy expenditure activity that promotes changes

Swimming involves most of the body's muscles. Swimming, with its rhythmic movements and prolonged elevated heart rate, gives more of a total conditioning effect than many other sports.

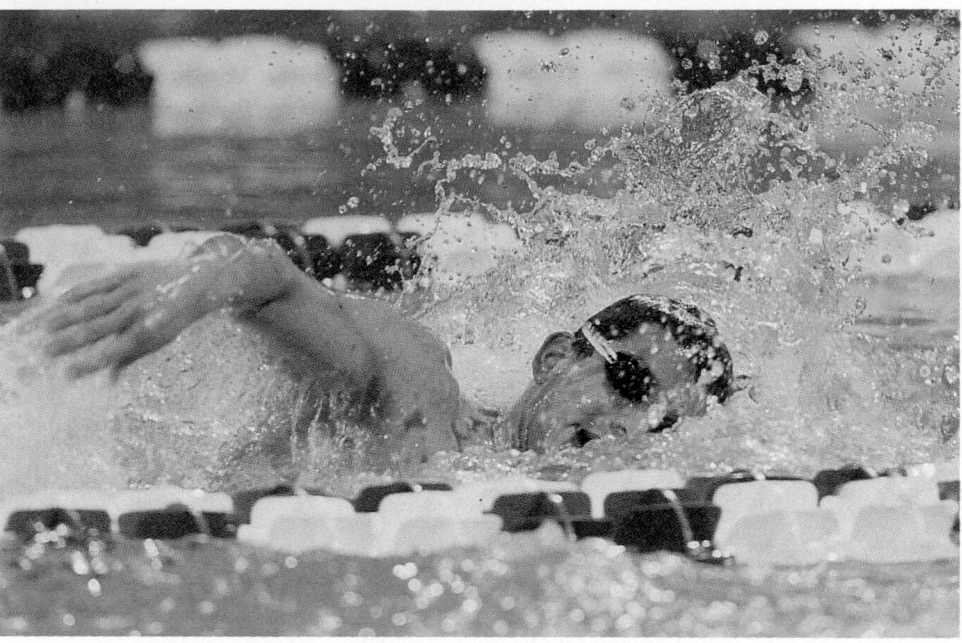

in body composition and weight control. Bicycling accidents are common; to avoid them, wear a helmet, use proper safety procedures, and avoid heavy traffic.

CROSS-COUNTRY SKIING

Cross-country skiing is another effective aerobic activity. As with swimming, the upper part of the body is used extensively. Cross-country skiing includes many of the same exercise-program guidelines as jogging and running and is used by many people as a wintertime replacement for these activities. The cost of the equipment will be more than for other sports. Cross-country skiers need to be cautious of potential avalanches, hypothermia, and frostbite.

STAIR CLIMBING

Another popular exercise choice is *stair climbing*. A high-intensity activity, if sustained for 20 minutes, stair climbing can be an excellent aerobic exercise. Because many people do not have access to enough flights of stairs for a 20-minute climb, stair-climbing machines are available. With some of these machines the feet never leave the ground, making it a low impact activity. Consequently, there are few strains of joints and ligaments. The

stair-climbing machines are programmable and can be adjusted to regulate the workload.

IN-LINE SKATING

A popular fitness activity since the early 1980s is *in-line skating,* also called *roller-blading* or *blading.* Similar to ice skating, blades are replaced by a line of wheels on hockey-type skates. In-line skating is an excellent activity to develop cardiovascular fitness and lower body strength. You set the intensity by how hard you blade. By maintaining a constant and rhythmic pattern, using arms and legs and minimizing the gliding phase, effective cardiovascular training can be achieved. In-line blading is also excellent for developing superior leg strength. Protective equipment is essential; a good helmet is important, and wrist guards and knee and elbow pads are recommended.

AEROBICS

One of the most common fitness activities for women in the United States is *aerobics* (also known as aerobic dance). Also enjoyed by men, it involves a series of routines, such as stepping, walking, kicking, skipping, jogging, and arm swinging performed to music. Aerobics can be performed in a class or along with videos. It is fun and promotes cardiovascular development. A version of this is the *aerobics program* developed by Dr. Kenneth Cooper, which uses common activities such as walking, running, and tennis. Based on a point system, Cooper's aerobics program categorizes and evaluates activities according to energy expenditure. It has been developed especially for cardiorespiratory development. Although aerobics has a low injury rate, shin splints, tendonitis, muscle strains, back strains, and fractures of foot bones can occur.

CIRCUIT TRAINING

Circuit training refers to a specific number of exercises arranged and consecutively numbered. The exercises can vary from calisthenics, or simple gymnastic exercises, to weight-training exercises, running stairs, or stretching. The size of the circuit is tailored according to the time, space, and equipment available. This program is self-paced; you move from station to station at your own speed, covering the entire circuit without resting. You perform a specified exercise at each station. Progress is based on completing the entire circuit in less time or in increasing the number of repetitions at each station. Circuit training may also concentrate on *calisthenics* in which a series of gymnastic, rhythmic exercises are performed without equip-

ment, or on weight exercises to increase muscular strength and endurance. Certain exercises may be harmful to your lower back and knees.

HIKING

Depending on the nature of the terrain, *hiking* can be a more intense activity than walking. A fine activity while on vacation, with or without the family, hiking combines the mind-refreshing benefit of the out-of-doors with an aerobic routine. It is important that proper footwear be worn. Depending on the terrain, it is also important to watch for loose soil on slopes and holes and stones.

RACQUET SPORTS

The aerobic benefits of racquetball, squash, tennis, and badminton depends on the intensity and length of time the game is played. Players need to run fast, hard, and as continuously as possible. Too many slowdowns in playing do not allow for maintaining the heart rate in the target zone for cardiovascular development. Although relaxing and socializing, people regularly using these activities may need to combine these activities with other aerobic exercises, such as jogging, cycling, or stair climbing. Usually low-impact sports, they may result in tendonitis, and back and muscle strains.

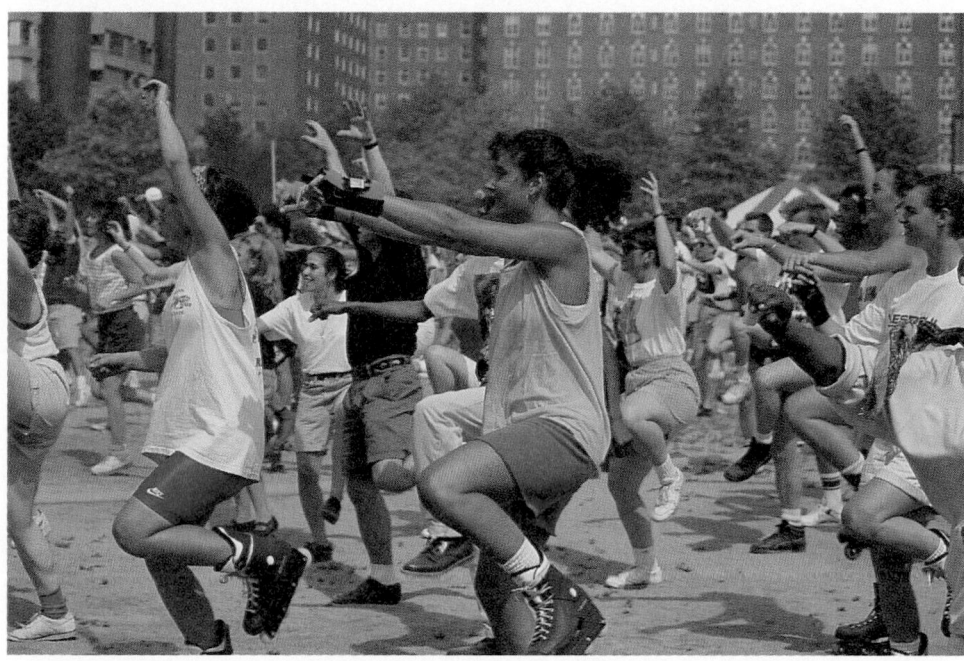

Aerobics is one of the most popular fitness activities in the United States.

SETTING YOUR OWN GOALS

One aspect of fitness training is designing a program to meet specific fitness goals. The goals you set will be based on your individual needs and the level of fitness you require. You will need to think about why you want to become fit. It may be to improve your ability to breathe properly after climbing a small hill, to lose weight, to find relief from backaches, or to prevent stiffness by staying limber (Feature 11.7). These fitness goals need to be translated into specific physical fitness components. To lose weight, you focus on body composition; to stay limber, you work on flexibility; to reduce breathlessness, you work on CRE. A program that stresses one component will probably improve other components as well.

If you are athletically inclined, you may want a training program that prepares you for a specific sport. If training for a skiing trip is what you have in mind, getting in shape for it would require a different program than what you would use to get in shape for varsity shot put. If you want to participate in aerobic exercises, anaerobic training would be inappropriate. Training is unique to a given sport or activity. A high level of conditioning acquired in one activity may not carry over to another. A football player who has just finished his season may not be conditioned for wrestling. An athlete, during the off season, wants to be certain to include in his or her exercise program those drills and movements used in the particular sport or activity.

FEATURE 11.7

FITNESS GOALS AND HEALTH INTEREST

The following are some specific fitness goals and fitness components involved in their achievement.

Goals	Cardiorespiratory Endurance	Body Composition	Muscular Strength	Muscular Endurance	Flexibility
Prevent, eliminate, or reduce low back pain	X	X	X	X	X
Make pregnancy and childbirth easier	X	X	X	X	X
Eliminate or reduce breathlessness brought on by climbing stairs	X	X		X	
Increase stamina in such activities as jogging, swimming, dancing, bicycling, long walks	X	X		X	
Increase resistance to muscle fatigue	X		X	X	
Increase muscular effectiveness for daily tasks and sports activities			X	X	X
Become more muscular; firm up muscle tone		X	X	X	
Lower high blood pressure	X	X			
Help to improve control of diabetes	X	X			
Prevent, eliminate, or reduce muscle and/or joint injury			X		X
Decrease muscle soreness due to physical activity				X	X
Reduce menstrual discomfort		X			X
Prevent heart attack at an early age	X	X			
Reduce asthmatic discomfort during exercise	X				
Improve fit of clothes		X			
Lose or gain weight		X			
Look trimmer by reducing the girth of waist, hips, thighs, arms		X			

Source: Kusinitz, I., and Fine, M. *Your Guide to Getting Fit,* 2nd ed. Mountain View, CA: Mayfield, 1991.

Table 11.3
Cardiovascular Exercise Prescription Guidelines

Activity: Aerobic (examples: walking, jogging, cycling, swimming, aerobics, racquetball, soccer, stair climbing)

Intensity: 50–85 percent of heart rate reserve

Duration: 20–60 minutes of continuous aerobic activity

Frequency: 3–5 days per week

*Source: "The Recommended Quantity and Quality of Exercise for Developing and Maintaining Cardiorespiratory and Muscular Fitness in Healthy Adults by the American College of Sports Medicine." Medicine and Science in Sports and Exercise **22** (1990), pp. 529–533*

A CARDIOVASCULAR EXERCISE PRESCRIPTION

The point of aerobic training is to improve the cardiorespiratory efficiency (CRE). To accomplish this, the heart muscle must be overloaded in order to increase its size, strength, and efficiency. This is done through improving the intensity, mode, duration, and frequency of exercise factors. The overall Cardiovascular Exercise Prescription Guidelines according to the American College of Sports Medicine (ACSM) are shown in Table 11.3.

Before starting on a program to improve CRE, you must pass an exercise stress test. The most common test used to determine cardiovascular fitness is the 1.5-mile run test or the 12-minute walking/running test. A stopwatch is used to time how long it takes to run (or walk) the course. From this, a cardiovascular fitness category can be determined (Tables 11.4 and 11.5). This test is only for conditioned persons. Unconditioned beginners should have at least six weeks of aerobic training before taking the test. Sedentary people and those over 30 years of age should receive medical clearance before taking this test. The test is not recommended for persons with cardiovascular disease or heart disease risk factors.

Table 11.4
1.5-Mile Run Test Time (Minutes)

Fitness Category	Age (Years)					
	13–19	20–29	30–39	40–49	50–59	60+
Very poor						
(men)	>15:31	>16:01	>16:31	>17:31	>19:01	>20:01
(women)	>18:31	>19:01	>19:31	>20:01	>20:31	>21:01
Poor						
(men)	12:11–15:30	14:01–16:00	14:44–16:30	15:36–17:30	17:01–19:00	19:01–20:00
(women)	18:30–16:55	19:00–18:31	19:30–19:01	20:00–19:31	20:30–20:01	21:00–21:30
Fair						
(men)	10:49–12:10	12:01–14:00	12:31–14:45	13:01–15:35	14:31–17:00	16:16–19:00
(women)	16:54–14:31	18:30–15:55	19:00–16:31	19:30–17:31	20:00–19:01	20:30–19:30
Good						
(men)	9:41–10:48	10:46–12:00	11:01–12:30	11:31–13:00	12:31–14:30	14:00–16:10
(women)	14:30–12:30	15:54–13:31	16:30–14:31	17:30–15:56	19:00–16:31	19:30–17:30
Excellent						
(men)	8:37–9:40	9:45–10:45	10:00–11:00	10:30–11:30	11:00–12:30	11:15–13:50
(women)	12:29–11:50	13:30–12:30	14:30–13:00	15:55–13:45	16:30–14:30	17:30–16:30
Superior						
(men)	<8:37	<9:45	<10:00	<10:30	<11:00	<11:15
(women)	<11:50	<12:30	<13:00	<13:45	<14:30	<16:30

< Means "less than"; > means "more than."

Source: Cooper, K., The Aerobics Program for Total Well-Being, 1982. Reprinted by permission of Bantam Books, a division of Bantam, Doubleday, Dell Publishing Group, Inc.

Table 11.5
12-Minute Walking/Running Test

Distances (miles) covered in 12 minutes

Fitness Category	Age (Years)					
	13–19	20–29	30–39	40–49	50–59	60+
Very Poor						
(men)	<1.30	<1.22	<1.18	<1.14	<1.03	<0.87
(women)	<1.0	<0.96	<0.94	<0.88	<0.84	<0.78
Poor						
(men)	1.30–1.37	1.22–1.31	1.18–1.30	1.14–1.24	1.03–1.16	0.87–1.02
(women)	1.00–1.18	0.96–1.11	0.95–1.05	0.88–0.98	0.84–0.93	0.78–0.86
Fair						
(men)	1.38–1.56	1.32–1.49	1.31–1.45	1.25–1.39	1.17–1.30	1.03–1.20
(women)	1.19–1.29	1.12–1.22	1.06–1.18	0.99–1.11	0.94–1.05	0.87–0.98
Good						
(men)	1.57–1.72	1.50–1.64	1.46–1.56	1.40–1.53	1.31–1.44	1.21–1.32
(women)	1.30–1.43	1.23–1.34	1.19–1.29	1.12–1.24	1.06–1.18	0.99–1.09
Excellent						
(men)	1.73–1.86	1.65–176	1.57–1.69	1.54–1.65	1.45–1.58	1.33–1.55
(women)	1.44–1.51	1.35–1.45	1.30–1.39	1.25–1.34	1.19–1.30	1.10–1.18
Superior						
(men)	>1.87	>1.77	>1.70	>1.66	>1.59	>1.56
(women)	>1.52	>1.46	>1.40	>1.35	>1.31	>1.19

< Means "less than"; > means "more than."

This simple exercise will help you assess your current level of aerobic fitness. Time yourself for 12 minutes. During that 12 minutes, run or walk as far and as fast as you can. You should try to pace yourself so that you are putting out your maximum effort at the end of the 12 minutes (i.e., you just can't go any further). Keep track of how far you go and then locate your distance, sex, and age on the chart above. Circle your fitness category.

Source: Cooper, K., The Aerobics Program for Total Well-Being, 1982. Reprinted by permission of Bantam Books, a division of Bantam, Doubleday, Dell Publishing Group, Inc.

The American College of Sports Medicine advises that a medical exam and a diagnostic exercise stress (tolerance) test, with a physician present be administered to apparently healthy men over age 40 and women over age 50, and to everyone with known medical conditions regardless of their age before engaging in any vigorous exercise.[22]

Intensity

Intensity refers to how hard you must exercise in order to improve CRE, or the ability of the lungs, heart, and blood vessels to deliver adequate amounts of oxygen to the cells to meet the demands of vigorous physical activity. Finding the right level of intensity for any exercise program depends on the individual. The heart and circulatory system are key players during any activity. The heart is a muscle and, like any other muscle, functions more efficiently as stress is placed on it. The level of stress, however, must be appropriate. If the stress is too light, the exercise benefits will be minimal; if the stress is too great, it may be dangerous and so uncomfortable that you may not be able to continue the program.

Cardiovascular development occurs when the heart is working in a range between 50 percent and 85 percent of **heart rate reserve (HRR).** This

heart rate reserve (HRR) the difference between the maximal heart rate (MHR) and the resting heart rate (RHR).

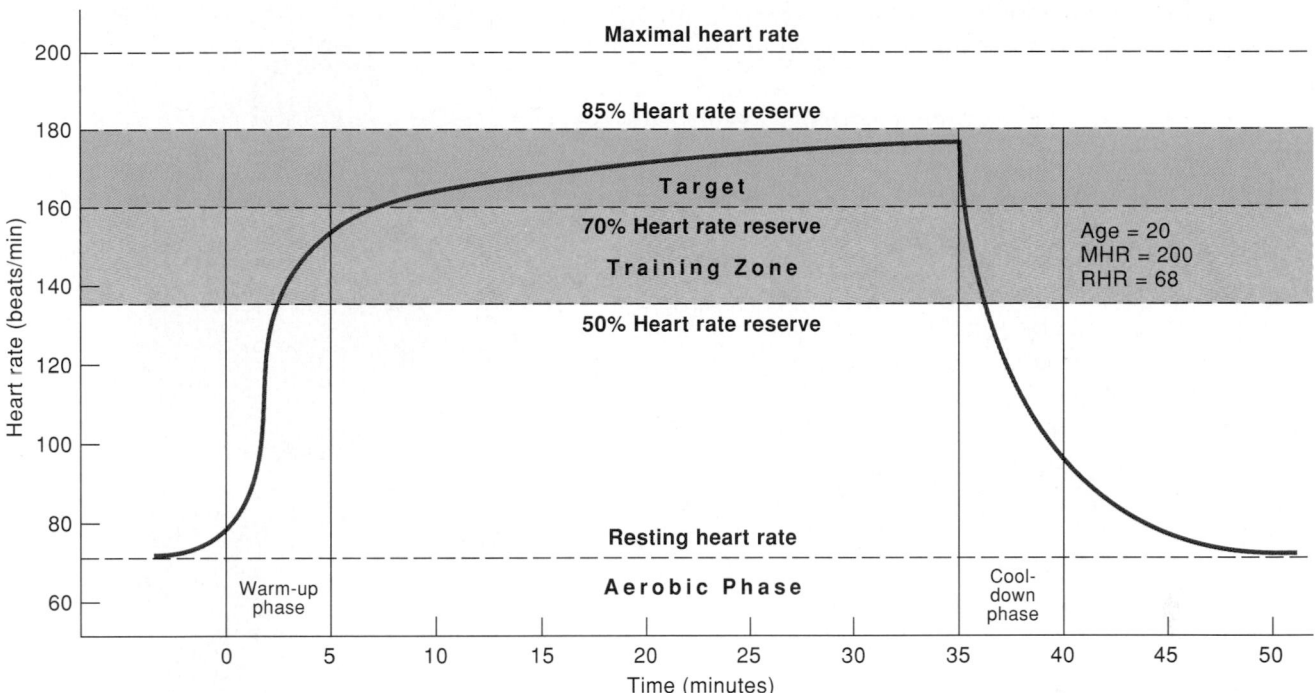

Figure 11.2

Typical Aerobic Workout Pattern

Source: Hoeger, W., and Hoeger, S. Fitness and Wellness, 2nd ed. Englewood, CO: Morton, 1993.

range is known as the **target training zone.** The Aerobic and Fitness Association of America recommends a target zone of 70–85 percent of the HRR. The positive response your body makes to increasingly vigorous aerobic exercise that falls within the target-zone heart rate is your **training effect.** The HRR is determined by:

1. calculating your **maximal heart rate (MHR).**

2. calculating your **resting heart rate (RHR).**

3. determining your HRR by subtracting the RHR from the MHR.

···

target training zone the rate at which the heart is beating to get the maximum aerobic effect.

training effect beneficial changes your body makes to aerobic exercise of sufficient intensity, duration, and frequency.

maximal heart rate (MHR) theoretical maximum rate at which your heart can beat for your age.

resting heart rate (RHR) the heart rate when the body is at rest.

4. calculating your training intensity (TI) at 50 percent, 70 percent, and 85 percent of the HRR (see Figure 11.2).

The maximal heart rate (MHR) is the theoretical maximum rate at which your heart can beat for your age. The MHR depends on a person's age and can be estimated by subtracting your age from 220:

MHR = 220 minus age (220 − age) = beats per minute (bpm).

The resting heart rate (RHR), or your heart rate when the body is at rest, can be determined after sitting quietly for 15–20 minutes. It can also be determined by taking your pulse the first thing upon awakening. The heart rate reserve (HRR) is determined by subtracting the RHR from the MHR (HRR = MHR − RHR). The HRR represents the amount of beats available when going from resting conditions to an all-out maximum effort.

As your physical condition improves, resting heart rate will drop. As the training effect strengthens the heart muscle, pulse rate and blood pressure decrease, and the oxygen transport system improves. To maintain your heart rate within the desired target zone you'll need to increase the **training intensity (TI)** of the exercise from time to time.

Cardiovascular development occurs faster when the heart is working close to 85 percent of the HRR; thus a HRR of 70 percent to 85 percent for young people is recommended. Exercising above the 85 percent rate does not give extra benefits and may even be hazardous for some persons. Orthopedic problems and abnormal heartbeats are much more likely when a person exercises at an intensity greater than 85 percent of HRR. Instead, working out at 80 percent HRR or less may be recommended. For people just beginning an exercise program, a target-zone heart rate of less than 70 percent is appropriate.

You can measure your heart rate by taking your pulse. This can be done by using either the radial artery in the wrist or the carotid artery in the neck (Figure 11.3). To locate the radial artery, place the middle three fingers of your right hand on your left wrist in the groove behind the thumb. The carotid artery is located by placing the tips of the three middle fingers of one hand on your neck under the jawbone about halfway between the chin and the ear. When pressure is applied, each pulsation felt signals one heartbeat. Count the number of beats in ten seconds and multiply this number by six to get a full minute count. To measure your exercise heart rate accurately, you must take your pulse within five seconds after you stop exercising.

Mode

The *mode,* or type, of exercise used to develop the cardiovascular system must be aerobic. Any exercise activity that raises your heart rate up to the target training zone and keeps it there for the duration of the exercise will give adequate development.

Duration

The recommended *duration* of the exercise activity should be between 20 and 60 minutes per ses-

....

training intensity (TI) how hard a person must train to achieve a given level of cardiorespiratory endurance.

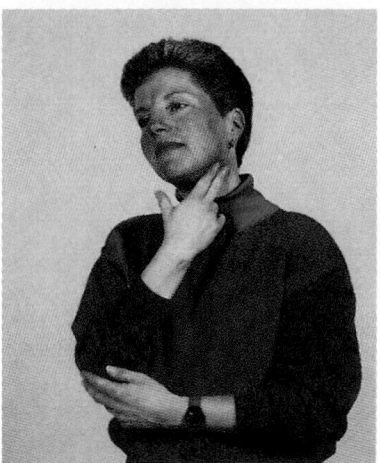
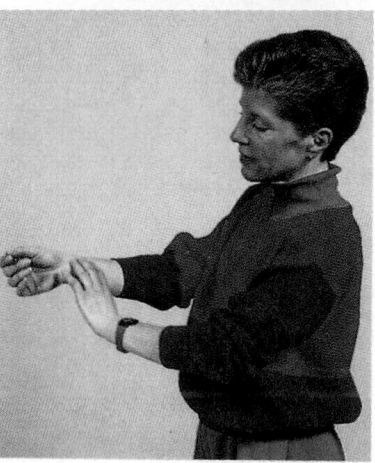

Figure 11.3
Measuring Heart Rate

Heart rate may be measured by taking a reading of your pulse. This is easily done by (a) placing the tips of your middle two or three fingers over the carotid artery on the side of the neck below the angle of the jaw bone, or (b) placing the tips of the middle three fingers on the radial artery on the inner side of the wrist behind the base of the thumb. Measured either way, when pressure is applied the pulsations of the arteries can be felt and counted.

sion. The higher the intensity, the less time required. If exercising is done around 85 percent, 20 minutes is adequate; the lower the intensity the longer the duration required. Unconditioned persons or older adults should train at a lower percentage of HRR, thus requiring a longer duration.

Frequency

Frequency refers to the number of exercise sessions per week. The ideal frequency of exercise should be three to five times a week. At least three times a week on nonconsecutive days maintains

CRE fitness. After a maximum strength workout, the muscles should be rested for about 48 hours to allow sufficient recovery. The musculoskeletal system is not able to properly adapt to daily hard exercising. It may lead to fatigue, soreness, and injury. Increasing the frequency to more than three to five times a week accomplishes little in training advantage.[23] With a frequency rate of *less* than three times a week, or more than two days between workouts, there are also reduced training benefits. If for some reason you are not completely recovered in two to three days, you may be overtraining in terms of some particular physical condition and may need to decrease the total length of intensity of the activity.

With this information in hand, the next step is to determine your own level of cardiovascular training by completing In Your Hands: Determining Your Cardiovascular Exercise Intensity.

TRAINING PRINCIPLES

Now that you have assessed your level of fitness, you are ready to examine some training principles. Your body has the ability to respond to physical demands placed on it if sound principles are used and if the level of demand is increased gradually. Individual muscles increase in strength and endurance as they increase in size. Sudden increases in levels of activity, however, may cause muscle and tendon injuries as well as stiffness and pain. Training principles to be considered are warm-up/cool down, finding your level of intensity, progressive overload, and setting a schedule.

WARM-UP/COOL DOWN

Before beginning a physical fitness activity, it is important to allow the heart and muscles to adjust

---

IN YOUR HANDS
DETERMINING YOUR CARDIOVASCULAR EXERCISE INTENSITY

1. Estimate your own maximal heart rate (MHR)

   MHR = 220 minus age (220 − age)

   MHR = _____ − _____ = _____ bpm

2. Resting Heart Rate (RHR) = _____ bpm

3. Heart Rate Reserve (HRR) = MHR − RHR

   HRR = _____ − _____ = _____ beats

4. Training Intensity (TI) = HRR × %TI + RHR

   50% TI = _____ × 0.50 + _____ = _____ bpm

   70% TI = _____ × 0.70 + _____ = _____ bpm

   85% TI = _____ × 0.85 + _____ = _____ bpm

5. Cardiovascular Training Zone. The optimum cardiovascular training zone is found between the 70 percent and 85 percent training intensities. Individuals who have been physically inactive or are in the poor or fair cardiovascular fitness categories, however, should follow a 50 percent training intensity during the first few weeks of the exercise program.

   Cardiovascular Training Zone:_____ (70% TI) to_____ (85% TI)

Mode of Exercise: List any activity or combination of aerobic activities that you will use in your cardiovascular training program:_____

Duration of Exercise: Indicate the length of your exercise sessions:_____ minutes.

Frequency of Exercise: Indicate the days on which you will exercise:_____

Student's Name:_____

Date:_____

Signature:_____

bpm = beats per minute

Source: Hoeger, W., and Hoeger, S. *Fitness and Wellness,* 2nd ed. Englewood, CO: Morton, 1993, p. 41.

Figure 11.4
Warm-Up/Cool-Down Exercises

Before and after exercising—especially walking, jogging, running, bicycling, and rope skipping—do these exercises to attain and maintain flexibility. Each should be done just once, except for the leg cross-overs, which should be done for 5–20 repetitions each.

Source: Kusinitz, I., and Fine, M. Your Guide to Getting Fit, 2nd ed. Mountain View, CA: Mayfield, 1991.

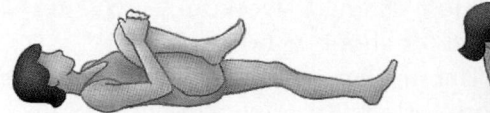
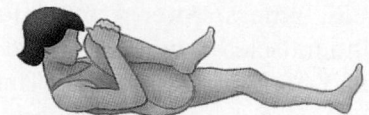

1. *Alternate knee-to-chest* (abdominals, hips, lower back)
Bend one knee up to your chest; raise your head and try to touch your knee with your chin. Hold the bent leg with both hands at the knee. Alternate first one leg and then the other.

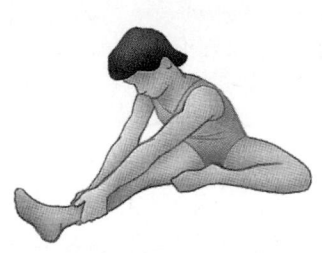
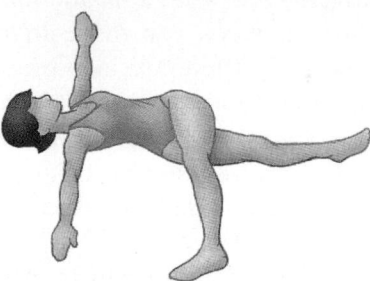

2. *Seated toe touch* (hamstrings)
Sit with your legs straight. Fold one leg in front and gradually reach for the toes of your other leg. Eventually you will be able to grasp your feet at the instep. Keep your head down. Alternate legs.

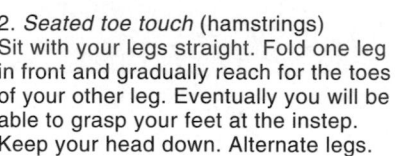

3. *Leg cross-overs* (hips, back)
Raise one leg and cross it over your body. Keep your upper back flat and your arms extended to the sides. Alternate first one leg and then the other. Turn only your hips.

gradually to the work increase. **Warm-up** prepares your body for vigorous exercise and increases the temperature of your muscles, allowing them to stretch and perform more easily (Figure 11.4). Each warm-up session should include three kinds of activity: stretching exercises to reduce resistance of the muscles to activity; calisthenics and jogging to increase body temperature and to stimulate the heart; and light exercise of the type of activity that is to follow to ensure the right muscle groups are stimulated and coordinated. Warm-up sessions should last at least ten minutes.[24]

The reason for stretching is to gradually loosen and lengthen the muscle group you're stretching. Stretch gently then hold for 6–10 seconds. You may be more flexible on some days than on others, so you may wish to vary your stretching routine to fit your needs. Stretching is particularly important before and after walking, jogging, bicycling, and rope skipping.

After finishing an activity, you need to **cool down** gradually by decreasing the intensity of the activity. Cooling down for five minutes or longer will allow your cardiovascular system and muscles to gradually return to their preexercise condition.[25] Without cool down, sudden and dangerous drops in blood pressure may occur.

PROGRESSIVE OVERLOAD

Muscles adapt to the workload to which they are subjected. Their strength and size increase as they work to their maximum limits. The first time you perform an activity, you may find it difficult, but as you repeat the activity, your body adapts to the increased workload.

As training increases muscle strength, the initial workload no longer provides sufficient work to further increase strength. Unless the workload is increased, the muscles maintain their existing level of strength. To continue to increase muscle strength, the intensity of the load must be progressively increased. This is known as **progressive overload.**[26]

Just as the body adjusts to increased demands, it also responds to reduced demands. If you reduce your workload, the overload becomes what had

warm-up exercises performed immediately before physical activity to prepare the body for rigorous exercise.

cool down continuation of exercise at a low intensity following a rigorous workout, to allow the body to adjust to a resting state.

progressive overload an increase in muscular strength by the progressive increase, over time, in the demands placed on a muscle.

previously been the acceptable workload. The following example demonstrates this: If you have a broken arm or leg in a cast, once the cast is removed, that muscle strength has been lost. Working gradually, the arm or leg can regain its prior abilities.

When training demands are excessive, the muscles and joints react, sometimes by aching or becoming painful. A gradual, or progressive increase in training demands may avoid such excessive overload. The goal of fitness training is to increase gradually the demands on your body so you get a training effect with little or no discomfort.

SETTING A SCHEDULE

The duration of one's exercise period depends on the intensity of the activity. Jogging allows a couple of options: You can run at a faster pace for a shorter time or at a slower pace for a longer time. Studies show that joggers who exercise at a low intensity for a longer time have fewer injuries and feel less discomfort.[27]

Beginners should start at a low intensity level, perhaps even below their target zone, to allow their muscles to adjust to the program. They should exercise no more than 15–20 minutes at a time. As they begin to feel comfortable, they should gradually increase the intensity and/or duration, eventually increasing to 20- to 30-minute sessions as fitness improves. The point is to maintain the heart rate within the target zone. Each activity period should include three segments: 5–10 minutes of warm-up, 20–30 minutes of exercise (as you adjust to the workload), and 5–10 minutes for cool down.[28]

Maximum cardiovascular fitness can be attained by exercising regularly between three and five days per week. Rest and recovery periods of one to two days are necessary between exercise sessions. Exercise sessions every day to every other day are within that range.

Exercising too frequently can result in consistent muscle soreness. Muscle soreness may also occur when you exercise strenuously only once or twice a week. If you miss a day of exercise in your routine, don't try to make up for it by exercising twice as hard the next time. More than 65 percent of those starting an exercise program drop out within six weeks because of injuries. Most of these can be avoided by exercising every other day rather than every day, and by stopping exercise when muscles hurt.[29]

It is essential that you maintain your exercise program. Studies show that when exercise is discontinued, deconditioning occurs within a few weeks. To maintain cardiorespiratory fitness, it is important that you maintain a workout program that falls within your target-zone heart rate about every other day.[30]

CHECKPOINT

1. What is the purpose of warming up before vigorous exercise? Cooling down afterward?

2. List the three activities that should be included in each warm-up session.

3. Explain target-zone heart rate and how it is determined.

4. What is the danger in exceeding 85 percent of the maximal heart rate while exercising?

5. Why is progressive overload necessary as part of a training program?

6. Discuss the reasons behind a fitness schedule of 20–30 minutes of exercise for 3–5 days each per week. What are the dangers of exercising too frequently?

GETTING STARTED

Once you have evaluated your level of fitness, chosen your fitness program, and become aware of some training principles, you are ready to begin. Pace yourself. Don't overextend. Remember that you need to build muscle strength and endurance gradually.

If your life-style has been one of physical inactivity, you should initially aim for a target zone heart rate of 60 to 70 percent (see discussion on finding your level of intensity on p. 354). After exercising at this level for several weeks, increase your target zone. Always begin your session with a set of warm-up exercises and end with cool-down exercises. Expect some initial muscular soreness; this is common if you have previously been inactive.

Check your heart rate periodically throughout your exercise sessions to make sure you are achieving your target-zone heart rate. If you are exceeding the target zone, slow down; if you are falling below the zone, speed up.

Try your routine for six to eight weeks, then reevaluate your CRE fitness level and replot your fitness paradigm and profile. Don't be discouraged by lack of immediate progress. If you stick with a fitness program, you will see and feel results; be patient.

While exercising, "listen" to how your body responds to exercise. Be sure your body feels right, and that you are not feeling continuing pain. If you are exercising with a group, listen to your body before reacting to the pressure you feel from the group. Set your own goals and pace. If at any point you feel ill or overly fatigued, stop exercising until you feel better. A good rule is: Don't push yourself to the point of exhaustion or pain. If your exercise is appropriate for you, you will feel tired, but refreshed, and you will not be in pain.

C H E C K P O I N T

1. List some precautions for starting your exercise program.

2. What is a safe target-zone heart rate for a relatively sedentary person?

3. How long should you continue a program before reevaluating your CRE fitness level?

4. During exercise, what should your response be to exhaustion or pain?

COPING WITH THE ENVIRONMENT

An increasing number of people live in areas with extreme climatic conditions and they participate in year-round sports. Activities such as mountaineering, skiing, and hiking are often done in cold weather and at higher altitudes; activities such as tennis, running, and water skiing are frequently done in hot climates. Both extremes call for precautions to avoid discomfort and/or injury.

HOT WEATHER EXERCISE

Exercising in hot weather can create stress on the circulatory system due to the high production of body heat. In hot weather the dilation of blood vessels in the skin diverts increased quantities of blood to the body surfaces, where heat is released. As the body sweats, skin heat evaporates the sweat, cooling the skin and the blood circulating near the skin.

During exercise in hot weather, the circulatory system must deliver large amounts of blood to the muscles, as well as to the skin. These competing demands may exceed the amount of blood the heart can pump, which may lead to circulatory shock or overload. The American College of Sports Medicine recommends that individuals not engage in strenuous physical activity when the temperature exceeds 82.5 degrees F.[31] Care must be taken in exercising when relative humidity is above 60 percent. Heat disorders may result. Mild heat fatigue may leave you very tired.

There are three major signs of trouble when exercising in the heat. **Heat cramps** are painful spasms of the voluntary muscles in the arms, legs, and abdomen. They may occur following a hard workout in a hot environment, without adequate fluid and salt intake. For relief, stop exercising, get out of the heat, massage the affected area, stretch slowly, and drink plenty of fluids. If exercise is continued, **heat exhaustion** can occur. A severe reaction to heat exposure, heat exhaustion is a condition of definite weakness brought on by the loss of normal fluids and sodium chloride by the body. Symptoms include dizziness, nausea, headache, and eventual collapse. The skin is cool and clammy, there is profuse sweating, body temperature is usually normal, and the blood pressure drops. Drinking fluids helps replace lost water. In extreme cases, **heat stroke** may result and require immediate medical attention. The skin is dry and hot, sweating stops, body temperature soars, and the person may suffer convulsions and/or loss of consciousness, and in extreme cases may die. Body temperature must be lowered by ice, cold

....

heat cramps painful spasms of voluntary muscles in the arms, legs, and abdomen following a hard workout in a hot environment, without adequate fluid and salt intake.

heat exhaustion severe reaction to heat exposure.

heat stroke a severe and dangerous reaction to heat exposure which requires medical attention.

water compresses, or other methods until professional help arrives.[32]

For exercising in hot weather, reduce your workouts by half, then gradually increase your exercise to the desired intensity and duration over the next week or so. As you become acclimated to hot, humid weather, you will sweat sooner and more profusely than before, and will lose less salt. Heavy sweating improves body temperature regulation, which slows down the heart rate and lessens the blood flow to the skin. By monitoring your exercise routine in hot weather, you will also experience less dizziness, fainting, and nausea.

Sweating and Water Loss

During extended rigorous exercise in hot weather, such as distance runs, you may sweat from one to three quarts of water per hour. In fact, under these conditions you can lose considerable amounts of water and not feel thirsty. It is essential that you replace this lost fluid by drinking adequate amounts of water so you will continue sweating and keep your body temperature from rising sharply. If lost fluid is not replaced you may become dehydrated by as little as one-half hour of rigorous exercise; body temperature may exceed normal limits. Distance runners are advised to drink water every 10–15 minutes.[33]

While exercising in hot weather, allow the body to lose a maximum amount of sweat. Wear shorts and light, loose-fitting clothing, allowing your skin to be exposed to the air. Avoid sweat suits, hoods, and towels around the neck.

Water Substitutes

Many professional and amateur athletes drink water substitutes when exercising in hot weather. Manufacturers claim that drinks such as Gatorade replace important minerals lost when you sweat.[34] While this may be true, the liquid is absorbed more slowly than water because of the glucose it contains.

For those drinking these commercial products, it is advisable to dilute them with water. The more water in the drink, the more rapid its absorption by the stomach. Other than plain water, a useful water replacement is a mixture of one pint of orange juice to four pints of water.[35]

COLD WEATHER EXERCISE

Regulating the body temperature is less difficult in cold weather than in hot weather, since the body's heating system is very efficient. Even so, it is important to dress warmly and to protect the hands and head. Dressing in layers usually keeps you warmer than dressing in one bulky coat or sweater. Warm air is trapped between layers that can be removed or added, depending on body temperature and changes in the weather. A good rule of thumb for cold weather exercise is to wear one layer less than you would for normal cold-weather activities.

Wear clothes that allow for heat and sweat to escape. Natural fabrics, such as wool and cotton, generally "breathe" better than synthetic fabrics, such as acrylic and polyester. A hat and scarf should also be worn at all times. Up to 40 percent of body heat is lost through the neck and head. Preventing

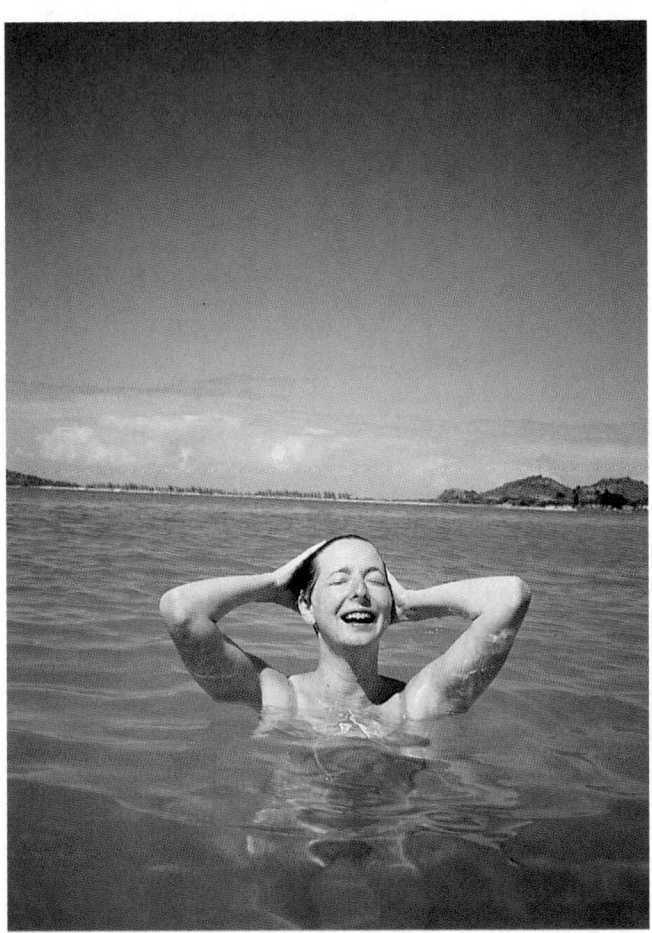

Exercising in hot weather places extraordinary demands on the circulatory system to supply both the muscles and the skin. Too great a demand can lead to a severe and dangerous reaction to heat exposure.

this heat loss with a hat actually keeps the torso and extremities warmer. If a scarf and hat are unavailable, use a hood, or even a towel around the neck.

When choosing cold-weather exercise gear, consider the type of sport, the temperature, and the wind-chill factor. Don't rely on a thermometer on a windy day, since wind always reduces the effective temperature substantially. Downhill skiing is artificially windy, and therefore makes it feel colder. While skiing, also remember that snow reflects most of the sun's brightness and can cause sunburn. Goggles, sunglasses, and a good sunscreen are extremely important when participating in all snow sports.

It is especially important to avoid excessive wetness from melted snow or soaking of clothes by perspiration. Wet socks and underclothing can freeze, presenting severe health risks. Modern cold-weather clothing is based on the principle of using inner layers of synthetic material that "wick" the sweat moisture away from the body. The outermost layer of clothing often contains a thin layer of membranous material, such as Gore-Tex, with microscopic pores that allow evaporated sweat to pass out of the garment but prevent drops of water from rain or melted snow from entering.

Frozen clothing or exposed skin can lead to **frostbite,** which can damage or destroy body tissues.[36] Length of exposure, the wind-chill factor, and the amount of moisture in the air and on the skin affect the risk of frostbite and its severity. Some parts of the body, such as ears, fingers, toes, and nose, need special protection. If skin becomes pale or white, or if it is numb, cover it right away and warm it gently. Very gentle massage will restore circulation to the warmed area. If frostbite is suspected, and if it seems severe, see a physician.

EXERCISING AT HIGH ALTITUDES

Exercising at altitudes over 6000 feet usually presents some risks if you do not normally live at that elevation. Above this altitude, the decreasing oxygen content of the air deprives working muscles of the oxygen they need. Light-headedness, headaches, and loss of appetite are some of the symptoms of altitude sickness.[37]

When ascending to higher elevations, do so gradually and at a rate of 2000–3000 feet a day.

....

frostbite the freezing or effect of freezing of body parts.

Delay vigorous exercise until you are used to the altitude. The body will adapt to elevational changes, and altitude sickness may disappear within two to five days. A diet high in carbohydrates and low in fats may reduce the severity of altitude sickness. After returning to a lower altitude, you may find the effect of high altitude training makes the same amount of work easier at lower altitudes and may temporarily increase the work output at the lower altitude due to the greater effort the body has been making to move a sufficient amount of air at higher altitudes.[38] This is a strategy used by world-class competitive athletes who train at high altitudes prior to competing at sea level.

EXERCISING IN POLLUTED AIR

Pollutants such as oxides and hydrocarbons, and particulates such as dust and soot, significantly reduce air quality. Auto exhaust fumes are particularly offensive to many. Exercising in polluted air not only creates eye irritation and respiratory discomfort; it also creates risks that may outweigh the advantages of exercising.

If air quality is poor, you may be better off exercising indoors. If you must exercise outdoors, do it in the early morning or late evening when traffic is lighter and air temperatures are cooler (see Chapter 24). Another option is finding some place that is away from heavy traffic.

CHECKPOINT

1. What are the additional demands on the circulatory system when exercising during hot weather?

2. Explain the difference between heat exhaustion and heat stroke.

3. What is the disadvantage of drinking drinks containing sugar when exercising in hot weather?

4. List ways in which a person can regulate body temperature during cold weather exercising.

5. Discuss the steps a person can take to reduce the chances of altitude sickness.

6. If living in an area in which the air is polluted, what time of the day may be the best time for exercising out of doors?

FACILITIES

There is no shortage of places to exercise. Your choices range from your home, neighborhood, schools, parks, and colleges and universities, to private and public health clubs. In deciding which option is best for you, consider factors such as weather and safety, expense, convenience, and availability of instruction and equipment.

If choosing a health club, be consumer smart. Visit the club, talk with the sales representative, and ask to be shown around. Ask about the certification of the trainers (Feature 11.8). Talk with members of the club to find out how satisfied they are with the services. You can also help yourself by reading a useful consumer booklet put out by the Wisconsin affiliate of the American Heart Association in Milwaukee, Wisconsin, entitled *How to Choose a Health Club*.[39] (It can be obtained by writing to the American Heart Association in Milwaukee, Wisconsin.) The booklet discusses the standards and guidelines you should look for and expect within the commercial fitness industry.

ATTIRE

When choosing exercise gear, comfort, freedom of movement, convenience and practicality, and safety must all be considered. In cool weather, you may want a sweat suit. In cold weather, mittens and a cap help to retain heat. Ski caps in very cold weather can also double as face masks. In warm weather, cotton shorts and T-shirts absorb sweat more effectively than nylon clothing; nylon, however, is easier to care for.

Choosing the right shoes/sneakers for your routine is probably the most important decision you must make. Jumping, running, jogging, and walking with improperly fitted or poor-quality shoes can lead to foot, ankle, knee, and back problems. In selecting a shoe, evaluate its characteristics (see Feature 11.6, p. 348).

You may or may not want to wear socks. Those who do usually prefer cotton or wool socks because they allow feet to "breathe" and stay drier. Nylon retains heat and moisture, and can cause blisters. Some athletes wear two pairs of socks—a lightweight cotton inner pair, and a thicker outer pair.

CHECKPOINT

1. List some important considerations in selecting a health club.

2. What are the recommendations for selecting attire for cold weather and hot weather exercising?

3. Explain the things to look for when selecting an athletic shoe.

GUIDELINES FOR MAINTAINING FITNESS

In *Dynamics of Fitness, A Practical Approach,* George McGlynn cites seven guidelines that will help you stick to your exercise program:[40]

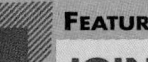

FEATURE 11.8

JOINING A HEALTH CLUB OR SPA

Before joining a health club, consider some guidelines:

- What hours is it open?
- Is the club overcrowded? Will you have to wait 15 minutes or more to use equipment?
- Are the facilities such as dressing rooms, showers, and lockers adequate?
- Is it a co-ed facility?
- Is the staff well qualified? As of now, no standards or certification of personnel are required or enforced.

- How does the cost compare to that of other clubs? (Ask for a copy of and carefully read any membership agreement.)
- Does the facility offer a reasonable trial or short-term renewable membership (such as for one month)?
- Is parking available?
- What do current members think of the club?

COMMUNICATION FOR WELLNESS

FITNESS AS A SOCIAL ACTIVITY

Too many people start a fitness program only to gradually slide back to their previous level of inactivity. What can be done to help maintain your initial enthusiasm over getting and staying in shape?

One approach that helps many people is to share their exercise, whatever form it may take, with one or more other people. There are several benefits:

• Exercise done as a shared experience is more interesting.

• The time passes much more quickly.

• People who exercise together encourage each other.

• "Peer pressure" makes it more difficult to drop out of an exercise program when it is being shared with one or more friends.

• Strong friendships can be built through the relaxed communication that can occur while exercising.

1. *Find a convenient location to work out.* Choose a place to exercise that is close to where you work or live. Don't depend on others for transportation.

2. *Vary your exercise.* To avoid boredom, don't get locked into one routine, whether jogging, swimming, or weights. Be creative.

3. *Stay within your limits.* Don't set goals that leave you exhausted.

4. *Record your progress.* If you keep track of what's happening to your body, heart rate, strength, and weight, you will be amazed at the changes. Such records also provide great feedback and reinforcement.

5. *Don't be obsessive about exercise.* Keep records, but don't keep score. You don't have to keep piling it on. Two miles of running a day is a lot safer and healthier for the average person than 20 miles, and besides, it's more enjoyable.

6. *Be patient, and stay with it.* The benefits do not come overnight. Generally, it takes a few months for physiological changes to become noticeable.

7. *Set your own time schedule.* It is important to organize a convenient schedule. Don't make it too rigid. Allow for some flexibility.

To these we can add:

• *Know how to exercise safely.* Learn which exercise movements are safe and which are hazardous. Don't overdo them. Control all of your movements and stop if any movement leads to continuing pain (see Features 11.9 and 11.10, p. 366).

• *Dress properly.* Be sure you are using proper shoes. Appropriate, stylish clothing also helps to add to your comfort and sense of self-image.

• *Find a friend.* Exercising with someone else makes the time go faster and adds motivation to maintain a schedule. Select a time or schedule for exercising and give that schedule first priority. Friends can help keep you on target, as pointed out in Communication for Wellness: Fitness as a Social Activity.

FEATURE 11.9

EXERCISING SAFELY

The human body improves with regular use, but not all exercises are good for you. Some exercises are bad, others are hazardous because they are performed incorrectly. To exercise safely, avoid overflexing a joint (such as a knee or an elbow), overarching the back or neck, sudden twisting or flexing, bouncing while stretching, excessive jumping or hopping, rapid swinging of arms or legs, and poor body alignment. Here are the right and wrong ways of performing several high-risk exercises.

DON'TS AND DOS

Straight-leg sit-ups arch the lower back and place excessive stress on it. Also, there's no need to sit up fully, since the abdominal muscles work only during the first part of the movement. After that the hip flexor muscles take over, and the shift to these muscles can pull the hip out of alignment and further arch the back.

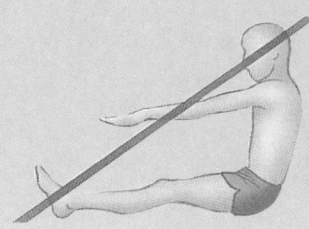

Bent-leg sit-ups, also called crunches, are the safest, most effective way to strengthen abdominal muscles. Keep your knees bent and come up only 30 degrees to 45 degrees. Always keep your lower back pressed into the ground to prevent arching. To prevent neck strain, cross your arms over your chest or cross them behind your head so that each hand rests on the opposite shoulder.

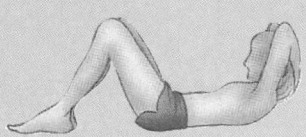

360-degree head rolls, in which you vigorously roll your head or bend your head back forcefully, may injure the disks in your neck.

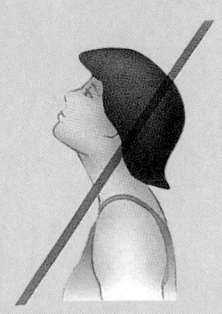

Side neck stretches—use the weight of your hand to pull your head gently to the side and then forward. Also pull it diagonally.

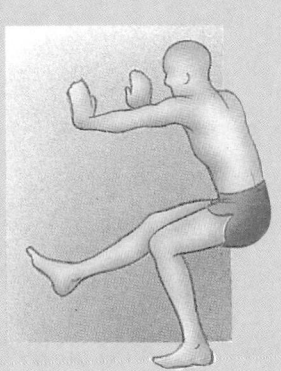

Locked-knee toe touches can overstress the back, knees, and hamstring muscles, especially when done quickly with a bouncing movement.

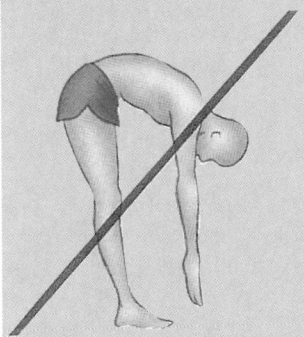

Bent-knee hang downs call for rolling down slowly with your knees slightly bent and abdominal muscles tight until you feel your hamstring and back muscles start to stretch. Hang over for 10–20 seconds. Don't use force, don't try to reach the floor, and don't bounce.

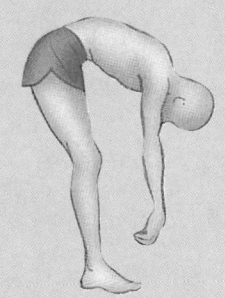

Full squats, like deep knee bends or squat thrusts, greatly increase stress on the knees.

Partial squats strengthen the muscles on the front of your thigh. Squat no more than one-quarter way down: Hold on to the wall for support as you extend one leg forward.

Double leg lifts can strain your lower back since raising both legs causes your back to arch. Leg scissors present similar risks.

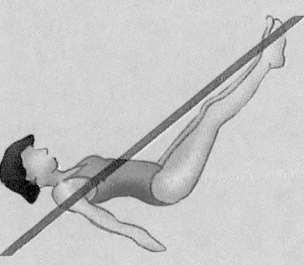

Raised-leg crunches are a safe way to strengthen abdominal muscles. Keep one leg bent with the foot on the floor; raise the other leg straight up. Raise your upper back and reach toward the lifted ankle.

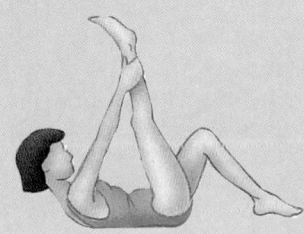

FEATURE 11.10

REFERENCE GUIDE FOR EXERCISE-RELATED PROBLEMS

Injury	Signs/Symptoms	Treatment[a]	Injury	Signs/Symptoms	Treatment[a]
Bruise (contusion)	Pain, swelling, discoloration	Cold application, compression, rest	Muscle cramps	Pain, spasm	Stretch muscle(s), use mild exercises for involved area
Dislocations/Fractures	Pain, swelling, deformity	Splinting, cold application, seek medical attention	Muscle soreness and stiffness	Tenderness, pain	Mild stretching, low-intensity exercise, warm bath
Heat cramps	Cramps, spasms and muscle twitching in the legs, arms, and abdomen	Stop activity, get out of the heat, stretch, massage the painful area, drink plenty of fluids	Muscle strains	Pain, tenderness, swelling, loss of use	Cold application, compression, elevation, rest, heat after 36–48 hours (if no further swelling)
Heat exhaustion	Fainting, profuse sweating, cold/clammy skin, weak/rapid pulse, weakness, headache	Stop activity, rest in a cool place, loosen clothing, rub body with a cool/wet towel, drink plenty of fluids, stay out of heat for 2–3 days	Shin splints	Pain, tenderness	Cold application prior to and following any physical activity, rest, heat (if no activity is carried out)
Heat stroke	Hot/dry skin, no sweating, serious disorientation, rapid/full pulse, vomiting, diarrhea, unconsciousness, high body temperature	Seek immediate medical attention, request help and get out of the sun, bathe in cold water/spray with cold water/rub body with cold towels, drink plenty of cold fluids	Side stitch	Pain on the side of the abdomen below the rib cage	Decrease level of physical activity or stop altogether, more gradually increase level of fitness
Joint sprains	Pain, tenderness, swelling, discoloration	Cold application, compression, elevation, rest, heat after 36–48 hours (if no further swelling)	Tendonitis	Pain, tenderness, loss of use	Rest, cold application, heat after 48 hours

[a]Cold should be applied three to four times a day for 15 minutes. Heat can be applied three times a day for 15–20 minutes.

Source: Hoeger, W. and Hoeger, S. *Principles and Labs for Physical Fitness and Wellness,* 3rd ed. Englewood, CO: Morton, 1994, p. 69.

• *Set goals and share them.* Tell someone you know what your goals are. Periodically assess your progress; this allows you to know when you are making progress toward your goals. When you reach a goal, you know you are ready to move to a higher fitness category. Reaching a goal is also a good excuse to indulge yourself in some rewards, such as a new jogging outfit or some piece of equipment.

SUMMARY

Fitness is the ability to carry out daily tasks with vigor and alertness, without undue fatigue, and with enough energy left for leisure pursuits. Exercise is muscular activity performed to maintain fitness. There are many physical and psychological benefits to exercising.

Physical fitness is more than having a muscular body. Its components include cardiorespiratory endurance, muscular strength and endurance, flexibility of joints, and balance in body composition.

An exercise program should include activities that are compatible with your interests, age, health, schedule, and finances. The same activities need not be in everyone's exercise program.

Certain training principles should be kept in mind while exercising. The body needs warm-up time before and cool-down time after full exercise. The exercise intensity, duration, and frequency must be enough to maintain a training effect.

Exercise precautions are appropriate in hot weather, cold weather, at high altitudes, and in polluted air. The right location and the proper attire helps make exercise enjoyable and comfortable.

Now you are about ready to commit yourself to the pursuit of fitness and wellness. More than this is a commitment to improving your total quality of life. Once you are into a new program of personal fitness and wellness the benefits of the new quality of life will become apparent before long, especially if you have been practicing a poor life-style. Being diligent in taking control of yourself will reward you with a life that is more productive, happier, and healthier. When you realize these benefits, you won't want to have it any other way.

REFERENCES

1. Hoeger, W., and Hoeger, S. *Fitness and Wellness,* 2nd ed. Englewood, CO: Morton, 1993.
2. American Heart Association. *1993 Heart and Stroke Facts, Statistics.* Dallas: The American Heart Association, 1992.
3. Whitney, E., and Rolfes, S. *Understanding Nutrition,* 6th ed. Minneapolis: West, 1993.
4. Centers for Disease Control. "Coronary Heart Disease Attributable to Sedentary Lifestyle: Selected States, 1988." *Morbidity and Mortality Weekly Report* (17 August 1990), Vol. 39, No. 32. U.S. Department of Health and Human Services, Centers for Disease Control, 541–544.
5. Tortora, G., and Grabowsky, S. *Principles of Anatomy and Physiology,* 7th ed. HarperCollins: New York, 1993.
6. Kash, F., et al. "The Effect of Physical Activity on Aerobic Power in Older Men (A Longitudinal Study)." *The Physician and Sports Medicine* 18 (1990), 73–83.
7. American Cancer Society. *Cancer Facts and Figures, 1993.* New York: American Cancer Society, 1993.
8. Enstrom, J. "Health Practices and Cancer Mortality Among Active California Mormons." *Journal of the National Cancer Institute,* 81 (1989), 1807–1814.
9. Hoeger, op. cit.
10. Blair, S. et al. "Physical Fitness and All-Cause Mortality: A Prospective Study of Healthy Men and Women." *Journal of the American Medical Association* 262 (1989), 2395–2401.
11. Kusinitz, I., and Fine, M. *Your Guide to Getting Fit,* 2nd ed. Mountain View, CA: Mayfield, 1991.
12. Whitney, op. cit.
13. Thygerson, A. *Fitness and Health, Life-Style Strategies.* Boston: Jones and Bartlett, 1989.
14. Saltman, P., et al. *The California Nutrition Book.* Boston: Little, Brown, 1987.
15. Kusinitz, op. cit.
16. Ibid.
17. Ibid.
18. Ibid.
19. Ibid.
20. Ibid.
21. Ibid.
22. American College of Sports Medicine. "Position Stand: The Recommended Quantity and Quality of Exercise for Developing and Maintaining Cardiorespiratory and Muscular Fitness in Healthy Adults." *Medicine and Science in Sports and Exercise* 22 (1990), 265–274.
23. Cooper, K. *The Aerobics Program for Total Well-Being.* New York: Bantam, 1982.
24. McGlynn, G. *Dynamics of Fitness,* 3rd ed. Dubuque, IA: Brown and Benchmark, 1993.
25. Kusinitz, op. cit.
26. Ibid.
27. Elmer-Dewitt, P. "Extra Years for Extra Effort." *Time* (17 March 1986), 66.
28. Hockey, R. *Physical Fitness: The Pathway to Healthful Living,* 6th ed. St. Louis: *Times-Mirror*/Mosby, 1989.
29. Mirkin, G., and Shangold, M. "Getting Back in Shape." *Nation's Business* (May 1983), 36.
30. Kusinitz, op. cit.
31. American College of Sports Medicine, op. cit.
32. Kusinitz, op. cit.
33. Ibid.
34. McGlynn, op. cit.
35. Kusinitz, op. cit.
36. Ibid.
37. McGlynn, op. cit.
38. Ibid.
39. Kelly, T., et al. *How to Choose a Health Club.* Milwaukee: American Heart Association of Wisconsin, 1988.
40. McGlynn, op. cit.

SUGGESTED READINGS

Alter, M. *Sport Stretch.* Champaign, IL: Leisure, 1990.
Althoff, S., Svoboda, M., and Girdano, D. *Choices in Health and Fitness,* 2nd ed. Scottsdale, AZ: Gorsuch Scarisbrick, 1992.
Cooper, K., and Cooper, M. *Aerobics for Women.* New York: Bantam, 1988.
Cooper, R. *Health, Fitness and Excellence.* Boston: Houghton Mifflin, 1989.
Darden, E. *The Nautilus Book.* Chicago: Contemporary, 1990.

Fox, M., and Broide, D. *Molly Fox's Step on It*. New York: Avon, 1991.

Gover, B., and Shepherd, J. *The Family Fitness Handbook*. New York: Penguin, 1989.

Hoeger, W., and Hoeger, S. *Fitness and Wellness,* 2nd ed. Englewood, CO: Morton, 1993.

Hoeger, W. *Principles and Labs for Physical Fitness and Wellness*. Englewood, CO: Morton, 1991.

Katz, J. *Swimming for Total Fitness*. New York: Doubleday, 1993

Kraemer, W., and Fleck, S. *Strength Training for Young Athletes*. Champaign, IL: Human Kinetics, 1993.

Leboey, F., and Averbuck, G. *The New York Runner's Club Complete Book of Running*. New York: Random House, 1992.

Meyers, C. *Aerobic Walking*. New York: Vintage, 1987.

Thygerson, A. *Fitness and Health*. Boston: Jones and Bartlett, 1989.

Vedral, J. *The 12-minute Total-body Workout*. New York: Warner, 1989.

White, T. *The Wellness Guide to Lifelong Fitness*. Staff of University of California at Berkeley Wellness Letter (eds.). New York: Rebus, 1993.

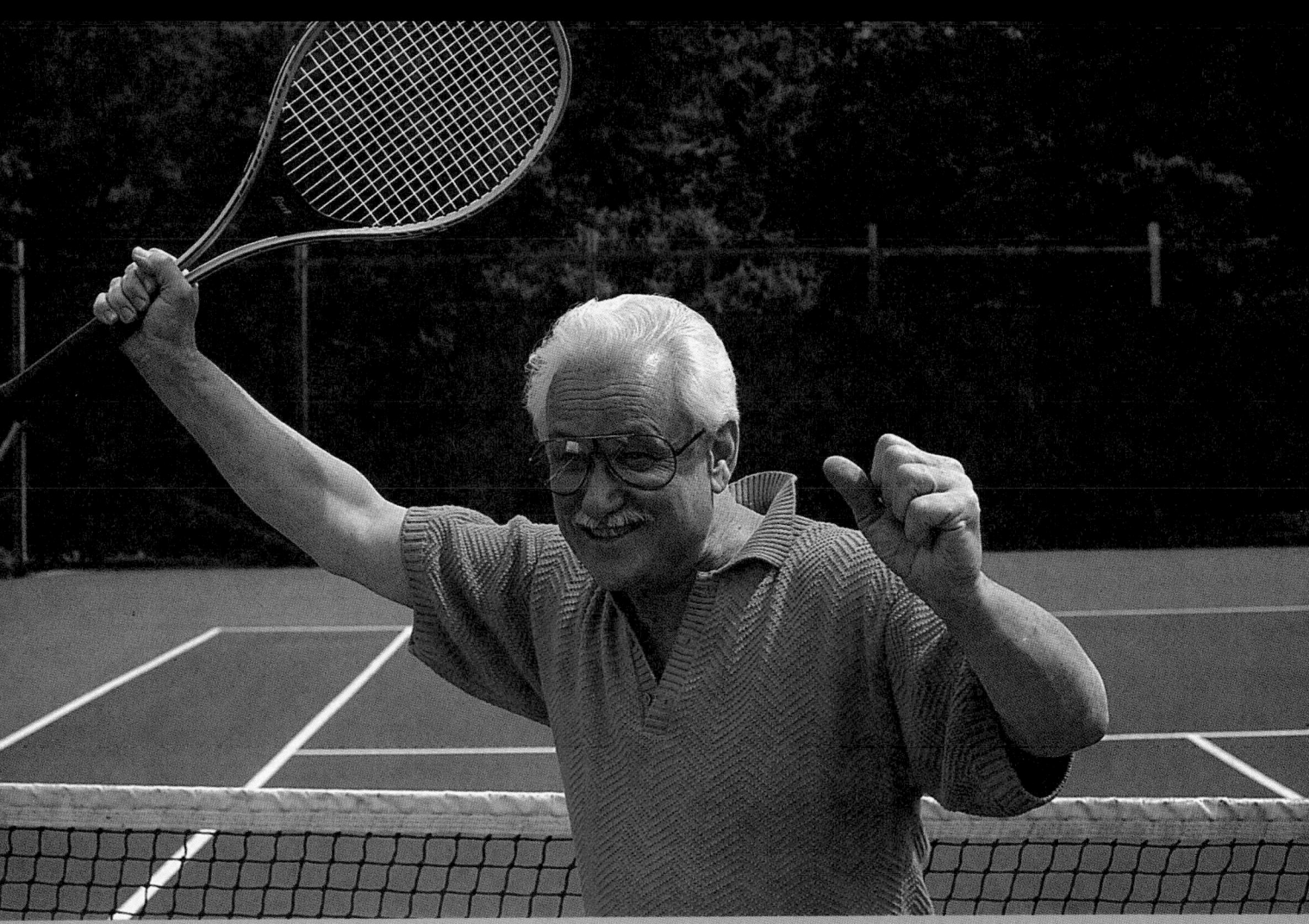

FIVE

AGING AND DEATH

Aging and death are not enemies to be conquered; they are integral parts of our lives, which help give meaning to human existence. They set a limit on our time in this life, urging us to make productive use of each precious moment.

Unfortunately, aging and death are subjects that are often evaded, ignored, and denied by our society. Aging and death remind us of our personal vulnerability and mortality, causing, for those of us who have not come to terms with these realities, an uncomfortable degree of anxiety.

Some of us would prefer to avoid confronting our feelings about aging and death. But we only begin to live our lives most fully after we come to terms with the finite nature of our existence. We don't have to wait until death seems imminent to start to really live. As soon as we come to view aging and death as invisible companions on our life journey, reminding us not to wait until tomorrow to do what we want and need to do, then we begin to *live* our lives rather than just pass through them.

Chapter 12, Aging, examines aging from multi-cultural, biological, psychological, social, family, and economic perspectives. Chapter 13, Dying and Death, explores how our attitudes about death affect our daily lives and how impending death affects a dying individual and his or her family. In these chapters, you will find a positive approach to aging and death. You will learn that there is no need to live in fear of growing old or of dying. When you feel comfortable with aging and death, you can live life at its very best. Explore your feelings about aging and death *now*. You will grow through the experience.

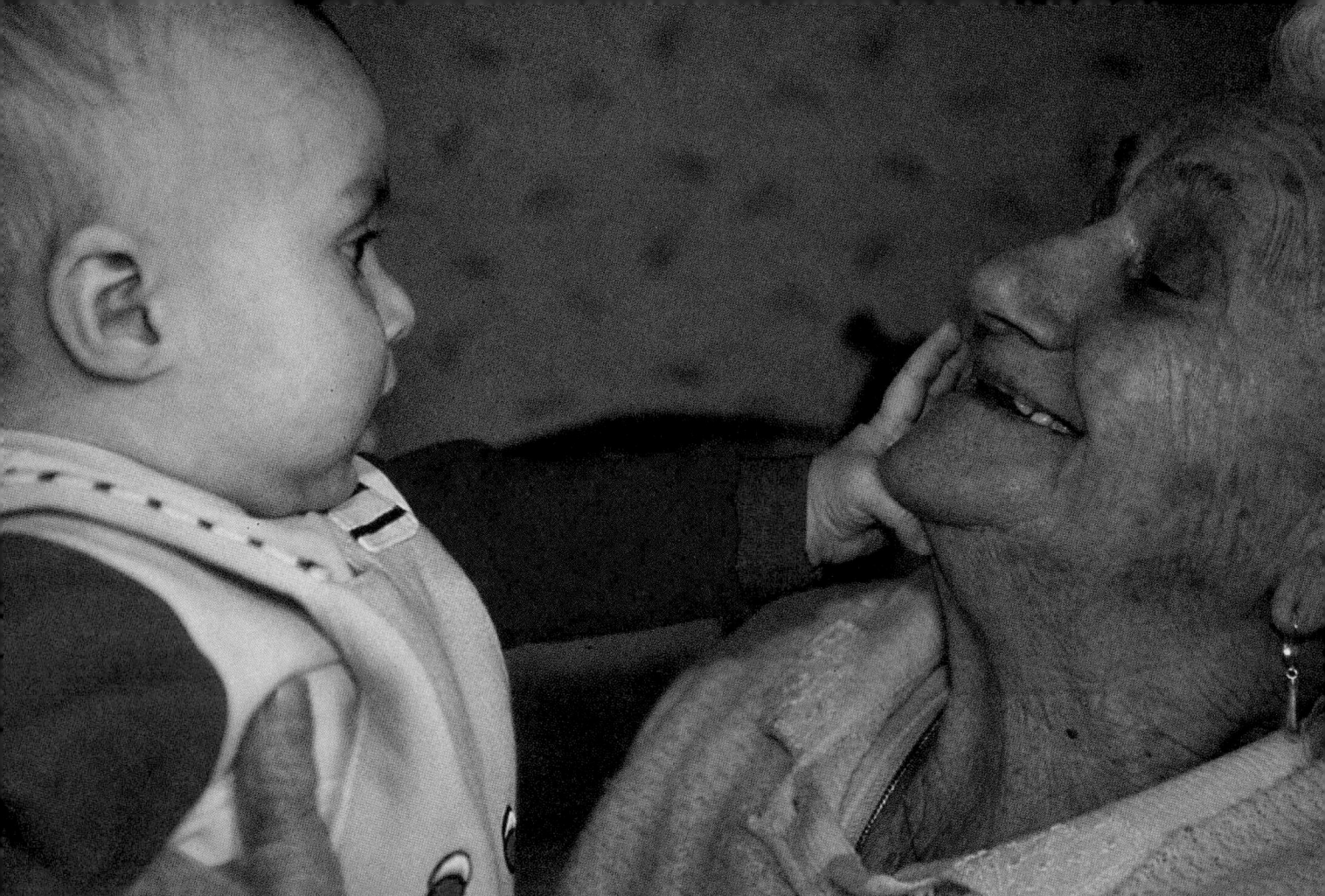

12
AGING

KNOWLEDGE

- Define the term *aging*.
- List six types of aging and explain how they influence each other.
- Define the term *ageism*.
- Explain how cultural factors influence the lives of older people.
- Contrast programmed versus stochastic aging theories.
- Explain the effects of aging on each body system.
- Explain the differences between normal aging and pathological aging.
- Describe the mental and social changes associated with aging.
- Explain the attitudes that can help make old age one of life's most rewarding experiences.

INSIGHT

- Identify ageism when it occurs in yourself and others.
- Outline a personal program for healthy aging.
- Explain how you might personally benefit from time spent with older people.

DECISION MAKING

- Make a commitment to develop more positive attitudes toward aging and older people.
- Make a commitment to live in ways that slow your biological aging process.
- Make a commitment to spend more time with older family members.

*I*n May 1993, Bob Hope turned 90 years old, celebrating the event with a three-hour television special. This was certainly an unusual way for a 90-year-old (or anyone, for that matter) to celebrate a birthday. However, for Bob Hope, staying mentally and physically active is a way of life, even at 90. To help him celebrate, his wife of over 60 years played a large part in the special day.

In his 60-plus years of radio, movie and television stardom, Bob Hope has "never retired and never made a comeback." It seems as if his life is lot like one of his comedy routines—if he fails on one joke, he moves on to another before anyone has a chance to think twice about it.

While everyone else seems to marvel at his longevity, Mr. Hope appears to prefer to avoid the issue altogether; in fact, he seldom even mentions his age in a joke. Those close to him recognize that Bob Hope has yet to reconcile himself to being 90. Maybe that is one of the reasons he keeps going so strong. He not only performs regularly (about twice a month), but he also takes part in most of his business matters and decisions. Mr. Hope is experiencing one noticeable problem that comes along with aging for many— a loss of hearing. This has been very frustrating for those around him because his pride keeps an expensive hearing aid in the drawer.

Bob Hope is a good example of how one can age gracefully, maintaining an active mental and physical life. Not everyone is blessed with the kindness nature has bestowed on Mr. Hope by helping him stay well throughout his years. However, health experts agree that the tendency to age well is closely related to maintenance of a high-level wellness life-style.

Source: The Wall Street Journal, *May 11, 1993, p. A16.*

Why study aging in a college health class? Isn't aging a rather distant concern for most college students? Why be concerned about it now? Here are some very good reasons:

- Aging is a lifelong process beginning at conception and taking place every day in every one of us.

- Our health habits influence the rate at which we age.

- There is a positive correlation between age and disease, but a healthful life-style can reduce the number and severity of diseases occurring with age.

- Our attitudes toward aging influence how we live every aspect of our lives.

- Most of us have older friends and relatives and we want to be able to relate to them.

- In time, each of us will be older and the quality of our lives will be influenced by the preparations we made while we were younger.

- Older people are forming an increasing percentage of the U.S. and world population.

- Our society's attitudes and political policies relating to older people are a critical concern for them and, in time, will be of equal concern to each of us. If we work to understand aging and the concerns of older people while we are young, we will pave the way for a more rewarding future for ourselves.

WHAT IS AGING?

Aging is the process of growing older. It is associated with gradually reduced functioning and adaptive abilities of most body systems. Gerontologist Robert Arking defines aging as "those series of cumulative, universal, progressive, intrinsic, and deleterious functional and structural changes that

....

aging the process of growing older; also defined as those series of cumulative, universal, progressive, intrinsic, and deleterious functional and structural changes that usually begin to manifest themselves at reproductive maturity and eventually culminate in death.

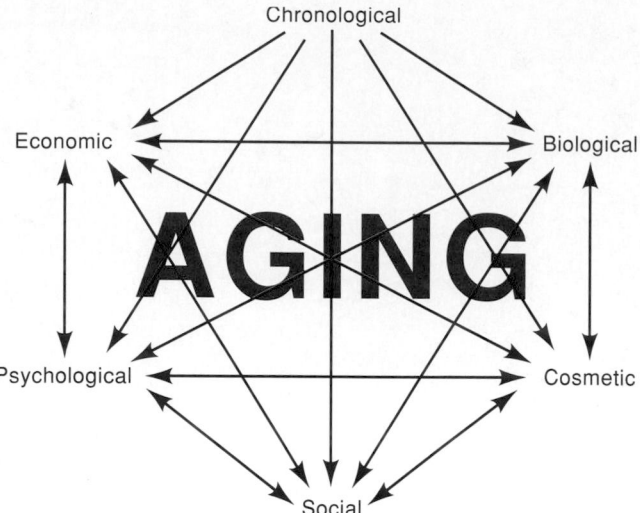

Figure 12.1

Interactions Among Types of Aging

There are six types of aging, each of which interacts with each of the others in obvious or subtle ways. Note that nothing affects chronological aging; it is simply the passage of time.

Source: "Interactions among Types of Aging" adapted from Human Aging by DiGiovanna & Augustine, 1994, p.8. Reprinted by Permission of McGraw-Hill, Inc.

usually begin to manifest themselves at reproductive maturity and eventually culminate in death."[1]

Gerontology (*je-ron-tol'ŏ-jē*) is the study of all aspects of aging, including the biological, psychological, sociological, and economic factors of advancing age. Only in recent decades has gerontology emerged as a major field of study in the United States. As older adults make up an increasing percentage of the U.S. population, this science will continue to grow in importance. **Geriatrics** (*jer-ē-at'riks*) is the branch of medicine that treats the health conditions and diseases associated with aging and old age.

Augustine DiGiovanna has identified six types of aging: chronological, biological, cosmetic, social, psychological, and economic.[2] A holistic view of aging shows us that each of these types of aging influences and is influenced by each of the others (see Figure 12.1). Note, however, that nothing affects chronological aging; it is simply the passage of time.

....

gerontology the study of aging.

geriatrics the branch of medicine that treats the conditions and diseases associated with aging and old age.

FEATURE 12.1

MYTHS OF SENILITY

Myths serve many purposes. They usually elevate one group—an ethnic group, nationality, religion, gender, or age group—at the expense of another. For the group that is elevated, there is an added sense of security and self-esteem. There may also be increased control over the other group.

For the older person, the most damaging myths are those that perpetuate the notion that most older people are dependent and most younger adults are independent. Some examples of these myths follow:

Myth: Most older persons are senile or demented (of unsound mind).

Fact: Senile is often used as a pejorative term. The vast majority of older people function very well mentally. They are neither senile nor demented. They are not emotionally disturbed; they are still intelligent; and fewer than 20 percent have any measurable memory impairment.[a]

Myth: Most older persons feel miserable most of the time.

Fact: The majority of older people are just as happy and satisfied with their lives as when they were younger.

Myth: Older people cannot work as productively as younger people.

Fact: Older workers are more consistent in their output, have fewer injuries, and less absenteeism than do younger workers.

Myth: Most older people are unable to care for themselves.

Fact: Eighty percent of people over age 65 are healthy enough to live independently and carry on their normal lifestyles. Less than 5 percent actually reside in nursing homes.

[a]Ebersole, P., and Hess, P. *Toward Healthy Aging*, 3rd ed. St. Louis: Mosby, 1990.

CHRONOLOGICAL AGING

Chronological aging is the passage of time since a person's birth. Your **chronological age** is how long you have lived. In this book, we have chosen to deemphasize chronological age as a measure of "oldness," because two people of the same chronological age may have aged at different rates and, thus, have very different biological ages (discussed in the following). Chronological age does, however, carry some social implications. Society holds expectations for behavior and function of persons having a certain chronological age although these expectations differ among cultures and change over time.

BIOLOGICAL AGING

Biological aging, which is far more significant than chronological aging, involves aging of a person's anatomy and physiology in ways that affect a person's appearance and abilities, including the ability to survive. The biological aging of different

people proceeds at very different rates. Some of this difference is genetically determined and beyond our control; much of it, however, relates to life-style factors that are very much within our ability to control. To some degree, each of us determines our rate of biological aging.

Senility refers to the physical and mental deterioration which is associated with advanced biological aging (see Feature 12.1). **Senescence** (*si-nes'ens* or *sē-nes'ens*) is the phase of old age, toward the end of the life span, during which functional deterioration of the body leads to an increased probability of death.

COSMETIC AGING

Cosmetic aging refers to the changes in outward appearance that occur with advancing age.[3] It includes changes in the body as well as culturally influenced changes in clothing and hair style. Cos-

. . . .

chronological aging the passage of time since a person's birth.

chronological age how long a person has lived.

biological aging aging of a person's anatomy and physiology in ways that affect a person's appearance and abilities, including the ability to survive.

senility the physical and mental deterioration that is associated with advanced biological aging.

senescence the phase of old age toward the end of the life span in which functional deterioration of the body leads to an increased probability of death.

cosmetic aging changes in outward appearance with advancing age.

metic aging is often used to estimate a person's chronological age or biological age, but it is an inaccurate indicator for either purpose. Even though cosmetic aging is an inaccurate indicator of chronological or biological age, it can have a powerful influence on a person's life. Right or wrong, people do judge us by our appearance and relate to us in different ways according to their estimate of our age. Further, we may judge ourselves by our appearance. If we believe that we look "old" we may think of ourselves as being "old" and withdraw from various physical and social activities. We may also begin to neglect our appearance, causing ourselves to look even "older."

SOCIAL AGING

Social aging consists of age-related changes in the interactions people have with each other. Each culture has its expectations for the behavior of people of different ages. As an example of how the types of aging interact, consider how being treated by others as being "old" causes a person to feel older, affecting psychological aging.

PSYCHOLOGICAL AGING

Psychological aging consists of age-related changes in how people think and act. It results partly from the biological aging of the brain, as well as from chronological, social, cosmetic, and economic aging. Whatever age you are right now, consider how many of your opinions and reactions have changed compared to those of ten years ago.

ECONOMIC AGING

Economic aging consists of age-related changes in a person's financial status. Up to a point, a person's economic position tends to improve with age, then, typically, to decline. Here is one type of aging where the effects of other types of aging can

social aging age-related changes in the interactions people have with each other.

psychological aging age-related changes in how people think and act.

economic aging age-related changes in a person's financial status.

be quite apparent. For example, biological, chronological, social, cosmetic, and psychological aging can all reduce a person's earning ability. Even though laws prohibit age-based employment discrimination, many older people find it difficult to obtain jobs or promotions because of their age or appearance of age.

LONGEVITY AND LIFE EXPECTANCY

Longevity is the duration of life of an individual. For humans, the maximum potential life span is about 115 years. The mean (average) longevity of a population is referred to as **life expectancy.** In the United States, life expectancy has increased from 35 years in 1776 to about 75.5 years now. Feature 12.2 explores increasing life expectancies on a world basis.

Life expectancies vary with gender and ethnicity. Life expectancy for women in the United States now is about 78.9 years, compared to 72.0 years for men. The difference in life expectancy between the genders widened from 2.0 years in 1900 to 7.8 years in the 1980s and has now narrowed somewhat to 7.0 years.[4]

Comparing ethnic groups in the United States, non-Hispanic white (Anglo) Americans tend to have the greatest life expectancy and African Americans and Native Americans the shortest, with Asian Americans and Hispanic Americans falling between. Anglo female life expectancy is 79.6 and African American female life expectancy is 73.8, a difference of 5.8 years. Anglo male life expectancy is 72.9 and African American male life expectancy is 64.6, a difference of 8.3 years.[5]

CHECKPOINT

1. Why is it useful to study aging?
2. Define the terms *aging, gerontology, geriatrics, senility,* and *senescence.*
3. What are six types of aging and what are some ways in which each interacts with the others?

longevity the duration of life of an individual.

life expectancy the mean (average) longevity of a population.

FEATURE 12.2

THE AGING HUMAN POPULATION: NOT JUST IN THE UNITED STATES

Most of this chapter focuses on the aging individual in the United States. Also significant is the worldwide aging of the entire human population. In every industrialized nation and in many developing countries, mean (average) life spans have sharply increased during this century. While in 1992 there were 342 million people age 65 or over in the world (6.2 percent of the population), by 2050 there will be at least 2.5 *billion* people over age 65 (about 20 percent of the world's population). This will be the greatest percentage of the population to reach that age in the entire history of humanity.

In past centuries, only a small segment of the population ever lived long enough to achieve what we think of as old age. You need only to read the headstones in any old cemetery to appreciate what life was like:

- The graves of many infants will be seen. Often almost one-third of the children born failed to live even one year.

- The graves of many women of childbearing age will be apparent. Many women died from causes directly related to pregnancy.

- Lines of graves containing all of the children in a family are common in every old cemetery. Diphtheria or other diseases would wipe out every child in a family within days of each other.

Much of today's extended life expectancy has come from eliminating most deaths of infants, children, and young adults. This has been accomplished through improved sanitation, immunization, and medications that have given a greater control over infectious and parasitic diseases. Now, more than 90 percent of the people born in any given year in an industrialized nation will live past the age of 65.

The decline in deaths of young people initially made the population younger, but this has been followed, in the industrialized nations, by a decline in births. Where six or seven children was once the norm, now most families are much smaller. So gradually the average age and the percentage of people who are over 65 has increased.

This changing age structure will have an impact on many aspects of society, including the job market, housing, transportation, patterns of retirement, and health care. If people continue to retire as young as they now do, many will spend as much as one-third of their lives in retirement. The current patterns of work and retirement will not be financially supportable in the future. With the improved health of older people, many will retire at older ages, enter new careers, or continue to work part-time. Also, there are and will be tax incentives for long-term savings to augment pensions.

Health care will be a special problem. Older people tend to use health services much more than younger people. With the older population growing larger and living longer, Medicare in the United States and similar programs in other countries face huge financial problems.

These demographic projections are not just speculation. They are based on the number of people of various ages that are already living. By 2010, when the "baby boomers" reach what we have thought of as "retirement age," the United States and other world governments will be forced to restructure their various old-age entitlement programs to accommodate the unprecedented number of older people.

Source: Kinsella, K., and Taeuber, C. *An Aging World II.* Washington, DC: Center for International Research, U.S. Bureau of the Census, 1993.

INCREASING PERCENTAGE OF OLDER PEOPLE IN U.S. POPULATION

Whether viewed in terms of absolute numbers or percentage of the U.S. population, the older population of the nation is increasing rapidly. By 2040, the population of Americans over age 65 may grow to 87 million, three times the current number. Based on estimates of the National Institute on Aging, the over-65 group will have grown from 4 percent in 1900 to 20 or 25 percent in 2040. Even more dramatic will be the number of people over age 85, of whom there may be nearly 24 million in 2040, ten times the current number (see Feature 12.2).

How does the National Institute on Aging know these things? These figures are based, in part,

on the known number of people of each age in our current population. (How old will *you* be in 2040?) Further, they are based on an expected increase in life expectancy from today's average of 72.0 years for men and 78.9 years for women, to a possible 85.9 for men and 91.5 for women by 2040. Of course, actual life spans could be either shorter or longer and, as we have pointed out, vary among the different ethnic groups.

To accommodate this increased older population, the availability of services required by older people will need to be greatly expanded. Housing, medical care, transportation, and other needs will have to be met and financed. There will be plenty of new jobs providing goods and services for older people. Will the increasing number of older people be viewed as a burden on society or as a financial boon for the younger population? What will be the effect of the larger percentage of people who will be retired being supported by the Social Security contributions of the smaller percentage of people who will be working? And what effect will the proposed advancement of the common retirement age from 65 to 67 or older have upon the supply of jobs available to younger workers?

C H E C K P O I N T

1. What are approximate current life expectancies for each gender in the United States?

2. What social, economic, personal, and health changes do you think will occur as a result of an increased percentage of older citizens in the United States?

AGEISM: OUR YOUTH-WORSHIPING CULTURE

Prevailing social attitudes and values regarding aging greatly affect the quality of life and the well-being of older people. Many of the world's cultures hold their older people in a position of high esteem. In the United States, however, there has been an erosion of the social foundations that once contributed to a sense of dignity and meaning in the lives of our older citizens, especially in the white, or Anglo, community. Among Native Americans, African Americans, Asian Americans, and Hispanic Americans the elders are usually revered more than in Anglo America and are more likely to be cared for within the family.

The term **ageism,** coined by Robert Butler in 1968,[6] refers to the stereotyping of and discrimination against people simply because they are old. Ageism deprives many older citizens of employment and other opportunities while decreasing their self-esteem. Ageism affects younger people as well, by magnifying their fears about growing older.

American society highly values youth, beauty, money, productivity, progress, speed, and independence. It associates few of these with the older population. Older people in the United States are often viewed as dependent, nonproductive, and a burden

to be borne by the younger members of society. Attitudes of younger people are powerfully influenced by the media, which too often present a negative picture of older people. Advertising, in particular, takes advantage of negative portrayals of aging to sell a wide range of products. The message is that to be old is to be ugly. Skin creams are promoted to hide "those *ugly* age spots and wrinkles." Gyms, spas, and diet plans tell us we must "keep that *youthful* figure." We must color our hair to "get rid of that *ugly* gray." Finally, greeting cards, such as birthday cards, are among the worst offenders in perpetuating negative stereotypes of aging.

Example: Front of card: "Aren't Birthdays Wonderful;" inside of card: "and root canals, aren't they great?"

The topic of death is implicit in any discussion of aging. In the United States, death is a culturally taboo subject. Most of us can talk easily about money, politics, and religion, but not about death. Aging brings us closer to death. The desire to avoid death, to separate it from everyday life and even to deny its inevitability is a major factor contributing to people's fear of aging. (Chapter 13 will help you feel more comfortable about death.)

Negative attitudes toward aging and older people are so pervasive that they are reflected in the attitudes of our children. This is especially true of young children who have not spent much time with grandparents.[7] Negative attitudes about aging are passed on to children from parents, peers, and the media, especially television.

Each of us needs to develop a better understanding of the older members of our society and to work to change society's attitudes toward them. It's only a matter of time before we are older and, unless attitudes change, we too will be victims of negative stereotyping. In order to start this crusade let's first examine our own attitudes toward aging. Take a moment right now to complete the In Your Hands: Your Attitudes Regarding Aging assessment.

C H E C K P O I N T

1. What is ageism?

2. In what ways can ageism be disadvantageous to older people?

3. What factors perpetuate ageism?

ageism stereotyping of and discrimination against people because they are old.

IN YOUR HANDS

YOUR ATTITUDES REGARDING AGING

Our attitudes toward aging influence not only our later lives, but our younger years as well. What are your attitudes regarding aging?

	Strongly Agree	Somewhat Agree	Strongly Disagree
1. I will start to think about aging when I get older.	0	1	2
2. I don't even like to think about aging.	0	1	2
3. I enjoy being around older people.	2	1	0
4. Older people make me feel uncomfortable.	0	1	2
5. Growing old is a natural part of life.	2	1	0
6. Being around older people makes me nervous.	0	1	2
7. I would rather die young than get old.	0	1	2
8. I can see some advantages in being old.	2	1	0
9. By living healthfully, I can slow the aging process.	2	1	0
10. Older people have a lot of good ideas.	2	1	0

Total points: _____

INTERPRETATION:

18–20 points: your positive attitudes toward aging will help you live your life with maximum fulfillment.

14–17 points: your attitudes toward aging are about typical of the population; there is room for improvement.

less than 14 points: if unchanged, your negative views of aging will cause problems throughout your life; read this chapter very carefully and try to apply it to your own life.

MULTICULTURAL PERSPECTIVES ON AGING

In response to a shortage of data on aging in specific ethnic groups, the American Association of Retired Persons (AARP) has commissioned research and sponsored conferences on this subject. The following information is based upon some of that research.[8, 9]

OLDER NATIVE AMERICANS

Older Native Americans tend to retain their cultural traditions. Long ago their parents taught them that the traditions of the Native American nations were more important than the complex and distant political systems of state and federal governments. Thus, older Native American people tend not to make effective use of government programs available for their benefit.

Older Native Americans are about as likely as older Anglo Americans to live with family members. They are, however, much more likely to live in poverty, in substandard housing lacking sanitary facilities, having poor heating, lacking telephones, and at great distances from health care providers. Even when health care is accessible, it is often avoided because of a preference for traditional, spiritually based healing and distrust of government sponsored programs.

Life expectancies for Native Americans are considerably shorter than those of Anglo Americans. In addition to inadequate health care, there are high death rates from diabetes and alcohol-related causes such as vehicle crashes, cirrhosis, and suicide.

OLDER ASIAN AMERICANS

The phrase *Asian Americans* throws together a diverse group of cultures including the Chinese, Japanese, Korean, Vietnamese, Laotian, Thai, Cambodian, Filipinos, Hmong, and more. Any generalizations made here may not be valid for all of these groups.

The older members usually play an important role in the Asian family and the obligation of the family to care for older members was formerly beyond question. With exposure to American society, however, many Asian Americans no longer feel so obligated to care for their older family members. Although the proportion of Asian American families taking care of their older members is greater than that of other groups, this gap is expected to close with time. Also, responsibility for caring for

Aging carries different meanings to people of different ethnicity in terms of health care, social status, and family relationships.

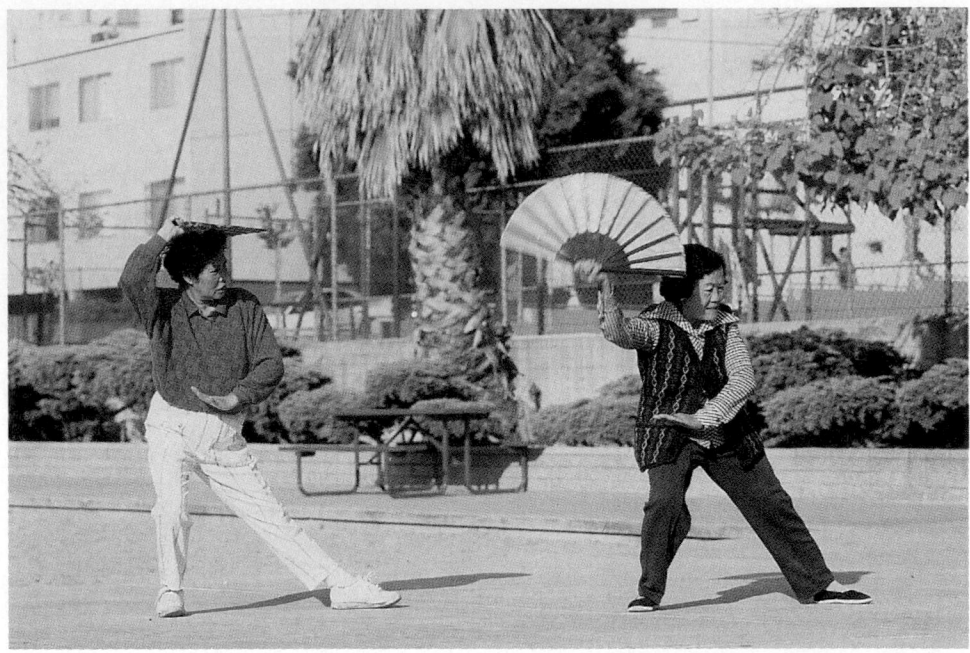

older parents is shifting from male children (the Asian tradition) to female children (the American tradition).

Despite a common perception of Asian Americans as being successful and wealthy, many older Asian Americans live in poverty or near poverty. Those who don't live with family may live in substandard conditions. Many do not qualify for Social Security or other entitlements or qualify for only minimal benefits. Often, newer immigrants do not know how to deal with a "new" health care system. Many rely on folk medicine and experience health problems that are debilitating and of long duration. Faced with events that seem beyond their control, many older Asian Americans react with a learned helplessness, assuming a passive role that precludes any effective resolution of their health problems. Some Asian cultures have high rates of smoking and the health effects of years of smoking are prevalent in older members.

OLDER AFRICAN AMERICANS

Older African Americans often have limited financial resources. Today's older African American people were educated at a time when schools were often segregated and those for African Americans were sometimes quite poor. Many have experienced unemployment and held low-paying jobs, resulting in low retirement income. African Ameri-

cans over age 65 are almost three times as likely as Anglo Americans to live in poverty.

The health status of older African Americans is often poor. Chronic illness strikes them more often and at a younger age than it does Anglo Americans. African Americans are less than half as likely as Anglo Americans to carry insurance to supplement their Medicare coverage.

A smaller percentage of older African Americans than of Anglo Americans live in nursing home facilities. Many who do live in nursing homes prefer a facility that is owned and operated by African Americans, where there is more opportunity to continue familiar cultural activities.

OLDER HISPANIC AMERICANS

As with the term *Asian Americans,* the term *Hispanic Americans* includes many subgroups—Mexican Americans, Puerto Ricans, Cubans, and people from many countries of Central and South America—for whom generalizations made about Hispanic Americans may not all hold true. Remember also that *Hispanic* is an ethnic designation, not a racial one. Hispanic people belong to all races.

Most older Hispanic people retain the traditional values and behaviors based on those of their countries of origin. Ethnic pride contributes to a strong self-image and social cohesion with other older Hispanic people. They also retain important social roles, such as passing on their history to younger persons and acting as arbitrators and facilitators for their families and communities. Family, religious beliefs, and church-related activities are major sources of social and emotional support for many older Hispanic people.

Hispanic people, collectively, are the nation's fastest-growing ethnic population. Hispanic Americans are a relatively young population, with a smaller percentage of older citizens (4.8 percent) than found in other ethnic groups (average of about 12 percent). The smaller numbers of older Hispanic people have made them an "invisible" group, taken care of primarily by their families.

Older Hispanic Americans have a high rate of poverty, over twice that of older Anglo Americans. Many are ineligible for Social Security, either because of citizenship issues or as a result of working in occupations not covered by Social Security. Compared to other ethnic groups, however, older Hispanic people are more likely to own their own homes and to remain in the same neighborhood where they have lived, even when their children move to other locations.

Older Hispanic people have high rates of chronic illness and disability, especially arthritis, hypertension, cardiovascular problems, and diabetes. Many are unable to afford adequate health services and others, through preference, depend on traditional ethnic cures and healers (*curanderos*) rather than on modern medicine.

CHECKPOINT

1. What are some reasons why older members of some ethnic groups receive inadequate health services?

2. What is meant by the phrase, "older Hispanic Americans are invisible?"

3. How does "learned helplessness" relate to older Asian Americans?

HEALTHY AGING

Picture yourself at your twentieth high school class reunion. Everyone there is about the same chronological age, mostly about 38 years old. Some of your classmates look almost the same as they did at graduation. Others look like they could be in their fifties. What has made the difference?

To a large extent, our genes determine how fast we age. This is why each species of animal has a fairly predictable maximum life span. The way we live, however, also has an effect on the speed and nature of our aging. If we adopt a life-style that promotes our well-being, we can slow down the process considerably. We cannot wait until we are 30, 50, or 70 to become concerned about aging. This is an ongoing process that begins at birth. The time to be concerned is now. How can we age most healthfully?

STRESS MANAGEMENT

High stress levels are among the greatest accelerators of the biological aging processes. The many physiological changes that comprise the stress response help prepare your body for emergency actions, but when maintained at high levels for long periods, stress speeds the aging of every part of your body. Effective stress management, as described in Chapter 4, is a *must* for slowing biological aging.

PROPER DIET

In order for body tissues to be maintained and for cells to be repaired and replaced as necessary, your diet must contain adequate amounts of essential nutrients. Extensive animal research indicates that a diet that restricts calories, but not essential nutrients, extends life spans.[10] It is still uncertain whether calorie restriction will do the same for humans (see p. 384). Overeating, however, has been associated with an increased speed of aging.

Statistical relationships between human weight and life expectancy are difficult to interpret. They do not necessarily prove a cause-and-effect relationship. In some cases, people may be slender because they have health problems. These people tend to die prematurely and thus bring down the average life expectancy for slim people.

Much has been written about life-extension diets. Can a particular diet or pill add years to your life? There is no evidence that any specific diet or pill is the answer. The life-extension diet appears to be the same diet recommended for the prevention of heart disease, cancer, and obesity. This diet emphasizes vegetables, fruits, and whole grains. It is low in fat, sugar, and salt; moderate in protein; low in calories; and adequate in all vitamins and minerals. Some authorities suggest taking supplementary vitamin C, E, and beta carotene (see p. 384).

AVOIDING HARMFUL SUBSTANCES

We age rapidly enough without doing anything to speed up the process. But that is exactly what people who are users of alcohol, tobacco, or other drugs are doing. Animal research and human autopsies indicate that the aging of virtually every organ of the body is accelerated by drinking, smoking, and other drug use. Since the damage usually occurs in small increments, we are rarely aware that it is happening. After a night or weekend of heavy drinking, we don't perceive ourselves as any less intelligent than we were before, but the fact is that about 10,000 of our irreplaceable neurons have been destroyed.

PHYSICAL ACTIVITY

Exercise is probably the single best strategy for slowing down biological aging. Between the ages of 30 and 70, the average sedentary (nonexercising) person loses 30–40 percent of his or her muscle mass. During this same time, the heart's pumping efficiency drops an average of about 30 percent. A lifelong program of regular exercise can delay these changes by as much as 20 years.[11]

Regular physical activity slows aging in many other ways. An ample supply of blood is essential to every part of the body and exercise improves the circulation of blood throughout the body. Active people stay more limber and experience less painful and disabling arthritis. Physical activity also:

- helps reduce stress levels
- contributes to a more positive state of mind
- helps maintain the calcium content of the bones, preventing osteoporosis in those with genetic vulnerability
- helps maintain proper body weight
- maintains muscle strength
- slows the pulse
- reduces blood pressure

- lowers overall blood cholesterol levels, while improving the ratio of high-density lipoprotein to low-density lipoprotein (see Chapter 20)

Many physical activities are especially appropriate for older people. Walking is one of the most recommended activities and many areas have organized walking clubs or groups. Swimming is also favored because it exercises the entire body and does not produce a jarring impact on the joints. Dancing is another excellent activity, providing social contact as well as exercise. Finally, many older people continue to ski or play racquet sports, such as tennis and racquetball, at very advanced ages.

Increasing numbers of authorities are emphasizing the benefits to older people, even those in their nineties, from working with weights or resistance. Muscle size and strength increase rapidly and walk-

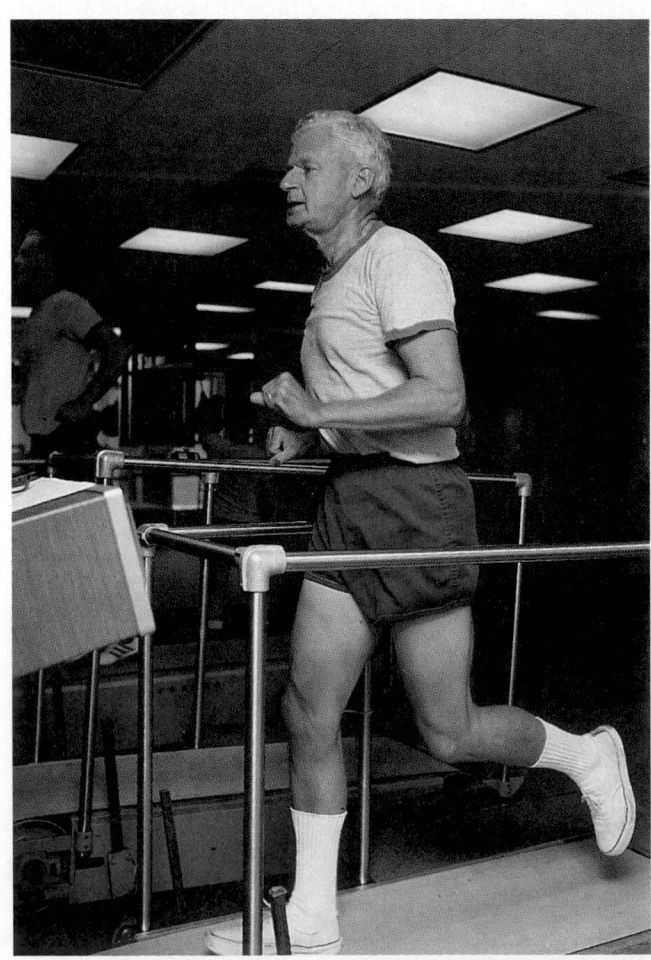

Regular physical activity helps maintain muscle mass, keeps the heart healthy, and slows aging in many additional ways.

ing ability and general mobility improve. William Evans and Irwin Rosenberg, in *Biomarkers,* recommend numerous exercise plans that can help to slow and reverse the physical effects of aging.[12]

Anyone over the age of 40 should consult with a physician before beginning an activity program or increasing his or her normal level of activity. At any age, to reduce the chance of injury, a person's activity level ought to be increased gradually, rather than suddenly.

MENTAL ACTIVITY

Staying mentally active is another key to slowing the aging process. Much of the mental deterioration that some older people experience is just the result of mental inactivity. To be mentally alert and sharp in your old age, you must remain mentally active throughout your life. If work does not provide enough mental stimulation, leisure activities should. Rather than spending evenings passively watching TV, you can take courses, read challenging material, and engage in thought-provoking games.

SOCIAL ACTIVITY

People with strong social support networks are reported to have a much lower risk of illness and death than socially isolated people.[13] One link between social contact and health may be the stress response. People with well-developed social support systems are able to experience life crises with lower stress levels. They are also less likely to rely excessively on alcohol or other drugs. Having adequate social contact is also associated with a greater sense of control over life, which, in turn, reduces stress.

ADEQUATE SKIN CARE

Most people judge someone's age by how wrinkled that person's skin is. Approximately 70 percent of the skin wrinkles that appear with age are a direct effect of the ultraviolet rays in sunlight.[14] People don't always associate wrinkling with sun exposure because the damage doesn't show until 10 or 20 years after exposure. Albert Kligman, a dermatologist at the University of Pennsylvania,

has spent 40 years studying the effects of sun on human skin and he urges minimizing exposure. If you must be in the sun, he recommends using a powerful sunscreen and wearing a hat to shade your face.

CHECKPOINT

1. When is a good time to try to start slowing down the aging process?

2. What type of diet appears to be associated with a long life?

3. In what ways does regular exercise reduce the effects of aging?

4. How can the loss of mental abilities with advancing age be minimized?

MIDDLE AGE

The boundaries of middle age are extremely vague and variable. Some people feel old at 35 while others still feel young at 60. Middle age is perhaps best defined not by years, but as a state of mind that accompanies the assumption of full adult responsibilities and the awareness of aging.[15] Most people enter this stage sometime between the ages of 35 and 45.

As a result of making healthful life-style choices, many of today's middle-aged people are less "old" for their age than were previous generations. By exercising more and being more careful about diet and other health habits, today's average 50-year-old looks, feels, and acts more like the 40-year-olds of his or her parents' generation.

Most of us expect a middle-aged person to experience a "midlife crisis," but midlife researchers now doubt that this is a universal event. Some middle-aged people do go through a period of questioning the validity of the lives they have led and are leading, perhaps making desperate efforts to recapture their lost youth. But most middle-aged people come to terms with their growing older in a gradual, decidedly noncrisis way. What does happen is a subtle acceptance of life's limitations. As in adolescence, one key task is to change your self-image. Those who most successfully move into middle and older ages are those with a strong internally based sense of self-esteem, as opposed to

Which of these people would you consider middle aged? Middle age is a very vague time of life, perhaps best defined as a state of mind, rather than a certain age bracket.

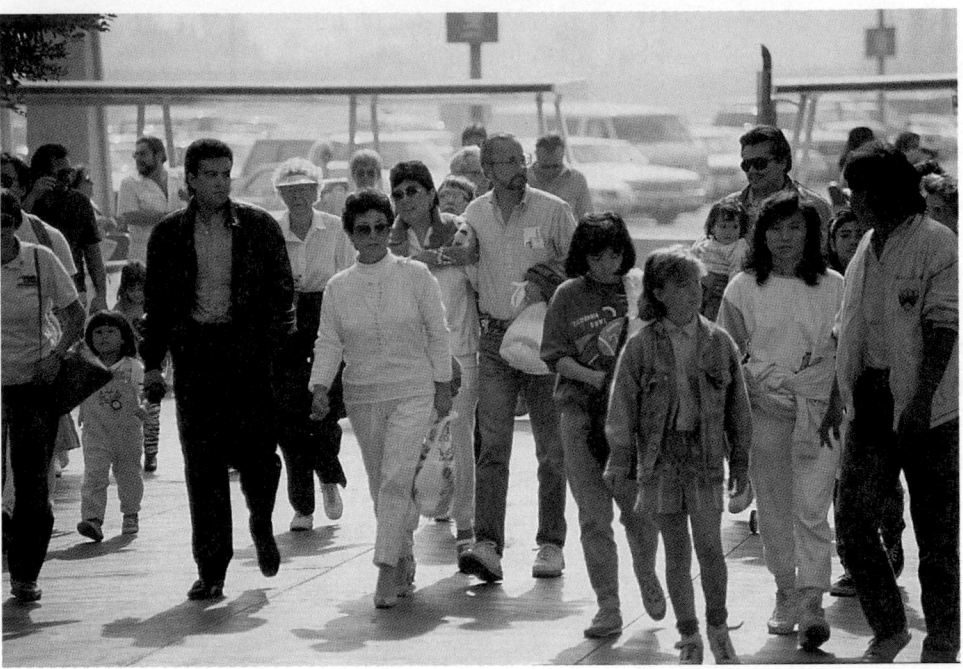

those who need constant external reinforcement regarding their worth.

Many gerontologists believe that a successful middle age is essential to a rewarding old age. Many adjustments are needed; the goals and rules that may have worked well in early adulthood may not work as well in middle age. A "successful" middle age involves accomplishing a number of tasks that help prepare you for a satisfying old age. Some of these tasks include:

- developing a new sense of identity
- coming to terms with your own aging
- renewing and perhaps redefining couple relationships
- discovering or rediscovering your creativity
- taking on added responsibility
- developing a more adult relationship with your parents and children
- accepting new family members such as in-laws and grandchildren
- coming to terms with the aging and/or death of your parents
- making preparations for retirement
- maintaining or establishing healthful living patterns

Each of us deals with these challenges in our own way and with our own degree of success.

Those who successfully face and deal with these issues are poised for a fulfilling old age.

CHECKPOINT

1. What is the psychological definition of middle age?

2. Does every middle-aged person experience midlife crisis?

3. What are the special challenges of middle age?

BIOLOGICAL THEORIES ON AGING

Sanitation, immunization, antibiotics, and other medical advances have eliminated many deaths of young persons, thereby increasing the *average* life expectancy in the industrialized countries. But these advances have had little effect on the *maximum* life span potential, the age at death of the longest-lived members of the population. Now, as thousands of years ago, the maximum longevity remains at between 110 and 120 years. So far, medical science has had little impact on the factors that limit maximum life span in humans. Life spans of other animal species have been extended by methods that may or may not prove successful in humans.

What causes aging and set limits on longevity? Many theories have been proposed and it is very unlikely that there is only one cause of aging; there are probably many factors involved and many valid theories. **Programmed aging theories** attribute aging to built-in mechanisms acting to ensure the finite lives of organisms. **Stochastic aging theories,** also called error theories, relate aging to external forces that damage cells until they can no longer function adequately; included here would be effects of environment factors such as diet, radiation, and harmful substances. The following are a few of the current biological theories on aging.[16]

PROGRAMMED AGING THEORIES

Since every species of animals has its own average and maximum longevity, there are strong arguments favoring the theory that aging is programmed into each species. Some biologists suggest that the control of aging is located in each cell of the body, while others suggest that there is one master control center for aging, possibly located in the hypothalamus of the brain. The thymus (discussed relative to immunity in Chapter 18) has also been mentioned as a possible control center for aging.

Most research appears to support the belief that each cell contains its own built-in program for aging. When normal human cells are cultured in the laboratory, they undergo a finite number of divisions, then they die, regardless of how carefully they are tended. Cells that have been removed from embryos undergo many more divisions before dying than do cells removed from adults.[17–19]

Gene Theories of Aging

Gene theories are foremost among the programmed theories on aging. Some suggest that the programming is due to one or more genes in each of us that become active only late in life and alter our physiology in ways that lead to our death. This suggests that longevity is an inherited trait; it is

....

programmed aging theories theories that attribute aging to built-in mechanisms acting to ensure the finite lives of organisms.

stochastic aging theories also called error theories, these theories relate aging to external forces that damage cells until they can no longer function adequately.

well-known that longevity does run along family lines. The best predictor of how long a person will live is how long his or her ancestors lived. Studies have also shown that the longevity of identical twins is more similar than the longevity of fraternal twins or other siblings who are not twins, lending further support to this theory.[20]

Another genetic theory relates aging to progressive damage to the ends (telomeres) of DNA molecules through repeated cell divisions. This theory holds that when damage is severe enough, cells cease dividing and die.[21]

Immunological Theories

At least two immunological changes are associated with aging, though it is unclear whether they are primarily causes or effects of aging. Some experts view declining immune function as a programmed aging event. First there is a gradual decline in the ability of the immune system to protect against invading disease germs (pathogens) and to recognize and destroy body cells that become cancerous. Second, there is an increase in autoimmune functions. As discussed in Chapter 18, an **autoimmune response** is a self-destructive process by which a person's immune system attacks his or her own body. Autoimmune theories of aging propose that, with advancing age, the immune system increasingly attacks a person's own self. One autoimmune theory holds that as we grow older, new antigens (body chemicals) appear and stimulate the autoimmune destruction of cells. Another autoimmune theory is that, with increasing age, the immune system is less able to discriminate between a person's own body chemicals and the foreign chemicals it is supposed to destroy.[22]

STOCHASTIC AGING THEORIES

Stochastic (error) theories suggest that aging is not an inherent characteristic of life, but is the result of the accumulation of injuries inflicted on cells and organisms by various environmental factors. These theories hold more promise for retarding the effects of aging through diet and other behavioral modifications than do the programmed theories.

....

autoimmune response a self-destructive process in which a person's immune system attacks his or her own body.

Gene Mutation Theory of Aging

The stochastic gene **mutation** theory suggests that mutations (genetic changes) accumulate in every cell, with the passage of time, until the cell can no longer function properly and it dies. Natural sources of radiation are presumed to be a major cause of mutations, with additional radiation exposure, as in x-rays, speeding the mutation process. Ultraviolet exposure is a major source of mutations in skin cells. Some chemicals, such as certain pesticides, also cause mutations.

Cells have several ways to repair damaged genes. The gene mutation theory assumes that with the passage of time these repair mechanisms become less efficient and allow mutations to remain uncorrected. The gene mutation theory is not among today's leading theories on aging.

Cross-Linkage Theory

Proteins are an essential part of every human cell and are composed of smaller molecules called peptides. Proteins can be permanently changed by the formation of chemical bonds (cross-links) between these peptides (see Figure 12.2).

The well-accepted **cross-linkage** theory, another stochastic theory, holds that with age, cross-links accumulate until the proteins can no longer function properly, causing the death of cells. The proteins most affected by cross-linking are said to be enzymes and collagen. Specific enzymes are necessary for the occurrence of most of a cell's chemical reactions. Collagen is a fibrous protein located between cells to hold them together. Cross-linkage in collagen is thought to contribute to the loss of elasticity of many body parts, such as the skin and blood vessels, that occurs with age.[23]

Free Radical Theory

Free radicals are highly reactive cell chemicals that are formed as by-products of normal chemical

....

mutation a change in a gene.

cross-linkage formation of chemical bonds between the peptide units of proteins.

free radicals highly reactive cell chemicals that are formed as by-products of normal chemical reactions within cells.

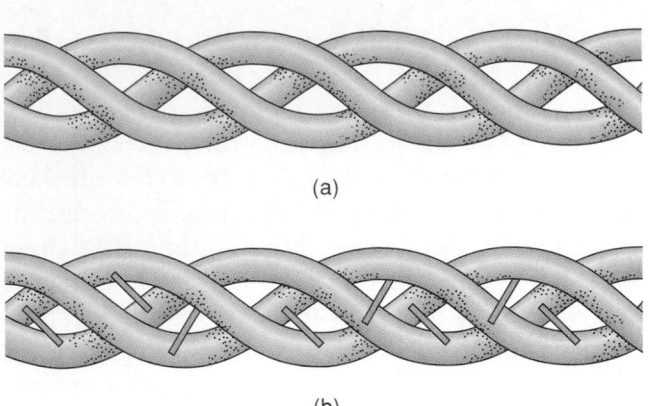

(a)

(b)

Figure 12.2
Cross-linkage

One theory of aging holds that with age, chemical bonds called cross-links form between the peptides of our body proteins. (a) Normal collagen, an important protein in skin, cartilage, and bone. Each collagen fiber consists of three peptide chains twisted into a helix. (b) Cross-links, shown in orange, reduce the flexibility of the collagen. In time, these cross-links interfere with the functions of the proteins, causing loss of elasticity of tissues and death of individual cells.

reactions within cells. Free radicals react quickly with other cell chemicals, especially fats. Because the membrane surrounding each cell contains much fat, it is thought to be progressively damaged when free radicals react with this fat. The function of the cell membrane, controlling the movement of chemicals into and out of the cell, is thus impaired. Free radicals also react with our genetic material, contributing to the accumulation of mutations. The stochastic free radical theory is currently widely accepted.[24]

One of the more controversial aspects of the free radical theory is the suggestion that aging might be delayed by consuming antioxidants such as vitamins C and E and beta carotene, which inhibit the formation of free radicals. Consumption of another antioxidant, the food preservative BHT (butylated hydroxytoluene), has also been suggested as a way of retarding aging, but this theory is also unproven.

Dietary Restriction

Dietary restriction is not so much a theory on aging as an *intervention* that has been shown to slow aging and extend life spans in a wide variety of vertebrate and invertebrate animal species. Countless animal experiments have led to the conclusion that diet restriction enhances longevity. Little of this research has involved humans, and, of course, it will take many years to know the outcome of any human research. The wide variety of animals showing life extension through dietary restriction, however, makes it likely that humans may also show this effect. Robert Arking has compiled information on dietary restriction, including the following:[25]

- The maximum life extension occurs when dietary restriction occurs early in life, before puberty, but there is some life extension when caloric restriction begins at any age.

- Caloric restriction before puberty retards growth to a degree that would probably be unacceptable to many people; a calorie-deprived person would always be small.

- It doesn't seem to matter whether it is protein, fat, or carbohydrate that is restricted; it is the total amount of calories consumed that matters.

- Working off the calories through exercise has no life-span-enhancing effect in animal species where this has been researched.

- The mechanism whereby dietary restriction extends life is unclear.

None of these theories on aging are mutually exclusive. Each of the processes mentioned could and probably does contribute to the physical effects of aging. The following section examines some of those effects.

CHECKPOINT

1. What does "programmed aging" mean? What are some forms of evidence in favor of this idea?

2. What is a stochastic theory on aging?

3. What is an autoimmune response?

4. To what extent would you be willing to go through life always hungry in order to live longer?

EFFECTS OF AGING

Physical, mental, and social changes are all important in the aging process. In the following sections we will consider how aging affects each of our body systems and how interaction with society changes with advancing age.

PHYSICAL CHANGES

Many physical characteristics change with age. Some of the changes we see are a normal part of the aging process; some are evidence of pathological aging. **Normal aging** consists of the gradual, inevitable changes that occur over time and that can be observed in all animal species. **Pathological aging** is marked by the presence of diseases that may result from unhealthful living habits. These diseases may be common in older humans, but are not seen in other animal species. They are the problems brought on by inactivity, dietary excesses, nutritional deficiencies, and abuse of harmful substances such as alcohol, tobacco, and other drugs. Sometimes problems are brought about by combinations or excessive doses of prescription medications (see Feature 12.3, p. 386).

Part of the negative view that people hold of old age stems from the prevalence of problems associated with pathological aging. With a lifetime of healthful living habits, many of these problems need not occur. The following aspects of normal aging are a gauge of what is and is not a normal part of the physical aging process:

Posture Changes

We lose about a half-inch of height every 20 years, mainly due to compaction of the cartilage disks between the vertebrae. After 40 years of age the cartilage shrinks as it gradually loses cells and water. A person's arms and legs begin to seem longer in relation to the shortened trunk of the body.

Posture often changes because of osteoporosis, degeneration of disks, and loss of muscle tone. These conditions can account for a stooped, forward-bent posture which develops in many older people. For those who have inherited the tendency to this condition, adequate physical activity,

normal aging the gradual, inevitable changes that occur over time and that can be observed in all animal species.

pathological aging aging marked by the presence of diseases that result from unhealthful living habits.

FEATURE 12.3

OVERMEDICATION: A PROBLEM FOR SOME OLDER PEOPLE

Prescribed medications play a major role in the longer lives enjoyed by today's older people. Many people today are able to live 20, 30, or more additional years because of the benefits of medical intervention. Yet no medication is without some potential hazards and side effects.

Physicians sometimes prescribe a drug for relief of an uncomfortable, but not life-threatening symptom. Often these symptoms could be reduced by increased exercise, modified diet, giving up alcohol and/or smoking, or other life-style changes. Sometimes a drug relieves one complaint, but its side effects create a new symptom. Problems start to snowball when the side effects of one drug are relieved by administering another drug.

Another potentially hazardous situation arises when a person is seeing several different physicians for different reasons. Not knowing what medications a patient is already taking, a physician may prescribe a drug that interacts with a drug prescribed by another physician. Older people often place a considerable confidence in their physicians and follow their orders unquestioningly.

People of any age who have more than one physician are advised to have all of their prescriptions filled by the same pharmacist. A pharmacist is trained to recognize potential problems associated with taking multiple medications. Taking your prescriptions to various pharmacies eliminates this protection.

If an older family member or friend develops a mysterious health problem, you might inquire about the medications he or she takes. It could be worthwhile to ask a physician or pharmacist to go over a list of the drugs. He or she may find several incompatible drugs or a single drug that could be causing the new health problem. Perhaps a drug being taken to relieve a minor complaint could be eliminated and the complaint tolerated or relieved by life-style changes.

---

proper diet, and hormone replacement therapy for postmenopausal women can often prevent or delay postural changes.

Redistribution of Fat Deposits

Some parts of the body accumulate fat, while other parts lose fat. The layer of fat behind the eyeballs thins, which gives a sunken appearance to the eyes. The layer of fat beneath the skin thins, which makes it harder for the body to stay warm and increases the risk of hypothermia. Conversely, fat tends to accumulate over the stomach and around the waist in males and in the hips and thighs in females if exercise is not maintained and calorie intake controlled.

Reduced Sweating

Sweat glands diminish in size, number, and activity, which can lead to overheating. Heat stroke is a common cause of death for older people in the summer.

Skin, Hair, and Nails

Cell division in the skin slows down with advancing age. The skin becomes thinner, more delicate, wrinkled, and dry. Pigment spots, similar to freckles, enlarge and become more numerous. Both genders experience thinning of hair on the head and body. Hair often becomes gray or white as pigment production in the hair follicles decreases. Finger- and toenails turn a yellowish color, develop ridges, and become thicker due to calcium deposition. This is especially noticeable in the toenails. Both fingernails and toenails grow more slowly.

Loss of Tissue Elasticity

As mentioned in the explanation of the cross-link theory of aging, tissues throughout the body become less flexible with age. This results in skin wrinkling and many internal changes. For example, increased blood pressure is often a result of loss of elasticity in the walls of the arteries. The entire body tends to lose flexibility, especially if the person has been inactive. Regular exercise helps to counteract this loss.

Cardiovascular Changes

The degree to which our heart and arteries (cardiovascular system) change as we get older depends largely upon how active we have been throughout our lives and what we have eaten. Changes often include decreased cardiac output, which means that less blood is pumped per heartbeat, unchanged or slightly slower resting pulse, slower elevation of pulse with exercise (may cause dizziness or fainting), and slower return to normal once the pulse is elevated. Blood pressure usually increases with age, especially in those who have been less active. *Arteriosclerosis* (hardening of the arteries) and *atherosclerosis* (thickening of the arterial walls), discussed in Chapter 20, are both nearly universal among older people in the United States.

Lung Function

The degree of change in lung function also depends upon how active we have been during our lives, whether or not we have been smokers, and how polluted the air has been where we have lived our lives. These changes are usually not obvious when a person is at rest, but they become evident during exercise or stress.

Our lungs do not shrink in size as we age, but they do become more rigid, perhaps because of cross-linkage. Although total lung capacity remains about the same, less air is moved into and out of the lungs with each breath. The vital capacity, the maximum amount of air that can be moved into and out of the lungs, is reduced.

Metabolic Rate

The rate at which the body uses energy, its metabolic rate, declines slightly with age. At age 80, metabolic rate is about 84 percent of what it was at age 30.[26] This decline is due to a reduction in the total number of body cells and a decline in the activity rate of each cell. The biggest loss of metabolic activity usually comes from loss of muscle tissue due to muscle disuse by inactive people. To prevent weight gain, some adjustments in calorie intake and/or caloric output through activity are necessary.

Hormonal Changes

During aging, the function of most endocrine (hormone-producing) glands usually declines only slightly. Little change is seen in the function of the pituitary gland, thyroid gland, parathyroid glands, and adrenal glands.

Although the ability of the pancreas to produce insulin is usually retained with age, there is a substantial increase in the incidence of diabetes after age 65. (Diabetes is discussed in depth in Chapter 21.) It is thought that this increase in diabetes is caused by a decline in the body cells' sensitivity to insulin, rather than in the pancreas's ability to produce insulin.

Following menopause, a woman's ovaries produce very little estrogen or progesterone. The greatly reduced estrogen level leads to thinner uterine and vaginal tissues, and an increased risk of heart disease and osteoporosis. Postmenopausal hormone replacement therapy has been controversial.[27] While taking hormone supplements following menopause is not entirely risk-free, many researchers and physicians believe that its benefits (reduced risk of heart attack and less-severe osteoporosis) greatly outweigh its risks (slight risk of uterine cancer). Taking a combination of estrogen and progesterone, rather than estrogen alone, reduces the risk of uterine cancer. The decision to take these hormones should be a joint decision between an informed woman and her physician.

Sexual Function

As men age, the testes become smaller in size, and the volume of ejaculate decreases. Ejaculation is less forceful. The penis becomes less hard when erect and the need to ejaculate seems less urgent. The refractory period, during which repeated erection and ejaculation is impossible, lengthens to as long as several days for men in their seventies, especially in men with infrequent sexual activity. Despite all of this, the majority of men remain sexually interested and competent and sex remains an important source of pleasure even at very advanced ages. Men who have always had a high level of sexual activity tend to continue to have higher levels of sexual desire and ability. Although the sperm count is reduced, most men remain fertile throughout their lives.

As women age, their ovaries become smaller, and the lining of the vagina gradually becomes thinner, resulting in decreased vaginal lubrication and less vaginal expansion with stimulation. A 70-year-old woman, however, is just as capable of multiple orgasms as a woman in her twenties. Female fertility ends with menopause.

Although sexual response in both genders slows down with age, most older people who are in good health remain sexually interested and active (see Feature 12.4, p. 388).

Society often stereotypes older people as asexual, but sexual interest and activity remain present in most healthy people until very advanced ages.

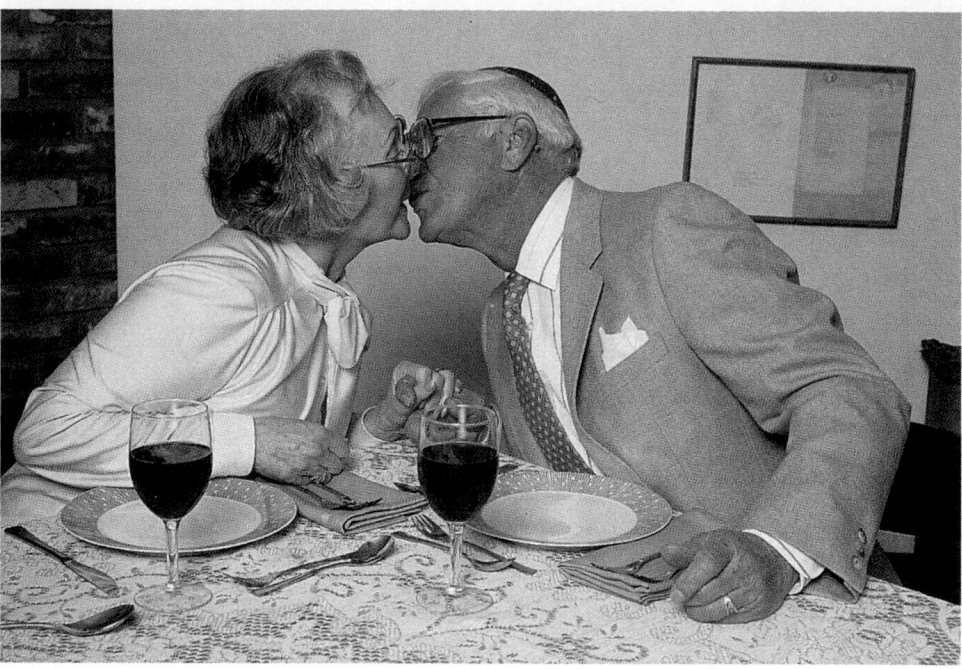

FEATURE 12.4

SEXUALITY AND OLDER PEOPLE

One of society's more damaging stereotypes of older people is that they become asexual. We say "damaging" because at any age a sense of sexual adequacy and attractiveness is an important part of a person's self-concept. We would even go so far as to suggest that one of the main reasons many peo-

ple fear aging is its perceived threat of loss of sexual attractiveness and ability.

How valid is this fear? We apparently have little to worry about:

	Age 50–59	Age 60–69	Age 70 and Older
Percentage of people remaining sexually active[a]			
Women	93	81	65
Men	98	91	79
Percentage of those still sexually active reporting sexual activity at least once a week			
Women	73	63	50
Men	90	73	58
Percentage of those still sexually active reporting a high level of sexual enjoyment			
Women	71	65	61
Men	90	86	75

[a]Includes sex with a partner and masturbation.

Source: Adapted from Brecher, E. *Love, Sex, and Aging.* Boston: Little, Brown, and Consumer Reports Books, 1984.

Unfortunately, our society has not dealt well with the sexuality of its older members. Families and senior-care facilities may ignore or deny the sexual needs of older persons. Soci-

ety needs to change some of its attitudes to recognize that older people also have needs for intimacy, companionship, and sexual fulfillment.

Digestive System

Age has little effect on the actions of the digestive system. Many people's eating habits change little as they grow older. The most frequent change is due to the loss of teeth, usually as a result of neglected oral hygiene and dental care. If dentures do not fit well, or if an older person cannot afford dentures or refuses to wear them, food may be chewed incompletely or some foods may be avoided. The senses of taste and smell decrease, making some foods less attractive. Also, the emotional state affects appetite; loss of a spouse or other loss may lead to loss of appetite and inadequate nutrition.

Many older people complain of constipation. This is usually caused by inadequate dietary fiber intake or exercise, both of which are necessary for proper intestinal mobility.

Sensory Perception

A number of sensory changes can be expected with age. Eyesight declines gradually. As the lens within the eye (Figure 12.3) loses flexibility, it becomes more difficult to focus on close objects, such as printed material. This condition is called **presby-opia** (*pres-bē-ō'pē-a*). Many people between the ages of 40 and 45 begin to need glasses for reading or other close work. The majority of older people need bifocal or trifocal lenses as their ability to focus at different distances is reduced. Bifocal lenses offer one focus for distance and one for close vision, while trifocal lenses add a third focus for intermediate distances. Other changes include reduced night vision, as the pupils become smaller, and reduced peripheral vision.

A **cataract** is clouding or opacity of the lens within the eye. About 90 percent of people over age 70 are said to have some degree of cataract formation, though not always severe enough to affect vision.[28] In many cases vision becomes blurred or dimmed and removal of the lens is recommended. After the lens is removed, vision is restored to almost normal by the use of lens implants, contact lenses, or eyeglasses. One factor in cataract devel-

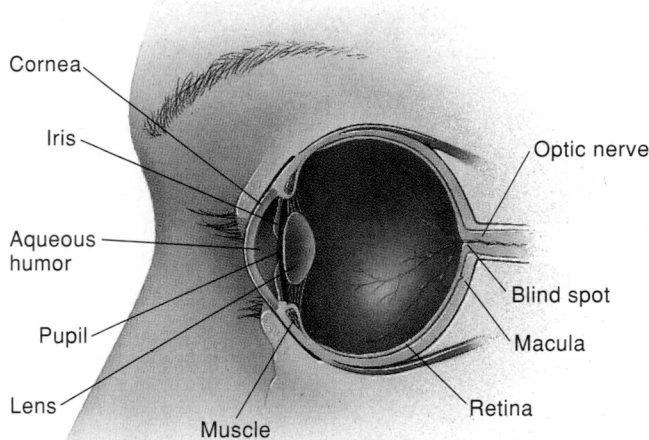

Figure 12.3
Cross-section of a Human Eye

With age, the lens, which enables the eye to adjust for close or distant vision, loses its flexibility and assumes a fixed focus, usually in the distance position. Reading glasses can easily correct this problem. The lens also frequently becomes cloudy with age, a condition called cataract. The retina, the light-sensitive membrane at the rear of the eye, may be damaged by glaucoma, the accumulation of excess pressure of the humors (fluids) within the eye. Finally, the macula, the area of sharpest vision in the retina, is subject to degeneration from disorders of the blood vessels supplying the retina.

opment is ultraviolet radiation in sunlight; wearing sunglasses can help prevent cataract development.

Glaucoma, increased pressure of the fluid within the eye, is the most serious eye disease associated with aging. The elevated pressure can squeeze shut blood vessels that nourish the light-sensitive retina of the eye, causing blindness. Glaucoma is treated by medication or by surgically providing a drainage pathway for the excess fluid within the eye. Everyone over the age of 40 should have periodic tests for glaucoma.

Macular degeneration is characterized by irreversible destructive changes in the **macula,** the area in the center of the eye's retina that functions as the eye's area of most acute or sharp vision. It is where our central vision occurs. Macular degeneration results from various disorders of the blood

---

presbyopia loss of ability to focus on close objects due to loss of elasticity of the lens of the eye.

cataract clouding or opacity of the lens within the eye.

glaucoma increased pressure of the fluid within the eye.

macular degeneration irreversible destructive changes in the macula.

macula the area in the center of the eye's retina that functions as the eye's area of most acute or sharp vision.

vessels supplying the retina, such as hardening of the arteries. It is the leading cause of blindness in people over age 75.

Hearing ability also usually declines with age (**presbycusis,** *pres-bē-ku'sis*), especially with regard to the high-pitched sounds that are essential to understanding speech. The extent of hearing loss depends on a person's history of exposure to loud noise, use of certain antibiotics or other drugs, and genetic factors. If hearing loss is of a type that cannot be corrected by a hearing aid, or if a person refuses to use a hearing aid, effective communication becomes difficult or impossible. The outcome may be considerable social isolation.

The senses of taste, smell, and touch can also suffer some degree of loss of acuity. In some older people the loss is severe and may cause serious problems. For example, a person may fail to eat because nothing tastes good. Or, he or she may fail to remove a hand from a hot stove or may turn a heating pad too high because it doesn't feel as hot as it is; or the person may fail to smell leaking gas or spoiled food.

The effect of aging on pain is unclear. Some research has indicated an increased sensitivity to pain, while other studies have shown a decreased or unchanged sensitivity to pain.[29]

Sleep Changes

Characteristically, older people do not sleep through the night and frequently comment on how poorly they have slept. Less time is spent in deep sleep and they are often awakened by the need to empty their bladder one or more times a night. Though insomnia is a great concern for some older people, it appears that most of them simply need less sleep than when they were younger. Also, some older people take one or more naps during the day, decreasing their need for and ability to sleep at night.

MENTAL CHANGES

Most research indicates that our cultural stereotype of older people exaggerates the mental decline associated with advancing age. The same behavior, such as forgetting something, may be attributed to the age of an older person, but is overlooked or justified in a younger person. This is not true for

those who develop Alzheimer's disease (discussed in Chapter 21 and Feature 12.5). People with Alzheimer's disease lose a great deal of their mental function. The information regarding mental changes that follows refers to that majority of older people who do not develop Alzheimer's disease.

Intellectual Abilities

In the brain, as in all organs, many cells die each day in the normal course of aging. In most parts of the body, however, the dying cells are replaced. This is not true in the brain. As its cells die, the brain may lose as much as 10 percent of its weight by the age of 90.

Fortunately, the brain has a large reserve capacity—it has more neurons than are needed to perform its many functions. Further, as neurons die, other neurons appear to grow new branches and form new connections with other neurons. This may make up for some of the neuron loss.

It is generally accepted that there is some decline in intelligence with aging as a result of the loss of neurons. This loss, however, varies widely among individuals. It appears to be least in those who remain intellectually active as they grow old and greatest in those who allow themselves to "vegetate." It seems as if using your brain helps to maintain its normal functioning. Thus, the key to maintaining keen mental abilities in your old age is to continue making full use of those abilities.

Memory

The suspicion that their memory is not as good as it used to be is a common complaint among older people. Considerable research has been done on memory and aging, though our understanding of the physiology of memory at any age is still quite incomplete. Most research has shown only minimal age-related differences in long-term memory, such as the recall of events from years ago. Substantial age-related differences are seen in the retrieval of new information from the short-term memory.[30] The reasons for this change are not yet known.

Problem-Solving Skills

In general, old and young adults perform differently on experimental problem-solving challenges.[31] Older adults tend to use less-efficient strategies and are less likely to change strategies when they are unsuccessful. There are indications that older peo-

presbycusis impairment of hearing with advancing age.

FEATURE 12.5

ALZHEIMER'S DISEASE

Alzheimer's disease is a degeneration of the brain that usually begins to develop prior to the age of 65. This diseased condition is not considered to be a normal part of the aging process, but its incidence is age-associated. The Alzheimer's Association (800-272-3900) estimates that about 10 percent of the population over the age of 65 is affected, and almost half of those over age 85. These figures are not precise because Alzheimer's is sometimes an uncertain diagnosis. The annual cost of caring for Alzheimer's patients is estimated at $90 billion. There is no known prevention or cure.

Among the earliest symptoms of Alzheimer's disease are impairment of recent memory, disorientation, and a lessening of spontaneous emotional responses. As the disease progresses, the abilities to read, write, and calculate deteriorate. The affected person becomes confused and eventually is unable to recognize his or her spouse or other family members. The affected person may speak constantly, though inappropriately. Ultimately he or she experiences seizures and dies. The span between early symptoms and death may be fairly short or may extend for many years.

The cause of Alzheimer's disease is still unknown, but its symptoms are produced by the death of brain cells that secrete acetylcholine, one of the neurotransmitters described in Chapter 14. In 1993, the FDA (Food and Drug Administration) approved a drug (tacrine hydrochloride, THA) that although it does not cure Alzheimer's disease, does provide some relief of symptoms for some patients. THA works by blocking the function of enzymes that break down acetylcholine, thereby making more of it available to brain cells.

Genes associated with Alzheimer's disease have been found on three different human chromosomes. It also seems very likely that yet-unidentified environmental factors are involved in producing Alzheimer's disease. It is possible that what we now call Alzheimer's disease will in time prove to be several different diseases with different causes.

Having a close relative with Alzheimer's disease can be emotionally, and often financially, very difficult. As the disease advances, the affected person may become totally dependent and his or her care become much like the care of an infant. Though family members may hate the idea of placing the affected person in a nursing home, this is often the best course of action for all concerned. About half of all nursing home residents are there because of Alzheimer's disease.

Sources: Faivelson, S., "Alzheimer's: Making Progress in This Progressive Dementia." *Medical World News*, September 1993, pp. 22–28; Pennisi, E. "A Molecular Whodunit, New Twists in the Alzheimer's Mystery." *Science News*, Vol. 145, 1 January 1994, pp. 8–11; Zittell, N. "Alzheimer's and Aging." *Medical World News*, September 1993, p. 2.

---

ple still possess the competence to solve experimental problems, but often fail to use their problem-solving skills. The reasons for this are unclear.

Self-Concept

How do older people view themselves? Most research suggests that older people are just as satisfied or dissatisfied with their bodies and body image as are younger people. Actually, many people in all age groups are dissatisfied with their body image because of the emphasis in our society, and especially the media, on physical perfection. Older people, however, do not consider themselves to be any less attractive than do younger people.[32]

Older people's gender-role self-concepts tend to shift away from the stereotypical gender roles of their youth—dominant, independent, assertive, and ambitious males and passive, dependent, nurturing, sensitive females—toward more **androgynous** (*an-droj'i-nus;* combining male and female

traits) concepts. Older women often view themselves as more independent, assertive, and dominant than they were in their youth, while older men view themselves as having become more nurturing, tender, and dependent.[33]

SOCIAL CHANGES

Aging changes social status in many ways. It affects position in the family as well as employment status, economic position, and social interactions.

Family Life

It is predicted that the family will become increasingly important to the older person as an emotional and economic support system during the remainder of this century.[34] This prediction is based on the fact that there will be an increased percentage of older people in the population and the likelihood that per capita government expenditures for programs for older people will be stagnant or reduced if current trends continue.

Alternatives to government-supported human services for older people lead directly to the fami-

androgynous combining male and female traits.

Unused mental skills decline, while frequently used skills are maintained. The key to mental sharpness in one's old age is to continue full use of one's mental abilities.

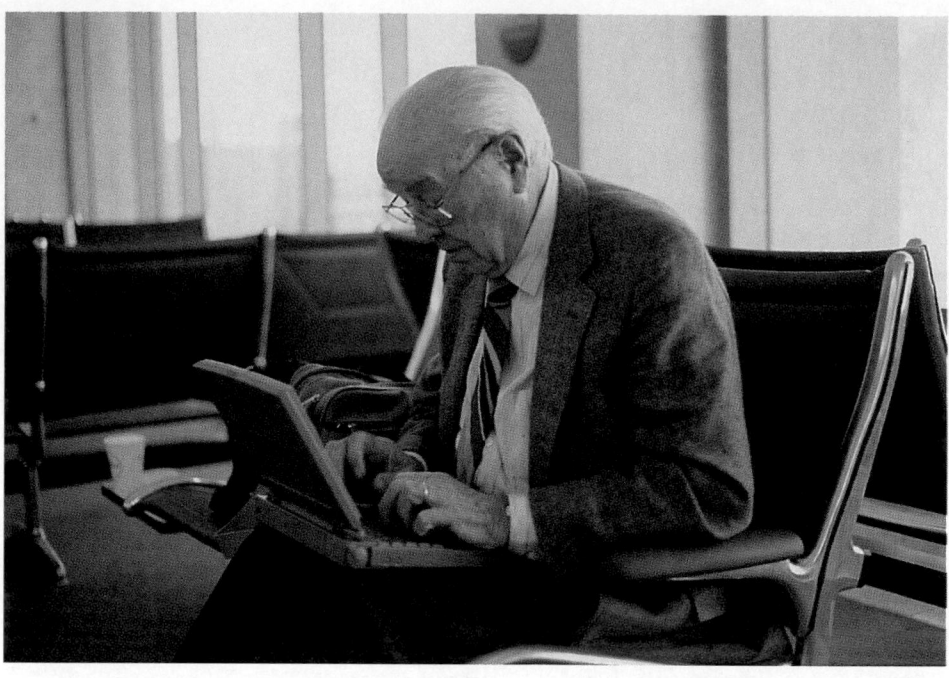

ly. There is nothing new about family responsibility for the care of older people—that is where the responsibility has lain throughout most of history—but it does represent a change from the philosophy of greater government involvement that prevailed during the 1960s and 1970s. Also, family care for older people has been complicated by our highly mobile society in which family members are often geographically separated.

And what about an older person who has never married or is widowed or divorced and who has no children or other family members to rely upon? Such people, and there are many of them, need to make special provisions for their advanced years. In addition to developing a strong social network, they will want to carefully consider how their financial needs will be met.

As long as an older person can meet his or her own needs for housekeeping, transportation, social interaction, grocery shopping and food preparation, and can perform unaided the activities of daily living such as walking, dressing, eating, bathing and grooming, the dependency on others is minimal. And we want to emphasize that more than 90 percent of all older people, excluding those with Alzheimer's disease, are able to live independently.

But when routine activities become difficult, family members are usually called on for help. This may create a crisis for both the older person and

his or her family members. Neither may be prepared for the increased degree of dependency. The older person may be distraught over loss of autonomy while family members, usually adult daughters and daughters-in-law, may suffer loss of freedom, privacy, free time, and, in some cases, money. Any smoldering long-term conflicts between family members may be brought to a head at this time. Outside help, such as a family counselor or social worker, is often necessary to enable the family to adjust to the new situation.

Retirement

For many people, retirement requires social, economic, and emotional adjustments. Some people respond well to these adjustments; others have a tougher time. Many social issues revolve around retirement. The age at which a person retires is an important concern. Many people hope to retire relatively young; but the younger a person retires, the longer he or she will draw retirement benefits, and the shorter he or she will have worked to earn those benefits. Thus, the smaller the pension check. Conversely, many people hope to continue working as long as their health allows. For those who are forced to retire while they would prefer to continue working, this change affects their income, health, and well-being. This will probably be affecting fewer people, as the government appears likely to increase the age at which people qualify for Social Security and other retirement benefits.

In a nation that defines individuals largely in terms of their occupation, retirement automatically places the retiree in a new social role. If the retiree has not developed any interests outside of his or her career, there may be little sense of identity or social role after retirement.

In planning for retirement, it is important to think not only in terms of what you are retiring *from*, but also in terms of what you are retiring *to*. For some people, it may be a mistake to retire to nothing. While the idea of having plenty of free time with no demands may initially seem appealing, some retirees who don't replace their career with other activites tend to deteriorate rapidly, both physically and mentally. A phased or gradual retirement, whereby a person works progressively fewer and fewer hours or days per week over a period of years, can ease the transition from career to retirement, as well as help with the financial aspects of retirement. Part-time work also helps maintain a social support system outside of the immediate family.

Many retirees become involved in volunteer work, which can provide activity, mental stimulation, social contact, and continued social usefulness. Others turn hobbies into businesses, which provides income as well as the other benefits mentioned previously. Many opportunities exist for part-time work, such as teaching, writing, consulting, store clerking, and so on. Money is only one reward. Part-time work may also provide an opportunity to continue in a related field or to fulfill a lifelong dream.

Housing

Where people live can have a great influence on the quality of their lives. People's housing needs often change considerably as they grow older. Almost every person or couple reaches a point in life when a decision must be made whether to remain in the same home or to relocate. Some of the options are:

- moving to a nearby retirement community
- moving away—to the sunbelt, to the city, to the country, or to be near children
- living with an adult child
- sharing housing with other older people
- remaining where you have been living

In general, older people usually decide to remain in place. Interviews have identified many reasons for remaining in place, including satisfaction with the place of residence, economic reasons, and, most of all, emotional attachment to a long-time home as a symbol of and a connection to past events and relationships.[35]

In addition to economics, a key factor that helps to determine whether to move or stay is the social support system. If the present living arrangement provides plenty of social opportunities, this may encourage a person to stay. If there is inadequate social interaction, an opportunity to find new companions may be a strong impetus to relocate.

CHECKPOINT

1. What effect does aging have on: height, fat deposits, sweating, tissue elasticity, metabolic rate, vision, and hearing?

2. How can a person increase the likelihood of a successful retirement?

RELATING TO OLDER PEOPLE

Most of us have older family members, friends, neighbors, and co-workers. Though we may care deeply for them, we may not always know how to talk to them because we believe we don't have a lot in common with them. How can we bridge this gap between generations?

SPENDING TIME WITH OLDER PEOPLE

One way to become more comfortable with aging is to spend time with older friends and relatives (see "Communication for Wellness: An Interview with a Parent or Grandparent," on p. 394). The benefits are mutual. As we come to terms with aging and share in the wisdom of age, we provide our older people with much wanted companionship, support, and contact with younger people.

Devoting our time may require making sacrifices, because each of us has our own busy life, with numerous conflicting demands on our time. Further, we may find that being with older people makes us uncomfortable. If this is the case, it may mean that we have not yet come to terms with our own aging. Being with an older person may thus create discomfort by reminding us of what our own future holds in store.

CARE-GIVING

"How is it that one parent can take care of ten children, but ten children cannot take care of one parent?" This question arises because there are many guidelines for parents as they raise children, but, in the United States, there are few guidelines for children who are taking care of their parents.

Almost everyone reaches a point in life when he or she needs help with some of the tasks of daily living. Family members are very likely to become involved in this process. At first, any family members who live nearby visit periodically to help their older relatives. Assistance commonly given includes:[36]

• providing transportation
• helping with personal finances
• doing household chores

When younger people spend time with older family members, both generations benefit. The older people enjoy the company of the young; the young gain in wisdom and improved attitudes toward aging.

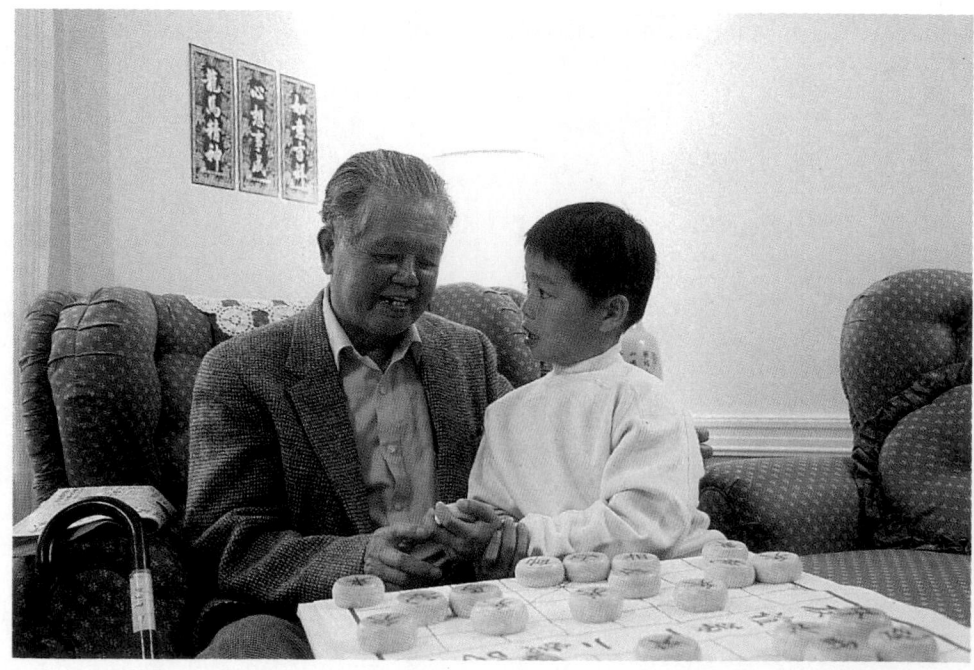

- running errands
- providing emotional support and
- including older relatives in family rituals such as birthdays and holidays

Eventually, some people reach a point where they can no longer live independently and other living arrangements must be made (see Feature 12.6). Sometimes, a live-in care-giver can be hired, though this is costly and a qualified person may be difficult to find. More often, however, the choice is either living with family members or entering a special care facility. When feasible, most older people who cannot live alone choose to live with family members. Only about 4–6 percent of people over age 65 live in nursing homes or similar facilities. Families, however, need to discuss some of the following questions before taking on the responsibility of caring for an older relative:[37]

- What are the needs of that person and of the family?
- Where will the new member sleep?
- How will the new member be included in family functions?
- How will care-giving responsibilities be shared?

- What community resources are available to assist everyone with the adjustment period?
- Is the home environment safe for the new member?
- Will use of adult day care be necessary? If so, is such care available in the community?
- How does the family feel about including the new member?

If all of these questions cannot be satisfactorily answered, other alternatives must be considered, such as a retirement home, nursing home, or similar institution. These facilities are also advisable for people who need round-the-clock health care. One million four hundred thousand Americans now inhabit these facilities and this number is likely to increase dramatically in the years ahead.

The quality of nursing home care ranges from excellent to very poor. To find one of the better nursing homes, the following points should be considered:

1. *Is 24-hour nursing care provided?* Approximately 28 percent of nursing homes, called intermediate-care facilities, do not offer this service. In most instances, it is better to choose a facility that

---

FEATURE 12.6

CARE-GIVER NEEDS HELP!

Most of us will find ourselves, at some time in our lives, deeply involved in caring for an older relative—often a parent or a parent of our spouse. As the health of the person deteriorates, we may reach a point where our own well-being begins to suffer and our own health is threatened. In these situations, many care-givers, possibly out of love, fear of admitting "failure," or a sense of guilt, continue trying to care for a relative until they, too, require care. Following are some signs indicating that other arrangements must be made:

- No matter what you do, it isn't enough.
- You no longer have any time or space to be alone.
- Family relationships are breaking down because of your obligation to your older relative.
- Your care-giving is interfering with your work and/or social life to an unacceptable degree.
- You have started overeating, undereating, abusing drugs or alcohol, or taking out your frustrations on your older relative.

- There are no more happy times. Loving and caring have given way to exhaustion and resentment and you no longer feel good about yourself or what you are doing.
- You would like to quit, but don't want to admit failure.

Some possible ways to reduce the stress include:

- Ask your doctor, health department, or local service agency about available health care and transportation services in your community.
- Ask other family members to help you in the care-giving process.
- Build a support system of friends or home care professionals you can call to help you when the need arises.
- Consider a nursing home or long-term-care facility instead of home care.

Source: Adapted from Wood, J., "Labors of Love." *Modern Maturity,* August–September 1987, pp. 28–91, and other sources.

does offer 24-hour nursing care, even though the cost is higher.

2. *Does the home participate in both Medicare and Medicaid?* Will the home allow residents to remain if they exhaust all of their funds and need to apply for Medicaid?

3. *How is the living environment?* Look for well-lit (older people need brighter lighting), cheerful, clean surroundings with sufficient privacy for residents. Some promising signs are a friendly, respectful staff and clean, active residents. Try to visit during a mealtime. Is the food attractive? Are there special diets for those who need them? Is help with eating available for those who need it?

4. *Are there recreational facilities and planned activities for those who are able to participate?* If the only recreation available is sitting in front of a television set, the lack of physical activity and mental challenge hastens the physical and mental decline of the residents.

5. *How are family inquiries met?* Hostile, sarcastic, or rude responses reveal an attitude that is certain to extend to the treatment of residents.

6. *Is there a council of family members of residents who meet on a monthly basis to express concerns and plan social programs with the help of the staff social worker?*

7. *How is the medical care and staff?* Does a physician visit regularly? Is at least one registered nurse (RN) on duty at all times? Is there at least one nurses' aide for every ten residents?

8. *Do the residents seem reasonably alert or do they seem to be highly sedated?* Some homes tend to keep their clients sedated to minimize the amount of attention they demand.

9. *Does the staff appear to be happy?* The happiness of the staff members reflects how they are treated by the management and predicts how they are likely to treat the residents.

10. *Is the location convenient for family members?* Regular visits from family and friends are important to residents and encourage quality care from the staff. A remotely located facility, no matter how good, is usually a poor choice.

Good nursing-home care is expensive. Though costs vary from area to area, a typical cost is about $2500–$3000 per month, plus medical expenses. Savings can be quickly exhausted. Medicaid will assume the cost of nursing-home care only after all of a person's resources are exhausted, and not before. If one spouse remains in good health while the other requires nursing-home care, an attorney can arrange to split their resources so that only half of the couple's assets must be exhausted before Medicaid begins to pay.

CHECKPOINT

1. What forms of assistance do family members often provide to older relatives?

2. What questions need to be addressed before an older person comes to live with family members?

3. What are some desirable characteristics of a nursing home?

AGING AS A POSITIVE EXPERIENCE

For those who have come to terms with aging, old age can be one of life's most rewarding experiences, one that can promote maximum self-actualization and provide a powerful sense of personal authenticity. **Self-transcendence** (the ability to rise above your own self, to extend your concern and efforts beyond the fulfillment of your own selfish needs), creativity, productive use of leisure time, courage, altruism, and humor can all help make aging a positive experience.

SELF-TRANSCENDENCE IN OLDER PEOPLE

The ability to rise above mundane self-concerns is helpful at any age. Many older people become actively involved in the important issues of society for the first time in their lives. Their activism provides the physical, mental, and social activity so essential to their well-being. With the primary focus off themselves, older people may find their aches and pains disappearing and their own problems less consuming. There are many issues to become involved in: education, consumer rights, politics, housing, crime, health care, transportation, environmental quality, economic development, handicapped access, and product safety, to name a few.

self-transcendence the ability to rise above your own self.

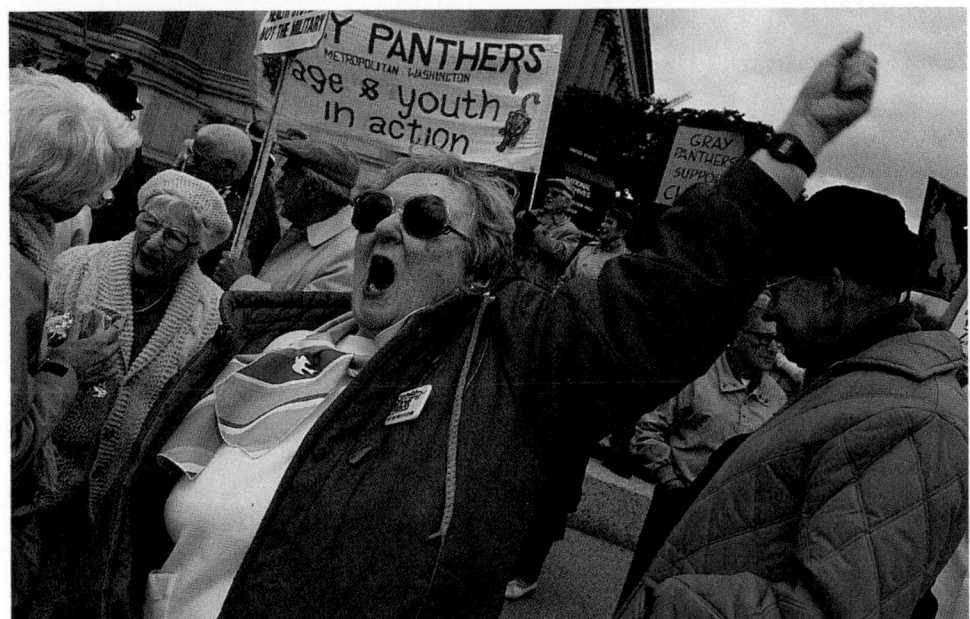

Social involvement helps one rise above the mundane concerns of one's self. It can provide older people with important physical, mental, and social activity and can add meaning and fulfillment to one's life.

CREATIVE SELF-ACTUALIZATION

Most older people have latent talents and interests that they have never had a chance to express. Perhaps they were too busy earlier in their lives or simply were not aware of their talents. We often don't know our ability to paint, write, or make music until we try. In light of the outstanding works of so many older painters, writers, and musicians, some authorities believe that human creativity reaches its peak late in life (see Feature 12.7, p. 398).

Consider some of the many ways that the needs of older people (and all of us) can be met through creative expression:

- clarification of thoughts and feelings
- communication of a message to others
- creation of a sense of balance and inner order
- a sense of being in control of the external world
- creation of something positive from defeating experiences
- enhancement of self-esteem
- contribution to self-actualization
- the pure joy of creative expression

PRODUCTIVE USE OF LEISURE TIME

Older people often have an increased amount of discretionary time—time to be spent in any way they wish. Those who use this time in stimulating, challenging, and rewarding ways almost certainly

view this phase of their lives as a positive experience. In addition to the self-transcendent and creative activities mentioned in the previous paragraphs, some rewarding activities include:

- volunteering
- spending time with grandchildren
- taking courses
- traveling
- walking
- taking retreats into wilderness areas
- reading
- bird watching
- fishing
- socializing

COURAGE, ALTRUISM, AND HUMOR

Courage is the quality of mind or spirit that enables a person to face difficulty, danger, pain, or the unknown with firmness and without fear. Growing old requires courage. Those who face old age courageously are able to make the most of each day. They view life as an adventure, and old age as simply a step along the way.

....

courage the quality of mind or spirit that enables a person to face difficulty, danger, pain, or the unknown with firmness and without fear.

FEATURE 12.7

ACHIEVEMENTS AT ADVANCED AGES

If you think older people aren't competent, think again. Consider these achievements:

- At 81, Benjamin Franklin organized the compromise that led to the adoption of the U.S. Constitution.
- At 82, Leo Tolstoy wrote *I Cannot be Silent*.
- At 82, Winston Churchill wrote *A History of English-Speaking Peoples*.
- At 84, W. Somerset Maugham wrote *Points of View*.
- At 85, Coco Chanel was the head of a fashion design firm.
- At 88, Michelangelo developed architectural plans for the Church of Santa Maria degli Angeli.
- At 89, Arthur Rubenstein gave one of his greatest recitals in Carnegie Hall.
- At 90, Pablo Picasso was actively producing drawings and engravings.

- At 91, Armand Hammer still actively headed Occidental Petroleum.
- At 93, George Bernard Shaw wrote the play, *Far-fetched Fables*.
- George Burns and Bob Hope are both still going strong into their 90s.
- Georgia O'Keeffe switched from painting to sculpting in her 90s.
- At 100, Grandma Moses was still painting.
- And also at 100, S. L. Potter, of Alpine, California, over the objections of his 68- to 74-year-old children, successfully executed a 210 foot bungee jump.

Add to this list some examples from your own family and community. Do we really need to fear aging?

Altruism is unselfish regard for the welfare of others. Altruism and rewarding old age go hand in hand. Those who care only for themselves wallow in self-pity at their loss of youth. Those who are helping others are happy that they can still help. They feel greater self-esteem and independence and find their lives meaningful.

Humor is the ability to laugh at ludicrous or ridiculous situations, sometimes even at our own expense. Older people, especially those who transcend themselves, frequently laugh at themselves. Perhaps having the perspective of a lifetime allows them to see more clearly the humor in human predicaments.

CHECKPOINT

1. What is self-transcendence and how does it relate to successful aging?

2. What is the significance of courage, altruism, and humor in aging?

altruism unselfish regard for the welfare of others.

humor the ability to laugh at ludicrous or ridiculous situations.

SUMMARY

Aging is the process of growing older. Aging is also defined as those series of cumulative, universal, progressive, intrinsic, and deleterious functional and structural changes that usually begin to manifest themselves at reproductive maturity and eventually culminate in death. Aging is an ongoing, life-long process. Types of aging include chronological aging, biological aging, cosmetic aging, social aging, psychological aging, and economic aging, all of which interact with each other.

Your attitude regarding aging influences how you live your entire life. Your health habits influence the rate at which you age. Biological age, the condition of your body, is usually more important than chronological age, how long you have lived.

An increasing percentage of the U.S. population is comprised of people over age 65. Ageism is stereotyping of and discrimination against people simply because they are old. In a youth-worshiping culture, ageism affects everyone; even young people worry about growing older.

People of different cultures experience aging and old age in different ways. Ethnic differences exist in the status of older people, their income levels, health problems, health care received, life expectancies, and housing arrangements.

The wellness life-style can slow the physical effects of aging. Stress management; proper diet; avoiding harmful substances; maintaining physical, mental, and social activity; and shielding the skin from ultraviolet all retard biological aging.

Middle age is best defined as a state of mind that accompanies the assumption of full adult responsibilities and the awareness of aging. Midlife researchers now doubt that "midlife crisis" is a universal event. People with adequate self-esteem usually move through middle age more easily than those who doubt their self-worth.

Although average life expectancies have increased considerably, the maximum human life span potential has changed little, suggesting built-in limitations. Biological theories on aging include programmed aging theories, which attribute aging to built-in mechanisms acting to ensure the finite lives of organisms. Various genetic and immunological theories are included here. Stochastic (error) aging theories relate aging to environmental forces that damage cells. Here is where the effects of diet and other environmental influences fit in. None of these theories are mutually exclusive; each probably contributes to the physical effects of aging.

Normal aging includes gradual changes in almost every body system, but older people usually are much more physically and mentally capable than many younger people presume. Important social changes with aging include family life, employment status, economic position, and social interactions.

Aging can and should be a positive experience in your life. It usually is such an experience for people who practice self-transcendence and creative self-actualization, make productive use of their leisure time, and who possess courage, altruism, and humor.

REFERENCES

1. Arking, Robert. *Biology of Aging.* Englewood Cliffs, NJ: Prentice Hall, 1991.
2. DiGiovanna, Augustine. *Human Aging: Biological Perspectives.* New York: McGraw-Hill, 1994.
3. Ibid.
4. National Center for Health Statistics. "Advance Report of Final Mortality Statistics." *Monthly Vital Statistics Report* Vol. 42, No. 2 (31 August 1993).
5. Ibid.
6. Butler, R. *Why Survive?: Being Old in America.* New York: Harper & Row, 1975.
7. Ebersole, P., and Hess, P. *Toward Healthy Aging,* 3rd ed. St. Louis: Mosby, 1990.
8. American Association of Retired Persons. *Empowerment of Minority Elderly.* Lakewood, CA: American Association of Retired Persons, 1990.
9. American Association of Retired Persons. *Aging and Old Age in Diverse Populations.* Lakewood, CA: American Association of Retired Persons, 1990.
10. DiGiovanni, op. cit.
11. Evans, W., and Rosenberg, I. *Biomarkers: The 10 Keys to Prolonging Vitality.* New York: Simon and Schuster, 1991.
12. Ibid.
13. Hafen, B., Frandsen, K., Karren, J., and Hooker, K. *The Health Effects of Attitudes, Emotions, Relationships.* Provo, UT: EMS Associates, 1992.
14. Kligman, A. Quoted in Smith, E. "Aging, Can It Be Slowed?" *Business Week* (8 February 1988), 58–64.
15. Ebersole and Hess, op. cit.
16. DiGiovanni, op. cit.
17. Hayflick, L. "The Limited *In Vitro* Lifetime of Human Diploid Cell Strains." *Experimental Cell Research,* Vol. 37 (1965) 614–636.
18. Hayflick, L. "Theories of Biological Aging." *Experimental Gerontology* Vol. 20 (1985), 145–159.
19. Hayflick, L. "Origins of Longevity." In H. Warner et al. (eds.). *Modern Biological Theories of Aging.* New York: Raven Press, 1987.
20. Spence, A. *Biology of Human Aging.* Englewood Cliffs, NJ: Prentice Hall, 1989.
21. Harley, C. "Loss of Telomeric DNA as a Marker and Possible Cause of Cellular Replicative Senescence." Presented at the Symposium on Cellular and Molecular Aspects of Aging, Beckman Research Institute, City of Hope, Duarte, California, 22 October 1993.
22. Arking, op. cit.
23. Ibid.
24. DiGiovanni, op cit.
25. Arking, op. cit.
26. Spence, op. cit.
27. Fackelmann, K. "Heart Findings Support Hormonal Therapy." *Science News* (17 April 1993), 246.
28. Spence, op. cit.
29. Ibid.
30. Poon, L. "Differences in Human Memory with Aging." In Birren, J., and Schaie, K. (eds.) *The Psychology of Aging,* 3rd ed. Plympton, MA: Academy, 1991.
31. Reese, H., and Rodeheaver, D. "Problem Solving and Complex Decision Making." In Birren, J., and

Schaie, K. (eds.) *The Psychology of Aging,* 3rd ed. Plympton, MA: Academy, 1991.

32. Bengston, V., Reedy, M., and Gordon, C. "Aging and Self-conception." In Birren, J., and Schaie, K. (eds.). *The Psychology of Aging,* 3rd ed. Plympton, MA: Academy, 1991.

33. Ibid.

34. Sussman, M. "The Family Life of Old People." In Binstock, R., and Shanas, E. (eds.). *Aging and the Social Sciences,* 3rd ed. New York: Van Nostrand Reinhold, 1990.

35. Lawton, M. "Housing and Living Environments of Older People." In Binstock, R., and Shanas, E. (eds.). *Aging and the Social Sciences,* 3rd ed. New York: Van Nostrand Reinhold, 1990.

36. Ibid.

37. Ibid.

SUGGESTED READINGS

Bass, S. *Achieving a Productive Aging Society.* Westport, CT: Greenwood, 1993.

DiGiovanna, A. *Human Aging: Biological Perspectives.* New York: McGraw-Hill, 1994.

Doress, P., and Siegal, D. *Ourselves, Growing Older: Women Aging with Knowledge and Power.* New York: Simon and Schuster, 1987.

Ebersole, P., and Hess, P. *Toward Healthy Aging,* 3rd ed. St. Louis: Mosby, 1990.

Evans, W., and Rosenberg, I. *Biomarkers: The 10 Keys to Prolonging Vitality.* New York: Simon and Schuster, 1991.

Friedan, B. *The Fountain of Age.* New York: Simon and Schuster, 1993.

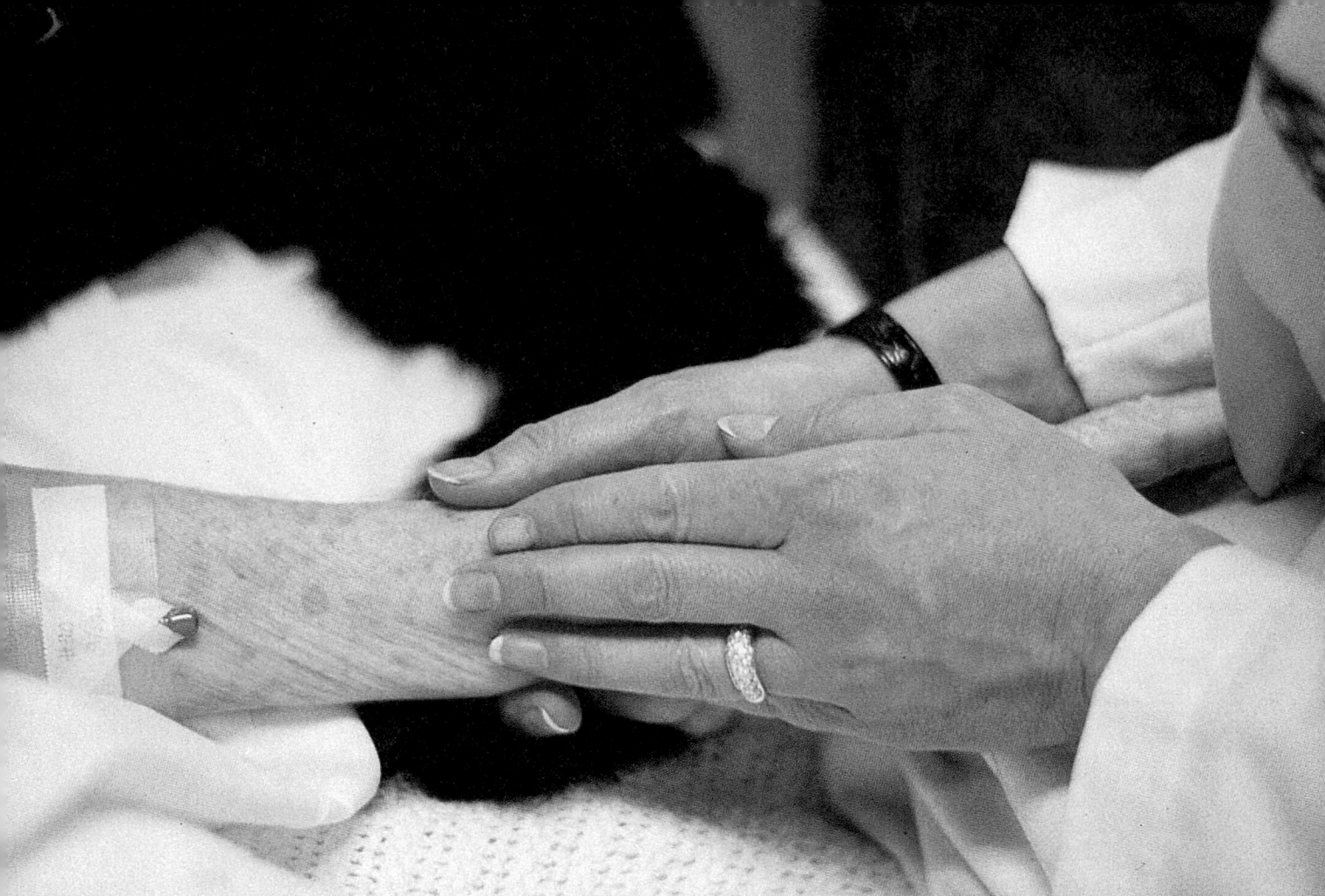

13
DYING AND DEATH

Upon completing this chapter, you will be able to:

KNOWLEDGE

- Explain why the study of death is important.
- Explain how the definition of death has evolved over the years.
- Explain the phrase "death as an organizer of time."
- Explain how a person's religious beliefs or nonreligious beliefs influence feelings about death.
- List the occurrences that are common in the near-death experience.
- List the emotions commonly experienced by people who know that they are dying.
- Explain hospice care.
- Describe the ten common emotional phases in grief.
- Contrast living wills and durable powers of attorney for health care.
- Explain the principles of organ donation and the need for donor organs.

INSIGHT

- Explain your own views of death and how they influence your daily life.
- Explain the mourning customs of your own ethnic group.
- Describe how you would give support to a grieving friend.

DECISION MAKING

- Make a commitment to view death as a part of life to be delayed as long as possible, but not feared.
- Make a commitment not to avoid interaction with dying people.
- Make a commitment to formalize your feelings about the kinds of health care you would want to receive by completing a living will and a durable power of attorney for health care.
- Make a decision about organ donation and make your wishes known to your health care provider.

Much controversy has surrounded the work of Dr. Jack Kevorkian, a physician who openly supports and actively engages in "assisted suicide." Dr. Kevorkian has helped cause the death of a number of patients who were, according to him, mentally competent to make the decision to die. In most cases, he has used a carbon-monoxide mask, allowing the patients to experience painless, quick deaths. Most of his patients were suffering from some painful, incurable disease or condition. However, he believes that the patient need not be suffering from a life-threatening illness to be a candidate for his help, nor does the person have to be in great pain. He believes that when the patient's quality of life is nil, then that person should have access to help in dying from a qualified physician. Dr. Kevorkian calls a physician who specializes in death an obitiatrist.

There are many opponents to Dr. Kevorkian's actions, including the courts—he has spent time in jail resulting from allegations that he broke the law by conducting assisted suicides. Some medical experts say that patients in this condition are not competent to make the decision to die because they are suffering from depression. These patients may be seeking suicide out of despair, not because of their disease. Others support the American Medical Association's philosophy that medicine is a profession dedicated to healing and its tools should not be used to kill people. Some believe that assisted suicide could become a tool to meet economic goals, given the tremendous pressure to reduce health care costs. Since people over 65 spend almost four times as much on health care as young people, a great burden could be placed on old, sick, and weak people who would be constantly asking themselves, "Is now the right time?"

Dr. Kevorkian has helped to stimulate discussion about this critically important issue. As medical technology advances in the area of life support for terminally ill patients, lawmakers and policymakers must make some very tough decisions about how to proceed. In the meantime, Dr. Kevorkian maintains that assisted suicide will ultimately become an accepted medical practice.

■ ■ ■

The study of death is called **thanatology** (*than-a-tol'ō-jē*). For the past several decades, death has been studied intensively by thanatologists, giving us valuable insights into this phase of life. This does not mean that all of us have come to terms with our own mortality—many people still feel quite uncomfortable with the topic of death. This chapter will examine death as it affects the dying person and loved ones. We will also take a broader look at how death is handled within various cultures.

WHY STUDY DEATH?

Don't think that you are all alone if this is the one chapter in this whole book that you least want to read. If that is the case, you probably share some attitudes and feelings about death with the majority of people in our society. It is one topic that many of us don't want to read about, to talk about, and, most of all, to think about.

Why don't we want to think about death? Mainly because focusing on death reminds us of our own personal vulnerability and mortality or reminds us of the loss of a loved one. For the many of us who have not yet come to terms with death, encountering it in any real way causes an uncomfortable degree of anxiety.

Only when we come to terms with the finite nature of our lives can we begin to live them fully.

Accepting the finite nature of life enables us to define clearly what we want to experience and accomplish before our death. When we see death as a possibility at any time, and an eventual certainty, we may begin to live our lives more fully, rather than just passing through them. We appreciate each day we have and do our best to make it a rewarding one.[1]

We live in less fear of death once we have come to terms with it. We take reasonable precautions to avoid a premature death, but we don't let the fear of dying take away the pleasure from those precious days that we do have to live.[2]

MEANINGS OF DEATH

What is death? The meanings of death are numerous and vary according to your culture, religion, age, health, mental capacities, and general life situation. Death can be viewed as a biological event, a transition, a rite of passage, an inevitability, a natural occurrence, a punishment, an escape (see discussion of suicide in Chapter 4), an extinction, God's will, a separation, a reunion, an outrage, or a time for judgment. Death can be a cause for anger, depression, denial, repression, guilt, frustration, relief, religious awakenings, or rejection of religion.

Death means one thing to a dying person and another to those who love that individual. For those who provide health care, conduct funerals, underwrite insurance, and administer estates, death has many other meanings.

One thing clear to all of us is that death is important. And so is the process of dying. Dying and death have an immense impact on every one of us, affecting all aspects of our lives, including our feelings, family relationships, social relationships, and spiritual well-being.

MEDICAL DEFINITIONS OF DEATH

A general definition of **death** is the cessation of life. The development of modern medical technol-

---

thanatology the study of death.

death the cessation of life.

ogy, though, has necessitated some refinement of this general definition. While, in the past, we thought of a person as being either alive or dead, this simple dichotomy is not always valid today. Thanatologists understand that there is no such thing as "the moment of death." In reality, the human body dies cell by cell. Dying is a process that occurs over a period of time, rather than at any one instant. Medical technology now makes it possible for many body systems to continue to live and function even after all brain activity has irreversibly ceased. The precise moment of death, once easily defined as the moment when breathing and heartbeat ceased, no longer applies, and has given way to a gradual and subtle ebbing of life processes.

The question of when death occurs has important psychological and economic implications for the friends and family of a dying person. It is emotionally difficult for a family when a member is "in limbo" for an extended period, perhaps in a coma and on life-support equipment, neither clearly alive nor clearly dead. Also, maintaining a person in this state can be very expensive and can quickly wipe out all of a family's financial resources.

There are also legal and ethical considerations about when death occurs. A physician could be accused of abandoning a patient by discontinuing treatment prematurely or criticized for persisting with treatment for too long.

Advances in medical technology have created an ever-increasing demand for lifesaving donor organs. Organs from one deceased person could possibly extend the lives of several recipients. Many people hope that when they die, their organs will help save the lives of others. For the organs to be of any value for transplant, however, they must be removed from a very recently deceased person while the organs are still alive and healthy. To accomplish this requires a clear definition of death.

Given the cell-by-cell manner in which death occurs, we can view death as a matter of degrees:

- *Cell death.* **Cell death** is the death of individual body cells. In most parts of our bodies, cells are constantly dying and being replaced. In unusual circumstances, such as ingestion or inhalation of a toxic chemical

or interruption of oxygen supply, cells may die rapidly and in large numbers.

- *Local death.* **Local death** is the death of a part of the body. For example, in some people with diabetes the circulation of blood into a foot becomes so impaired that the tissue may die. The death of such areas of tissue is called **necrosis** or **gangrene.** Toxin-forming bacteria often become established in such areas, causing further death of tissue. Sometimes only amputation of the affected body part will stop this infection from spreading.

- *Death of individual brain cells.* Of all of our cells, brain cells are the most sensitive to lack of oxygen and to many drugs and other toxic chemicals. Further, brain cells that die are never replaced. When a person's oxygen supply is interrupted, as in electric shock, drowning, strangulation, or a heart attack, cells of the higher, conscious part of the brain, the cerebrum, begin to die within just a few minutes. In a few more minutes, cells in the reflex centers of the brain start to die. Muscle cells, in contrast, survive for several hours without oxygen. Kidney cells survive for about seven hours, making the kidney ideal for transplantation.

Death of brain cells tends to progress from the "higher," conscious areas of the brain to "lower" parts of the brain that control basic body functions. Thus a person might lose all potential for regaining consciousness while retaining the ability to physically survive for a long time if nourishment is provided, even without life support equipment.

- *Brain death.* **Brain death** is the cessation of all brain function. It produces a deep coma, with total unresponsiveness to painful stimuli and the absence of reflexes. The **electroencephalogram (EEG)** (*e-lek-trō-en-sef´-a-lō-gram*), a diagnostic test that records the

---

cell death death of individual body cells.

local death death of a part of the body.

necrosis or **gangrene** death of an area of tissue surrounded by healthy tissue.

brain death cessation of all brain function.

electroencephalogram (EEG) a test that records the electrical activity of the brain.

brain's electrical activity, becomes "flat," meaning that no electrical activity can be detected (see Figure 13.1). Today, the death of a person being maintained on life-support equipment is usually defined in terms of flat electroencephalograms, lack of reflexes, and lack of response to painful stimuli over a 24-hour period. If the life-support equipment being used to maintain heartbeat and breathing of such a patient were turned off and he or she did not continue to breathe or maintain a heartbeat spontaneously, he or she would be considered dead.

In cases where brain activity has been suppressed by a drug overdose or hypothermia (very low body temperature), a longer period may pass before death is declared. Further, a child under six months of age may have a flat EEG for an extended period and not be brain dead.[3]

To resolve the question of when death occurs, the President's Commission for the Study of Ethical Problems in Medicine and Biomedical and Behavioral Research developed the Uniform Determination of Death Act in 1981. This act states that "An

Figure 13.1

Electroencephalogram

(a) Recording the electrical activity of the brain is called electroencephalography. (b) The tracing of brain waves produced through electroencephalography is called an electroencephalogram (EEG). (c) Part of the definition of death includes the absence of brain activity (a flat EEG such as this) for 24 hours.

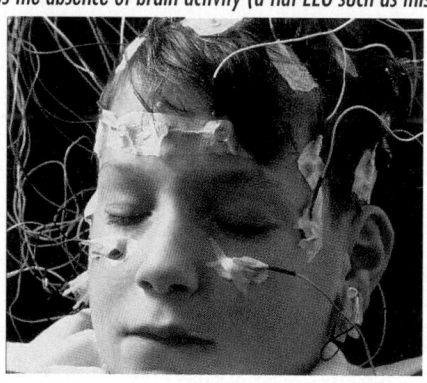

(a)

(b)	(c)
LF-P	LF-P
RF-P	RF-P
LP-O	LP-O
RP-O	RP-O
LF-T	LF-T
RF-T	RF-T
LT-O	LT-O
RT-O	RT-O

individual who has sustained either (1) irreversible cessation of circulatory and respiratory functions, or (2) irreversible cessation of all functions of the entire brain, including the brainstem, is dead. A determination of death must be made in accordance with accepted medical standards."

CHECKPOINT

1. What is the study of death called?

2. What are some reasons why a precise definition of death is needed?

3. How is death now defined?

VIEWS OF DEATH

Humans are probably the only living organisms that can anticipate and plan for their own death. Our awareness is based, either directly or indirectly, on our experiences with the deaths of others. It is through these experiences that we each develop our own views of death. Television is a powerful vehicle by which people vicariously experience death. Children who watch television witness hundreds or thousands of deaths, mostly by violence. Psychologists point out that this lowers a child's sensitivity to death, making death seem less significant and less real.

Because we are all aware, to some degree, that our death could come at any moment, death has meaning for people of all ages and affects the feelings and behavior of all of us, and not always positively. Richard Kalish, a noted sociologist, has summarized some of our views of death into three categories: death as an organizer of time, religious views of death, and death as loss.[4]

DEATH AS AN ORGANIZER OF TIME

Our awareness that life is finite affects the way we use time. If life went on forever, there would be no limit to the things we could do and we would not need to establish priorities for our time. Because we must set priorities, however, we formulate a general mental agenda for our lives and make decisions accordingly. Research shows that as we age, our perception of the time we have left changes.

The prospect of death thus organizes time differently for people of different ages.[5]

RELIGIOUS VIEWS OF DEATH

Every religion has among its doctrines some view of death. Some religions view death as a punishment for sins, as a release from pain, or as a transition to a better existence. Other religions view death rather neutrally, as a passage from one incarnation to another. Few, if any, religions view death as the final end of a person's existence in any form. Almost all promise some form of afterlife or reincarnation (see Feature 13.1, p. 408).

DEATH AS LOSS

Death brings numerous losses: the loss of all conscious awareness; of all further experiences; of all

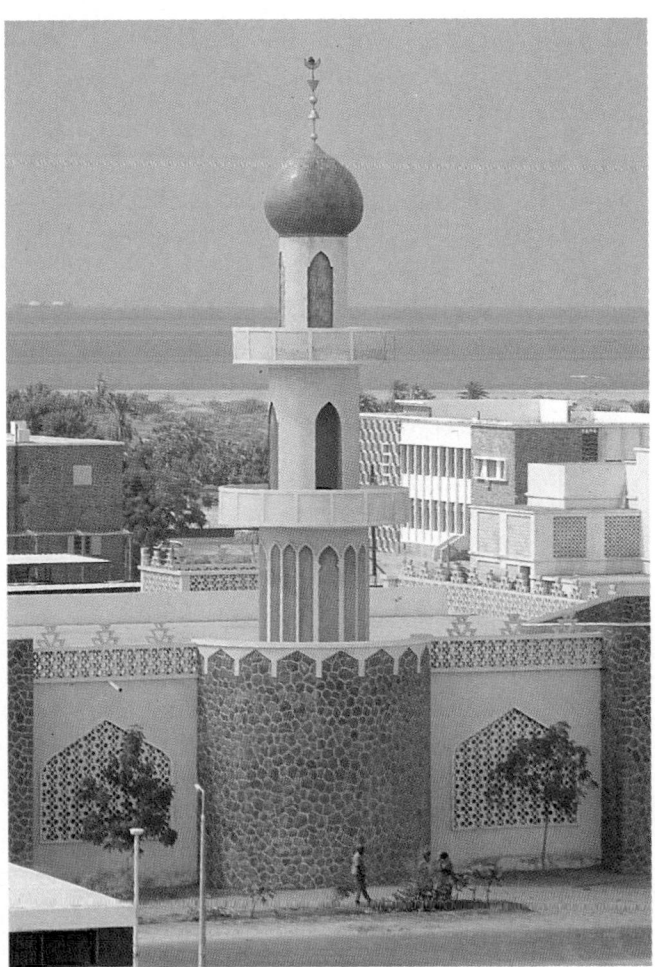

Every religion has among its doctrines some view of death. Few religions view death as the final end of a person's existence in any form.

MULTICULTURAL PERSPECTIVES: SOME OF THE WORLD'S CULTURAL TRADITIONS

Our religious beliefs (or nonreligious beliefs) have a major influence on how we deal with death. Death means something very different to a person who strongly believes in an afterlife compared to what death means to a confirmed atheist. Let's compare the Roman Catholic, Protestant, Jewish, Traditional Chinese religions (Taoism and Buddhism), Hindu, Muslim, and atheist answers to some questions concerning death.

1. WITHIN EACH RELIGION, HOW UNIFORM ARE BELIEFS ON THE THEOLOGY OF DEATH?

Roman Catholicism: Beliefs about death among Roman Catholics are more uniform than are those of Protestants or Jews.

Protestantism: There are vast differences among Protestants regarding the theology of death.

Judaism: There is some variation among Orthodox, Conservative, and Reform beliefs.

Traditional Chinese Religions: Traditional Chinese religions have roots in Taoism, Buddhism, and other sects. China is officially an atheistic country and most Chinese are not religious. Ideas regarding death, burial, and afterlife are dictated more by social customs than by religious beliefs. Traditional practices and beliefs are described in the following.

Hinduism: There is a nearly infinite variety of rites, attitudes, beliefs, and practices, but all varieties aim for one end, the individual's liberation into Brahman (absolute reality).

Islam (Muslims): Several sects (Sunnis, Shi'ites, etc.) disagree on some beliefs about death.

Atheists: The main unifying element among atheists is their disbelief in supernatural beings.

2. WHAT SPECIAL CUSTOMS ARE ASSOCIATED WITH DEATH?

Roman Catholicism: When someone is near death a priest performs a special final communion called *Viaticum,* more commonly known as the last rites.

Protestantism: There are no universal Protestant customs regarding death. Each denomination has its own customs.

Judaism: A person becomes a mourner upon death of a father, mother, husband, wife, son, daughter, brother, or sister. Mourning rituals include tearing of a garment. The tearing can take place at either the moment of hearing of the death, immediately prior to the funeral service (the most common time), or at the cemetery, prior to interment. For a parent, the tear is made on the left side over the heart; for all others, it is on the right.

The first seven days of mourning, beginning immediately after the funeral, is called Shiva. The bereaved remain at home receiving condolence calls. Following Shiva comes Sh-loshim, a 30-day period of normal activity, but no entertainment. Mourning for a deceased parent continues for an entire year. Mourning beyond the prescribed periods is taken as a lack of trust in God. A child under age 13 does not have to observe mourning rituals.

Traditional Chinese Religions: Traditionally, when a death occurred in China, one of the older relatives would rush to the nearest temple to inform the local gods of the death. (Information on traditional Chinese religions is in the past tense because China is officially an atheistic country and religious practices are forbidden.) The family of the deceased would hang blue and white or blue and yellow lanterns from the door to inform others that a death has occurred. The family wept in the room where the death had occurred. The body was wrapped in cotton sheets and clothed. The feet were tied together to keep the body from jumping about due to evil spirits. The body was placed in a large, heavy coffin and clothing was packed around it.

Hinduism: Hindus place great importance on ceremonial preparation of the body and other ceremonies. The body is laid out, draped with flowers, and a lamp placed at its head. The navel is smeared with oil, cotton is placed in the nostrils, the big toes are tied together, the eyelids are closed, and the hands are folded across the chest. Women are expected to mourn more than men and to follow certain steps, including anointing rituals.

Islam: Muslims usually say "It is the will of Allah" to the deceased person's family. It is not proper to keep the body in the house very long. Burial is usually the day of or the day after a death. In some groups, all curtains are immediately taken off windows as a sign of mourning. Mourners wail and scream to express grief. Relatives remain awake until the deceased is buried.

Atheism: No special customs.

3. HOW IS THE FUNERAL CONDUCTED?

Roman Catholicism: There are three phases: the wake, the funeral Mass, and the burial. The wake was formerly an all-night or several-day vigil held in the family home of the deceased prior to the funeral. Wakes are now more often for shorter periods and held at funeral homes. The funeral Mass is held a few days after the death. It begins at the funeral home with a procession to the church. The casket is covered with a white cloth pall and the priest wears white vestments, emphasizing the joy of faith overcoming the sadness of death. A candle is placed at the casket as a sign of Christ's presence. At the cemetery, the official ritual is quite brief. The priest blesses the grave, reads scripture, and offers several prayers. The mourners may or may not remain while the body is lowered into the grave.

Protestantism: The funeral may be at the local church, a funeral home, or at a private home. The service is often 15–20 minutes long. Some denominations have an open casket, some have the casket closed. Funeral music is an important part of the service. The funeral usually ends with a brief service at graveside. In some cases a memorial service with no casket present is held in place of a funeral.

Judaism: The funeral is nearly always held within a day after death. The funeral is a rite of separation where denial is transformed to acceptance. The casket is present and in Orthodox services is plain wood without adornment. At most Jewish funerals, flowers are not permitted and music may not be played, since they are both considered symbols of joy inappropriate during mourning. Attendance at the graveside portion of the service is considered the ultimate demonstration of honor and respect.

Traditional Chinese Religions: Religious authorities were summoned to the home to carry out ceremonies. All relatives attended the mourning ceremonies. Special clothing and hairstyles demonstrated mourning. The funeral procession involved many people and many symbols to glorify the dead. Three days after the burial, mourners returned to give food and burn money for the spirit. Ceremonial mourning behavior of the family continued for a year.

Hinduism: Prior to cremation, the body is placed on a framework called a *bier.* A procession forms at the house of the deceased to take the body to where cremation will take place. Cremation is ceremonial, on a *pyre* of combustible materials. Prayers are recited as the body burns.

Islam: There is no embalming. The service is not in the cemetery, but in an open spot near the graveyard or in the home of the deceased. No singing or music is permitted before or during the service. At the cemetery, the body is lowered into the ground in the presence of the relatives. If a coffin is used, the lid is left off so the person's soul can rise. The body is placed on its back with the head to the north and the face turned east toward Mecca.

Atheism: If any service is held, it is a memorial service honoring the life of the deceased.

4. WHAT ABOUT CREMATION?

Roman Catholicism: Cremation was not allowed in the past as it was viewed as denying the possibility of resurrection of the dead. It is now allowed. The funeral Mass is still held.

Protestantism: Cremation is permitted.

Judaism: Cremation is opposed by Orthodox Jews as being the deliberate destruction of God's creation. Cremation is practiced by some liberal Jews.

Traditional Chinese Religions: Not a traditional practice.

Hinduism: Cremation of the body on a funeral pyre accompanied by mantras and expiation rites is customary.

Islam: Cremation is not used.

Atheism: Cremation is often favored over burial by atheists.

5. WHAT ARE THE CONCEPTS OF AN AFTERLIFE?

Roman Catholicism: Catholics believe in "life" beyond death. The deceased first enters purgatory for purification before entering heaven. "Life" is experienced without a body until the day of final judgment.

Protestantism: Many Protestants believe in an afterlife, though beliefs vary among denominations. Some Protestants believe in a heaven and a hell, some in a heaven only (no hell), and some believe that heaven and hell are experienced only during a person's earthly life (no afterlife).

Judaism: Beliefs vary. Immortality is usually seen in earthly or natural (rather than supernatural) terms. Jews believe that we live on in body through our children; we live on in thought through those who remember us; and we live on in our influence on those who follow us. Jews have always been more concerned with this world than the next and have always concentrated their religious efforts toward building an ideal world for the living. The ideal world functionally serves as a "Heaven on Earth." Few Jews accept any literal concept of heaven or hell.

Traditional Chinese Religions: There is belief in reincarnation here on earth and spirits that reside here on earth. Taoism views death as part of the yin-yang harmony that governs the universe. Buddhism, in one perspective, offers a view of the afterlife as "ultimate reality" or Nirvana, in which all personal identity is lost with the transition into ultimate reality.

Hinduism: Hindus strive for immortality through emancipation from mortal life. Mortal life is considered as an expression of the cycle of rebirth to death. Emancipation from mortal life means breaking out from the cycle of rebirth to death.

Islam: The spirit of the deceased is said to roam for 40 days. On the fortieth day the spirit finds joy in heaven or pain in hell. Pain in hell, however, is a period of purification and not forever. The more corrupted the spirit, the longer it remains in hell. Once purified, the spirit is allowed to enter heaven.

Atheism: Atheists do not believe in an afterlife.

Source: Hardt, D. *Death, the Final Frontier.* Englewood Cliffs, NJ: Prentice Hall, 1979; Hutchinson, John, *Paths of Faith,* 4th ed. New York: McGraw-Hill, 1991; Kertzer, Morris, *What Is a Jew?* New York: Macmillan, 1965; Kung, Hans, *Eternal Life?* New York: Crossroad, 1991; and other sources. Special thanks to Rudy Saldana, Professor of World Religions, Mt. San Antonio College, for sharing his expertise.

loved people, places, and things; of control; of productivity; and of your very being. No other life event carries the assurance of such total loss. When we think about death it is primarily in terms of these losses.

When death comes slowly or at an advanced age, many people have already begun to lose much of what they had valued in life. With a progressive illness such as AIDS, emphysema, or cancer, a person gradually loses health, productivity, control, social contact, positive experiences, and many other important aspects of life. Advancing age brings many of the same losses and these losses accelerate in a person's later years. Friends and loved ones are lost through death with increasing frequency. Regardless of whether death comes suddenly or gradually, in a person's youth or old age, it is the anticipation of total loss that most affects our attitudes about death. Let's examine some of these attitudes.

CHECKPOINT

1. What is the meaning of the phrase "death as an organizer of time?"

2. What losses do we associate with death?

ATTITUDES TOWARD DEATH

Throughout our lives, we have experiences that shape and influence our attitudes toward death. We hear death discussed at home and in the media reports. Violent crimes fill the media reports. Famous people die. Our pets die. People we love die. We have illnesses, injuries, or near accidents that remind us of our own vulnerability. How we perceive these events is influenced by society's attitudes toward death; our society is one that does not always deal well with death.

Death has traditionally been a taboo subject for discussion in our culture. This is because many of us have not come to terms with our own feelings about death. Even talking about it causes discomfort and anxiety for many people. If we must speak of death, we tend to use euphemisms. For example, we say that people "pass away," or that we visit the "slumber room" at the mortuary. We try to keep death a step removed from reality. This avoidance of the subject of death, however, keeps us from dealing with it realistically.

Only when we come to terms with death are we able to live our lives most rewardingly. Confronting death contributes to our total plan for life. Facing the inevitability of our own death forces us to see our lives in a totality that includes our past, our present, and the indefinite portion of life remaining ahead of us. Many people think of death as unreal, or as something in the very distant future about which they can postpone thinking. As a result, they are incapable of forming any total life plan.

Despite our resistance to death, it affects each of our lives. The more we are willing to face death, the less helpless we will feel when death strikes those near to us. Our ability to deal with death will also make it easier for us to communicate with those who are dying and with their survivors. Psychiatrists believe that our unresolved feelings about death affect our daily living more than we realize.

How can we develop more positive attitudes toward death? We might start by analyzing the emotions that death evokes in us. We must become consciously aware of our suppressed fears of death if we are to deal with them. When there is an occasion to visit a dying person or to be in contact with persons who have recently encountered death, we should not avoid these people. Feeling comfortable around reminders of death is not easy. Yet, if we are ever to achieve a healthy attitude toward death, we must dispel our feelings of helplessness and fear. Take a minute right now to complete the assessment, In Your Hands: Your Attitudes Regarding Death.

CHECKPOINT

1. Why do some people avoid talking about death?

2. What are the advantages of coming to terms with death?

THE NEAR-DEATH EXPERIENCE

As we have discussed, there is no single moment of death. Many people, as a result of heart attacks, electrical shock, drowning, strangulation, and other injuries and illnesses, have been in a condi-

IN YOUR HANDS

YOUR ATTITUDES REGARDING DEATH

Our attitudes regarding death are important because they influence how we live our entire lives. Circle the number of points for the response that best represents your reaction to each of the following statements:

	Strongly agree	Somewhat Agree	Strongly disagree
1. I do or would feel uncomfortable around a dying person.	0	1	2
2. I try to avoid funerals if at all possible.	0	1	2
3. I might go to a funeral, but if the casket was open, I would not look at the body.	0	1	2
4. I don't like to think about death.	0	1	2
5. It makes me feel uncomfortable when people discuss death.	0	1	2
6. I hope that during my lifetime, science will overcome death.	0	1	2
7. Death is probably the most painful human experience.	0	1	2
8. Society would be better off if science overcame death.	0	1	2
9. I would like to have my body frozen when I die and brought back to life when a cure is found for the cause of my death.	0	1	2
10. If I had a life-threatening illness, I would want to be told of my condition.	2	1	0
11. I have written a will.	yes = 2		no = 0
12. I have executed a living will and durable power of attorney for health care if they are valid in my state.	yes = 2		no = 0
13. I would like to make my organs available for transplantation, and I carry a signed Uniform Donor Card.	yes = 2		no = 0

Total points: _____

INTERPRETATION

22–26 points: You understand that dying is a normal part of living. Your positive attitudes toward death enable you to live your life more fully.

17–21 points: Your attitudes toward death are about average.

16 points or less: You may not have come to terms with death. Your negative attitudes toward death may be adversely affecting your day-to-day life.

tion in which their pulse and breathing have stopped. That condition would have been considered death at one time. Today, many of these people are resuscitated and survive. This is called the **near-death experience.** It is estimated that about 1 in 20 people will, at some time, have a near-death experience.[6]

There are many ways to interpret the near-death experience, depending on the interpreter's frame of reference. The same experience, for exam-

ple, might be explained spiritually, psychologically, or physiologically. Regardless of the explanation, the conclusion reached by most who study death is that it is *not an unpleasant experience.*

About a dozen occurrences are frequently reported during and following the near-death experience. The average person reports about eight of these occurrences. They do not necessarily occur in this exact sequence:

1. *Hearing the news.* Many people remember hearing themselves spoken of as being dead by those present. They may recall exact words used and their accuracy may be confirmed by those who said them.

near-death experience when a person is resuscitated and survives after his or her pulse and breathing have stopped.

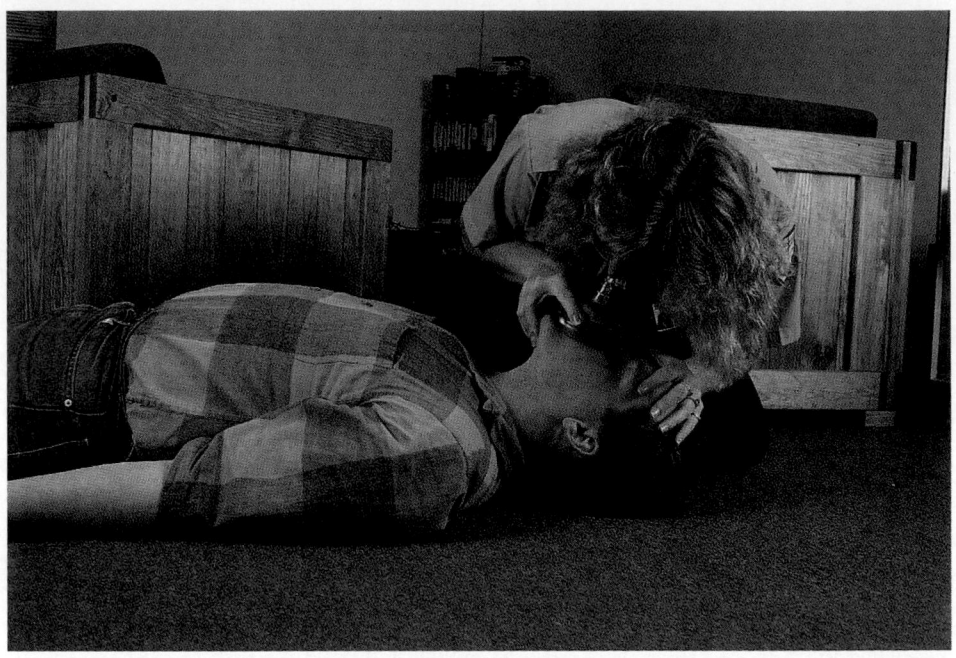

A near-death experience. Many people today are resuscitated after what would once have been considered death (no pulse or breathing). Most survivors of near-death experiences report that death is apparently not an unpleasant experience and, though they have a renewed appreciation for being alive, they feel less fear of death than before.

2. *Feelings of peace and quiet.* This is often described as a sensation of extreme comfort and relief.

3. *Hearing an unusual sound.* The sound is often described as a very loud ringing, buzzing, or clicking, or as beautiful or strange music.

4. *Passing through a dark tunnel.* The passage is described as traveling through a tunnel, a well, a cave, a vacuum or void, or through a valley.

5. *Out-of-body experience.* Many people report memories of standing or floating a few feet away from their bodies and looking at their bodies and at the other people present.

6. *Meeting others.* After leaving their bodies, many people remember being aware of the presence of spiritual beings, either deceased persons they have known or strangers.

7. *Seeing a bright light.* The light is described as very bright but not so bright that it hurts the eyes.

8. *The life review.* This is probably the most well-known occurrence in the near-death experience. Most of us have heard the statement, "My whole life flashed before my eyes."

9. *Coming back to life.* There is usually little memory of this process, other than that of waking up or regaining consciousness. The moods and feelings associated with the near-death experience, however, linger on for some time.

10. *Telling others.* People who have been through a near-death experience have no doubt about its reality and importance to them. Some are eager to talk about it if they find a receptive listener. Others are reluctant to share this experience for fear of being perceived as peculiar or mentally unstable.

11. *Effects on lives.* As might be expected, people who have survived near-death experiences feel extremely lucky to be alive. The experience often gives a person's life more meaning and he or she makes the most of every remaining day.

12. *New views of death.* Almost without exception, when someone has a near-death experience, he or she no longer fears death. Death is no longer seen as an unpleasant event. While most people who have had near-death experiences want to continue to live as long as possible, they are able to do so with a new freedom from the fear of death.

CHECKPOINT

1. What is a near-death experience?

2. List as many of the 12 common occurrences in the near-death experience as you can.

3. Some people interpret the near-death experience spiritually. What are some other ways of interpreting the 12 occurrences?

FACING YOUR OWN DEATH

Recent years have brought a dramatic increase in the number of seriously ill people who are aware that they are probably not going to live longer than a few months or years. Some of this increase can be attributed to advances in life-sustaining medical technology for people with cancer or heart conditions and some to the spread of AIDS in the population. Also, unlike the past, there are very few patients who are not made aware of their diagnosis. AIDS is just one of many conditions that medicine cannot yet cure, but for which life-prolonging treatments are available that can give people an extended time to prepare for death.

While the physical care needs of those dying slowly are often great, the emotional needs of the dying and those close to them are usually even greater. Those who are dying and their families and friends often need special help in coping with their emotions. Thanatologists such as Dr. Robert Kavanaugh[7] and Dr. Elisabeth Kübler-Ross[8-11] have devoted much time and energy to helping people who are dying and studying how dying people and those close to them can best handle this part of life. Their efforts have given us valuable insights into death, and have helped the dying to realize that their feelings are normal and somewhat predictable. This research has also enabled care-givers to realize that there is more to dying than the physical manifestations.

EMOTIONS EXPERIENCED BY THE DYING

Kübler-Ross describes five emotional states or stages commonly experienced by the dying. When someone is dying, he or she may or may not experience all of these stages or experience them in any particular sequence. A person may shift between emotional states and may feel several of them simultaneously. Kübler-Ross's five stages include the following:

1. *Denial and isolation.* This follows a person's initial awareness that he or she is dying. The patient may go from doctor to doctor looking for a more favorable diagnosis and may isolate him- or herself from relatives and friends.

2. *Anger.* This is a very difficult time for those who are close to the dying person because he or she may take anger out on anybody. Everyone is blamed for the situation, including loved ones, doctors, and the dying person's own self.

3. *Bargaining.* After the anger subsides, the dying person may try to bargain with him- or herself, God, or fate for a longer life. Frequently, these bargains are based on feelings of guilt: "God, if you'll just let me live, I'll never smoke again."

4. *Depression.* Depression is a predictable psychological state associated with any loss. A person who is dying feels sad about leaving family behind, not seeing children or grandchildren grow up, and all of the personal losses involved in dying. A person who is dying also mourns his or her own impending death. This is a vital emotional adjustment in preparation for final separation.

5. *Acceptance.* Often the last emotional state is acceptance. During this stage, the dying person has already mourned the loss of self, other people, and all earthly possessions. It is usually not a state of happiness, but one that is nearly devoid of feelings. A dying person, however, often clings to hope until the very end, and only wavers when death is imminent. Some dying people *never* reach the acceptance stage.

These stages often coexist and are often repeated. The amount of time it takes for a person to progress through these stages varies greatly and depends on how much time a person has left to live. Some may go through all of the stages and reach acceptance in a matter of days; for others, it may take many months.

LETTING GO

Family members and friends need to understand that acceptance of a person's own impending death often involves the **letting go** of family and friends. This is necessary in order to accept death and it should not be construed as rejection. Family members also need to let go of the dying person. Ties to earthly life must be broken so that a person can die in peace.

Another example of letting go is when a dying person gives away prized possessions. When such gifts are offered, they should be graciously received.

....

letting go breaking ties to earthly life so a person can die in peace.

As death draws near, it is very important for the dying person to receive permission to die from those who are closest to him or her. This permission is tacitly granted when those who are held dear accept the impending death themselves. They will no longer plead with him or her to try to hold on to life or complain about the hardship his or her death is going to impose on them. Once permission is granted, the dying person may slowly let go of all of the people and possessions held dear until everything except his or her own person has been relinquished. Not everyone takes this step; as mentioned, some never reach the acceptance stage and fight death until the very end.

CHECKPOINT

1. What five emotional stages do dying people often experience?

2. Do these emotions always occur in the same sequence?

3. What is meant by a dying person's "letting go" of family and friends?

REACTIONS OF A DYING PERSON'S FAMILY

The presence of a slowly dying family member causes many changes in a household. Normal activities are interrupted. Emotional, financial, and interpersonal difficulties may result. Depending on how well the family copes with the situation, relationships between the survivors may be strengthened or hostilities may disrupt family ties for years.

Open communication can alleviate problems for both the dying person and for family members. To achieve open communication, the family members, including the person who is dying, must share their feelings. This open communication is not always easy, however, because our attitudes toward death often make it extremely difficult or impossible.

The family members of a dying person often pass through stages of adjustment that are very similar to those of the dying person:

- They typically begin by denying that the person is dying. As long as people are in this stage of *denial,* they will not be able to communicate about the impending death.

- Family members often feel *anxiety* in response to the many uncertainties associated with the situation.

- As with any anticipated loss, *depression* is a common and natural emotional response.

- Those who are close to the dying person often feel and express *anger.* Anger is often directed at health care personnel for not doing more for the patient or for failing to keep family members informed about the patient's condition. Anger may also be directed at the dying person, whose illness may be interpreted as his or her own fault or as a hostile act.

- Many people who are close to a dying person may feel extreme *guilt.* They may feel guilty because they resent having to care for the dying person. They may also feel guilty for not having treated the person better in years past. Other reasons for guilt come from not having urged the person to seek treatment earlier. A person may even feel guilty because he or she will survive and enjoy life after the dying person is gone. Young children often feel guilt because they believe that they may have in some way caused a person to die.

- As is true with the dying person, the final emotion reached by family members may be *acceptance.* Just as some dying people never accept the likelihood of their death, some family members refuse to accept the inevitability of an impending death. This stage is more likely to be achieved when family members openly share emotions. Kübler-Ross[12] notes that it is easier for the dying person to accept death if he or she senses that family members and health care personnel have reached this point. If the people surrounding the dying person support the acceptance process instead of insisting that the patient "fight it out to the end" or that health personnel prolong life as long as possible, the patient's acceptance of impending death might be made easier. Once the likelihood of death has been accepted, it opens the possibility of the hospice approach to care, discussed in the following section.

HOSPICE CARE

A **hospice** is a program or organization that provides care and support for dying people and their families. Hospice care comes in several forms: it might be a place, called a hospice, where the dying person resides. More commonly, hospices are organizations that support the home care of the dying person by aiding family members, and provide emotional support for the dying person and his or her care-givers.

A hospice openly accepts that a person is probably going to die. The goal of the hospice is to keep the patient free of pain, comfortable, and alert throughout the final stages of life. Pain is recognized as a state arising from physical, psychological, social, or spiritual sources or any combination of these causes. Pain is controlled by carefully analyzing its source, by administering combinations of medications, and by offering psychological support. Heroic life-sustaining measures such as resuscitations and heart stimulation are not part of the hospice concept.

Family members are included in the hospice program, whether the patient is at home or in a hospice facility. Services to families typically include the following:

- Training family members to participate in the patient's care.
- Encouraging family members to do such things as cooking special meals for the patient (favorite foods stimulate the appetite and are psychologically beneficial).
- Offering unlimited visiting hours so that the entire family, including children, can visit the dying person at any time.

hospice a program or organization that provides care and support for dying people and their families.

- Promoting or facilitating communication of feelings regarding the dying experience by both the dying person and family and friends.
- Providing social and educational programs for the patient and family before and after the patient dies.

Most deaths in the United States occur away from home, sometimes because high-technology treatment of the severely ill requires hospitalization and sometimes because family members are unable or unwilling to administer the kinds of care severely ill persons may require. Yet when asked where they want to die, most people of any age state that they would prefer to die at home.[13] Further, the majority of family members of people who do die at home are glad that the death took place where it did, even though the burden on the home caretakers of a dying person is very heavy. This is where the hospice can be especially useful. Additional hospice services may include the following:

- Arranging patient transportation, special beds, and other equipment.
- Arranging visits by volunteers or health care professionals to the patient's home at regularly scheduled times for patient care, and/or psychological support for the patient and family members.
- Maintaining a staff of professionals on call 24 hours a day to assist the patient or family with any crises that may arise.
- Providing respite care—temporarily relieving family members of their responsibilities so they can take care of their own needs.
- Providing counseling services for family members following the death.

Most of us fantasize or hope that we are going to have a quick, painless, and unexpected death: "I just want to be perfectly healthy until I'm about 80 years old, and then one night, suddenly die in my sleep." While this makes a fine fantasy, it is seldom a reality. As a result, we do nothing to prepare ourselves psychologically for the much more likely event of a slow death from a chronic (long-term) illness. One way to help ourselves, while performing a great service to others, is to do volunteer work in a hospice program. Such work is emotion-

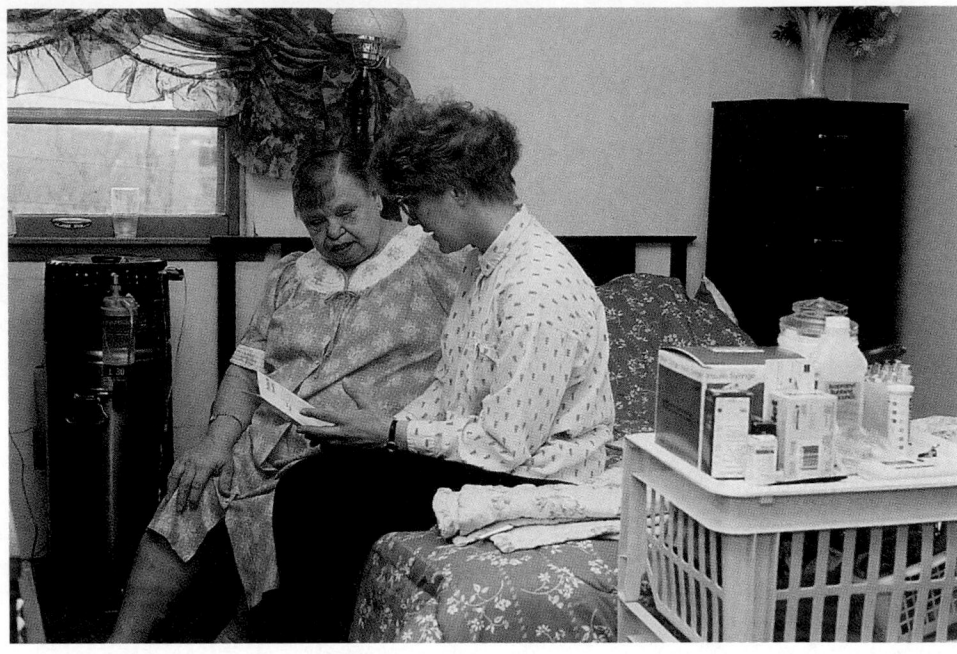

A hospice is a program that provides care and support for dying people and their families. Hospice care might involve a place where a dying person resides or it might, as in this photo, support the home care of someone who is dying.

ally demanding, but highly rewarding, both in the immediate term and in preparing to face our own eventual death. No special qualifications are usually needed, as volunteers are trained for the work they will do.

CHECKPOINT

1. What are the forms of hospice care?

2. What are the characteristics of residential (in-patient) hospice care?

3. What services does a hospice typically offer to help with home care of a dying person?

GRIEF AND LOSS REACTIONS

The emotional reactions following any major loss are rather predictable and are surprisingly similar for different forms of losses. The death of a loved person, a divorce, and the loss of a body part or function are examples of losses that can precipitate very similar **grief** responses. The emotional stages experienced in these diverse losses tend to be similar, as are the methods of treatment, should grief

....

grief the distress occurring as a result of any serious loss.

be prolonged and disabling. Here, we will specifically consider the grief associated with the loss of a loved person.

The **bereavement** period begins after the death of a loved one. There is no universal pattern of events and emotions during this period. Most survivors experience grief—a deep sense of loss, and a feeling of extreme sadness. When the death was expected, the period of grief is usually shorter than in the case of an unexpected death. In either case, even when all grief is apparently finished, it frequently reappears.

In addition to extending the period of grief, a sudden, unexpected death, as from an injury or sudden heart attack, leaves the survivors with uncomfortable feelings regarding not having been able to say goodbye and not having had the chance to resolve any conflicts that may have existed with the deceased. Also, financial and other personal affairs are often left in a state of disarray, creating an additional burden for the survivors.

Mourning is the culturally sanctioned expression of grief. It is how the survivors are expected to behave following a death. Mourning customs vary

....

bereavement the state of having lost a loved one through death.

mourning the culturally sanctioned expression of grief.

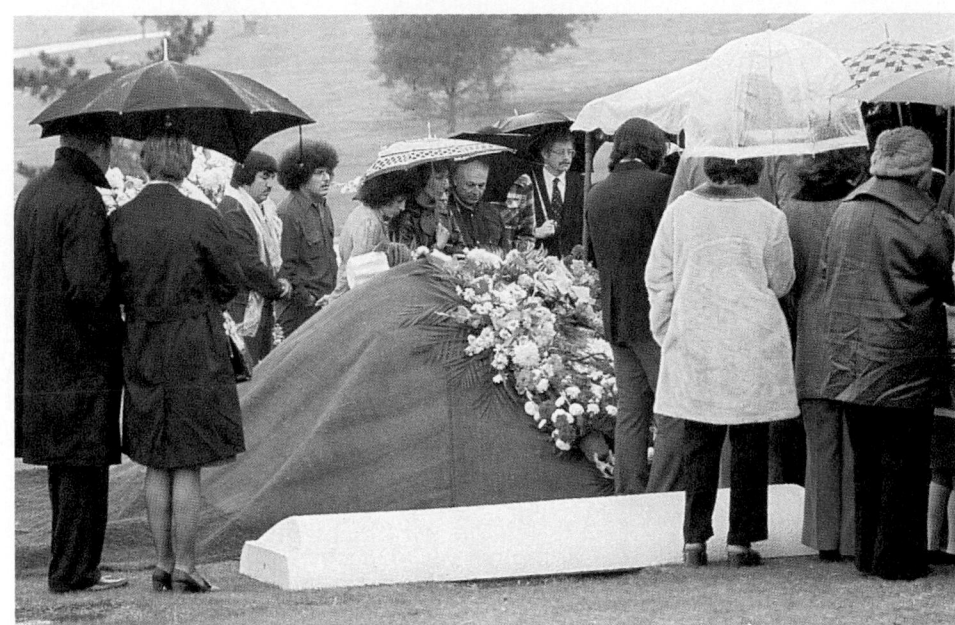

Following a death, the survivors usually experience grief, a deep sense of loss and a feeling of sadness. Grief can last a year or longer and is gradually replaced with acceptance. Years later, grief may still be felt on anniversary dates such as the deceased person's birthday or date of death.

widely among different cultures. They may involve the type of clothing to be worn. For example, black clothing is expected in some cultures and white in others. Mourning customs also suggest appropriate periods before remarriage, and may influence many other aspects of daily life.

EXPERIENCING GRIEF

Every person experiences the death of a loved one in a unique way. Ernest Morgan has identified ten typical emotional phases in the grieving process.[14] These phases are sequential, although several can occur at the same time and earlier phases can reappear. At one time or another, most survivors will experience each of these emotions, some of them many times, and even after years have passed.

1. *Denial, shock, and numbness* protect us from fully realizing the magnitude of our loss, especially in the case of a sudden loss.

2. *Emotional release* begins with the full realization of the loss and often includes a flood of tears. This is the necessary beginning of healing.

3. *Depression, loneliness, and isolation* are quickly felt and may continue to be felt for years.

4. *Physical expressions of grief,* ranging from minor discomforts to potentially fatal physio-

logical disruptions, are common. In older couples, the death of one spouse is often soon followed by the death of the other.

5. *Panic* may occur when a survivor feels unable to cope with an uncertain future.

6. *Remorse* or *guilt* is nearly universal among survivors who may believe that they have in some way contributed to the death or that they could in some way have prevented the death, or who wish they had spent more time with the deceased or had resolved conflicts with them.

7. *Anger* is almost always felt—at the deceased for dying, at health professionals for not preventing the death or making it more comfortable, at a person's self, or at God. This anger is often displayed indiscriminately and misdirected at inappropriate targets.

8. *The need to talk,* to express feelings, share memories, and to find meaning in the deceased person's life is nearly universal.

9. *Taking positive actions in response to the death,* like working to avoid similar deaths of others, reaching out to other grieving persons, and completing projects for the deceased is important in the healing process.

10. *Readjustment* is the final step, in which a survivor reaches out in new relationships and new experiences. We never totally overcome

the loss of a loved one, but eventually we need to get on with the business of living our own lives.

These experiences overlap and a survivor may move backward to a previous experience from time to time. Sometimes, when a survivor denies or represses the reality of the death, the entire grieving process is postponed, possibly for many years. Eventually the survivor must deal with emotions surrounding the loss. Feature 13.2 offers some suggestions for dealing with grief.

Other authorities[15, 16] have described three time-related stages in grief:

- *Stage 1.* This stage includes first few days after the death, including the time of the funeral. The bereaved family members are in a state of numbness and shock. Activity pre-

vails—the phone rings constantly; friends and family arrive to express condolences; funeral arrangements must be made; papers located; and bills paid.

- *Stage 2.* This stage is the letdown. The phone stops ringing. Friends start to disperse, and grief begins in earnest. During this period the survivors become aware of the immensity of their loss. Stage 2 can last a long time—six months to a year is common, and for some people it can go on for years. This is a period of disorientation, despair, bewilderment, worry, and depression. The thought of the dead person may become obsessive: Many times a day he or she is remembered. Depression may lead to physical apathy. The bereaved may feel drained of energy and lack motivation to do anything. A lot of tears may be shed.

FEATURE 13.2

DEALING WITH GRIEF

Most of us face periods of bereavement as we go through life. Grandparents die, parents die, spouses die, and sometimes we even lose children. Here are some suggestions for how to deal with the grief that almost always accompanies the death of a loved one.

- Grief can last far longer than most people expect. Be patient with yourself.

- Crying is an acceptable and healthy expression of grief; crying is a stress reliever.

- Common reactions to death include eating disorders, loss of energy, sleep disorders, inability to concentrate, and sexual difficulties. Healthful living habits such as maintaining a balanced diet and getting adequate amounts of sleep and exercise are important at this time. *Avoid using alcohol and other drugs.* They interfere with necessary grieving processes and you are especially vulnerable to developing chemical dependency at this time.

- Friends and relatives may feel uncomfortable around you, not knowing just what to say. Initiate conversations. Talk about the deceased person so others will know that this is appropriate.

- Put off major life changes—remarriage, moving, or career changes—for at least a year. Each of these is stressful and stress is cumulative. Also, acting in haste can lead to regrets later on.

- Don't feel rushed to dispose of the belongings of the deceased. You can do it little by little as you feel ready.

- Feelings of guilt are often a problem for the bereaved. Guilt is a normal part of grief. Feelings may surface in the form of regrets such as: "If only. . . ." Share these feelings with others and learn to forgive yourself.

- Anger is also very common, and may be vented indiscriminately. Again, share your feelings of anger with others and learn to be forgiving of others.

- Don't forget that any children in the family are feeling powerful grief too. They need to be encouraged to talk about their feelings and they also need plenty of love and attention.

- Consider contacting a grief support group. Most areas have such groups; some are specifically for those who have lost a child or a spouse, some are for those dealing with any death. You can obtain information about support groups from your physician or through a local service agency or house of worship. Those who have lost a child may wish to contact The Compassionate Friends, P. O. Box 3696, Oakbrook, IL 60522; (708) 990-0010.

- Feelings of grief can be expected to return year after year with holidays, birthdays, and the date of death of the deceased. Consider the feelings of the entire family in planning for such days and allow each person the time and space for his or her personal emotional needs.

- *Stage 3.* This stage, characterized by resignation and acceptance, develops gradually. It typically starts six months to a year after the death and lasts for approximately six months. The pain subsides; the death is accepted with some composure; sleep patterns, appetite, and energy all make a gradual return; and a survivor gets on with life. Periodically, however, features characteristic of Stage 1 and Stage 2 may recur, particularly on dates of special significance and when survivors engage in various activities without the deceased person for the first time.

GRIEF FOLLOWING A SUICIDE

Grief is especially powerful when a friend or family member has died by suicide (suicide is discussed in depth in Chapter 4). In addition to all of the usual feelings surrounding a death, there is the feeling that the death was unnecessary and there is often the added burden of powerful guilt feelings. Even though there may have been nothing that you could have done to prevent the suicide, it is common to feel guilty for "letting it happen." Some people become so depressed over the suicide of someone close that they consider or actually attempt suicide. It is important to understand that suicide is a result of severe emotional problems and the total failure of coping mechanisms and that intensive professional help is usually necessary to resolve such extreme problems. It does

no one any good to blame yourself when a suicide has occurred.

SUPPORTING GRIEVING FRIENDS

Most bereaved people pass through the stages of grief successfully. Though life may never be quite the same as before the death, overall functioning often stabilizes after about a year. Those who are unable to cope with their loss, however, may become seriously ill or deeply depressed and possibly even suicidal (see Chapter 4).

In addition to encouraging a grieving friend to follow the suggestions given in Feature 13.2, you can help by being a sympathetic listener and providing essential emotional and social support (see Communication for Wellness: Expressing Condolences). Grieving people need to know that their feelings of sadness, anger, and guilt are normal and will pass. They may also need to be encouraged to carry on with social activities and contacts, rather than isolating themselves.

CHILDREN AND GRIEF

Children have more awareness of death than many adults realize. Even by age 2, their play demonstrates an awareness of death. Children up to about age 5 tend to see death as temporary and reversible. By age 10, most children understand the reality of death much as adults do.[17]

Acceptance of death as a part of life begins with adults being honest with children about death. On occasions of deaths in a family, children need to be honestly informed and given age-appropriate roles to carry out in family activities relating to the deaths. Adults need not try to conceal their emotions from their children. This is part of an honest approach to death. Children also benefit from knowing that death is not painful and that dead people feel no pain. It is useful to explain that people are part of nature and that the natural cycle is to be born, grow, mature, and die. Most parents will also explain death to their children in terms of their religious beliefs.

C H E C K P O I N T

1. Distinguish between the terms *bereavement, grief,* and *mourning.*

2. What are Robert Kavanaugh's seven phases in the grieving process?

3. What are other authorities' three stages of grief?

4. How should parents explain death to their children?

DEATH OF A YOUNG PERSON

The most difficult of all deaths to accept is the death of a young person. Whether it is a sudden injury death, a suicide (see Chapter 4), or a gradual death from disease, there is a powerful feeling that the loss is greater than when an elderly person dies. And rightfully so, as the years of potential life lost are much greater and we are much less emotionally prepared for the death of a young person.

Every year in the United States, about 37,000 infants under 1 year of age and about 54,000 people between the ages of 1 and 24 die.[18] Each of these deaths affects a family in ways that are difficult for outsiders to comprehend. Often, grieving continues for years; some families never find their way out of the emotional turmoil of their bereavement.

FEELINGS OF A DYING CHILD

Terminally ill children, even if they are very young, are acutely aware of their condition and perceive death in many of the same ways as adults.[19] Forms of denial and bargaining are common. Anger, depression, fear, and withdrawal are frequent reactions. They may be very concerned with not wasting their limited remaining time.

The dying child's world is filled with images of disease and death. There is intense awareness of how medications and other treatments work or fail to work. Dying children are less concerned with the possibility of an afterlife than with what they are leaving behind on earth.

Terminally ill children are acutely aware of their condition and perceive death in many of the same ways as adults. Home care, whenever possible, is vastly superior to the unfamiliar environment of a hospital.

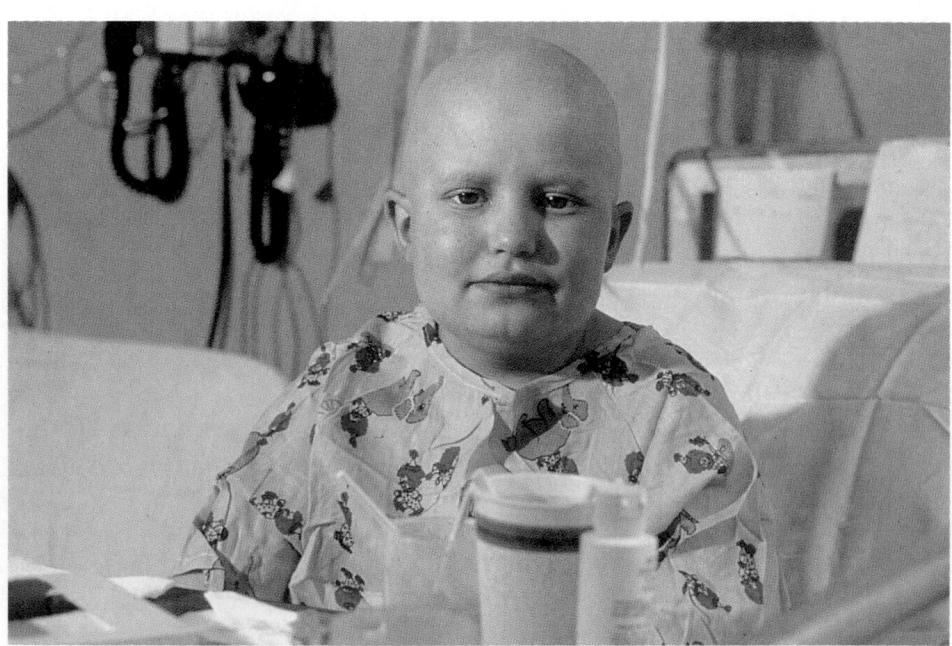

CARING FOR A DYING CHILD

Hospitalization can be extremely frightening to a child. The first thing a parent can do for the dying child is to consider the possibility of caring for him or her at home. If this is feasible, there is no question that the sick child is more comfortable in familiar home surroundings than in a hospital. Although it is harder work to keep a child at home and requires a greater commitment, in the long run, it is better for the child and the parent(s).

Home care is not always possible. Often tests, operations, and procedures require hospitalization. When this is the case, it is crucial to the child's morale that the parent(s) spend as much time with him or her as possible. Some hospitals even allow a parent to stay overnight in the same room with the child. Other family members should also visit regularly. The child should be kept well supplied with books, toys, and other diversions.

GRIEVING FOR A CHILD

Few experiences in life are as potentially shattering as the death of a person's child or young sibling. Yet, as with any death, bereaved family members can eventually heal and find hope for the future as they reorganize their lives in a positive way.[20] The suggestions in Feature 13.2 on grief may be especially useful for those who have lost a child.

CHECKPOINT

1. Why is the death of a child often seen as a greater loss than the death of an aged person?

2. Are dying children usually aware of their situation?

3. How can hospitalization be made less frightening for a child?

IMPORTANT ARRANGEMENTS

Each of us needs to make some advance preparations regarding our own death. Many people fail to make these preparations, primarily because they are not ready to face the possibility of their own death. Considerable difficulty can be avoided, both for the dying person and the survivors, by having a will and by making other arrangements well in advance.

MAKING A WILL

Should everyone, even college-age people, have a will? With very few exceptions, the answer is yes. If you die without a will, your property will pass to certain survivors as designated by state laws. These laws vary from state to state and may not reflect your desires.

In addition, every estate requires an administrator, or executor, who is usually named in a will. If you haven't drawn up a will, the executor is named by the court, usually from among family members. Again, this may not reflect your desires.

A will is a highly technical document. Its preparation requires considerable skill and, except in the simplest cases, is best executed by an attorney. If a person's estate is modest and he or she has no unusual requests for its disposition, a *handwritten* (it must be handwritten by the individual) and unwitnessed will, called a **holographic will,** might suffice. Holographic wills, however, are not honored in all states. Computer-generated wills, signed by three witnesses, are legal in most states. They can be completed by most people with simple estates in about 20 minutes.

FUNERAL PLANNING

We need to clear up some common misconceptions about funerals and related topics. A *funeral* is a ceremony with a body present. After the funeral there is a disposition of the body, usually either by earth burial, cremation (burning to ashes), or entombment in an above-ground vault or chamber. A *memorial service* is a ceremony without the body present. It usually occurs at some time following the disposition of the body.

There are two schools of thought on funeral planning. One holds that there are both practical and psychological advantages to preplanning a funeral and the disposal of a person's remains. Advance planning can save considerable amounts of money. Survivors often, in their grief, plan very expensive funerals, trying to "do what's best" for the deceased, though the deceased might have preferred much more modest arrangements. Also, prepaying funeral expenses can avoid the effects of inflation.

holographic will a handwritten and unwitnessed will.

Preplanning one's own funeral is helpful in coming to terms with death. It is also reassuring to know that one's funeral will be what one would want. Advance planning takes considerable pressure off the survivors during the difficult period immediately following a death.

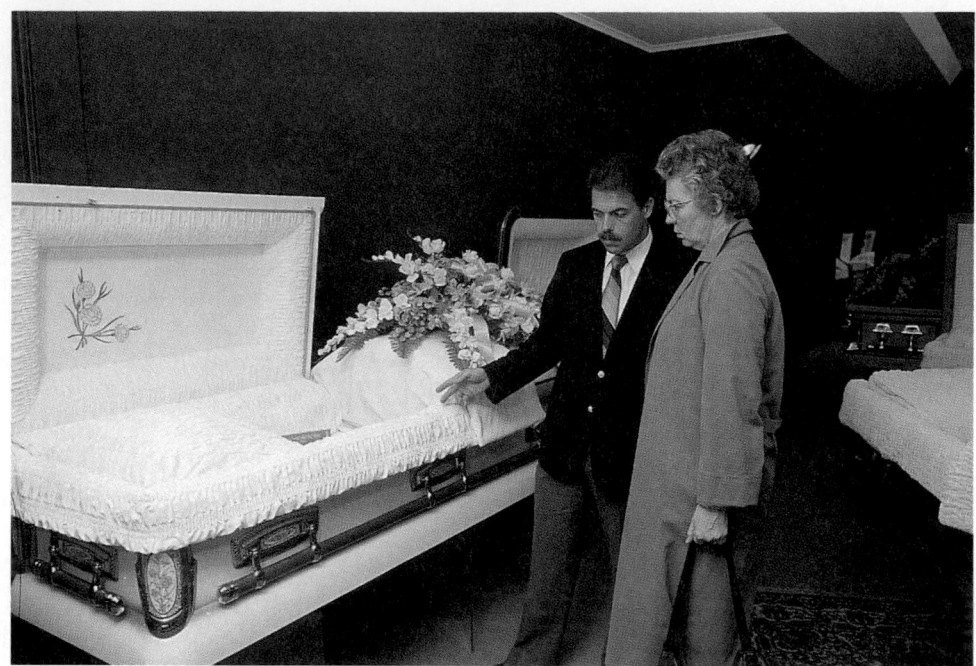

Memorial societies are cooperative, nonprofit consumer organizations that help their members to obtain simple, dignified, and economical funerals through advance planning. Memorial societies do not themselves provide funeral services, but act in an advisory capacity and often have contracts with funeral directors on behalf of their members, who commonly save 50–75 percent over usual funeral costs.[21] Information on memorial societies can be obtained from the Continental Association of Funeral and Memorial Societies at 2001 S Street N.W., Washington, DC 20009; (202) 462-8888.

Psychologically, planning your own funeral and/or disposition helps you to accept the inevitability of death. It is also reassuring to know that your arrangements will be exactly as you want. Another advantage to advance planning is that it takes considerable pressure off your survivors during the difficult period immediately following your death.

The other school of thought is that at least part of the funeral planning ought to be left to the survivors. There are significant psychological advantages to their being involved at this time. Their participation helps them overcome their emotional denial and accept the reality of death. It helps reduce their feelings of helplessness and gives them the satisfaction of "doing something" for the deceased. Funerals, after all, exist solely to meet the needs of the survivors, not the person who has died.

CHECKPOINT

1. What happens when a person dies without a will?

2. What is a holographic will? Is it always valid?

3. What are the advantages of preplanning your own funeral? What are the advantages of the survivors being involved in funeral planning?

THE RIGHT TO DIE

Now that medical technology can keep a severely ill person alive long after any hope of recovery has vanished, many people want to have some control over the point at which drastic treatments are discontinued. They would like to be allowed to die with dignity, in peace, and in comfort.

EUTHANASIA

The word **euthanasia** (*ū-tha-nā′zē-a*) is derived from the Greek words *eu,* meaning "good," and *thanatos,* meaning "death." Definitions of euthana-

euthanasia (1) dying easily or painlessly; or (2) the act of willfully ending life in someone with an incurable disease.

sia vary. The most controversial interpretation involves administering a painless death to someone suffering from an incurable disease who wants to die and is *not yet close to death*. This "assisted suicide" or "active euthanasia" is sometimes requested by someone who does not wish to experience the long period of decline and suffering expected as a result of his or her disease or is experiencing intolerable pain and suffering and pleads to die. Assisting in a suicide is illegal in most states.

More commonly, euthanasia is interpreted as helping those who are near death to die with as little anguish as possible. The medical profession approaches this in four ways:[22]

1. *Keep the patient as happy and free of pain as possible.* Nothing is done that would hasten death.

2. When pain is very severe, *administer therapy that, in the process of providing pain relief, could shorten life.* Quality of life is chosen over length of life.

3. *Acknowledge the inability to heal the patient, stop therapy, and allow the forces of nature to take place.* This is sometimes called "passive euthanasia."

4. *Participate in terminating the life of someone who is near death and who pleads for release from a painful and hopeless situation.* (See Feature 13.3.) This "active euthanasia" might take the form of a lethal injection. Even though the patient may be near death, this is still illegal in the United States. Active euthanasia is more common and is legally more acceptable in some countries, such as The Netherlands.[23, 24]

Once a patient starts receiving medical care, the right to decide his or her own fate often seems to be given up to the physician. Older people, in particular, often believe that the physician knows all the answers and they are therefore the most likely to abdicate their rights.[25] They often look to the physician, just as a child looks to a parent, for permission—in this case, to die. To die in peace, the patient needs to hear from the physician and other care-givers that it is all right, when the patient feels ready to give up, let go, and die.

LIVING WILLS AND DURABLE POWERS OF ATTORNEY FOR HEALTH CARE

Any one of us could, through an injury or illness, be in a position where we could be kept alive for

---

FEATURE 13.3

THE "RATIONAL SUICIDE" AND ASSISTED SUICIDE DILEMMAS

A popular young professor with a brain tumor is admitted to a hospital because of her rapidly deteriorating condition. A few days later, she is found unconscious in her bed with an empty container of unprescribed pain pills, from an unknown source, at her side. Should she be resuscitated? If it was found that her physician had provided the pills, should the physician be prosecuted for assisting in a suicide, currently illegal in most states? Should state laws be changed to allow such aided suicide, as Oregon did in 1994?

The suicide of a healthy person is usually considered to be the result of emotional illness. The suicide of a dying person, in contrast, is often referred to as "rational suicide."

Public opinion is increasingly supportive of someone who wants to end a hopeless, joyless, and painful existence through suicide. There also appears to be increasing support for making it legal for a physician to assist in the suicide of a dying person, though only Oregon had changed its law as of 1994. Public opinion regarding assisted suicide such as that practiced by Dr. Jack Kevorkian is quite mixed. (Dr. Kevorkian, a Michigan pathologist, assisted in 19 suicides of seriously ill people between 1990 and 1993, when he

agreed to discontinue that activity. In May, 1994, Dr. Kevorkian was acquitted of violating Michigan's ban on assisted suicide. The same week, a federal judge in Seattle overturned Washington state's ban on assisted suicide, ruling that dying people have just as much right to overtly end their lives as they do to refuse medical care.)

Laws in many states grant people the right to refuse medical treatment if they believe the benefits of the treatment do not justify the pain or prolonged suffering resulting from the treatment. This, in a sense, allows a passive form of suicide.

Should further legal provisions be made to assist those who desire "rational suicide?" Should physicians, for example, be allowed to provide lethal pills for dying patients as they are in Oregon? Another issue is which principle takes precedence in a case where a dying person has attempted suicide. If a living will or a similar document has been completed and the patient's chart is marked "do not resuscitate," doesn't resuscitation conflict with that desire? But doesn't the failure to resuscitate constitute assisting in a suicide, which is illegal? What do you think?

months or even years in an unconscious condition with no hope of recovery. Depending on our cultural and religious beliefs, many of us would not want a prolonged survival in this hopeless condition.

Under common law, any adult *of sound mind* has the right to refuse medical treatment necessary to sustain life. Once a person is mentally incapacitated or unable to communicate, however, discontinuing treatment requires previously prepared written proof of that person's wishes. A proper document or documents must be prepared *while a person is still of sound mind.*

The Natural Death Act, passed by the California State Legislature in 1977, has served as a model for legislation in other states. This Act states that: "Adult persons have the fundamental right to control decisions related to the rendering of their own medical care, including decisions to have life sustaining procedures withheld or withdrawn in instances of a terminal condition."

Laws regulating the care of severely ill people vary from state to state and are subject to change. Thus, the counsel of an attorney who specializes in health care is essential in drawing up documents that can effectively direct the forms of care you receive.

The American Medical Association has addressed several issues related to the right to die. A clear definition of the condition, called **persistent vegetative state (PVS),** has been determined. The distinguishing feature of PVS is "chronic wakefulness without awareness," which can be accompanied by spontaneous eye opening, unintelligible sounds, reflex movement of the head toward a noise or movement, or even brief smiles. PVS patients, however, demonstrate no coherent speech, comprehension, or capacity to make purposeful movement. The diagnosis of PVS is confirmed by a highly technical form of brain scan called *positron emission tomography.* This can confirm that, although the more primitive parts of the brain remain functional, the cerebral cortex, where consciousness lies, is no longer capable of functioning. A conservative criterion for PVS is lack of awareness for at least 12 months. "If any doubt

exists, the diagnosis of PVS should be avoided or deferred."[26]

A diagnosis of PVS could form the basis for a decision to withdraw or withhold treatment, if documents instructing physicians to do so had been prepared before the patient became incapacitated. For example, should a patient with PVS develop pneumonia, it might not be treated with antibiotics. Should a cardiac arrest occur, there might be no resuscitation.

Pain upon treatment withdrawal in PVS is, "by definition," impossible, because in PVS the capacity to perceive stimuli is destroyed. Physicians personally opposed to participating in withdrawal of treatment are obligated to transfer the patient to a physician who isn't, according to the AMA.

Such withdrawal of treatment is likely to occur only when a patient has previously prepared the proper documents to direct that action. Two documents are often necessary: a **living will** and a **durable power of attorney for health care.** Under the laws of increasing numbers of states, both of these documents are needed. Those who desire to have control over the forms of medical care they receive should have these documents executed by an attorney according to the laws of their particular state, signed and witnessed, and copies given to their physician and close family members. The living will, or Directive to Physicians (Figure 13.2), makes your specific desires clearly known. The specific language of the living will, however, can be a significant problem when circumstances arise that were not anticipated when the living will was written.

A durable power of attorney for health care enables you to appoint a trusted person to make health care decisions when you are incapacitated. This arrangement can avoid the living will's potential limitations of overly specific instructions or ambiguous directions. Physicians can rely upon the

....

persistent vegetative state (PVS) chronic wakefulness without awareness.

living will a document instructing one's physician to withdraw or withhold treatment under certain specified conditions.

durable power of attorney for health care a document appointing a trusted person to make health care decisions should a person become incapacitated; such decisions might involve withdrawing or withholding treatment.

Figure 13.2

The Living Will or Directive to Physicians

As authorized by the model California Natural Death Act, this document allows you to describe the forms of care you would want when in a terminal condition. Another document, the Durable Power of Attorney for Health Care, is also needed to allow a designated person to make decisions in situations not specified in the living will.

NATURAL DEATH ACT
(Section 7185, et seq, California Health & Safety Code)

DECLARATION OF _____

If I should have an incurable and irreversible condition that has been diagnosed by two physicians and that will result in my death within a relatively short time without the administration of life-sustaining treatment or has produced an irreversible coma or persistent vegetative state, and I am no longer able to make decisions regarding my medical treatment, I direct my attending physician, pursuant to the Natural Death Act of California, to withhold or withdraw treatment, including artificially administered nutrition and hydration, that only prolongs the process of dying or the irreversible coma or persistent vegetative state and is not necessary for my comfort or to alleviate pain.

If I have been diagnosed as pregnant, and that diagnosis is known to my physician, this declaration shall have no force or effect during my pregnancy.

Signed this _____ day of _____, 199__.

_____	_____
Signature	Residence Address
_____	_____
(Print Name)	City State Zip

The declarant voluntarily signed this writing in my presence. I am not a health care provider, an employee of a health care provider, the operator of a community care facility, an employee of an operator of a community care facility, the operator of a residential care facility for the elderly, or an employee of an operator of a residential care facility for the elderly.

_____	_____
Signature	Residence Address
_____	_____
(Print Name)	City State Zip
_____	_____
Signature	Residence Address
_____	_____
(Print Name)	City State Zip

(AT LEAST ONE OF THE ABOVE WITNESSES MUST ALSO SIGN THE FOLLOWING DECLARATION.)

I further declare under penalty or perjury under the laws of California that I am not related to the principal by blood, marriage, or adoption, and to the best of my knowledge I am not entitled to any part of the estate of the principal upon the death of the principal under a will now existing or by operation of law.

_____
Signature

_____
Signature

A physician or other health care provider who is furnished a copy of this declaration shall make it a part of the declarant's medical record and, if unwilling to comply with the declaration, promptly so advise the declarant.

---

appointed agent's decisions even when your desires were not clearly expressed. A living will and a durable power of attorney for health care document can protect you and your family from the emotional and financial devastation of your protracted existence.

Living wills are only binding in the states that have legislated their legality. Their powers do not extend across state lines. If a person is in a terminal condition outside of his or her own state of residence, such as after an injury, his or her living will is invalid.[27] Even in states where living wills are not legally recognized, the completion of such a document fosters serious thinking and discussion among the physician, patient, and family about the forms of care to be given.

Communication between a patient and his or her physician about the forms of care to be given is critical. In addition, this information needs to be available to other physicians in a group practice or HMO who may be providing care. Further, the philosophies and policies of the hospital to which you are admitted will affect the kinds of care given. Information about this should be collected *before* admission to a hospital and, when you have options, should be considered in hospital selection.

CHECKPOINT

1. What are the various interpretations of the term *euthanasia?*

2. What does the Natural Death Act state?

3. What is a living will? What is a durable power of attorney for health care?

ORGAN DONATION

One of the most remarkable advances in medicine has been the development of methods to transfer healthy organs or parts of organs from one person to another. Organ transplants become appropriate when one organ, such as the heart, liver, or both kidneys, of a person is severely diseased while the remainder of the body is in relatively good health. This situation has become more common as medical advances have made survival possible for many people with severe health problems. Other commonly transplanted body parts are skin, bone, bone marrow, corneas, and heart valves.

The first successful kidney transplant was done in 1954. Since that time, improved methods have greatly increased the success rate of transplants. The ability to match potential donor organs with transplant recipients has improved, as has the ability to overcome rejection reactions. Rejection happens because the immune system recognizes the organ as being foreign to the body and destroys the transplanted organ.[28]

The possibility of transplant rejection is greatly reduced by a variety of immunity-suppressing drugs, none of which is perfect. Some are directly toxic to the recipient and some, by nonspecifically suppressing immunity, promote viral, bacterial, and fungal infections. One of the most useful drugs at this time is cyclosporine. It is derived from a fungus and works by rather selectively blocking the rejection reaction. It is usually used with corticosteroids.

An even bigger problem than rejection is the shortage of organs available for transplantation. Over 25,000 Americans are currently waiting to receive lifesaving heart, kidney, liver, pancreas, or heart and lung transplants.[29–31] Only about 16,000 per year are lucky enough to receive such transplants. Thousands more, whose lives might have been extended, die for lack of a suitable organ.

Year by year the waiting list grows. Improving medical technology is increasing the demand for organs while decreasing the supply by prolonging the lives of many who might have become donors. The decision as to who receives an organ and who does not is literally a decision as to who will live and who will die.

Why aren't more organs available? Several factors contribute to the shortage:[32]

- Physicians are not taking a strong enough stand favoring organ donation. Sometimes they feel uncomfortable asking for permission from the patient before his or her death or from the family after a death.

- Some physicians have social, religious, or moral objections to transplantation.

- People may be afraid that they or their loved ones may be prematurely declared dead due to the need for their organs.

- Some physicians are reluctant to declare a patient brain dead because they see it as a sign of their failure.

Aware of the possibility of extending the lives of others, many concerned people want to make their organs available for donation in the event of their death. The Uniform Anatomical Gift Act, or similar legislation allowing the donor's wish to be binding after his or her death, has been adopted by all 50 states. Potential donors may carry wallet-sized donor cards (see Figure 13.3), which are widely available through many organizations, such as the American Medical Association, Kidney Foundations, The Living Bank (P. O. Box 6725, Houston, TX 77265) and state Departments of Motor Vehicles (they are often printed on the back of a driver's license).

Even more significant than the donor card is the Required Request legislation passed by most states during the 1980s. In most states, the hospital is now required to ask survivors about organ donation if the deceased falls within certain guidelines. The family makes the decision and it doesn't matter whether or not there was ever a donor card signed. The donor or donor's family is *not* responsible for donation-related costs, all of which are assumed by the nation's organ procurement organizations.

In order to facilitate the matching of available organs to potential recipients, the United Network

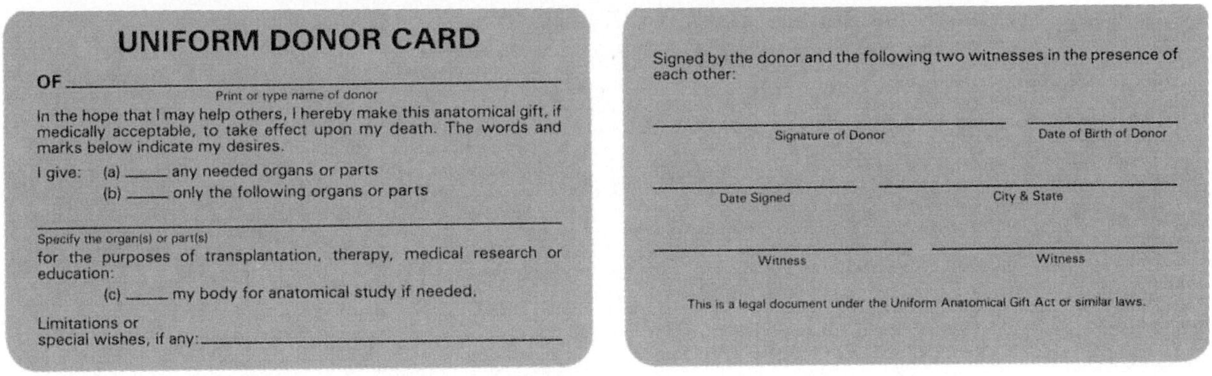
UNIFORM DONOR CARD

OF ______________________
Print or type name of donor

In the hope that I may help others, I hereby make this anatomical gift, if medically acceptable, to take effect upon my death. The words and marks below indicate my desires.

I give: (a) ____ any needed organs or parts

(b) ____ only the following organs or parts

____
Specify the organ(s) or part(s)

for the purposes of transplantation, therapy, medical research or education:

(c) ____ my body for anatomical study if needed.

Limitations or special wishes, if any: ______________________

Signed by the donor and the following two witnesses in the presence of each other:

Signature of Donor ____ Date of Birth of Donor ____

Date Signed ____ City & State ____

Witness ____ Witness ____

This is a legal document under the Uniform Anatomical Gift Act or similar laws.

Figure 13.3
A Sample Donor Card

Uniform Donor Card adopted under the Uniform Anatomical Gift Act that has been adopted in all 50 states. These widely available cards make it possible to remove lifesaving organs immediately from a body in the event of sudden death.

for Organ Sharing (UNOS) was established during the 1980s as a national listing of persons in need of specific organs. Priorities for allocating organs to those in need are determined by a point system that includes how critical the need is, how long the potential recipient has been on the waiting list, closeness of matching of blood and tissue antigen types to minimize problems of rejection, and the geographic distance of the potential recipient from the available organ.

Sometimes there are religious concerns about organ donation—some religions require the burial of an intact body—but most major religions in the United States now encourage organ donation. Consulting with a member of the clergy often helps to reassure family members of the religious acceptability of organ donation.

CHECKPOINT

1. What principle relating to the death of a person makes organ donation a possibility?
2. Have you discussed with your family members your feelings about organ donation?

SUMMARY

Death is just as much a part of the human life cycle as birth; however, many of us tend to deny the inevitability of death. Consciously accepting that we will eventually die causes many of us anxiety; yet, unconsciously, we are all aware of our mortality and this awareness affects every aspect of our lives. Only when we come to terms with the finite nature of life can we live our lives to the fullest.

The definition of death has changed over the years. Today there is no "moment of death." Death is a gradual and subtle ebbing of life processes. We die cell by cell. Brain death is the cessation of all brain function and is the basis of today's definition of death. Even though the rest of the body may be alive, once someone's brain is dead, most people believe that all meaningful life has ended.

Death can be viewed as an organizer of time, forcing us to set priorities; as a passage to another existence, as in some religious beliefs; and as loss, both for the dying person and for survivors. Many people do not deal well with death. They may try to keep it a step removed from reality. More positive attitudes about death can help us to live our lives more rewardingly. People who have been resuscitated following apparent death, report having many similar experiences and that their near-death state was not an unpleasant event.

People who know that their illnesses are terminal pass through predictable psychological stages: denial and isolation, anger, bargaining, depression, and acceptance. Similar stages are experienced by their loved ones. Dying people may feel the need to let go of people and possessions that have been held dear.

A hospice is a program or organization that provides care and support for dying people and their families. Family members are included in the hospice program, whether the patient is at home or in a hospice facility. Following a death, the survivors usually experience rather predictable emotional stages. Grief following a suicide is especially powerful. Death should be handled honestly with children, who by age 10 understand death in the same ways as adults do.

The death of a young person is especially difficult to accept, because the loss, in years of potential life lost, is greater and we are less emotionally prepared for such a death. Children who are gradually dying are aware of what is happening and need much support.

Each of us should have a current will and, if desired, a completed organ-donor card. Many people are concerned that medical technology will keep them alive against their will when they reach the late stages of an incurable disease or have been severely brain-injured in a vehicle crash. In many cases, this can be avoided by completing the proper documents—a living will and a durable power of attorney for health care—while still in good health.

REFERENCES

1. Morgan, E. *Dealing Creatively with Death,* 12th ed. Bayside, NY: Excelsior, 1990.
2. Ibid.
3. Jenks, S. "The Lingering Image of Life." *Medical World News* (28 April 1986), 77–96.
4. Kalish, R. "The Social Context of Death and Dying." In Binstock, R., and Shanas, E. (eds.). *Handbook of Aging and the Social Sciences,* 3rd ed. New York: Van Nostrand Reinhold, 1990.
5. Ibid.
6. Gallup, G. *Adventures in Immortality.* New York: McGraw-Hill, 1982.
7. Kavanaugh, R. *Facing Death.* Baltimore: Penguin Books, 1974.
8. Kübler-Ross, E. *On Death and Dying.* New York: Macmillan, 1969.
9. Kübler-Ross, E. *Questions and Answers on Death and Dying.* New York: Macmillan, 1974.
10. Kübler-Ross, E. *Death: The Final Stage of Growth.* Englewood Cliffs, NJ: Prentice-Hall, 1975.
11. Kübler-Ross, E., and Warshaw, M. *To Live Until We Say Goodbye.* Englewood Cliffs, NJ: Prentice-Hall, 1978.
12. Kübler-Ross, 1974, op. cit.
13. Kalish, op. cit.
14. Morgan, op. cit.
15. Carrol, D. *Living with Dying,* revised ed. New York: Paragon House, 1991.
16. Martel, L, and Adis, A. "Bereavement: Coping with Widowhood." *Medical Aspects of Human Sexuality* 23, No. 2 (February 1989), 96–101.
17. DeSpelder, L., and Strickland, A. *The Last Dance: Encountering Death and Dying,* 3rd ed. Palo Alto, CA: Mayfield, 1991.
18. National Center for Health Statistics. "Annual Summary of Births, Marriages, Divorces, and Death: United States 1991." *Monthly Vital Statistics Report* Vol. 40, No. 13 (30 September 1992).
19. Carrol, op. cit.
20. Knapp, op. cit.
21. Morgan, op. cit.
22. Ebersole, P., and Hess, P. *Toward Healthy Aging,* 3rd ed. St. Louis: Mosby, 1990.
23. Parachini, A. "The Netherlands Debates the Legal Limits of Euthanasia." *Los Angeles Times* (5 July 1987) Part VI, 1–9.
24. Jones, T. "Setting a Date for Death." *Los Angeles Times* (14 March 1993) Sect. A, 1.
25. Ebersole and Hess, op. cit.
26. Cotton, P. "AMA Pushing Living Wills, Guide to Life-Support Use." *Medical World News* 26–27 (24 July 1989).
27. Ebersole and Hess, op. cit.
28. Coleman, R., Lombard, M., Sicard, R., and Rencricca, N. *Fundamental Immunology.* Dubuque, IA: Wm. C. Brown, 1989.
29. Kott, A. "Organ Procurement Programs in State of Emergency." *Medical World News* (February 1992), 15–16.
30. Shaffer, M. "Baboon Liver in Man: the Beginning of the Xenograph Era?" *Medical World News* (August 1992), pp. 27–28.
31. Sloan, B. "Triumph, Tragedy Envelop Transplant Recipients and Those Who Wait." *Los Angeles Times* (24 October 1992), J1–J4.
32. Kott, op. cit.

SUGGESTED READINGS

Aiken, L. Dying, *Death, and Bereavement,* 2nd ed. Boston: Allyn and Bacon, 1991.

Anderson, P. *Affairs in Order: A Complete Resource and Guide to Death and Dying.* New York: Macmillan, 1993.

Carroll, D. *Living with Dying,* Revised ed. New York: Paragon House, 1991.

DeSpelder, L., and Strickland, A. *The Last Dance: Encountering Death and Dying,* 3rd ed. Palo Alto, CA: Mayfield, 1991.

Kastenbaum, R. *Death, Society, and Human Experience,* 4th ed. Columbus, OH: Merrill, 1991.

Kung, H. *Eternal Life?* New York: Crossroad, 1991.

Morgan, E. *Dealing Creatively with Death,* 12th ed. Bayside, NY: Excelsior, 1990.

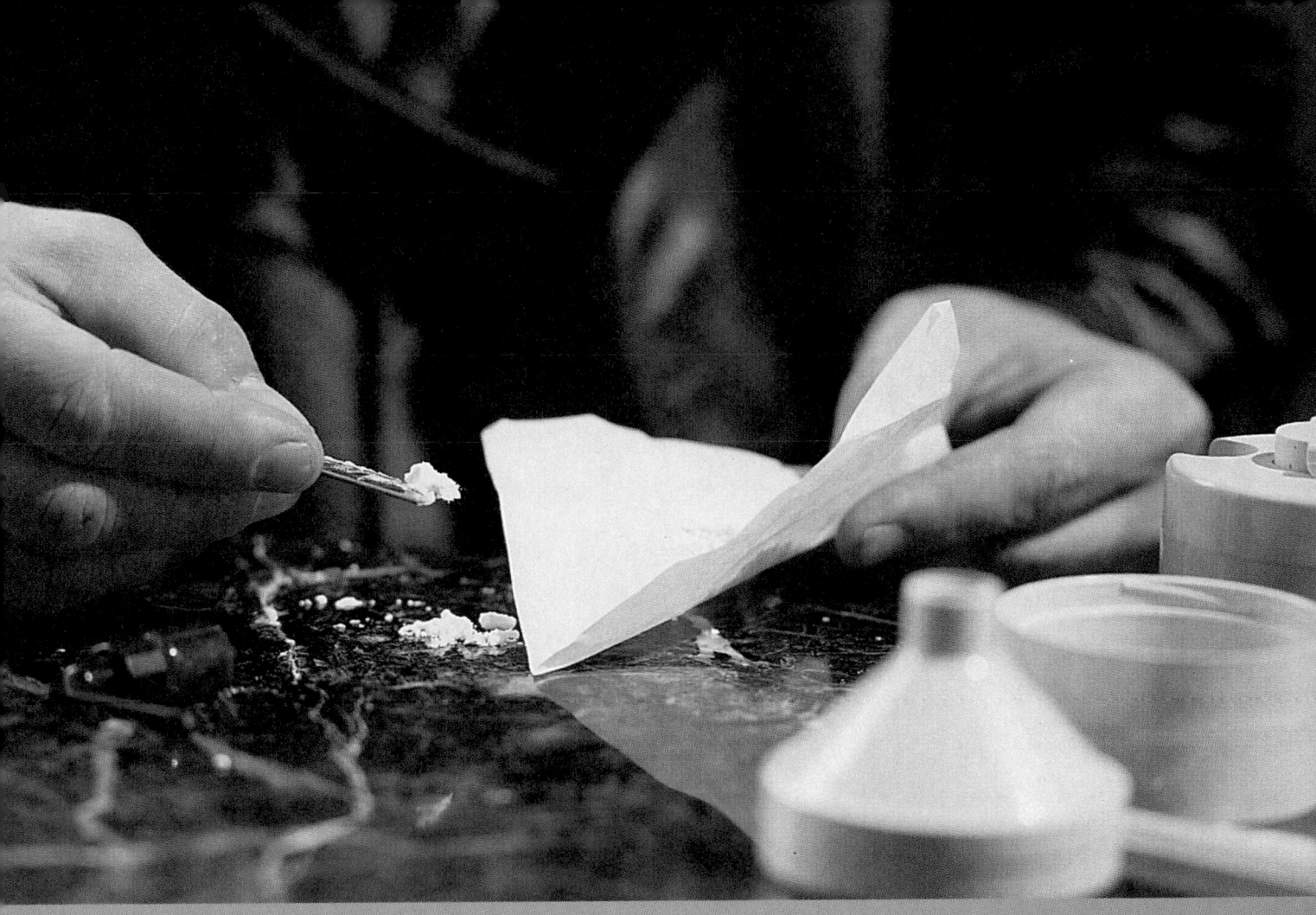

SIX

SUBSTANCE USE AND ABUSE

Alcohol, marijuana, tobacco, cocaine—these and other drugs are a common part of life on and around most college campuses, high schools, and even junior high schools. Some students develop severe substance-abuse problems that interfere with their success in school and may continue to plague them years later.

Using drugs to make life more pleasurable, or at least more tolerable, is nothing new. This has been a part of human existence throughout history. It is apparently part of human nature to search for something—anything—to enhance the quality of life.

Underlying all discussion in this unit is the philosophy that substance abusers are not terrible people, but that substance abuse is an unhealthful and unrewarding life-style. This unit explains why drugs are *not* the key to an enhanced quality of life. It shows how, because of basic human physiology, it is impossible to achieve the benefits people seek from psychoactive drugs over any extended period of time.

The use of drugs is an emotionally charged issue that is difficult to discuss in an objective manner because everyone has individual values and biases. We doubt that any individual reader will agree with everything we say on this subject.

In this unit, we take a family and social systems approach to drug abuse. Our discussion will emphasize how families and society affect drug abuse and how drug abuse affects families and society. Because drug abuse in the United States starts at very young ages, much of the material in these chapters is presented to assist you as a caring adult who wants to help your children and other young people avoid the traps of substance abuse. Finally, for those of you for whom chemical dependency is or may be a personal problem, we will describe the many resources that are available to help with your recovery.

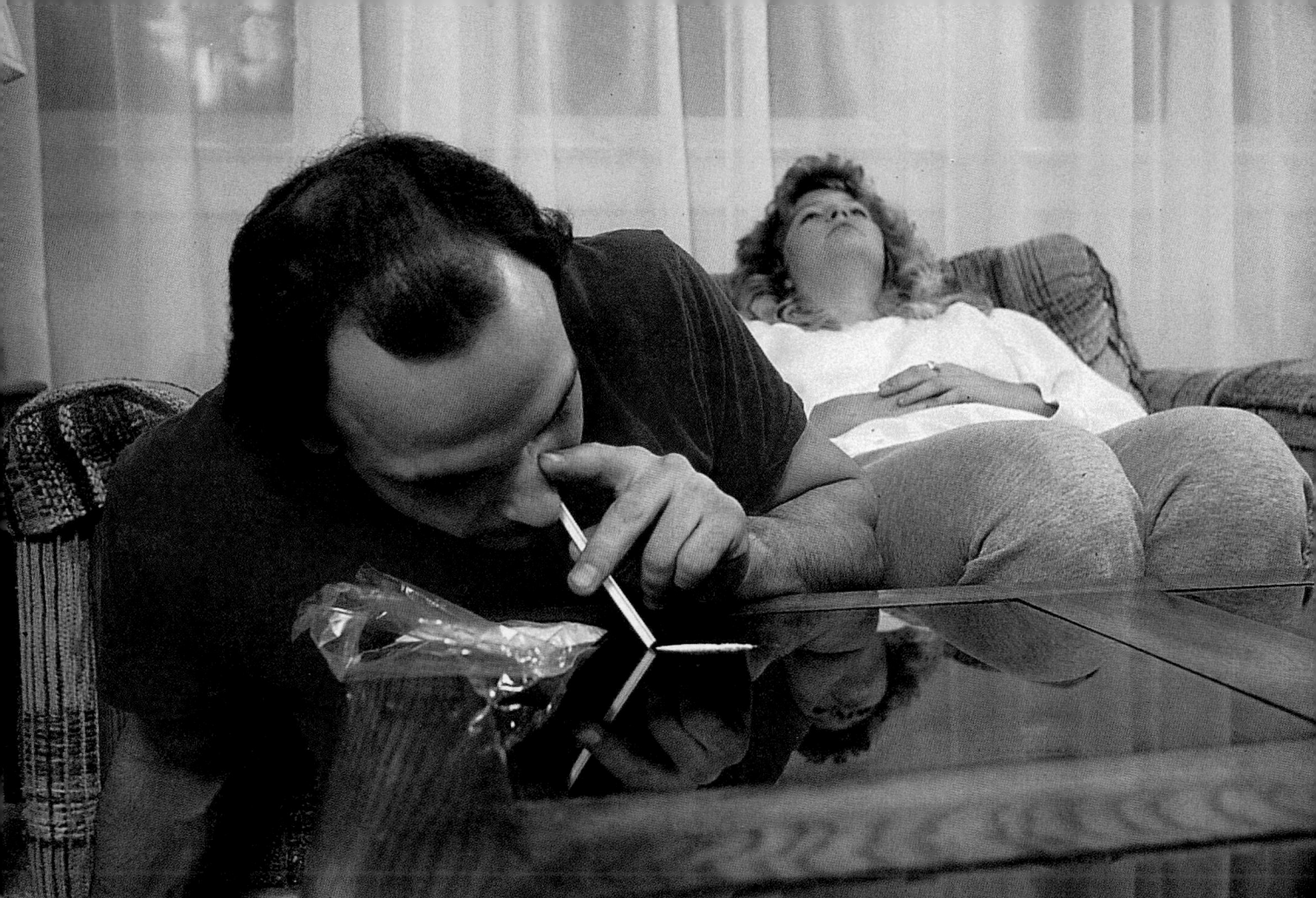

14

DRUGS IN AMERICAN FAMILIES AND SOCIETY

KNOWLEDGE

- Explain the characteristics of American society that promote substance abuse.
- Explain how family dynamics affect substance abuse and how substance abuse affects family dynamics.
- Describe the five survival roles assumed by some family members of drug abusers.
- Describe codependency and enabling behavior.
- Explain the psychological, cultural, and biological factors motivating use of psychoactive drugs.
- Describe the continuum of drug use from abstinence to overwhelming drug involvement.
- Explain why substance-abuse programs need to target young people.
- Identify signs of possible substance abuse in young people.
- Explain different approaches to substance-abuse prevention.
- Explain what is meant by intervention in substance abuse.
- Describe the different types of recovery programs.
- List the traits associated with a drug-free life-style.

INSIGHT

- Identify the role(s), if any, that psychoactive drugs play in your own life.
- Identify how your childhood family life has influenced you to use or avoid psychoactive drugs.
- Identify where you fit along the continuum of drug use.
- Identify any adverse effects (past, present, or future) that your own drug use may have or have had on your life.

DECISION MAKING

- Make a commitment to a drug-free life-style for yourself.
- Make a commitment to parent your children in ways that lower their risk of drug involvement.

orey Feldman began acting at the young age of 3, when he had his first professional gig in a Welch's grape juice advertisement. He grew up in Los Angeles with a father who was a musician and a mother who was a part-time cocktail waitress. As a young child, he felt that acting was an escape from his feelings of low self-worth. His parents split up when he was 11. He lived with one parent, then the other, then his grandparents. His near constant depression as a teenager was to some extent related to a feeling of being torn between his parents. Drug use began at age 14, with marijuana. While his acting career escalated as he starred in several movies (Stand by Me, The Lost Boys, The Goonies, to name a few), his drug-abuse experiences escalated as well. He began using alcohol and cocaine.

At age 15, he left his parents when he discovered that they had spent almost all of the money he had earned acting. At only 16 years of age, he was on his own, with lucrative movie contracts, and running with a fast crowd in Hollywood. He was soon introduced to heroin by a young man who Corey says abused him sexually. The heroin was a powerful escape for Corey; he became addicted to heroin and *cocaine. A turning point in his out-of-control life occurred when he was arrested for speeding and heroin and cocaine were discovered in his car. He spent that night in jail. Corey now recognizes that his arrest, and the ensuing embarrassing and painful publicity, was probably the best thing that could have happened to him. It might even have saved his life. He entered an intense rehabilitation program and committed himself to staying sober. At age 20, he is experiencing a new-found freedom from drugs and working to put his life in order. He admits that he occasionally has that urge to get high. However, he knows that he could end up back in jail, and for him, getting high is just not worth it. As he said, "I don't want to live in hell anymore."*

Corey Feldman's experiences reflect those of many who grow up in broken homes and feel the pressure of society to fit in and to be accepted. Fortunately, he was able to afford treatment and had the support of others who cared enough to push him in that direction. For many others, however, poverty, lack of support, and lack of available treatment programs combine to prevent the rehabilitation and starting over that Corey Feldman has been fortunate enough to be able to achieve.

Source: **People Weekly,** *1992 February 10, pp. 38–41.*

This, the first of four chapters on substance use and abuse, explores the behavioral side of the use of alcohol, tobacco, and other drugs. Emphasis will be on why people use and abuse drugs; how drug use affects and is affected by family dynamics; and the prevention, intervention, and treatment for drug abuse problems. The next chapter will examine the biological side of drug action and briefly survey some of the commonly used and abused substances. The final two chapters in this unit focus in on America's two most prevalent drug problems: tobacco and alcohol.

WHAT IS A DRUG?

A **drug** is any substance, other than a food, that modifies any function of the body. The word *drug*

can have different connotations depending on the context in which it is used. Often the word is laden with emotion—either positive or negative. A drug can be used to save your life or it can be abused and destroy your life.

We discuss many categories of drugs throughout this book: birth control pills, antibiotics, blood pressure medications, and cancer drugs, which are each covered in appropriate chapters. This unit, however, focuses on the **psychoactive** (*sī'kō-ak'-tiv*) **drugs:** those that affect moods, emotions, perceptions, and behavior and may be used specifically for their mind-altering effects. They are the drugs with the greatest potential for abuse and the development of dependency.

CHECKPOINT

1. Define the word *drug*.
2. What effects do psychoactive drugs have on the human mind?

DRUG USE AND ABUSE

Not everyone in our society agrees on what constitutes drug abuse. For example, though many people do not consider moderate alcohol consumption to be drug abuse, others believe that it is. In the case of other psychoactive drugs, there is also disagreement. While some people approve of moderate recreational use of these drugs, the majority of people believe that any nonmedical use constitutes abuse.

Even drug experts have different views on what constitutes abuse. Some typical definitions include the following:

- Drug abuse is drug use that is not consistent with accepted medical practice. This could be in terms of dosage, administration (whether the drug is taken orally or injected), or your reason for taking it.
- Drug abuse occurs when a drug is taken for some purpose that the drug cannot fulfill (such as using a drug in an effort to solve your problems).

drug any substance, other than a food, that modifies any function of the body.

psychoactive drugs drugs that affect moods, emotions, perceptions, and behavior and may be used specifically for their mind-altering effects.

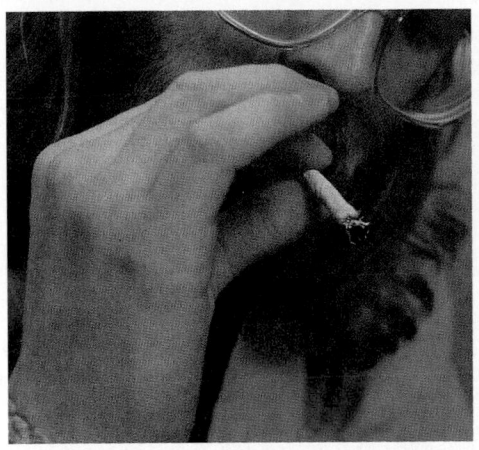 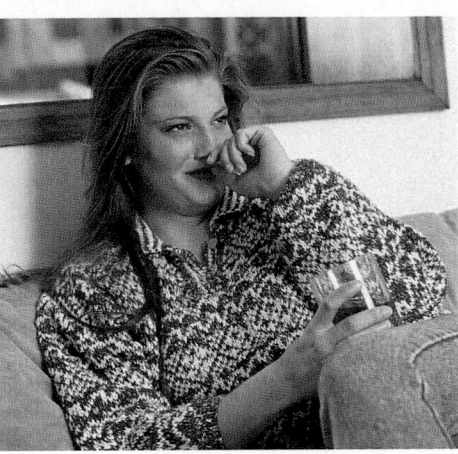

What is drug abuse? Does either, both, or neither of these photos represent drug abuse?

- Drug abuse is using a drug that threatens your health, family relations, social relations, educational progress, job efficiency, economic well-being, or that causes you to have legal difficulties (defining drug abuse not in terms of dosage or frequency of use, but in terms of potential effects on your life).

In addition to these definitions, see In Your Hands: Evaluating Your Own Drug Use, on p. 434, which helps clarify the distinction between drug use and drug abuse. Take a minute right now to complete this assessment.

CHECKPOINT

1. What are three definitions of drug abuse?
2. Which of these most closely represents your view?

DRUGS IN AMERICAN SOCIETY: AN OVERVIEW

Throughout our four chapters on substance use and abuse, our focus will be on the relationships of social and family structure to substance abuse. Richard Fields, Director of Family and Addiction Conferences and Educational/Counseling Services in Bellevue, Washington, has identified some characteristics of American society that promote the unhealthful use of alcohol and other drugs:[1]

- *Powerful drive to seek pleasure and avoid pain at almost any cost.* We see this value demonstrated every day of the year in ads for nonprescription (and increasingly for prescription) medications offering instant re-

lief for every ailment. The message: No one should have to suffer the slightest pain or inconvenience.

- *Unrewarding and **dysfunctional** (functioning with difficulty) relationships between spouses, parents and children, friends, neighbors, and co-workers.* Rather than working through problems in relationships, we seek to reduce the pain caused by our relationships by using alcohol and other drugs.

- *Widespread physical inactivity and lack of a regular, balanced exercise program.* Regular exercise is an excellent pain reliever and has many mental benefits that reduce your desire to use psychoactive drugs.

- *Inability to "self-entertain" by means such as enjoying nature, taking a long walk, meditating, or quietly reading a good book.* We need to be constantly entertained by TV, parties, or chemically induced mental states. True happiness comes from within.

- *Tendency to be self-centered and uninvolved in altruistic activities that promote self-esteem and other positive feelings.* When we focus entirely on ourselves, every minor physical and emotional pain becomes magnified and we may seek to reduce such pain through chemical means. Doing for others provides abundant rewards and helps us keep our own pains and problems in perspective.

- *Narrowly focused lives.* Being involved in a variety of friendships, interests, hobbies, and

....

dysfunctional functioning with difficulty.

IN YOUR HANDS

EVALUATING YOUR OWN DRUG USE

Answer each question with yes, no, or maybe. Whenever the word drug *appears, remember that alcohol and tobacco are drugs.*

1. Do you use drugs because of feelings of hopelessness? _____
2. Do you use drugs because you feel lonely? _____
3. Do you use drugs because you are angry or frustrated? _____
4. Do you use drugs to build up courage? _____
5. Do you use drugs to get you through the day? _____
6. Are you unable to enjoy a party if drugs are not present? _____
7. Do you prefer the company of people who use drugs? _____
8. Do you think you are more fun to be with when you are using drugs? _____
9. Do you feel more competent when you are using drugs? _____
10. Do you have difficulty finishing projects because of drugs? _____
11. Have you gotten low grades at school because of drugs? _____
12. Have drugs created problems in any of your relationships with other people? _____
13. Have you had any legal problems because of drugs? _____
14. Have you had any financial problems because of drugs? _____
15. Have you had any medical problems because of drugs? _____
16. Do you worry about being caught with drugs in your possession? _____
17. Do you feel physically or mentally bad following drug use? _____
18. Do you use one drug to counteract any unpleasant or undesired effects of another drug? _____
19. Do you have any close relatives who have chemical dependency problems?[a] _____
20. Do you sometimes feel guilty about your drug use? _____

There is no definite scale to this inventory. If you answered yes or maybe to one or more questions, please give serious consideration to the possibility that drugs may be creating problems in your life. There are many effective ways to reduce or eliminate the impact of drugs on your life.

[a]The tendency toward chemical dependency has been shown to have genetic elements. If you answered yes to this question and one or more of the other questions, you should be aware that you are at above-average risk of developing a chemical dependency.

activities provides the positive mental state that many of us seek through chemicals.

- *Ongoing feelings of anger, anxiety, or depression.* Rather than attacking the sources of these feelings, perhaps through talking them out with a friend or counselor, we try to block out these painful feelings chemically.

- *Feelings of lack of meaning in life.* Many of us experience a general feeling of despair because we see no meaning or value in our work, relationships, or elsewhere in our lives. This often is the result of an inability to transcend ourselves and develop a feeling of

connection to humanity and the world in which we live. Some people use drugs in an effort to gain insights and add a sense of meaning to their lives.

- *Tendency to deny that there is a problem.* Members of even the most dysfunctional families often deny that there is any problem. People with severe chemical dependency problems usually deny that they have a problem. And on a broad social and political scale, we deny that there are characteristics of U.S. society and family life that promote drug abuse. Thus, the government has traditionally focused its efforts on reducing the supply of drugs, rather than on programs that would effectively reduce the demand.

MULTICULTURAL PERSPECTIVES

Drug abuse cuts across all boundaries of race and ethnicity. Present knowledge of alcohol and other drug use patterns among specific ethnic groups is limited. Most studies have been school-based and focused on younger people; less is known about use patterns of adults of each gender and of special populations such as recent immigrants, the homeless, and pregnant women within each ethnic group.[2]

Much of what we think we know about drug use in various ethnic groups may be inaccurate. Researchers and counselors must consider the values, norms, life conditions, history, heritage, and adaptive challenges of each group. There has been some tendency to consider the values and behavior of middle-class, white, non-Hispanic Americans as the norm against which to judge other ethnic groups. Differences between other groups and such white Americans are often attributed to economic and social oppression. The assumption has been that if oppression were eliminated, the other groups would become more like whites. A cross-cultural approach that views behaviors of individuals in terms of the values and traditions of their ethnic groups would probably lead to development of more culturally relevant and, thus, more effective drug-abuse-prevention programs.[3]

CHECKPOINT

1. What nine characteristics of U.S. society promote the unhealthful use of alcohol and other drugs?

2. Which of these relate to you personally?

3. In what ways do you think your ethnic affiliation(s) has influenced your attitudes about alcohol and other drugs?

FAMILY DYNAMICS OF SUBSTANCE-ABUSE PROBLEMS

Having an alcohol or other drug abuser in a family is among the most disruptive influences on family life. Every member of the family feels the effects of the problem and is powerfully influenced by it. This is true whether the abuser is an adult or a younger member of the family. Throughout this unit we will be emphasizing how family life affects and is affected by the abuse of alcohol and other drugs. The following are some of the ideas we will be examining:

- Chemically dependent people exhibit many chemically induced behavioral changes. Other family members may not fully attribute these behaviors to the substance abuse, but instead may believe that they are in some way responsible. This leads to feelings of embarrassment, shame, fear, confusion, anger, and guilt. These other family members may, in fact, develop behaviors as impaired as those of the drug abuser. Therefore, family life becomes severely dysfunctional.

- Dysfunctional families are *not* uncommon in the United States. Richard Fields[4] estimates that only 20 percent of U.S. families function well; 30 percent are somewhat dysfunctional; and 50 percent are severely dysfunctional.

- Most members of dysfunctional (Fields prefers the term *imbalanced*) families deny that there is any problem in their family. Parents with alcohol or other drug problems deny that their behavior has any impact on their children. Other family members deny their feelings of shame, abandonment, and rejection.

- Many U.S. parents are severely deficient in parenting skills. They expect too much or too little of their children because they have no idea of what is appropriate behavior for their child's age. They practice damaging or ineffective disciplining techniques, with behavioral boundaries that are too rigid, too loose, inconsistent, or ambiguous.

- The longer a family denies it has problems, the more vulnerable its members become to abuse of alcohol or other drugs. Children of chemically dependent parents are at a four- to eightfold increased risk of becoming chemically dependent themselves.[5]

- Children who grow up being physically, emotionally, or sexually abused are at increased risk of chemical dependency.

Chemical dependency and family dysfunction form a vicious cycle in which each contributes to the other.

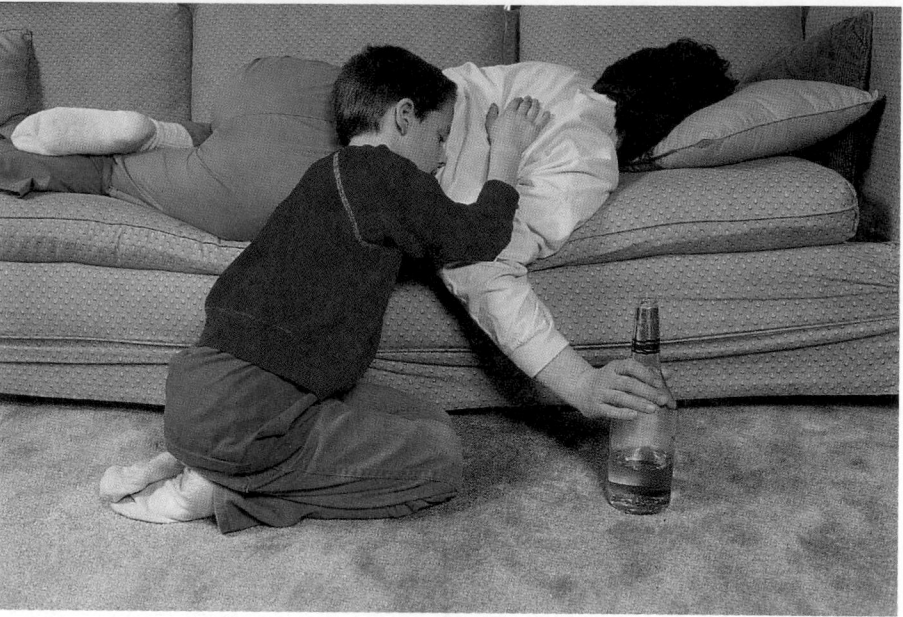

Most substance-abuse counselors take a **family systems approach** to therapy. This approach views a family as a system that seeks to maintain balance, with other family members altering their behavior in an attempt to compensate for the altered behavior of the chemically dependent person. When a substance abuser is part of a family, the prospects for his or her long-term recovery from dependency are influenced by family factors such as *enabling* (see p. 438). If only the abuser enters recovery, and other family members do no recovery work, the dysfunctional family system will not change. Continuing the same old dysfunctional styles of family interaction places the recovering family member at great risk for relapse into substance abuse or the development of a new dysfunctional behavior.

RELUCTANCE OF FAMILY MEMBERS TO PARTICIPATE IN RECOVERY

Family members may avoid becoming involved in the recovery of a chemically dependent family member for several reasons:

- They may fear getting in touch with painful feelings that have been repressed and might

family systems approach an approach to therapy that views a family as a system that seeks to maintain balance, with other family members altering their behavior in an attempt to compensate for the altered behavior of the chemically dependent person.

seem overwhelming if brought to the surface (see Communication for Wellness: Family Patterns of Communication).

- They may resist looking at their own behavior and any role it may play in the family's difficulties.
- They may believe that if the substance abuser would just stop using alcohol or other drugs then everything would be OK.
- They may fear that the family unit could not survive an examination of its difficulties and that the result would be one or more members leaving the family. In any case, it is essential for the entire family to become involved in recovery. Old, ineffective, or damaging methods of family interaction need to be revised. Recovery from chemical dependency is a long-term process that can seldom succeed without the active participation of the entire family unit.

CHECKPOINT

1. What is a dysfunctional family?
2. What roles does denial play in dysfunctional families?
3. Why are other family members often reluctant to participate in the recovery of a chemically dependent family member?

FAMILY PATTERNS OF COMMUNICATION

Virginia Satir's[a] theories on communication within families are widely applied in substance abuse counseling and in family counseling. She identifies the following four dysfunctional communication styles:

1. *Placaters* Placaters *discount themselves* in order to avoid conflict and the anger of other family members. They agree with anything or do anything in order to avoid conflict. Their self-esteem is very low. Placaters feel trapped in dependent, dysfunctional relationships because they see no way out.

2. *Blamers* Blamers elevate themselves by *discounting others*. They try to avoid looking at themselves and their own responsibility in the family situation. The feelings, opinions, and abilities of others are discounted. Blamers are critical, judgmental, and place blame and shame on others.

3. *Intellectualizers* Intellectualizers *discount their own feelings*. They try to avoid painful feelings by being rational, intellectual, and nonemotional. Their communication deals with logic rather than feelings. Intellectualizers hope to solve family problems by ignoring their feelings and those of others, but it never works because feelings are real, valid, important, and won't go away just because they are ignored.

4. *Distracters* Distracters *discount context*. They are escape artists. They try to keep themselves and others away from painful feelings by distracting attention away from the real family issues. Their communication is confusing and irrelevant. This pattern of communication is common among chemically dependent people who want to distract attention from their dependency.

Satir describes healthy family communication as "**leveling**," meaning when your words, actions, nonverbal communication, and feelings are all consistent with each other. It is, in essence, *honest communication*. Only with honest communication, in which feelings are freely revealed, can families become functional. At first this kind of communication seems painful and threatening, but as feelings that have been concealed for years are brought forth, many families, for the first time ever, begin to provide the nurturing and support needed. Only with honest communication can the chemical dependency or other individual problem be dealt with in any lasting beneficial way.

[a]Satir, V. *Conjoint Family Therapy.* Palo Alto, CA: Science Behavior Books, 1967. Satir, V., Stachowiak, J., and Taschman, H. *Helping Families to Change.* Northvale, NJ: Aronson, Jason, 1976; Satir, V., and Baldwin, M. *Satir—Step by Step—A Guide to Creating Change in Families.* Northvale, NJ: Aronson, Jason, 1983.

FAMILY SURVIVAL ROLES

When one or both parents in a family are chemically dependent, there are powerful effects on every family member. One widely accepted model of family adjustment to dependency has been proposed by Sharon Wegscheider-Cruse.[6] According to this model, in order to survive in a dysfunctional family, each member may adopt a "role" in family interaction. Please understand, however, that the roles Wegscheider-Cruse described are just some of the possible roles and should never be used to stereotype a person. Most members of families of abusers of alcohol or other drugs exhibit traits from several or even all of the roles and may fall into different roles in different situations. Wegscheider-Cruse's roles include the following:

1. *Chief enabler.* **Enabling** behavior, discussed on p. 438, is any behavior that in any way allows or makes it easier for another person to continue substance abuse or other undesirable behavior. The chief enabler assumes primary responsibility for the chemically dependent family member. The chief enabler makes excuses to the user's boss and friends, bails the user out of jail, supplies the user with money, shields the user from crises, and so on. The chief enabler will often be a spouse or equivalent, but can be an offspring.

2. *Family hero.* The family hero is the "good kid." He or she excels at school, never gets in trouble, assumes responsibility for the family's sense of worth. Everything is done for the family, but at a great personal cost. Personal feelings and needs are ignored. Despite apparent success, the family hero continues to feel empty inside and, as an adult, will be vulnerable to chemical dependency and may have difficulties in relationships.

3. *Family scapegoat.* A scapegoat is a person who bears the blame for others. The role of the family scapegoat is to divert attention away from

enabling any behavior that in any way allows or makes it easier for another person to continue substance abuse or other undesirable behavior.

leveling honest communication.

the family's real problem, such as a parent's alcoholism. The scapegoat does this by his or her own misbehavior, which might include behavioral problems at school or at home or alcohol or other drug abuse. The other family members then can blame the scapegoat for all of the family's problems.

4. *Lost child*. The lost child becomes almost invisible in the family. The lost child tries to decrease the family's pain by taking on the pain of the other family members. The lost child tends to be very quiet, denying his or her feelings and needs, and becoming emotionally isolated from other family members. Because of their isolation and unexpressed feelings, lost children are at risk of chemical dependency, emotional breakdown, and suicide.

5. *Family mascot*. Like the scapegoat, the family mascot tries to divert attention away from the real family issues and family pain. The mascot does this through being funny and silly. In school, he or she may be the class clown. Unfortunately, the mascot lacks self-esteem and, as an adult, may feel unworthy of being loved by a fully functional person. He or she, like other family members, is likely to find a relationship with a chemically dependent or otherwise "damaged" person.

ENABLING

Enabling, as previously defined, is any behavior that in any way allows or makes it easier for another person to continue substance abuse or other undesirable behavior. There are various motivations for enabling. Sometimes it is motivated by love, sometimes by fear or guilt, and sometimes as a way of keeping the chemically dependent person in an impaired condition, perhaps so he or she will be less likely to leave or form a new relationship. Even when enabling is motivated by love, it is doing the chemically dependent person no favor, as it only serves to prolong the dependency. Charles Nelson[7] described five forms of enabling behavior:

1. *Any behavior that prevents the user from experiencing the full impact of his or her drug use.* This would include calling in "sick" for the user, shielding the user from a situation that would send him or her into therapy or into legal difficulty, making excuses for the user, or bailing him or her out of jail.

2. *Any behavior that attempts to take control over the user's drinking or other drug use.* This would include hiding or throwing away the user's alcohol or other drugs or his or her paraphernalia, threatening to hurt the user or self if she or he does not quit using, using sex or other favors as a bargaining tool to control drinking or other drug use, and screaming or crying to try to make the user quit. Although such controlling behaviors might seem to be the opposite of enabling, they are ineffective because they move the locus of control over the substance abuse away from the abuser. Only when the control lies within the abuser can substance abuse be overcome effectively.

3. *Any behavior that attempts to take over the user's personal responsibilities.* This would include taking a second job to make up for money that is going for alcohol or other drugs, covering the user's debts, waiting hand and foot on the user, making sure the user gets to work or takes care of other responsibilities, or missing work or school to take care of responsibilities the user is neglecting.

4. *Any behavior that communicates an acceptance of or rationalization for the alcohol or other drug abuse.* Examples include believing or communicating that the user "really doesn't use that much" of the substance or believing or communicating that the substance abuse is in some way beneficial to the user or to the family.

5. *Any behavior that contributes to the user's supply of drugs.* Examples include providing the substance itself, giving the user money that is likely to go to purchase the substance, and selling or helping in any way with the sale of drugs.

Enabling only serves to prolong the user's dependency and the family's dysfunction. Sometimes it is painful for the enabler to accept that his or her behavior is harming rather than helping the user, but the enabling must stop before the user and family can begin their recovery.

CODEPENDENCY

Codependency is a term that has become quite popular for describing the effects of chemical dependency on family members of a substance

....

codependency the effects of chemical dependency on family members of a substance abuser.

abuser. *Codependent* is the term used for the affected individual. If the substance being abused is alcohol, the term *coalcoholism* or *para-alcoholism* is sometimes used.[8]

There is no single definition for codependency. Some people define the term broadly to mean the simple fact of being a family member of a chemically dependent person. This definition is based on the belief that there is no way a family member can avoid being affected by the presence of chemical dependency in the family.

Other authorities[9, 10] believe that such labeling of every family member can itself be damaging, as some family members do develop effective coping strategies and suffer little from their codependency. Following the lead of Timmen Cermak,[11] some experts prefer to use the term codependency only when specific behavioral criteria characterize the family member of a substance abuser. Cermak defines codependency in terms of the following five criteria:

1. Basing your self-esteem on the ability to influence or control your own and others' feelings and behaviors in the face of obvious adverse consequences.

2. Assumption of responsibility for meeting others' needs to the exclusion of (and with the denial of) your own needs.

3. Anxiety and boundary distortions regarding intimacy and separation.

4. Enmeshment in relationships with chemically dependent, codependent, or personality-disordered people.

5. Maintaining a primary relationship with an active substance abuser for two years or longer without seeking counseling or other outside support, *and/or* three or more of the following:

- excessive reliance on denial
- constriction (holding in) of emotions
- depression
- hypervigilance (constantly watching for danger)
- compulsive behaviors
- anxiety
- substance abuse
- being a past or current victim of physical or sexual abuse
- stress-related illnesses

Codependency and enabling are separate, though often related, behaviors. Codependent people may or may not also be enablers. Frequently, through the use of denial, the codependent begins to accept the substance abuse as normal behavior and may participate in the family's elaborate system of rationalization to explain the substance abuse and its consequences.

Chemically dependent people tend to pass the blame for their problems on to others and true codependents tend to accept that blame. The outcome of this is to delay the intervention (see p. 451) that is needed to get the substance abuser into recovery. The substance abuser often holds other family members as psychological hostages by threatening them with all kinds of tragedies—suicides, abandonment, beatings, and so forth—unless the abuser gets his or her way.

Living with this oppression, codependents may develop emotional and spiritual deterioration and stress-related physical disorders such as asthma, allergies, ulcers, and high blood pressure.

Codependents often assume a martyr role, becoming selfless to the point of hurting themselves by giving service to other family members or friends, without taking care of their own human needs. They feel no internal sense of self-esteem, but depend on their relationships to provide them with some sense of self-worth. Thus, they will do almost anything to maintain a relationship.[12]

Codependents tend to develop relationships that provide opportunities for martyrdom, but little growth. Often, these relationships are with chemically dependent or otherwise dysfunctional people. Because of his or her own psychological abandonment, the codependent partner tends to take on the other's unhappiness, depression, anxiety, fears, or confusion. Because the effects of codependency can be lifelong, counseling is often needed to provide the insights and new behaviors necessary for the codependent to develop rewarding, functional relationships (see Adult Children of Alcoholics on p. 454).

SOCIAL ISOLATION

Most families of alcohol or other drug abusers are deprived of needed social interaction for a variety of reasons. There may not be money for participation in recreational or other social activities. The children may be ashamed or forbidden to bring friends home because of the presence of the

Social isolation is characteristic of family members of substance abusers. Children are often ashamed or forbidden to bring friends home because of the family's impairment.

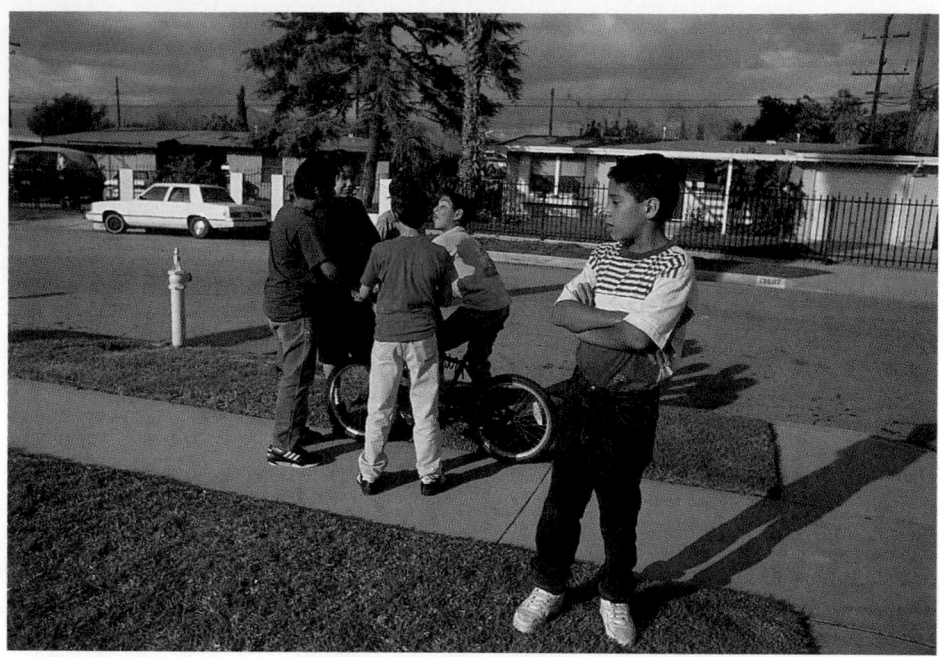

impaired parent. A couple may avoid parties, or may not be invited, because of the likelihood of unpleasant alcohol-induced behavior.

Inadequate social interaction causes problems beyond just the lack of companionship. Family members develop a sense of shame, as if the substance abuse somehow were a personal reflection on them. In fact, other children can be quite cruel to the children of substance abusers if they are aware of the problem. The sense of isolation becomes intense and often leads to deeply ingrained psychological problems.

SUBSTANCE ABUSERS' MARRIAGES

Many studies indicate that while a non-substance-abusing woman will often remain with a substance-abusing man, serving as his enabler, the reverse is seldom true.[13] When a man remains with a substance-abusing woman, he also is likely to be dependent on alcohol or another drug. If two substance-abusing partners stay together, the potential for recovery for either of them as individuals is not promising unless both work at recovery.

CHECKPOINT

1. What does enabling mean?

2. Name and describe each of Sharon Wegscheider-Cruse's five family survival roles.

3. Give five examples of enabling behaviors.

4. What are two meanings of the term *codependency?*

5. What are Cermak's five behavioral characteristics of codependent people?

WHY PEOPLE USE AND ABUSE PSYCHOACTIVE DRUGS

At a superficial level, the reason people use psychoactive drugs seems simple: It's fun, enjoyable, stimulating, and relaxing. At a greater depth, however, drug use and abuse can be viewed from many different perspectives. Biological, psychological, cultural, legal, ethical, political, and economic factors are all involved. Drug use can rarely, if ever, be attributed to just one cause. Let's look at some of the more important motivating factors of psychoactive drug use.

PSYCHOLOGICAL FACTORS

Human use and abuse of psychoactive drugs is certainly not a recent development. Throughout recorded history, people have experimented with various plants and chemicals in search of something to make life seem more pleasant.

Today some people still see drugs as the best means of relief from pain (physical or emotional), boredom, frustration, loneliness, anxiety, depression, and every other form of unhappiness. Further, some believe that drugs promise a higher level of pleasure or consciousness than is otherwise possible. The fact that psychoactive drugs only temporarily produce the effects for which they are taken, then often produce the opposite effects, and the fact that the desired effects often become increasingly difficult to repeat, have not discouraged people from seeking pleasure through drugs.

Self-esteem

One factor that contributes to substance abuse is the lack of self-esteem. People who feel a sense of shame about themselves may try to block it out by abusing alcohol or other drugs. People with poor self-esteem are less concerned with the harmful effects of substance abuse. This disregard for the inherent risks of drug abuse, such as injuries, AIDS, and overdoses, is self-destructive behavior. These people need expert counseling as well as support from their friends and family. If parents want to help "drug-proof" their children, one of the most useful things they can do is to contribute to the development of their children's self-esteem by praising them and making them feel loved and valuable as individuals. Schools, too, can help fight substance abuse through policies and programs that are concerned with the self-esteem of every student.

Dependency-prone Personality?

The importance of dependency-prone personality types remains controversial. Over the years, many efforts have been made to describe a certain personality type that increases the likelihood of chemical dependency. Some of the personality traits that have been associated with dependency-proneness have included difficulty in handling frustration, a need for immediate gratification, difficulty relating to others, low self-esteem, impulsiveness, and a resistance to authority.

The problem with this hypothetical dependency-prone personality is that many drug dependent people lack some or all of these traits, while many people who have such traits do not become dependent. In prospective studies, in which people's personalities have been evaluated and follow-

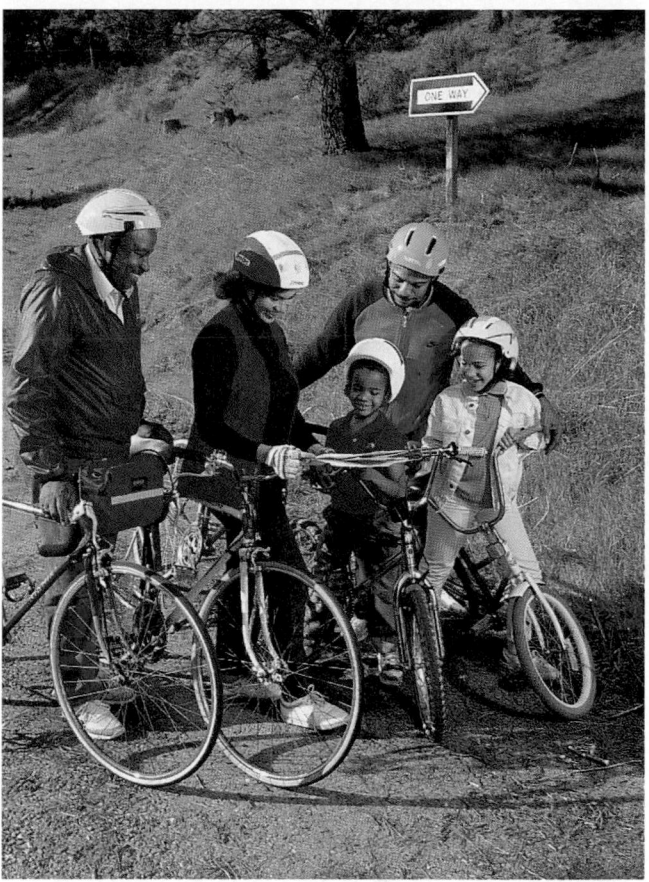

If parents want to help "drug-proof" their children, one of the most useful things they can do is to contribute to the development of their children's self-esteem by praising them and making them feel loved and valuable as individuals.

up checks for chemical dependency made years later, it has been impossible to predict which people will develop chemical dependencies.[14]

SOCIAL AND CULTURAL FACTORS

Cultural influences affect drug use, just as they affect every aspect of our lives. Some specific factors we will discuss include our society's attitudes toward drugs, peer influences, and the mass media.

Cultural Attitudes Regarding Drugs

While psychoactive drugs are abused worldwide, certain attitudes prevail in the United States that contribute to our drug problems. Among these are the following:

- the belief that there should be a drug to solve every problem
- a readiness to use drugs as problem solvers

- the expectation of a "quick fix" for any problem
- the belief that alcohol is not a drug

In general, our society is ambivalent and hypocritical about drugs. On the one hand, a large portion of society doesn't approve of the user of illicit or "street" drugs; at the same time, the concept of the "miracle drug" is held dear. The same person who takes tranquilizers at dosages much higher than prescribed by his or her physician may be highly vocal in pushing for stricter drug laws and enforcement.

Multicultural Perspectives

These comments generalize U.S. beliefs regarding alcohol and other drugs. Specific attitudes, however, are influenced by ethnic and socioeconomic affiliations as well as by age group. For example, different drugs tend to be prevalent within different ethnic groups, with more favorable views being held of the more familiar drugs.

In some cultures, such as certain Native American nations, specific substances, such as peyote (see p. 484) play clearly defined, ritualistic roles in spiritual/religious ceremonies. These substances are held sacred and are used very differently than the same substances might be used by members of other cultures. Such ritualistic use is far removed from "recreational" use and should not be viewed as substance abuse.

Drug Subcultures

We often hear about "the" drug subculture as if it were a single entity. In reality, there is not just one drug subcultural group, but many of them.[15] Some are characterized by ethnicity; for example there are white, African American, Asian American, and Hispanic drug subcultures. Some are characterized by age group; there are high school, college, young adult, and older adult drug subcultures. Finally, there are subcultures revolving around specific drugs, such as the alcohol subculture, the marijuana subculture, the cocaine subculture, and so on. Some experts emphasize the role of the subculture in perpetuating drug abuse, noting that the subculture provides peer support for drug use and helps ensure the uninterrupted supply of a drug.[16]

Peer Influence

Peer pressure influences everyone's behavior in ways that can be either positive or negative. For young people, peer pressure is especially strong. One welcome trend in many regions is the increasing peer pressure *not* to use drugs. In some peer groups, however, part of the price of admission to the group is using alcohol and/or other psychoactive drugs. The use of alcohol or other drugs has become a "rite of passage" in some parts of our society, in a sense comparable to the initiation rites of preindustrial societies.

The very fact that using psychoactive drugs other than alcohol and tobacco is counter to the laws and conventions of adult society and thus involves risk-taking, makes it an appealing entrance requirement for some peer groups. For minors, this risk-taking is also true for alcohol and tobacco. Risk-taking offers a thrill that may initially be more rewarding than the effects of the drug used. It also forms a common bond between members of the drug-using group. Effective drug-abuse-prevention programs must address this important motivation for drug use. Peer pressure can work just as effectively against drug use as for it.

Influence of Popular Media and Advertising

Over the years, many films, TV programs, and popular songs have glorified the abuse of alcohol and other drugs. When the associated risks are mentioned, the risk-taking behavior is often glorified. Antidrug groups are exerting pressure to discourage glorification of drug abuse; however, there are still numerous songs and films that do the opposite.

Advertising is an especially powerful tool for promoting alcohol and tobacco use. Almost every possible medium is used, from billboards to skywriting. Advertisers are always quick to state that they are not trying to encourage people to drink or smoke, only to buy their brand. But drinking and smoking are portrayed as being positive and social, with a special effort often made to appeal to young people. Models used in alcohol and tobacco advertising often look young, sexy, popular, and healthy, and often appear to be involved in sports. Alcohol and tobacco are portrayed as being part of an exciting, sophisticated life-style.

Advertising is increasingly "targeted" to catch the attention of specific groups. Much alcohol and tobacco advertising is targeted at young people and African American or Hispanic ethnic groups. Neighborhoods with large African American or Hispanic populations almost always contain billboards with targeted messages promoting alcohol and tobacco. Twenty-four hours a day the message is: smoke and drink.

Malt liquors, which feature a high alcohol content at a low price, are especially targeted at African Americans and Hispanics. Malt liquor ads not-too-subtly emphasize the high alcohol content of these products and tell young men that drinking them is the key to fun and sexual success.[17] This is a powerful message that is hard to ignore.

BIOLOGICAL FACTORS

Biological explanations for chemical dependencies are gaining favor among authorities.[18–22] Many cases of alcoholism and other chemical dependency can now be traced to inherited deficiencies or other disorders in certain brain chemicals.

To trace the development of this theory briefly, it was first noticed that alcoholism and other chemical dependencies seemed to run along family lines. Chemically dependent parents often pro-

duced chemically dependent children. This in itself did not prove any genetic basis for chemical dependency, as the environmental influence of being raised by chemically dependent parents might well lead to chemical dependency in the offspring. Recent research has provided evidence that both heredity and environment are involved in the development of chemical dependency.

Twin studies have been useful in quantifying the genetic component in many human conditions.[23, 24] Comparisons are made of the rate of occurrence of a specific trait, such as alcoholism, in pairs of identical twins versus pairs of fraternal twins. This type of information helps separate the genetic component of a behavior from the environmental influences on that behavior. If genetics were to play a role in the condition, then the condition should occur much more frequently among both members of a pair of identical twins, who have identical genes, than among both members of a pair of fraternal twins, who share only some genes. This is what has been observed in studies of alcoholism among both male and female twins.[25]

Researchers at Virginia Commonwealth University studied 1300 pairs of female twins and found that if one member of a set of identical twins had a problem with alcohol, her twin was four to five times more likely to have the same problem than

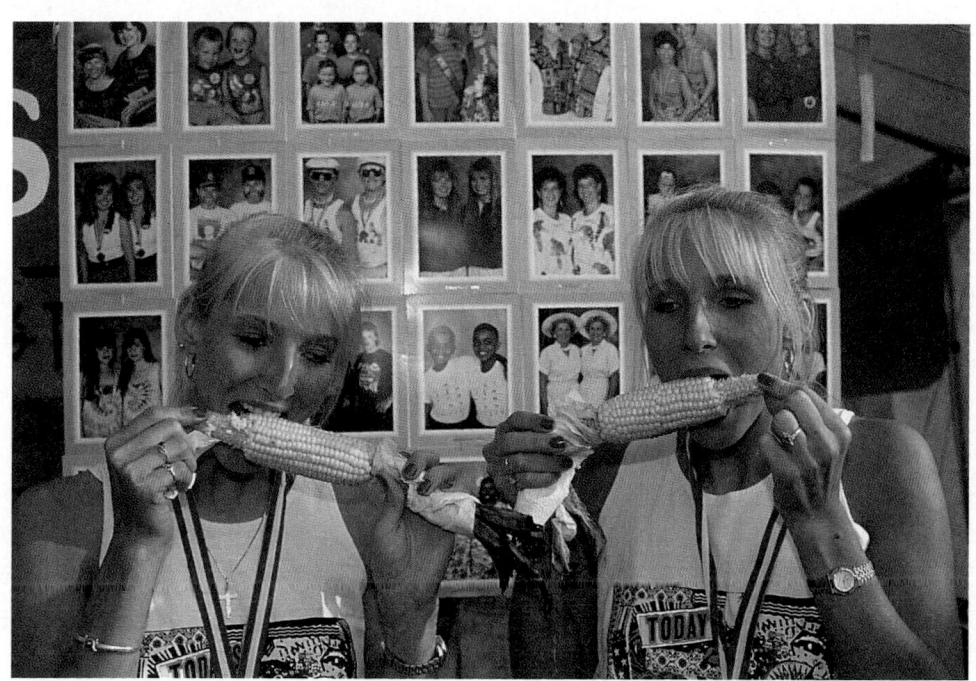

Through studies of identical (such as these) versus fraternal twins, researchers have concluded that genes control 50 to 60 percent of a woman's susceptibility to alcoholism.

were women in the general population. If one member of a set of fraternal twins had an alcohol problem, the second twin was only one-and-a-half to two times as likely as other women to have the problem. It was concluded that genes control 50–60 percent of a woman's susceptibility to alcoholism, with cultural and environmental factors accounting for the rest. Other studies have shown similar results for males. This means that genes are very important in determining susceptibility to alcoholism, but do not dictate completely whether you will or will not become an alcoholic.[26]

Studies of children raised as adoptees have also been useful in clarifying the role of heredity in the risk of alcoholism. Among adopted children, sons of alcoholic biological fathers have shown about three times the rate of alcoholism as sons of nonalcoholic biological fathers. Similarly, daughters of alcoholic mothers have shown about three times the alcoholism rate of daughters of nonalcoholic mothers. Alcoholism in the parent of the other gender also increased the risk of alcoholism, but not to the degree that alcoholism in the parent of the same gender did.[27]

Animal studies have revealed a genetic element in the preference for alcohol among mice. Using selective breeding, strains of mice might show either a strong preference for or an aversion to alcohol. This difference in alcohol preference can then be associated with a difference in the brain cells' receptor sites for alcohol.[28] Brain cells of alco-hol-loving mice have more alcohol receptors than do the brain cells of alcohol-avoiding mice.

Studies of human brain chemistry have further confirmed the presence of inherited brain differences between people who do and do not become alcoholic.[29, 30] Alcoholism and other chemical dependencies have been related to deficiencies in brain chemicals such as the endorphins. Alcoholism, specifically, has been related to a deficiency in an enzyme found throughout the body that converts acetaldehyde (the toxic first breakdown product of alcohol) to harmless carbon dioxide and water.

It would be erroneous to conclude, however, that every alcoholic carries genes for alcoholism. Numerous alcoholics have no alcoholic relatives and many children of alcoholic parents have no problem with alcoholism. It is still valid to think that many cases of alcoholism arise from psychological, social, and cultural causes, rather than genetic ones (see Feature 14.1).

Hereditary factors do not appear to motivate your first use of alcohol or any other drug *directly;* for example, someone who has never tasted alcohol does not feel an inherited craving for a drink. People with certain inherited characteristics, however, may be more likely than other people to find the effects of alcohol or other drugs to be especially pleasant. Others may experience a rebound effect (see p. 468) that is much greater than that of other people. This could contribute to a rapid development of chemical dependency.

FEATURE 14.1

"DON'T BLAME ME—IT'S IN MY GENES"

In emphasizing the role of genetics in chemical dependency, it is important to realize that even though genetics is important, *it is not the whole story.* Other factors are also quite important in determining who does and does not become chemically dependent.

As more is learned about the genetic elements in chemical dependency, we can expect accurate tests to become available to identify those who are at greatest risk. Effective and ethical ways of counseling these people will have to be developed. To be of value, detection and counseling will be needed at a very young age, as many people become chemically dependent during or even prior to adolescence.

There are several implications of the theory that chemical dependency has a genetic basis. First, it helps legitimize, in the minds of many people, the concept of chemical depen-

dency as a disease. For some chemically dependent people, this makes it easier to acknowledge and seek help for their dependency because they view it as a health problem, rather than as a lack of willpower.

At the same time, there are those who will probably use the disease concept as a rationalization for their continued drug use: "It's not my fault I do drugs, it's in my genes." These people need to understand that just as people with diabetes are responsible for taking care of themselves even though their disease may be genetic, so is the person who carries the genetic tendency toward chemical dependency. Whether chemical dependency is primarily psychological, sociological, or biological in its origin, the responsibility for its prevention or recovery ultimately lies with the individual.

One theory is that some people tend not to "feel good" because of an inherited low endorphin level. These people are more depressed than other people, less tolerant of pain, and able to tolerate less frustration than other people. According to this theory, alcohol or other psychoactive drugs make these people feel *very good;* but the rebound effect, as drugs wear off, makes them feel *very bad.*[31] This creates a powerful compulsion for repeated drug use and a high risk of chemical dependency.

CHECKPOINT

1. What is the relationship of self-esteem to drug use?

2. How valid is the concept of the dependency-prone personality?

3. What are four cultural attitudes that contribute to drug problems?

4. What types of evidence point to a genetic factor in chemical dependency?

PATTERNS OF DRUG USE AND ABUSE

Before discussing any specific patterns of drug use, we must emphasize that every person is unique and has his or her own pattern of drug use. We can gain some insights, however, by generalizing some drug use patterns that may approximate those of many people.

One approach to describing drug use is the following continuum:

abstinence → experimentation → occasional use → frequent use → mild psychological dependence → severe psychological dependence → compulsive drug use → overwhelming drug involvement

This continuum emphasizes the *potential* for escalating drug use, but is not intended to imply that everyone makes the full progression to dependency. Over a period of time, people move up and down through these levels of use and may "plateau" at any level for an extended time. A very unlikely movement, however, is downward from any of the three highest use levels to a more moderate use level. Once a person becomes highly dependent on a drug, it is very difficult to return to moderate use of that drug. A much more realistic and attainable goal for persons at these levels is to return all the way to abstinence.

Another way to describe patterns of drug use is by the *context* and *motivation* of the use. One or more of the following patterns may apply to a particular individual:

1. *Experimentation.* Curiosity is a basic part of human nature; sometimes this curiosity leads to experimenting with alcohol, tobacco, and other psychoactive drugs. If a friend is enthusiastic about a particular drug or if there is a lot of hype about a particular drug, it may be tempting to try out the drug just to see what that experience is like. Most people, having satisfied their curiosity, may try a drug once or twice and that's it. Some people, though, because of their physiological or psychological makeup, will find a particular drug that produces a very pleasant feeling. These people are likely to continue using that drug and to progress, to some extent, through the continuum described earlier. Maybe they will become occasional users; maybe they will become dependent. The possibility of progressing to dependency is what makes experimentation potentially dangerous.

2. *Social use.* The key element defining social use of alcohol or other drugs is that the effect of the drug use is secondary to the companionship, ceremony, and other social associations that become tied to its use. Alcohol, marijuana, and cocaine are examples of drugs that are likely to be used socially. People often rationalize their drug use as "social" when in fact they have other motives. Here is a simple test: It is Wednesday afternoon and you are looking forward to Friday night's party. You know that there will be plenty of alcohol or another drug available. As you anticipate Friday night, what looms larger in your mind, the opportunity for companionship and socialization or the fact that there will be plenty of this drug available?

3. *Use-for-escape or other effects.* Psychoactive drugs offer many mood modifications—relaxation, escape, decreased inhibitions, stimulation, perceptual modifications, and so on. A great deal of drug use is specifically motivated by the desire for such

Is it social use? A simple test, as you look forward to the next party, is: Is it the companionship or the chance to drink or use some other drug that you are looking forward to?

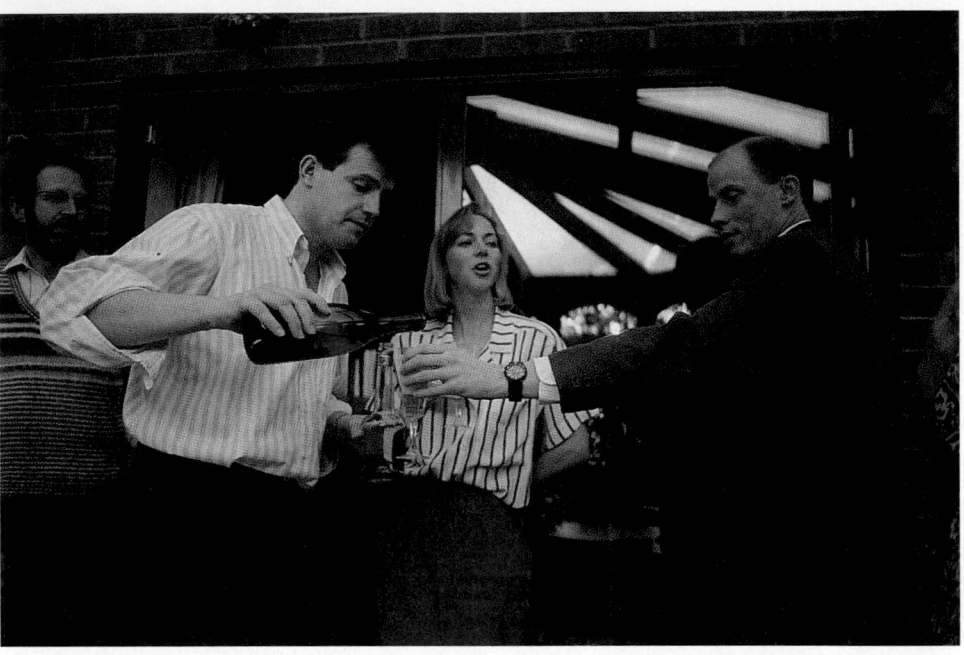

effects. Use-for-effect can take place at any step on the continuum of use. The majority of American society can probably be classified as occasional users-for-effect of alcohol. At times they drink specifically for relaxation, escape, or decreased inhibition and never experience any serious problems as a result. If, however, use-for-effect becomes more frequent or escalates to higher dosages, this becomes a cause for concern, as it may lead to chemical dependency.

4. *Chemical dependency.* **Chemical dependency** can be a purely psychological phenomenon, in which a substance is compulsively and repeatedly used for its psychological effects. It can also include physiological dependency, in which high levels of tolerance develop and the body actually comes to require the presence of the substance in order to function normally. Discontinuing drug use at this point results in unpleasant symptoms known as a **withdrawal syndrome** or **abstinence syndrome.** The kind of symptoms and their duration depend on the drug. Not every

....

chemical dependency the compulsive abuse of one or more drugs, despite the adverse consequences of this drug abuse.

withdrawal syndrome or **abstinence syndrome** a group of symptoms that occur when a drug that causes physiological dependence is no longer taken.

psychoactive drug produces physiological dependency. Drugs that clearly do, however, include alcohol, cocaine, opiates, barbiturates, and nicotine. Physiological dependency has also been called addiction.

ADDICTION

Drug experts don't agree on how or even whether to use the term *addiction*.[32–34] Some use the term for any powerful dependency or compulsive behavior, even extending its use to nondrug dependencies such as "sexual addiction." Others reserve the term addiction for those chemical dependencies that involve physiological dependency. Still others refuse to use the term at all, feeling that its meaning is unclear and that "chemical dependency" or "drug dependency" is preferable.

Those involved in many drug recovery programs, either as participants or as professionals, do use the word addiction to describe chemical dependency. It is used intentionally and emphatically as an open, straightforward way of labeling the difficulty that a person has had with drugs.

In this text, we most often use the phrase *chemical dependency*. We do sometimes use the term addiction, but only in reference to a dependency that has a physiological component. We emphasize here and elsewhere that whether or not a drug produces physiological dependency is of limited importance in determining how powerful its hold over a person can become and the impact the drug can have on a person's life.

YOUTH AND SUBSTANCE ABUSE

Substance abuse among young people has special significance for many reasons:

- Using alcohol or other drugs before age 15 greatly increases the risk of later substance abuse.[35]

- Adolescent drinking or other drug abuse is often the beginning of a lifelong struggle with chemical dependency.

- Substance abuse in young people can interfere with important developmental tasks such as identity, emotional and social maturity, education, and career preparation.

- Substance abuse can alienate a young person from the rest of society.

- Substance abuse can involve a young person in illegal and dangerous activities such as prostitution, theft, and drug dealing.

- Young people are easily manipulated and exploited.

- Young people metabolize drugs differently from older persons and may experience greater damaging effects from drugs.

Substance use and abuse often starts at a *young* age. Young people often want to feel and be perceived as older and more mature than they really are. Regardless of age, they tend to imitate the behavior of those who are slightly older. Thus, drug use trickles down through the grades, sometimes beginning at age 8 or 9. Children of this age have little concept of the dangers inherent in psychoactive drugs and have little idea of their own vulnerability and mortality. Many become severely and permanently damaged by drug use.

Some young people are at greater risk of substance abuse than others. Factors that have been associated with high-risk youths include the following:

- disrupted or dysfunctional family (see Communication for Wellness: Family Communication and Substance Abuse, p. 448)

- parent or older siblings who abuse alcohol or other drugs

- permissive parental attitude toward alcohol or other drugs

- victims of sexual, physical, or emotional abuse

- absence of caring parents

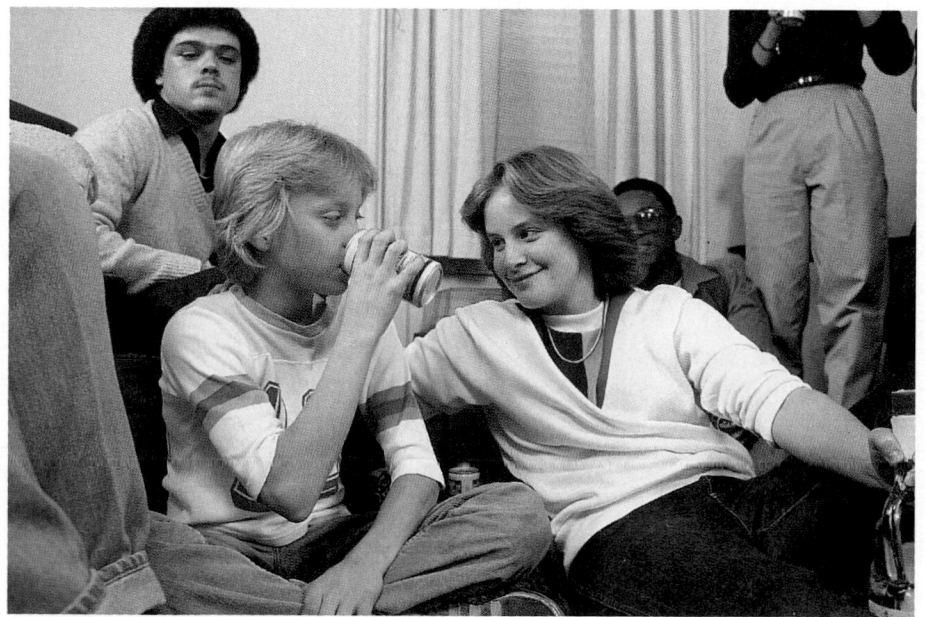

Drug use starts young, sometimes as young as eight or nine. Using alcohol or other drugs before age fifteen greatly increases the risk of later drug abuse.

FAMILY COMMUNICATION AND SUBSTANCE ABUSE

As the text points out, dysfunctional family life is frequently associated with chemical dependency and growing up in a healthy, strong family is the best prevention for substance abuse. What characterizes a healthy family? Every expert who studies this issue concludes that the number one trait of a healthy family is the ability to communicate.

Children in dysfunctional families do not feel free to talk to their parents about difficult subjects such as using alcohol or other drugs, or about sexual issues. Instead of relying on their parents for help, they turn to equally confused peers or just try to work things out on their own. Efforts to communicate with parents turn out unhappily. Some parents turn a "deaf ear" to their children's concerns, while others interrupt their children with angry and judgmental responses, quickly ending the possibility of any effective interaction. Parents jump to conclusions and overreact on the basis of incomplete information. Following their example, the children jump to their own conclusions and overreactions. Soon everyone is yelling and nobody is really listening to anyone else.

Healthy families gather around the table at mealtime and talk and really listen to each other. In addition to the day's events, feelings and concerns are shared. Children feel free to be open because they are confident that they will receive an understanding and supportive response. Parents listen in a way that encourages more communication. Instead of jumping to conclusions they listen attentively and draw out more information.

When parents communicate there is a sense of equality. They don't bully their children or force children into a position of subordination or submission. Members of healthy families don't use silence as an expression of hostility or a means of punishment. When disagreements occur, as they will in any family, communication continues. Issues are talked out, feelings are explored, and a mutually acceptable conclusion is reached. Children growing up in such families feel worthy and competent. They might "sample" drugs with their friends, but their self-esteem and sense of responsibility will almost always protect them from the overwhelming drug involvement characteristic of so many children of unhappy families.

- alcohol or other drug use by peer group
- availability of drugs at school or in the neighborhood
- feelings of anger, frustration, isolation, and hopelessness
- early antisocial behavior in school, especially aggressiveness
- alienation and low commitment to getting an education
- academic failure in school

- rebellion against rules at home and/or school
- withdrawing from family and friends
- acquiring new friends with different values
- narrowing interests
- constant need for money with little to show for it
- secretiveness
- declining appearance
- legal problems

SIGNS OF POSSIBLE SUBSTANCE ABUSE IN YOUNG PEOPLE

There are usually many signs indicating that a young person may be involved with alcohol or other drugs. Parents often either fail to see these signs or they deny that their child might be a user. A young person showing one or more of these signs might have an emotional problem rather than a chemical involvement, but he or she still is in trouble and needs help. The signs include the following:

- declining grades
- attendance problems at school
- conflict with school authorities

One of the most basic health principles is that prevention of a problem is always preferable to trying to cure it. In view of the effects substance abuse can have on young people, it is obvious that effective prevention programs are vital.

CHECKPOINT

1. Why is substance abuse by young people a special concern?

2. What are some factors associated with young people at high risk of substance abuse?

3. What are the signs of possible substance abuse in a young person?

SUBSTANCE-ABUSE PREVENTION

It is "human nature" to seek simple solutions for complex problems. This has certainly been the case with substance-abuse prevention. Preventing substance abuse, however, requires many different types of efforts targeted at every segment of the population. Further, these efforts need to be chosen and evaluated scientifically, not politically, as has too often been the case.

FAILED APPROACHES

From the 1930s through the 1960s, the main approach to drug education was to use scare tactics.[36] It was assumed that if people were told horror stories about a drug, they would be too frightened to try it. This approach proved ineffective because the information presented was exaggerated, sensationalized, or false. What people heard bore no resemblance to what they observed in themselves and their friends. As a result, the sources of information, mainly the federal government, lost credibility. Scare tactics tended to increase curiosity about drugs and increased, rather than decreased, experimentation.[37]

By the early 1970s, substance abuse had become epidemic. Network TV shows, such as "Laugh-In," openly glorified drug use. President Richard Nixon declared war on drugs. Plenty of federal money was made available for drug-treatment programs, but many programs of that era were ineffective. When no progress was evident, much of the funding was cut.

By the late 1970s, emphasis was on highly drug-specific drug education. For each drug, physical and psychological effects, routes of administration, dose levels, tolerance potential, withdrawal symptoms, and so forth were taught. The assumption was that if people knew enough about a drug, they would leave it alone. Even today this is a common form of drug education. There is evidence, however, that rather than discouraging drug use, this mass of specific information increases drug experimentation, at least by some people.[38]

In recent years, government efforts have been focused on the "supply side" of the problem, rather than on the "demand side." The theory has been that if no drugs are available because of mas-

sive enforcement efforts, there will be no drug abuse (see Feature 14.2 on p. 450). We all know that this approach has failed. Anyone who wants to buy a particular drug will have no trouble finding it in most U.S. cities.

FAMILY SYSTEM APPROACH

As this chapter has tried to make clear, substance abuse is best viewed as a family problem that spreads from generation to generation. The most promising approach to reducing substance abuse appears to be well-developed, scientifically based, family-oriented prevention, intervention, and treatment programs. When we refer to families, we do not mean only the traditional two-parent family, but include all types of families, such as those that consist only of one parent and one or more children.

There is no simple solution. Efforts to control the supply side, even though of limited effectiveness, should be maintained. Schools and teachers should continue their efforts to reduce substance abuse. Physicians should be well informed and proactive on substance-abuse identification, intervention, and treatment. The media should portray drugs in a factual way and certainly not glorify drug use.

Improved family function can be a major factor in combating substance abuse. Families need assistance in developing communication skills, relationship skills, and parenting skills. Families need to view chemical dependency realistically, not as a source of shame, but as a problem to be recognized and dealt with. Effective intervention and recovery programs need to be readily and immediately available to any family members who need them.

MULTICULTURAL PERSPECTIVES

The cultural diversity of the United States suggests the need for some prevention programs tailored to the cultures and values of specific ethnic groups. Studies show that members of different ethnic groups use alcohol and other drugs in different ways and for different reasons and that, to be effective, prevention programs need to reflect these differences.[39] Programs must also address basic survival needs, such as housing, employment, health care, and social services. Health and drug abuse educators Dorothy Dusek and Daniel Girdano

FEATURE 14.2

SHOULD DRUGS BE LEGAL?

In the 1960s, some people advocated legalization of psychoactive drugs because they were enthusiastic about drug use or felt it was not the role of government to regulate that aspect of people's lives. In recent years, some people have advocated legalization, not because they endorse drug use or see it as an issue of individual rights, but because they believe that the nation's efforts to control drug abuse through regulation have not worked and will not work.

ARGUMENTS THAT HAVE BEEN MADE IN FAVOR OF LEGALIZATION INCLUDE THE FOLLOWING:

1. Legal drug sales would eliminate the criminal element in drug distribution.
2. Prices would be lower, reducing the need for drug addicts to resort to crime to support their dependencies.
3. Taxes could be collected on legal drug sales, as they are on sales of alcohol and tobacco.
4. The huge current expenditure of tax money for drug enforcement would no longer be necessary.
5. The purity and strength of drugs sold could be checked by federal and/or state agencies.
6. Chemical dependency would be a medical problem, rather than a legal problem.

ARGUMENTS THAT HAVE BEEN MADE AGAINST LEGALIZATION INCLUDE THE FOLLOWING:

1. There is no successful world model for legalization.
2. Alcohol is legal and many millions of Americans have alcohol dependencies.
3. Many drugs, such as cocaine, are more addictive than alcohol.
4. Many more people would become addicted to cocaine and other currently illegal drugs.
5. Legalization of psychoactive drugs would be seen by many people as a government endorsement of their use.
6. Just as alcohol abuse is a problem among children today, there would be no way to prevent other legal psychoactive drugs from reaching the younger population.

Which side is "right" in this controversy? In the sense that all of the pros and cons presented are probably true, both sides are "right." What do you think is the best course of action for the nation, legalization or strict prohibition?

have compiled information on multicultural substance abuse prevention programs.[40] Some of their findings on selected ethnic groups follow:

- *Native Americans* Native Americans may have a strong genetic susceptibility to alcoholism (see p. 443). Alcohol is the most widely abused substance among Native American nations. A higher percentage of high-school-age Native Americans drink than of most other ethnic groups, and a higher percentage drink very heavily.[41] Heavy drinking is cited as the main reason why many Native Americans fail to finish high school. Many young Native Americans die in alcohol-related vehicle crashes. There appear to be no universal explanations for alcohol and other drug abuse among Native Americans.

- *African Americans* Drug-abuse-prevention programs in the African American community are being targeted toward the very young. There is evidence that African American parents are well aware of the hazards of drug use, but are more reluctant to voice disap-

proval to their children than are other parents.[42] Messages are thus directed at parents to encourage them to keep their children away from drug-using peers. Messages to older teenagers try to convince them to actively discourage younger brothers and sisters from using drugs. TV, radio, and billboard ads are also directly targeting preteens for messages designed to deglamorize drug use and portray nonusers as winners.

- *Pacific and Asian Americans* This category actually includes 32 highly diverse ethnic groups. The non-Pacific or Asian American public tends to stereotype Pacific or Asian Americans as being immune from alcohol and other drug abuse, so few prevention programs have targeted these ethnic groups specifically. Dusek and Girdano report that drug abuse among Asian and Pacific Americans is more widespread than is commonly believed and that additional culturally sensitive, bilingual prevention programs for specific Asian and Pacific American ethnic groups need to be developed.[43]

- *Hispanic Americans* Hispanic Americans are a diverse group with roots in Cuba, Puerto Rico, Mexico, and many Central and South American countries. Generalizations about Hispanic Americans do not necessarily apply to all of these groups. Some Hispanic ethnic groups are associated with high rates of drug abuse and HIV infection. Prevention programs targeted at Hispanics take advantage of a strong sense of ethnic identity and ethnic pride. The message, a universally applicable one, is "Drugs are uncool, they're unacceptable, drug abuse disgraces your ethnic heritage and increases your risk of contracting AIDS."[44]

CHECKPOINT

1. What are three failed approaches to preventing substance abuse?

2. What is the family system approach to substance-abuse prevention?

INTERVENTION

In years past it was generally believed that before a chemically dependent person could be helped, he or she had to "hit bottom." Only when everything was lost—family, home, job, and health—would the person be ready to accept rehabilitation. Fortunately, this idea has been disproved and the emphasis is now on early treatment—the earlier, the better.[45]

Because of today's greater openness and awareness concerning chemical dependency, many chemically dependent people initiate their own rehabilitation at a relatively early stage in their disease. Others, using the rationalization and denial characteristic of chemically dependent people, maintain that they have no problem and resist any efforts or suggestions for help. This is when **intervention** (a structured, confrontational technique used to help drug abusers overcome their rationalization and denial and accept the reality of

....

intervention a structured, confrontational technique used to help drug abusers overcome their rationalization and denial and accept the reality of their drug problems.

their drug problems), as pioneered by Vern Johnson, founder of a successful treatment program, may be appropriate.[46]

Every situation is unique and every intervention must be individually planned. The following is a typical intervention:

John's drinking has become progressively worse over the past ten years. He is missing more and more days of work when he is too drunk or too sick. His wife, Mary, always calls in for him, making up excuses, such as the flu. At work, his efficiency has dropped sharply. His co-workers suspect that he sneaks drinks during the work day and have complained to his boss, Fred.

At home John is a tyrant. He alternates between yelling at Mary and the children, sulking by himself, and being overly nice to everyone when he starts to feel guilty. He is rarely sober. John and Mary never make love any more. The family finances are a disaster. Many bills are unpaid. The mortgage company is threatening to foreclose on the house.

One day while John is at work Mary receives a call from Fred. Fred explains that he is concerned about John's drinking and asks if Mary believes that John might be an alcoholic. At first, Mary acts irate and denies that there are any problems at home. Then, as Fred tells of all of John's problems at work, Mary begins to cry and admits that there are many problems at home as well.

With Mary's approval, Fred talks to the EAP (Employee Assistance Program) officer in the corporation and together they arrange an intervention. One afternoon at work, Fred calls John to a sudden meeting in a small, private room where, to John's surprise, he finds Mary and the children, along with Fred and the EAP officer.

Each speaks in turn. Fred tells John his concerns about John's poor job performance and his belief that alcohol is the problem. Mary and the children each tell John of their unhappiness at home and their belief that alcohol is the problem. The EAP officer tells John that he has already made arrangements for John to enter a local hospital-based rehabilitation program.

John denies vigorously that he drinks too much, blaming everyone but himself for the problems he has just heard described. At this point, several ultimatums are made: Fred says that if John does not enter the program, he is

In the past, it was believed that a chemically dependent person had to "hit bottom" before starting recovery. Today, interventions such as this are often planned to apply pressure toward recovery before the abuser's condition deteriorates too severely.

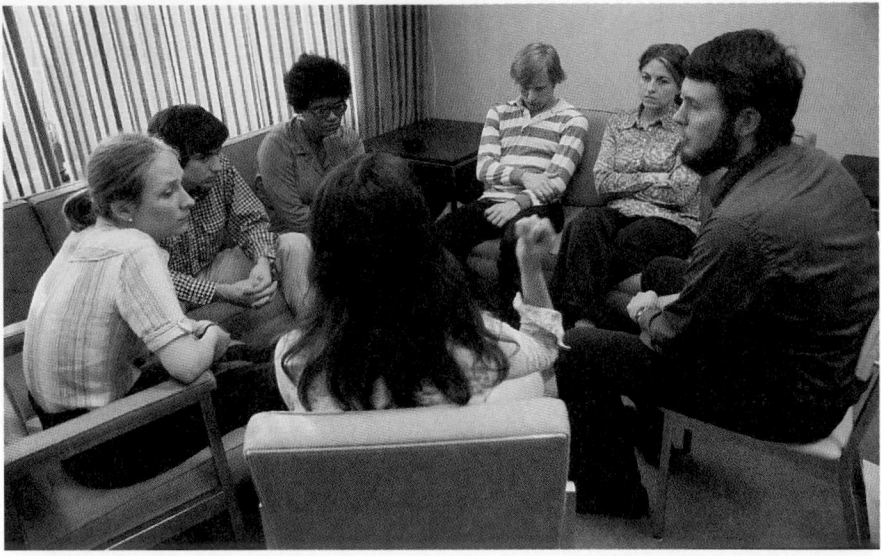

fired. Mary says that if John does not enter the program, he is not welcome to come home that evening. Taken aback, John asks for a few days to think about it. Mary and Fred say that John must decide right now. Mary says that the clothes and toiletries John will need for his hospital stay are packed and out in the car. Reluctantly, John agrees to enter the program.

Not every intervention turns out successfully. John might have told them all good-bye, quit his job, and left his family. But he eventually would have lost his job, home, and family anyhow.

The majority of well-planned interventions do succeed. When it is not possible or appropriate to involve an employer, intervention can usually be arranged by contacting a local alcohol/drug counselor or program. It may seem cruel or an invasion of the dependent person's privacy, but not to intervene is to enable his or her continued progression in the disease of chemical dependency.

RECOVERY FROM CHEMICAL DEPENDENCY

Because recovery from chemical dependency can be extremely difficult, many abusers of alcohol or other drugs eventually require the help of others in conquering their dependencies. The terms *rehabilitation, recovery,* and *treatment* are all used rather interchangeably. Some people prefer *rehabilitation* or *recovery,* as these terms imply a more active role of the chemically dependent person, while

treatment may imply a more passive role. All of these terms, though, are acceptable.

GOALS IN RECOVERY

The goals of chemical dependency recovery are straightforward. The drug abuser is expected to stop or greatly decrease drug abuse, find a job (if unemployed), stop committing crimes (if this has been the case), stabilize his or her personal life, and become a useful and productive citizen.[47]

Evaluating the success of recovery programs, however, is difficult.[48] *When* do you evaluate success? After a drug-free month? Six months? Ten years? *How* do you evaluate success? Do you require total abstinence for success? This all-or-nothing approach may give the perception of failure when, in fact, a considerable improvement (decrease in drug abuse) has occurred. Or, conversely, a recovery may be called a success, when in fact, the original problem drug has simply been replaced by another. For example, an alcohol abuser may have stopped drinking, but begun heavy pill abuse. These and other issues have made comparing the success rates of various recovery programs quite difficult.

UNDERLYING CONCEPTS IN CHEMICAL DEPENDENCY TREATMENT

Though many types of programs address chemical dependency, successful programs are usually based on the following underlying concepts:[49]

1. In chemical dependency treatment, *there are no hopeless cases.*

2. Chemical dependency is a complex *disease* having unknown or incompletely known causes.

3. Chemical dependency can be successfully arrested and controlled, but *cannot be cured*. The goal of treatment is not to reduce the use of the problem drug(s) to a lower level, but to abstain completely from psychoactive drug use.

4. Chemical dependency is to be regarded as the primary problem that needs to be treated. A host of contributing or resulting problems must also be addressed in treatment, but are to be regarded as secondary in importance to the individual's chemical dependency.

5. Denial of a chemical-abuse problem is the norm. Defense mechanisms such as projection, avoidance, and **passive-aggressive** behaviors are used by almost all chemically dependent people.

6. Successful recovery involves a broad-based change in life-style. Eliminating drug-centered behavior leaves an enormous hole in a person's life that must be filled with other **adaptive behaviors** (behaviors that enable a person to interact with his or her environment efficiently) or drug abuse will resume.

7. Chemical dependency is a family disorder; therefore treatment programs should involve the whole family.

8. Many personality traits that are common in chemically dependent people require long-term treatment:

- lack of assertiveness
- dependency
- negative self-image
- fear of rejection
- feelings of isolation and alienation
- immaturity in social interaction
- inadequate coping mechanisms

9. Intense initial involvement in a treatment program is desirable, followed by long-term participation in a 12-step program (see p. 454).

10. Some resumption of drug use following treatment is not uncommon. The recovering person who never has a slip or relapse is rare.

passive-aggressive a personality behavior characterized by both excessive passivity and aggressiveness.

adaptive behavior behavior that enables a person to interact with his or her environment efficiently.

LAPSE VS. RELAPSE

There is an important distinction between a lapse and a relapse in recovery from chemical dependency. Although the goal of most rehabilitation programs is abstinence from drugs, it doesn't always work that way at the beginning. The fact is that the majority of recovering persons will have "slips" or **lapses** (brief returns to drug use). This does not have to put them back to square one in their recovery. Even if a recovering person does lapse, he or she should be encouraged to keep fighting the chemical dependency. The distinction between lapse and **relapse** (recurrence of a disease after apparent recovery) is that the recovering person, by viewing his or her slip as only a lapse, is less likely to give up hope for a drug-free life. It has not been a total failure in his or her recovery, just a temporary setback.

TYPES OF RECOVERY PROGRAMS

Many types of recovery programs are available. Five sets of opposing elements can be used to describe recovery programs.[50] Each program represents some combination of these elements:

1. *Medical versus social model programs.* The medical model program makes a clear distinction of roles between the therapist, who is often a physician, and the client. In the social model, on the other hand, the roles are less clearly defined. The setting in the social model is nonmedical and the staff members themselves are often recovering from chemical dependencies. The medical model emphasizes the individual client, while the social model emphasizes the group. The medical model tends to make use of medications, while the social model uses little or none. In the medical model, chemical dependency is viewed as a symptom of an underlying mental disorder. In the social model, dependency is seen as the problem.[51]

2. *Residential versus outpatient programs.* In residential programs, the chemically dependent person resides for a period, perhaps 28 days, in a facility. In outpatient treatment, the person visits the facility at designated intervals.

lapses brief returns to drug use.

relapse recurrence of a disease after apparent recovery.

3. *Drug-free versus maintenance programs.*
Drug-free programs start with **detoxification** (the process of removing the physiological effects of a drug from an addicted person). Then, progress toward a long-term drug-free life-style can begin. Maintenance programs, to prevent withdrawal symptoms, provide a substitute for the drug that has been abused. For example, heroin addicts may be given methadone (trade name Dolophine), which prevents withdrawal symptoms while blocking the pleasurable effects of heroin or other opiates.[52]

4. *Selective versus nonselective programs.*
Selective programs screen prospective clients and accept only those whom they judge are likely to benefit. Nonselective programs accept all who apply or are sent there.

5. *Voluntary versus involuntary programs.*
The term *voluntary* may be a little misleading, as practically all drug treatment involves some degree of coercion from family and/or employer. Involuntary, in this context, means treatment under court order as an alternative to jail or prison.

Twelve-Step Self-Help Programs

Twelve-step programs, such as Alcoholics Anonymous, Narcotics Anonymous, Cocaine Anonymous, and many others, are major resources in chemical-dependency rehabilitation. Twelve-step programs succeed for many people, alone or integrated into other treatment models.

Alcoholics Anonymous (AA), the original 12-step program (see Feature 14.3), had its origin in 1935 in Akron, Ohio, when two alcoholics, Bill W. and Dr. Bob, met together. Today, with over a million active members worldwide, AA is generally recognized as the most effective road to long-term sobriety.

AA meetings are readily available throughout the United States (look up Alcoholics Anonymous in the white pages of the phone book). Membership is very loosely structured and the only requirement for membership is a desire to stop drinking. Larger cities have many meetings each day, including some specifically for younger persons, for women, for nonsmokers, and so on. The atmosphere is comfortable and nonthreatening, and new

members are always welcome. The people attending these meetings will be just like the people you know at school, at work, or in your neighborhood. If you want to just sit and watch, they will let you do it without even asking your name.

Al-Anon is an affiliated organization for family members of alcoholics. Meetings are similar to AA meetings. The main difference is that in Al-Anon the members are there to deal with their being powerless over *others'* alcohol use rather than their own. Members gain an understanding of their responses to the drinking behavior, learn ways of dealing with their alcoholic family member, and learn how to live their own lives more effectively.

Al-Ateen is an organization for young people with an alcoholic parent or parents. Children of alcoholics must deal with many special problems. They feel a sense of stigma attached to alcoholism. Because young people are reluctant to talk about a parent's alcoholism, most believe that they are the only ones with this problem and they feel all alone in the world. One of the greatest benefits of Al-Ateen is that it lessens the sense of shame and isolation.

Adult Children of Alcoholics

Self-help groups for adult children of alcoholics (ACAs) are a fairly recent development. These groups help ACAs deal with the ongoing problems many experience. Although not everyone who grows up in an alcoholic home develops lasting problems, many characteristics are common among ACAs:[53]

- *Fear of abandonment,* which may either cause clinging, dependent behavior, or the inability to form intimate relationships.
- *Sense of personal failure,* from being unable to control the parent's drinking.
- *Strong need for outside approval,* causing obsessive striving for success.
- *Intense guilt feelings,* left from hating the alcoholic parent or from a sense of having been the cause of the family problems.
- *Victim mentality,* in which the feeling of being a victim of life prevents a person from taking charge of his or her life.
- *Great confusion over a person's feelings.*
- *Many other problems.*

detoxification process of removing the physiological effects of a drug from an addicted person.

FEATURE 14.3

THE 12 STEPS OF AA

Alcoholics Anonymous and other 12-step programs have some of the best success rates in combating chemical dependencies. The 12 steps were first published in 1939 in the book, *Alcoholics Anonymous* (the *Big Book*). They are in the past tense because they describe what the by-then 100 members of AA had done to maintain their sobriety. Perhaps this approach is so successful because the 12 steps were written not by theoretical research scientists, but by sober alcoholics. The comments in parentheses are by the authors of this text.

1. *We admitted that we were powerless over alcohol— that our lives had become unmanageable.* (Acknowledges that you are an alcoholic and that alcoholism is the source of your problems.)

2. *Came to believe that a Power greater than ourselves could restore us to sanity.* (Recognizes the irrationality of your drinking behavior and the need for reliance on an outside agent—God, AA, and so on, for support.)

3. *Made a decision to turn our will and our lives over to the care of God as we understood Him.* (Each member makes his or her own interpretation of "God" and need not be conventionally religious for AA to succeed.)

4. *Made a searching and fearless moral inventory of ourselves.* (Allows a close look at the ways of thinking and acting that encouraged drinking.)

5. *Admitted to God, to ourselves, and to another human being the exact nature of our wrongs.* (This gets the guilt-causing behavior out into the open instead of keeping it destructively inside.)

6. *Were entirely ready to have God remove all of these defects of character.* (Recognizes the alcoholic's tendency to hold onto unhealthy behavior patterns.)

7. *Humbly asked Him to remove our shortcomings.* (Instills hope that change is possible.)

8. *Made a list of all persons we had harmed and became willing to make amends to them all.* (A guide to sorting out injury done to others and deciding how best to deal with it; also gets the alcoholic away from blaming others for his or her difficulties.)

9. *Made direct amends to such people wherever possible, except when to do so would injure them or others.* (Helps improve strained relationships with others and eliminate some of the guilt the newly sober alcoholic is likely to feel.)

10. *Continued to take personal inventory and when we were wrong, promptly admitted it.* (Helps prevent slips back to old ways of living.)

11. *Sought through prayer and meditation to improve our conscious contact with God as we understood him, praying only for knowledge of His will for us and the power to carry it out.* (Helps maintain the spiritual basis for sobriety.)

12. *Having had a spiritual awakening as the result of these steps, we tried to carry this message to alcoholics and practice these principles in all our affairs.* (One of the most important steps; people in 12-step programs help themselves by helping others.)

These ACA characteristics, coupled with the genetic risk factor inherent in being a child of alcoholic parents, present a strong rationale for self-help groups for ACAs.

CHECKPOINT

1. Explain the concept of intervention in chemical dependency.

2. Why is it difficult to evaluate the success rate of recovery programs?

3. What are ten underlying concepts in chemical dependency treatment?

4. What is the difference between a lapse and a relapse during recovery and what is the psychological significance of this?

5. Contrast a medical model and a social model program.

6. What is a 12-step program?

7. Why do 12-step programs have a good success rate?

8. What is an ACA and what traits are common among ACAs?

ALTERNATIVES TO DRUG USE

Drug use occurs for many reasons that are unique to each individual. One thing that all drug users have in common, however, is that they are trying to fulfill basic human needs. How can you satisfy these needs without using drugs? Some traits associated with a drug-free life-style include the following:

- *Strength from within:* believing that true happiness and fulfillment can only come from within the individual.

- *Strength from without:* believing in something larger than yourself. This may be a religious belief or other strongly held value system.
- *An other-centered life-style:* recognizing that other people are important to our happiness and we are important to theirs.
- *Recognition of the futility of drugs:* understanding that whatever drugs seem to promise is unattainable in the long run. Rebound effects and tolerance, discussed in

Chapter 15, guarantee that long-term drug-induced satisfaction is impossible.

How can a drug user reach such a state of mind? A starting point is to explore your expectations from drugs and to consider other possible ways to fulfill these needs (see Table 14.1). For people whose drug use is well established, professional help or organized self-help (such as a 12-step program) is usually necessary in making the transition away from a drug-centered life-style. Conquering chemical dependency is rarely easy, but it is *always* worth the effort.

Table 14.1
Expectations from Drug Use and Possible Alternatives to Drug Use

Drug Expectation—Physical needs: relaxation, more energy, feel better physically
Drug-free Alternatives: sports, dance, exercise, hiking, walking, running, more sleep, better diet

Drug Expectation—Sensory needs: more powerful sensory stimulation
Drug-free Alternatives: sensory awareness training, sky diving, SCUBA diving, rock climbing, appreciation of the beauty of nature, intellectually stimulating companionship

Drug Expectation—Emotional needs: pain relief, escape from problems, relief from bad moods, escape from anxiety
Drug-free Alternatives: individual or group counseling, psychology course, deal with problems, stress management

Drug Expectation—Interpersonal needs: peer acceptance, communicating more easily, breaking down of barriers
Drug-free Alternatives: organized group sports, common interest groups, social clubs, group therapy, volunteer work, helping others

Drug Expectation—Intellectual needs: escape from boredom, curiosity, gaining new understanding, exploration of your own awarenesses
Drug-free Alternatives: reading, debating, discussion, special interest groups, games, puzzles, college courses

Drug Expectation—Aesthetic needs: improvement of own creative performance, enhancement of enjoyment of art or music
Drug-free Alternatives: courses in performing or art, music, or drama appreciation

Drug Expectation—Philosophical needs: discovery of new values, finding meaning in life, establishment of personal identity, organization of a belief structure
Drug-free Alternatives: discussions, seminars, courses, and literature that explore value systems; investigating various religions

Drug Expectation—Spiritual needs: transcending existing religious beliefs, developing new spiritual insights, reaching higher levels of consciousness
Drug-free Alternatives: exploration of various religions, study of world religions and mysticism, meditation, yoga

Source: Modified from Cohen, A. Alternatives to Drug Abuse: Steps Toward Prevention. Washington, DC: National Institute on Drug Abuse (No. 14), Department of Health, Education, and Welfare, 1973.

CHECKPOINT

1. What are four traits associated with a dependency-free life-style?
2. What are some specific needs that motivate drug use and some possible alternative ways to fulfill these needs?

SUMMARY

A drug is any substance, other than a food, that modifies any function of your body. Psychoactive drugs are those that affect your moods, emotions, perceptions, and behavior. These are the drugs with the potential for abuse and dependency. Drug abuse has various definitions, but can be defined as misuse or excessive use, usually by self-administration, of any drug.

There are many characteristics of American society that promote unhealthful use of drugs: seeking pleasure and avoiding pain at any cost; dysfunctional relationships; physical inactivity; inability to be self-entertaining; tendency to be self-centered; narrowly focused lives; feelings of anger, anxiety, or depression; feelings of lack of meaning in life; and the tendency to deny that there is a problem. Drug use and abuse is influenced by the values and traditions of each ethnic group.

Chemical dependency is both a cause and a result of dysfunctional family life. Family members, however, are often reluctant to become involved in the recovery of a chemically dependent family member. Each member may adopt a role in family interaction such as the chief enabler, the family hero, the family scapegoat, the lost child, or the family mascot.

Enabling is acting in a manner that allows a chemically dependent person to continue his or her substance abuse. Codependency is defined either as having a chemically dependent family member or in terms of personality traits developed as a result of being a member of such a family. The effects of codependency can be lifelong.

Drug use and abuse are motivated by psychological factors such as boredom, frustration, loneliness, anxiety, depression, and low self-esteem, though no dependency-prone personality has been identified. Social and cultural factors influencing drug use include ethnic affiliation, peer influence and the media. Biological factors include genetic traits such as the levels of certain brain chemicals.

Patterns of drug use range from abstinence to overwhelming drug involvement. Chemical dependency can be a purely psychological phenomenon or may also include physiological dependency, in which high levels of tolerance develop and the body comes to require the presence of the drug in order to function normally. Discontinuing a drug in the latter case results in an unpleasant withdrawal syndrome. Drug experts don't agree on how or whether to use the term addiction, but many use it in cases of physiological dependency.

Substance abuse by young people is of special concern because of its many serious psychological and physiological effects and its potential to spawn a lifelong struggle with chemical dependency. Some young people are at greater risk than others because of family or social factors.

Failed approaches to substance-abuse prevention include scare tactics, highly drug-specific drug education, and focusing on controlling the supply of drugs rather than the demand for them. The family system approach is viewed as more promising. Because members of different ethnic groups use alcohol and other drugs in different ways and for different reasons, prevention programs need to reflect these differences.

Intervention is a structured, confrontational technique used to help drug abusers overcome their rationalization and denial and accept the reality of their drug problems by applying family, peer, or work-related pressure. Many types of programs are available to help in a person's recovery. Twelve-step programs have a good success rate, alone or incorporated into other treatment models. Adult children of alcoholics or other chemically dependent people may have lasting problems and may benefit from counseling or self-help groups. Keys to living your life without drugs include strength from within, strength from without, an other-centered life-style, and recognition of the futility of drugs.

REFERENCES

1. Fields, Richard. *Drugs and Alcohol in Perspective.* Dubuque, IA: Wm. C. Brown, 1992.
2. Dusek, D., and Girdano, D. *Drugs, A Factual Account,* 5th ed. New York: McGraw-Hill, 1993.
3. Ibid.
4. Fields, op. cit.
5. Ibid.
6. Wegscheider-Cruse, S. *Another Chance: Hope and Health for the Alcoholic Family.* Palo Alto, CA: Science and Behavior Books, 1981.
7. Nelson, C. "The Style of Enabling Behavior." In Smith, D., and Wesson, D. (eds). *Treating Cocaine Dependency.* Center City, MN: Haselden Foundation, 1988.
8. Carroll, C. *Drugs in Modern Society,* 3rd ed. Madison, WI: Brown & Benchmark, 1993.
9. Kinney, J., and Leaton, G. *Loosening the Grip, A Handbook of Alcohol Information,* 4th ed. St. Louis: Mosby, 1991.
10. Avis, H. *Drugs and Life,* 2nd ed. Madison, WI: Brown & Benchmark, 1993.
11. Cermak, T. *Diagnosing and Treating Co-dependence: A Guide for Professionals Who Work with Chemical Dependents, their Spouses, and Children.* Minneapolis, MN: Johnson Institute Books, 1986.
12. Carroll, op. cit.
13. Kirkpatrick, J. *Goodbye Hangovers, Hello Life: Self-help for Women.* New York: Ballantine, 1987.
14. Kinney and Leaton, op. cit.
15. Goode, E. *Drugs in American Society,* 4th ed. New York: McGraw-Hill, 1993.
16. Ibid.
17. Taylor, Patricia. "Should Alcohol Advertising Be Limited?" In Goldberg, R. (eds.). *Taking Sides: Clashing Views on Controversial Issues in Drugs and Society.* Guilford, CT: Dushkin, 1993.
18. Gordis, E. "The Genetic Paradigm: Implications for Research and Treatment." *Alcohol Health and Research World* 12, No. 2 (Winter 1987/88), 96–97.
19. Dietrich, R., and Erwon, G. "The Drinker's Tail: Animal Genetics in Alcohol Research." *Alcohol Health and Research World* 12, No. 2 (Winter 1987/88), 98–101.
20. Stoil, M. "The Case of the Missing Gene: Hereditary Protection Against Alcoholism." *Alcohol Health and Research World* 12, No. 2 (Winter 1987/88), 130–136.

21. Cowley, G. "The Gene and the Bottle." *Newsweek* (30 April 1990), p. 59.
22. Maugh, T. "Study Finds Genetic Link to Alcoholism in Women." *Los Angeles Times* (14 October 1992), p. A1.
23. Cowley, op. cit.
24. Maugh, op. cit.
25. Ibid.
26. Ibid.
27. National Institute on Alcohol Abuse and Alcoholism. *Sixth Special Report to the U.S. Congress on Alcohol and Health*. Rockville, MD: National Institute on Alcohol Abuse and Alcoholism, 1987.
28. Dietrich and Erwin, op. cit.
29. Stoil, op. cit.
30. Cowley, op. cit.
31. Brennan, W. "Are You Disposed at Birth Towards Addiction/Alcoholism?" Lecture presented at Charter Oak Hospital, Covina, California, 26 May 1988.
32. Fields, op. cit.
33. Carroll, op. cit.
34. Witters, W., Venturelli, P., and Hanson, G. *Drugs and Society,* 3rd ed. Boston: Jones and Bartlett, 1992.
35. National Institute on Drug Abuse. *Drug Abuse and Drug Abuse Research*. Rockville, MD: National Institute on Drug Abuse, 1987.
36. Fields, op. cit.
37. Ibid.
38. Ibid.
39. Dusek and Girdano, op. cit.
40. Ibid.
41. Ibid.
42. Ibid.
43. Ibid.
44. Ibid.
45. Dykman, B. In Felsted, C. (ed). *Youth and Alcohol Abuse: Readings and Resources*. Phoenix, AZ: Oryx Press, 1986.
46. Johnson, V. *I'll Quit Tomorrow*. New York: Harper & Row, 1973.
47. Witters, Venturelli, and Hanson, op. cit.
48. See the entire issue of *Alcohol Health and Research World* 12, No. 3 (1988).
49. Van Ness, M. Introduction to Drug and Alcohol Counseling course at the University of California, Riverside, Fall Quarter, 1987.
50. Witters, Venturelli, and Hanson, op. cit.
51. Van Ness, op. cit.
52. Ray, O., and Ksir, C. *Drugs, Society, and Human Behavior,* 5th ed. St. Louis: Mosby, 1989.
53. Kinney and Leaton, op. cit.

SUGGESTED READINGS

Avis, H. *Drugs and Life,* 2nd ed. Madison, WI: Brown & Benchmark, 1993.
Carroll, C. *Drugs in Modern Society,* 3rd ed. Madison, WI: Brown & Benchmark, 1993.
Fields, R. *Drugs and Alcohol in Perspective*. Dubuque, IA: Wm. C. Brown, 1992.
Kinney, J., and Leaton, G. *Loosening the Grip, A Handbook of Alcohol Information,* 4th ed. St. Louis: Mosby, 1991.
Kirkpatrick, J. *Goodbye Hangovers, Hello Life: Self-help for Women*. New York: Ballantine, 1987.
Satir, V., and Baldwin, M. *Satir—Step by Step—A Guide to Creating Change in Families*. Northvale, NJ: Aronson, Jason, 1983.
Venturelli, P. (ed.). *Drug Use in America*. Boston: Jones and Bartlett, 1994.
Witters, W., Venturelli, P., and Hanson, G. *Drugs and Society*. Boston: Jones and Bartlett, 1992.

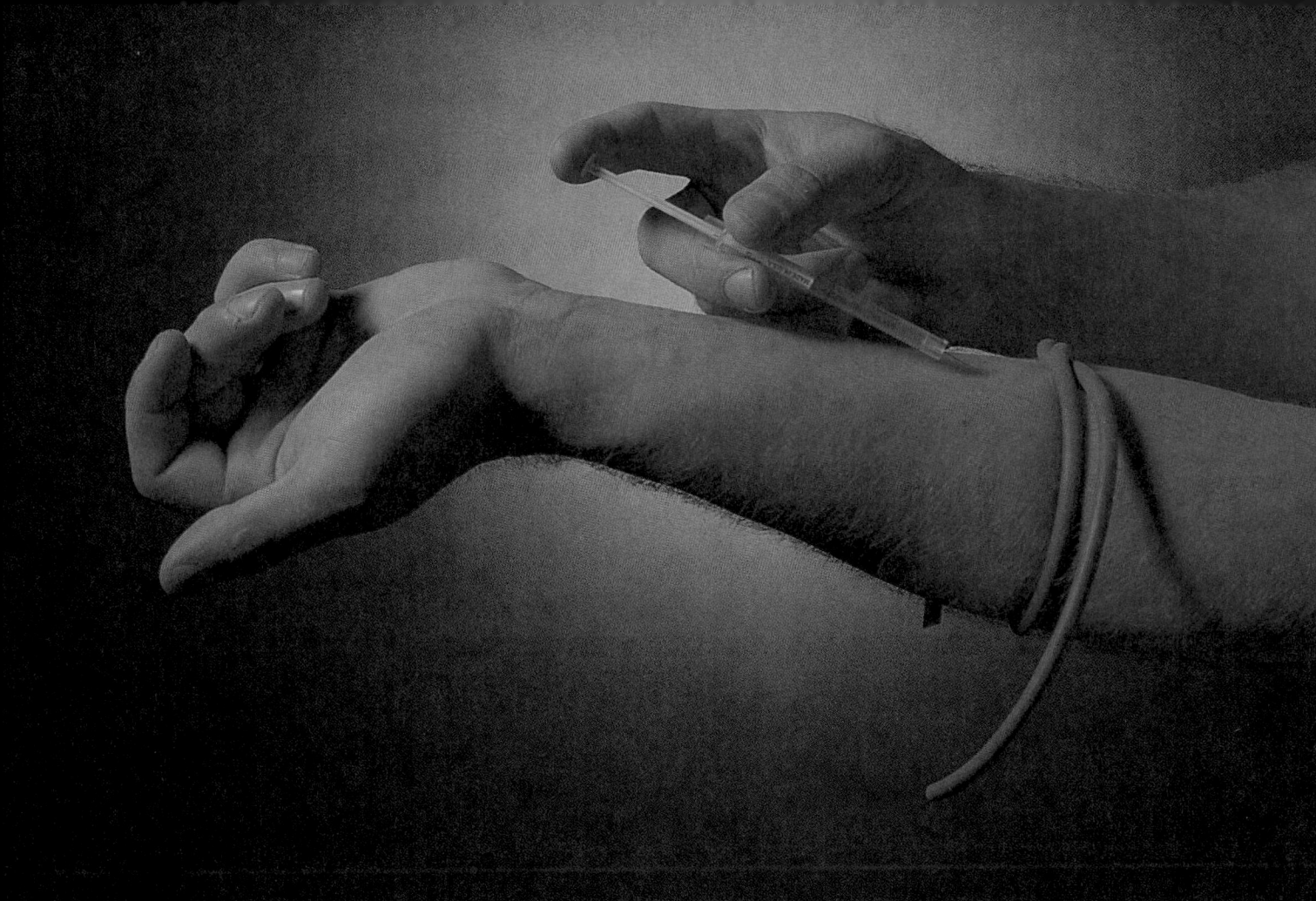

15
PSYCHOACTIVE DRUGS

KNOWLEDGE

- Explain how drugs enter and become distributed throughout the body.
- Explain neurotransmitters and receptor mechanisms and how psychoactive drugs relate to these.
- Describe endorphins and their relationship to psychoactive drugs.
- Explain the logarithmic breakdown rate applicable to most drugs versus the arithmetic breakdown rate of alcohol.
- Describe the rebound effect of a drug.
- Explain the hazards inherent in polydrug abuse.
- Describe the general characteristics of each psychoactive drug discussed in this chapter.

INSIGHT

- Explain the reasons you think psychoactive drugs are not the road to long-term human happiness.

DECISION MAKING

- Make a commitment to maintain a drug-free life-style.

B asketball star Len Bias was in the public eye one minute for his slam dunks, the next for his untimely death. Why might a strong athlete in the prime of his youth die so suddenly? The nation was shocked to learn that cocaine use had ended the successful basketball career of this University of Maryland star who had been selected by the Boston Celtics in the first round of the NBA draft and had agreed to a $1.6 million, five-year endorsement contract with Reebok.

Len Bias's death came in a dormitory room, early in the morning, where Bias and three friends had been snorting a shared half-cup of cocaine. His friends were alarmed at the amount of cocaine Bias was snorting and cautioned him against using so much. He continued, however, and soon he experienced a series of violent seizures as the toxic effects of cocaine set in. He never regained consciousness after the seizures, and was officially pronounced dead at a nearby hospital later that morning.

A thorough investigation of Bias's death followed with unpleasant repercussions. His coach at the University of Maryland resigned after accusations of a cover-up and a friend—one of the three witnesses to the death—went to court on charges of cocaine possession and distribution. On the more positive side, stricter drug-testing procedures went into effect and task forces on campus drug use were appointed at the University of Maryland and at many other universities.

Probably no event has had a greater impact on the way young people in the United States view drug use, particularly cocaine use, than the death of this rising young star. Cocaine had been viewed as a relatively "safe" drug. Sadly, it has taken the tragic deaths of people like Len Bias to make us realize the deadliness of cocaine use.

Source: Sports Illustrated, *10 November 1986, pp. 76–92.*

■   ■   ■

In Chapter 14, we explored some of the social and psychological aspects of substance abuse. Now let's turn our attention to some of the biological aspects. After a brief look at how drugs interact with the human body, we will examine some of the commonly abused psychoactive drugs. Tobacco and alcohol, the two most widely abused drugs in the United States, are discussed in Chapters 16 and 17.

HOW DRUGS ENTER THE BODY

Before any psychoactive drug can produce its effects, it must enter the body, be absorbed into the blood, and be carried to the brain. Drugs can enter the body in a number of different ways. The manner in which any drug enters the body will affect the body's reaction. The way a drug is taken also affects how quickly the drug takes effect, the duration of its action, and its potency. Ingestion, inhalation, and injection are the most common methods of taking drugs.

INGESTION (ORAL DRUG USE)

Drugs are most commonly taken into the digestive system by swallowing them, in either a solid or liquid form. Following ingestion, it can take 20–40 minutes for the drug to enter the bloodstream and reach the brain. An overdose may occur when a drug user, impatient for the drug's effect or thinking the dosage has been too small, takes additional doses during this period of delay.

Some drugs, such as insulin, cannot be taken orally as they are broken down by the digestive juices or have molecules that cannot be absorbed into the blood from the digestive system.

INHALATION INTO THE LUNGS

Inhaling a drug usually leads to rapid absorption into the bloodstream because of the rich supply of blood vessels in the lungs. Medications for asthma and other respiratory problems are often taken in this manner. Inhalation of smoke, such as that of tobacco or marijuana, presents a hazard independent of the psychoactive ingredients of the smoke, for all smoke contains cancer-causing chemicals.

MEMBRANE ABSORPTION

Almost any body membrane can be used for rapid drug absorption. Cocaine is commonly absorbed through the nasal membranes. Some drugs, such as the nicotine in chewing tobacco and nitroglycerin tablets for heart patients, are absorbed through the lining of the mouth. Even the lining of the vagina or rectum can be used for drug absorption. Some prescription drugs are incorporated into rectal or vaginal suppositories. Increasing numbers of prescription drugs are available in "patches" worn on the skin, through which they are readily absorbed into the blood.

INJECTION

Drugs can be injected in several ways: into or just beneath the skin, into a muscle, or directly into a vein (**intravenously**). Psychoactive drugs are most commonly injected intravenously, giving a very rapid effect.

In addition to any hazards the drug itself may present, injection carries hazards all its own. Foremost is the risk of infection when people share needles. In addition to the traditional risks of hepatitis and bacterial blood infections (septicemia), AIDS has emerged as an often fatal risk for people who share needles. In some cities, up to 70 percent of those who inject illicit drugs are infected with HIV, the AIDS virus.[1]

The possibility of contracting AIDS, hepatitis, and other diseases is not limited to chronic abusers. Even the occasional recreational drug user or the steroid user who shares a needle or syringe is at risk. The total number of Americans who occasionally or regularly inject drugs has been estimated at several million.[2]

One of the many controversies surrounding AIDS concerns the legal availability of sterile injection equipment. One argument holds that laws restricting sale of injection equipment to those with medical prescriptions forces the sharing of needles and syringes by users of illegal drugs, thereby contributing to the spread of AIDS. The opposing argument is that easing the availability of injection equipment would seem to condone and encourage drug abuse.[3] Actually, whether or not an individual is a drug abuser is likely to hinge upon much more basic issues. See Communication for Wellness: Drugs as a Substitute for Communication for one example.

....

intravenous into a vein.

DRUGS AS A SUBSTITUTE FOR COMMUNICATION

People abuse drugs for a wide variety of reasons. One common reason is to try to block out what seems to be unbearable emotional pain. Those who abuse drugs for this reason are often people who keep their feelings hidden inside and may even take pride in their ability to "suffer in silence." But feelings kept inside don't just go away. And painful emotions kept inside tend to grow ever more powerful until they become just too much to bear.

Effective substance-abuse-prevention and recovery programs emphasize learning how to open up to others and share painful feelings. Communicating painful emotions with supporting friends helps us to keep problems in perspective so they don't seem so overwhelming. For many people this can make the difference between depending on drugs to blot out pain and being able to live a rewarding, satisfying, drug-free life.

DISTRIBUTION OF DRUGS THROUGHOUT THE BODY

Once a drug is absorbed into the blood, the circulating blood distributes it throughout the body. This distribution usually takes no more than one minute. Then virtually all drugs begin to move out of the bloodstream into the fluid surrounding the cells of the many body tissues. The concentration of a drug in the blood and the tissue fluid usually reaches an equilibrium. If the drug is capable of penetrating body cells, as many are, it moves next into the actual body cells. Those drugs that do not penetrate cells affect the outer membrane of the cell.

MEMBRANES AND DRUG ACTION

The absorption and distribution of a drug is influenced by how the drug interacts with the body's membranes. We will discuss several membranes that are especially important in this respect.

Cell Membranes

Every human body cell is contained within its individual **cell membrane,** also called the **plasma membrane.** This membrane is composed of fat and protein and is permeable to some drugs and impermeable to others. The ability of a drug to penetrate this membrane depends on the solubility of that drug in fat. **Fat-soluble** drugs enter cells

....

cell membrane or **plasma membrane** the delicate membrane, made of fat and protein, enclosing a cell and regulating the movement of all materials into and out of the cell.

fat-soluble dissolving in fat.

much more freely than those that are not fat-soluble. Tiny pores present in the cell membrane allow the passage of a few small, fat-insoluble drug molecules. For example, alcohol, being a small molecule and being soluble in both fat and water, enters body cells very freely.

Walls of Blood Capillaries

Blood capillaries are tiny tubes that have walls formed by a single layer of very thin cells. Between the cells are minute pores connecting the interior of the capillary with the exterior. These pores are larger than most drug molecules. Thus, drug molecules can pass out of the capillaries with little difficulty.

Placental Membranes

Most psychoactive drugs pass freely through the placental membranes, within minutes reaching levels in the fetal blood that are as high as in the mother's blood. The fetus is much more vulnerable to drugs than the mother as its organs are in the critical process of formation and are highly susceptible to drug damage, and its liver is not yet able to eliminate drugs from its blood. This is why it is important for expectant mothers to abstain from the use of drugs. There are numerous cases of drug-dependent mothers giving birth to drug-dependent babies. The effects of nicotine and alcohol on a developing fetus are described in Chapters 16 and 17.

The Blood-Brain Barrier

The brain is very sensitive to drugs and other chemicals. The movement of chemicals from the blood to the brain is regulated by the **blood-brain barrier.** Capillaries serving the brain lack the pores characteristic of other capillaries, forcing chemicals leaving the blood to pass directly through the cells of the capillary wall. Fat-soluble drugs are able to move through these capillary walls much more readily than are water-soluble drugs for the reasons explained earlier. Thus, most psychoactive drugs are fat-soluble.

CHECKPOINT

1. Outline the different ways that drugs can be taken and any special hazards of each method.

2. Which route of drug administration produces the fastest effects? Which is the most common?

3. How long does it take for a drug to be distributed throughout the body?

4. Which types of drugs can penetrate cell membranes with the greatest ease?

5. Explain the importance of the blood-brain barrier.

NEUROTRANSMITTERS AND RECEPTOR MECHANISMS

Though a psychoactive drug is typically distributed throughout the body, its effects on mood, emotions, and behavior result from the drug's effects on the brain. Psychoactive drugs often work by attaching to specific **receptor sites** (see Figure 15.1) on the brain cells. These receptor sites are present for the purpose of interacting with natural body chemicals, such as the **neurotransmitters** (*nū-rō-trans'mit-ters*). Neurotransmitters are chemicals released from one brain cell to stimulate or inhibit another brain cell. Neurotransmitters play an essential role in transmitting nerve impulses

blood-brain barrier a barrier membrane between the circulating blood and the brain that prevents some harmful substances from entering brain tissue.

receptor site a special protein on the surface or within a cell with which a drug, neurotransmitter, or hormone interacts.

neurotransmitter a chemical released from one brain cell to stimulate or inhibit another brain cell.

from one neuron to another by bridging the gap in the **synapse** (*sin'aps*), the junction between two neurons (Figure 15.2).

Psychoactive drugs often work by mimicking the normal action of neurotransmitters. Drugs attach to receptor sites when their chemical structures are similar to neurotransmitters. The effects of a drug will be similar to those of the body chemical it resembles.

Because receptor sites are specific for different body chemicals or drugs, taking a stimulant drug to cancel a depressant or vice versa is ineffective. The drug originally taken would continue to exert its action and problems could be compounded by the effects of the second drug. *If someone has overdosed, instead of trying to counteract the overdose with another drug, immediately take the person to a hospital emergency room or call paramedics so that proper care can be provided.*

ENDORPHINS

Endorphins have been called "the body's own narcotics." (A **narcotic** is a drug that can relieve pain and cause sleep. The natural and synthetic opiates, such as morphine and heroin, are the only drugs that are medically classified as narcotics.) Research done in the 1960s revealed that nerve cells in parts of the brain, spinal cord, and intestines carried highly specific receptors for opiate drugs. Experts thought this strange at the time—why would our cells carry receptors for chemicals that are not normally present in the human body?

The answer came in 1975 when Dr. John Hughes and Dr. Hans Kosterlitz of the University of Aberdeen, Scotland, found opiatelike chemicals in the brains of pigs and eventually in all vertebrates.[4] These chemicals were named **endorphins** (*endor'fins*), from the words "**endogenous** (*en-doj'e-nus;* originating within) morphine." To date, a total of 18 opiatelike chemicals have been identified in the human brain.

Endorphins work like neurotransmitters and appear to have many effects, the most important of

synapse the junction between two neurons.

narcotic a drug that can relieve pain and cause sleep.

endorphin an endogenous opiatelike chemical.

endogenous originating within a cell or organism.

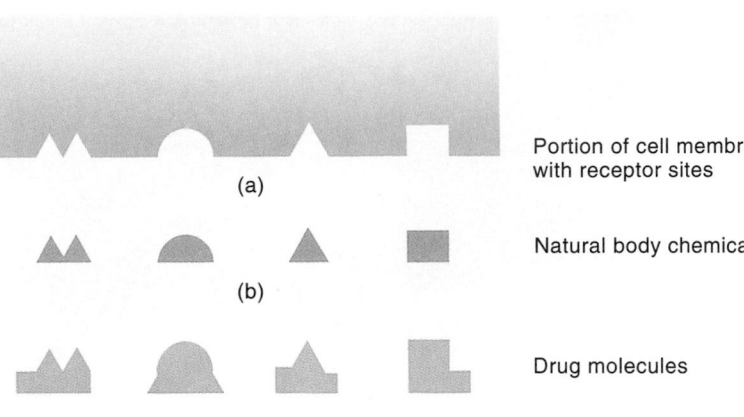

Portion of cell membrane with receptor sites

Natural body chemicals

Drug molecules

Figure 15.1
Receptor Sites

Many psychoactive drugs mimic normal body chemicals and occupy receptor sites on the surface of brain cell membranes intended for the body chemicals. (a) A portion of cell membrane illustrating microscopic receptor sites. (b) Natural body chemicals intended to react with each receptor site; note their complementary shapes. (c) Psychoactive drug molecules; note how the shapes of the drug molecules closely resemble those of the natural body chemicals.

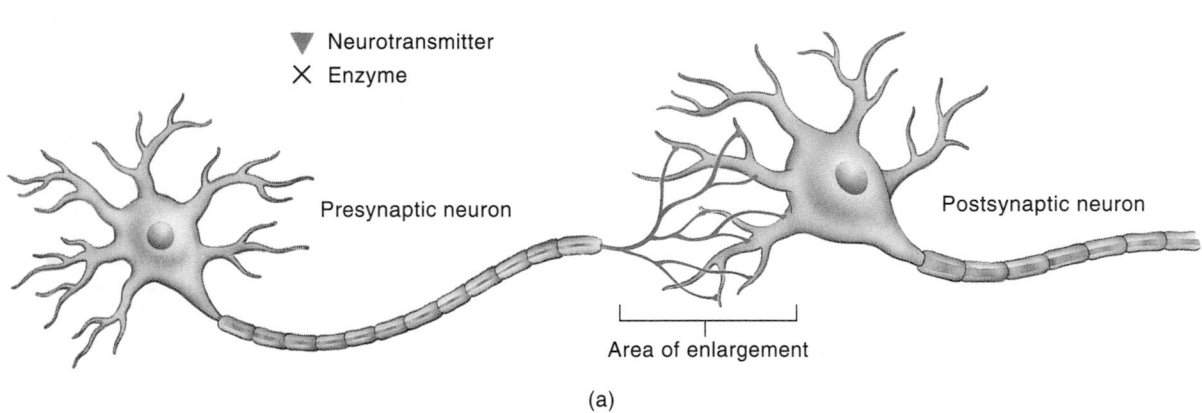

▼ Neurotransmitter
✕ Enzyme

Presynaptic neuron

Postsynaptic neuron

Area of enlargement

(a)

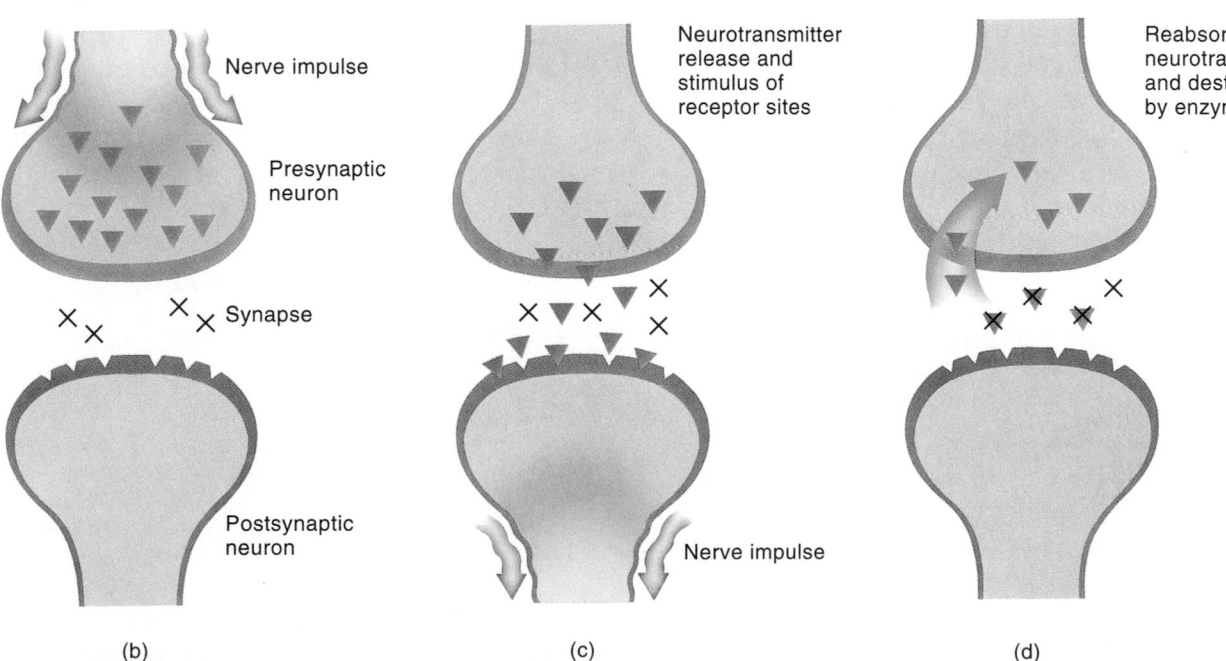

Nerve impulse

Presynaptic neuron

Synapse

Postsynaptic neuron

Neurotransmitter release and stimulus of receptor sites

Nerve impulse

Reabsorption of neurotransmitter and destruction by enzymes

(b)

(c)

(d)

Figure 15.2
The Synapse

A synapse, the junction between two neurons (nerve cells). When a nerve impulse reaches the end of the first neuron, that neuron releases a neurotransmitter substance that simulates an impulse to start down the second neuron. The neurotransmitter is then reabsorbed or destroyed by enzymes (Xs in sketch).

which may be regulating the sense of pain. In essence, endorphins block nerve impulses that the brain would perceive as pain. Endorphins also appear to modulate emotional responses, producing feelings of pleasure. They also are believed to be involved in hunger, memory, stress, seizures, emotional disorders, and the response to alcohol.[5, 6]

Raising Endorphin Levels

The pain relief obtained from acupuncture is believed to work by stimulating nerves that cause the increased release of endorphins.[7] Pain relief achieved through the *placebo effect* (the use of inert pills or other treatments that work through the power of suggestion) may also be due to an increased release of endorphins. It is possible that the mere suggestion that pain will be relieved causes endorphins to be released, producing pain relief. Devices that relieve severe pain by applying small amounts of electric current to the skin also work by stimulating endorphin release.

It is also believed that the euphoria many people feel from running and other vigorous exercise results from increased endorphin release during exercise.[8] This is one reason why a regular exercise program is so valuable in the prevention of and rehabilitation from chemical dependency.

The **narcotic-antagonist** drug naloxone, used in treating narcotic overdoses, also blocks the action of endorphins and has been shown to eliminate the pain-relieving effects of acupuncture, placebo treatments, and electric skin stimulation.[9, 10]

Endorphins and Psychoactive Drugs

How does all of this relate to the use or abuse of psychoactive drugs? The most obvious relationship occurs with opiate drugs such as morphine and heroin. The pain relieving and **euphoria**-producing action of opiates occurs when these drugs attach to the brain's endorphin receptors. Euphoria is an exaggerated feeling of well-being. The presence of an opiate drug, however, causes the endorphin regulatory mechanism to shut off the normal release of endorphins. Then, as the drug breaks down, the brain is left with an abnormally low

....

narcotic-antagonist a drug that prevents or reverses the action of a narcotic.

euphoria an exaggerated feeling of well-being or elation.

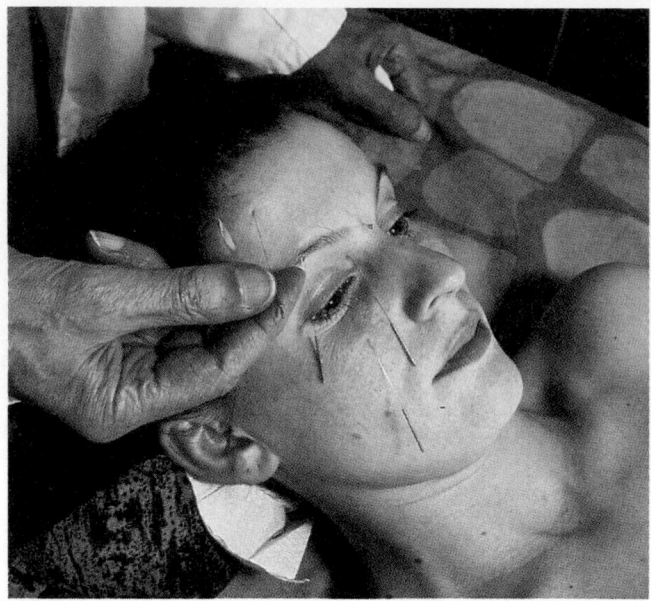

Acupuncture is believed to relieve pain by stimulating the release of endorphins.

endorphin level, causing both physical and emotional pain. To relieve the pain, the user feels compelled to take more of the drug. This is the basis of opiate dependency. When a frequent opiate user stops taking the drug, there is an adjustment period of a few days before the brain resumes endorphin production. This unpleasant adjustment period is called withdrawal.[11]

It has been suggested that some people are genetically prone to alcoholism and other chemical dependencies because of an inherently low endorphin level.[12] These people feel more physical and emotional pain than do other people and find a much greater satisfaction in psychoactive chemicals.

CHECKPOINT

1. What are the roles of neurotransmitters?

2. In what ways can drugs affect the actions of brain cells?

3. What roles do endorphins play in the brain?

4. What occurs when an opiate abuser stops taking the drug?

ELIMINATION OF DRUGS FROM THE BODY

There are several ways for the human body to eliminate drugs. Although the kidneys are the main excretory organs, they do not function well in elim-

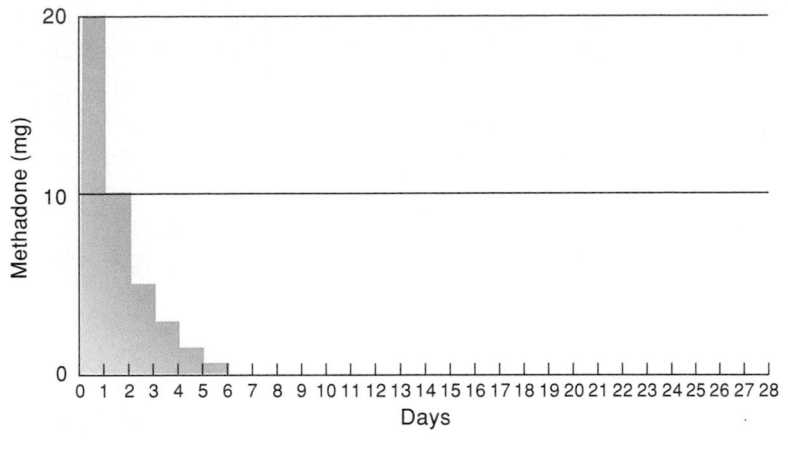

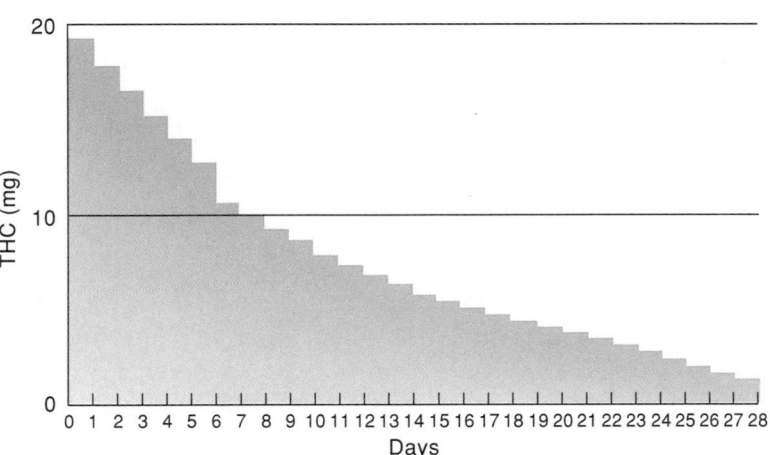

Figure 15.3
Half-Lives of Drugs

The half-life is the time required for half of the drug present in the body to be eliminated. (a) The breakdown in the body of methadone, which has a half-life of 24 hours. (b) The breakdown in the body of the THC from marijuana, which has a half-life of 7 days.

inating most psychoactive drugs from the body, at least in the drugs' original forms. Most drugs are first modified by enzymes in the liver; their metabolic products are then excreted in the urine or feces. The enzymes of the liver usually decrease the psychoactive effect of a drug, though there are drugs, such as Valium, that become active (or develop increased activity) as a result of modification of the drug by the liver.

Small amounts of some drugs are lost through breathing, sweating, saliva, and other secretions, although these are seldom main paths of drug elimination. Breast milk is one secretion that can be a source of drug elimination. Many drugs, if taken by a breastfeeding mother, will be present in her milk at levels that may be very harmful to her infant.

Different drugs are eliminated from the body at very different rates. Most drugs are broken down by the liver at a **logarithmic rate**, meaning that

the same *percentage* of the remaining drug is broken down during each equal time period. For example, if 50 percent of a drug dosage was broken down in the first 24 hours, then 50 percent of what remained would be broken down in the second 24 hours, and so on. The **half-life** (Figure 15.3) is the time period needed for the breakdown of one-half of the drug remaining in the body. Half-lives of common drugs range from minutes to days. Table 15.1 compares the half-lives of some psychoactive drugs.

Drug Myth:
When the effects of a drug are no longer felt, it means that the drug has been cleared from the body.

logarithmic rate of drug breakdown the same *percentage* of the remaining drug is broken down during each equal time period.

half-life the time needed for the breakdown of one-half of the amount of a drug remaining in the body.

Table 15.1
Half-lives of Some Common Drugs

Drug	Half-life[a]
Cocaine	1–5 hours[b]
Fentanyl	45 minutes[c]
Heroin	2–5 hours[b]
Librium	5–30 hours[b]
LSD	1.5 hours[b] (mental effects continue for 8–12 hours)
Marijuana	1 week[d]
Methadone	24 hours[d]
Methamphetamine	5–20 hours (highly variable)[b]
Methaqualone	18–24 hours[b]
Valium	20–50 hours[d]
Xanax	12–19 hours[e]

[a]Half-life is the time required for half of the drug present in the body to be eliminated.
[b]Radcliffe, A. *The Pharmer's Almanac.* New York: Ballantine, 1991.
[c]Julien, R. *A Primer of Drug Action,* 6th ed. New York: Freeman, 1991.
[d]Liska, K. *Drugs and the Human Body,* 3rd ed. New York: Macmillan, 1989.

Drug Reality:
Many drugs remain in the body at high concentrations long after their obvious effects have disappeared. There is the potential for dangerous interactions when another drug is taken during this period.

Alcohol differs from most drugs in that it breaks down at an **arithmetic rate,** rather than a logarithmic rate. This means that the same *amount,* rather than percentage, of alcohol will be broken down in each hour, regardless of how many drinks have been consumed. Thus, the more alcohol you have consumed, the more time you must allow for sobering up. People vary in the speed at which they break down alcohol. In general, the average person can break down the alcohol in one can of beer in one hour. If a person metabolized the alcohol in one can of beer in one hour, then that person would break down the alcohol in five cans of beer in five hours, and so on. We must emphasize that some people require considerably more than the average time to metabolize alcohol.

arithmetic rate of drug breakdown the same *amount* of a drug will be broken down in each equal time period.

Some drugs remain in the body long after their effects are no longer felt. This occurs, for instance, when a drug moves from the blood into storage in the body's fatty tissues. Fentanyl ("China White"), for example, produces a euphoria lasting for only about 15 minutes, whereas the drug remains in the body fat for several hours. Similarly, the active ingredient in marijuana is present in the body for weeks after its use.

CHECKPOINT
1. Explain the term *half-life.*
2. List the various pathways by which the body eliminates drugs.
3. Contrast a logarithmic versus an arithmetic breakdown of a drug.

REBOUND EFFECTS

A **rebound effect,** sometimes called the paradoxical effect, of a drug means that after the drug has been eliminated from the user's body, he or she experiences effects that are the opposite of the original effects of the drug. For example, if a drug has sedative effects, its rebound effect is nervousness and agitation. If a drug is a stimulant, its rebound effect may include feelings of depression and fatigue (for example, the "cocaine blues" or "crashing"). Rebound effects are characteristic of drugs that cause physical dependence and are usually very unpleasant. To eliminate this unpleasant feeling, people will often take another dose of the drug. This cycle of using a drug to eliminate the unpleasant feelings produced by that same drug can easily lead to chemical dependency. The withdrawal illness experienced when heavy use of certain drugs is discontinued is in a large part caused by the rebound effect.[13]

DEVELOPMENT OF TOLERANCE

Many of the psychoactive drugs are tolerance-forming. **Tolerance** is the body's ability to adjust to

rebound effect the development of effects opposite to those of the drug as a drug is eliminated from the body.

tolerance the body's ability to adjust to increasing levels of a drug.

increasing levels of a drug. Heavy users of some drugs may take doses that are many times the dose that would be fatal to a nonuser or an infrequent user of the same drug. The degree of tolerance and the rate at which it develops depends on the drug, the person using the drug, and the frequency and dosage with which the drug is used. In some cases, tolerance develops to only some of the effects of a drug. For example, a drug might no longer produce the same degree of euphoria, but still carry the same threat of fatal overdose. A period of abstinence from a drug usually reduces a person's tolerance to it.

DRUG DOSAGES

Even though drug dosage levels alone do not form a basis for distinguishing between drug use and abuse, the quantity of any drug taken at one time *is* highly significant. It *does* make a difference if you take one pill or many pills. It *does* matter whether you drink one beer or many beers. Beer may be "the beverage of moderation," but only if it is consumed *in* moderation.

Comparisons of the strengths of various drugs are not as significant as they might seem. Even the mildest drugs, if taken in large dosages, can have extremely powerful effects. People tend to adjust the dosage of psychoactive drugs to achieve the effects they seek.

C H E C K P O I N T

1. Explain rebound or paradoxical effects of drugs.

2. What is tolerance to a drug?

POLYDRUG ABUSE

A dangerous development in recent years has been **polydrug abuse:** the simultaneous abuse of more than one drug. Today, relatively few drug abusers use only a single drug.[14] There are few "pure" alcoholics, cocaine abusers, marijuana smokers, or other drug abusers. People often drift into polydrug abuse by using one drug to overcome an unpleasant or unwanted effect of another drug.

Almost every possible combination of psychoactive drugs has been used at some time or place. Among more common examples are alcohol and marijuana or alcohol and pills of various kinds. The combination of alcohol and barbiturates is especially dangerous. In recent years, drug experts have been dismayed by the reemergence of the old combination of cocaine and heroin, sometimes called speedball. This combination produces an extremely powerful physiological dependence.

Sometimes a person is unaware that he or she is actually using several drugs at the same time. Some drugs have long half-lives and remain in the body for days or weeks, even though their noticeable effects may have lasted only a few hours. When a second drug is introduced into the body while residues of the first remain, interactions between the two drugs may occur.

Polydrug abuse can have unknown and unpredictable effects, which can be immediate and/or long term. The effects of a single psychoactive drug are complex and not completely understood, but when several psychoactive drugs are in the body simultaneously, they may interact in extremely complex, dangerous, and unpredictable ways. Polydrug abusers risk severe, and possibly permanent, damaging effects. We cannot emphasize strongly enough the inadvisability of polydrug abuse.

DRUG INTERACTIONS

Since many people today use more than one psychoactive drug, or use "street" drugs in addition to medically prescribed drugs, it is important to consider how different drugs simultaneously present in the body may interact. Table 15.2, on p. 470, lists some representative drug interactions.

Enhancing Interactions

The interactions between drugs can either enhance or inhibit the effects of the interacting drugs. **Enhancing interactions** are those in which the effects of one drug increase the effects of another. There are several types of enhancing interactions (though some authorities and some medical dictio-

---

polydrug abuse the simultaneous abuse of more than one drug.

enhancing interactions drug interactions in which the effects of one drug increase the effects of another.

Table 15.2
Some Representative Drug Interactions

Note: This is only a sample of drug inter-actions. Omission of a combination does not imply that it is safe. Do not use any combination of drugs without first check-ing with your physician.

Alcohol combined with:	may produce this effect:
barbiturates	severe depression of brain function, with possible respiratory failure
tranquilizers	greatly increased sedation
antihistamines	greatly increased sedation
chloral hydrate	greatly increased sedation
MAO inhibitors	depression of central nervous system
Barbiturates combined with:	**may produce this effect:**
alcohol	severe depression of brain function, with possible respiratory failure
MAO inhibitors	depression of central nervous system
tranquilizers	increases effects of both drugs
oral contraceptives	inhibition of contraceptive action
male hormones	decreased action of sex hormones
antidiabetic drugs	increased barbiturate activity
antihistamines	first, severe depression of central nervous system, then they neutralize each other
Dilantin	diminished anticonvulsant activity
Tranquilizers combined with:	**may produce this effect:**
alcohol	greatly increased sedation
MAO inhibitors	greatly increased sedation
barbiturates	increases effects of both drugs
Demerol	increases sedation

Source: FDA Consumer, *various issues.*

naries view the following two terms as synony-mous and interchangeable).

Synergism (*sin'er-jism*) produces effects that are more powerful than the sum of the effects of each drug if taken individually. Synergism can be represented by the formula $2 + 2 = 8$. Meant as an example only, this formula would indicate that the combined effect of two drugs would be double the sum of their individual effects.

One of the most dramatic and dangerous exam-ples of synergism is the combination of alcohol and barbiturates. Even when moderate amounts of each

....

synergism when two drugs produce effects that are more powerful than the sum of the effects of each drug if taken individually.

are used, the combined effect may result in a severe depression of brain function, with possible respira-tory failure. Alcohol is also dangerous in combina-tion with tranquilizers, cold medications, antihista-mines, and any form of sedative.

Potentiation (*pō-ten-shē-ā'shun*) describes a situation in which a drug enhances a certain effect of another drug, but does not have that effect by itself. Potentiation can be represented by the for-mula $0 + 2 = 4$. For example, isopropyl (rubbing) alcohol by itself, although toxic in many other ways, does not cause liver damage. But rubbing alcohol combined with the fumes of carbon tetra-chloride (a solvent formerly used in fire extin-guishers) causes severe liver damage.[15]

Antagonism

Antagonism (*an-tag'ō-nizm*) means that one drug reduces the effect of another drug or two drugs may mutually inhibit each other. Like potentiation, antagonism can be caused by various physiological mechanisms. An example is when one drug increases the level of liver enzymes that break down the other drug.

The effects of a medically prescribed drug may in many cases be increased or decreased by alco-hol or another psychoactive drug. When taking any prescribed medication, it is important to check with the prescribing physician or pharmacist before using alcohol or any nonprescribed drugs. Even prescribed drugs may affect each other. A physician or dentist who is about to prescribe a drug for you should always be made aware of any other medications you are taking. It is also impor-tant to have all of your prescriptions filled at the same place so the pharmacist can detect any incompatible drugs.

CHECKPOINT

1. What is polydrug abuse and what are its spe-cial hazards?

2. Define the terms *synergism, potentiation,* and *antagonism.*

....

potentiation when a drug enhances a certain effect of another drug, but does not have that effect by itself.

antagonism one drug prevents or reduces the effect of another or two drugs mutually inhibit each other.

SOURCES AND CLASSIFICATION OF PSYCHOACTIVE DRUGS

Psychoactive drugs can be derived from natural sources such as fungi and other plants or synthesized from purely chemical sources. A semisynthetic drug has a molecule taken from a natural source, then chemically altered. Some examples within each category are listed in Table 15.3.

Over the years, advocates of various natural source drugs, such as marijuana, cocaine, and opium, have argued that such drugs, as products of nature, are inherently safer than synthetic drugs. Unfortunately, an organically produced drug is not necessarily safe. The safety or hazard of each drug must be judged by its effects, not by its source.

CLASSIFICATION OF PSYCHOACTIVE DRUGS

Many systems of classifying psychoactive drugs have been proposed; almost every book on the subject has its own system of classification. There are many reasons for this diversity:[16]

- A drug usually affects a number of brain functions simultaneously and may act in different ways with each.
- Varying dosage levels of a drug may result in different behavioral effects.
- The same drug may affect each individual differently.

Despite the limitations of any system of classification, it is useful to have an organized basis for our discussion of drugs. Table 15.4 presents the classification system we will follow in this chapter.

Table 15.3
Some Examples of Natural and Synthetic Psychoactive Drugs

Some Drugs from Natural Sources

1. Opium, codeine, and morphine—from the opium poppy
2. Cocaine—from coca shrub
3. Marijuana and hashish—from *Cannabis* plants
4. Psilocybin—from *Psilocybe* mushroom
5. Mescaline—from peyote cactus
6. Alcohol—from yeast

Some Synthetic Drugs

1. Valium and Xanax
2. Amphetamines
3. Barbiturates
4. MDMA (ecstacy or XTC)
5. PCP

Semisynthetic

1. Heroin—diacetyl morphine
2. LSD—a modification of a chemical produced by a fungus.

Table 15.4
A Classification of Some Common Psychoactive Drugs

Stimulants

Cocaine
Amphetamines
Caffeine
Nicotine

Sedative-Hypnotics (Depressants)

Barbiturates
Nonbarbiturate hypnotics: glutethimide, methaqualone, and so on
Minor tranquilizers (ataraxics or antianxiety agents): Librium, Valium, Xanax, Equanil
Alcohol

Opiate Narcotics

Opium
Codeine
Morphine
Heroin
Synthetic opiates: Percodan, Demerol, Methadone, Dilaudid

Psychedelics and Hallucinogens

LSD
Mescaline
Psilocybin
PCP
Substituted amphetamines: DOM (STP), MDMA (ecstasy), and so on

Marijuana and Other *Cannabis* Derivatives

Marijuana, hashish, THC

Inhalants (Volatile substances)

Glues, gasoline, thinners, cleaning fluids, toluene, benzene, nitrous oxide, amyl nitrite, butyl or isobutyl nitrite, and so on

Note: This is a partial listing, containing only drugs that are most commonly abused.

Before we begin our survey of specific drugs, take a minute right now and complete the assessment In Your Hands: Evaluating Your Own Drug Use.

SPECIFIC PSYCHOACTIVE DRUGS

The balance of this chapter will survey many of the specific psychoactive drugs to be found on the street today. We will begin with the stimulants.

STIMULANT DRUGS

The principal action of these drugs is stimulation of the central nervous system. We will consider cocaine, amphetamines, and caffeine in this chapter and nicotine in Chapter 16.

Cocaine

Cocaine is a natural ingredient found in the leaves of the coca shrub, *Erythroxylon coca,* native to South America. There, the leaves, containing about 1 percent cocaine, are chewed, providing stimulation and essential vitamins and minerals.

Although drug-use statistics are, of necessity, estimates, it appears that cocaine use is on a downward trend in the United States.[17] At one time, cocaine use was associated with high income levels, and as such, gained an aura of high status. Today, cocaine use is found in all strata of U.S. society and carries no enhanced status. One estimate is that about 8 million people used cocaine in some form at least once during the most recent year, and just under 3 million used it at least once the most recent month. Estimates of the number of Americans who are cocaine-dependent range from 862,000 to 2.4 million.[18]

Cocaine Myth:
You can't become dependent on cocaine.

Cocaine Reality:
Cocaine is highly dependence forming. Ten percent or more of those who repeatedly snort coke and perhaps 50 percent of those who smoke it become dependent.

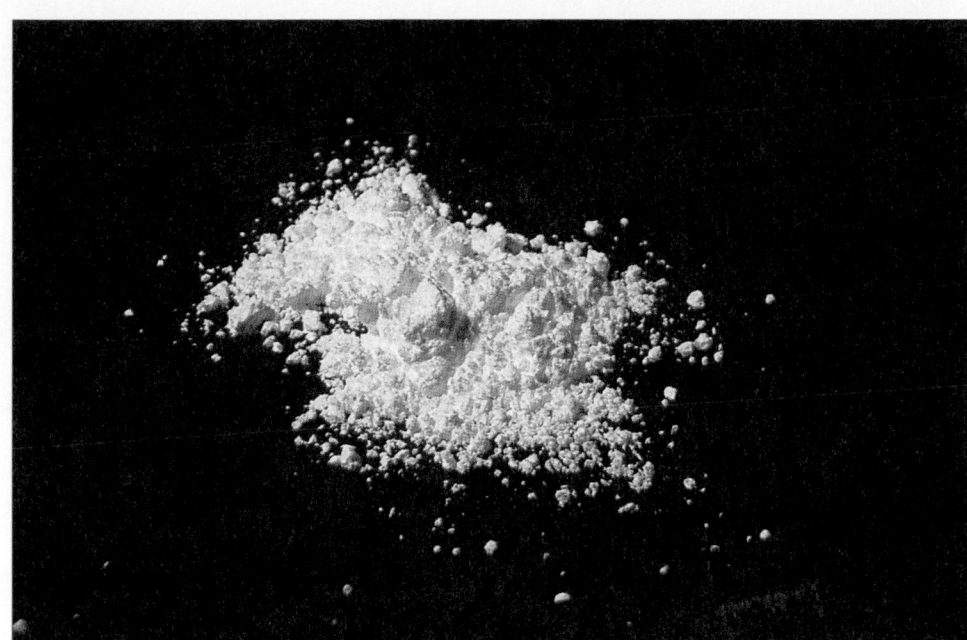

Most cocaine enters the United States as cocaine hydrochloride, a white powder. This powder usually is diluted considerably before it is sold on the street.

Forms and Effects of Cocaine   Cocaine is used on this continent in several forms, including cocaine hydrochloride, freebase, and crack or rock. Most common is **cocaine hydrochloride,** a white powder that is sniffed ("snorted") into the nose and absorbed through the nasal membranes or is injected intravenously. Most cocaine hydrochloride is diluted or "cut" considerably before it is sold on the street. *As with almost all street drugs, the ultimate user receives a product of uncertain identity, at an unknown concentration, diluted with unknown and possibly hazardous **adulterants*** (less valuable substances used to dilute a product). Cutting agents include sugars, caffeine, and the local anesthetics, lidocaine and benzocaine. Most of these chemicals have physiological effects of their own, which compound the dangers of street cocaine.

When cocaine is snorted, effects begin within a few seconds to several minutes and peak at about ten minutes. Cocaine's immediate effects include euphoria, increased self-confidence and self-esteem, increased talking, a sense of increased mental clarity, hypersexuality, insomnia, and loss of appetite. Although some users feel no adverse effects afterward, many experience a rebound effect, feeling anxious, depressed, and irritable (the "crash" or "cocaine blues"). There is often a craving for more cocaine within about 30 minutes to an hour after snorting. This is why cocaine has such a high potential for producing dependency.

When cocaine hydrochloride is injected intravenously, it produces a faster and more pronounced, but shorter-lived, effect. Euphoria occurs within about 15 minutes after injection. Because of the intense and brief euphoria, followed quickly by a severe "crash," injecting cocaine carries a great risk of dependency.

Another method of using cocaine is by smoking it. Cocaine is prepared for smoking in one of several ways. Freebasing is a solvent-extraction method using ether or a similar solvent. The product is called **freebase.** Cocaine can also be prepared for smoking by the chemical reaction that results when it is combined with a strong base, such as ammonia or baking soda. The product is called **crack** or **rock.** Smoking cocaine produces almost instant effects: an intense euphoria within 8–12 seconds, accompanied by a rise in pulse,

cocaine hydrochloride the hydrochloride form of the alkaloid cocaine derived from the leaves of the coca shrub.

adulterants inert or less valuable substances used to dilute a product.

freebase cocaine that has been converted from the stable hydrochloride form to the less stable but more potent basic form.

crack or **rock** freebased cocaine made by mixing cocaine hydrochloride, sodium bicarbonate (baking soda), and water.

"Crack" or "rock" cocaine is produced by treating cocaine hydrochloride with an alkaline substance such as baking soda. Crack is smoked and is much more addictive than snorted cocaine hydrochloride.

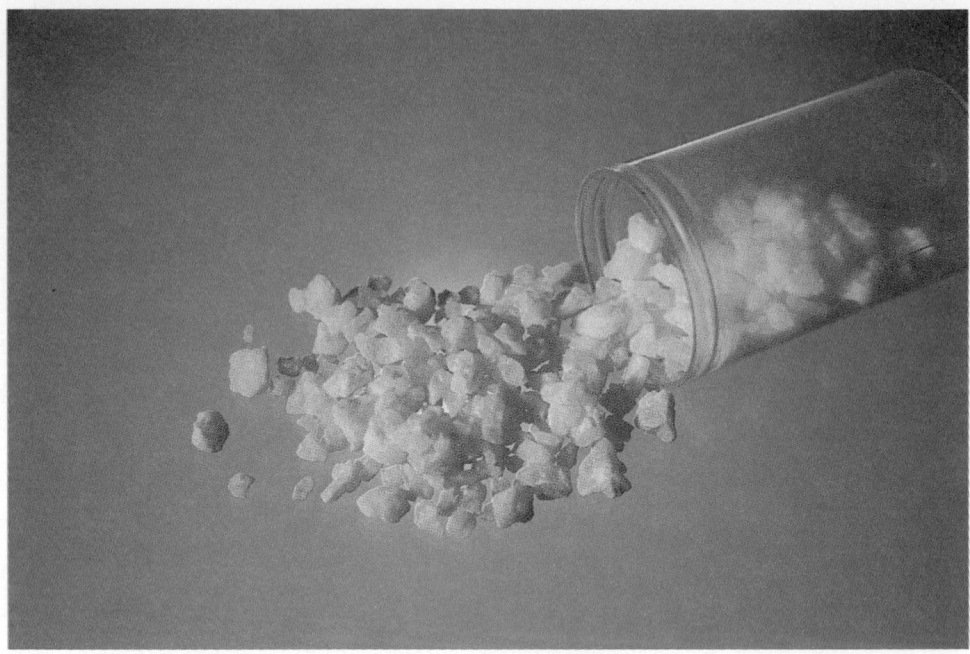

blood pressure, body temperature, and respiratory rate. The euphoria ends within 10–20 minutes, followed by a more intensive craving for cocaine than that following intranasal or intravenous use.[19] *The faster a drug gets into the brain, the higher its potential for dependency.* The dependency-producing potential of smoked cocaine is extreme.

Coca paste is a very impure form of cocaine that is a serious problem in some countries and a potential problem in the United States because of its low cost. Coca paste is made by pouring sulfuric acid over coca leaves, converting the cocaine in the leaves to cocaine sulfate, which is collected as a paste. Coca paste is very inexpensive and can be smoked or eaten. Cocaine sulfate can cause dependency in as little as four or five days. Cocaine sulfate also causes more brain damage than other cocaine forms, perhaps due to its high content of impurities.[20]

How Cocaine Works and Causes Dependency

Cocaine causes a buildup of neurotransmitters in the brain, thereby increasing nerve transmission and producing euphoria and mood elevation. As the cocaine wears off, however, the rebound effect causes depression and fatigue.

....

coca paste an impure, cocaine-containing product made by pouring sulfuric acid over coca leaves.

Cocaine is among the most dependency-forming of the psychoactive drugs, as is reflected in the large number of dependent persons. Animals, in experiments, develop such strong cravings for cocaine that, given their choice, they will take cocaine instead of food, even to the point of starvation.

Cocaine dependency was formerly viewed as primarily psychological, rather than physical. Now it is recognized as being physiologically based.[21] Withdrawal symptoms include depression, social withdrawal, tremors, severe drug cravings, muscle pains, eating and sleeping disturbances, and changes in a person's EEG (electroencephalogram).

Medical Uses of Cocaine Cocaine is a local anesthetic, used during some eye, ear, nose, and throat surgery. It also reduces bleeding during surgery by narrowing blood vessels. In Canada and England, cocaine is one of the ingredients in Brompton's cocktail, a mixture given to relieve the severe pain of terminal cancer.

Dangers of Cocaine Use Several hundred deaths per year are associated with cocaine use, usually from heart failure, respiratory paralysis, or prolonged convulsions. Cocaine has been shown to block the transmission of impulses from the heart's natural pacemakers (the sinoatrial and atrioventricular nodes) to the heart muscle.[22] Other serious risks include constricted blood vessels, increased heart rate, elevated blood pressure, convulsions, and coma. Complications include nasal tissue damage, anorexia, nausea, diarrhea, liver damage, headaches, severe fatigue, and depression.

Cocaine Use in Pregnancy   Cocaine or crack use by a woman during pregnancy has been blamed for causing a multitude of adverse effects on her baby.[23] Many babies of cocaine users are born prematurely or have low birthweights, do not cuddle or nurse well, and are generally irritable and unresponsive. Many other effects have also been associated with cocaine use. Cocaine users' babies are at increased risk of **sudden infant death syndrome (SIDS).** Long-term, they may have an increased rate of respiratory and kidney disorders, and lasting neurological damage, as evidenced by behavioral difficulties (impulsiveness and moodiness), learning disorders, impaired vision, and lack of motor coordination.

It is unclear to what degree these problems are direct results of cocaine use. Some experts now wonder whether there really is a "cocaine baby" or "crack baby" syndrome.[24] These authorities suspect that some of the effects that have been attributed to cocaine use actually may be caused by other behaviors that are common among cocaine-using women. For example, many women who use cocaine also drink alcohol, smoke cigarettes, and/or use other drugs while pregnant, neglect proper nutrition, have sexually transmitted diseases, and fail to obtain prenatal care. Each of these factors is definitely associated with a poor outcome of a pregnancy.

Whether or not there proves to be a true "crack baby" syndrome, we can't repeat often enough the importance of *avoiding nonprescribed drugs during pregnancy*. Both parents also need to be drug free for a few months *before* conception. It is now clear that sperm are also damaged by drug use.

Amphetamines

Amphetamines (*am-fet'a-mēnz*), such as amphetamine sulfate (Benzedrine), dextroamphetamine sulfate (Dexedrine), and methamphetamine

(Methedrine), are synthetic stimulants. Street names include Whites, Speed, Crank, Ice, and Crystal. Amphetamines are similar to the neurotransmitter norepinephrine and the hormone used in the fight or flight response, epinephrine (adrenalin). They produce an arousal response similar to your normal reactions to emergency situations or at high levels of stress. Amphetamines are taken in pill form or by intravenous injection.

A relatively new form of methamphetamine called *ice* first emerged in Japan, Hawaii, and California. It is inexpensive and easy to manufacture. Ice most often exists as small, clear chunks and is usually smoked. It is more expensive than crack cocaine, but provides a much more prolonged effect of up to 24 hours. Many overdoses are presently occurring in areas where ice has become prevalent. Users sometimes become very aggressive and difficult to control.

Moderate doses of amphetamines make some people feel quite good—alert, talkative, and "turned on." Other people find that amphetamines just make them feel nervous. Even those who enjoy the effects of amphetamines may also take a depressant, such as a barbiturate, to relieve their nervous feelings. Like cocaine use, amphetamine use is often followed by a period of depression.

Frequent users develop tolerance to amphetamines, so they often progress to very high dosages. Psychological dependence to amphetamines can be very strong. For years it was argued whether or not physiological dependency occurs. It is now clearly known that when large doses are used for a

Dexedrine (whites), sometimes abused by students, truck drivers, athletes, or purely recreational users. Frequent users may develop a strong psychological dependency.

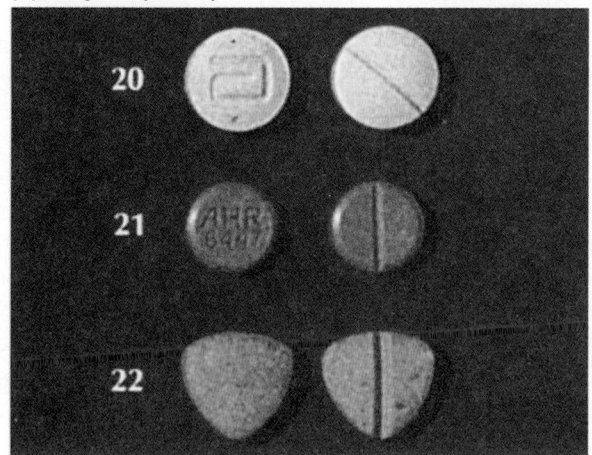

....

sudden infant death syndrome (SIDS) the completely unexpected and unexplained death of an apparently well infant.

amphetamines a group of synthetically produced nervous system stimulants.

long time, physiological dependency does develop, producing definite physical withdrawal symptoms when amphetamine use is discontinued.[25]

Amphetamine Myth:

Amphetamines can safely improve the performance of athletes.

Amphetamine Reality:

Amphetamines can, under some circumstances, improve athletic performance, but not safely. Athletes, for many reasons, such as performance pressure, wanting to play while injured or at loose ends while sidelined by injuries, having plenty of money and free time, and feelings of invulnerability, are highly prone to chemical dependency, especially when drugs are easily available. Anyone who follows sports can cite many examples of tragedies including ruined careers and deaths of drug-dependent athletes.

Intravenous Abuse A few very heavy amphetamine abusers do "speed runs," in which they may inject several thousand milligrams a day for several consecutive days. By comparison, most legally manufactured amphetamine tablets range in potency from 5 to 15 milligrams and most illegally manufactured tablets in street trade contain only 1–2 milligrams.

During a speed run, amphetamine abusers do not sleep and they eat very little. Very early in the run they feel happy, confident, talkative, and energetic. After a day or so, they become confused and disorganized, compulsively repeat meaningless acts, and become paranoid, aggressive, and antisocial. Prolonged sleep follows the run.

Continued use of massive amphetamine doses leads to severe weight loss, sores that don't heal, high blood pressure, strokes, kidney damage, and brain damage.

Prescription Use Medical prescription of amphetamines has declined over the years because of the hazards that have been discovered. Currently accepted uses include the treatment of narcolepsy (a rare condition in which a person falls asleep up to 50 times a day), the treatment of hyperactive children (amphetamine-like Ritalin is used to stimulate inhibitory areas of the brain), and in *short-term* weight-reduction programs.

Table 15.5
Caffeine Content of Some Frequently Used Products

Product	Amount	Milligrams of Caffeine
Brewed coffee	5 fl. oz.	90–150[a]
Instant coffee	5 fl. oz.	14–93[a]
Decaffeinated coffee	5 fl. oz.	1–6
Tea	5 fl. oz.	30–70[b]
Cola beverages	12 fl. oz.	30–50
Chocolate bar	1 oz.	20–22[c]
No-Doz	one tablet	100
Anacin	one tablet	32

[a]Amount depends on type of coffee, strength, and brewing method.
[b]Tea also contains the related stimulant *theophylline*.
[c]Chocolate also contains the related stimulant *theobromine*.

Caffeine

Caffeine is America's most commonly used stimulant drug, and is present in coffee, tea, cola drinks, chocolate, and nonprescription stimulant tablets. Table 15.5 compares the caffeine content of some common products.

Caffeine, along with *theophylline* from tea and *theobromine* from chocolate, belong to the **xanthine** (*zan'thēn*) group of alkaloid stimulants. Xanthines have many physiological effects, most notable of which is stimulation of parts of the brain. Caffeine, at 125–250 milligrams (one or two cups of coffee or tea), produces an arousal pattern in the cerebral cortex, with some people experiencing increased speed and clarity of thought. Higher caffeine doses (over 500 milligrams) increase pulse and breathing rates.

All xanthines, especially theophylline, act as diuretics, increasing the flow of urine. Theophylline also relaxes the lungs' bronchi and bronchioles, easing breathing in some forms of asthma or bronchial spasms.

Heavy use of xanthines can lead to various symptoms, such as extreme nervousness, inability to sleep, irregular heartbeat, and ringing in the ears. Conflicting research results have been published concerning links between caffeine and pancreatic cancer, as well as between caffeine and noncancer-

---

xanthine chemical substance in the alkaloid family with stimulant properties; for example, caffeine.

ous breast cysts in women. Enough is known to indicate that caffeine should be used in moderation.

Tolerance and Dependence Caffeine users tend to develop a tolerance to and a dependence upon caffeine. Regular caffeine users are less affected by a given dose than are occasional users. Abrupt termination of caffeine intake in a heavy user will often lead to mild withdrawal symptoms including headaches, lethargy, depression, and inability to concentrate.

CHECKPOINT

1. What is the principal action of stimulant drugs?

2. List and briefly describe the various methods of abusing cocaine.

3. What are the pharmacological effects of cocaine?

4. Explain some of the dangers connected with cocaine use.

5. Explain the physiological and psychological effects of amphetamines.

6. List some of the symptoms resulting from heavy caffeine use. ✔

SEDATIVE-HYPNOTICS (DEPRESSANTS)

Sedative-hypnotic drugs are central nervous system depressants, including barbiturates, nonbarbiturate hypnotics such as methaqualone, all tranquilizers, and alcohol. Use of any of these drugs is characterized by the following:[26]

1. Increasing dosages produce progressive central nervous system depression, ranging from mild sedation to sleep to death.

2. Increasing dosages progressively cause mental clouding, loss of muscular control, and respiratory arrest.

3. Chronic use leads to the development of tolerance, but a level of intoxication can always be reached if the dose is high enough.

4. There is **cross tolerance** (an increased tolerance to one class of drugs following exposure to a different class) between the groups. For example, an alcoholic may be somewhat tolerant to the effects of tranquilizers.

5. Chronic use of large doses leads to physiological dependence and withdrawal if use is suddenly stopped. Sedative-hypnotic withdrawal can be dangerous as it may include convulsions. Withdrawal symptoms can be lessened to some extent if another sedative-hypnotic is substituted under medical supervision. For example, alcohol withdrawal symptoms can be prevented or lessened by substituting barbiturates during alcohol withdrawal.

6. When two drugs from this group are taken together, the result is synergism, with a far greater depressant effect than would be predicted by adding the individual effects of each drug.

Barbiturates

More than 2500 **barbiturates** (*bar-bit'ū-rāts* or *bar-bi-tū'rāts;* a group of central nervous system depressant drugs derived from barbituric acid) have been synthesized, and about 50 of these have been marketed. Barbiturates' names end in *-al,* indicating their relationship to barbital, the first one made. A few of these are listed in Table 15.6 on p. 478. Barbiturates are mainly taken in pill form or injected. Medical uses of barbiturates include:

- sleeping pills
- sedation (relaxation)
- preanesthesia
- anesthesia
- anticonvulsant use

Effects of Barbiturates

Barbiturates depress functions of all body cells, but the central nervous system is more sensitive than other body systems to barbiturates. At dosages

---

cross-tolerance an increased tolerance to one class of drugs following exposure to a different class.

barbiturates a group of central nervous system depressant drugs derived from barbituric acid.

sedative-hypnotic drugs drugs that depress the central nervous system.

Table 15.6
Some Common Barbiturates

Generic Name	Trade Name	Street Name
Thiopental	Sodium Pentothal	
Amobarbital	Amytal	Blues, Blue Heavens
Pentobarbital	Nembutal	Yellow Jackets, Yellows
Secobarbital	Seconal	Reds, Red Devils
Amobarbital plus Secobarbital	Tuinal	Rainbows, Tooeys

where sedation or sleep occurs, there are few effects on other body systems.

Barbiturates and alcohol have some similar effects. To an observer, barbiturate intoxication would appear the same as alcohol intoxication. Also, like alcohol, barbiturates disrupt the normal sleep cycle. Both drugs reduce the amount of time spent in rapid eye movement (REM) sleep (dreaming). With chronic barbiturate use, though, dreaming climbs back to a normal level (about 20 percent of the time you are asleep). Upon discontinuing barbiturates or alcohol, a rebound effect occurs in which REM sleep can go as high as 100 percent and nightmares and troubled dreams occur.

Although the sedation caused by barbiturates may last only a few hours, mood distortions, impaired judgment, and impaired muscular coordination can persist for 10–22 hours after a single dose of a barbiturate. It is unknown whether this is a result of some active barbiturate **metabolite** (a product of metabolism; in this case, the body's breakdown of the barbiturate) in the body or an effect of reduced REM sleep.[27]

Barbiturate Myth:
Barbiturates provide a good night's sleep.

Barbiturate Reality:
Barbiturates interfere with REM sleep and the sleep they produce is less effective than natural sleep.

Intravenous Use   Some barbiturate abusers inject the dissolved contents of capsules or tablets

metabolite a product of metabolism.

into their veins. The sudden rapid peak in blood barbiturate level produces a "rush" (a rapid, intense high). The intravenous abuse of any drug involves risks of infection (including AIDS if needles or syringes are shared) and damage to blood vessels. Barbiturates are alkaline (caustic) compounds and are highly irritating to the blood vessels. If the drug is accidentally injected into an artery, the artery will go into spasm and may collapse. If this happens, the loss of blood supply can result in permanent damage to a body part.

Tolerance Formation   Like all sedative-hypnotics, barbiturates are tolerance-forming. The time required to develop tolerance depends on the doses being used. The higher the daily dose, the shorter the time required to develop tolerance. As people become tolerant, they tend to increase their dosages so the same high can still be achieved. Yet in doing this, they come closer and closer to the lethal level; eventually there is only a very narrow margin between the dose at which effects are felt and the dose that causes death. Death from barbiturate overdose occurs when the respiratory centers of the brain are depressed by high doses of barbiturates and breathing stops. The synergistic action between barbiturates and any other sedative-hypnotic drug, including alcohol,

Barbiturates interfere with normal sleep patterns, are addictive, and carry the risk of overdose, especially when combined with alcohol.

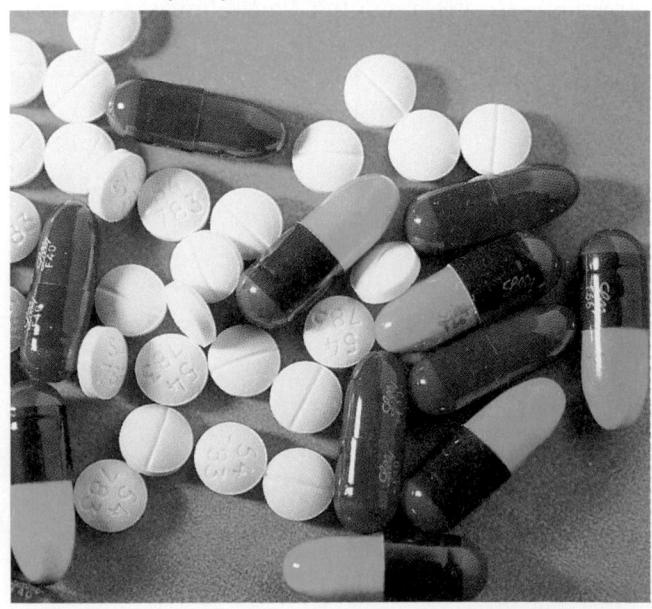

greatly increases the risk of a fatal overdose when these drugs are taken at the same time.

Withdrawal Withdrawal from barbiturates is among the most hazardous of all drug withdrawals. Symptoms include shaking, sweating, sleeplessness, restlessness, and nervousness or irritability. Life-threatening convulsions may occur suddenly, with no warning. This withdrawal may be prompted by sudden discontinuance or lowering of a dosage of barbiturate dosage. It is important that anyone withdrawing from heavy barbiturate use be carefully monitored in a hospital setting.

Methaqualone

Methaqualone (*meth-ak'kwa-lōne*) is an example of a nonbarbiturate sedative-hypnotic. It was formerly prescribed in the United States as a sedative (under the trade names Quaalude, Mequin, Sopor, and Parest), but because of high levels of abuse, its legal U.S. manufacture and distribution was discontinued in 1985. Since that time, illegal methaqualone, imported from Colombia, Mexico, and Canada, has remained available in the United States. Street names of methaqualone include "Qs," "'ludes," "Lemmons," and "Sopors." Methaqualone has been responsible for many overdoses and accidents, and has a severe withdrawal syndrome that can include seizures.

Methaqualone, taken orally, is rapidly absorbed into the bloodstream and produces a "rush." This, plus its reputation as an aphrodisiac, probably accounts for methaqualone's street popularity. As with alcohol, the supposed aphrodisiac effect is, in reality, a release from inhibitions. Methaqualone produces temporary feelings of euphoria, confidence, and relaxation. Because of the association of these pleasant feelings with this drug, it is highly dependency-forming.

Tolerance and physiological dependence can develop within a month if the drug is taken regularly. As with barbiturates, withdrawal carries the risk of fatal convulsions and should be monitored in a hospital. Also like barbiturates, the combination of methaqualone with alcohol carries a high risk of fatal overdose.

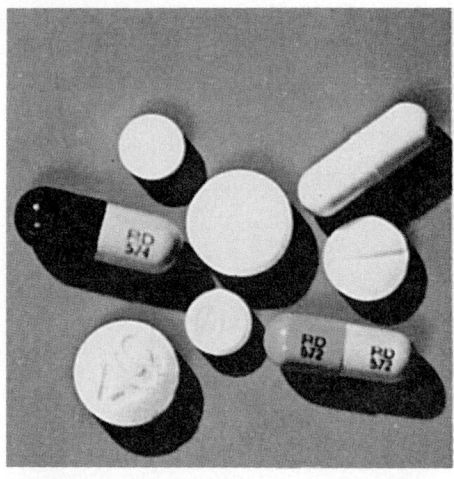

Methaqualone. This powerful depressant drug was originally prescribed as a sedative, but is no longer legally manufactured in the United States because of many problems associated with its abuse.

Antipsychotics and Tranquilizers (Antianxiety Agents)

Two broad categories of drugs prescribed for emotional problems are the antipsychotics, prescribed for severe emotional illnesses, and the tranquilizers (antianxiety agents), prescribed for anxieties. Table 15.7, on p. 480, gives some examples of each.

Antipsychotics are drugs that produce emotional quieting and relative indifference to the user's surroundings. Such drugs have been extremely valuable in treating **psychotic** people, those affected by psychosis—severe personality disintegration and loss of contact with reality. Antipsychotics do not cure psychological problems, but they do relieve symptoms and facilitate psychotherapy by putting disturbed people back in touch with reality. Antipsychotics can reduce hallucinations and delusions, calm agitated persons, and bring out severely withdrawn people. There is relatively little abuse of the antipsychotics because they require three weeks or longer to take effect.

It is important to note that the use of antipsychotic drugs can result in serious, permanent aftereffects, possibly even requiring prolonged hospi-

methaqualone a powerful sedative drug.

antipsychotics drugs that produce emotional quieting and relative indifference to one's surroundings.

psychotic affected by psychosis—severe personality disintegration and loss of contact with reality.

Table 15.7
Examples of Antipsychotics and Tranquilizers

A. Antipsychotics
  1. Phenothiazines
      a. Chlorpromazine (Thorazine)
      b. Trifluoperazine (Stelazine)
  2. Thioxanthenes
      a. Thiothixene (Navane)
  3. Butyrophenones
      a. Haloperidol (Haldol)
B. Tranquilizers
  1. Benzodiazepines
      a. Alprazolam (Xanax)
      b. Chlordiazepoxide (Librium)
      c. Diazepam (Valium)
      d. Flurazepam (Dalmane)
      e. Triazolam (Halcion)
  2. Propanediol carbamates
      a. Meprobamate (Equanil, Miltown)
      b. Carisoprodol (Soma, Rela)

talization of the patient. These drugs must be used very cautiously and only when really necessary.

Among **tranquilizers,** also called **antianxiety drugs,** the benzodiazepines (*ben-zō-dī-az'e-pēnz*) are currently used most often. In fact, they are among the most prescribed of all drugs in the United States. Clinical uses of benzodiazepines include reducing anxiety, inducing sleep, causing muscle relaxation, and helping to control seizures. When used for sleep induction, these drugs, unlike barbiturates, cause little or no REM suppression. The muscle relaxant dose is large enough to cause sedation.

Tranquilizer use for anxiety reduction is most appropriate when anxiety is transient and related to some unusual, temporary life situation. It is less appropriate for long-term management of the anxieties of everyday living. In the latter case, it is better to come to terms with the source of the anxiety and either resolve the problem or develop more-effective stress-management methods to reduce the need for tranquilizers.

....

tranquilizers or **antianxiety drugs** drugs with sedative and antianxiety effects, also used as muscle relaxants and anticonvulsants.

Possible adverse reactions to benzodiazepines include oversedation, slurred speech, dizziness, obesity, decreased muscle tone, tolerance, and physical dependence. Benzodiazepines must not be used during pregnancy or by mothers who are breastfeeding.

Tolerance to the benzodiazepines develops more slowly than barbiturate tolerance, but can reach high levels. As with all sedative-hypnotics, physical dependence can occur. Due to the long half-life of most benzodiazepines (20–50 hours for Valium), signs of withdrawal do not appear until three to seven days after cessation of drug use and last for one to three weeks. The nature of the withdrawal depends on the dose level. Following lower dosages, withdrawal is mild, characterized by some sleep disturbance and anxiety. Withdrawal from higher dosages may result in definite psychotic behavior or potentially fatal seizures.[28]

Nonprescribed use (abuse) of benzodiazepines has decreased in recent years. Those people who do abuse benzodiazepines are usually polydrug abusers who also abuse alcohol, opiates, barbiturates, and other drugs.

Overdoses of benzodiazepines, alone or in combination with other drugs, still rank among the most common of all drug overdoses in the United States. They are used in many suicides and suicide attempts. As with other sedative-hypnotics, overdoses suppress the breathing control centers, and may result in death from respiratory arrest.

Tranquilizer Myth:

Tranquilizers such as Valium and Xanax are mild drugs which carry little danger of dependency or overdose.

Tranquilizer Reality:

Many people are dependent upon tranquilizers and every year tranquilizers are among the top several causes of drug overdoses.

CHECKPOINT

1. List the various pharmacological effects of sedative-hypnotic drugs.

2. Explain the term *cross-tolerance.*

3. What are the medical uses of barbiturates?

4. Explain the relationship of barbiturate use and sleep patterns.

5. Explain the seriousness of tolerance and withdrawal in barbiturate use.

6. What medical purpose do tranquilizers serve?

7. What are the possible adverse effects of tranquilizers?

OPIATE NARCOTICS

Though the legal system has historically called any illegal drug a narcotic, only those drugs that produce sleep or stupor and also relieve pain are actually narcotics. This definition limits the use of the word narcotic to the **opiates:** opium and its natural and synthetic derivatives. The word **opioids** is used by some drug experts to include all natural and synthetic opium derivatives, while other experts use opioid only in reference to the synthetic opiates, such as Demerol and methadone.

Sources of Opiates

Opium is the dried sap from the green seed pods of the opium poppy, native to Turkey, northern India, Burma, Thailand, and northern Laos. The pods are slit and a white milky sap oozes out, dries, and turns brown. This substance is opium. In this crude form, opium can be smoked or ingested, or its active ingredients, morphine and codeine, can be extracted and purified. Of opium's two active ingredients, morphine is 6–12 times as strong as codeine in relieving pain and in its other effects. Heroin, not a natural ingredient in opium, is diacetylmorphine, morphine that has been slightly altered. Synthetic opiates, such as hydromorphone (Dilaudid), oxycodone (Percodan), meperidine (Demerol), methadone (Dolophine), and propoxyphene (Darvon), are not made from opium, but are synthetic (made from chemicals).

Absorption

Morphine, heroine, and some other opiates are poorly absorbed when taken orally. For this rea-

opiates opium and its natural and synthetic derivatives.

opioids opiumlike substances.

son, they are often injected, either for clinical use or for abuse. Morphine, for example, is only one-fifth to one-third as effective when taken orally as when it is injected. Many of the synthetic opiates are effective in tablet or capsule form.

Effects of Opiates

Opiates all have similar effects, though different dosages may be required to achieve these effects:

1. Opiates are sedatives (depressants) and produce pain relief, cough suppression, drowsiness, mood changes, and mental clouding or impairment of intellectual processes. Many people experience a sensation of well-being and euphoria from opiates. These people are more likely than others to become dependent on these drugs. Other people feel "drugged" and are not likely to abuse opiates.

2. Opiates depress the respiratory centers of the brain. Many deaths from respiratory arrest are associated with opiate abuse.

3. Some, but not all opiates cause the pupils of the eyes to constrict (pinpoint pupils).

4. Some opiates, whether taken orally or intravenously, cause nausea and possible vomiting soon after being taken. Later, following the same drug dose, the vomiting center is suppressed and it becomes difficult to induce vomiting, as might be desired in an overdose situation.

5. Taken in very high doses, the opioids Demerol, Darvon, and Talwin can cause convulsions.

6. Total sleep time can be increased or decreased, but REM sleep time is usually decreased.

7. Constipation often results.

Tolerance and Physical Dependence

A high degree of tolerance develops with regular opiate use. Those who are seeking euphoria or escape from everyday reality must constantly increase their dosages to achieve this effect. Many regular users of opiates require doses that would be fatal to someone with no tolerance.

Strong physiological dependency to opiates develops in as little as two weeks of daily use. Withdrawal from morphine or heroin will begin 8–12 hours after the last dose. Early symptoms include yawning, sweating, teary eyes, and runny nose. As withdrawal progresses, pupils dilate, one loses one's appetite, and the person becomes restless and irritable. Withdrawal reaches full intensity in two or three days, with increasing irritability, insomnia, violent yawning, severe sneezing, teary eyes, runny nose, weakness, depression, vomiting, and diarrhea. Bone and muscle pain and involuntary muscle jerks and kicks also occur (hence the phrase "kicking the habit"). As unpleasant as these symptoms may be, in adults they do not involve convulsions and they present no threat of death. However, withdrawal *can* cause convulsions and possible death in infants born addicted to opiates (see Feature 15.1). Most withdrawal symptoms abate in seven to ten days, but irritability, low self-esteem, and low pain tolerance may continue for several weeks.

Heroin

Heroin is a very powerful drug that was first produced from morphine in 1898 in an effort to reduce morphine's addictive effects. That goal was not achieved. Heroin is not only a more powerful pain reliever than morphine, but it is also much more dependency-producing. As a result, in the United States, heroin is illegal, even for clinical use (it is used for pain relief in other countries).

Heroin Myth:
Heroin withdrawal is the most dangerous of all drug withdrawals.

Heroin Reality:
Heroin causes a powerful physiological dependency and its withdrawal is quite unpleasant; however, withdrawal from alcohol or barbiturates is much more dangerous.

Many heroin-related problems revolve around its illicit production and distribution network. Heroin enters the United States from Asia, Mexico, and other sources. It then passes through an elaborate criminal distribution system, during which time it is diluted from its original 95 percent level of purity down to perhaps 3–5 percent. *As previously mentioned, with almost all street drugs, the ultimate user receives a product of uncertain identity, at an unknown concentration, diluted with unknown and possibly hazardous adulterants.*

Becoming involved with heroin automatically places you at risk of serious legal problems. It is illegal to possess; its purchase requires dealing with criminals; and as tolerance develops, it becomes very difficult to support a heroin dependency with a legitimate job. Many users eventually support their dependency by dealing drugs; others turn to robbery, car theft, prostitution, or other illegal activities.

Further heroin-related problems stem from its injection, the most common way of taking heroin. Only small amounts of heroin are absorbed if it is taken orally. Heroin can be absorbed through sniffing, but if this is done often, it causes considerable damage to the nasal membranes. Heroin can be smoked if its potency is up around 7 percent. People just starting to use heroin may inject it just under the skin ("skin popping"), but regular users almost always inject intravenously ("mainlining"), producing a more immediate effect.

Because injection syringes and needles are often shared, the viruses that cause AIDS and hepatitis B have infected a large proportion of the heroin users in the United States. In some cities, the majority of users are now infected. One reason drug abusers share needles is that injection equip-

---

FEATURE 15.1

DRUG ABUSE IN PREGNANCY

Most psychoactive drugs taken during pregnancy cross the placenta. Babies born to mothers who are dependent on cocaine, opiates, or other drugs producing physiological dependency are born with a physiological dependency. Drugs usually leave infants' bodies slowly, as their livers have only low levels of the enzymes that break down drugs. Thus, the onset of withdrawal may be slower than in an adult.

Withdrawal in an infant can also be more hazardous than the same withdrawal in an adult. For example, while convulsions are uncommon in an adult during opiate withdrawal, they are not unusual in infants. Many withdrawing infants need medical assistance, including gradual withdrawal with declining drug doses. Long-term psychological and physical effects of fetal drug exposure are not yet fully known. Perhaps the best understood example is Fetal Alcohol Syndrome, discussed in Chapter 7.

ment requires a prescription for purchase. Beyond that, many heroin and other drug abusers have little regard for their own well-being, which contributes to their lack of motivation to use sterile equipment.

Methadone and Opiate Antagonist Programs

There are several drug-based approaches to treating heroin use. The most common is methadone (Dolophine) maintenance, which dates back to 1965. Methadone is a synthetic opioid, taken daily in pill or liquid form. It is available in special methadone clinics in many major cities. Methadone is a synthetic narcotic and has most of the same effects as morphine or heroin. Like other opioids, it is tolerance-forming and produces physiological dependency. When taken orally, however, it produces little euphoria and, most importantly, it blocks heroin induced euphoria. Methadone prevents heroin or other opiate withdrawal. In essence, it is a substitute dependency, but to society, a more acceptable dependency than heroin or morphine.

Though controversial, methadone maintenance programs have been successful. Many "hard-core" heroin users voluntarily accept methadone treatment, with a resultant 55–80 percent retention in treatment for two years or longer.[29] Methadone offers many advantages over heroin. It is medically safe, with very few side effects found in people taking it for as long as ten years. It "normalizes" behavior of former heroin users, allowing them to hold jobs and to function well in society. It avoids such problems as AIDS and hepatitis B, and it takes the heroin user away from the criminal element of society. Methadone is used only to treat opiate abuse; methadone does nothing to treat alcohol, marijuana, cocaine, or other drug abuse.

Another drug-based approach to treating heroin use is taking **narcotic antagonists,** drugs that block the effects of opiates. These drugs do not substitute one dependency for another, as methadone does. The heroin or other opiate-dependent person is first withdrawn from physical dependency on opiates, then maintained on a narcotic antagonist. These drugs block the opiate receptors on cells, but produce little or no behavioral effect. The success rate of this treatment method (about 20 percent) has not approached that of methadone.[30] Narcotic antagonists are, however, ideal for highly motivated individuals because they do not produce a substitute addiction.[31]

C H E C K P O I N T

1. List the various physical effects of opiates.
2. Describe the aspects of tolerance and withdrawal in the use of opiates.
3. Why is heroin not used medically in the United States?
4. What are the dangers in injecting heroin?
5. What are the positive and negative aspects of methadone treatment programs?

PSYCHEDELICS AND HALLUCINOGENICS

The principle action of drugs in this category is producing **hallucinations,** or false sensory perceptions. In addition to psychedelics (*sī-ke-del'iks*) and hallucinogens (*ha-loo'si-nō-jens*), these drugs are called "perceptual distorters" and "psychotomimetics" (*sī-kōt'ō-mi-me'tiks*). We will define each of these terms:

- **psychedelic:** a substance producing a mental state of great calm and intensely pleasurable perception.
- **hallucinogens:** substances producing false sensory perceptions.
- **perceptual distorter:** substance that distorts perceptions.
- **psychotomimetic:** mimicking a psychosis.

Taken together, these definitions give a good idea of the effects of this drug group.

---

narcotic antagonists drugs that block the effects of opiates.

hallucination a false sensory perception.

psychedelic a substance producing a mental state of great calm and intensely pleasurable perception.

hallucinogens substances producing false sensory perceptions.

perceptual distorter a substance that distorts sensory perceptions.

psychotomimetic mimicking a psychosis.

LSD (Lysergic Acid Diethylamide)

LSD is a semisynthetic hallucinogenic derivative from an alkoloid in ergot fungus. Ergot grows on grains such as rye and wheat. LSD is one of the most potent of all drugs, with most doses in the range of 50–300 micrograms. LSD equaling the weight of a paper clip would provide from 3,333 to 20,000 doses.[32]

LSD is usually taken orally. Within approximately one hour after ingestion, perceptual alterations begin. Although all of the senses are involved, vision is usually most affected. Color and texture become more vivid. **Afterimages** (images that persist in the mind after their stimuli have ceased) are prolonged and may be superimposed one upon another. Senses overlap and people "see" music or "hear" color (**synesthesia**). There are feelings of **depersonalization** (the belief that you no longer exist, but are instead something inanimate or unreal), a loss of body image, and a loss of the sense of reality. The perception of time is altered and past, present, and future become jumbled together. Concentration is difficult and vague ideas flow. The user may believe that he or she has discovered new insights, but these discoveries seem unintelligible or nonsensical to others. Emotions shift quickly and unpredictably during LSD use. A mood can shift from intense euphoria to deep despair for little or no reason.

Two phenomena—"bad trips" ("bummers") and "flashbacks"—are special causes of concern with LSD and some other hallucinogens. A "bad trip" is an acute panic reaction. It may become an intense and prolonged drug-induced psychosis lasting up to several *years*.[33] The mechanism of this action of LSD is unknown. It is impossible to predict when and to whom such reactions will occur. "Flashbacks" are spontaneous reoccurrences of an LSD (or other hallucinogen) experience that can occur without warning for up to a year or longer after the last drug use. The flashback can be as vivid as if the drug had just been taken. The exact mechanism of flashbacks is not known, but the fact that they occur is a good reason to avoid using LSD or similar drugs.

Tolerance to LSD develops rapidly with repeated use. Cross-tolerance among LSD, mescaline, and psilocybin indicates the possibility of a similar mechanism of action in these drugs. There is no evidence of physiological dependency on LSD.[34]

> ### LSD Myth:
> LSD and similar hallucinogens provide the user with new insights into reality and the meaning of life.
>
> ### LSD Reality:
> While affected by hallucinogens, users often believe that they have discovered new insights, but when their trip is over, they find that they have somehow lost these insights or are unable to articulate them in a rational manner to anyone else.

Mescaline (Peyote)

Mescaline (*mes'ka-lēn*) is an amphetamine-like hallucinogenic compound contained in the peyote (*pāy-ō'te*) cactus, which grows in parts of northern Mexico and the southwestern United States. Peyote is ingested legally in the religious ceremonies of many Native Americans, including 250,000 members of the Native American Church of North America.

The actions of pure mescaline are similar to those of LSD, though a much larger dose is required (LSD is about a thousand times as potent). Mescaline is more likely to produce euphoria. The psychological effects of mescaline begin 1–2 hours after ingestion and are usually preceded by nausea and vomiting. Effects continue for up to 12 hours. When the peyote cactus is ingested, instead of the purified mescaline, additional effects occur, due to the presence of over 30 other psychoactive agents.[35]

Repeated mescaline use causes tolerance and physiological dependency to develop, as well as

---

LSD lysergic acid diethylamide, a hallucinogenic derivative of an alkaloid in ergot fungus.

afterimages images that persist in the mind after their stimuli have ceased.

synesthesia when the stimulus of one sense (such as hearing) produces the perception of another sense (such as smell).

depersonalization the belief that you no longer exist, but are instead something inanimate or unreal.

mescaline an amphetamine-like hallucinogenic compound contained in the peyote cactus.

cross-tolerance to LSD. Very little true mescaline is available in illegal trade. Most samples (98 percent) of street "mescaline" that have been analyzed have proved to be LSD or PCP.[36]

Psilocin and Psilocybin

Over two thousand years ago, natives of parts of Mexico and Central America were already aware that some species of mushrooms had hallucinogenic properties. As with peyote, religious rituals developed around the consumption of these "sacred mushrooms," called the "flesh of the gods." The hallucinogenic chemicals in these mushrooms, **psilocin** (*sil'ō-sin*) and **psilocybin** (*sil-ō-sī'bin*), are somewhere between mescaline and LSD in strength.

After these mushrooms are eaten, their effects begin within 10–15 minutes, peak at about 90 minutes, and last for 5–6 hours or longer. The effects are similar to those of LSD. Tolerance to psilocin and psilocybin develops rapidly and includes cross tolerance to LSD and mescaline, indicating a similar mode of action of these drugs.

Synthetic Amphetamine-like Hallucinogens

A great many hallucinogenic amphetamine derivatives (Table 15.8) have found their way into street trade. Their molecules are similar to amphetamines and to mescaline. There are unlimited variations on this chemical theme. Many of these drugs were legal until the Anti-Drug Abuse Act of 1986 (Public Law 99-570) was passed (see Feature 15.2, p. 486).

All of these **designer drugs** are taken orally. Some of their actions are similar to those of amphetamines. They all cause extra release of the neurotransmitter norepinephrine and depletion of the brain's dopamine. Beyond that, each drug appears to modify brain activity in its own specific way. All are tolerance-forming. All share the hazard of being manufactured in illicit laboratories, meaning that their identity, purity, and content is unreliable.

Though classified as hallucinogens, designer drugs have additional effects, including stimulant

Table 15.8
Some Amphetamine-Derived Hallucinogens

Street Name	Chemical Name
STP or DOM	4-methyl-2, 5-dimethoxyamphetamine
MDA	3,4-methylenedioxyamphetamine
MDM	N-methyl-3, 4-methylenedioxyamphetamine
MDMA or MMDA (ecstasy, XTC, Adam)	2-methoxy-3, 4-methylenedioxymethamphetamine

action and euphoria. MDA (methylenedioxyamphetamine) is sometimes called "the love drug" because people taking it often experience a sense of well-being along with increased tactile (touch) sensations, which result in increased sexual pleasure. People under the influence of MDA often have a powerful need to be with or talk to other people.

MDA overdoses can cause convulsions and death. Moderate doses leave the user physically exhausted for up to two days, probably due to depletion of the neurotransmitters norepinephrine and dopamine.[37] As with all hallucinogens, there is the possibility of a "bad trip," the effects of which may require medical attention.

MDMA (methylenedioxymethamphetamine), also known as ecstasy, XTC, or Adam, has been widely used during the past few years. It can produce euphoria, increased sensitivity to touch, and lowered inhibitions. Many users claim that MDMA intensifies their emotional feelings and body awareness without producing sensory distortion.[38] Drug experts point out that it may also cause agitation and panic anxiety, which can be intense and unpredictable. There is also evidence that MDMA and MDA can cause permanent brain damage in frequent users.

Phencyclidine (PCP)

Phencyclidine (*fen-sī'kli-dēn*) (**PCP**) was first developed in the 1950s as an intravenous anesthetic. It was used only briefly in human medicine because sometimes people awoke from the anesthetic in states of delirium and excitation lasting up to 18 hours. It remained in use in veterinary medi-

....

psilocin and **psilocybin** two hallucinogenic chemicals produced by mushrooms.

designer drugs hallucinogenic amphetamine derivatives.

phencyclidine (PCP) an anesthetic formerly used in veterinary (and briefly in human) medicine.

FEATURE 15.2

DESIGNER DRUGS

Until the Anti-Drug Abuse Act was passed in 1986, to be legally controlled each drug had to be specifically mentioned in a law as being illegal. In order to skirt the drug laws, "designer drugs" similar to, but not identical to, regulated drugs were produced. These designer drugs defied the spirit, but not the letter of the law, so they were impossible to regulate. Though designer drugs are now illegal, they remain available on the street.

Designer drugs include amphetamine derivatives such as MDMA (Ecstasy), heroin-related drugs such as China White,

and many others. The dangerous nature of designer drugs was exemplified by MTPT, sold in California as China White in the early 1980s. Some of the users of this drug were left with permanent brain damage resembling late-stage Parkinson's disease and are now permanently and severely paralyzed.

The risks posed by designer drugs point out the hazards of all street drugs: uncertain chemical identity, unpredictable strength, and unknown diluents and contaminants. Anyone contemplating purchasing street drugs should ask themselves: Is it worth the risk?

---

cine longer, but was phased out because of adverse reactions in animals. Legal manufacture of PCP was discontinued in 1985.

PCP remains in street trade, where it has been called "Hog," "Peace Pill," "Angel Dust," "Dust," or when sold in cigarettes, "Sherms." PCP is easily produced from readily available chemicals and is often misrepresented as being mescaline, THC, cannabinol, LSD, hash oil, or some other drug.

PCP can be taken orally, but it is more commonly smoked or snorted (sniffed like cocaine). After smoking or snorting, the effects begin within 1–5 minutes, peak within another 5–30 minutes, and last 4–6 hours. It takes 24–48 hours or longer for a complete return to normal. When PCP is taken orally, it takes effect more slowly, requiring at least 15 minutes. Because it takes so long to go into effect, the user may think more is needed and this can lead to an overdose. Overdose with oral use is more likely than with other modes of use.

PCP produces severe perceptual distortions. The body may feel like it is several feet off the floor, or an arm or leg may feel foreign or unattached. The user cannot coherently grasp what is going on inside or outside of the body. At low doses, a person may appear drunk, exhibiting staggering, slurred speech, trembling, muscle weakness, and decreased pain sensitivity. At slightly higher doses, there may be increased blood pressure, shivering, muscle rigidity, vomiting, and drooling. High doses may cause seizures and severe hallucinations. The effects of PCP are usually not remembered by the user. Chronic users develop memory disorders, disorientation, and commonly have difficulty with speech.

Severe adverse reactions are quite common with PCP. Extreme psychosis may develop and last for days or months. This happens in people with no previous history of mental disorders and antipsychotic medications have no effect on this condition.[39] Violent behavior is a trademark of PCP. It often requires several strong people to restrain one violent PCP user.

Many deaths are associated with PCP use. Causes of death include uncontrollable seizures, cardiac or respiratory arrest, and rupture of blood vessels in the brain due to high blood pressure. Because of PCP-altered perceptions of reality, deaths may also result from accidents such as drowning, walking in front of vehicles, falling from buildings, and so on.

CHECKPOINT

1. List the various definitions of the psychedelics and hallucinogens.

2. Why is LSD considered such a powerful and dangerous drug?

3. Compare the effects of mescaline and psilocin.

4. What are the additional effects of the designer drugs beyond their hallucinogenic effects?

5. What are the serious health consequences designer drug users may experience?

6. Which definition of psychedelics would best describe PCP?

7. Describe the physical and psychological effects of PCP.

MARIJUANA AND OTHER *CANNABIS* DERIVATIVES

No other psychoactive drug has evoked as much controversy as marijuana. A large percentage of the North American population, and especially the younger population, have tried marijuana.

Forms of *Cannabis*

Marijuana ("pot") consists of the dried leaves and flowers of the hemp plant, *Cannabis sativa*. The main psychoactive ingredient in marijuana is delta-9-tetrahydrocannabinol, usually called **THC. Sinsemilla** (Spanish for "without seeds") is an especially strong form of marijuana produced from the flowering tops of unfertilized female plants (*Cannabis* plants have separate sexes). **Hashish** is a resinous substance obtained from the flowers by dragging a chamois or cloth over the tops of *Cannabis* plants. It is much higher in THC content than marijuana.

Pure THC can be made synthetically, but it is very expensive. Anything sold on the street as "THC" or "THC oil" is very likely some other drug, often PCP.

Medical Uses

Marijuana has been used for medicinal purposes for thousands of years. Marijuana or THC can be useful for the following conditions.[40]

- *Glaucoma* (*glaw-kō'ma*): THC can lower pressure within the eye in some cases of glaucoma.

- *Asthma:* THC causes dilation of the airways and has been used for centuries in primitive

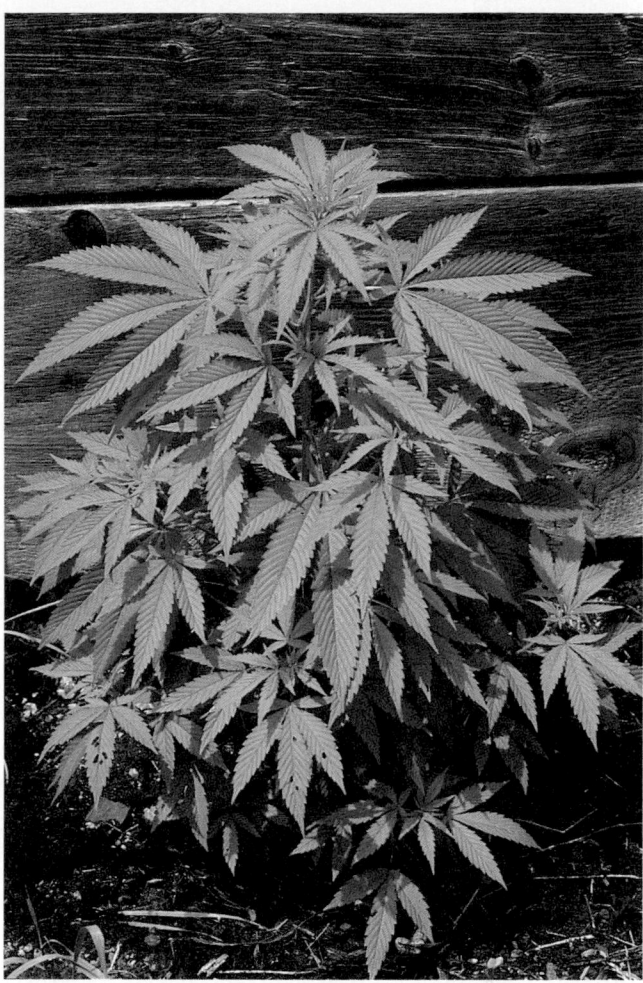

Cannabis sativa. The dried leaves and flowers constitute marijuana. Hashish is produced by rubbing a chamois or cloth over the tops of Cannabis plants.

cultures to treat asthma. The smoke from marijuana is irritating to the lungs, however, and is therefore not a good means of delivering THC to the lungs.

- *Seizure disorders:* THC increases electrical thresholds of brain cells so it may be useful in treating certain seizure disorders.

- *Nausea and vomiting:* THC can be very useful in suppressing the nausea and vomiting that are frequent side effects of radiation and drug treatments of cancer patients. This suppression of vomiting can be hazardous when marijuana and alcohol are abused together, as it may block the vomiting that usually helps prevent fatal overdoses of alcohol.

---

marijuana the dried leaves and flowers of the hemp plant.

THC tetrahydrocannabinol, the active ingredient in marijuana.

sinsemilla "without seeds"; marijuana produced from unfertilized female plants.

hashish resinous substance obtained from the flowers of *Cannabis* plants.

Action of THC

Cannabis products are usually smoked in cigarette form (a "joint") or in a pipe. The drug action begins within a few minutes, peaks in 20–30 minutes, and lasts from one to two hours. When marijuana is eaten, such as in cookies or brownies, it takes longer to go into effect and the effects are more prolonged. THC persists in the body long after its psychoactive effects have worn off. It can be detected in urine for weeks after the last use.

THC's effects on individuals are very complex and depend on dosage. At low doses, marijuana has a stimulantlike effect and results in mild euphoria, increased sensory awareness, and altered time perception. With increasing doses, a sedativelike effect, characterized by impaired memory, lapses of attention, disturbed thought patterns, and passivity occurs. With very high doses, perceptual distortions (hallucinations), such as changes in body image, depersonalization, and marked sensory distortion, occasionally occur. For this reason, some experts classify *Cannabis* as a hallucinogen.

Many physical changes accompany marijuana use. The pulse speeds up, blood pressure may be raised or lowered, blood vessels dilate (visible as red eyes), tear and saliva production decrease, appetite (especially for sweets) increases, and REM sleep is suppressed.

Marijuana Myth:

Marijuana is harmless because it is a natural plant product.

Marijuana Reality:

Smoking *anything* is damaging to the lungs. Marijuana impairs driving performance and many harmful physical effects have been documented.

Tolerance and Dependence

Neither tolerance nor dependence develops for light or moderate marijuana users. People who repeatedly use very high doses do develop a tolerance, and psychological dependency can be strong. Physiological dependency rarely develops. Withdrawal symptoms include sleep disturbances (rebound of REM sleep, with nightmares), irritability, restlessness, sweating, and loss of appetite.

Harmful Effects

There is strong evidence that marijuana use impairs driving ability. This is confirmed by laboratory tests of reaction time, coordination, and similar driving skills. As with alcohol, most people whose driving is impaired by marijuana use do not recognize their impairment.[41]

Marijuana smoke is damaging to the lungs, as is any smoke. It may cause lung cancer, bronchitis, asthma, and reduced lung capacity. Because joints have no filter tip and most people smoke them to the very end, they receive a full dose of tars. Marijuana has been shown to impair immunity and heavy users tend to have an increased number of infections. Like tobacco smoke, marijuana smoke is rich in carbon monoxide and can also contribute to heart disease.

Reproductive function may be impaired in frequent marijuana users of either gender. In males, THC may reduce testosterone levels and heavy marijuana use can cause abnormal sperm, as well as reduced sperm count and decreased sperm motility (swimming ability).[42] In females, gonadotropic (ovary-stimulating) hormone levels may be reduced and ovulation may not occur. Women who use marijuana during pregnancy may have increased rates of stillbirth and infant mortality. Effects similar to fetal alcohol syndrome have also been reported.[43]

CHECKPOINT

1. Describe the various forms of *Cannabis* products.
2. What is the main active ingredient in *Cannabis?*
3. What are the physical and psychological effects of marijuana?
4. List the harmful physical effects of marijuana.

INHALANTS (VOLATILE SUBSTANCES)

Any hardware store, paint store, or grocery store contains many products with vapors that could be

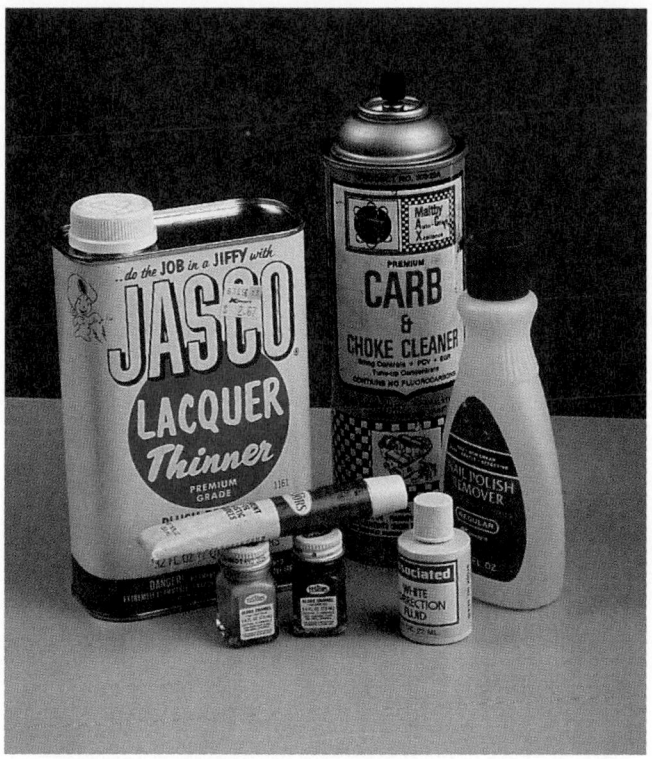

Volatile substances that can be inhaled for psychoactive effects are not difficult to obtain, but their use is very dangerous.

concentrated and inhaled for their psychoactive effects. These products include gasoline, paint and lacquer thinners, solvents, degreasers, adhesives, aerosol products, and many more. **Volatile** (easily vaporized or evaporated) substances are often abused by soaking a rag or spraying the product in a bag and deeply inhaling the fumes.

Inhalants are classified into four groups:

1. *Volatile solvents* such as those in gasoline, glues, paint thinners, and many common household and commercial products.

2. *Aerosols* such as hair sprays, deodorants, spray paints, and so on.

3. *General anesthetic agents* such as nitrous oxide in pressurized whipped cream and trichloroethylene in typing correction fluid.

4. *Volatile nitrites* such as amyl nitrite and butyl nitrite.

volatile easily vaporized or evaporated.

The first three groups listed are similar in their effects and will be discussed together. A brief discussion on the volatile nitrites will follow.

Volatile Solvents, Aerosols, and General Anesthetic Agents

Volatile substances or inhalants are abused mainly by young children, low-income persons, and prison inmates because these intoxicants are cheap and widely available. There are two types of inhalant abusers: experimenters and chronic abusers. Inhalant experimentation is common among the young, many of whom try some form of inhalant. Chronic abuse is found primarily among young people from the most unstable, disorganized, and dysfunctional families. Chronic inhalant abusers are usually socially isolated individuals and are solitary in their inhalant abuse. Such individuals are not part of any drug-abusing subculture.[44]

Inhalants work as nervous system depressants. Their immediate effects are similar to those of alcohol or barbiturates: slurred speech, staggering gait, mental confusion, emotional instability, and drowsiness, and, in high doses, stupor or coma. Sudden death due to cardiac arrhythmia (loss of the normal heart rhythm) or to respiratory depression may occur.

Long-term damage from chronic inhalant use may be severe. Formation of blood cells by the bone marrow may be suppressed, causing anemia, loss of ability to fight infection, and/or inability of the blood to clot. Serious, even fatal, liver and kidney damage is possible. Permanent damage to the brain and peripheral nerves is common. Finally, an increased cancer rate appears some 10–30 years after inhalant abuse.

Inhalant Myth:
The fumes from volatile substances provide a good, cheap, legal high.
Inhalant Reality:
Volatile substances can cause very serious physical damage and serve no benefit to the user.

Volatile Nitrites

Volatile nitrites, such as amyl, butyl, or isobutyl nitrite dilate blood vessels. For this reason, they are medically prescribed for use by people with chest pains to increase the blood supply to the heart. Butyl nitrite has been sold in "head shops" (stores that sell drug paraphernalia) and through mail order under names such as "Locker Room" and "Rush." Amyl nitrite is formulated in small crushable capsules called "poppers."

Volatile nitrites are inhaled in an effort to increase the length and intensity of orgasm, possibly due to a dilation of genital arteries. As blood pressure drops, the blood flow to the brain is reduced, which can cause dizziness and euphoria. This may also contribute to increased sexual intensity. With regular use, tolerance may develop.

Side effects include flushing of the skin, severe headaches, nausea, dizziness, and weakness. More serious side effects are known to occur, such as the reduced immune response that occurs in frequent users. An occasional severe side effect is the dissolving of massive numbers of red blood cells. As we have noted, the benefit-to-risk ratio of inhalants is very unfavorable.

CHECKPOINT

1. What does *volatile* mean?

2. Why are volatile substances abused and what are their harmful effects?

ANABOLIC STEROIDS

Anabolic steroids are synthetic versions of male hormones, such as testosterone. About 20 steroids are available through black market sources, at gyms or schools, or through some physicians. These drugs mimic the effects of testosterone in the body, causing the development of male secondary sex traits—deep voice, facial hair, and muscle building. They are named anabolic steroids for their ability to build muscle mass.

Steroids are used legitimately for the treatment of breast cancer and anemia and in rehabilitation of people who have become physically weakened because of serious long-term injury or illness. They have become, however, a serious drug-abuse problem among professional and amateur athletes of both genders, and among young people who just want to appear more muscular.

Though steroids are usually taken for their muscle-building effects rather than for their psy-

choactive effects, mental disorders are among their many adverse effects. These may take the form of aggression, violence, paranoia, delusions of grandeur, irritability, and depression. Steroids also have a hormonal stimulant effect that creates an adrenaline-like high that can cause dependency. Losing that stimulant effect after quitting steroids can produce a withdrawal-like depression.

Many other adverse, even fatal, effects of steroid use are known or suspected. Feature 15.3 lists some of these effects.

It is clear that the short-term benefits of steroids are not worth their dangers. Why, then, do people use them? In the case of young people who just want to look better, the reasons may include lack of knowledge of the possible adverse effects of the steroids and the sense of immortality felt by some young people. In the case of athletes, the tremendous competitive pressure to win at any cost may override any concern about the potential dangers of these drugs. Top athletes, accustomed to hours of strenuous training, know that there is a "price to pay" for success; they may view the effects of steroids as part of that price. They also often know or believe that their competitors are using steroids and believe that if they do not do the same, they will be unable to win. Further, tolerance or even encouragement of steroid use is said to come at times from self-serving coaches and managers, who put their own careers ahead of the long-term well-being of their athletes.

CHECKPOINT

1. What are anabolic steroids?

2. Though steroids are taken for muscle-building effects, what are some of their potential mental effects?

3. List five proven harmful effects of steroids that occur in both genders and three specific effects for each gender.

SUMMARY

Drugs can enter the body by ingestion (oral use), inhalation into the lungs, membrane absorption, or injection. Once absorbed into the blood, a drug is distributed throughout the body in no more than one minute. Some drugs enter body cells; some work on their outer membranes.

FEATURE 15.3

ADVERSE EFFECTS OF STEROIDS

The harmful effects of steroid abuse have been well documented. Here are just a few of the known or suspected effects.

PROVEN EFFECTS IN BOTH GENDERS INCLUDE:

acne

cancer

edema (water retention)

heart disease

high blood cholesterol levels

liver disease

liver tumors

mental disorders

sterility

strokes

stunted growth (if taken before growth has ceased)

PROVEN EFFECTS IN FEMALES INCLUDE:

enlargement of clitoris

fetal damage if taken during pregnancy

hirsutism (increased hairiness)

male pattern baldness

oily skin

PROVEN EFFECTS IN MALES INCLUDE:

unwanted erections

painful, prolonged erections

prostate enlargement

testicular atrophy

SUSPECTED EFFECTS INCLUDE:

abdominal pains

allergic reactions

bone pain

male breast development

chills

fever

diarrhea

frequent urination

gallstones

headache

high blood pressure

male impotence

increased frequency of sports injuries

insomnia

kidney disease

listlessness

female menstrual irregularities

muscle cramps

nausea

vomiting blood

purple or red spots on body and inside mouth

rash

bloody noses

sexual problems

darkening of skin

weight loss or gain

unnatural hair growth

bad breath

unusual bleeding

Source: Miller, R. "Athletes and Steroids: Playing a Deadly Game." *FDA Consumer* November 1987, pp. 17–21.

Psychoactive drugs often work by attaching to specific receptor sites on brain cells. The normal function of these sites is to interact with neurotransmitters. The effects of a drug are similar to the neurotransmitter it resembles. Endorphins are natural brain chemicals that block pain and produce feelings of pleasure. Some drugs work by attaching to the brain's endorphin receptors.

Most drugs are broken down by liver enzymes. Different drugs are eliminated from the body at very different speeds. After a drug is eliminated, people often experience a rebound (paradoxical) effect, which is the opposite of the drug's effect. This is usually perceived as unpleasant, leading to repeated use of the drug. Frequent use of some drugs leads to tolerance, causing the dosage to be increased to achieve the same effect. People tend to adjust the dosage of psychoactive drugs to achieve the effects they seek.

Many people abuse more than one drug. Certain drugs can interact in very dangerous ways. Drugs come from both natural and synthetic sources. Naturally occurring drugs are not necessarily safer than synthetically produced drugs.

This chapter surveys many specific psychoactive drugs. Although some drugs are more hazardous than others, none is totally free of risk to the abuser. Street drugs are especially hazardous because of their uncertain identity, unpredictable strength, and unknown contaminants and diluents. Sharing drug-injection equipment carries the additional risk of infection by HIV (AIDS virus), hepatitis, and other diseases.

People use psychoactive drugs with expectations of fulfilling certain needs, but because of rebound effects, tolerance, and development of dependency, drugs are unable to meet these expectations in the long run. There are, however, actually many ways to achieve the benefits that drugs falsely promise. We sincerely hope that you will choose drug-free routes to fulfillment.

REFERENCES

1. Goode, E. *Drugs in American Society,* 4th ed. New York: McGraw-Hill, 1993.
2. National Institute on Drug Abuse. *Drug Abuse and Drug Abuse Research.* Washington, DC: National Institute on Drug Abuse, 1987.
3. Singer, M., Irizarry, R., and Schensul, J. "Needle Access as an AIDS Prevention Strategy for IV Drug Users: A Research Perspective." In Goldberg, R. *Taking Sides.* Guilford, CT: Dushkin, 1993.
4. Liska, K. *Drugs and the Human Body, With Implications for Society,* 3rd ed. New York: Macmillan, 1989.
5. Ibid.
6. Hopson, J. "A Pleasurable Chemistry." *Psychology Today* (July/August 1988), 29–33.
7. Witters, W., Venturelli, P., and Hanson, G. *Drugs and Society,* 3rd ed. Boston: Jones and Bartlett, 1992.
8. Hopson, op. cit.
9. Witters, Venturelli, and Hanson, op. cit.
10. Hopson, op. cit.
11. Doweiko, H. *Concepts of Chemical Dependency.* Pacific Grove, CA: Brooks/Cole, 1990.
12. Brennan, W. "Are You Disposed at Birth Toward Addiction/Alcoholism?" Lecture at Charter Oak Hospital, Covina, California, May 26, 1988.
13. Witters, Venturelli, and Hanson, op. cit.
14. Ibid.
15. Payne, W., Hahn, D., and Pinger, R. *Drugs: Issues for Today.* St. Louis: Mosby, 1991.
16. Julien, R. *A Primer of Drug Action,* 6th ed. New York: Freeman, 1991.
17. Goode, op. cit.
18. Carroll, C. *Drugs in Modern Society,* 3rd ed. Madison, WI: Brown & Benchmark, 1993.
19. Weiss, R. "The Physician Cocaine User." *Medical Aspects of Human Sexuality* 21, No. 9 (September 1987), 67–73.
20. Witters, Venturelli, and Hanson, op. cit.
21. Doweiko, op. cit.
22. Radcliffe, A. Pharmacology of Psychoactive Drugs, a course at the University of California, Riverside, California, Fall 1987.
23. Carroll, op. cit.
24. Goode, op. cit.
25. Witters, Venturelli, and Hanson, op. cit.
26. Radcliffe, A., Rush, P., Sites, C., and Cruse, J. *The Pharmer's Almanac.* New York: Ballantine, 1991.
27. Ibid.
28. Ibid.
29. National Institute on Drug Abuse, op. cit.
30. Ibid.
31. Carroll, op. cit.
32. Radcliffe et al., op. cit.
33. Ibid.
34. Ibid.
35. Witters, Venturelli, and Hanson, op. cit.
36. Liska, op. cit.
37. Witters, Venturelli, and Hanson, op. cit.
38. Ibid.
39. Ibid.
40. Radcliffe et al., op. cit.
41. Witters, Venturelli, and Hanson, op. cit.
42. Radcliffe et al., op. cit.
43. Liska, op. cit.
44. Witters, Venturelli, and Hanson, op. cit.

SUGGESTED READINGS

Carroll, C. *Drugs in Modern Society,* 3rd ed. Madison, WI: Brown & Benchmark, 1993.
Julien, R. *A Primer of Drug Action,* 6th ed. New York: Freeman, 1991.
Liska, K. *Drugs and the Human Body, With Implications for Society,* 3rd ed. New York: Macmillan, 1989.
Radcliffe, A., Rush, P., Sites, C., and Cruse, J. *The Pharmer's Almanac.* New York: Ballantine, 1991.
Witters, W., Venturelli, P., and Hanson, G. *Drugs and Society,* 3rd ed. Boston: Jones and Bartlett, 1992.

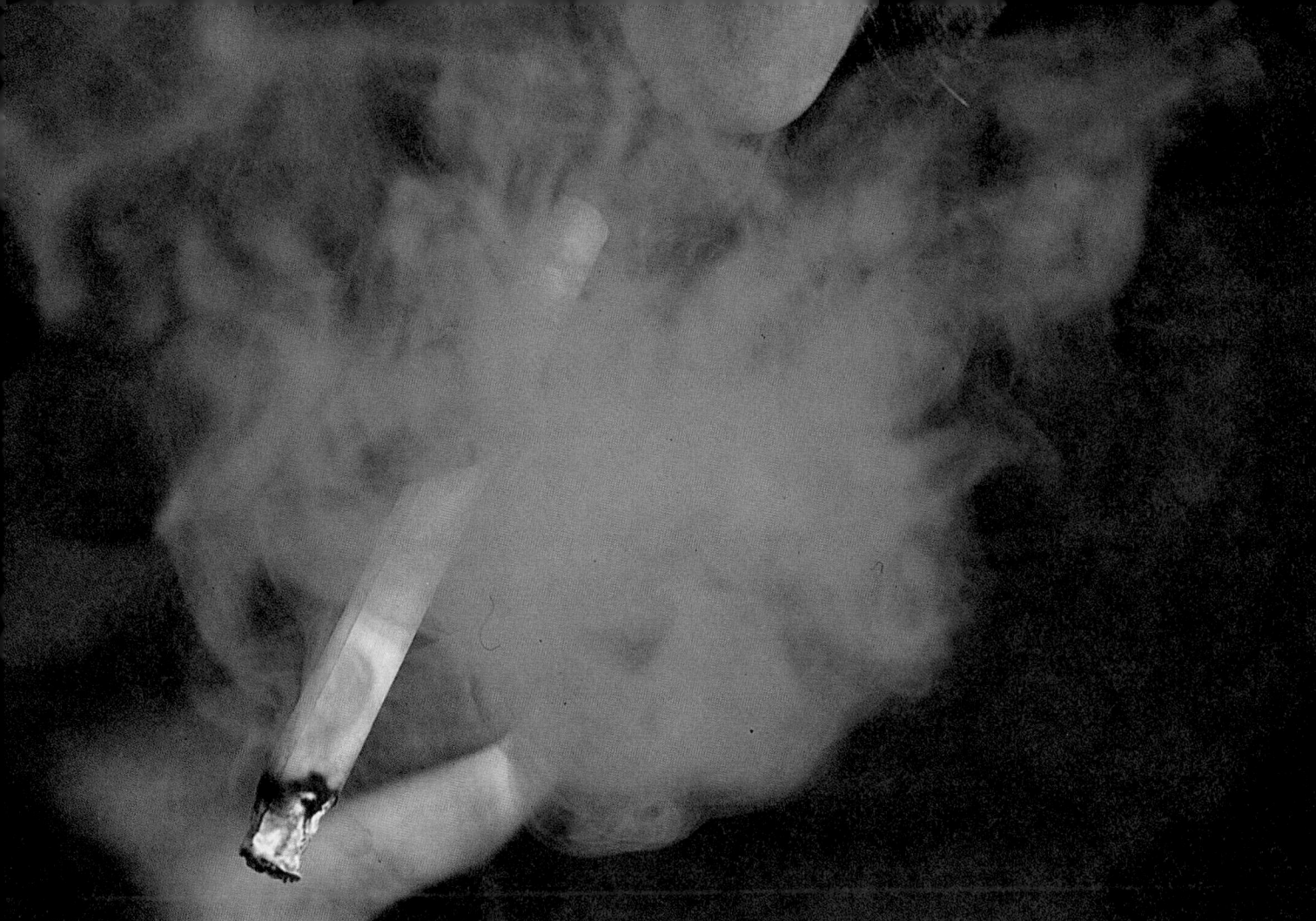

16
TOBACCO

Upon completing this chapter, you will be able to:

KNOWLEDGE

- List the harmful chemicals contained in tobacco smoke.
- Describe the harmful effects of each component of tobacco smoke.
- Describe the harmful effects of smokeless tobacco use.
- Explain how tobacco smoke can harm even those who don't smoke.
- List reasons why smoking by adolescents is considered to be a serious problem.
- List the factors that increase a young person's likelihood of becoming a smoker.
- Describe smoking's special harmful effects on women.
- Compare the various methods of quitting smoking.

INSIGHT

- If you are a smoker, identify the reasons why you started smoking and why you continue to smoke.
- Explain your position on the issues involved in conflicts between the rights of smokers and nonsmokers.

DECISION MAKING

- Make a commitment to minimize your own exposure to tobacco smoke and smokeless tobacco use.
- Make a commitment to encourage your friends to remain or to become nonsmokers.

Babe Ruth, Charles Lindbergh, Nat "King" Cole, and John Wayne had something in common—they all died of lung cancer and they all were cigarette smokers. When these men began smoking it was considered safe. In fact, advertisements appeared in the Journal of the American Medical Association (JAMA) up until 1953 stating, for example, that "More doctors smoke Camels than any other cigarette." At present, tobacco companies spend about $6.5 million to promote characters such as Joe Camel and his partner, Josephine.

Joe Camel, or "Old Joe" as he is sometimes called, and Josephine are cartoon characters that have become a symbol of the battle between antismoking activists and tobacco companies. In December 1991, a study was published in JAMA reporting that 6-year-olds find Joe Camel as easy to recognize as Mickey Mouse. Moreover, the study reported that since Joe Camel was introduced, Camel's share of the illegal cigarette market, comprised of those cigarette buyers under age 18, has increased dramatically, from 0.5 percent to 32.8 percent, representing a rise in sales from $6 million to $476 million. Other studies have provided evidence that these types of ads actually entice young people to smoke. The tobacco companies counter this claim by arguing that they are only trying to persuade adults to switch brands.

The battle against Old Joe is particularly significant because most smokers begin smoking as teenagers. Since nicotine has been recognized as an addictive drug, many of those who begin smoking as teens will continue to smoke as adults. Each day about 5000 children light up for the first time. Many of those children may be influenced by advertisements such as those featuring youth-appealing Joe Camel.

Several significant blows to the tobacco industry have occurred recently, including the EPA's report that identified environmental tobacco smoke (passive smoke) as a Class A carcinogen, the finding that *tobacco companies manipulate the amount of nicotine in cigarettes to maintain addiction, and the decision by public agencies (such as the U.S. military) and private businesses (such as McDonald's) to ban smoking in their workplaces. However, the battle is not over; the tobacco companies are a powerful political force because of the jobs created by this profitable industry. The best way to protect our children from the harmful influence of tobacco and tobacco advertisements is by setting a good example—make a commitment to quit now!*

Source: Breo, D. Journal of the American Medical Association, October 27, 1993.

▪   ▪   ▪

Tobacco, when used in any form, poses severe health risks to its user. When smoked, it also threatens the health of those nonusers who are exposed to its fumes. Few behaviors have as many—and as detrimental—effects upon a person's health as tobacco use. In fact, when the *Surgeon General's Report on Health Promotion and Disease Prevention* was released in 1979, tobacco use was identified as "the single most important preventable cause of death."[1] Though a smaller percentage of Americans use tobacco now than in 1979, that statement remains true today. Tobacco still causes over 400,000 premature deaths every year and causes debilitating chronic diseases in millions of Americans.[2]

In this chapter, we will examine how tobacco is used, the composition of tobacco as a drug, the harmful effects of tobacco on its users and others, why people start using tobacco, why it is addictive, and how this addiction can be overcome.

FORMS OF TOBACCO CONSUMPTION

Tobacco is the dried leaves of the native American tobacco plant, *Nicotiana tabacum*. The mature leaves are one- to two-and-a-half feet long. Hundreds of years before the arrival of European explorers, Native Americans from Paraguay to Quebec were smoking tobacco in cigars and pipes, drinking it as a syrup, chewing it, sniffing it, and using it in ceremonial enemas.[3] When Columbus returned to Europe, he and his crew introduced tobacco to that continent.

CIGARETTES

To make cigarettes, mature tobacco leaves are harvested, dried, shredded, remoisturized with glycerine or other chemicals, and packed in huge wooden barrels to age for one to two years. After this aging process, the tobacco is again remoisturized and different types of tobacco are blended together to produce the proper balance of flavor and mildness. Up to 25 percent of the tobacco in a cigarette comes from stems and other scraps of tobacco leaves, which are ground up and rolled into thin sheets of reconstituted tobacco, then shredded and mixed with regular tobacco. Many chemicals are added, including natural and synthetic flavoring agents as well as chemicals to keep the tobacco burning between puffs. This mixture is then rolled up in thin paper. Over 90 percent of the cigarettes sold in the United States are fitted with filters that remove some, though not all, of the harmful substances in the smoke. Most people who smoke cigarettes deeply inhale the smoke to allow maximum absorption of nicotine into their blood.

CIGARS AND PIPES

Cigars are made from rolled, unshredded tobacco leaves, wrapped with a special leaf of tobacco instead of paper. Pipe tobacco is a shredded tobacco that is usually highly flavored with aromatic substances. The tobacco in cigars and pipes is more irritating to the smoker (and to the nonsmoker!) than that in cigarettes, so most cigar or pipe smokers do not inhale the smoke (see Feature 16.1, p. 497).

SMOKELESS TOBACCO

Smokeless tobacco forms include chewing tobacco and snuff. Chewing tobacco is shredded tobacco, heavily treated with moisturizing and flavoring agents. A "plug" of chewing tobacco is often held inside the cheek. Chewing tobacco stimulates the flow of saliva and its use usually involves frequent spitting.

Snuff is a preparation of finely pulverized tobacco. It can be inhaled through the nostrils or a pinch can be placed between the lower lip and the gum. In both cases, nicotine is absorbed through the oral membranes (see Feature 16.2, p. 498).

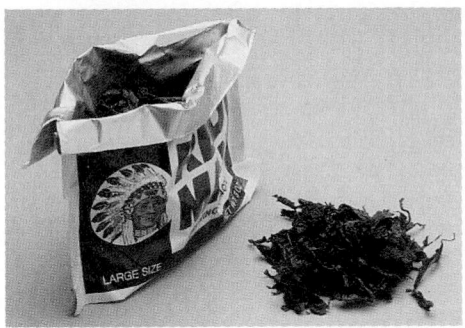 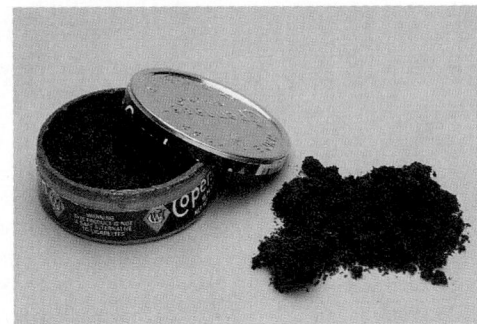

Smokeless tobacco. On the left, chewing tobacco; on the right, snuff.

FEATURE 16.1

CIGARS? PIPES? CLOVES?

How do the risks presented by cigars, pipes, and clove cigarettes compare to the hazards of ordinary cigarettes?

Compared with regular cigarettes, pipes and cigars are more hazardous in some ways, but less hazardous in others. The overall risk for the average pipe or cigar smoker is less than that for the average cigarette smoker. Because pipe and cigar smoke is quite strong, most pipe or cigar smokers do not inhale much smoke. For those who don't inhale, the risks of circulatory or respiratory diseases are less than for cigarette smokers. For those who do inhale, however, these risks are higher than for cigarette smokers.

Whether the pipe or cigar smoker inhales or not, some risks are higher than for cigarette smokers. Specifically, the incidence of cancers of the lip, mouth, throat, larynx, and stomach are higher for pipe and cigar smokers than for cig-

arette smokers because of the increased contact of these body parts with carcinogens.

Clove cigarettes or "cloves," which peaked in popularity in the early 1980s, contain an average of 60 percent tobacco and 40 percent ground cloves, clove oil, and other flavoring ingredients. The smoke they produce is higher in tar, nicotine, and carbon monoxide than most regular cigarettes. Clove cigarettes cause more allergic reactions than regular cigarettes. In addition, the clove oil has many harmful effects, such as stimulating the central nervous system, which can cause delirium, hallucinations, and seizures. Clove oil lowers blood pressure and can cause sweating, weakness, dizziness, and ringing in the ears. Clove oil severely irritates the respiratory membranes, but because clove oil is an anesthetic, the smoker may not feel this irritation. The long-term effects of clove cigarettes are even more harmful than those of regular cigarettes.

CHECKPOINT

1. For how long has tobacco been used in the Americas?

2. Is a cigar simply a giant cigarette? If not, how do they differ?

3. List the various types of smokeless tobacco and briefly describe how they are used.

TOBACCO AS A DRUG

Tobacco is a psychoactive, addictive drug. In this section we will examine some of the **pharmacology**

....

pharmacology the study of the properties and reactions of drugs.

(*far-ma-kol'ō-jē*), the study of the properties and reactions of drugs, of tobacco such as its composition, how it is administered and absorbed into the body, its physical and psychological effects, and how the body rids itself of the drug.

COMPOSITION OF TOBACCO

Tobacco, in its raw form, is a complex mixture of chemicals that becomes increasingly complicated as it is processed into cigarettes or "smokeless tobacco" forms. The smoke from burning tobacco is the most complex form of all. Tobacco smoke contains about 3000 chemical substances that have the ability to harm living tissue.[4] Among these substances are tars and related compounds, nicotine, and toxic gases, including carbon monoxide (CO), hydrogen cyanide (HCN), and nitrous oxide (N_2O).

FEATURE 16.2

SMOKELESS TOBACCO: AN UNSAFE SUBSTITUTE FOR CIGARETTES

Smokeless tobacco products include chewing tobacco (tobacco in leaf or compressed brick form) and snuff (powdered tobacco). Chewing tobacco is usually held inside the cheek in a large wad. Snuff is usually used by placing a pinch between the cheek or lip and the gum.

In response to heavy advertising, featuring macho sports figures and entertainment personalities, and possibly in response to the increasing social pressure against smoking,

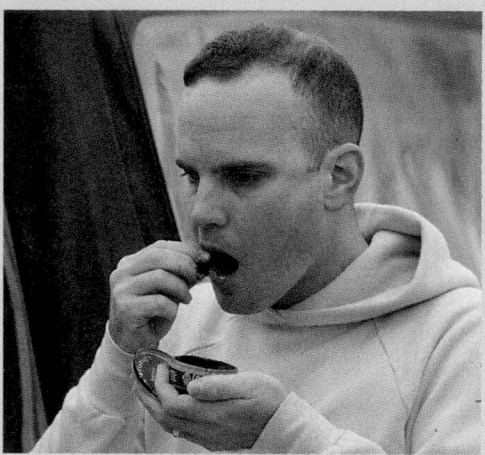

Chewing tobacco has been popularized with young males by its common use among professional baseball players.

the use of smokeless tobacco has increased sharply in recent years. Advertising for smokeless tobacco is designed to appeal to impressionable young males, extending down to those in elementary school. Because of the success of this advertising, many millions of young males are now daily users of smokeless tobacco products. Smokeless tobacco is just as addictive as smoking tobacco.

Although some of the hazards of smoking, such as carbon monoxide and inhaled tars, are absent, smokeless tobacco users absorb massive doses of nicotine. Studies show that within 20 minutes of using snuff, young healthy males (under age 20) experience increases in average pulse rates from 69 to 88 per minute, while their average blood pressure increases from 118/72 to 126/78.°

Leukoplakia (*lū-kō-plā'kē-a*), very common among users of smokeless tobacco, is the formation of white spots or patches on the mucous membrane of the tongue or cheek. The spots are smooth, irregular in size and shape, hard, and occasionally fissured. *These are precancerous lesions that may become malignant.* Other damaging effects of smokeless tobacco include reduced sense of taste and smell, bad breath, stained teeth, receding gums, greater wear on tooth enamel, and tooth decay.

Smokeless tobacco is *not* a safe alternative to smoking.

°Schlaadt, R., and Shannon, P. *Drugs of Choice,* 3rd ed. Englewood Cliffs, NJ: Prentice Hall, 1990.

TARS

Tars are thick, black, sticky materials produced when tobacco is burned. Tars act as the carriers for **carcinogenic** (*kar-si-nō-jen'ic*)—cancer causing—chemicals in tobacco smoke. Tars also contribute to the development of chronic bronchitis and "smoker's cough" (see Figure 16.1).

NICOTINE

An **alkaloid** is an alkaline (caustic) organic substance obtained from a plant. **Nicotine,** a poisonous alkaloid found in tobacco leaves, is one of the

tars thick, black, sticky materials produced when tobacco is burned.

carcinogenic producing cancer.

alkaloid an alkaline (caustic) organic substance obtained from a plant.

nicotine a poisonous alkaloid found in tobacco leaves.

most toxic and addicting of all poisons. It is also the most abundant psychoactive ingredient in tobacco.

Nicotine is rapidly absorbed into the blood from the lungs upon inhalation and from the mouth and stomach linings with smokeless tobacco use. It is distributed throughout the body within seven seconds, penetrating all body organs including the brain and, during pregnancy, all organs of the fetus.

Nicotine leaves the body by first being metabolized (changed) by enzymes in the liver; it is then excreted by the kidneys. Nicotine is present in the milk of breastfeeding women who smoke. In fact, the breastfed infant may have a blood level of nicotine as high or even higher than that of the mother.[5]

Effects of Nicotine

Nicotine is a powerful stimulant that affects the brain, the spinal cord, the entire nervous system,

leukoplakia formation of white spots or patches on the mucous membrane of the tongue or cheek.

FEATURE 16.3

WHAT ABOUT LOW-NICOTINE, LOW-TAR CIGARETTES?

Over 70 percent of today's cigarettes fall into the low-nicotine, low-tar category, with advertised nicotine and tar levels much lower than some other brands. Are they really that much safer to smoke? Couldn't a smoker just switch to a low-nicotine, low-tar brand instead of quitting?

The answer to both of these questions is *no*. Many people who switch to low-nicotine cigarettes adjust their smoking habits so that they still absorb approximately the same amount of nicotine as before and avoid a reduced nicotine intake which triggers the unpleasant symptoms of nicotine withdrawal. When smokers switch to low-nicotine cigarettes, changes in their smoking patterns may include:

- smoking more cigarettes per day
- taking bigger puffs and/or holding the smoke in the lungs longer
- taking more frequent puffs on each cigarette
- leaving a shorter butt (the last puffs on each cigarette contain the most nicotine and tar)

Low-nicotine cigarettes are *not* a risk-free alternative to other cigarette brands. The best course of action for any tobacco user is to quit tobacco use altogether.

the heart, and many other body organs. Nicotine directly stimulates neuron receptors that are sensitive to the neurotransmitter **acetylcholine** (*as-e-til-kō'lēn*), a chemical that plays an important role in the transmission of nerve impulses at synapses. Nicotine's many effects include increased blood pressure, increased pulse rate, lowered skin temperature due to constriction of blood vessels, release of epinephrine (adrenalin) from the adrenal glands, and increased intestinal activity (occasionally causing diarrhea). Urine formation is reduced for two to three hours, causing the smoker to retain fluid. Saliva flow is first increased and then decreased. A nicotine user's tendency to develop blood clots increases, while the effectiveness of his or her immune mechanism is reduced. Muscle tone is reduced, which gives some smokers a feeling of relaxation, despite the fact that nicotine is a stimulant.[6]

Nicotine stimulates the entire nervous system and can cause tremors and, in very large doses, convulsions. As with all stimulant drugs, stimulation of the brain is followed by a period of depression, which creates the desire for more nicotine. Repeated use of nicotine increases tolerance and can lead to one of the strongest physical and psychological chemical dependencies.

Not everyone who smokes is addicted to nicotine. There is no exact number of cigarettes a person must smoke each day to be considered an addict, but anyone who smokes 15 or more (a pack

contains 20) is very likely addicted to nicotine.[7] For those who are addicted, discontinuation of nicotine use may result in withdrawal symptoms including restlessness, anxiety, irritability, depression, headache, stomach pain, insomnia, and dizziness (see Feature 16.3). Though nicotine withdrawal is never fatal, it can be extremely unpleasant and prolonged.

GASES IN CIGARETTE SMOKE

Carbon monoxide (CO), a poisonous component of automobile exhaust, is also a major ingredient in cigarette smoke. Carbon monoxide is colorless, odorless, and has no taste, so the smoker does not notice its presence in tobacco smoke. Nonsmokers are also affected when there is heavy smoking in a poorly ventilated space.

Carbon monoxide has a strong affinity for the red blood cells' oxygen-carrying pigment, **hemoglobin** (*hē'mō-glō'bin*), bonding with the sites on the hemoglobin molecules that normally carry oxygen. **Carboxyhemoglobin** (*kar-boks'i-hē-mō-glō'bin*), the compound formed by carbon monoxide and hemoglobin, cannot carry any oxygen. Thus, the blood's ability to supply oxygen to the brain, heart, muscles, and every other part of the body is reduced. The exact degree of reduction depends, of course, upon the number of cigarettes

acetylcholine a chemical that plays an important role in the transmission of nerve impulses at synapses.

hemoglobin the oxygen-carrying pigment of the red blood cells.

carboxyhemoglobin the compound formed by carbon monoxide and hemoglobin.

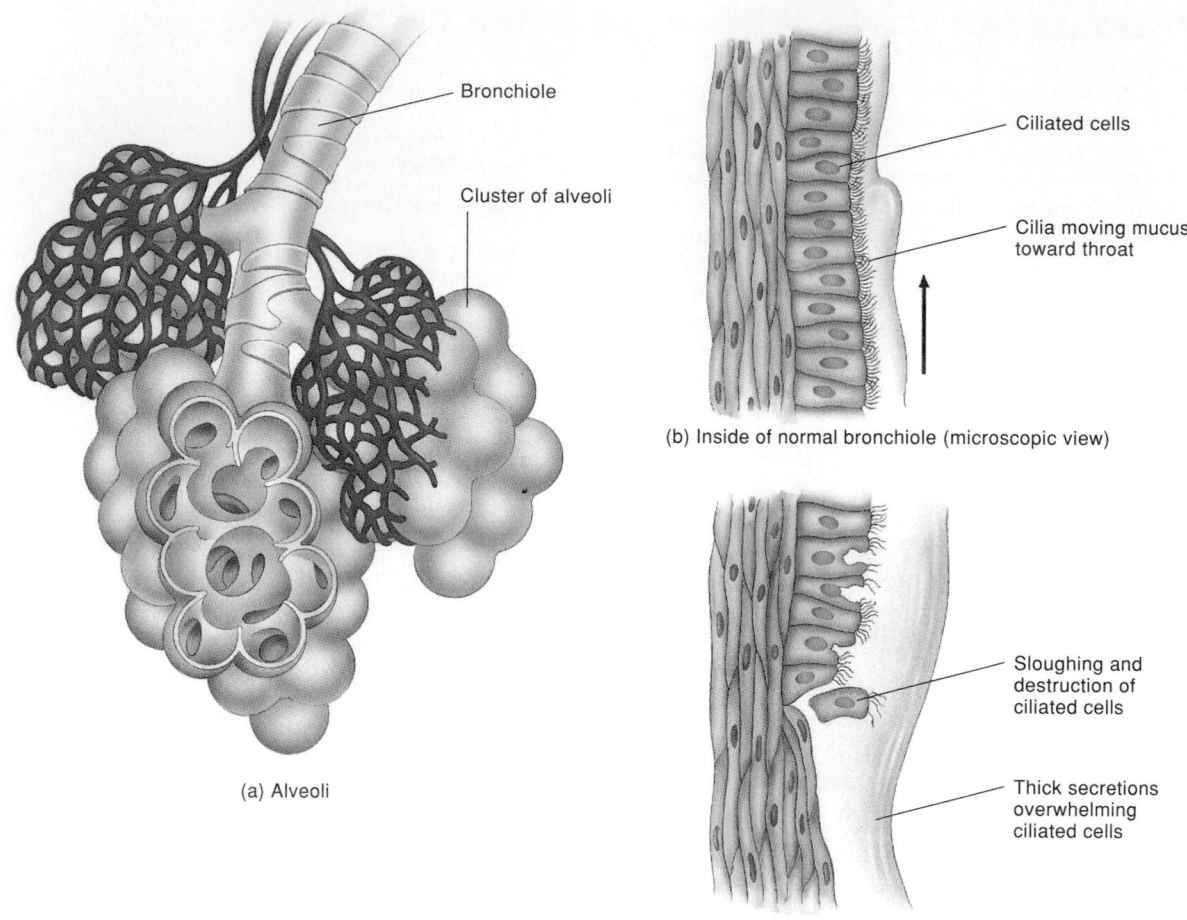

(a) Alveoli

(b) Inside of normal bronchiole (microscopic view)

(c) Chronic bronchitis (microscopic view)

Figure 16.1

Microscopic Human Lung Structure

(a) Each lung consists of millions of microscopic air sacs (alveoli) from which oxygen is absorbed into the blood. The alveoli are supplied with air by small ducts called bronchioles. (b) Internal view of healthy bronchiole. In nonsmokers, microscopic, hairlike cilia convey mucus, disease germs, dust, pollen, and other contamination from the lungs to the throat where this material is harmlessly swallowed. (c) In smokers, chronic bronchitis develops when smoke irritates the bronchioles, causing swelling of their lining, loss of cilia, and increased production of mucus.

smoked per day and the manner in which they are smoked (number of puffs per cigarette, how deeply they are inhaled, and how long the smoke is held). A smoker's oxygen shortage becomes most obvious during periods of increased oxygen demand, such as during vigorous exercise.

Hydrogen cyanide (HCN), another poisonous gas present in tobacco smoke, is the chemical in smoke most responsible for impairing the function of the lung's cilia. This impairment is responsible for the accumulation of mucus, tar, and infection-causing bacteria.

Another compound in cigarette smoke is nitrous oxide, a toxic gas that is also present in smog. Nitrous oxide decreases the effectiveness of the **macrophages,** special white blood cells that patrol the inner surfaces of the lungs and destroy bacteria and other disease agents.[8] Therefore, this

....

macrophages special white blood cells that patrol the inner surfaces of the lungs and destroy bacteria and other disease agents.

IN YOUR HANDS

TOBACCO USE ASSESSMENT

This is one of the shorter self-assessments in this book, as no "safe" level of tobacco use has been identified. Thus, tobacco use behavior is not seen as a matter of degrees—any tobacco use must be viewed as excessive and as a matter of concern.

If you never use tobacco in any form, give yourself 10 points right here _____

QUESTIONS FOR EVERYONE TO ANSWER:

	Almost Always	Usually	Almost Never
1. I try to avoid situations in which I have to breathe other people's smoke	2	1	0
2. I actively try to discourage other people from smoking in my presence	2	1	0
3. I actively try to discourage other people from using tobacco at any time	2	1	0

INTERPRETATION:

14–16 points: Excellent. By not using tobacco, you are healthier, look better, smell better, feel better, enjoy food more, enjoy greater social acceptance, and save a lot of money. By avoiding the smoke of others, you further increase the benefits of avoiding tobacco. By encouraging others not to use tobacco, you demonstrate your concern for their health.

10–13 points: Very good. Don't underestimate the harmful effects of secondhand smoke.

Less than 10 points: The sooner you quit using tobacco in any form, the better. Many of its harmful effects are reversed within a few months after quitting.

---

gas contributes to smokers developing chronic respiratory infections.

Are you minimizing your exposure to the hazards associated with tobacco use? Take a minute right now to complete In Your Hands: Tobacco Use Assessment.

CHECKPOINT

1. How many potentially harmful chemicals are contained in tobacco?

2. How many premature deaths are caused by tobacco use each year?

3. What health hazards are associated with tars in cigarettes? Nicotine? Carbon monoxide?

✓

HARMFUL EFFECTS OF TOBACCO

Few cause-and-effect relationships are as well documented as the harmful effects of tobacco. Tobacco use is recognized by health authorities as the chief avoidable cause of death in the United States.

Over 400,000 Americans die each year as a result of tobacco use (see Table 16.1, p. 502).[9] (Published estimates vary considerably because of different research methodologies used.)

Another way to look at the toll taken by tobacco is the years of potential life lost. Years of potential life lost because of a tobacco-related death can be calculated by subtracting the age of the person at the time of death from the life expectancy for his or her gender. Nationally, the total years of potential life lost from tobacco use each year is over 5 million.[10]

EFFECTS OF TOBACCO ON THE CARDIOVASCULAR SYSTEM

The amount of tobacco-induced damage to the **cardiovascular** system (the heart and blood vessels) is directly proportional to the number of cigarettes smoked or other tobacco used.[11] Nicotine and carbon monoxide are responsible for tobacco's

....

cardiovascular pertaining to the heart and blood vessels.

Table 16.1

Relative Risk of Death (Current Smokers[a] vs. Never Smokers) and Numbers of Smoking-Attributable Deaths from Various Causes

Cause of Death	Male		Female		Total Deaths
	Relative Risk	Number of Deaths	Relative Risk	Number of Deaths	
Cancers					
Lip, mouth, throat	27.5[b]	5,033[c]	5.6	1,442	6,475
Esophagus	7.6	5,668	10.3	1,616	7,284
Pancreas	2.1	2,667	2.3	3,447	6,114
Larynx	10.5	2,379	11.9	611	2,990
Lungs and trachea	22.4	81,179	4.7	35,741	116,920
Cervix	—	—	2.1	1,294	1,294
Urinary bladder	2.9	3,046	1.9	980	4,026
Kidney	3.0	2,866	1.2	353	3,219
Circulatory Diseases					
High blood pressure	1.9	3,299	1.2	2,151	5,450
Ischemic heart disease[d]					
age 35–64	2.8	26,431	1.4	7,701	34,132
age 65+	1.6	38,918	1.3	25,871	64,798
Other heart diseases	1.9	23,295	1.2	12,019	35,314
Stroke					
age 35–64	3.7	4,557	4.8	4,114	8,671
age 65+	1.9	10,421	1.0	4,189	14,610
Atherosclerosis[e]	4.1	3,737	3.0	2,675	6,412
Aortic aneurysm[f]	4.1	5,913	1.3	1,382	7,295
Other arterial disease	4.1	2,032	1.3	1,115	3,147
Respiratory Diseases					
Pneumonia, influenza	2.0	11,191	2.2	7,881	19,173
Chronic bronchitis and emphysema	9.7	9,324	7.0	5,541	14,865
Chronic airway obstruction[g]	9.7	30,385	7.0	18,597	48,982
Other respiratory diseases	2.0	787	2.2	668	1,455
Infant deaths (under one year old)[h]					
Low birthweight	1.8	285	1.8	222	507
Respiratory disorders	1.8	433	1.8	301	734
Sudden infant death syndrome	1.5	288	1.5	182	470
Burn Deaths		863		499	1,362
Deaths of Nonsmokers[i]		1,055		1,945	3,000
Total		276,153		142,537	418,690

[a]Risk of death for those who have quit smoking is lower in each case.

[b]Risk of death for smokers relative to those who have never smoked (e.g., 27.5 means 27.5 times as much risk of dying from this specific cause).

[c]Number of deaths from this specific cause that are directly attributable to smoking.

[d]Ischemic (is-kē'mik) heart disease occurs when there is an insufficient blood supply to the heart muscle due to obstruction of the blood vessels serving the heart.

[e]Atherosclerosis is thickening and hardening of the arterial walls.

[f]Aortic aneurysm is a balloonlike bulge on the major artery leaving the heart. Its rupture may cause a fatal hemorrhage.

[g]Chronic airways obstruction, also called chronic obstructive lung disease (COLD) or chronic obstructive pulmonary disease (COPD), is the reduced ventilating capacity of the lungs. Its causes include chronic bronchitis, emphysema, and chronic asthma.

[h]Infant deaths are those that relate to smoking by the pregnant mother or by people in the home of the infant.

[i]Deaths among nonsmokers from lung cancer attributable to environmental tobacco smoke.

Source: Centers for Disease Control. "Cigarette Smoking-Attributable Mortality and Years of Potential Life Lost—United States, 1990." Morbidity and Mortality Weekly Report 42, No. 33, 27 August 1993, pp. 645–649.

cardiovascular effects. While carbon monoxide reduces the amount of oxygen available to the heart muscle, nicotine increases the heart's need for oxygen. The elevated heart rate and blood pressure caused by nicotine increase the amount of work the heart must perform and, thus, its requirement for oxygen. Further, both carbon monoxide and nicotine increase the incidence of *atherosclerosis* (narrowing of the arteries) and **thrombosis** (*throm-bō'sis*) (clot formation) in the small coronary arteries serving the heart muscle. These actions result in a sharp increase in the risk of death from heart attack in smokers as compared to nonsmokers. If a smoker also has high blood pressure or diabetes, the risk of heart attack is even greater.[12]

Smoking causes changes in the blood chemistry that contribute to the development of *plaque* deposits that narrow the coronary arteries and lead to heart attacks. A strong correlation exists between tobacco use and the development of atherosclerosis which may become severe enough to require coronary bypass surgery (see Chapter 20). Reports indicate that 92 percent of people requiring coronary bypass surgery before the age of 40 are smokers.[13]

Another circulatory problem aggravated by nicotine is **Buerger's disease.** Buerger's disease causes inflammation and blockage of blood vessels. It occurs mainly in young males and impairs the flow of blood through the blood vessels of the extremities, especially in the feet and legs. When combined with the **vasoconstrictive** (blood vessel narrowing) effects of nicotine, **gangrene** (death of tissue) often develops, necessitating amputation of one or both legs.

Tobacco users also have an increased risk of **strokes,** or blockage of blood flow to the brain, which can lead to death or disability. Nicotine,

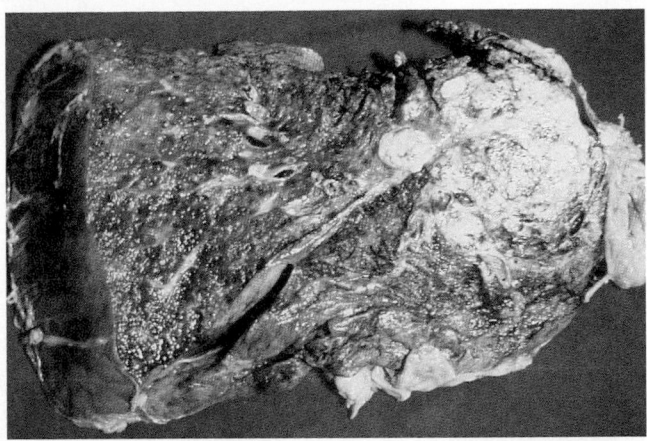
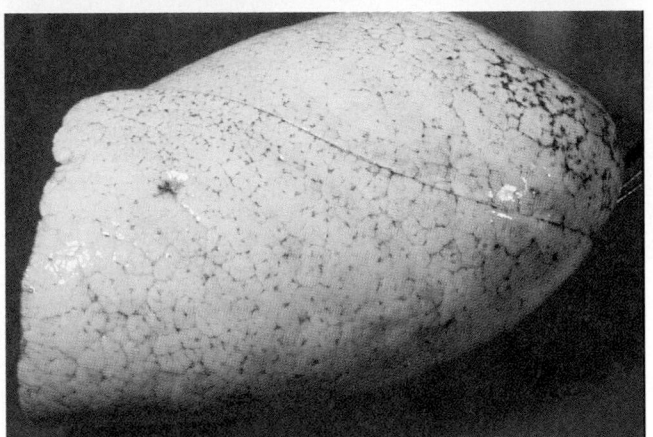

Smoking takes a terrible toll on the lungs. Autopsy specimens of (top) a lung from a smoker and (bottom) a lung from a nonsmoker.

again the culprit, causes arteries supplying the brain with blood to become hard and narrow. Both the carbon monoxide and the nicotine in tobacco promote the formation of blood clots, which are the most common cause of stroke.

RESPIRATORY DISORDERS

Some smokers are so accustomed to coughing that they view their coughing as normal rather than as a warning sign of lung damage. Similarly, some smokers attribute their shortness of breath to their age or to being "out of shape." A smoker's coughing and shortness of breath are in fact often symptoms of **chronic bronchitis** (*brong-kī'tis*) (see Figure 16.1) or **emphysema** (*em-fi-sē'mah*), known collectively

....

thrombosis formation of blood clots.

Buerger's disease an inflammatory disease blocking the flow of blood through the arteries and veins of the extremities.

vasoconstrictive causing blood vessels to constrict.

gangrene death of tissue, usually due to deficient blood supply.

stroke a cerebrovascular accident in which the blood supply to part of the brain is interrupted through rupture or blockage of a blood vessel supplying the brain.

....

chronic bronchitis inflammation of the mucous membrane of the bronchial tubes.

emphysema breakdown and increase in the size of the alveoli (air sacs) in the lungs.

Not many endurance athletes are smokers. Smoking reduces one's vigor and endurance and is incompatible with any sport that requires great stamina.

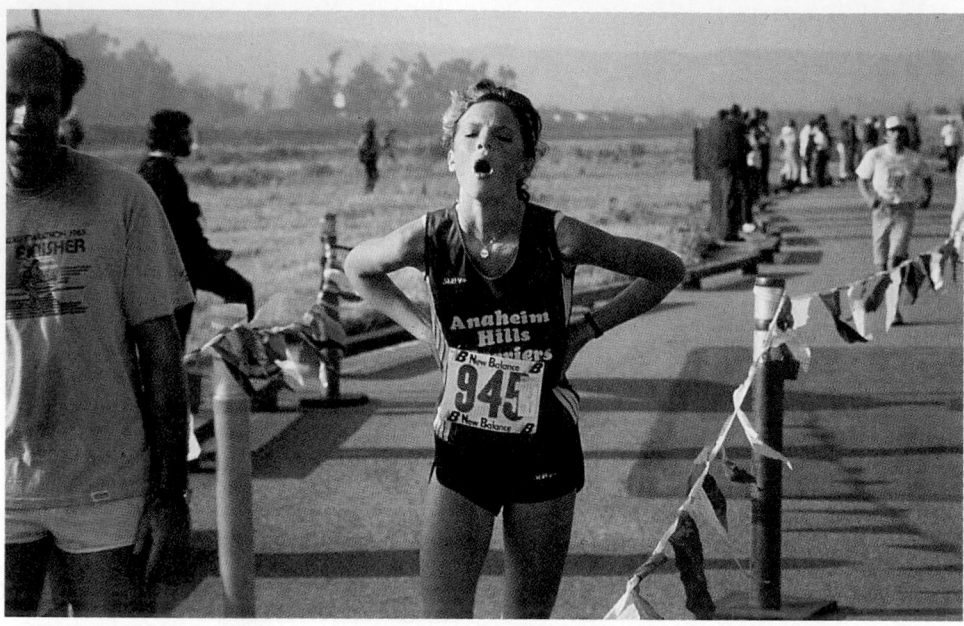

as **chronic obstructive pulmonary disease (COPD).** These conditions are described and illustrated in Chapter 21. According to the U.S. Public Health Service, smoking is the most common cause of COPD for both genders in the United States.[14]

CANCERS

Tobacco use contributes to cancers of not just the lungs, but of the lips, mouth, throat, larynx (voice box), trachea, esophagus, stomach, pancreas, cervix, urinary bladder, and kidneys as well (see Table 16.1). The carcinogens resulting from tobacco use enter the blood and circulate throughout the entire body. Tobacco use is associated with about 30 percent of all cancer deaths in the United States.[15] Each year, about 148,000 people die of cancers that are the direct result of tobacco use. This is especially tragic because cancers associated with tobacco are preventable.

The risk of developing this type of cancer is directly related to the number of years a person has smoked and the number of cigarettes smoked each day during that period. If tobacco use is discontinued before cancer has developed, however, the cancer risk gradually declines almost to that of a person who has never smoked.[16]

chronic obstructive pulmonary disease (COPD) a group of respiratory disorders characterized by obstruction of the airflow in the lungs.

SMOKING AND STAMINA

Smoking reduces vigor and endurance. Several factors are involved. First, the smoker's lungs are less able to **oxygenate** blood, owing to accumulation of mucus and tar in the lungs, loss of elasticity of the lungs, and the frequent presence of chronic bronchitis. The swollen, constricted bronchioles create a high resistance to the movement of air into and out of the lungs. Because breathing is harder work for a smoker, a smoker's breathing process uses up far more oxygen and energy than a nonsmoker's. With all of the limitations that the smoker endures, the result is reduced capacity for enjoying life.

SMOKING AND NUTRITION

Nicotine affects stomach contractions and blood sugar levels, both of which influence hunger. Smoking suppresses the stomach's hunger contractions for 15–60 minutes per cigarette. Nicotine also causes the liver to release sugar into the blood, which decreases hunger.[17]

Many smokers are reluctant to quit smoking for fear they will gain weight. This fear is not unfounded. Many people who quit smoking tend to replace cigarettes with food. Studies indicate that one-third

oxygenate to supply with oxygen.

of these people gain weight, one-third remain the same, and one-third lose weight. They may eat more, partially to fulfill the oral need they had been satisfying with cigarettes, but also to satisfy an increased appetite that occurs due to the lack of nicotine, which had acted as an appetite suppressor. This is a poor rationale for continuing to smoke, however.

Smoking also affects how a person's body uses vitamins. Blood levels of vitamins B_6, B_{12}, and C are reduced as increased amounts of these vitamins are used in the process of detoxifying chemicals in cigarette smoke.

CHECKPOINT

1. How does nicotine affect the cardiovascular system?
2. What occurs when carbon monoxide is present in the blood?
3. How does nicotine help promote strokes?
4. Indicate the possible health hazards of smoker's cough.
5. Define the terms *bronchitis* and *emphysema*.
6. List some of the cancers associated with smoking.
7. How many people die of smoking-related cancers per year?
8. Describe the factors involved in reduced stamina in smokers.
9. Which vitamins are reduced in the blood due to cigarette smoking?

PASSIVE SMOKING

The right of nonsmokers to a smoke-free environment has become an emotional issue. The controversy centers around how seriously the nonsmoker is threatened by **passive smoke,** also called "second-hand" or "side-stream" smoke.

Studies have shown that the danger from passive smoking is very real. The smoke rising from a burning cigarette resting in an ashtray or in a smoker's hand is *not* the same as the smoker is inhaling. The smoker is inhaling smoke that has been filtered through the tobacco along the length of the cigarette (and usually by its filter) while the nonsmoker is inhaling smoke that is totally unfiltered. Of course, the smoker also inhales this unfiltered smoke. Unfiltered "side-stream" smoke contains 50 times the amounts of carcinogens, is twice as high in tar and nicotine, has 5 times the carbon monoxide, and has 50 times as much ammonia as smoke inhaled through the cigarette.[18] Although the nonsmoker does not usually inhale side-stream smoke in the concentration that the smoker inhales the **mainstream smoke,** the concentration inhaled still amounts to, for the average person in the United States, the equivalent of smoking one cigarette per day. For people working in very smoky places, such as a bar or office, passive smoking can reach the equivalent of 14 cigarettes per day.[19]

CANCER AFFECTING PASSIVE SMOKERS

In January 1993, a long-awaited Environmental Protection Agency (EPA) report classified passive cigarette smoke as a human carcinogen that causes lung cancer in nonsmokers. According to the report, passive smoking causes somewhere between 700 and 7000 lung cancer deaths a year in the United States. The agency said that the most likely number is about 3000 deaths a year. This report is expected to result in additional limits on smoking in public places and federal regulations on smoking in the workplace. Predictably, the tobacco industry said that the report was based on inadequate scientific data.

OTHER EFFECTS

Passive tobacco smoke is a major lung irritant. At the very least, breathing second-hand smoke causes discomfort and coughing. Research has demonstrated that children raised in homes of smokers show early signs of conditions known to lead to

passive smoke exposure to smoke from other people's cigarettes; also called second-hand or sidestream smoke.

mainstream smoke smoke inhaled directly from a cigarette by its smoker.

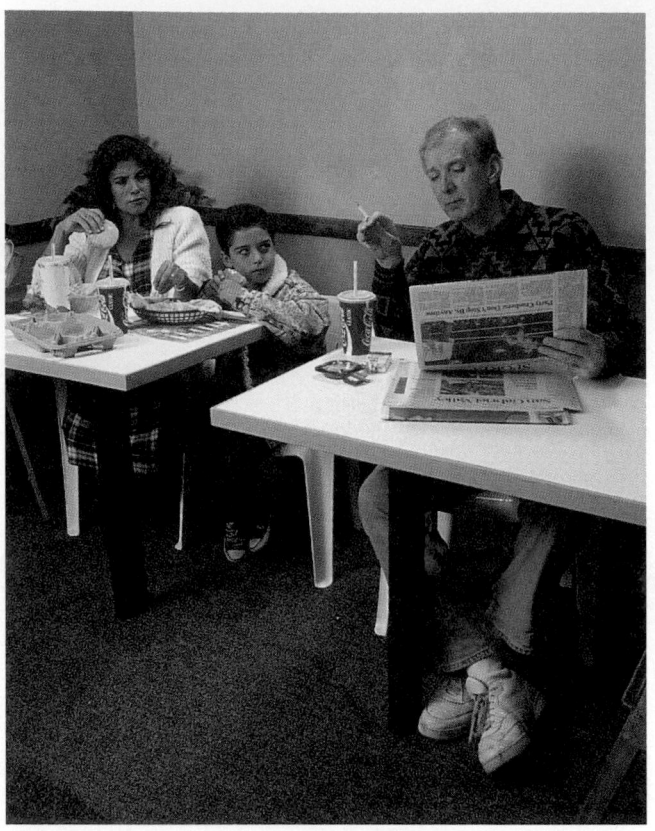

When there is heavy smoking in a poorly ventilated space, the carbon monoxide level also affects nonsmokers. Passive smoking is also a proven cause of cancer.

heart disease in adulthood.[20] For example, they show increased stiffness of the arteries, thickened walls of the heart chambers, and an unfavorable change in the blood's ratio of high-density lipoprotein to low-density lipoprotein (see Chapter 20, p. 638).

For people susceptible to **asthma** (attacks of difficult breathing caused by narrowing of the bronchioles), passive smoking can bring on a full-blown asthma attack. This is especially true for children. The incidence of asthma is higher among children who live in homes where someone smokes than among those from homes in which no one smokes. One estimate is that passive smoking may cause up to 100,000 new cases of childhood asthma in the United States each year.[21] Further, asthmatic children from homes in which someone smokes are likely to be in poorer health than asth-

....

asthma attacks of difficult breathing accompanied by wheezing and caused by spasm of the bronchioles or swelling of their lining.

matic children from homes where no one smokes.[22] Infants living in homes with smokers also experience twice as many respiratory infections as other infants.

SOCIETAL ISSUES

In addition to the health effects of passive smoking, there are major social objections to subjecting nonsmokers to the smoke of others. With fewer people smoking and more homes and offices becoming smoke-free, nonsmokers are becoming increasingly sensitive to the smell of tobacco smoke. Many people do not enjoy the smell of burning tobacco, do not want to have the taste of their dinner spoiled by the smell of smoke, do not want their clothing or hair contaminated with the smell of stale smoke, and consider it very rude to be subjected to these intrusions.

Conversely, many smokers are addicted to nicotine and are thus uncomfortable if required to forego smoking for extended periods. Many have tried to quit smoking without success. To be denied the right to smoke in public places makes it difficult or impossible for them to enjoy restaurant dining and other activities. As long as there are both smokers and nonsmokers we can expect to see conflicts regarding the rights of each group.

SMOKING IN THE WORKPLACE

Not only is passive smoking a now-proven cause of lung cancer, it also is very irritating to many people. For many people, the smoking of others irritates the conjunctiva (membrane of the eyes), causing reddening, itching, and increased tear flow. Also irritated are the mucous membranes of the nose, throat, and lungs, causing itching, sore throat, and coughing.

In one large survey,[23] 85 percent of people who had never smoked and 74 percent of former smokers reported that the smoke from another person's cigarette was annoying to them. When asked about smoke at their workplace, 64 percent of people who had never smoked and 51 percent of former smokers reported some degree of discomfort from people smoking at work. Even 15 percent of *current* smokers reported at least some discomfort caused by the smoke of others at their workplace.

Now that EPA has declared second-hand smoke a carcinogen, we can expect a continued

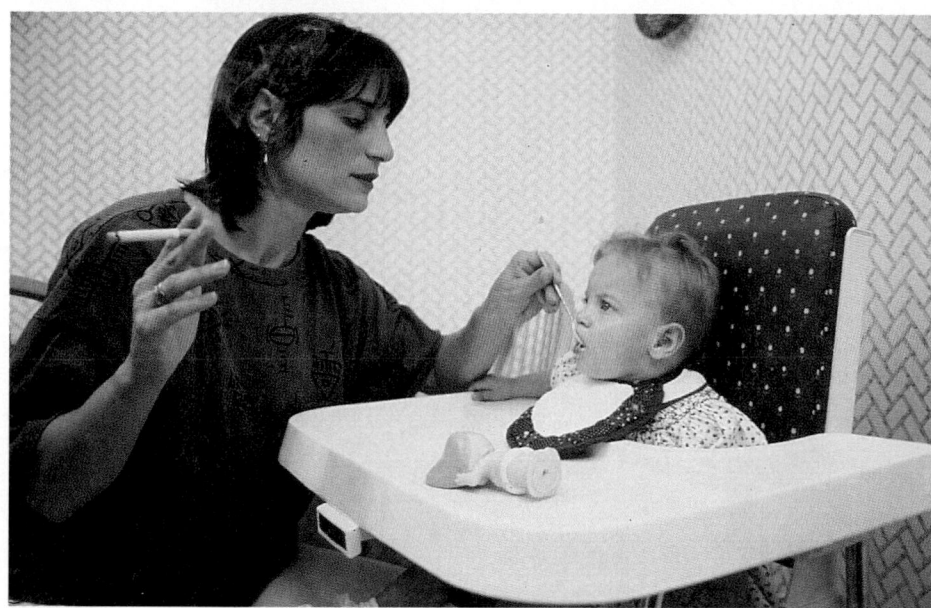

Infants and children living in homes where someone smokes have more respiratory problems than children living in smoke-free homes.

tightening of city, state, and federal laws regarding smoking in the workplace and other enclosed public places. As of 1992, 44 states and the District of Columbia, as well as hundreds of cities, had some form of restriction on smoking in public places (see Feature 16.4).[24] In 1992, 85 percent of employers had workplace smoking policies, compared with 54 percent in 1987. With ever-fewer people smoking, social pressure will also dictate an end to smoking in most work environments. Even the

majority of smokers now support limiting smoking in a wide range of locations.[25]

CHECKPOINT

1. Define the terms *passive smoke* and *mainstream smoke*.
2. Discuss the differences in levels of dangerous materials between passive and mainstream smoke.

FEATURE 16.4

THE GOVERNMENT AND TOBACCO

Many people wonder why a product that kills about a thousand people a *day* remains available to the public. Certainly, many products that have injured or killed far fewer people have been instantly removed from the marketplace. But when it comes to tobacco, the federal government has maintained an oddly ambivalent stance. Consider:

- The first *Surgeon General's Report on Smoking and Health* issued 30 years ago—in 1964—declared smoking to be the main cause of lung cancer and other disorders.
- Many subsequent *Surgeon General's Reports* have implicated tobacco as the cause of an ever-increasing list of major health problems.
- Since 1970, the government has required cigarette packs and cartons to carry labels warning of the dangers of smoking.
- Since 1971, tobacco advertising on radio and TV has been prohibited.

Yet also consider:

- Tobacco advertising in the print media is allowed, with many ads designed to appeal to youth and women. Smoking is associated with status, glamour, good times, masculinity or femininity (depends on the brand) and independence (interesting in an ad for a dependency-forming product).
- The U.S. Department of Agriculture aids tobacco growers in numerous ways.
- Little effort is made to control sales to minors, as cigarette vending machines are widespread and unsupervised.
- The U.S. government has encouraged the export of American cigarettes by threatening sanctions against some countries that have tried to restrict the importation of tobacco.

DECLINING TOBACCO USE

As Americans have recognized that the risks in tobacco use outweigh its benefits, and as they have felt a dramatic increase in social pressure against tobacco use, millions of people have given up tobacco.

As reported in 1992, 50.1 percent of U.S. adults had been smokers at some time in their lives, but only 25.5 percent of adults (28.4 percent of males and 22.8 percent of females) were current smokers (Table 16.2). This means that 49.1 percent of those who had ever smoked had quit.[26]

Comparing smoking rates of different categories of people, more males than females in every age group smoked, though in the youngest groups the margin was narrow. Smoking declines sharply as educational levels increase: 31.8 percent of those with less than 12 years of education smoked, while only 13.5 percent of those with 16 years or more of education smoked.

Even with the decline in tobacco use, the survey showed that millions of Americans, age 18 or older (plus millions who are younger), still smoke cigarettes. Additional millions use the various forms of "smokeless tobacco" such as snuff and chewing tobacco. Thus, tobacco use remains a problem in society and is considered one of the most hazardous, unhealthful behaviors.

Adolescent tobacco use is a special concern. In the next section we will examine when and why people begin to use tobacco.

CHECKPOINT

1. About what percent of people who have ever smoked have quit?

2. How does the percentage of males and females who smoke compare?

3. What is the correlation between smoking and educational level?

TOBACCO USE AMONG ADOLESCENTS

Lifelong smoking patterns are usually formed during adolescence. The majority of adults who smoke began smoking when they were teenagers. There-

Table 16.2
Percentage of U.S. Adults Currently Smoking Cigarettes by Year

Year	Persons of ____[a] years or below	Percent Currently Smoking	
		Men	Women
1944	18	48.0	36.0
1965	17	51.1	33.3
1970	17	43.5	31.1
1980	20	38.3	29.4
1986	17	29.5	23.8
1990	18	28.4	22.8

[a]Surveys in different years defined "adult" at various ages, ranging from 17 to 20.

Source: Centers for Disease Control. "Cigarette Smoking Among Adults—United States, 1990." Morbidity and Mortality Weekly Report 41, No. 20, May 22, 1992, pp. 354–361.

fore, smoking and other tobacco use among adolescents is of special concern. In fact, only 10–15 percent of today's smokers began smoking after the age of 19.[27] Thus, tobacco use prevention efforts must concentrate on preadolescents and adolescents to be most effective.

Further, measurable physiological effects of tobacco use become rapidly evident when adolescents smoke. At least three risk factors for cardiovascular disease increase in adolescents who have been smoking less than a pack a day for less than two years.[28] These include the following:

- Increased white blood cell counts that correlate closely with carbon monoxide levels in smokers' blood.

- Levels of high density lipoprotein, believed to help protect the body from cardiovascular disease, decline within two years after smoking begins.

- The ability to exhale rapidly (as in blowing out a candle) decreases within two years after smoking begins, indicating impaired lung function.

FACTORS ASSOCIATED WITH ADOLESCENT SMOKING

For adolescent antismoking programs to be effective, they need to address emotional, social, and familial factors that lead to tobacco use. Several recent research projects have attempted to identify such factors.

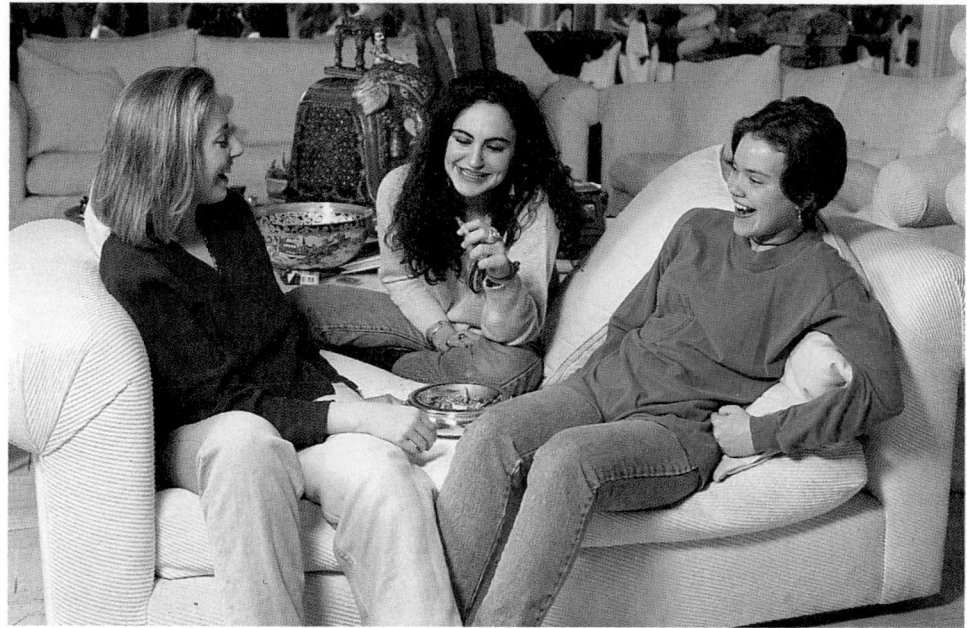

The majority of adults who smoke began smoking when they were teenagers. Peer pressure is one of the leading reasons why people start to smoke.

One carefully designed study analyzed the factors predicting cigarette smoking in adolescents in Southern California.[29] The following factors were found to increase a person's likelihood of becoming a smoker:

- smoking by parents and peers (a very important factor)
- having cigarettes easily accessible
- having trouble turning down offers of cigarettes
- having the intention of starting to smoke
- perceiving that parents and peers approve of smoking
- holding a positive image of smokers
- having a preference for taking risks
- having low self-esteem
- doing poorly in school

Note that knowledge or lack of knowledge of health consequences is not listed as a significant influence on smoking. Simply knowing the harmful effects of smoking does not, in itself, prevent young people from smoking. Smoking-prevention programs must go beyond simply teaching facts.

In a University of Minnesota study, adolescent smokers were found to hold the following views regarding smoking:[30]

1. It is a coping mechanism for dealing with boredom and frustration.

2. It is enjoyable and a way to have fun.

3. It is a strategy to reduce stress.

4. It is a transition marker or a claim on a more mature, adult status.

5. It is a way to gain admission into a peer group (if you accept instead of refuse a cigarette, it signals mutually acceptable behavior).

6. It is a way to maintain personal energy and to feel centered or renewed.

Since 85–90 percent of all current smokers began smoking prior to age 20, effective smoking-prevention programs must be directed at the preadolescent and early adolescent population. The Minnesota Smoking Prevention Program consists of six 45-minute sessions held in seventh-grade classes. This program enables students to identify what influences tobacco use and to deal with those influences. Within the program, the six views of smoking just discussed are addressed by the following:

1. Small group discussions on why people of their age group start smoking.

2. Interviews with parents, which focus on their perceptions of why adolescents smoke and how the things they say and do influence their children's smoking behavior.

3. Sessions that educate adolescents about how to identify the sources of their perceptions

Simply knowing the harmful effects of smoking has not been shown to prevent young people from smoking. Effective smoking prevention programs must deal with the attitudes of young people and their parents.

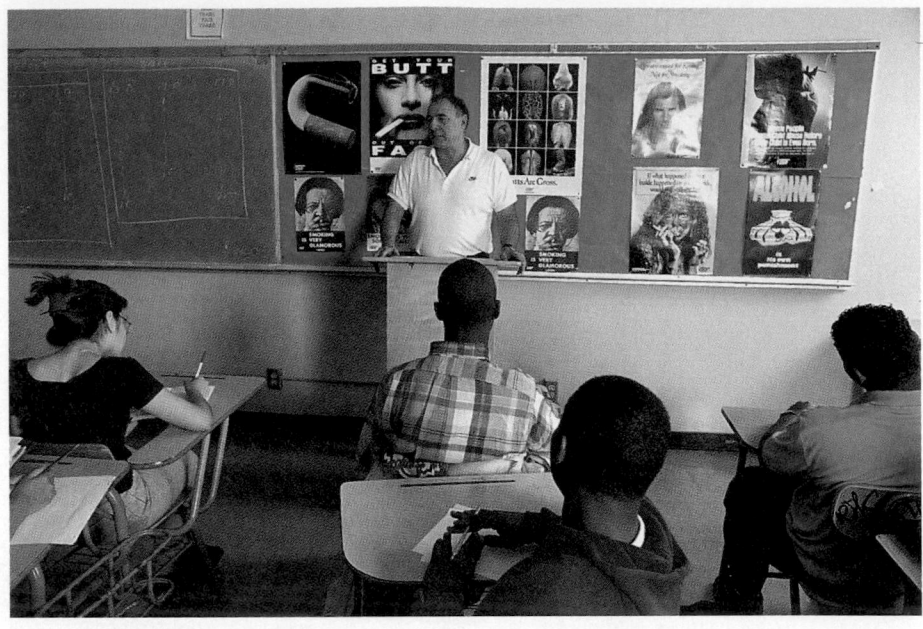

regarding the benefits of smoking, including peers, adults, and the mass media.

4. Comparisons of what adolescents perceive as advantages of smoking with the actual effects of smoking and discussions about the discrepancy.

5. Training sessions where students are taught effective ways to resist pressure from their peers to smoke cigarettes. Students are taught how to analyze advertising techniques and to give counterarguments (see Communication for Wellness: Issues on Regulation of Tobacco Advertising). They also learn how to approach their parents and other adults who smoke about quitting smoking.

6. Sessions in which each student prepares a statement explaining his or her reasons for remaining a nonsmoker; these explanations provide counterarguments to the reasons to begin smoking.

CHECKPOINT

1. What percent of smokers began smoking before the age of 20?

2. What are the risk factors associated with adolescent smoking?

3. For adolescent antismoking programs to be effective, what needs to be addressed?

4. List the six strategies of the Minnesota Smoking Prevention Program.

COMMUNICATION FOR WELLNESS
ISSUES ON REGULATION OF TOBACCO ADVERTISING

One of the controversies surrounding tobacco has been the extent, if any, to which advertising of tobacco products should be regulated. On the one hand are those who believe that prohibiting advertising of tobacco, a legal product, is an infringement on our rights of free speech. On the other hand are those who believe that tobacco advertising is too often influential on young people who may not yet have decided whether or not to smoke.

This latter point does have some validity. In the first place, a large percentage of those who ever become smokers do begin to smoke at a young age, usually before age 20. And tobacco ads do often associate smoking with fun, sophistication, sexual attractiveness, and other themes that appeal to young people. Also, while tobacco ads do include the government mandated warning statement, it is usually

inconspicuous and weak in comparison to the powerful message of the ad.

Radio and TV advertising of tobacco has been prohibited for many years. Tobacco companies have, to some degree, gotten around this prohibition by sponsoring sporting events. The name of the product is closely associated with the name of the event, providing lots of exposure and adding status to the product. People are hired to ensure that the product name is boldly emblazoned in positions where it will receive a lot of camera coverage when the event is televised.

What should be the policy on tobacco advertising? Should the print media, billboards, and buses continue to carry tobacco ads? Should we go back to allowing radio and TV ads? What do you think?

SMOKING AND WOMEN

Women who smoke experience all of the problems that affect male smokers—lung cancer, heart disease, emphysema, strokes—but they also face additional medical risks related to reproduction.

The combination of smoking and birth control pill use poses a serious health threat to women. For nonsmokers, today's oral contraceptives are quite safe. For smokers, however, using oral contraceptives is dangerous because the combination of smoking and pill use produces blood changes that increase the risk of blood clot formation within blood vessels. The results of these blood clots include heart attacks and strokes. The risk increases after the age of 30. Although the combination of smoking and birth control pill use is not recommended at any age, it is especially important if you are on the pill to discontinue smoking before age 30. If it is impossible to quit smoking, then use of the pill should be discontinued.

Smoking affects a woman's reproductive capacity in many ways. It takes women who smoke an average of 25 percent longer to conceive than nonsmokers because smoking decreases levels of estrogen and other female reproductive hormones.[31] Substances absorbed from cigarette smoke into the blood may also alter the critical environment within the fallopian tubes, where conception occurs.

If a woman smokes during pregnancy, her risk of miscarriage is up to ten times higher than that for a nonsmoker.[32] One possible reason is that the embryo or fetus receives less oxygen, because the carbon monoxide in the cigarette smoke inhaled by the mother reduces the oxygen-carrying capacity of the maternal and fetal bloodstreams. Other toxic chemicals absorbed from smoke may also be involved.

Infants born to smokers weigh an average of one-half pound less than the babies of nonsmokers. Lower birthweight is responsible for an increased first year infant death rate from a variety of causes. Smokers' babies run an increased risk of respiratory and intestinal problems. In a study of 53,000 births, smokers' infants had a 50 percent higher risk of developing sudden infant death syndrome (SIDS).[33]

There is also evidence of mild, but long-term, intellectual impairment in children of mothers who smoke during pregnancy. This may be another result of carbon-monoxide–induced oxygen depri-

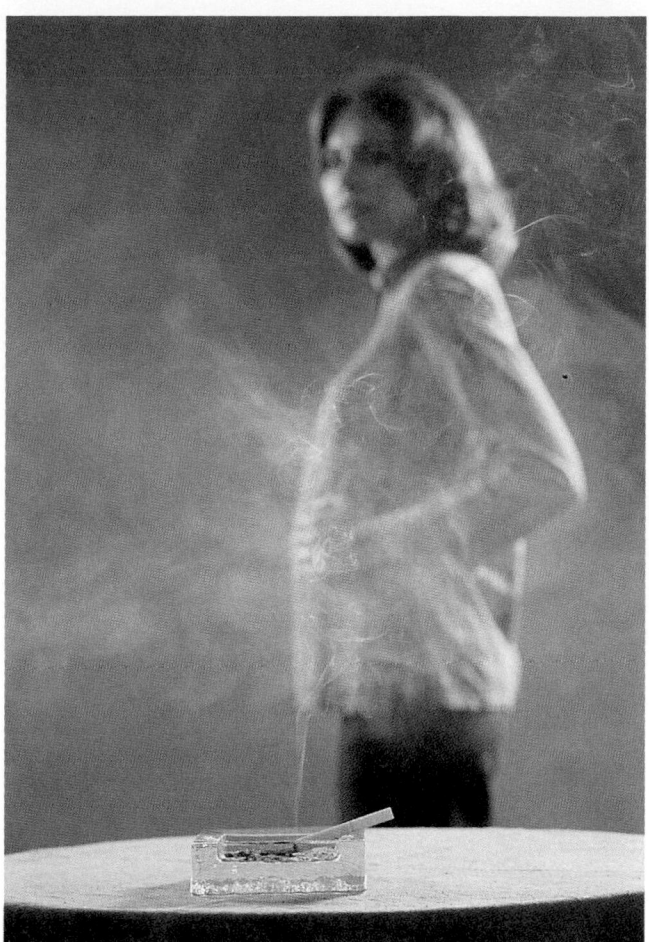

NO SMOKING. If a pregnant woman smokes, her risk of miscarriage is up to ten times higher than for a nonsmoker, her baby has an increased risk of infant death, and the baby's intellectual development will lag behind the baby of a nonsmoking mother.

vation. In a study of 13,000 children whose mothers smoked at least ten cigarettes per day during pregnancy, reading and math skills for children tested at ages 7 and 11 were found to average 3–5 months behind children of nonsmokers.[34]

Osteoporosis, the loss of bone density, is more prevalent among women who are or have been long-term smokers.[35] Osteoporosis causes a hunched posture and bone fractures, especially of the hip bones. For women who smoke, menopause begins an average of one- to one-and-a-half years earlier than for nonsmokers. Estrogen helps prevent osteoporosis; however, during menopause, a woman's production of estrogen decreases. The increased prevalence of osteoporosis among women smokers is partially due to their earlier menopause and partially due to the fact that smoking lowers estrogen levels during the reproductive years.

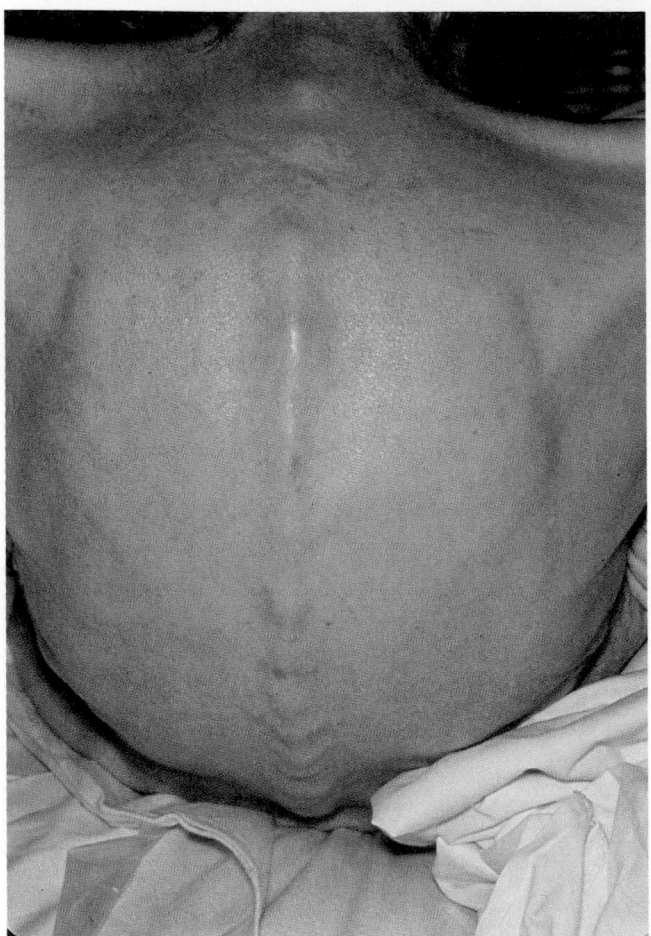

Because of an earlier menopause (with resulting decrease in estrogen levels) and because smoking lowers estrogen levels during the reproductive years, osteoporosis, the loss of bone density, is more prevalent among genetically susceptible women who are or have been long-term smokers.

CHECKPOINT

1. List the ways smoking affects a woman's reproductive capacity.
2. Why is osteoporosis more prevalent in smoking women?

QUITTING SMOKING

Quitting smoking is a very difficult task for most smokers. When a smoker is giving up cigarettes, that means breaking a dependency that has both physiological and psychological components. Nicotine dependency, though incredibly powerful, is not the only reason people continue to use tobacco. Successful programs to help people stop smoking must address all of the reasons people smoke.

OBSTACLES TO QUITTING

Nicotine provides psychological stimulation, which is the cause of many smokers' dependency. Tolerance and physiological dependency (addiction) develop as tobacco use becomes more frequent. A physiologically dependent smoker who tries to quit will experience withdrawal symptoms, which range from nervousness to severe headaches and the inability to concentrate.

Routine behaviors and effects of smoking are major factors in a smoker's continuing dependency. For example, smoking provides repetitious hand-to-mouth activity, which becomes routine and habit-forming. Smoking provides relaxation, oral gratification, and appetite suppression. Knowing your reasons for smoking is helpful in the process of quitting.

WAYS OF QUITTING

Methods of quitting smoking range from "cold turkey"—crushing out a cigarette and never lighting up again, without the help of anyone or any product—to lengthy, elaborate, and expensive commercial programs. The difficulty many people experience in quitting smoking has attracted many quacks with unproven products and programs into the "stop smoking" industry. Some methods work for some smokers and fail for others. The outcome with any method will depend on the degree of addiction and the strength of the smoker's motivation to quit. Feature 16.5 offers some tips for quitting smoking.

Nicotine Gum

One way to stop smoking, yet to avoid the distress caused by nicotine withdrawal, is to obtain nicotine from some other source. Nicotine gum, available only by a physician's prescription, is one possible source of nicotine. Though still temporarily exposed to the harmful effects of nicotine, the former smoker is able to escape the other harmful elements in smoke, such as tar and carbon monoxide. The amount of gum chewed daily should gradually taper off and the use of nicotine gum should be totally eliminated by the fourth to sixth month. In order for nicotine gum to be effective, the former smoker must completely abstain from smoking, as even one cigarette carries the risk of resuming the smoking habit.

FEATURE 16.5

TIPS FOR QUITTING SMOKING

Regardless of the method you use to quit smoking, the following suggestions will improve your chances of success.

1. Plan a meaningful date for stopping if such a date is coming up soon. You might choose your birthday, your spouse's or child's birthday, New Year's Day, or your anniversary. If you smoke under stress at work, pick a date for stopping when you will be away from work. Don't choose a date so far in the future that you will lose momentum.

2. Make an agreement with a smoking friend or spouse to quit together, so you can support each other.

3. Ask to move to a nonsmoking part of your workplace so that the temptation to smoke is reduced.

4. Tell everyone you know that you have quit smoking. They will give you plenty of support.

5. Form a support group of people you can call any time you feel the urge to smoke.

6. Try various substitutes for smoking, such as exercise, a new hobby or activity, chewing gum, or low-calorie snacks. Avoid eating high-calorie foods; many people gain weight when they stop smoking.

7. It is usually best to quit suddenly and totally. Gradually phasing out the smoking habit is less successful. Those who are nicotine addicts, however, may have to taper off (or use nicotine gum) to avoid withdrawal symptoms. If you are going to stop gradually, work out a scheduled plan in advance and stick to it.

8. Never light up until at least five minutes have passed since you got the urge to smoke. During that five minutes, attempt to change your emotional state or become involved in another activity. Telephone a member of your stop-smoking support network.

9. Make smoking as inconvenient as possible. Buy only one pack at a time and only after you have finished the previous pack. Never carry cigarettes around with you at home or at work. Never carry matches or a lighter with you.

10. Make a list of things you could buy with the money saved by not smoking. Convert the price of each item to days of not smoking.

11. Always ask yourself: Do I really need this cigarette or is it just a reflex response?

12. Remove all ash trays from your home, car, and workplace.

13. Find activities to keep your hands occupied.

14. As soon as you quit, visit a dentist to have your teeth cleaned of tobacco stains.

15. Devote your spare time to new activities; avoid the types of activities you associate with smoking (drinking in bars, watching TV, and so on). Become a more physically active person.

16. If you're having trouble quitting on your own, check with the American Cancer Society, American Heart Association, or American Lung Association in your area (check your phone book). They are very likely to offer effective programs to help you quit.

Nicotine gum is not recommended for everyone. It must be avoided by heart patients, breastfeeding mothers, and women who are pregnant or planning to become pregnant. Some users find that nicotine gum causes nausea, hiccups, or sore throats.

Nicotine Patches

Like nicotine gum, nicotine-releasing skin patches allow a person to stop smoking immediately but to taper off gradually from his or her addiction to nicotine. The patch is effective because nicotine, like many other chemicals, is readily absorbed through the skin into the blood.

Patches are used in an 8–20 week program, during which the dosage of nicotine is gradually reduced from 15–21 milligrams per day down to 5–7 milligrams, depending on the brand. For lasting cessation of smoking, it is important for the smoker to participate in some type of behavioral smoking-cessation program. Patches are obtained through a physician's prescription.

Aversion Therapy

Aversion therapy is a type of behavior therapy that uses negative conditioning to take the fun out of smoking and make it repulsive to the smoker. One form of therapy requires the participant to draw on a cigarette every six seconds until smoking becomes very unpleasant. Another technique used is accompanying each puff on a cigarette with a mild electric shock.

Hypnosis

Hypnosis is used in smoking-control programs to lull the conscious mind into a passive condition,

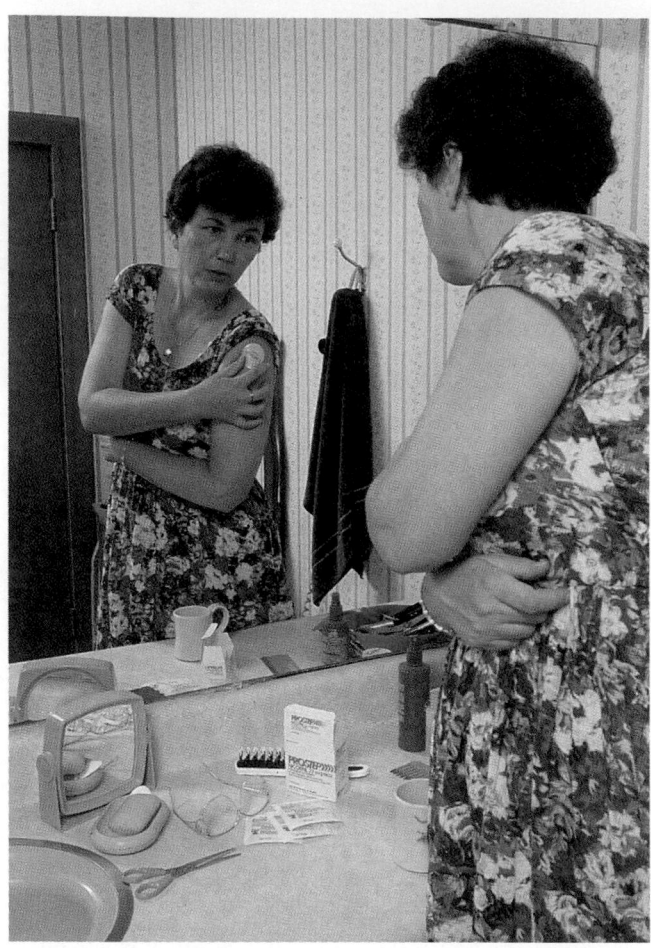

Nicotine-releasing skin patches do not allow a person to stop smoking immediately, but to taper off gradually from his or her addiction to nicotine. These patches also serve as a demonstration of how chemicals can enter the blood through one's skin.

allowing the subconscious mind to accept the suggestions of the hypnotist to stop smoking. This process is most likely to succeed with highly motivated people who are receptive to the concept of hypnosis. Anyone considering hypnosis should choose their practitioner carefully, as some poorly trained people enter this field. For names of certified hypnotists in your area, write to the American Society of Clinical Hypnosis.

Group Programs

A wide range of nonprofit and commercial organizations offer group programs to help people stop smoking. The American Cancer Society, American Heart Association, and American Lung Association all offer excellent programs. Most of these programs are based on the concept of mutual support

in reaching a common goal. A few include some or all of the elements common to the 12-step programs based on Alcoholics Anonymous. Some other programs offer weight-management assistance to help counteract the tendency to gain weight after quitting smoking (see Feature 16.6). Smokers in most areas will also find that local hospitals, colleges, and health departments sponsor stop-smoking clinics.

EFFECTIVENESS OF DIFFERENT SMOKING CONTROL STRATEGIES

Smoking-cessation methods fall into one of two categories:

- *Self-help strategies,* such as quitting abruptly and completely, or using nonprescription drugs.
- *Assisted strategies,* such as smoking-cessation clinics, hypnosis, acupuncture, or medically prescribed nicotine gum or patches.

As in all chemical-dependency recovery, there is no universal agreement on how to evaluate the success of different methods. For example, is a program a success if a smoker goes from smoking 40 cigarettes (two packs) a day to just 10 cigarettes? And how soon do we evaluate success? Many who have quit smoking return to smoking at some later date. Being abstinent from smoking for one year is a common measure of success. By this measure:

- The 12-month abstinence rates for people using self-help methods have ranged from 8 to 25 percent, compared to 20–40 percent of people who used assisted strategies.[36]
- Twelve-month success rates are higher for programs with an ongoing maintenance component.
- The success rate for males is consistently higher than for females, but only minimally so if adjusted for people who switch to smokeless tobacco.
- The success rate is higher for whites than for blacks, for older smokers than for younger smokers, and for college graduates than for people with less than a high school education.
- Least successful at quitting are young females who have not completed high school.

FEATURE 16.6

HOW TO QUIT SMOKING AND NOT GAIN WEIGHT

When you stop smoking, three things begin to happen:

1. Your body's metabolism begins to work to its optimum capacity. Thus, you utilize food more efficiently.

2. For years your taste buds have been deadened by smoking. Once you quit smoking, your taste buds become more keen and food tastes better, so you are tempted to eat more.

3. For years you have been used to having a cigarette in your mouth. Now you are tempted to enjoy between-meal snacks to replace the cigarettes.

Here are some tips to help you stay healthy and keep your weight down after you quit smoking:

1. Eat three regular meals a day.

2. Eliminate between-meal snacks (they are eaten mainly out of habit).

3. Eat one normal serving at a meal. If you are still hungry, wait 20 minutes before having a second helping. You will probably no longer feel hungry.

4. Remove high-calorie items from your diet. Eliminate or reduce:

   High-fat foods such as fried foods, margarine, butter, rich cheeses, many desserts, fatty meats, snack foods, and mayonnaise.

   Sugars—desserts, jams and jellies, sweetened cereals, soft drinks.

5. Exercise regularly—regular exercise burns calories, reduces stress, and serves as an activity to replace smoking.

These women are of special concern because they have a high pregnancy rate and tend to smoke during pregnancy, the period of breastfeeding, and in the presence of their children. Even though fewer people smoke than in the past, over one million young people begin smoking every year. Given the low success rate of young people at quitting smoking, intensive efforts must be made to discourage young people from beginning to smoke.[37]

CHECKPOINT

1. What are some reasons, in addition to nicotine dependency, that people continue to smoke?

2. What are some different ways of quitting smoking?

3. Which ways of quitting are more effective?

✓

SUMMARY

Although a smaller percentage of Americans use tobacco now than in the past, it still causes over 350,000 premature deaths every year and debilitating chronic diseases in millions of Americans.

No form of tobacco use is without some hazards. Harmful chemicals in tobacco smoke include nicotine, tars, carbon monoxide, hydrogen cyanide, and nitrous oxide. Among the harmful effects of tobacco are cardiovascular disorders, respiratory diseases, cancers, reduced stamina, and vitamin deficiencies. "Second-hand smoke" affects nonsmokers by causing cancer, asthma, and irritation of the eyes, nose, and throat.

About half of those Americans who have ever smoked have quit. Among those who still smoke, smoking is more prevalent in males than in females and in people with a lower level of education. Adolescent smoking is a special concern because most people who become smokers do so before the age of 19.

Women who smoke experience all the problems that affect male smokers as well as increased risk of blood clots if they take birth control pills. They miscarry more often and their babies weigh less at birth, have more respiratory and intestinal problems, and an increased risk of sudden infant death syndrome. Women who smoke are also at a greater risk for osteoporosis.

There are many ways of quitting smoking. Assisted strategies such as clinic programs, hypnosis, acupuncture, or prescribed nicotine gum or patches have a higher success rate than self-help strategies such as quitting abruptly. The success rate is lowest for people who are young, female, and have a lower level of education.

If you don't use tobacco, don't start. If you do use tobacco, quit. If people who are important to you use tobacco, encourage them to quit. Minimize your exposure to other people's smoke. Nonsmokers feel better, look better, smell better, and enjoy longer, more active lives.

REFERENCES

1. U.S. Public Health Service. *Healthy People: The Surgeon General's Report on Health Promotion and Disease Prevention*. Washington, DC: U.S. Department of Health, Education, and Welfare, 1979.
2. Centers for Disease Control. "Cigarette Smoking-Attributable Mortality and Years of Potential Life Lost—United States, 1990." *Morbidity and Mortality Weekly Report* 42, No. 33 (27 August 1993), 645–649.
3. Witters, W., Venturelli, .P, and Hanson, G. *Drugs and Society,* 3rd ed. Boston: Jones and Bartlett, 1992.
4. Schlaadt, R., and Shannon, P. *Drugs of Choice,* 3rd ed. Englewood Cliffs, NJ: Prentice Hall, 1990.
5. Centers for Disease Control. "Smoking-Attributable Mortality and Years of Potential Life Lost, United States, 1984." *Morbidity and Mortality Weekly Report* 36, No. 42 (30 October 1987), 694–697.
6. Schlaadt and Shannon, op. cit.
7. Julien, R. *A Primer of Drug Action,* 5th ed. New York: Freeman, 1988.
8. Schlaadt and Shannon, op. cit.
9. Centers for Disease Control, 1993, op. cit.
10. Ibid.
11. Schlaadt and Shannon, op. cit.
12. Julien, op. cit.
13. Schlaadt and Shannon, op. cit.
14. U.S. Public Health Service. *1984 Surgeon General's Report, Health Consequences of Smoking: Chronic Obstructive Disease.* Rockville, MD: U.S. Department of Health and Human Services, Public Health Service, Office on Smoking, 1984.
15. American Cancer Society. *Cancer Facts and Figures—1993.* New York: American Cancer Society, 1993.
16. Schlaadt and Shannon, op. cit.
17. Ibid.
18. Chandler, W. "Banishing Tobacco." *Society* 18, No. 3 (May/June, 1981), 56–64.
19. Ibid.
20. Moskowitz, W. Associated Press report of paper presented at annual meeting of American Heart Association, November 18, 1987.
21. Fackelmann, K. "Passive Smoking Risk Proves a Family Affair." *Science News* Vol. 141 (25 January 1992), p. 54.
22. Ellis, E. Interview in *U.S. News and World Report,* 2 June 1986, 60.
23. Centers for Disease Control. "Discomfort from Environmental Tobacco Smoke Among Employees." *Morbidity and Mortality Weekly Report* Vol. 41, No. 20 (22 May 1992), 351–354.
24. Ibid.
25. Ibid.
26. Centers for Disease Control. "Cigarette Smoking Among Adults—United States, 1990." *Morbidity and Mortality Weekly Report* Vol. 41, No. 20 (22 May 1992), 354–362.
27. Kreuter, M., and Powell, K. "Psychosocial Predictors of Smoking Among Adolescents." *Morbidity and Mortality Weekly Report* 36, No. 4s (4 September 1987), 1–2.
28. Dwyer, J., Lippert, P., Rieger-Ndakarerwa, G., and Semmer, N. "Some Chronic Disease Risk Factors and Cigarette Smoking in Adolescents: The Berlin-Bremen Study." *Morbidity and Mortality Weekly Report* 36, No. 4s (4 September 1987), 35–40.
29. Sussman, S., Dent, C., Flay, B., Hansen, W., and Johnson, C. "Psychological Predictors of Cigarette Smoking Onset by White, Black, Hispanic, and Asian Adolescents in Southern California." *Morbidity and Mortality Weekly Report* 36, No. 4s (4 September 1987), 11–16.
30. Perry, C., Murray, D., and Klepp, K. "Predictors of Adolescent Smoking and Implications for Prevention." *Morbidity and Mortality Weekly Report* 36, No. 4s (4 September 1987), 41–45.
31. Seligmann, J. "Women Smokers: The Risk Factor." *Newsweek* (25 November 1985), 76–78.
32. Ibid.
33. Ibid.
34. Ibid.
35. Ibid.
36. Centers for Disease Control. "Effectiveness of Smoking—Control Strategies—United States." *Morbidity and Mortality Weekly Report* Vol. 41, No. 35 (4 September 1992), 645–647.
37. Ibid.

SUGGESTED READINGS

Avis, H. *Drugs and Life,* 2nd ed. Madison, WI: Brown and Benchmark, 1993.
Schlaadt, R., and Shannon, P. *Drugs of Choice*, 3rd ed. Englewood Cliffs, NJ: Prentice Hall, 1990.
Surgeon General's Reports on Smoking, various periodic reports.
U.S. Public Health Service. "Health Consequences of Smoking," various periodic reports.
Witters, W., Venturelli, P., and Hanson, G. *Drugs and Society,* 3rd ed. Boston: Jones and Bartlett, 1992.

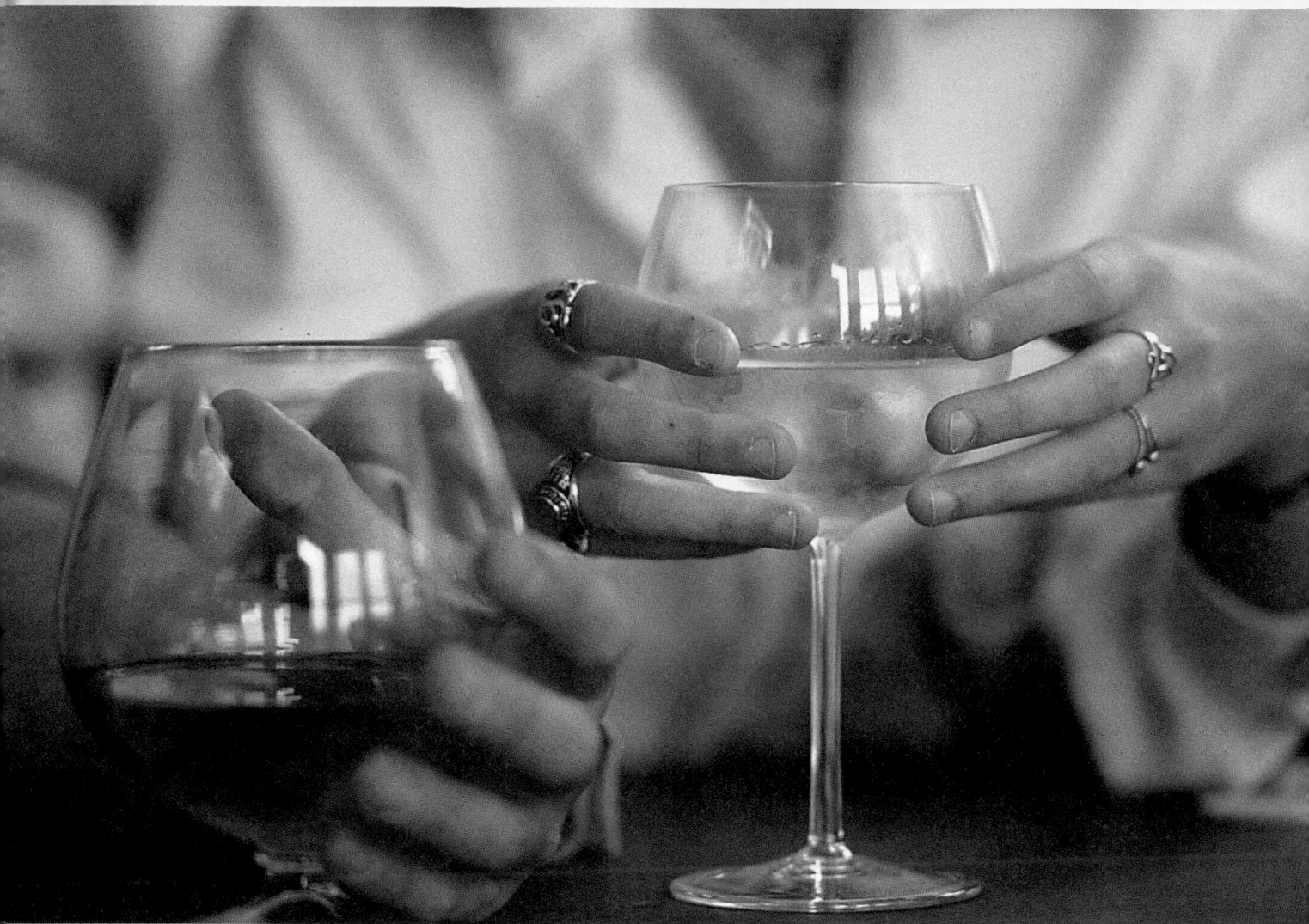

17
ALCOHOL AND HEALTH

KNOWLEDGE

- List the ways alcohol abuse hurts individuals, families, and society.
- Describe the relative alcohol content of common alcoholic beverages.
- Explain the effects of alcohol on each body system.
- Describe fetal alcohol syndrome.
- Define the terms *problem drinking* and *alcoholism*.
- Explain blackouts and alcoholic loss of control.
- Outline the factors that cause or contribute to alcoholism.
- Explain how cultural customs and attitudes regarding alcohol use influence the development of alcoholism.
- List factors that promote adolescent drinking.
- Explain why most experts believe that alcoholics should not attempt to return to social drinking.

INSIGHT

- Recognize any signs that your own drinking may be causing problems for you.
- Explain how many drinks a person of your own body weight can take and still remain under the legal blood alcohol limit for driving a vehicle.
- Manage alcohol in such a way that it does not threaten your success in college.

DECISION MAKING

- Make a commitment to be alert for any signs of developing an alcohol problem yourself.
- Make a commitment never to use rationalization and denial regarding your drinking.
- Promise yourself to stop drinking immediately if you start having any problems as a result of your drinking.

I n late March 1993, a tragic boating accident resulted in the deaths of two Cleveland Indian baseball players, Tim Crews and Steve Olin. Investigators found that Crews, who was piloting the boat at the time of the accident, had a blood alcohol level of 0.14. At this time, a blood alcohol content (BAC) of 0.10 was considered legally drunk in Florida, where the accident occurred. (BAC is a measure of the amount of alcohol in the blood. A BAC of 0.10 means that one-tenth of 1 percent of the blood content is comprised of alcohol.) Apparently, it was just after dark and the boat rammed a pier at high speed. While it was impossible to determine just how fast the boat was going, experts estimated that it had to be travelling at least 25 miles per hour. The two players who died were killed from "blunt force trauma to the head." The survivor, Bob Ojeda, another Cleveland Indian player, also suffered head injuries in the crash, and has no recollection of either seeing or hitting the pier.

The medical examiner who performed the autopsy on Crews said that the amount of alcohol he had consumed was in the range of six to seven beers for a man of his size (6 ft., 195 lbs.). While we often hear about the perils of drinking and driving an automobile, there is too little emphasis on drinking and driving boats and other recreational vehicles. Many deaths and injuries occur each year when people drink and engage in recreational sports, especially water-related activities. The tragic deaths of these young *men in the prime of their lives is a solemn reminder that drinking and engaging in recreational sports, such as boating, has as much potential to kill or cause permanent injury as drinking and driving an automobile.*

∎ ∎ ∎

As mentioned in previous chapters, alcohol is a psychoactive drug. Alcohol plays more varied roles in American society than any other drug. It is used to celebrate special occasions, to mourn losses, to reduce anxiety, to escape reality, to relax, and to enhance the enjoyment of a gourmet meal. Alcohol is legal, is used by about 60 percent of the adults in the nation (about 43 percent in any given week),[1] is a major industry that provides the incomes of many people, *and is America's number one drug problem.*

The costs of alcohol abuse can be measured in many ways:[2]

- About 10 percent of all deaths in the United States each year are alcohol-related.
- Lives of heavy drinkers are shortened by an average of 15 years.
- About 38 percent of all traffic fatalities involve alcohol.
- In over half of all murders, the assailant, victim, or both, have been drinking.
- Alcohol is estimated to add about $15 billion to the nation's annual health care bill.
- The annual cost of alcohol-related loss of productivity (days lost from work and unemployment) is estimated at over $71 billion.
- Alcohol is involved in about two-thirds of all family violence.
- Alcohol abuse severely reduces the quality of life of the abuser.

In this chapter we will explore the nature of alcoholic beverages, how alcohol is absorbed and processed by the body, its physical effects, alcohol and driving, patterns of alcohol use and abuse, the effects of alcohol abuse on families and in young people, and programs for recovery from alcohol abuse.

CHECKPOINT

1. List some of the many ways alcohol hurts individuals and society.

A BRIEF HISTORY OF ALCOHOL USE

The production of alcohol requires only that a solution of any form of sugar or starch be exposed to a few cells of yeast. After a few days of fermentation, an alcoholic beverage will be present. No one knows when humans first noticed this fact, but the consumption of alcohol began very early in human history. The early Egyptians, Greeks, and Romans all had their gods of wine and the Bible is full of references to wine.

Many early customs developed around the use of alcohol. In some cultures, alcohol was viewed as a staple and essential part of the daily diet. By the Middle Ages, alcohol accompanied birth, courting, marriage, the crowning of kings, and death. It was seen as the cure for most illnesses and a source of good cheer; indeed, it was viewed as a gift from God.

European explorers and colonists brought many forms of alcohol to North America, including beer, wine, brandy, rum, and whiskey. From the beginning of European colonization, the production and importation of alcoholic beverages have been important industries here. Today, alcohol is deeply ingrained in American social customs.

CHECKPOINT

1. Can you visualize the first time someone unknowingly drank some fruit juice that had fermented? Would they want to drink more the next day?

2. What do you think would happen if alcohol were to be discovered today for the first time? Would it be seen as a miracle drug or a threat to society?

AMERICA'S NUMBER ONE DRUG PROBLEM

The main factor that distinguishes alcohol from other drugs is its legal availability and its acceptability by most members of American society. About 60 percent of the adult population are at least occasional users of alcohol. Many people who use alcohol experience few, if any, problems as a result. For some of its users, however, the resulting problems are as severe as those from the abuse of any drug. How can a substance that causes little trouble for some of its users cause such severe problems for others?

Some insight on drinking in the United States can be gained from looking at the distribution of alcohol consumption through the U.S. population. Suppose that all of the alcohol consumed in the United States in a year were represented by ten cans of beer. And suppose that the entire adult population of the nation were represented by ten people. Here, based on figures compiled from a variety of sources, is what would become of the ten beers:[3]

four people drink none (40 percent of the population does not drink)

four people share two cans of beer (40 percent of the population are light drinkers and share only 20 percent of the alcohol used)

one person drinks two cans of beer (10 percent of the population are heavy drinkers and drink 20 percent of all alcohol used)

one person drinks six cans of beer (10 percent of the population are alcoholics and drink 60 percent of all alcohol sold in the United States)

Recent studies provide slightly different statistics on alcohol consumption, which is declining in the United States, but confirm the fact that a small percentage of the population accounts for most of the alcohol consumed.[4] In addition to how much or how often a person drinks, other factors, explored throughout this chapter, also determine whether or not a person's alcohol use creates problems. Where do you fit in? Take a minute right now to answer the questions in In Your Hands: An Assessment of Drinking Patterns.

IN YOUR HANDS

AN ASSESSMENT OF DRINKING PATTERNS

Give a simple yes or no answer to each question:

1. Do you sometimes drink to escape from disappointment, anger, boredom, or loneliness? _____
2. Do you sometimes take a drink *before* you go out on a date or to a party or other social event? _____
3. When you look forward to a party or other social event, does the opportunity to drink seem more important than the chance for socializing and companionship? _____
4. Do you choose your friends on the basis of whether or not they drink? _____
5. Do you drink more than most of your friends? _____
6. Does it bother you if someone suggests that maybe you drink too much? _____
7. Do classes or lectures on alcohol irritate you? _____
8. Are there times when you can't remember part of an evening of drinking, though you did not pass out? _____
9. Do you find it difficult to stop after two drinks? _____
10. Do you sometimes drive after having more than two drinks? _____
11. Have you had financial problems because of drinking? _____
12. Have you had school or job problems because of drinking? _____
13. Have you had any trouble with the law because of drinking? _____
14. Do you have a strong urge for a drink at any certain time of the day? _____
15. Do you sometimes sneak drinks, hoping that others will not notice? _____
16. Do you sometimes feel guilty or sorry about drinking too much? _____
17. Do you sometimes gulp down drinks to get a rapid effect? _____
18. Do you avoid certain situations if you know alcohol will not be available? _____
19. Did answering these questions make you feel uncomfortable? _____

If you answered yes to any two of these questions, you probably have a drinking problem. Being able to handle alcohol well is not a matter of willpower. It has nothing to do with masculinity or femininity.

Some people just do not handle alcohol well and never will. For those people, the only answer is to stop drinking.

CHECKPOINT

1. What percent of the U.S. population ever uses alcohol?

2. What percent of the U.S. population can be considered heavy drinkers and what percent are probably alcoholics?

CHECKPOINT

1. What are several names for the type of alcohol in alcoholic beverages?

2. Describe the fermentation process and the distillation process of producing alcoholic beverages.

ALCOHOLIC BEVERAGES

The chemical name for the form of alcohol in alcoholic beverages is ethanol or ethyl alcohol; its common name is grain alcohol. Alcohol consists of very small molecules and it is soluble in both water and fat. This accounts for its rapid absorption into the blood and easy movement into every organ of the body, including the brain (refer back to Chapter 15).

Alcohol is produced by the **fermentation** of sugar by yeast. Different sugar sources result in the various beverages: beer is made from malted barley; wine is fermented grape juice; rum is fermented molasses. Fermentation stops when the alcohol reaches 12 percent. Stronger beverages are produced by **distillation.** Alcohol boils at a lower temperature than water, so alcohol-containing mixtures (see Table 17.1) can be boiled in a still and the alcohol-rich steam cooled and condensed to yield a stronger beverage. The alcohol content of distilled beverages is usually expressed as "proof," which is double the percentage. Thus, 100 proof vodka is 50 percent alcohol.

People often make a distinction between drinking beer or more highly alcoholic beverages. "I couldn't be an alcoholic, I only drink beer." "But officer, I only had a few beers." The fact is that beer, even "light" or reduced calorie beer, contains plenty of alcohol—enough to make you legally drunk. Some alcohol abusers drink no alcoholic beverage other than beer.

Now we will examine how alcoholic beverages are absorbed into the blood and how they rate nutritionally.

fermentation process by which yeast converts sugar into alcohol.

distillation condensation of a vapor that has been obtained from a liquid heated to its boiling point.

Alcohol Myth:
Drinking is one of the social graces. You have to drink if you want to get along socially in the United States.

Alcohol Reality:
Millions of people have full and rewarding social lives without any use of alcohol. In fact, abstainers now make up 40 percent of the U.S. population. Many people who say they are **social drinkers** (those who drink only in a social context) are actually **problem drinkers** (those whose drinking causes interpersonal, family, or work problems) who often drink alone.

ABSORPTION AND NUTRITIONAL VALUE OF ALCOHOL

Because an alcohol molecule is small and easily absorbed into the blood, no digestion of alcohol is necessary before its absorption begins. Absorption is rapid, with a small amount absorbed even through the lining of the mouth. More alcohol, about 20 percent of the total, is absorbed through the stomach lining. The majority, about 80 percent, is absorbed in the small intestine.

The presence of food in the stomach slows the absorption of alcohol; alcohol consumed on an empty stomach is absorbed quite rapidly. The more alcohol is diluted—mixed with nonalcoholic liquids as in mixed drinks—the more slowly it is absorbed, even though the same amount of alcohol is consumed. Carbonation (the presence of carbon diox-

social drinkers those who drink only in a social context.

problem drinkers those whose drinking causes interpersonal, family, or work problems.

Table 17.1
Source and Alcohol Content of Alcoholic Beverages

Beverage	Source of Sugar	Distilled?	% Alcohol (proof)
Beer	Malted barley	No	3–6 (mostly 4–4.5)
Light beer	Malted barley	No	3.2–3.3
Malt liquor	Malted barley	No	4–8
Ale	Malted barley	No	6–8
Wine coolers	Grape juice	No	5–9
Table wine	Grape juice	No	12–14
Fortified wine	Grape juice	No	19–21 (fortified with brandy)
Brandy	Grape juice	Yes	40–50 (80–100 proof)
Whiskey	Malted grains	Yes	40–50 (80–100 proof)
Gin	Various	Yes	40–50 (80–100 proof)
Tequila	Cactus juice	Yes	40–50 (80–100 proof)
Vodka	Various	Yes	40–50 (80–100 proof)
Rum	Sugar cane	Yes	40–50 or higher (80–100 or higher proof)

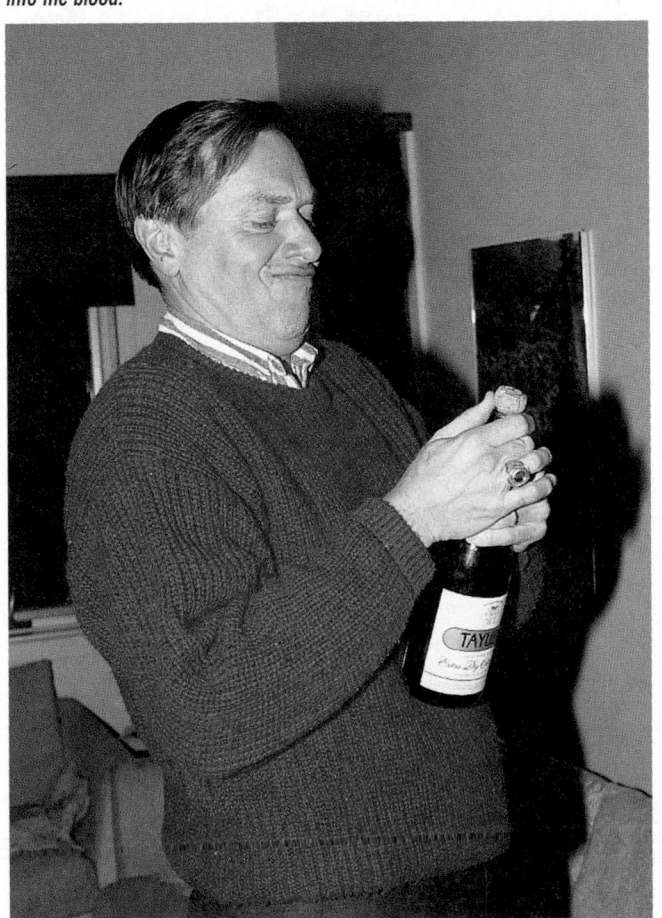

Champagne earns its reputation for quick intoxication on the basis of its high degree of carbonation. The presence of CO_2 speeds the absorption of alcohol into the blood.

ide) tends to speed absorption. This is why the alcohol in champagne is absorbed faster than the same amount of alcohol in noncarbonated wine.

Most alcoholic beverages have very little nutritional value. Although they contain calories (Table 17.2, p. 524), they contain little or no protein, vitamins, or minerals. Thus, the calories in alcoholic drinks are "empty calories." Many alcohol abusers derive most of their calories from alcohol, while neglecting good nutrition. Severe malnutrition may result from this pattern.

CHECKPOINT

1. What accounts for the rapid absorption of alcohol into the bloodstream?
2. Why is the alcohol in champagne absorbed faster than the alcohol in drinks with fruit juice?
3. What are empty calories?

BLOOD ALCOHOL LEVELS

The most objective legal measure of the degree of intoxication is the **blood alcohol level,** the percentage of alcohol circulating within the blood. A

blood alcohol level the percentage of alcohol circulating with one's blood.

Table 17.2
Calorie Content of Some Alcoholic Beverages

Beverage	Amount (oz.)	Calories
Beer	12	150
Light beer	12	70–134
Table wine	4	100
Fortified wine	2.5	100
80 proof liquor	1.25	88
100 proof liquor	1.25	100

blood alcohol level of 0.10 percent (meaning one part alcohol in a thousand parts blood) renders a person legally too drunk to drive in any state in the United States. Some states, such as California, Maine, Oregon, Utah, and Vermont, have lower blood alcohol limits—0.08 or 0.05 percent—for driving. It is expected that more states will follow this trend. Some states are also establishing a zero tolerance (blood alcohol limit of 0.00 percent) for drivers under age 21.

Blood alcohol levels are not a perfect way of measuring intoxication because alcohol is a tolerance-forming drug, and frequent, heavy drinkers are affected less at a given blood alcohol level than are light or occasional drinkers. Thus, in many states a person may be convicted of drunk driving with blood alcohol levels lower than 0.10 or 0.08 percent if the arresting officer testifies that the person's driving was affected by alcohol. For many people, driving becomes impaired at blood alcohol levels as low as 0.03 percent.

Because alcohol diffuses throughout the body, a major factor in determining your blood alcohol level when you drink is your body weight. A given amount of alcohol will produce about twice the blood alcohol level in a 100-pound person as it will in a 200-pound person. Table 17.3 gives the maximum number of drinks that people of different body weights can consume and keep blood alcohol levels below the various legal limits.

Another important factor affecting the blood alcohol level is the amount of time that passes after alcohol consumption. Alcohol is eliminated from the bodies of different people at different rates. Alcohol elimination occurs at the *average* rate of about one typical drink (such as a 12-ounce beer) per hour. A common "rule of thumb" is to allow at least one hour for each drink consumed before dri-

ving or operating any dangerous machinery. This may be misleading and possibly dangerous because "one drink" can contain a widely varying amount of alcohol and some people sober up more slowly than the average. You should always allow plenty of time before driving. The following section explains how alcohol leaves the body.

CHECKPOINT

1. What does 0.10 percent blood alcohol level mean?

2. What is the average length of time it takes for one drink to be eliminated from the body?

BREAKDOWN AND REMOVAL OF ALCOHOL FROM THE BODY

Some alcohol is broken down by an enzyme in the stomach and never enters the bloodstream. Males appear to have more of this enzyme than females, who thus absorb a greater percentage of the alcohol they consume. Of the alcohol that is absorbed, small amounts leave the body unchanged with the sweat, breath, and urine. This is the basis of breath and urine tests for alcohol. At most, however, only 5 percent of the alcohol absorbed leaves the body in this manner. The remainder must be metabolized (broken down within the body).

The first step in breaking down alcohol—its conversion to **acetaldehyde** (*as-e-tal'dah-hīd*)—can occur only in the liver. The second step—acetaldehyde to **acetic acid** (vinegar)—also occurs only in the liver. The final step—acetic acid to carbon dioxide and water—can occur throughout the body. To summarize these steps:

Alcohol → acetaldehyde → acetic acid → CO_2 + H_2O

One treatment to alleviate the urge to drink works by interfering with this pathway (see Feature 17.1).

acetaldehyde an intermediate product in the metabolism of alcohol.

acetic acid the acid in vinegar.

Table 17.3
What's Your Limit?

*A blood alcohol level of 0.08 percent makes you a **drunk driver** under the laws of some states, while 0.10 percent makes you a drunk driver in every state. Further, in many states, you may also be convicted of drunk driving at blood alcohol levels as low as 0.05 percent if the arresting officer testifies that your driving was impaired. How many drinks can you take and remain below these limits? Remember that for drivers under age 21, many states are now enforcing a zero tolerance (0.00 percent) for blood alcohol.*

	Maximum Drinks One Can Take and Remain Under a Blood Alcohol level of:		
Weight	0.05%	0.08%	0.10%
90–109 pounds	0	1	2
110–129 pounds	1	2	2
130–149 pounds	1	2	3
150–169 pounds	1	3	3
170–189 pounds	1	3	4
190–209 pounds	2	3	4
210–229 pounds	2	4	5
230 pounds and up	2	4	5

   1. "One drink" is a 12-ounce beer, or a 4-ounce glass of dry (12 percent alcohol) wine, or a 1¼-ounce shot of 80-proof liquor.
   2. This chart assumes that the drinks have been consumed over a period of one hour. For each drink beyond the above numbers, allow one additional hour of sobering up time before driving. For example, if you weigh 140 pounds and have had four drinks in a one-hour period, you must wait one hour after the last drink to go below 0.10 percent blood alcohol level and three hours after the last drink to get below the more desirable maximum 0.05 percent blood alcohol level.
   3. You can be unsafe with fewer drinks if they are larger drinks, if you drink on an empty stomach, or if you are tired, sick, upset, or have taken medications or other drugs.
   4. This table is valid for over 95 percent of people; less than 5 percent will exceed the legal limits when drinking the stated amounts on an empty stomach. Actual blood alcohol levels can vary by body type, gender, health status, and other factors.

Source: Information from the California Department of Motor Vehicles, California Highway Patrol, and other government agencies.

FEATURE 17.1

HOW ANTABUSE WORKS

Antabuse (disulfiram) is a drug sometimes taken by alcoholics to help them resist any urge to have a drink. Taken daily in pill form it works by blocking the conversion of acetaldehyde to acetic acid within the liver:

$$\text{alcohol} \rightarrow \text{acetaldehyde} \rightarrow \text{acetic acid} \rightarrow CO_2 + H_2O$$
$$\text{enzyme blocked}$$
$$\text{by Antabuse}$$

If the Antabuse taker should go ahead and drink even a small amount of alcohol, high levels of acetaldehyde accumulate in the blood, causing severe toxic illness. Effects may include headache, nausea, vomiting, fever, facial flushing, and a decrease in blood pressure. Drinking large amounts of alcohol can cause convulsions and even death.

   Obviously, Antabuse will only work for someone who is motivated to stay sober. Someone who really wants to drink will simply stop taking the pills.

The speed at which you will sober up is determined by enzyme levels in your liver (see Features 17.1 and 17.2). As we have mentioned, the average speed of breaking down alcohol is about one typical drink per hour, though the actual rate varies considerably from person to person. *Nothing can be done to speed this process.* Coffee or other stimulants don't do it. Exercise doesn't do it. No pill will do it. Only time will do it.

The livers of heavy drinkers convert alcohol somewhat faster than those of occasional drinkers, allowing heavy drinkers to drink more with less effect than occasional drinkers—up to a point. Once heavy drinking causes significant liver damage, sobering up occurs more slowly because of the liver's reduced capacity to convert alcohol.

After alcohol is eliminated from a person's body, an uncomfortable "hangover" commonly follows. Feature 17.2 explains the causes of hangovers.

CHECKPOINT

1. What percent of alcohol is eliminated through sweat, urine, and breath? Why are these routes of elimination important in determining blood alcohol levels?

2. What determines the speed of sobering up?

3. Why are heavy drinkers able to drink more and feel it less?

PHYSICAL EFFECTS OF ALCOHOL

Alcohol affects the functions of many parts of the human body. We will first examine its effects on the nervous system and then its effects on other parts of the body.

EFFECTS ON THE NERVOUS SYSTEM

Alcohol is a nervous system depressant that slows down and interferes with the normal activity of the brain. Not all parts of the brain are equally affected, however. Small amounts of alcohol depress the areas of the brain that control inhibitions. This results in a loss of inhibition, causing some people to think of alcohol as a stimulant. As alcohol levels increase, progressively more primitive portions of the brain (those that control basic body function) are depressed. At very high blood alcohol levels, the part of the brain that controls breathing is affected and death from respiratory failure may occur.

Alcohol appears to exert its effects on the brain in several ways. Both the structure and function of brain cell (neuron) membranes, along which nerve impulses travel, are affected by alcohol, causing the behavioral changes associated with intoxication. Alcohol also appears to affect the neurotransmitter substances that carry impulses from neuron to neuron.[5]

Alcohol is highly tolerance-forming. Frequent drinkers are much less impaired at a given blood alcohol level than are occasional drinkers. This tolerance is thought to result from adaptation within the membrane surrounding each neuron (brain cell). This is an adaptive mechanism apparently serving to counteract the toxic effect of alcohol. Frequent drinkers are also at risk of developing physiological dependency upon alcohol. Then, if drinking is discontinued or reduced, withdrawal symptoms may develop.

FEATURE 17.2

WHAT CAUSES HANGOVERS?

Typical hangover symptoms include headache, nausea or a "tender" stomach, generalized flulike aching, irritability, and trembling hands. Several factors contribute to this unpleasant condition. First, most alcoholic beverages contain fermentation by-products, called *congeners,* that give each type of drink its characteristic flavor. Congeners are one cause of hangovers. In general, the darker the beverage, the higher its congener level. But drinking even pure laboratory alcohol will still cause a hangover, because the first step in the liver's breaking down of alcohol is *acetaldehyde,* a toxic chemical that also causes hangovers. *Dehydration,* caused by alcohol's

diuretic effect, is another cause of hangovers. (Chronic alcohol abusers, however, tend to retain water.) Finally, the *irritating effect of alcohol* on the stomach lining and nervous system causes the nausea, irritability, and trembling hands.

The *best* hangover prevention is to drink moderately. Drinking a lot of water before going to bed will help prevent dehydration. Aspirin before bed may help prevent the morning headache, but it may add to stomach irritation.

The *worst* hangover remedy is to take another drink. The person who drinks to relieve the unpleasant effects of previous drinking is starting a "vicious cycle" that can lead to alcoholism.

What are the permanent effects of heavy drinking on the brain? Even after detoxification, some evidence of impaired brain function may remain, due to damage to cells of the cerebral cortex, the "thinking" part of the brain.[6] Autopsies of even relatively young alcoholics often show a dramatic wasting away of the brain, especially the cerebral cortex.

The peripheral nervous system (the nerves running throughout the body) also may show damage from alcohol (called **alcoholic neuropathy** [*nū-rop'ah-the*]). A common symptom is numbness, especially in the legs.

Alcohol Myth:

Alcohol is a stimulant.

Alcohol Reality:

Alcohol depresses the function of the nervous system; any feeling of stimulation is from loss of inhibition.

EFFECTS ON THE DIGESTIVE SYSTEM

No part of the body is immune to the damage caused by alcohol. In the *digestive system,* alcohol can erode the stomach lining, contributing to the development of stomach **ulcers.** Bleeding of the stomach lining often occurs. Heavy drinking also impairs the absorption of vitamins and minerals from your food. This is especially true of Vitamin B_1, the deficiency of which is quite common among alcoholics. Depending on the type of beverages consumed and dietary factors, alcohol use is associated with both diarrhea and constipation.

EFFECTS ON THE LIVER

The organ most often and most severely damaged by alcohol abuse is the liver. As the body's main "chemical factory," the liver processes about 95 percent of the alcohol absorbed into the blood, converting it into the toxic compound acetaldehyde. In the process, fatty compounds are deposited in the liver, causing a condition called *fatty liver,* which is very common in alcoholics. Fatty liver by itself is reversible if alcohol intake stops, but with continued drinking it progresses to **alcoholic hepatitis** and on to cirrhosis.

Cirrhosis is characterized by the replacement of functional liver cells by nonfunctional scarlike tissue. About one in every ten long-term heavy drinkers will eventually develop cirrhosis. Fifty to 80 percent of those who develop alcoholic hepatitis will progress to cirrhosis if they continue to drink.[7] The cirrhotic liver is unable to perform the liver's many duties properly. Among the many problems caused by cirrhosis are:

- inability of the liver to remove toxic substances from the blood
- buildup of blood pressure in portal veins going from intestines to liver, with the possibility of hemorrhaging
- large amounts of fluid accumulation in the abdominal cavity
- inability of the liver to store sugar and maintain a stable blood sugar level
- 30 percent risk of liver cancer

Among people who continue to drink after developing cirrhosis, more than half are dead within five years.[8]

Loss of liver function in long-term heavy drinkers eventually results in loss of tolerance to alcohol. Now that the liver has lost much of its ability to process chemicals, alcohol is broken down more slowly. People at this stage get drunk on less alcohol than before and sober up more slowly.

EFFECTS ON MUSCLES AND SKIN

Chronic alcohol abuse often results in weakness and wasting of the muscles. Alcohol may damage the muscles directly, or damage the peripheral nerves that control the muscles. Poor nutrition is another potential factor in muscle loss in alcohol abusers.

---

alcoholic neuropathy any disease of the nerves that is associated with heavy drinking.

ulcer an open lesion (sore).

alcoholic hepatitis inflammation of the liver produced by alcohol.

cirrhosis the replacement of functional liver cells by nonfunctional scarlike tissue

Skin disorders are visible in 30–50 percent of alcohol abusers. These disorders result from poor nutrition, the direct effects of alcohol, and impaired liver function. Alcohol dilates blood vessels in the skin, causing a flushed appearance of the face and nose. Among heavy drinkers, chronically dilated blood vessels are often visible on the nose and chest. The lower part of the nose may become bulbous (enlarged) and red.

Alcohol Myth:

Alcohol use does not hurt your appearance; just look at all of the good-looking people in the alcohol ads.

Alcohol Reality:

Alcohol use causes dehydration and premature aging of the skin, hair, and nails. It dilates blood vessels in the skin, causing permanent reddening and enlarged veins. It aggravates acne and other skin problems. It causes a bulbous nose.

SEXUAL EFFECTS OF ALCOHOL

Chronic alcohol abuse affects the *reproductive system* in both genders. Women may skip menstrual periods or fail to ovulate. In men heavy drinking may have feminizing effects. (This is ironic in view of the "macho" image associated by some with heavy drinking.) First, the testes shrink and produce less of the male hormone testosterone. At the same time, the liver's ability to break down female hormones is reduced by alcohol. (The adrenal glands of all males produce some female hormones.) The result is a definitive feminization: Breasts enlarge, body hair thins or is lost, and sexual drive and erectile ability decrease. Many men who drink heavily become partially or totally impotent.

How did alcohol gain its reputation as an aphrodisiac (sexual stimulant)? The majority of occasional, moderate drinkers do, in fact, report that alcohol increases both their sexual interest and sexual pleasure (based on surveys of thousands of the authors' students). These effects result from alcohol's disinhibiting effects, rather than direct sexual stimulation. Heavy drinking, either chronic or occasional, is sexually disastrous. Males may become impotent and females unable to reach orgasm.

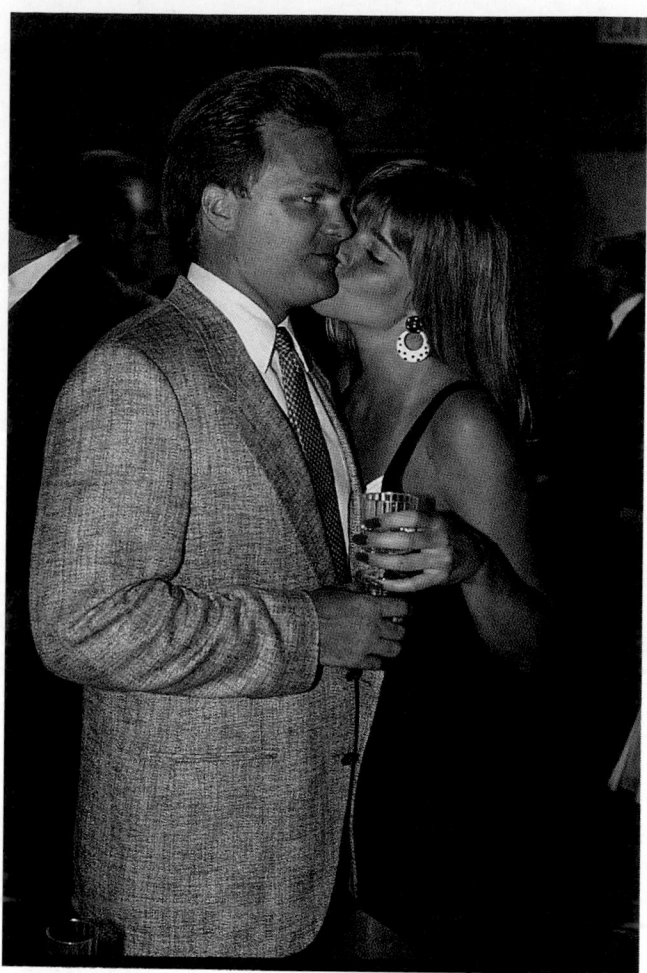

Alcohol is commonly viewed as a sexual stimulant because, for many people, it decreases inhibitions. Heavy drinking, whether chronic or occasional, actually impairs sexual responses.

Alcohol Myth:

Alcohol enhances sexuality.

Alcohol Reality:

For men, heavy drinking causes a drop in male hormone levels, which reduces sex drive and can cause impotence. Women who are heavy drinkers experience increased rates of gynecological problems, such as infertility and menstrual disorders.

EFFECTS ON CIRCULATORY SYSTEM

Heavy drinking affects the circulatory system by causing direct damage to the heart muscle, which

FEATURE 17.3

DRINK FOR YOUR HEALTH?

Numerous studies in recent years have concluded that moderate (one or two drinks a day) drinking reduces your risk of heart attack by 20–40 percent. This is a significant decrease, comparable to what you might achieve by exercising regularly or by maintaining a strict low-fat diet. Alcohol apparently produces its protective effect in two ways: It raises blood levels of high-density lipoproteins (HDL, the "good" cholesterol) while reducing the tendency for blood clots to form in arteries. Can alcohol actually be good for your health?

To answer this question we must weigh risks against benefits. The benefit is that moderate drinkers suffer fewer heart attacks and, as a result, enjoy a slightly longer lifespan. Among the risks associated with *moderate* drinking are:

- chance of moving from moderate to heavy or problem drinking
- increased risk of breast cancer in women (25–30 percent increase by drinking just one or two drinks a day)
- birth defects caused by drinking during pregnancy
- impaired driving ability

Of these risks, the most significant is the chance of moving beyond moderate drinking. At even three drinks a day for men or two for women, the risks associated with drinking exceed the benefits. Among the risks from heavier drinking are:

- cirrhosis of the liver
- heart damage

- cancers in many parts of the body
- osteoporosis in women
- damage to the nervous system

This is, of course, only a partial listing.

Some people should not drink at all. For them, the risks of drinking far outweigh the benefits. If they currently drink, they should stop. If they don't currently drink, they should not start. Among these people are:

- those who have ever had a chemical dependency problem
- those who have a family history of alcoholism (the tendency, you will remember from Chapter 15, is inherited)
- those who tend to have emotional health problems such as depression or anxiety
- those who have any existing health problem and have not obtained the specific approval of their physician for moderate drinking
- those who take any medication with which alcohol may react

Bottom line: Those who enjoy moderate drinking, have no trouble keeping their drinking moderate, and who do not fit in any of the mentioned categories can continue their moderate drinking with little overall risk to their health. Others are advised to abstain from alcohol completely.

---

results in reduced pumping of blood, enlargement of the heart, and shortness of breath with the least exertion. Heavy drinkers are also susceptible to irregular heartbeat and strokes.

Moderate drinking, in contrast, has actually been shown to reduce the risk of heart attack. This benefit, however, must be weighed against alcohol's many harmful effects (see Feature 17.3).

Alcohol causes the peripheral blood vessels to dilate, bringing more blood into the skin and making people feel warmer. For centuries, people have consumed alcohol in cold weather for this reason. Actually, alcohol sharply increases the risk of fatal **hypothermia,** because, by bringing more blood into the skin, an increased amount of body heat is

lost to the air, even though it makes people feel warmer.

EFFECTS ON IMMUNITY, CANCER PRODUCTION, AND KIDNEYS

Heavy drinking has long been known to increase susceptibility to diseases and is listed as a specific risk factor for many. In the past it was assumed that this was a result of malnutrition and other unhealthful living habits. Now alcohol is recognized as having many direct effects on the immune mechanism. Both the humoral and cell mediated components are impaired.[9]

Alcohol use has been associated with an increased incidence of many cancers, including cancers of the liver, breast, skin, and thyroid gland.

Alcohol's *diuretic* (stimulation of urine production) effect on the kidneys is legendary. Alcohol

---

hypothermia a body temperature below normal.

Alcohol makes one feel warmer in cold weather because it dilates the peripheral blood vessels. Unfortunately, this increases heat loss from the body and increases the risk of fatal hypothermia.

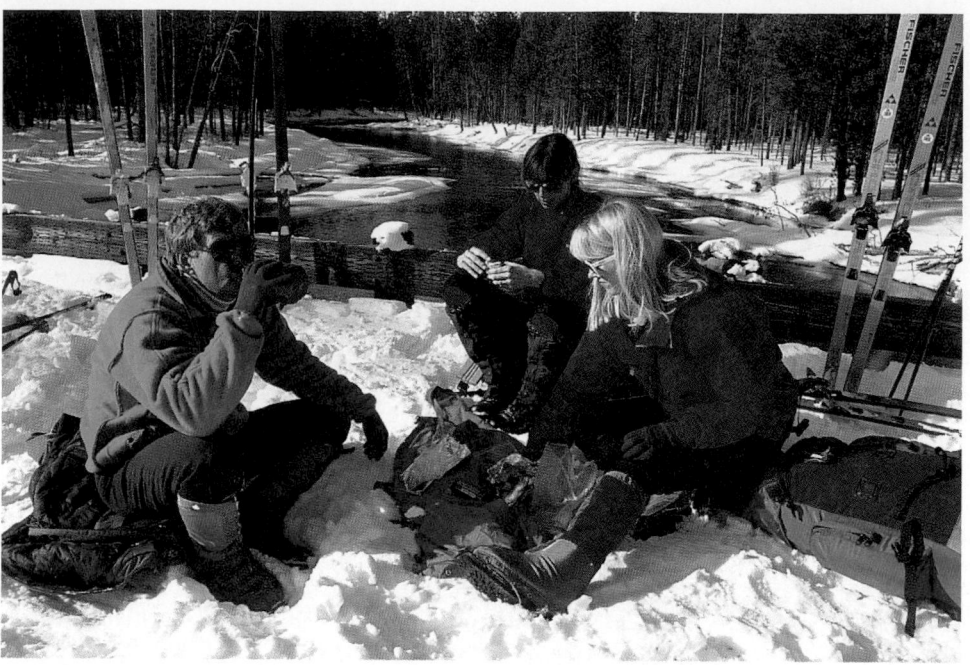

apparently inhibits the pituitary gland's release of **antidiuretic** hormone. This inhibition only occurs while blood alcohol levels are rising—not when they are stationary or falling. In chronic heavy drinkers, alcohol itself has an antidiuretic effect, causing problems of water retention—swollen ankles and general bloating.

CHECKPOINT

1. Why does alcohol sometimes seem like a stimulant when it is really a depressant?

2. What is alcoholic neuropathy?

3. What vitamin appears to be most deficient in heavy drinkers?

4. Which organ is most often and most severely damaged by alcohol?

5. Describe the stages of alcohol-associated liver damage.

6. What are the sexual effects of alcohol?

7. Why do people feel warmer after drinking alcohol?

8. Which cancers are associated with drinking alcohol?

antidiuretic lessening urine secretion.

PHYSICAL DEPENDENCY AND WITHDRAWAL

Not every alcohol abuser becomes physically dependent (addicted), but for those who do, daily drinking becomes a must in order to prevent unpleasant withdrawal symptoms. With very heavy drinking—about a quart of distilled liquor a day—physical dependence can develop in as little as one week.[10]

The withdrawal symptoms for any drug are usually the reverse of the effects of the drug itself. Since alcohol is a depressant, its withdrawal is characterized by overactivity of the nervous system. Four different alcohol withdrawal syndromes have been described, though often these syndromes occur in various combinations.[11] They are as follows.

1. **Hyperarousal.** This, the most common sign of alcohol withdrawal, can include shaking, anxiety, agitation, rapid pulse, irritability, loss of appetite, and insomnia. Usually these symptoms diminish after two or three days, but some may persist for 2 or 3 weeks or longer. Avoiding this

hyperarousal a sign of alcohol withdrawal characterized by symptoms including shaking, anxiety, and insomnia.

condition is what drives many alcoholic people to have a morning drink and further drinks during the day and evening.

2. **Alcoholic hallucinosis.** This condition occurs in about 25 percent of those withdrawing from alcohol.[12] It includes true hallucinations, both auditory and visual, as well as nightmares, illusions, and misperceptions of real stimuli. Alcoholic hallucinosis usually ends within a week, but in a few cases may last for weeks or months.

3. **Convulsive seizures** ("rum fits"). Seizures that occur during alcohol withdrawal are usually of the generalized tonic-clonic, formerly called grand mal (see p. 685), type. There is loss of consciousness and powerful muscle contractions. Although very frightening to see, these seizures are usually not dangerous and usually only one or two occur during the withdrawal period. They can occur anywhere from 12 hours to one week after the last drink.

4. **Delirium tremens (DTs)** (*dē-lir'i-um trē'menz*) is the most serious form of alcohol withdrawal. With intensive medical treatment, there is a 1–2 percent death rate. Without treatment, the death rate can reach 20 percent. The word *delirium* refers to hallucinations, confusion, and disorientation. *Tremens* refers to shaking, agitation, rapid pulse, high blood pressure, and fever. Many alcohol-dependent people require access to medical help during their detoxification ("drying out") period. This period can range from a day or two up to a week.

C H E C K P O I N T

1. What are four different types of alcohol withdrawal syndromes and the symptoms of each? ✓

....

alcoholic hallucinosis a form of alcohol withdrawal including hallucinations, nightmares, illusions, and misperceptions of reality.

convulsive seizures repeated involuntary contraction of all of the body's muscles.

delirium tremens a disorder including trembling and hallucinations; usually occurs during alcohol withdrawal.

FETAL ALCOHOL SYNDROME (FAS)

Fetal alcohol syndrome (FAS) is a group of birth defects that occur in infants born to mothers who drink during their pregnancy. At birth FAS infants are smaller than average, both in weight and length. The head is smaller than normal. Facial characteristics include small eyes, fat cheeks, a short nose with a low bridge, thin red portion of the upper lip, indistinct groove in the center of the upper lip, and other unusual features. At birth the infants are "jittery" (hyperreactive to sounds and other stimuli) and shaky. Almost half of these infants have heart problems and/or mental retardation. FAS is the third leading cause of mental retardation.[13]

Fetal Alcohol Syndrome. At birth, infants with FAS tend to have a small head, small eyes, fat cheeks, a short nose with a low bridge, a thin red portion on the upper lip, and an indistinct groove in the center of the upper lip. Brain damage is evidenced by poor coordination and/or mental retardation. Even moderate drinking by a pregnant woman can damage a fetus.

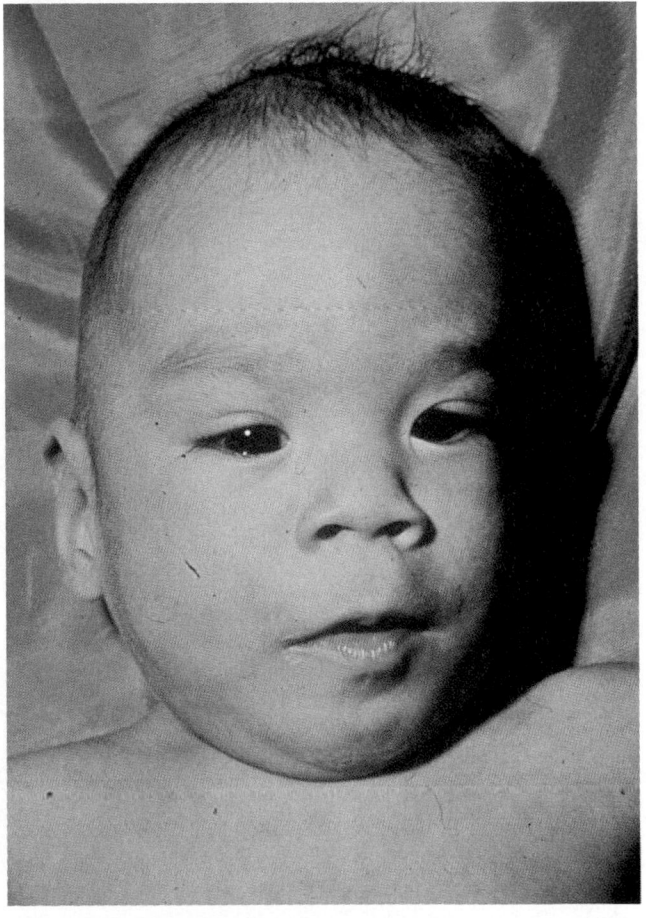

A mother does not have to be a chronic alcohol abuser to expose her fetus to the risks of alcohol during pregnancy. There are documented reports of fetal damage caused by social levels of drinking.[14, 15] As is true with most drugs, the damaging effects of alcohol are greatest during the first three months of pregnancy. During the first weeks the mother may not even be aware that she is pregnant. Since no birth control method is 100 percent effective, some people question the wisdom of any drinking by a sexually active woman of reproductive age.

How much alcohol is it safe to drink during pregnancy? The risk to an embryo or fetus is in proportion to the quantity of alcohol consumed, but some risk exists at any level of alcohol consumption. To quote the National Institute on Alcohol Abuse and Alcoholism: "The data so far do not suggest a threshold level of drinking below which there is no effect on the unborn child. . . . Pending the clarification of susceptibility factors, all women are advised to avoid drinking during pregnancy."[16]

CHECKPOINT

1. Define FAS.

2. How much drinking during pregnancy is considered safe?

ALCOHOL AND DRIVING

One encouraging alcohol-related statistic is the percent of motor vehicle fatalities involving alcohol. Since 1980, when half of all traffic deaths involved alcohol, the percentage has dropped to about 38 percent.[17] This decline is attributed to stricter enforcement of "drunk driving" laws, lowering of the maximum legal blood alcohol level in many states, and raising of the drinking age in many states.

Still, drinking and driving remains a major cause of preventable deaths in the United States. The incident rate starts to climb with the first drink. By the time a blood alcohol level of 0.10 is reached, the chances for a fatal crash are eight times higher than for a nondrinking driver. At low blood alcohol levels, the chief effects on driving are a reduced level of judgment, increased risk-taking, and reduced peripheral (side) vision. As blood alcohol levels rise, care and judgment continue to decline, vision and coordination are progressively impaired, and the crash rate skyrockets. Drinking drivers seldom realize how much their driving ability has deteriorated, because the effects of alcohol on the brain that cause them to be dangerous drivers also make them unaware of how poor their driving has become. People who drink must plan

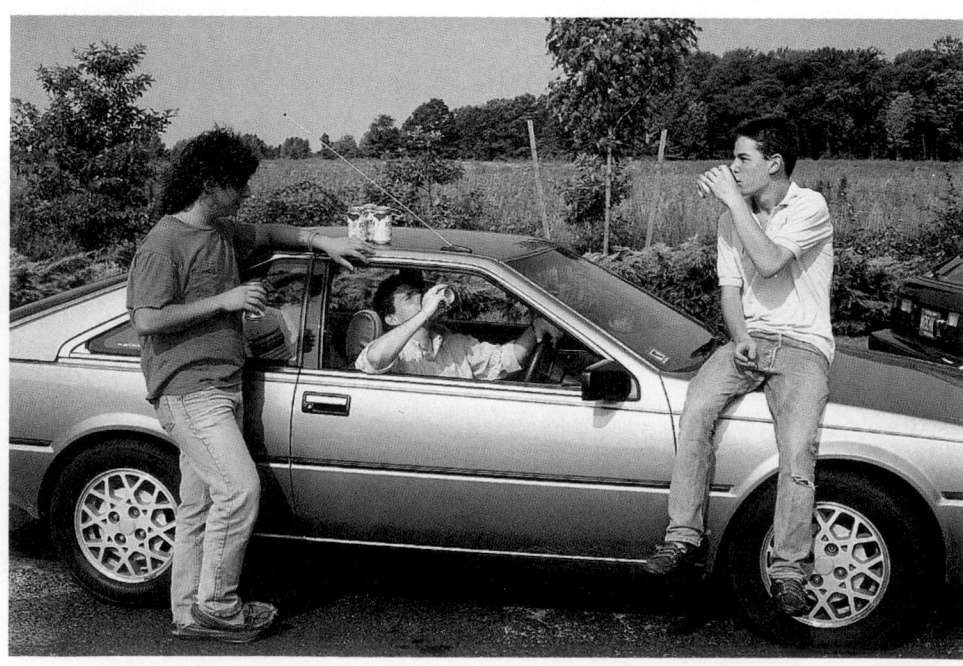

Careful! Driving begins to be impaired with the first drink. Even below the legal blood alcohol limit, reflexes, vision, and judgment are affected.

FEATURE 17.4

BE A RESPONSIBLE HOST

How would you feel if a friend were killed while driving home after drinking too much at a party you hosted? Chances are, you would feel terrible and wonder whether anything you could have done might have prevented such a tragedy. In some states you might even be held liable for incidents resulting from drinks served in your home.

In some cases, nothing you could have done would have mattered. Some people will drive drunk despite your best efforts. But for the majority of people, being a responsible host will make a difference. Responsible hosts do the following:

1. Never serve drinks without food available to slow the absorption of alcohol.

2. Always have alternative, nonalcoholic beverages easily available and as attractively presented as the alcoholic drinks.

3. Have a responsible person tend bar to measure the alcohol content of drinks and to discourage excessive drinking.

4. Never pressure anyone to drink alcohol or to drink more than he or she wishes.

5. Always have plenty of planned activities at your party. Keep people busy with games, dancing, or other activities rather than just drinking.

6. Decide in advance when you want the party to end and close the bar to allow some nondrinking time before guests leave.

7. Do everything you can to discourage anyone who has had too much to drink from driving. Offer them a ride, call a cab, or urge them to stay over. Remember that most people do not realize how drunk they are. You may have to be very insistent.

ahead. While still sober, they should arrange for a means of transportation home other than driving a car (see Feature 17.4).

Who are the alcohol-impaired drivers? To answer this question and to find a solution to deter such drivers, the U.S. Department of Justice has studied those arrested for drunk driving. First of all, 95 percent of arrested drunk drivers are male. There are many reasons for this. More males drink heavily. And males are much more likely than females to insist on driving when they have been drinking because they want to preserve their "macho" images. Being able to "hold your liquor" is viewed as masculine, as is being in control, which, in this case, means driving.

The median age of drunk drivers is 32. From 1983 through 1987, 26 states raised their alcohol purchase age from 18 or 19 to 21. During this span, the number of drunk-driving arrests among 18- to 21-year-olds dropped by 24 percent, more than twice the decline seen in any other age group during that period. This provided a powerful argument in favor of raising the drinking age to 21 years. In 1988, Wyoming became the last of the 50 states to raise its drinking age to 21.[18]

Arrested drunk drivers are mostly people who drink very heavily. Half of those arrested had consumed the equivalent of at least 12 bottles of beer before their arrests and over a quarter had consumed the equivalent of at least 20 beers before

driving, based on their blood alcohol levels. Almost half were repeat offenders, and about half had previously been in alcohol-abuse treatment programs.[19]

None of this means that social or occasional drinkers can safely drive after drinking. Even a single occasion of alcohol-impaired driving by the most infrequent drinker can result in a serious crash. *No one,* whether a frequent or occasional drinker, can safely drive after drinking large amounts of alcohol.

One of the most successful ways of avoiding drunk driving is the consistent use of a **designated driver**—someone who, before any drinking begins, agrees to abstain from drinking alcohol and to drive the other members of the party home safely. One of the reasons this program works so well is that it enhances the status of the abstainer. It also makes it much easier to abstain when you can say, "No, thank you, I'm the designated driver tonight." If you and your friends are not already using designated drivers, we urge you to do so. You will be pleased with the results.

designated driver the person who agrees to abstain from drinking and to drive the other members of the party home.

Alcohol Myth:

"I drive better after a couple of drinks."

Alcohol Reality:

Driving performance begins to decline with the first drink. People often think they drive better after drinking because the same brain effects that impair driving also impair your perception of driving ability.

LEGAL REGULATION OF ALCOHOL-IMPAIRED DRIVING

What can be done to decrease the number of drinking drivers on our roads? As we have seen, the typical alcohol-impaired driver is a repeat offender and has not responded to previous attempts to change this behavior. Many persist in driving even after their licenses have been suspended or revoked.

Because of pressure from citizen groups such as Mothers Against Drunk Driving (MADD) and Students Against Drunk Driving (SADD), drunk driving has captured the public's attention. Millions of people have demanded stricter penalties for alcohol-impaired driving and their lobbying has, for the most part, been successful.

Most alcohol authorities appear to favor stricter law enforcement, stiffer penalties, and better education programs. Drunk-driving laws are believed to be effective deterrents only if they result in certain, severe, and swift punishment. Unfortunately, this is often not the case. Drunk drivers in many areas of the country correctly perceive that their chance of arrest is small and that their chance of going to jail for drunk driving is smaller still. Any program that increases the rate of drunk-driving arrests must be supported by a judicial system that can handle the increased burden of cases and an availability of jail space for those convicted.

How effective are laws in reducing alcohol abuse? Many legal approaches to alcohol regulation have been tried, ranging from limiting hours of sale and setting a minimum drinking age up to total prohibition of all sale and possession of alcoholic beverages. While no approach has been totally successful in eliminating alcohol abuse in the United States, laws have been shown to have at least some impact on the problem.

The most extreme example of regulation occurred in the United States from 1920 to 1933.

During this period, called **Prohibition,** all alcohol sales were outlawed. Even though anyone who really wanted alcohol was probably able to find a **bootlegger** (a person who manufactures or sells alcohol illegally) eager to sell it, evidence indicates that there was some decline in alcohol consumption, though no one knows how much alcohol was sold illegally. There was no apparent decline in drinking by problem drinkers and alcoholics. The prohibition of alcohol fostered the same type of illegal activity characteristic of street drugs today. Prohibition was a boon to organized crime while creating enforcement problems for law agencies and legal problems for drinkers.

Alcohol use continues to be a political and social issue. Most Americans want alcohol to remain legal, yet pressure is mounting for people to use it more responsibly. However, effective methods for ensuring responsible use have yet to be established.

CHECKPOINT

1. At alcohol blood levels below 0.10, what are the impairments experienced by drinking drivers?

2. What is the profile of the typical drunk driver?

3. In your opinion, what could be done to decrease alcohol-impaired driving?

PATTERNS OF ALCOHOL USE

Kinney and Leaton[20] have compiled some demographic associations with drinking. Among the influences on alcohol consumption are gender, age, ethnicity, and income level.

- *Gender* Women are less likely to drink than are men. Women who do drink consume less than men who drink. This has been changing, however. Recent studies indicate that among women below age 30, drinking patterns are approaching those of men.[21]

- *Age* Older people are less likely to drink than are younger people.

Prohibition a period in the United States from 1920 to 1933 during which all alcohol sales were outlawed.

bootlegger a person who manufactures or sells alcohol illegally.

FEATURE 17.5

AM I AN ALCOHOLIC?

There are many alcoholism screening questionnaires being used today, ranging from as few as 4 questions to as many as 25. No questionnaire is perfect; the same person might be classified as alcoholic on the basis of some tests, but not by others. This is because there is no clear line between alcoholism and nonalcoholism. One test that is used frequently consists of only four questions:

1. Have you ever felt you should cut down on your drinking?

2. Have people annoyed you by criticizing your drinking?

3. Have you ever felt bad or guilty about your drinking?

4. Have you ever had a drink first thing in the morning to steady your nerves or to get rid of a hangover?

Two or three yes answers indicates a high probability of alcoholism. Four yes answers definitely indicates alcoholism. Refer also to the alcohol-use assessment earlier in this chapter.

Source: Ewing, J. "Detecting Alcoholism, the CAGE Questionnaire." *JAMA* 252, No. 14 1984, pp. 1905–1907.

- *Ethnicity* Non-Hispanic whites are more likely to drink than are African Americans or Hispanics.

- *Education* The percentage of people who use alcohol increases with education level, although the rate of heavy drinking is not associated with education level.

- *Income* The proportion of drinkers increases with increasing income.

No two people are exactly alike in their drinking patterns. Alcohol use falls along a continuum ranging from strict abstinence to daily heavy drinking. Classifying people as light, moderate, or heavy drinkers is a matter of subjective judgment—even experts don't agree on where to draw the lines between different levels of drinking. Further, how much or how often you drink is less important than the effects of your drinking (Feature 17.5). The following section will examine problem drinking and alcoholism.

CHECKPOINT

1. What is the relationship to alcohol consumption of:

    gender?

    age?

    ethnicity?

    education?

    income?

2. How accurately can people be classified as light, moderate, or heavy drinkers?

ALCOHOL ABUSE

What is alcoholism? How does it differ from problem drinking? Is it a disease? How common is alcoholism? What causes alcoholism? How can I know if I'm an alcoholic or a problem drinker? Is alcoholism curable? How can I help my friend who is an alcoholic? The questions seem simple enough, but the answers can be complex. The following sections consider these and some other questions about alcohol use.

DEFINING PROBLEM DRINKING AND ALCOHOLISM

Many definitions of problem drinking and alcoholism have been proposed over the years, but none has gained universal acceptance. This may be because different experts tend to view alcohol problems from different perspectives—mental health, physical health, social health, and so on. Some alcohol experts make no distinction between problem drinking and alcoholism; others see them as quite different. Some do not even use the terms problem drinking or alcoholism, preferring to use phrases such as alcohol abuse and alcohol dependence.

Those who distinguish between problem drinking and alcoholism usually define **problem drinking** as drinking that causes problems in any area of a person's life or causes problems for other people. This would include problems with a per-

....

problem drinking drinking that causes problems in any area of a person's life or problems for other people.

son's health, job, school, or home life; drunk driving; legal, financial, or social problems; or any other kind of problems. There are several key elements in this definition.

This definition of problem drinking does *not* mention how much or how often you drink. Problem drinking is defined in terms of the results of the drinking, not the quantity. Thus, it is possible that of two people who drink the same amount with the same frequency, one may be a problem drinker and one may not.

Alcoholism can be defined as a disease characterized by strong psychological and, in severe cases, physiological dependency on alcohol and the inability to drink in moderation (loss of control). This definition embraces the disease concept of alcoholism. Most experts view alcoholism not as a sin, moral weakness, or lack of willpower, but as a chronic, progressive disease. As a chronic disease, alcoholism develops slowly. For this reason, it is impossible to pinpoint an exact time at which a nonalcoholic person becomes alcoholic.

Viewing alcoholism as a disease does *not* relieve the alcoholic of responsibility for continued drinking behavior. Just as a person with diabetes must assume responsibility for eating correctly and possibly using insulin or another medication, so must a person who is an alcoholic assume the responsibility for achieving and maintaining sobriety.

INCIDENCE OF ALCOHOL ABUSE

Figures on the incidence of alcohol abuse are inexact. For one thing, the variety of definitions of alcohol abuse results in varying estimates of its incidence. Further, many alcohol abusers deny their abuse, do not enter rehabilitation programs, and are never officially recognized as abusers of alcohol.

The National Institute on Alcohol Abuse and Alcoholism (NIAAA) estimates that 18 million Americans 18 years old and older "experience problems as a result of alcohol abuse." NIAAA estimates that 10 percent of all adults who use alcohol

are alcoholics. In addition, many persons below age 18, some as young as 8 or 9 years old, have severe alcohol-abuse problems.[22]

A higher percentage of men than women are alcohol abusers: 14–16 percent of men who drink have alcohol-abuse problems compared to about 6 percent of women who drink. Whether this difference can be attributed to basic biological dissimilarities or to psychological and cultural factors is unknown.

Let's now focus our attention on the disease of alcoholism.

BLACKOUTS

A **blackout,** not to be confused with losing consciousness or passing out, is a period when a person is conscious and drinking, but later will have no memory of that period. During the blackout, the drinker may seem fine to others, who later may be surprised when the drinker does not remember where he or she has been or what he or she has done. The "missing" period of time can range from several hours to several days.

Blackouts are often characteristic of alcoholism. Most alcoholics experience blackouts; most nonalcoholics do not. There are exceptions: Kinney and Leaton report that up to a third of alcoholics state that they have never had a blackout and that some nonalcoholics do have blackouts when they drink very heavily.[23]

The mechanism of blackouts is not fully understood, but it appears that during blackouts, alcohol interferes selectively with the memory functions of the brain to a greater degree than with other functions. Blackouts may be caused by alcohol's interference with the chemical events of long-term memory.

ALCOHOLIC LOSS OF CONTROL

Loss of control, perhaps the most characteristic feature of the disease of alcoholism, is the inability

---

alcoholism a disease characterized by strong psychological and, in severe cases, physiological dependency on alcohol and the inability to drink in moderation (loss of control).

blackout period during which a person is drinking, but later will have no memory of that period.

loss of control the inability to drink in moderation.

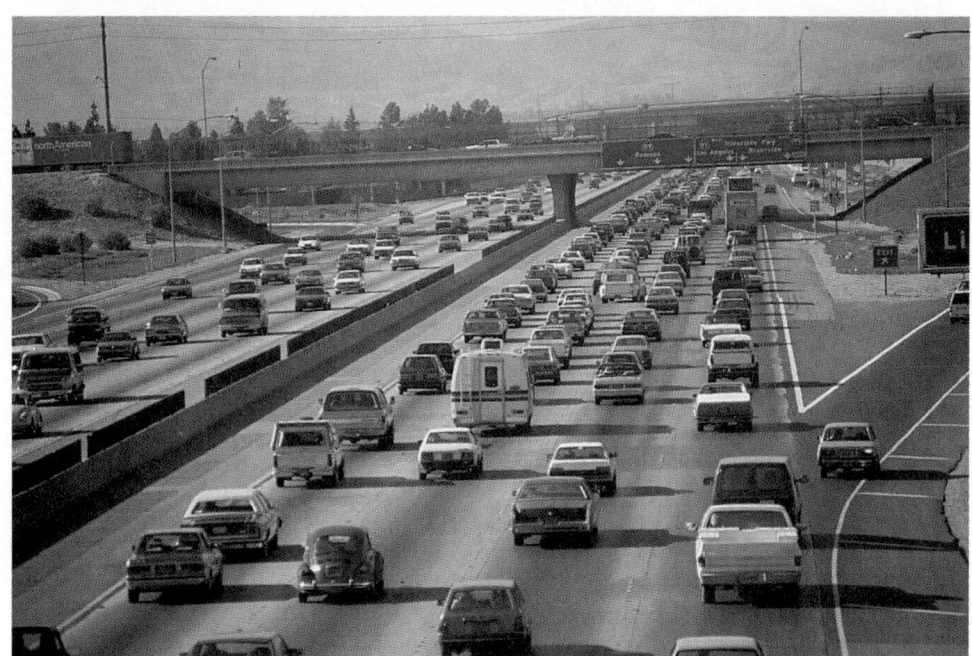

About two-thirds of alcoholics experience blackouts when they drink. People in blackouts still function, but have no memory of what they did during the blackout. Many alcoholics have had the experience of finding themselves in a new location and having no idea of how they got there.

to drink in moderation. Unless an alcoholic has reached the point of physiological dependency, which would require daily drinking to prevent withdrawal symptoms, he or she still has the option of drinking or not drinking on any particular day. What is impossible is drinking in a controlled manner. Once an alcoholic takes the first drink, he or she is likely to drink to excess.

Many alcoholics, called binge drinkers, may go for several months without drinking any alcohol. Once the first drink is consumed, however, it is impossible for them to drink only a moderate amount. This is the problem that many alcoholics fight year after year. Only when an alcoholic accepts this inability to drink in moderation can the road to recovery begin.

One of the controversies in alcohol recovery programs has been about the advisability of alcoholics attempting to return to controlled drinking. This goal has been promoted by a few therapists and programs. The great majority of alcohol experts, however, believe that the potential for an alcoholic to return successfully to controlled drinking is so slim that it is foolish to attempt to do so. Total abstinence from alcohol is seen as the only reasonable goal for an alcoholic.

Even after an alcoholic has remained sober for many years, it remains dangerous to attempt controlled drinking. The opinion of most experts is:

Once an alcoholic, always an alcoholic. Thus, it is possible to be a sober alcoholic, but not a former alcoholic.

CAUSES OF ALCOHOLISM

Some people use alcohol for most of their lives without developing any alcohol-related problems. Others become alcoholics. Why? The causes of alcoholism are complex and include many factors. This public health or **epidemiological** (relating to disease frequency and distribution) model of alcoholism integrates these factors, and in viewing alcoholism as a disease, includes the disease agent (alcohol), the host (the drinker), and the environment (social and cultural factors).

The Disease Agent (Alcohol)

Several characteristics of alcohol as a drug increase the likelihood of its abuse. The rewards in alcohol use are immediate; the negative effects or penalties occur later. Alcohol can make you feel better immediately, especially while your blood alcohol level is rising. Alcohol produces relaxation and a

....

epidemiological relating to disease frequency and distribution.

more carefree feeling. Tensions are relieved. Inhibitions are forgotten. These positive effects provide reinforcement of drinking behavior. On the other hand, a declining blood alcohol level produces unpleasant feelings of nervousness, agitation, fatigue, and irritability. Now the drinker feels worse than before he or she started drinking. To find relief, many people take another drink.

The Host (The Drinker)

What individual factors in people, as disease hosts, promote alcoholism? In recent years, a considerable shift in opinion on the personal causes of alcoholism has occurred. In the past, psychological factors were seen as most important; currently, genetic factors are more strongly emphasized.

Many early reports on alcoholism described an "alcoholic personality" that predisposed people to alcoholism. The problem was that the research leading to this conclusion involved people who were already alcoholics. The personality being described was the *result* of alcoholism, rather than the cause. In prospective studies, such as those of Vaillant, in which the personalities of many people are evaluated at a young age and the people followed for a period of years, *no prealcoholic personality has been identified.*[24] No personality factors have been identified that will predict whether or not alcoholism will develop.

Genetic factors have been shown to play a major role in the development of alcoholism in people of both genders. One approach to research on the influence of genes on alcoholism has been studying the rate of alcohol problems in pairs of identical twins versus pairs of fraternal twins. Most studies have shown that when one twin has a problem with alcohol, the second twin is much more likely to also have such a problem if the twins are identical rather than fraternal. Research at Virginia Commonwealth University has even quantified the effect of genes as making a 50–60 percent contribution to the development of alcohol problems in women.[25] Other research has led to similar conclusions for males.

No research has indicated that genes are the only factor dictating whether or not a person will become an alcoholic. People whose family members tend to have alcohol problems are not doomed to being alcoholics, but should be aware that they are at an increased risk of alcoholism and should handle alcohol with care. If they do choose to drink, they need to be alert to the early signs of a developing alcohol problem and to understand that if such signs appear, their best course of action is to abstain from alcohol.

> ### Alcohol Myth:
> Alcoholism is entirely the result of psychological causes; certain personality types lead to alcoholism.
>
> ### Alcohol Reality:
> Many experts now believe that the so-called "alcoholic personality" is the result, rather than the cause, of alcoholism.

The Environment (Multicultural Perspectives)

Your risk of alcoholism is influenced by your social and cultural affiliations. Alcohol abuse rates vary considerably from society to society and culture to culture. Customs, attitudes, religious influences, and laws within each society and culture influence how its members deal with alcohol.

Following are some examples of cultural and societal views toward alcohol use and how each affects the incidence of alcohol abuse:

- *The expectation of abstinence,* characteristic of Mormons, Muslims, Mennonites, Seventh Day Adventists, and others, is associated with the lowest incidence of alcohol abuse in a population.

- *Ritual use,* primarily in religious ceremonies and on special occasions, with drinking on other occasions frowned upon, is also associated with a low incidence of alcohol abuse.

- *Convivial use,* on social occasions, with the emphasis on companionship and camaraderie, results in a somewhat higher incidence of alcohol abuse.

- *Utilitarian use,* characteristic of the majority of U.S. society, allows people to drink for any reason—to celebrate, to lose inhibitions, to relax, or to forget—and is associated with the highest incidence of problem drinking and alcoholism.

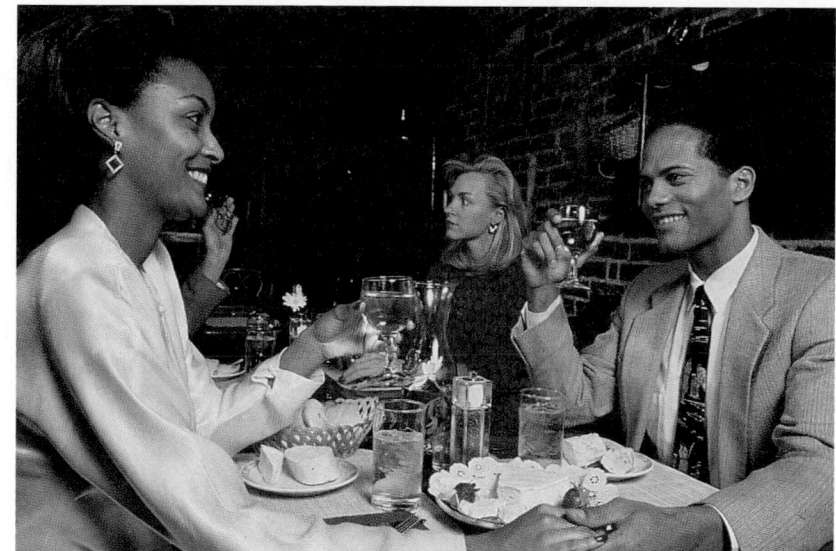
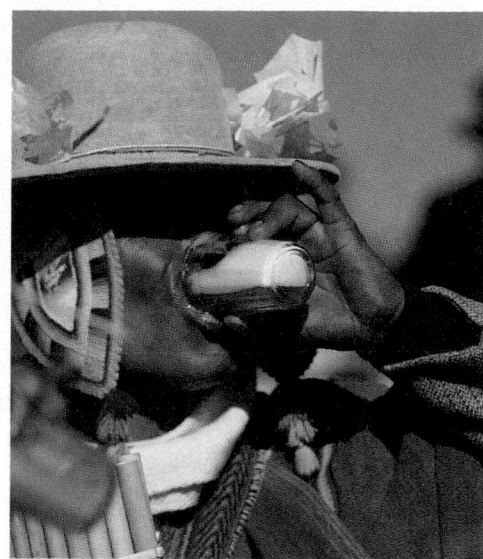
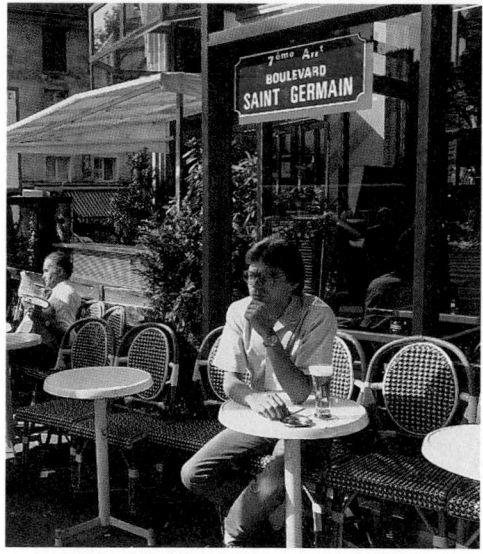
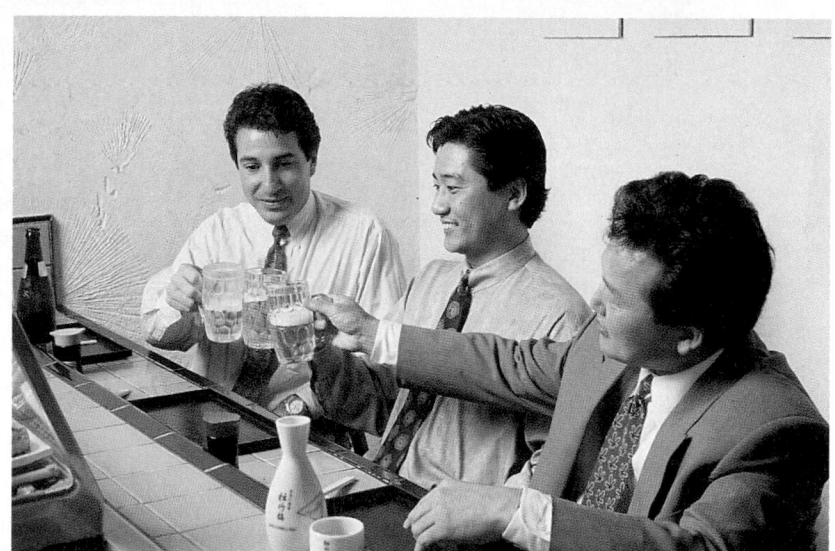

Alcohol abuse rates vary considerably from society to society. Customs, religious influences, and laws greatly influence how people deal with alcohol.

Lower rates of alcoholism are found in cultures characterized by the following:[26]

- Children observe their parents drinking in moderation, primarily with meals.
- There is strong disapproval of intoxication.
- There are clear cultural guidelines on when, where, and how much to drink.
- Drinking is not seen as a sign of masculinity.
- Abstinence is totally acceptable.
- Drinking is seen as neither a virtue nor a sin.
- Drinking is not a primary activity, but accompanies other activities.

High rates of alcoholism are associated with the opposite of these patterns. In the absence of clear rules on how to drink, conflicting or ambiguous guidelines lead people into destructive drinking patterns.

Because of increased world travel and communication, drinking differences among different ethnic groups are less pronounced than in the past.[27] However some generalizations about the role of alcohol in some specific cultures follow.

Some Native American nations (tribes) suffer from high rates of alcohol-abuse problems. It is commonly supposed that the bodies of Native Americans don't "handle" alcohol well and that this leads to their alcoholism. Different Native American nations, however, have widely differing rates of alcoholism, favoring a cultural explanation for the high alcoholism rates of some.[28]

As pointed out in Chapter 14, Asians and Asian Americans include at least 32 different ethnic groups. In most of these groups the rate of alcohol abuse is low. One notable exception is Japanese males in corporate management positions, who tend to drink quite heavily.

Among Hispanic Americans, a low percentage of women drink, but a high percentage of men drink, and among those who do, the rate of alcohol abuse is high. Heavy drinking by males is encouraged by the idea that drinking together is an important way of identifying with other members of the social group. Also, heavy drinking is seen as a masculine behavior. There is evidence that the Hispanic cultural values, which reduce alcohol use by women, gradually break down with exposure to Anglo society.[29]

Overall, the rate of alcohol use among African Americans is lower than among white Americans. African American men, women, and youths are more likely to abstain from alcohol than are the corresponding white Americans. But those who do drink are more likely than white Americans to drink heavily, to use other drugs as well, and to experience health or other problems because of drinking. In fact, alcohol abuse is one of the most important health problems in the African American community, contributing to high rates of homicide, liver disorders, heart disease, and certain cancers.[30]

CHECKPOINT

1. Discuss the different views of problem drinking and alcoholism.

2. How many people does the National Institute on Alcohol Abuse estimate as being alcohol abusers?

3. Define the term *blackout*.

4. Define the term *loss of control*.

5. Do you believe that alcoholics can become successful social drinkers after a long period of abstinence?

6. Discuss the characteristics of alcohol that enhance the likelihood of its abuse.

7. Is there an "alcoholic personality"?

8. Which sociological factors contribute to a climate for alcohol abuse?

ALCOHOL AND YOUTH

Alcoholic beverages have become an established part of the youth culture in the United States. Each year, the National Institute on Drug Abuse conducts a nationwide survey of thousands of high school seniors regarding their use of alcohol and other drugs. This survey shows that youthful alcohol use, after peaking in 1979, has declined somewhat, but remains very high. Some recent statistics follow:[31]

- Seventy-six percent of eighth-graders and 87 percent of tenth-graders have tried alcohol.

- Five percent of eighth-graders and 13 percent of tenth-graders are frequent drinkers.

- Forty percent of male tenth-graders and 33 percent of female tenth-graders had consumed five or more drinks consecutively on at least one occasion during the two weeks before the survey was taken.

- Twenty-one percent of male tenth-graders and 16 percent of female tenth-graders had consumed alcohol in combination with other drugs on at least one occasion during the month before the survey was taken.

Drinking five or more drinks at one time and combining alcohol with other drugs are dangerous behaviors. Even though adolescent drinking has decreased somewhat, as has drinking in all age groups, it still remains an extremely serious problem that threatens the health, safety, and futures of millions of young people. The disease of alcoholism can progress very rapidly in young drinkers; an estimated three million American adolescents are alcoholics.

Alcohol Myth:

Drinking is a normal part of growing up.

Alcohol Reality:

Alcohol is causing severe problems for millions of young Americans. It is a factor in 60 percent of all attempted teen suicides.

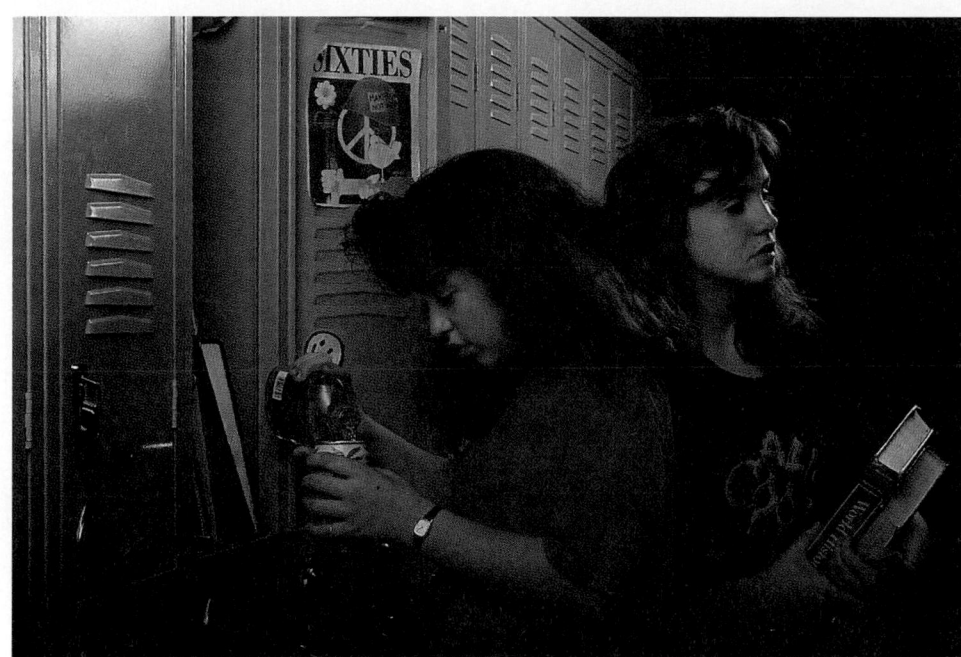

According to recent statistics, 76 percent of eighth graders have used alcohol at least once and 5 percent are already frequent drinkers.

WHY DO YOUNG PEOPLE START USING ALCOHOL?

There is no simple answer to why young people start to drink. Felsted reports that adolescent drinking is related to all of the following:[32]

- the belief that their friends drink and expect them to drink
- accessibility of alcohol and social settings where unsupervised drinking can take place
- low levels of self-esteem
- the belief that drinking is a sign of adulthood
- the belief that experimenting with alcohol is a normal part of adolescent development
- the drinking habits of their parents
- the belief that their parents approve of their drinking
- having low expectations of academic achievement
- rebelliousness

EFFECT OF ALCOHOL ADVERTISING

Alcoholic beverages are heavily advertised everywhere, using every possible medium from television to bus stop benches. Alcohol advertisers use people in their ads who are attractive and appear to be wealthy, sexy, healthy, and friendly, and living exciting lives. They are often well-known per-

sonalities. The advertisers prey on people's fantasies of "the good life," of which alcohol is shown as being an essential part. In ads, drinking is shown to be appropriate in a wide variety of situations and the negative consequences of drinking are overshadowed. The message, repeated thousands of times over, is that drinking is OK. By age 21, the average young person will have seen tens of thousands of beer and wine ads on TV alone.

What effect does alcohol advertising have on young people? Research indicates that exposure to alcohol advertising is closely linked with drinking behavior.[33] Alcohol advertising has a more powerful effect on adolescent drinking habits than does parental influence or social status. The relationship is especially strong for distilled liquors such as vodka and tequila. The question that remains unanswered is how can alcohol-abuse-prevention programs, with their limited resources, combat the powerful pro-drinking effects of alcohol advertising and peer pressure?

Alcohol Myth:

Alcohol advertising doesn't affect young people's drinking behavior.

Alcohol Reality:

Alcohol advertising has a more powerful influence on young persons' drinking than does parental influence or social status.

ADOLESCENT ALCOHOLISM

Not only do the majority of adolescents use alcohol, but many of them become alcohol-dependent at very early ages. Every alcohol counselor, school nurse, and psychologist can tell stories of even preadolescent alcoholics, some as young as 8 or 9 years old.

Parents are usually unaware of their children's drinking habits. Here are some common signs of an adolescent's alcohol or other drug problems (in a recent survey, 76 percent of adolescent Alcoholics Anonymous members said that they had been abusers of other drugs as well):[34]

- avoidance of family members and long-term friends
- irritability with family members and friends
- suspiciousness of family, friends, and others
- falling grades at school
- poor attendance record at school
- constant need for money and vagueness about how it is spent
- shortened attention span
- inability to cope with frustration
- rebelliousness
- mood swings
- lying
- secretiveness
- impulsive behavior
- new friends not known to the family
- narrowing of interests, abandoning former interests
- loss of motivation and perseverance

How can parents or friends help an adolescent alcohol abuser, who may seem so hostile and remote? The following are some suggestions:[35]

1. *Express concern.* Tell the young person that you care about him or her and are concerned over the changes in his or her behavior.

2. *Point out the offensive behavior.* Young alcohol abusers use denial just as older ones do. The young person may not be aware of how great a problem his or her drinking or other drug use

can become. Reflect upon changes in his or her attitudes, values, and behavior.

3. *Don't accept excuses.* Just like older alcohol abusers, young people develop excuses, rationalizations, and ways to avoid talking about or to divert attention from their problem. Don't fall for this; keep the discussion on track.

4. *Confront the alcohol abuse.* Make it clear that you are rejecting the drinking behavior, but not the person. "I love you, but I don't love your drinking."

5. *Seek expert help.* Enlist the aid of a professional alcohol counselor, a local council on alcoholism, Alcoholics Anonymous, or a local youth chemical-dependency program.

Helping a young alcohol abuser is often difficult and frustrating. Lies and rationalizations are to be expected. Alcoholism is an illness and denial is part of that illness. Often, though, by receiving simultaneous acceptance and support as a loved person, coupled with the rejection of his or her drinking behavior, the adolescent alcohol abuser may accept that drinking has become a problem and start on the road to recovery.

CHECKPOINT

1. Briefly discuss the scope of the problem of alcohol abuse among youth.

2. What effect does alcohol advertising have on young people?

3. What are some of the common signs of adolescent alcohol abuse?

4. List some of the suggestions made to help adolescent alcohol abusers.

ALCOHOL AND COLLEGE STUDENTS

Alcohol has long been very much a part of life on most college campuses, where it is included in social events of all kinds. Many students believe that alcohol helps to facilitate social interaction and helps relieve the unrelenting pressures of exams and other college demands. Alcohol consumption is far greater among college students than among the general population. This is true regarding both the percentage of people who drink and for the amount of alcohol each person who does drink consumes.

For many students, alcohol is just another aspect of the college experience. But for some, it causes serious problems that interfere with academic success or other aspects of their lives. After college, many graduates' alcohol consumption drops. Some, though, leave college with drinking problems that will plague them for many years.

How can you function socially in the alcohol-centered college environment without having alcohol-associated problems or developing an alcohol dependency that will persist long beyond your college years? We can offer some suggestions:

- Ask for an alternative beverage (See Communication for Wellness: 22 Ways to Say No to a Drink, on p. 544).

- If you're going to drink, drink in ways that minimize the effects of alcohol (see Feature 17.6).

- When you are the host, make sure that your guests don't drink too much (refer back to Feature 17.4).

If alcohol is becoming a problem for you, as it does for many college students, don't wait too long to do something about your drinking. We will conclude this chapter with a look at some ways of overcoming alcohol-abuse problems.

CHECKPOINT

1. How does alcohol consumption by college students compare to that of the general population?

2. Do college-acquired drinking problems end when you leave college?

ALCOHOL-ABUSE RECOVERY

The only realistic goal for anyone having a problem with alcohol is total abstinence from alcohol and other psychoactive drugs. This is true regardless of the form of treatment used. We cannot emphasize this point strongly enough. Perhaps a few—a very few—alcoholics have returned to controlled drinking (the experts debate this point). Odds are overwhelming that, even with the greatest motivation and best available treatment, efforts to drink or use other drugs in a controlled manner will only result in continued problems. For this reason, most alcohol experts avoid using terms such as "former alcoholic," "ex-alcoholic," or "recovered alcoholic." The prevailing opinion is: "Once an alcoholic, always an alcoholic." Thus, the phrases "recovering alcoholic" or "sober alcoholic" are preferred. The physiological changes associated with alcoholism remain with a person even after years of sobriety. If drinking resumes, it *will* be in an uncontrolled manner. *It is never safe for a recovering alcoholic to have a drink.*

FEATURE 17.6

HOW TO MINIMIZE THE CONSEQUENCES OF ALCOHOL USE

As you might expect, the authors of this text do not recommend drinking alcohol. We have seen much harm caused by it and very little benefit. But we have spent enough years around colleges to know that many students *will* drink. If you are going to drink, here are some steps you can take to minimize the harmful effects of alcohol:

1. Drink diluted forms of alcohol—the more diluted, the better. Avoid undiluted hard liquor, such as straight shots or shooters.

2. Pace your drinking. Learn to hold a full glass, bottle, or can. Drink slowly so that you don't exceed one drink per hour.

3. Never drink without consuming some food to slow the absorption of alcohol. Tell your friends you're starving and must have something to eat.

4. *Never* get involved in drinking games. When you play these games you surrender control over your drinking. Drinking games are most popular with people who don't want to assume responsibility for their own heavy drinking.

5. If driving will be involved, make certain that there is an alcohol-free designated driver.

6. Don't be afraid to say "I've had plenty" and mean it. People with drinking problems often try to validate their drinking behavior by encouraging other people to also drink heavily along with them. True friends don't push you to drink more than you should.

22 WAYS TO SAY NO TO A DRINK

Peer pressure can make it difficult for both young persons and adults to say no to a drink. When you have a drink, you validate the drinking behavior of those around you, which, in essence, tells them that their drinking is OK. Some people need this validation. Thus, they can be quite insistent upon your having a drink, and then encourage you to have another, and another. Saying no can require a lot of maturity, thought, and practice. Try out some of these suggestions to see which ones you feel most comfortable using. Then practice saying them a few times.

1. No, thanks, I don't drink.
2. No, thanks, I don't enjoy alcohol.
3. No, thanks, I don't enjoy drinking.
4. No, thanks, it's just not for me.
5. No, thanks, I don't like the taste.
6. No, thanks, I feel fine already.
7. No, thanks, I want to keep a clear head.
8. No, thanks, I've got to study later.
9. No, thanks, I've got some work I have to do.
10. No, thanks, I have to get up early.
11. No, thanks, I have to pick up a friend.
12. No, thanks, I like to stay in control.
13. No, thanks, I'm driving.
14. No, thanks, I don't want to get into trouble with my. . . .
15. No, thanks, I don't want to embarrass myself.
16. No, thanks, drinking makes me feel tired.
17. No, thanks, I don't need the calories.
18. No, thanks, I'm in training.
19. No, thanks, my coach wouldn't approve.
20. No, thanks, I'm trying to lose some weight.
21. No, thanks, what else do you have?
22. No, thanks.

It is entirely possible that you might lose a "friend" by refusing to drink or by stopping at one or two drinks. If the "friendship" is based upon your validating that person's drinking habits, however, it's a friendship you can well do without.

There are no "quick fixes" for alcoholism. The road to recovery can be long and difficult, but it is *always* worth it in the end. Some form of ongoing supportive therapy or attendance at meetings is usually necessary if sobriety is to be maintained.

Alcohol Myth:
With enough willpower, an alcoholic should be able to return to controlled, social drinking.

Alcohol Reality:
Few if any alcoholics have ever returned to controlled drinking for any period of time. Once an alcoholic, always an alcoholic.

CHECKPOINT
1. What is the goal in alcohol-abuse recovery?
2. Is it accurate to say "former alcoholic?" Why?

SUMMARY

Alcohol is legal, is used by about 60 percent of the adults in the United States, is a major industry, and is America's number one drug problem. Ten percent of Americans are alcoholics and drink about 60 percent of all alcohol sold in the nation.

Alcohol is produced by fermentation, and concentrated in stronger beverages by distillation. Other than calories, alcoholic beverages offer little or no nutritional value.

Intoxication is measured by blood alcohol levels, though frequent, heavy drinkers are less affected by a given blood alcohol level than are occasional drinkers. Alcohol is mainly removed from the body by breakdown in the liver. The liver of the average person breaks down the alcohol from about one drink per hour.

Alcohol is a nervous system depressant, is highly tolerance-forming, and causes a physiological dependency. Harmful physical effects include alcoholic neuropathy, stomach ulcers, liver damage (alcoholic hepatitis and cirrhosis), weakness and wasting of muscles, skin disorders, irregular menstrual cycles, feminization in men, sexual dysfunction, birth defects if consumed during pregnancy, heart damage (though moderate drinking is associated with reduced risk of heart attack), cancers, osteoporosis, and impaired immunity. Other harmful effects include traffic deaths and injuries, family dysfunction, and work, school, social, and legal problems.

Many drinkers become physically dependent on alcohol. If drinking is discontinued, withdrawal can take one or more of four forms: hyperarousal, alcoholic hallucinosis, convulsive seizures, and delirium tremens (DTs).

Fetal alcohol syndrome (FAS) is a group of birth defects in infants whose mothers drank during pregnancy. No amount of alcohol is considered safe to consume during pregnancy.

Although alcohol-related traffic fatalities have decreased, alcohol remains a major cause of vehicle crashes. Driving begins to be impaired with the first drink. One of the most successful ways to avoid alcohol-related crashes is the use of a designated driver. Strict enforcement of drunk driving laws is also effective.

Various definitions of problem drinking and alcoholism are used. We have defined problem drinking as drinking that causes problems in any area of your life or problems for other people (how much or how often you drink is not part of this definition). Alcoholism is a disease characterized by strong psychological and, possibly, physiological dependency on alcohol and the inability to drink in moderation. Heredity is now recognized as an important factor in alcoholism, though the importance of cultural factors is also recognized.

Drinking is very prevalent among high school age and younger people and is a special concern because of the potential impact on their lives. Among college students, both the percentage who drink and the amount each consumes are greater than among the general population.

In alcohol-abuse recovery, the only realistic goal is total abstinence from alcohol and other psychoactive drugs. Few if any alcoholics are able to return to controlled social drinking.

The bottom line: Not everyone can drink successfully. If you choose to drink, be alert for the early signs of developing alcohol-related problems in your life. If you detect any sign that alcohol is beginning to cause school, family, health, legal, social, or financial problems for you, please stop drinking—immediately and totally. If you are unable to do this by yourself, please contact AA or another alcoholism recovery program. Don't let alcohol control your life.

REFERENCES

1. Kline, H., and Pittman, D. "The Distribution of Alcohol Consumption in American Society." In Venturelli, P. (ed.). *Drug Use in America: Social, Cultural, and Political Perspectives.* Boston: Jones and Bartlett, 1994.
2. Goode, E. *Drugs in American Society,* 4th ed. New York: McGraw-Hill, 1993.
3. Based on an idea from Kinney, J., and Leaton, G. *Loosening the Grip, A Handbook of Alcohol Information,* 4th ed. St. Louis: Mosby, 1991, and updated with data compiled from many sources.
4. Kline and Pittman, op. cit.
5. Kinney, J., and Leaton, G. *Loosening the Grip, a Handbook of Alcohol Information,* 4th ed. St. Louis: Mosby, 1991.
6. Radcliffe, A., Rush, P., Sites, C., and Crusek J. *The Pharmer's Almanac.* New York: Ballantine, 1991.
7. Kinney and Leaton, op. cit.
8. Ibid.
9. Roselle, G. "Alcohol and the Immune System." *Alcohol Health and Research World* 16, No. 1 (1992), 16–22.
10. Kinney and Leaton, op. cit.
11. Ibid.
12. Ibid.
13. Ibid.
14. Ibid.
15. National Institute on Alcohol Abuse and Alcoholism (NIAAA). *Sixth Special Report to the U.S. Congress on Alcohol and Health from the Secretary of Health and Human Services.* Rockville, MD: National Institute on Alcohol Abuse and Alcoholism: 1987.
16. Ibid.
17. Kinney and Leaton, op. cit.
18. Lichtblau, E. "Higher Age Limit Tied to Drop in Drunk-Driving Arrests" *Los Angeles Times,* (29 February 1988) Sec. 1, 5.
19. Ibid.
20. Kinney and Leaton, op. cit.
21. Maugh, Thomas. "Study Finds Genetic Link to Alcoholism in Women." *Los Angeles Times* (14 October 1992), A1–A17.

22. National Institute on Alcohol Abuse and Alcoholism, op. cit.

23. Kinney and Leaton, op. cit.

24. Vaillant, G. *The Natural History of Alcoholism.* Cambridge: Harvard University Press, 1983.

25. Maugh, op. cit.

26. Kinney and Leaton, op. cit.

27. Ibid

28. Avis, H. *Drugs and Life,* 2nd ed. Madison, WI: Brown & Benchmark, 1993.

29. Ibid.

30. Ibid.

31. Windle, Michael. "Alcohol Use and Abuse: Some Findings from the National Adolescent Student Health Survey." *Alcohol Health and Research World* Vol. 15, No. 1 (1991), 5–10.

32. Felsted, C. (ed.). *Youth and Alcohol Abuse: Readings and Resources.* Phoenix, AZ: Oryx Press, 1986.

33. Ibid.

34. Kinney and Leaton, op. cit.

35. Dykman, B., in Felsted, op. cit.

SUGGESTED READINGS

Alcohol Health and Research World, a quarterly magazine published by the National Institute on Alcohol Abuse and Alcoholism. Subscriptions are available through the Superintendent of Documents, Government Printing Office, Washington, D.C. 20402-9371.

Alcoholics Anonymous World Services, Inc. publishes a variety of books, booklets, and pamphlets. The book *Alcoholics Anonymous,* published in 1939, is a basic reference.

Johnson, V. E. *I'll Quit Tomorrow.* New York: Harper & Row, 1973. A classic.

Kinney, J., and Leaton, G. *Loosening the Grip, A Handbook of Alcohol Information,* 4th ed. St. Louis: Mosby, 1991, or most recent edition.

Kirkpatrick, J. *Goodbye Hangover, Hello Life; Self-help for Women.* New York: Ballantine, 1987.

Venturelli, P. (ed.). *Drug Use in America: Social, Cultural, and Political Perspectives.* Boston: Jones and Bartlett, 1994. An anthology on U. S. drug and alcohol issues.

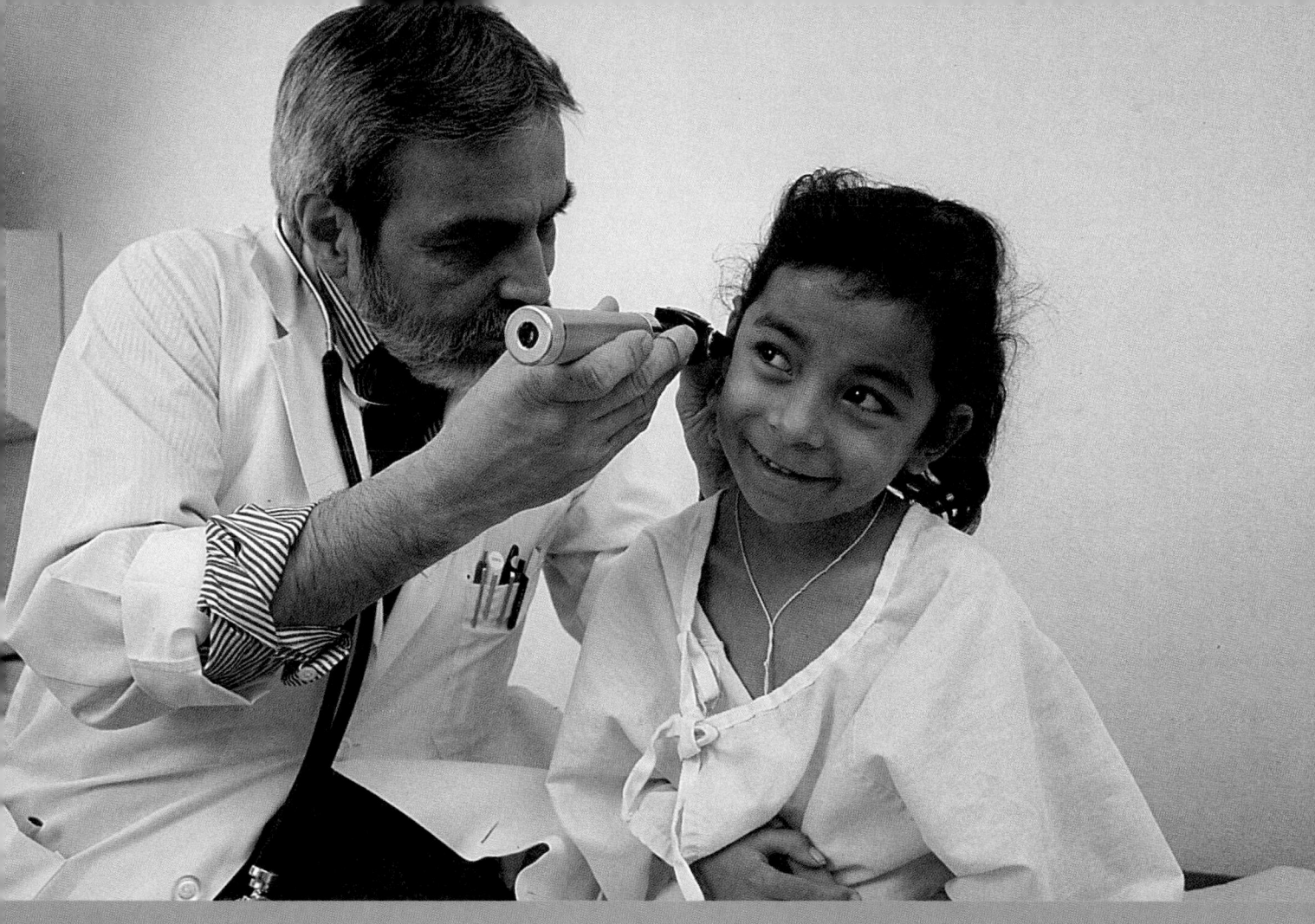

SEVEN
DISEASES

In this four-chapter unit we explore infectious diseases, heart conditions, cancer, and other major health problems. Even these seemingly negative topics can be approached in a positive manner. Although genetic and environmental factors can contribute to these problems, individual health behaviors are the single most important contributing factor. Many of the conditions we will examine can be prevented, postponed, or minimized by adopting healthful living habits. Individual responsibility for your health is essential for the prevention, early detection, and effective treatment of each of these disorders.

Chapter 18 presents the basic concepts relating to the communicable diseases—those caused by infectious agents. Chapter 19 applies this information to an important group of communicable diseases,

those that are sexually transmitted. In Chapter 20, we examine the nation's leading causes of death, cardiovascular disorders (diseases of the heart and blood vessels), which currently kill almost as many people in the United States as all other causes of death combined. To complete the unit, Chapter 21 discusses cancer and some other serious health problems, including diabetes, arthritis, neurological disorders, and disorders of the urinary and respiratory systems.

Throughout these four chapters, we emphasize preventing illness by taking personal responsibility for your health. By applying information that is now available about preventing diseases through diet, exercise, and other life-style elements, you can feel optimistic about avoiding many of the problems described in this unit.

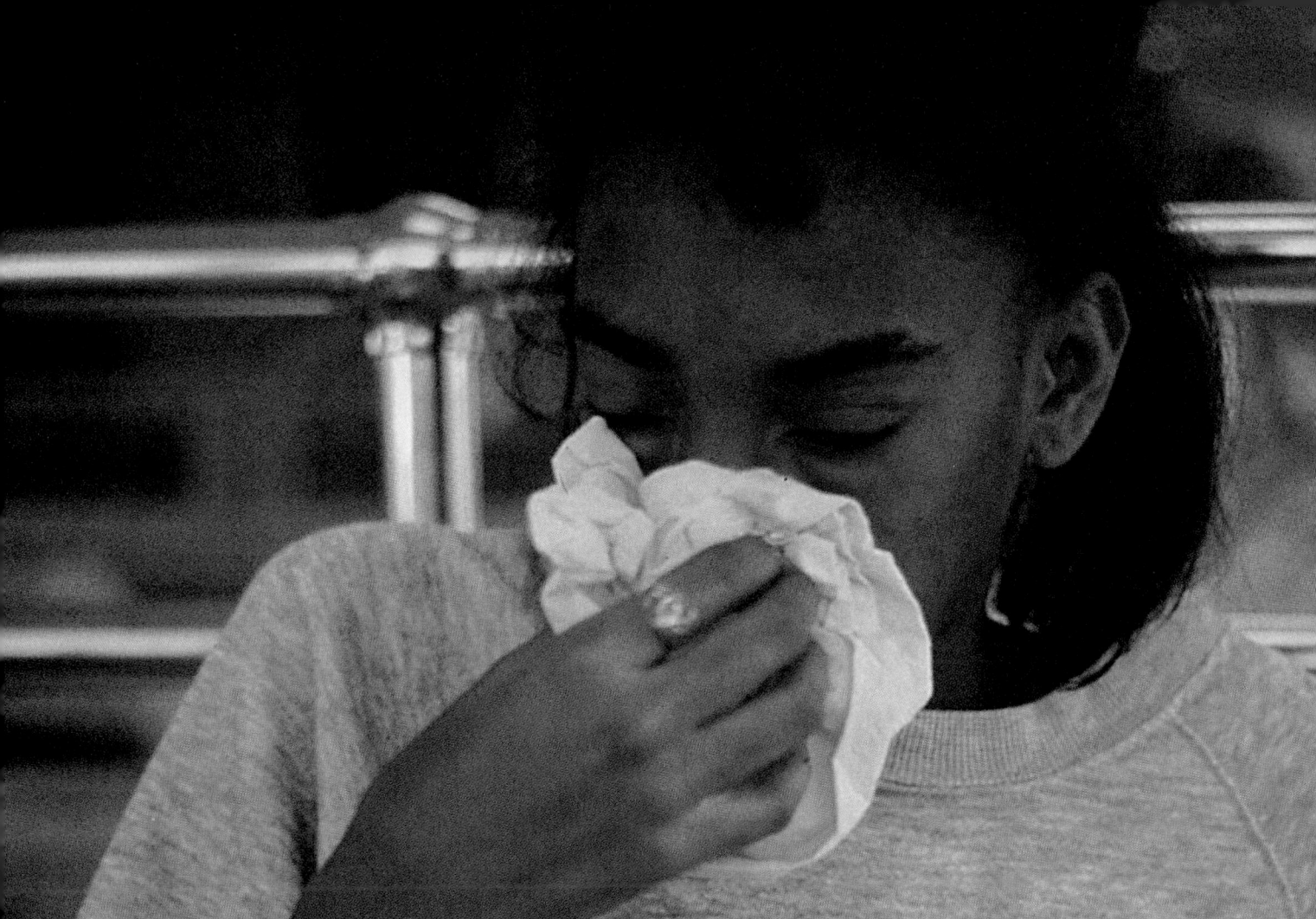

18

COMMUNICABLE DISEASES

CHAPTER OBJECTIVES

Upon completing this chapter, you will be able to:

KNOWLEDGE

- Explain the basic characteristics of viruses, bacteria, fungi, protozoa, and parasitic worms.
- Describe each link in the chain of infection.
- Explain the infective dosage of a pathogen.
- Describe each step in the course of a communicable disease.
- Contrast specific and nonspecific body defenses against disease.
- Explain cell-mediated and humoral immunity.
- Contrast active and passive immunity.
- Explain how vaccines protect against disease.
- List the causes of immune deficiency.
- Explain allergies and autoimmune disorders.
- Explain the salient features of Lyme disease, colds, influenza, bacterial pneumonia, measles, mononucleosis, and hepatitis.

INSIGHT

- Explain how your living habits can affect your risk of infectious disease.
- Explain which vaccines you, as an adult, might need.
- Explain the life-style factors that influence resistance to diseases and how they relate to your current life.

DECISION MAKING

- Make a commitment to ensure full immunization for yourself and any children you may have.
- Make a commitment to a life-style that ensures maximum resistance to disease.

The lifetime of Arthur Ashe was characterized by triumphs over situations in which he faced huge odds. As a youngster, growing up in segregated Richmond, Virginia, he excelled at tennis, a sport that was almost exclusively played by whites. At only 37 years of age, while he was at the top of his professional tennis career, he suffered from the first of several heart attacks. He was able to overcome all of these problems. He could not overcome AIDS, however; at the age of 49, he succumbed to that disease.

The cause of Arthur Ashe's HIV infection was a tainted blood transfusion that he received after his second coronary bypass operation in 1983. Nine years later, in 1992, he stunned people who watched as he announced, under the pressure of a possible newspaper story, that he had AIDS. Yet Arthur Ashe was not the type of person to withdraw or expect pity. Soon after that announcement, he became active in promoting AIDS research and set up an AIDS foundation. He spoke at many gatherings about his disease and about other issues of importance, such as race relations.

Less than one year after announcing that he had AIDS, Arthur Ashe died. Blood supplies are now screened and blood and blood products are tested to ensure that HIV is not transmitted. Sadly, these *techniques were not available when Ashe received his transfusion. The world will miss this great man whose graceful style on and off the court was combined with a strong dedication to improving life for others.*

    Source: Time *15 February 1993, p. 70.*

                        ■   ■   ■

Communicable diseases are caused by microscopic, parasitic **organisms** that invade the body. These diseases are also called infectious diseases. Diseases are referred to as being **contagious** if they can be passed from person to person.

    Throughout history, communicable diseases have threatened human lives and have in some cases altered the course of entire civilizations. Diseases such as plague, malaria, smallpox, leprosy, syphilis, polio, and AIDS are examples of the immense power that microscopic disease agents hold over human well-being. In this chapter we will explore the basic nature of communicable diseases, how the body combats them, and some of today's more prevalent diseases. The sexually transmitted diseases, because of their importance, will be treated in a separate chapter, Chapter 19.

    Throughout the four chapters in this unit the terms *prevalence* and *incidence* often appear. **Prevalence** refers to the number of cases of a disease present in a specified population at a given time. **Incidence** is the frequency of occurrence of a disease over a period of time, usually a year, in relation to the size of the population in which it occurs. Incidence figures are often expressed as cases per 100,000 population per year.

communicable disease one that is due to an infectious agent.

organism any living thing.

contagious capable of being passed from person to person.

prevalence the number of cases of a disease present in a specified population at a given time.

incidence the frequency of occurrence of a disease over a period of time, usually a year, in relation to the size of the population in which it occurs.

PATHOGENS

Disease-causing organisms are called **pathogens** (*path'ō-jenz*), or more commonly, *germs*. Most pathogens are microscopic and are referred to as **microbes,** or **microorganisms.** Relatively few microorganisms cause human disease. Many others are actually beneficial, while some cause diseases in plants and animals other than humans. We will look at five major categories of pathogens, in order of increasing size:

1. *Viruses:* ultramicroscopic, simple, semiliving (Feature 18.1) particles.
   Examples of diseases caused: AIDS, colds, influenza, and herpes.
2. *Bacteria:* microscopic, single-celled organisms.
   Examples of diseases caused: strep throat, gonorrhea, and tuberculosis.
3. *Fungi* (molds and yeasts): single-celled or multicellular plantlike organisms.
   Examples of diseases caused: athlete's foot and "yeast" infections.
4. *Protozoa:* microscopic, single-celled, animal-like organisms.
   Examples of diseases caused: malaria and vaginal *Trichomonas.*
5. *Parasitic worms:* multicellular true animals.
   Examples: tapeworms, pinworms, and liver flukes.

VIRUSES

Viruses, which are among the smallest of the pathogens, cause numerous minor and major diseases, including colds, influenza, hepatitis, herpes, and AIDS. Viruses are visible only through powerful electron microscopes having many thousands

pathogen disease-causing organisms.

microbes or **microorganisms** microscopic living things.

viruses infectious particles consisting of nucleic acid (either DNA or RNA) and protein, and, in some cases, an outer envelope of protein and fat.

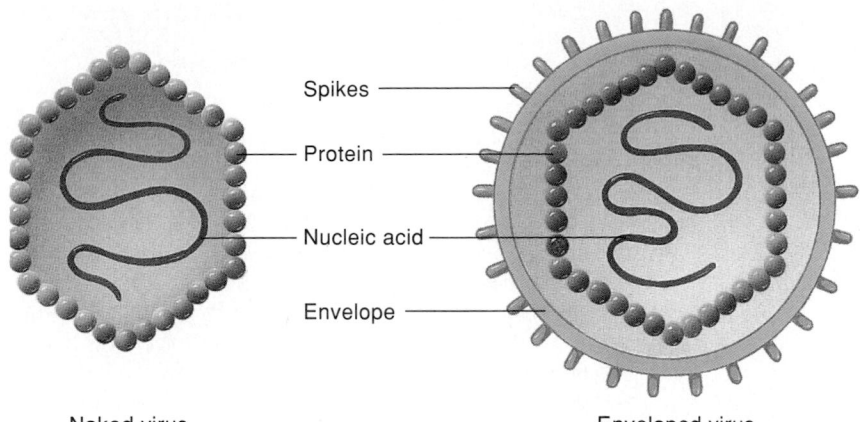

Spikes

Protein

Nucleic acid

Envelope

Naked virus

Enveloped virus

Figure 18.1
Typical Virus Particles

"Naked" viruses (left) consist only of nucleic acid and protein. Enveloped viruses (right) have an additional layer of mainly fat derived from the host cell. Because of their simple structure, viruses are quite difficult to control.

of times magnification. What viruses lack in size, they make up for in **virulence** (degree of disease-producing ability). In fact, viruses are the most challenging group of pathogens to control.

Viruses are difficult to control because of their simplicity. They lack the many vulnerabilities inherent in the complex structures and functions of other kinds of pathogens. Viruses consist mainly of a central core of nucleic acid (either DNA or RNA) enclosed within a protein coating (see Figure 18.1). Some viruses have an additional outer envelope of fat and protein. Thus, their structure is much less complex than even the simplest cell (see Feature 18.1).

Viruses are intracellular parasites. Reproduction, or **replication** of viruses occurs only within living host cells. The **host** is the organism that is infected by a parasite. The genetic material of the virus takes control of the host cell and directs the manufacture of more virus particles. The normal functioning of the host cell is thus disrupted, often with serious consequences.

Some viruses, notably those in the herpes group, have the ability to lie **latent** (dormant) in host cells for many years, periodically reactivating to produce their diseases. Between attacks, these latent viruses reside within the human nervous sys-

tem, where they are protected from the body's defenses.

Going even further to avoid destruction by body defenses, some viruses insert their genes into the host's own chromosomes, becoming, in effect, part of the host's genetic makeup.[1] HIV (the AIDS virus) is one example.

Another alarming ability of some viruses is to cause healthy host cells to become cancerous. Research indicates that some human cancers are the result of viruses working in conjunction with harmful environmental forces.[2] This concept will be examined in more depth in Chapter 21.

Development of effective antiviral drugs has been complicated by the simple structure and function of the viruses. None of the antibacterial drugs, such as antibiotics and sulfa drugs, exerts any effect against viruses, because viruses lack the metabolic processes that these drugs block.[3] In some cases, drugs are available to slow or moderate the course of viral diseases. For example, attacks of genital herpes can be made less frequent and less severe with oral acyclovir, and the symptoms of HIV infection can be delayed and their severity decreased by drugs such as zidovudine (Retrovir or AZT) and dideoxyinosine (Videx or ddI). In both cases, however, the virus is not actually destroyed.

Many viral diseases can be effectively prevented (as opposed to cured) by immunizations. The human immune mechanism works well against many types of viruses. *Even when more effective antiviral drugs become available, prevention by vaccines will remain far superior to treatment of diseases after they develop.*

....

virulence degree of disease-causing ability.

replication the process of reproduction.

host an organism that is infected by a parasite.

latent dormant or inactive.

FEATURE 18.1

VIRUSES: ARE THEY ALIVE?

When the nature of viruses first became understood in the 1950s, these minute particles presented quite a dilemma to science. Were they living or nonliving? The question is still not entirely resolved.[a] Before viruses were known, there seemed to be two distinct conditions: life and nonlife. Other than viruses, every known entity was either living or nonliving. Viruses defied such classification. They clearly had *some* characteristics of life: They were parasitic, they had genetic material, they mutated (experienced genetic changes), and they increased in numbers. But other features shared by all living things were missing: Viruses did not consist of cells, they had no metabolism (ongoing chemical processes), and they were only able to reproduce with considerable involvement of their host organisms.

Eventually, many scientists revised their view of life as an either-or phenomenon. Viruses are now recognized by such scientists as being *semiliving*. Viruses fall in the "gray area" between life and nonlife. Other biologists have concluded that viruses are living organisms and that our definition of life needs revision. Richard Novick,[b] for example, has suggested that any nucleic acid system controlling its own replication should be considered a living organism.

Are there other kinds of semiliving entities? So far, two types have been identified. **Viroids** are infectious particles consisting of nucleic acid (RNA) only, with no protein. (Viruses consist of both nucleic acid and protein.) It is not yet known how many human diseases are caused by viroids. **Prions** (prē'onz) are infectious particles consisting of protein only, with no nucleic acid. Several rare degenerative conditions of the human brain, such as kuru and Cruetzfeldt-Jakob disease (CJD) are thought to be caused by prions. Perhaps as more knowledge of these and possibly other semiliving pathogens develops, the causes of some of today's "mystery" diseases will become known.

[a]Morello, J., Mizer, H., Wilson, M., and Granato, P. *Microbiology in Patient Care*, 5th ed. Dubuque, IA: Wm. C. Brown, 1994.

[b]Novick, R. "Plasmids." *Scientific American* 243, 1980, pp. 103–127.

BACTERIA

Bacteria are microscopic, single-celled organisms (see Figure 18.2). Although larger than viruses, bacteria are still microscopically small. Not all bacteria are harmful; in fact, many are quite beneficial. For example, the human vagina contains millions of acid-forming bacteria that help prevent yeast and other vaginal infections.

Pathogenic bacteria usually produce their harmful effects by releasing poisons called **toxins** and by releasing tissue-damaging enzymes. Some of the bacterial toxins are among the most poisonous substances known—the most minute trace of tetanus toxin, for example, can be fatal.

Bacteria occur in many shapes, but three shapes are most common. **Cocci** (*kok'sē*), which are spherical, may occur singly, in pairs (*diplococci*), in chains (*streptococci*), or in grapelike clusters (*staphylococci*). Some diseases caused by cocci include gonorrhea, meningitis, strep throat, boils, and scarlet fever. The **bacilli** (*ba-sil'ē*) are rod-shaped bacteria that cause diseases including

tuberculosis, diphtheria, and tetanus. Finally, **spirilla** (*spī-ril'la*) are spiral in form. Long spirilla having many twists are called **spirochetes** (*spī'rō-kēts*). The best-known spirochetes are the ones causing syphilis and Lyme disease.

Rickettsia and *Chlamydia* are unusually small bacteria that, like viruses, reproduce only within living host cells. Their size is also similar to that of large viruses. In other respects, however, they are more like bacteria and are now classified as such.[4] One distinguishing feature of most rickettsia (though not *Chlamydia*) is that they are transmitted to humans by insects and ticks. An example of a disease caused by a rickettsia is Rocky Mountain

---

toxins poisons produced by bacteria.

cocci spherical bacteria.

bacilli rod-shaped bacteria.

viroids infectious particles consisting of nucleic acid (RNA) only, with no protein.

prions infectious particles consisting of protein only.

spirilla spiral bacteria.

spirochetes long, slender, coiled bacteria.

rickettsia unusually small bacteria that reproduce only in living host cells; most are carried by insects or ticks.

Chlamydia unusually small bacteria that reproduce only in living host cells; have no ability to break down foods for energy.

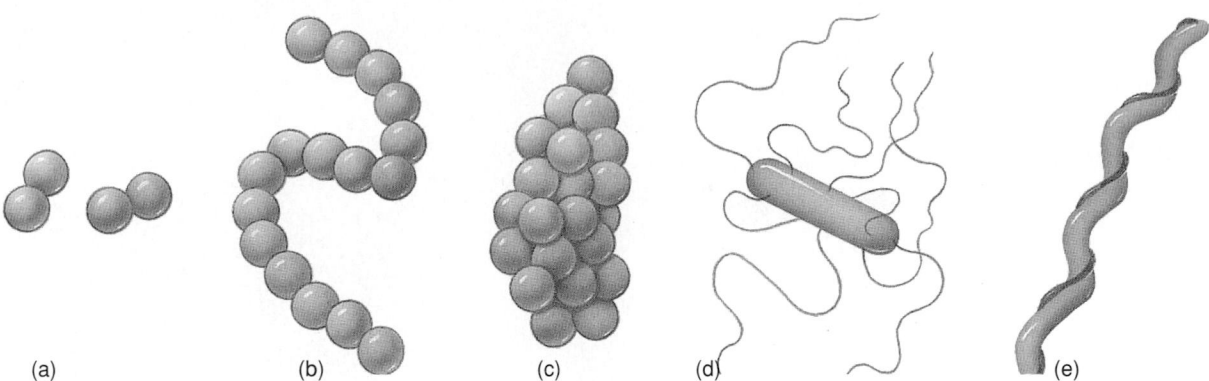

Figure 18.2
Some Important Bacterial Pathogens

(a) Neisseria gonorrhoeae, *the cause of gonorrhea; (b)* Streptococcus pyogenes, *the cause of strep throats, scarlet fever, and rheumatic fever; (c)* Staphylococcus aureus, *which causes infections and food poisoning; (d)* Salmonella, *a common cause of food-borne diarrhea; and (e)* Treponema pallidum, *the spirochete that causes syphilis.*

spotted fever, transmitted by ticks. A distinguishing feature of Chlamydias is that they have no ability to break down foods for energy; they must absorb their energy from a living host cell. An example of a disease caused by a *Chlamydia* is genital *Chlamydia* infection, currently the most common sexually transmitted disease.

Bacteria respond well to drugs such as sulfonamides (commonly called sulfa drugs) and antibiotics. Bacterial physiology is sufficiently different from our own that drugs can interfere with their physiology without interfering with ours. However, some people develop severe allergies to some of these drugs and must take alternative drugs.

FUNGI

Fungi are primitive spore-forming plantlike organisms. Common examples include yeasts, mushrooms, and bread and cheese molds. Relatively few fungi cause human diseases. Fungal infections are most commonly associated with the skin (ringworm, athlete's foot), nails ("fungus nails"), and lungs (histoplasmosis, coccidiodomycosis). The common vaginal "yeast" infection is caused by a form of fungus called *Candida*. Effective drugs are available to control fungal infections.

....

fungi primitive, spore-forming plantlike organisms.

PROTOZOA

Protozoa are microscopic, single-celled animal-like organisms (see Figure 18.3). Protozoa differ from both bacteria and fungi in that they lack rigid cell walls around each cell. Some diseases caused by protozoa include amoebic dysentery, malaria, African sleeping sickness, and a form of vaginitis called trichomoniasis. Many protozoan diseases tend to be recurrent. Between attacks the pathogen remains dormant in the body. Protozoan infections can usually be controlled with drugs, although the treatment can be quite prolonged for some diseases, such as malaria.

PARASITIC WORMS

The **parasitic worms** (see Figure 18.4) are multicellular true animals (true animals have specialized tissues and organs) ranging in size from microscopic, such as the worm causing trichinosis, to many feet long, such as some tapeworms. Parasitic worms often have complex life cycles that include other animals as well as humans. Some worms,

....

protozoa microscopic, single-celled animal-like organisms.

parasitic worms multicellular true animals that draw nourishment from living hosts such as humans.

Fungi are composed of thread-like filaments and reproduce by forming huge numbers of spores. This is the fungus called Penicillium, which often grows on cheese and bread and is the source of penicillin antibiotics.

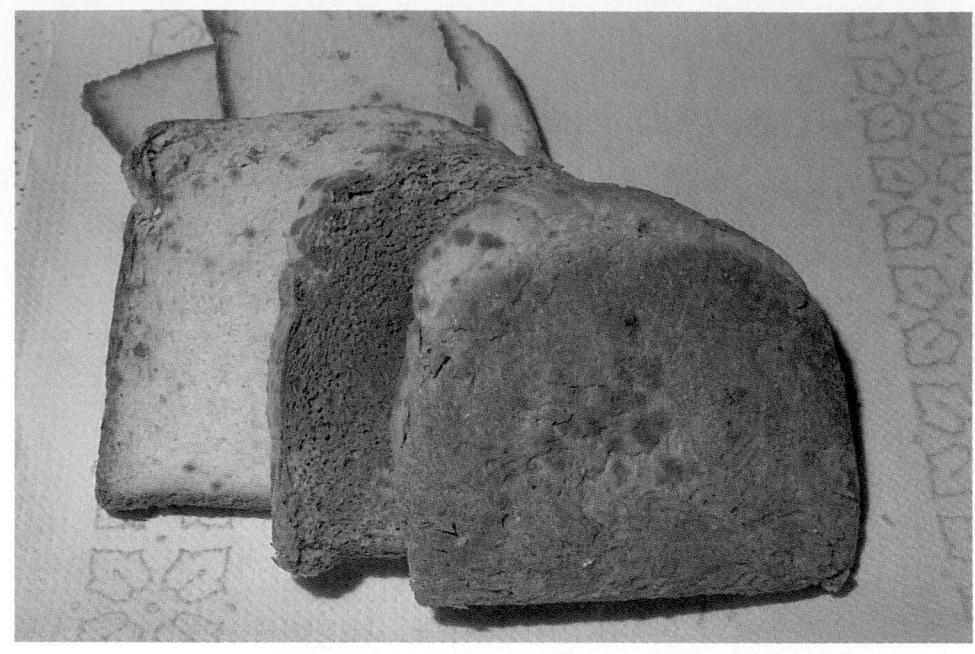

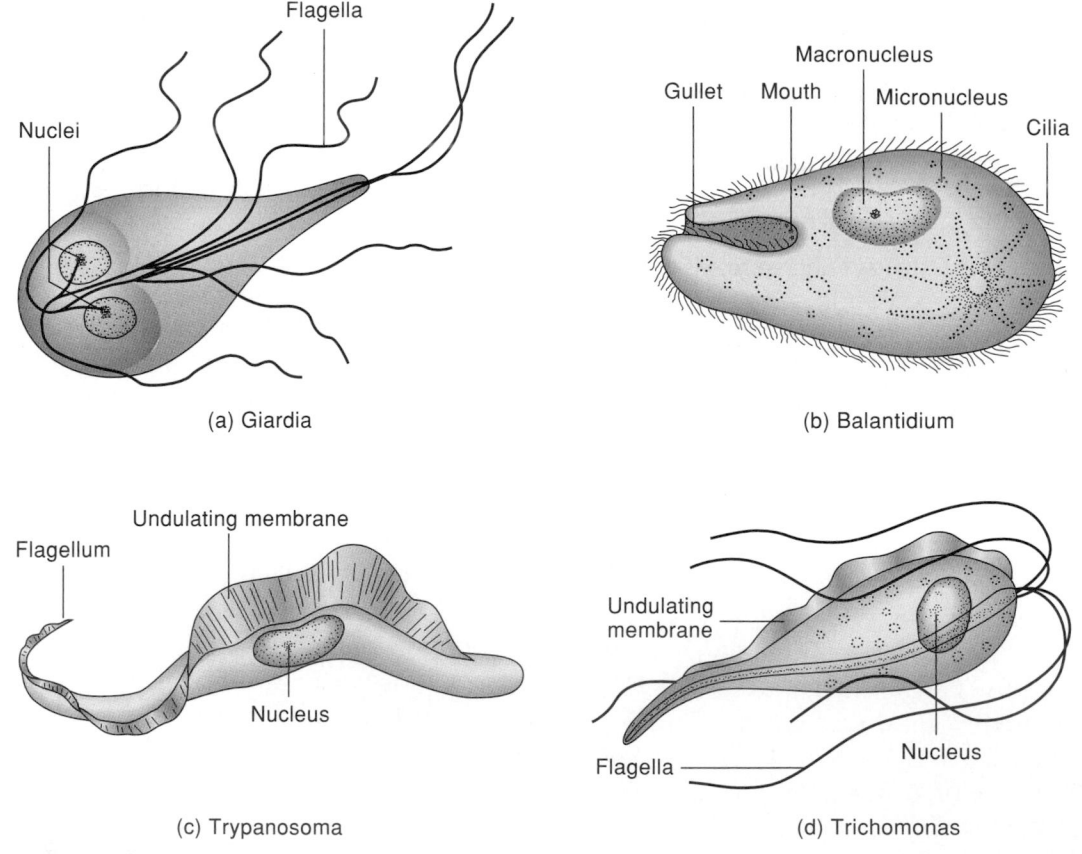

(a) Giardia

(b) Balantidium

(c) Trypanosoma

(d) Trichomonas

Figure 18.3

Protozoa

Protozoa are microscopic, single-celled animal-like organisms. (a) Giardia, a common water-borne intestinal pathogen; (b) Balantidium, another intestinal parasite; (c) Trypanosoma brucei gambiense; the pathogen of African sleeping sickness; (d) Trichomonas, the pathogen of a form of vaginitis called trichomoniasis.

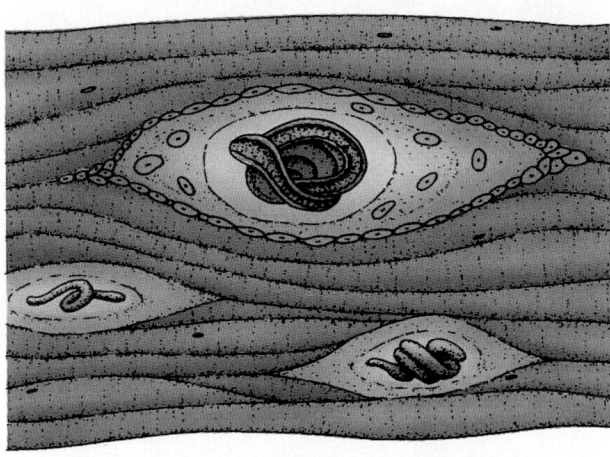

(a) Trichinella larvae in human muscle

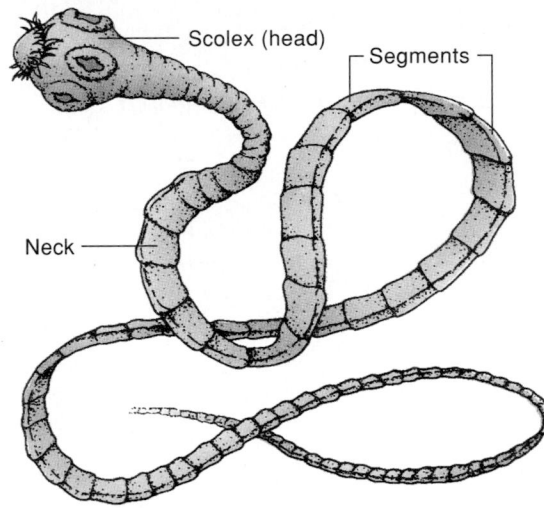

Scolex (head)

Segments

Neck

(b) Adult tapeworm

Figure 18.4
Parasitic Worms

The largest of the pathogens, parasitic worms range from microscopically small up to many feet long. (a) Drawing of microscopic worm of trichinosis in human muscle; (b) Drawing of an adult tapeworm, removed from the human intestine (actual size 10–20 feet long); (c) elephantiasis, the result of long-term infection of the blood and lymph vessels by filaria worms.

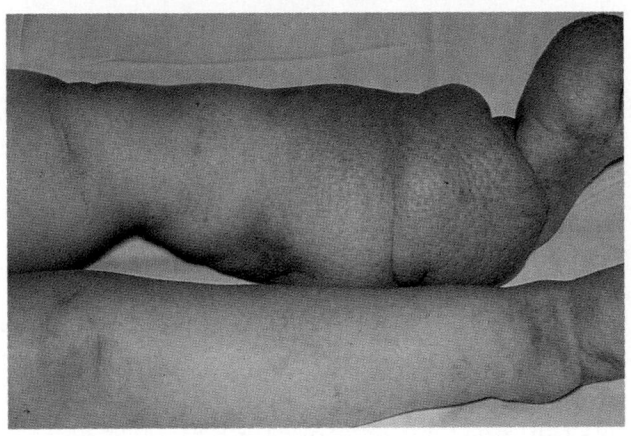

(c) Elephantiasis

such as trichinosis and tapeworms, are acquired by humans through eating raw or incompletely cooked meats. Most worm infections are curable with specific antiworm medications.

CHECKPOINT

1. Briefly contrast viruses, bacteria, fungi, protozoa, and parasitic worms.

2. Which group of pathogens is most difficult to control with drugs? Why is this so?

THE CHAIN OF INFECTION

Epidemiologists are scientists who study the dynamics of disease frequency and distribution.

....

epidemiologist scientist who studies the dynamics of disease frequency and distribution.

These specialists sometimes refer to the series of events necessary to spread disease as the **chain of infection** (see Figure 18.5). This is the series of events necessary to transmit disease from one host to another. Its links are as follows:

reservoir (source of pathogen) → portal of exit (avenue by which pathogen leaves reservoir) → transmission (transfer of pathogen to new host) → portal of entry (avenue by which pathogen enters new host) → infection of **susceptible** (having little resistance to a disease) host (pathogen overcomes host defenses and establishes parasitism)

....

chain of infection series of events necessary to transmit disease from one host to another.

susceptible having little resistance to a disease.

Figure 18.5
The Chain of Infection

A key idea in epidemiology is that if any one link in this chain can be broken, the spread of a disease will be prevented.

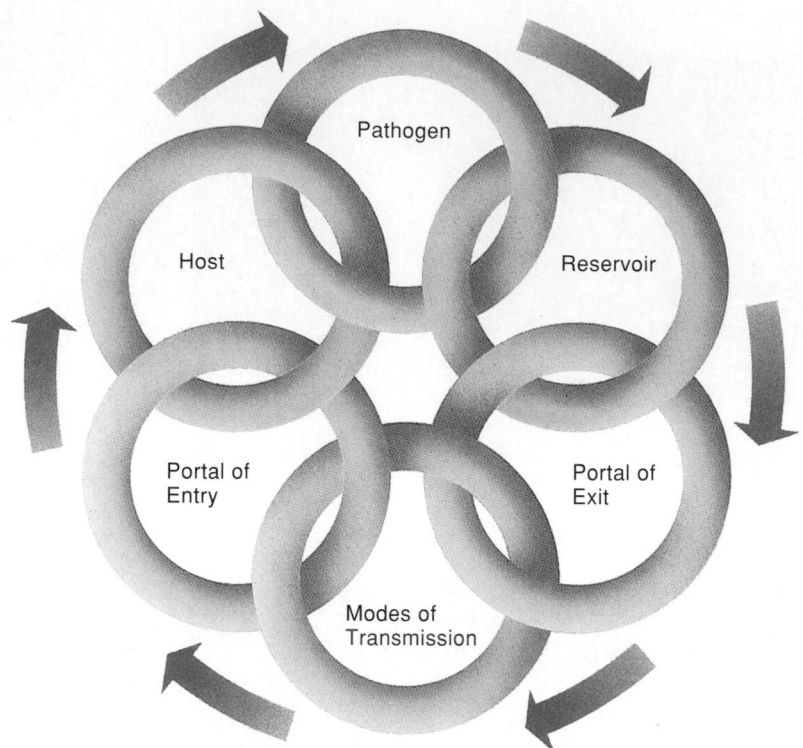

A key idea is that if any one link in this chain can be broken, the spread of a disease will be blocked.

RESERVOIR

The **reservoir** is the source of the pathogen. The reservoir for many human diseases is humans, who may either be ill, or who may be **asymptomatic carriers** of a pathogen. These people harbor a pathogen without symptoms and are capable of transmitting it to other people. For some diseases, the reservoir is an animal or contaminated soil or water.

PORTAL OF EXIT

Pathogens leave the body of an infected person or other host through the **portal of exit.** They leave

....

reservoir the source of a pathogen.

asymptomatic carrier a person who harbors a pathogen without symptoms and is capable of transmitting it to other people.

portal of exit the avenue by which pathogens leave the body of an infected host.

the human body through the skin and mucous membranes (in the case of many sexually transmitted diseases), feces (for intestinal infections), semen and vaginal secretions (for HIV and hepatitis B), blood (also for HIV and hepatitis viruses), saliva (mumps and mononucleosis), and nose and throat discharges (colds and influenza).

TRANSMISSION

Transmission is the transfer of a pathogen to a new host. Different authorities use different systems of classifying the methods of disease transmission. The following is one widely used system of classifying transmission of human diseases:[5]

1. *Contact Transmission*

   Direct contact transmission Also called person-to-person transmission. No intermediate object is involved. Examples include touching, kissing, or sexual contact.

   Indirect contact transmission The pathogen is transmitted from its reservoir to a host by

....

transmission transfer of a pathogen to a new host.

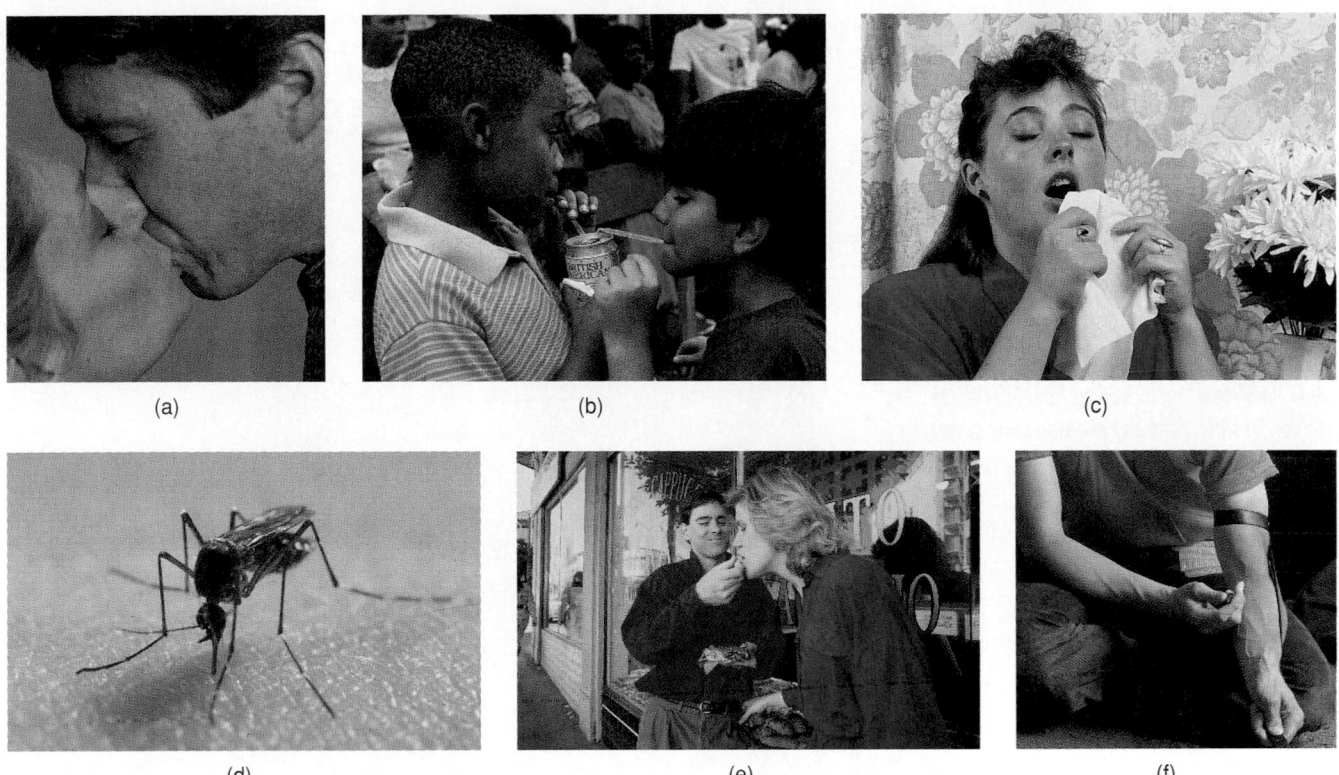

Common methods of disease transmission include (a) by direct contact with an infected person; (b) and (e) through contaminated food or water; (c) through droplet infection; (d) through insect carriers (vectors); and (f) through contaminated objects such as shared injection equipment (indirect contact).

means of a nonliving object. Examples include tissues, towels, bedding, diapers, syringes and needles, cups, and eating utensils.

Droplet infection Pathogens are spread through the air for a distance of *less than one meter* in droplets of saliva, mucus, or sputum discharged into the air by coughing, sneezing, laughing, or talking.

2. *Common Vehicle Transmission* Transmission of disease agents to many people by a common nonliving source such as food, water, or a drug.

3. *Airborne Transmission* Spread of pathogens through the air for a distance of *greater than one meter.* The source of the pathogens could be an infected person or contaminated soil.

4. *Vector Transmission* Insects, ticks, and similar carriers of pathogens are referred to as **vectors.**

....

vector insect or similar carrier of a pathogen.

PORTAL OF ENTRY

The **portal of entry** is where the pathogen enters its new host. Each pathogen has its own specific portal or portals of entry—skin, mucous membrane, digestive system, lining of the respiratory tract, and so forth. Infection can occur only if the pathogen finds its appropriate portal of entry.

INFECTIVE DOSAGE

Exposure to a pathogen does not necessarily mean that you will become infected. Your body's nonspecific defense mechanisms can overcome a certain number of most pathogens. The **infective dosage** is the number of pathogens necessary to overwhelm your body defenses and initiate an

....

portal of entry where the pathogen enters its new host.

infective dosage the number of pathogens necessary to overwhelm body defenses and initiate an infection.

Figure 18.6

Typical Course of a Communicable Disease

Many communicable diseases pass through a series of predictable stages. The incubation period stretches from infection to the appearance of symptoms; the prodromal period includes non-specific symptoms; the typical illness period brings specific disease symptoms, and during the convalescence period one recovers from symptoms, though a relapse of symptoms may occur. Note the dotted line extending from infection to the carrier state. For many diseases, some people become carriers without exhibiting any symptoms.

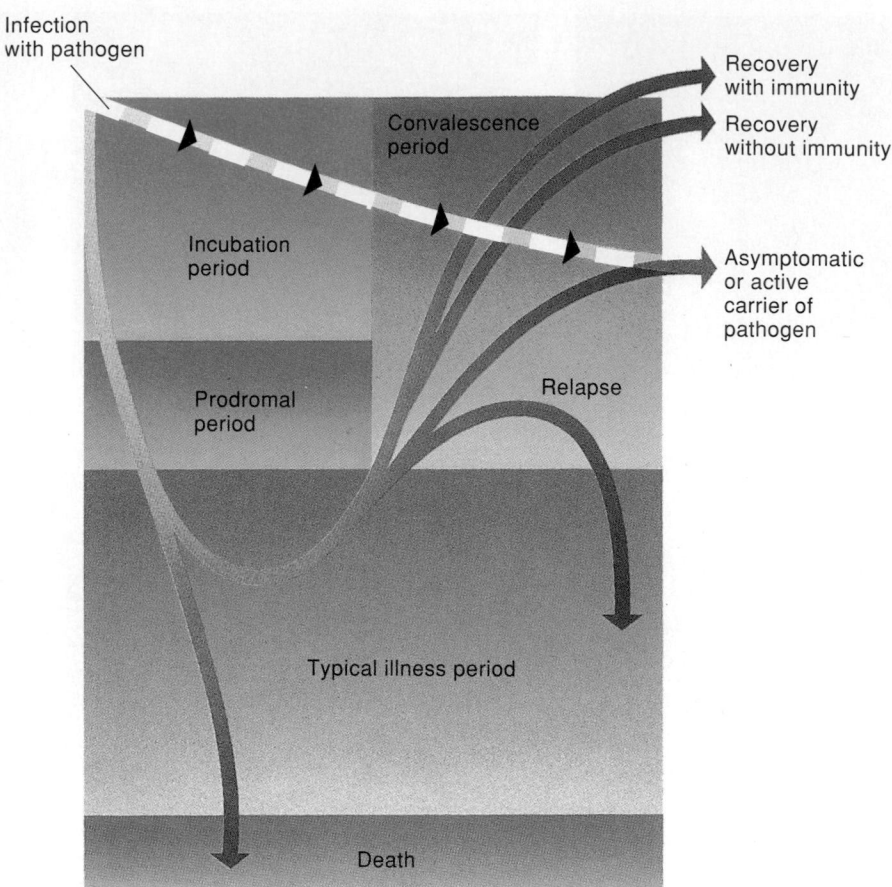

Infection with pathogen

Convalescence period

Incubation period

Recovery with immunity

Recovery without immunity

Asymptomatic or active carrier of pathogen

Prodromal period

Relapse

Typical illness period

Death

infection. The better your body's defenses, the higher this number will be. Thus, a dosage of pathogens that might infect one person might not infect another. Further, for the same person and the same pathogen, the infective dosage varies from day to day depending on life-style factors such as diet, rest, and stress management.

CHECKPOINT

1. What are the links in the chain of infection?

2. What does the term *infective dosage* mean?

COURSE OF A COMMUNICABLE DISEASE

Many (though not all) diseases pass through the following sequence of events (see Figure 18.6). This sequence is especially characteristic of **acute**

diseases, those with a sudden onset and a short duration. **Chronic** communicable diseases, those with a gradual onset and a long duration, tend not to follow such a distinctive course.

INCUBATION PERIOD

After a pathogen has entered the body, there is a period of time before any symptoms appear: This is the **incubation period.** During this time, the pathogen is multiplying, adapting to its new host, and sometimes migrating to a specific part of the body.

Incubation periods can be as short as a few hours (for food poisoning) or as long as many years (for AIDS and Hansen's disease [leprosy]). They are typically a few days to a few weeks.

acute having a sudden onset and a short duration.

chronic having a gradual onset and a long duration.

incubation period interval between infection and appearance of symptoms.

HELP YOUR PHYSICIAN HELP YOU

When you visit your physician because you are feeling ill, you can expect certain questions to be asked as an aid to diagnosis. A little forethought and your full cooperation will help your physician make an accurate diagnosis. Before your visit, become familiar with your family health history. The tendency toward many health conditions is inherited and it will help the physician to know what conditions have been present in your family. Your own health history is also important. In addition, you will likely be asked:

1. When did your symptoms first appear?
2. Did your symptoms develop suddenly or gradually?
3. Are you, or have you been, in a sexual relationship (if a sexually transmitted disease is a possibility)? It is imperative to be honest about this.

4. Have you had a fever? If so, has it been continuous or intermittent, and how long has it lasted?
5. Do you know or suspect that you have been exposed to an illness?

If you have traveled recently, especially if you have been hiking, camping, or traveling out of the country, this information may be very helpful for your physician to make an accurate diagnosis. If your occupation involves any unusual exposure to pathogens, such as working with animals, this information should also be presented. Even the best physician needs complete information to make an accurate diagnosis.

PRODROMAL PERIOD

The **prodromal** (*prō-drō'mal*) **period** is the phase during which nonspecific symptoms appear following the incubation period. The first symptoms to appear tend to be similar for many diseases—fever, headache, aching body, and a vague feeling of discomfort or **malaise** (*ma-lāz'*). It is usually impossible to diagnose a disease by its prodromal symptoms. Most people in this stage of disease will continue with their normal routine of work or school activities, which is unfortunate, because *the late incubation period and prodromal period are the most contagious times for many diseases.*

TYPICAL ILLNESS PERIOD

After a few hours to several days of prodromal symptoms, the more specific symptoms of a disease appear. Now, diagnosis on the basis of symptoms is possible in the case of some diseases (see Communication for Wellness: Help Your Physician Help You), though many illnesses are best diagnosed using laboratory tests. During the typical illness period, the pathogen and the body defenses are engaging in a life-or-death battle. Usually the body defenses, possibly aided by antimicrobial drugs, are victorious and recovery begins.

CONVALESCENCE OR RECOVERY PERIOD

Convalescence is the period of recovery after a disease. As a person is regaining health, even though most disease symptoms may have abated, *some of the pathogens remain alive in the body,* and are held in check by the body's defenses. Improper diet or lack of rest may weaken the body defenses, allowing the pathogen to break free and multiply once again. This causes disease symptoms to return, and is known as a **relapse.** Following any illness, it is advisable to resume normal activities gradually, allowing the body defenses to eradicate the pathogen completely.

TERMINATION OF ILLNESS

The convalescence period is followed by one of three possible states: immunity, resusceptibility, or the carrier state.

Immunity, discussed later in this chapter, is protection from a repeated attack of a disease, lasting anywhere from a few months to a lifetime. This type of immunity is highly specific and often does not even extend to closely related forms of the

prodromal period the initial stage of a disease.

malaise discomfort or uneasiness.

convalescence the period of recovery after a disease.

relapse recurrence of a disease after apparent recovery.

immunity state of being protected from a disease; body defenses that act against specific pathogens.

same illness. For example, having influenza confers immunity only to the specific strain of virus that was involved.

Recovery without immunity means that a person may become infected again by any new contact with the pathogen. This is the case for diseases such as gonorrhea, for which no immunity usually develops.

Someone who has recovered from a disease, but still harbors a pathogen, is called an **active carrier.** This active carrier state occurs with many diseases, such as hepatitis B, mononucleosis, and typhoid fever. For many pathogens, including those causing gonorrhea and genital *Chlamydia,* a person may pass directly from infection to the carrier state, without experiencing any symptoms (see the dashed line in Figure 18.6).

CHECKPOINT

1. What is taking place during the incubation period of a disease?

2. When are many diseases most contagious?

3. What is a relapse and why is it possible?

BODY DEFENSES AGAINST DISEASE

Every day, you are exposed to potentially lethal pathogens. You carry many of them on and in various parts of your body at all times. Yet most of the time you are protected by your many effective body defenses and as a result, you remain healthy. Some of these defenses, the nonspecific defenses, act against pathogens in general, rather than against any one specific pathogen. Collectively, these nonspecific defenses are called **resistance.** Other defenses act against specific pathogens and are called *immunity.* The effectiveness of both resistance and immunity depends on your heredity and on your living habits. Both suffer when you are excessively stressed, when you neglect proper

nutrition or rest, or when you abuse alcohol or other drugs. Among today's greatest threats to your immune system is being infected with HIV, the virus that causes AIDS.

NONSPECIFIC DEFENSES: RESISTANCE

Nonspecific body defenses include the skin and mucous membranes, respiratory cilia, acidic gastric juices, white blood cells, inflammation, and interferons. Healthy skin and mucous membranes, commonly referred to as the "first line of defense," form an effective barrier against many pathogens.

Lining the respiratory tract are **cilia,** countless microscopic hairlike projections (see Figure 16.1 on p. 500) that clear pathogens and other foreign matter from the lungs. These cilia, which wave constantly and rhythmically, carry dust and pathogens (on a layer of mucus) from the lungs to the throat to be swallowed. The cilia are destroyed or paralyzed in heavy smokers, who as a result develop a "smoker's cough" to clear the lungs of mucus and foreign matter.

Many pathogens may be ingested with food or beverages. The highly acidic digestive juices in the stomach kill many, but not all, pathogens.

Our eyes are protected against infection by their constant flow of tears which washes away many bacteria and contains an enzyme that kills bacteria by dissolving away their cell walls.

Many forms of white blood cells (**leukocytes**) are capable of engulfing, killing, and digesting pathogens. This process, called **phagocytosis** (*fāg'ō-sī-tō'sis*) (see Figure 18.7), is highly effective in protecting against infection. White blood cells that are capable of phagocytosis are called **phagocytes.**

Any tissue injury initiates a process called **inflammation.** The injured cells release a chemi-

active carrier someone who has recovered from a disease, but still harbors the pathogen.

resistance the nonspecific defenses against disease.

cilia microscopic hairlike projections that clear pathogens from the lungs.

leukocyte a white blood cell.

phagocytosis engulfing of solid particles by a cell.

phagocytes white blood cells that are capable of phagocytosis.

inflammation tissue reaction to an injury including dilation and increased permeability of capillaries.

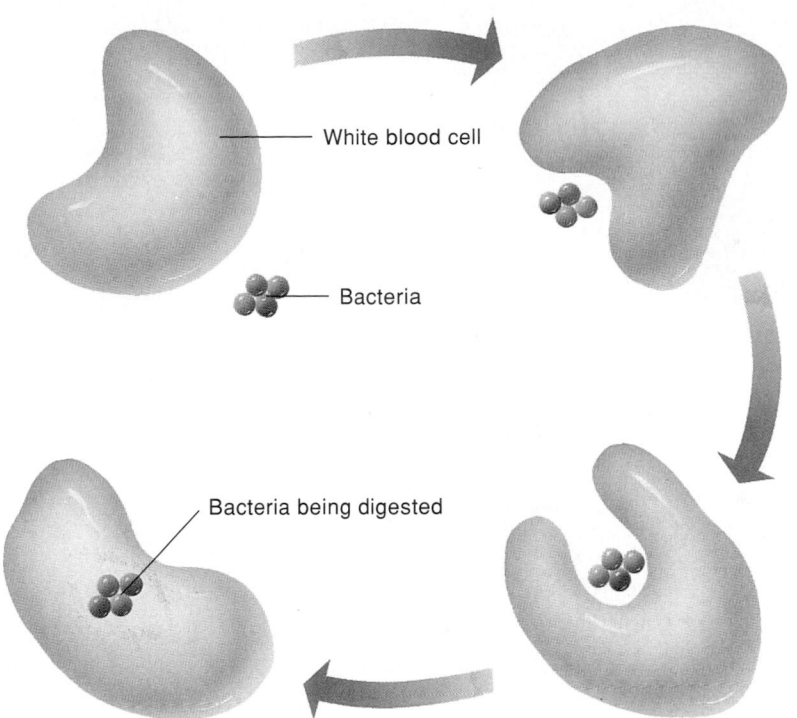

White blood cell

Bacteria

Bacteria being digested

Figure 18.7
Phagocytosis

Phagocytosis, one of our most effective defenses against infection. A white blood cell is attracted to a pathogen, engulfs it, and kills it with powerful digestive enzymes.

cal called **histamine** (*his'-ta-mēn*) that causes dilation and increased permeability of the capillaries (microscopic blood vessels). Inflammation brings more blood into the area of the injury and makes it easier for the phagocytes to squeeze out of the capillaries and attack any bacteria present. Familiar symptoms of inflammation include redness, pain, heat, and swelling. While inflammation can be a painful problem in disorders such as arthritis, it is usually highly beneficial in preventing and combating infections. Terms describing inflammation end in **-itis,** as in *arthritis* (inflammation of joints) and *vaginitis* (inflammation of the vagina).

Interferons (*in-ter-fer'onz*) are a group of proteins released from virus-infected body cells. In several ways, they protect healthy cells from being taken over by viruses. Some interferons prevent viruses from entering healthy cells, while others block viral replication within the cell. Interferons are not specific: They act against viruses in general, rather than just any one type of virus.[6]

----

histamine chemical released from injured cells to cause inflammation; also important in allergic reactions.

itis suffix meaning inflammation of.

interferons proteins released from virus-infected cells to protect healthy cells from viral damage.

Interferons have also shown some promise in preliminary experiments in treating cancers. Only in recent years have the necessary quantities of human interferons become available to allow in-depth research into the role of interferons in cancer control and to determine the potential uses of interferons in preventing and treating viral diseases. Now produced by genetically engineered microorganisms, interferons may have an important future in medicine.

Fever, an increase in body temperature, can slow or halt the replication of some pathogens. Efforts to reduce a fever are thus inadvisable unless the fever is high, perhaps over 101°F. It is always important when you have a fever to drink plenty of nonalcoholic liquids, as you can quickly become dehydrated.

SPECIFIC DEFENSES: IMMUNITY

The human immune mechanism is an important defense against infectious diseases. It plays a central role in a wide range of disorders, including allergies, arthritis, and cancers. AIDS is a disorder of the immune mechanism.

The Immune Mechanism: Stimulus

The purpose of the immune mechanism is to detect the invasion of the body by some harmful outside

Figure 18.8
Development of the Human Immune Mechanism

Development of the human immune mechanism occurs in late fetal development and early infancy. Stem cells from the bone marrow are processed by either the thymus or the bone marrow, to become, respectively, T lymphocytes (T cells) or B lymphocytes (B cells). Upon exposure to antigens, B cells release antibodies to attack pathogens (humoral immunity), while T cells produce cell-mediated immune responses and regulate the B cells.

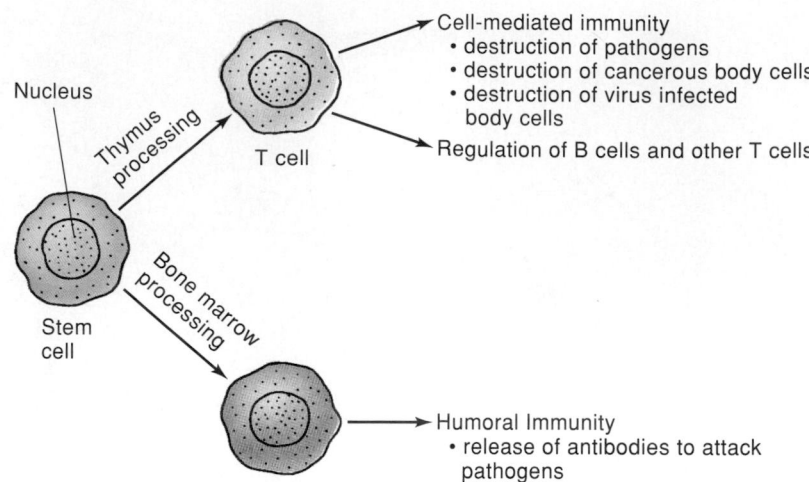

agent and to destroy or inactivate that agent. Any substance that stimulates an immune response is called an **antigen** (*an'ti-jen*). Chemically, most antigens are large molecules such as proteins, carbohydrates, and nucleic acids. Smaller molecules may become antigenic when they enter the body and attach to proteins in the blood.

Antigens occur in many forms. They can be parts or products of pathogens, such as the protein coats of viruses or the toxins of bacteria. Any vaccine is a preparation of antigens. Anything causing an allergic reaction is acting as an antigen (the allergic symptoms result from the immune response). Also, every cell in your body contains chemicals that would be antigenic to someone else, as in organ transplants. Some people even produce immune responses against their own tissue antigens, causing autoimmune disorders, discussed later in this chapter.

The Immune Mechanism: Response

The human immune response is carried out by special white blood cells called **lymphocytes** (*lim'fō-sītz*). These lymphocytes are produced in the bone marrow as immature **stem cells,** not yet capable of an immune response (see Figure 18.8). Some of the stem cells are processed by the thymus (a gland

lying just under the sternum, or breast plate, in the chest). These stem cells become **T lymphocytes (T cells),** which produce a type of immunity called **cell-mediated immunity.** Other stem cells are processed by the bone marrow. These stem cells become **B lymphocytes (B cells),** which produce another form of immunity called **humoral immunity.**

Cell-Mediated Immunity T cells respond to antigens by producing cell-mediated immunity. In general, the target of a cell-mediated immune response is a cell—either the cell of a pathogen or an abnormal human body cell. The latter include cells infected with intracellular pathogens, such as viruses, and cells that have become cancerous.

T cells act in various ways.[7] Some, called T-helper or T-4 lymphocytes, activate B cells and other T cells. T-4 lymphocytes are of special significance as they are infected and destroyed by the AIDS virus. This loss of T-4 lymphocytes impairs the function of both humoral and cell-mediated immunity. Other T cells, called T-suppressor lymphocytes, sup-

---

antigen any substance that stimulates an immune response.

lymphocyte type of white blood cell involved in producing immunity.

stem cell immature lymphocyte.

T lymphocyte or **T cell** lymphocyte processed by the thymus and capable of producing cell-mediated immunity.

cell-mediated immunity the immune responses produced by T lymphocytes.

B lymphocyte or **B cell** lymphocyte processed by the bone marrow and capable of producing humoral immunity.

humoral immunity the immune responses produced by the release of antibodies by B lymphocytes.

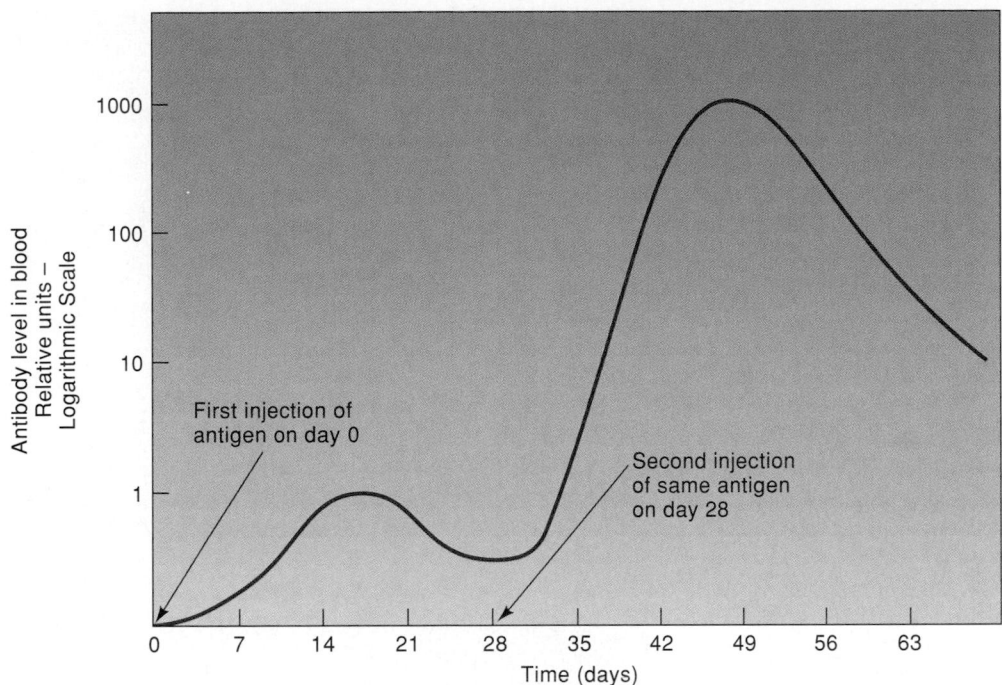

Figure 18.9
Primary and Secondary Immune Response

Upon first exposure to an antigen (by either natural exposure or injection), the immune response is slow and weak. Upon a subsequent exposure to the same antigen, the response is rapid and strong because of B and T memory cells, so the same disease usually does not recur.

press the activity of the B cells, preventing undesirable immune responses. Still other T cells, called T-killer or T-cytotoxic cells, dissolve abnormal cells, such as cancerous cells or virus-infected cells. A final type of T cell releases inflammation-producing chemicals in response to specific antigens.

Humoral Immunity The word *humoral* refers to a fluid. This form of immunity is called humoral because, upon exposure to antigens, B cells release **antibodies,** also called **immunoglobulins,** to circulate in the blood and to be present on the surface of mucous membranes. Antibodies are Y-shaped proteins that chemically bond to specific antigens. In this way, antibodies inactivate or destroy antigens. For example, viruses and bacterial toxins may be inactivated by antibodies. Other types of antibodies clump bacteria together, making it easier for *phagocytes* to clean up an infection.

Active Immunity

When first exposed to any particular antigen, such as a pathogen, the immune response is slow and weak. If other body defenses are unable to overcome the pathogen, disease will occur before immunity can develop. Upon future exposure to the same

antigen, however, the immune response will be rapid and strong, so the same disease usually does not recur (see Figure 18.9). There are some diseases for which immunity usually does not develop, however. In other cases, there are some individuals who will fail to develop immunity to a disease for which most people do develop immunity.

The mechanism of **immune memory** is that once B cells or T cells "learn" a certain immune response, some of them settle down in the lymph nodes and spleen as **memory cells.** When memory cells sense the presence of "their" antigen in the body, they rapidly spring into action, multiplying and destroying the pathogen before it has a chance to develop.

The form of immunity we have just described, in which long-term immune memory develops, is called **active immunity.** If immunity results from a natural exposure to an antigen, such as having a disease or symptomless infection, it is called *nat-*

antibodies or **immunoglobulins** Y-shaped protein molecules produced by B lymphocytes to destroy or inactivate antigens.

immune memory memory of a specific immune response, allowing a rapid immune response upon repeated exposure to an antigen.

memory cells B or T cells that retain the memory of a specific immune response.

active immunity immunity that develops from exposure to an antigen and produces immune memory of that specific immune response.

ural active immunity. Fortunately, you don't always need to have a disease in order to develop immunity. You can often gain immunity through a **vaccine**, which is a preparation of one or more antigens used to stimulate the development of active immunity. Immunity resulting from a vaccine is called *artificial active immunity*. It is often as effective as the immunity you build after having the disease and it is much safer.

Artificial Active Immunity (Vaccines) The concept of a vaccine is to expose a person to an antigen, such as might be found in a pathogen, but in a harmless form. This will lead to the development of active immunity as if the person had been exposed to the actual pathogen, but without the risks involved in experiencing the disease.

Vaccines contain various types of antigens, including dead or inactivated pathogens, living modified strains of pathogens, **toxoids** (modified bacterial toxins), chemicals derived from pathogens (such as viral protein), and genetically engineered organisms. As an example of the latter, at least one type of experimental AIDS vaccine has been produced by splicing genes from the AIDS virus into the virus formerly used as smallpox vaccine.

From time to time the safety of some particular vaccine is publicly questioned. While no medical procedure, even taking an aspirin, is totally free of risk, the benefit-to-risk ratio of most immunizations is quite favorable. Interesting social issues arise from the fact that while all of society benefits from the use of a vaccine, including those members who fail to be immunized, the risk falls only on those who receive the immunization.

Unfortunately, the potential for expensive lawsuits associated with vaccine use (either because a vaccine has failed to protect, has caused an adverse reaction, or has been perceived to do so) has greatly dampened the enthusiasm of corporations for developing and producing vaccines. In at least one case (diphtheria-pertussis-tetanus vaccine) the federal government has had to assume the product liability in order to ensure the nation of an adequate supply of vaccine.

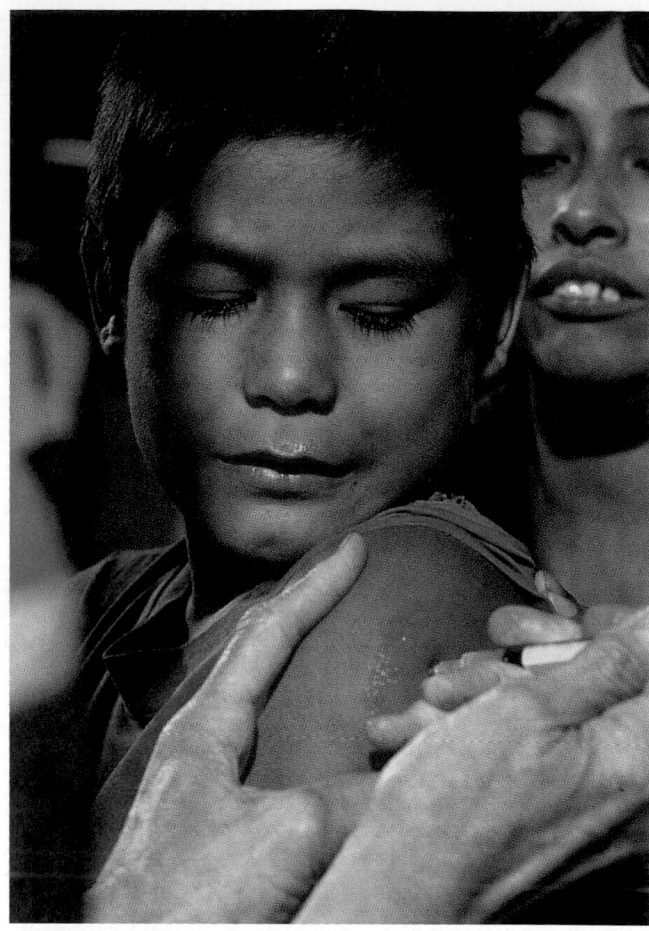

Childhood immunization saves lives and prevents damaging illnesses. Vaccines are preparations of antigens that stimulate development of specific immune responses (active immunities) without one having to experience the diseases.

Table 18.1 presents a suggested immunization schedule for children in the United States. Physicians, schools, and health departments all actively encourage immunization of children, but the ultimate responsibility falls on parents. Some states assign this responsibility to the schools instead of the parents. In such cases the principal may go to jail if a child is not immunized. Adults have a lifelong responsibility to themselves to obtain appropriate immunizations (see Feature 18.2).

Passive Immunity

Passive immunity results when someone receives antibodies that have been produced by another person or by an animal. Passive immunity provides

---

vaccine preparation of one or more antigens used to stimulate the development of active immunity.

toxoid modified bacterial toxin used as a vaccine.

passive immunity short-term immunity that results from receiving preformed antibodies.

Table 18.1
Recommended Schedule of Immunizations for Children in the United States

Vaccine	Birth	2 Months	4 Months	6 Months	12 Months	15 Months	4–6 Years[a]	14–16 Years
DTP: Diphtheria, Tetanus, and Pertussis Vaccine		✔	✔	✔		[b]	✔	
TD: Adult Tetanus-Diphtheria Booster								✔[c]
POLIO: Live Oral Polio Vaccine Drops (OPV) or Killed (Inactivated) Polio Vaccine Shots (IPV)		✔	✔			[b]	✔	
MMR: Measles, Mumps, and Rubella Vaccine						[d]	[e]	
HIB: Haemophilus b Option A[f]		✔	✔	✔		✔		
Conjugate Vaccine Option B[g]		✔	✔		✔			

Vaccine		Birth	2 Months	4 Months	6–18 Months
HB: Hepatitis B Vaccine	Option A		✔	6	6
	Option B	6	6		6

[a]Vaccine to be given before school entry.
[b]Many experts recommend these vaccines at 18 months.
[c]Adult tetanus-diphtheria booster should be given every 10 years throughout life for people at high risk of tetanus.
[d]In some areas this dose of MMR vaccine may be given at 12 months.
[e]Many experts recommend this dose of MMR vaccine be given at entry to middle school or junior high school.
[f]HIB vaccine is given in either a four-dose schedule (A) or a three-dose schedule (B), depending on the type of vaccine.
[g]Hepatitis B vaccine can be given simultaneously with DTP, Polio, MMR, and Haemophilus b Conjugate Vaccine at the same visit.

Note: These recommendations are for the United States. In recent years, this schedule has changed frequently. For example, it is likely that chicken pox vaccine will have been added before this text is published.

Source: Compiled from various issues of U.S. Public Health Service, Centers for Disease Control, Morbidity and Mortality Reports.

FEATURE 18.2
WHAT IMMUNIZATIONS DO *I* NEED?

Immunization does not end with childhood. Assuming that you have completed your basic childhood immunizations, here are some immunizations that you may still need.

- *Adult Tetanus-Diphtheria Booster* The tetanus bacterium grows in wounds, releasing a deadly nerve poison that causes constant muscle contraction (tetanus). The spores of the tetanus bacterium are very widespread and contaminate wounds. Various types of injury are associated with tetanus, not all of which may appear important when they occur. In general, puncture-type wounds are most likely to become contaminated with the spores of tetanus and provide the oxygen-free habitat in which those spores can flourish. People who have a relatively high risk of injury should receive adult tetanus diphtheria booster vaccine every ten years. Others should receive this vaccine if any injury has occurred and more than ten years has passed since the last booster.

- *Hepatitis B Vaccine* Now a routine infant immunization, this vaccine is also highly recommended for adults who have occupational exposure to blood or other body fluids. It is further recommended for people who

have multiple sex partners. It is administered in three injections over a period of several months.

- *Influenza Vaccine* Annual influenza immunization is recommended for all people age 65 or older, as well as people of any age who have chronic respiratory or circulatory disorders.

- *Pneumococcal Pneumonia Vaccine* (Pneumovax) A one-time immunization, recommended for the same people as influenza vaccine. Repeated immunization at six- or seven-year intervals is recommended for certain high-risk individuals.

- *Travel Vaccines* People preparing to travel to certain parts of the world (usually developing countries) should check with their physician or public health department for current recommendations for immunizations needed against diseases that are prevalent in those areas.

- *New Vaccines* New genetic-engineering techniques make possible vaccines against additional diseases. Considerable effort is being devoted to the development of safe and effective new vaccines for diseases such as AIDS and hepatitis A.

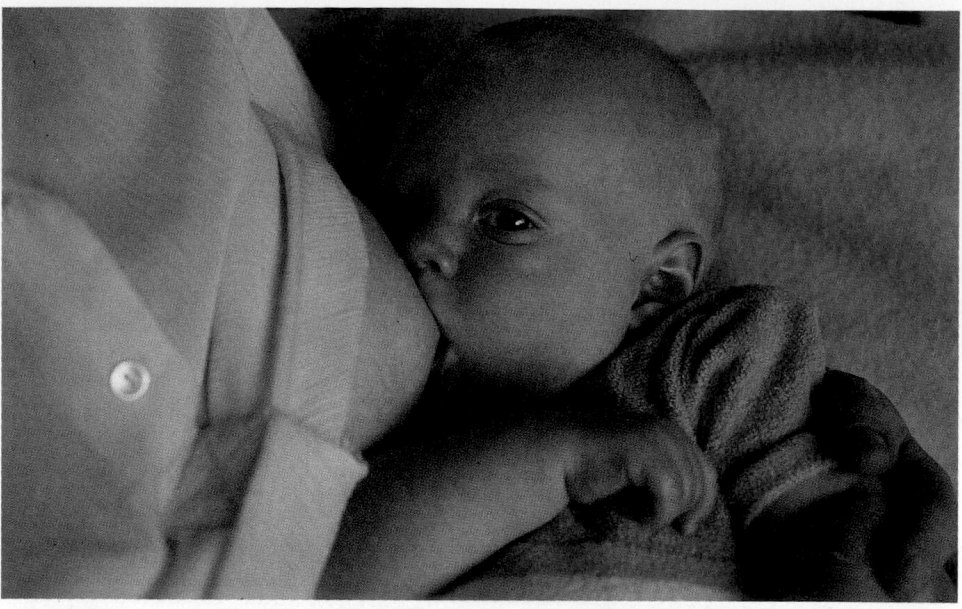

Human milk contains antibodies that help protect an infant from infections such as infant diarrhea.

instant protection, but it is short term as no immune memory develops.

Natural passive immunity results from antibodies that are passed from a mother to her baby. This occurs in two ways. First, antibodies cross the placenta from mother to fetus, producing **congenital immunity.** The newborn infant needs this protection because at birth his or her own immune mechanism is still poorly developed. Half of the antibodies that have crossed the placenta break down within the first 21 days following birth; three-quarters are gone after 42 days. But the need for protection remains. Continued passage of immunity from mother to child takes place through breastfeeding. The *colostrum* produced by the breasts the first day or two following birth is very rich in antibodies. Human milk also contains antibodies that help prevent infections in infants.

Artificial passive immunity is immunity resulting from the injection of antibodies isolated from human or animal blood or produced by genetic engineering (see Feature 18.3). Injections of anti-

natural passive immunity immunity resulting from antibodies that are passed from a mother to her baby, across the placenta and in breastfeeding.

congenital immunity immunity resulting from antibodies crossing the placenta.

artificial passive immunity immunity resulting from the injection of antibodies.

bodies are given when a person is at risk of some disease to which he or she is not immune. Some of these injections are known as gamma globulin, immune globulin, antitoxin, and antivenin. Some specific examples include tetanus antitoxin (tetanus immune globulin), for injured persons who have not been adequately immunized against tetanus; hepatitis immune globulin, for people exposed to hepatitis; rabies immune globulin, for people bitten by rabid animals; and snake antivenins, for snakebite victims.

CHECKPOINT

1. What are some important nonspecific body defenses against disease?

2. What is an antigen?

3. What is in a vaccine?

4. What kind of immunity do T cells produce? What about B cells?

5. What is the difference between active immunity and passive immunity?

IMMUNE DISORDERS

Many things can go wrong with a person's immune mechanism. Immune disorders range from rare to common and from minor to life-threatening. They

FEATURE 18.3

MONOCLONAL ANTIBODIES

Traditionally, when antibodies have been needed for disease prevention or treatment or for laboratory diagnostic purposes, they have been derived from human or animal blood. The problem with this is that blood-derived antibodies are never pure—blood always contains a mixture of many kinds of antibodies and there is no way to separate out one particular kind. This can cause adverse reactions when the antibodies are injected into a person and can reduce the reliability of diagnostic tests.

In recent years, extremely pure preparations of single types of antibodies have become available—these are *monoclonal antibodies.* B cells can be "taught" to produce a certain antibody (one B cell produces only one kind of antibody) and, in a broth culture, will divide and produce their anti-

body for a period of time; then they will die. Apparently a genetic "counter" keeps track of their cell divisions and only allows a certain number of cell generations.

Cancer cells have no genetic limitation on their reproduction—they can go on dividing forever. Monoclonal antibodies are commercially produced by fusing together a "trained" B cell and a lymphatic cancer cell. The resulting hybrid cell, called a *hybridoma* (hi-brid-ō'mah) cell, will produce the desired antibodies and will continue to divide and produce antibodies indefinitely, given proper care. The availability of monoclonal antibodies has made possible a great number of new diagnostic tests and holds considerable promise for new disease treatments.

---

include immune deficiencies, allergies, and autoimmune disorders.

IMMUNE DEFICIENCIES

Immune deficiency can affect cell-mediated immunity, humoral immunity, or both. An inadequate immune response leads to frequent and/or severe infections and an increased risk of cancer.

Some forms of immune deficiency are inherited. Typically, genes for immune deficiency are recessive, meaning that two normal parents can have a child with an immune deficiency disorder if both carry the recessive gene for this trait. As yet, there is no fully satisfactory method of treating inherited immune disorders.

Radiation also causes immune deficiency. A radiation accident, excessive exposure to x-rays, or intensive doses of radiation given as treatment for cancer can damage the bone marrow and lymphocytes (see Chapter 24).

Chemicals can destroy lymphocytes and thus damage the immune mechanism. These chemicals include certain medically prescribed drugs such as the antibiotic chloramphenicol, some street or recreational drugs such as butyl nitrate (poppers), and certain industrial chemicals. Chemotherapy for cancer can also suppress the formation of new white blood cells, resulting in immune deficiency.

Finally, *viruses* can infect the lymphocytes, causing immune disorders such as HIV infection (AIDS). (HIV infection is discussed at length in Chapter 19.)

ALLERGY

Although they are not communicable diseases, allergies do involve the immune mechanism. An **allergy,** also called **hypersensitivity,** is an immune response against an otherwise harmless substance, called the **allergen.** Some allergies, such as "hay fever," are produced by humoral immune responses, in which case they become evident within a few hours after exposure to the allergen. Other allergies, such as poison ivy, are caused by cell-mediated immune responses and become evident in a day or two after exposure to the allergen. The unpleasant symptoms associated with allergies are "side effects" of the immune responses, caused by histamine and a variety of other chemicals released from cells during immune responses.

It is unclear why people develop allergies, though heredity and stress are known to play roles. Common symptoms in allergies include respiratory problems such as asthma and hay fever; skin problems such as rashes, itching, and hives; red, watering eyes; and occasional unusual symptoms, such as headaches or arthritis, that may not be recognized as allergy symptoms.

Skin tests, laboratory tests, and diets in which various foods are eliminated for periods of time, are often used to identify the substance causing an

....

allergy or **hypersensitivity** immune response against an otherwise harmless environmental substance.

allergen the substance causing an allergy.

allergy. If that substance cannot be avoided, it is sometimes possible to reduce the allergic symptoms by using antihistamines or other drugs. A last resort in treating an allergy is desensitization through a series of injections of tiny amounts of the substance causing the allergy. This may require hundreds of injections, costing hundreds or thousands of dollars, but is often successful.

Some allergic reactions to insect bites or certain drugs, such as penicillin, may be fatal. These severe reactions, called **anaphylaxis** (*an-a-fil-lak'sis*) or **anaphylactic shock,** require immediate emergency treatment. Immune responses include the release of chemicals that cause excessive dilation (opening) of blood vessels and constriction (closing) of bronchioles (air ducts) in the lungs. The results may include severe lowering of blood pressure, stagnation of the blood flow, and extreme difficulty in breathing. Anaphylaxis is usually characterized by redness and swelling or puffiness of the face, difficulty in breathing, and a rapid, weak pulse. Death may occur. Part of the treatment is injection or inhalation of epinephrine (commonly called adrenaline), which people with severe insect sting allergies are advised to carry at all times.

AUTOIMMUNE DISORDERS

Like allergies, autoimmune disorders are noncommunicable disorders of the immune mechanism. **Autoimmune disorders** may occur when the immune mechanism fails to recognize a person's own body cells and attacks that person's own body tissues. The result is the gradual, progressive degeneration of tissues or organs, under the attack of either cell-mediated or humoral immune processes.[8] Any part of the body can be damaged. Some possibly autoimmune disorders include systemic lupus erythematosis (lupus), rheumatoid arthritis, Type I diabetes, and some types of degeneration of the kidneys or thyroid gland. We say "possibly autoimmune" because there is also the possibility that what appears to be an autoimmune disorder actually results from infection of the

affected tissue by an unrecognized intracellular pathogen, such as a virus or prion. Treatment of autoimmune disorders usually involves suppressing the immune response. Current treatment methods usually just slow the disease process, rather than curing it. Several of the autoimmune disorders are discussed in Chapter 21.

CHECKPOINT

1. What are three major causes of immune deficiency?
2. What causes an allergic reaction?
3. What is an autoimmune disorder?

PREVENTION AND CONTROL OF COMMUNICABLE DISEASES

Even though communicable diseases are no longer the leading cause of death in the United States, their pathogens are still prevalent. Only unrelenting efforts keep them from reemerging as major killers. Efforts to control communicable diseases can be grouped into four general categories: leading a healthful life-style, immunization, treating diseases when they occur, and public health efforts.

HEALTHFUL LIFE-STYLE

You encounter potentially lethal disease agents every day of your life. Yet, most of the time, you successfully resist invasion by these organisms and remain healthy. Your ability to do this depends, to a great extent, on a healthful life-style, including proper diet, sufficient rest, adequate exercise, avoiding harmful substances, stress management (see Feature 18.4), avoiding possible exposure to diseases (see Feature 18.5), and obtaining needed immunizations (review Feature 18.2).

Diet and Disease

Optimum effectiveness of pathogen-fighting body defenses requires adequate nutrition. Various unusual "immunity-boosting" diets have been suggested over the years, but none has stood the test of critical scientific examination. Certain nutrients have, however, been identified as helping to maintain a strong immune system. Among them are the following:

anaphylaxis or **anaphylactic shock** a massive, potentially fatal allergic reaction.

autoimmune disorder an immune response against part of your own body.

FEATURE **18.4**

PSYCHONEUROIMMUNOLOGY: STRESS AND COMMUNICABLE DISEASES

The many links among the mind, nervous system, hormonal system, and immune system form the basis of the field of medicine called *psychoneuroimmunology*. Since psychologist Robert Adler's pioneering experiments on psychoneuroimmunology at the University of Rochester in the 1970s, a huge body of evidence has been amassed to demonstrate the concepts of psychoneuroimmunology.[a] Among this evidence is the following:

- Nerve endings are present in the organs of the immune system, including the thymus, lymph nodes, spleen, and bone marrow.

- The circulating immunity-producing lymphocytes respond directly to hormones produced by the nervous system and released into the bloodstream.

- Changes in hormone levels and neurotransmitter (see Chapter 15) levels affect immune responses and vice versa.

- Immune system cells carry on their surface specific receptors for endorphins and many other hormones.

- Lymphocytes produce tiny amounts of the same neurotransmitters and hormones produced by the nervous system and the pituitary gland.

- Intensive or prolonged stress reduces the ability of immune cells to produce immune responses.

- Psychoactive drugs (drugs that affect the nervous system), including alcohol, marijuana, cocaine, heroin, and nicotine, also affect the immune response, generally suppressing it.

As we learned in Chapter 4, moderate amounts of stress may *increase* your resistance to stressors, including pathogens. But when stress levels are too high for too long, body defenses become exhausted, and both specific and nonspecific defense mechanisms become impaired. Pathogens that are ordinarily held under control are then free to produce disease.

The common cold is a good indicator of excessive stress. You are frequently—perhaps daily—exposed to the viruses that cause colds. Most of the time you successfully resist these viruses. During periods of increased stress, however, you are much more likely to develop colds. If you were to keep a record for a year or so of every cold or other health problem you developed, with notations on concurrent life events, it would probably become quite evident that most of your illnesses were stress related.

This record-keeping technique can help you recognize your limits. If certain life events stress you to the point where disease is predictable, it is obvious that these events exceed your ability to cope with stress. If you apply the information on stress management that you learned in Chapter 4, you may be able to deal with these situations in less stressful ways. If stress remains a problem, you may find it beneficial to eliminate one or more highly stressful activities. Not only will you avoid the inconvenience and discomfort of frequent minor ills such as colds, but in the long run, you will help prevent more serious problems such as heart disease and cancer.

[a]Kiecolt-Glaser, J., and Glaser, R. "Mind and Immunity." In Goleman, D., and Gurin, J. (eds.), *Mind/Body Medicine*. Yonkers, NY: Consumer Reports Books, 1993.

FEATURE **18.5**

WASH YOUR HANDS!

The simple act of washing your hands is one of the most effective disease-preventing methods. Many pathogens can be carried in great numbers on the hands. Though hand washing can't remove every single pathogen, it can reduce their number to below that which is necessary to cause infection.

Some specific reasons for hand washing are:

- Most colds are caught when you rub your eyes or nose with hands that are contaminated with a virus that has been acquired through shaking hands or touching contaminated objects.

- Many forms of diarrhea can be caught by eating with hands that have been contaminated with human or animal feces.

- Many cases of *Salmonella* infection are transmitted when someone cuts up poultry (which often carries *Salmonella*) and then handles other foods without hand washing.

- Hepatitis A is very commonly transmitted when infected food-handlers fail to wash their hands after using the toilet.

- Many infections of hospital patients occur because health personnel fail to wash their hands between patients.

Though it's some of the world's oldest advice, it's well worth repeating: wash your hands before eating, cooking, or handling food; after using the toilet; and after being around someone with a cold. Further, those who work in health care must be very thorough in washing their hands between patients.

One last bit of advice: When for any reason, such as at an accident scene, you have contact with blood or other human body fluids, wear latex gloves. AIDS and hepatitis viruses may enter the skin through small abrasions before they can be washed off.

- beta-carotene (precursor to Vitamin A), acts as an antioxidant and stimulates certain pathogen-fighting white blood cells
- Vitamin B₆, necessary for production of white blood cells
- folic acid, increases the activity of white blood cells
- Vitamin C, antioxidant and necessary for healthy barrier membranes, also an immune stimulant
- Vitamin E, antioxidant and immune stimulant
- selenium, a micronutrient (required in very small amounts) that appears to help defend from bacteria
- zinc, another micronutrient, small amounts promote wound healing, large doses impair immunity

The ideal quantities for these nutrients are still uncertain and may, in fact, vary considerably from person to person. An optimal level for one person might be too much for another. And as large doses of some of these nutrients have actually been found to impair body defenses, they must be taken with caution. The best approach may be a varied diet with plenty of fresh fruits and vegetables and whole grains. Make sure that you meet the Recommended Daily Allowances of all the essential nutrients. If "vitamin pills" are necessary to achieve these allowances, it is best to avoid taking really large dosages of any nutrients until further research establishes their value and safety.

Alcohol, Tobacco, and Other Drugs

Toxic substances clearly impair your body's ability to fight pathogens. Alcohol has been proven to suppress both the humoral and cell-mediated branches of immunity. Tobacco smoke paralyzes or destroys the respiratory cilia, leading to frequent or chronic respiratory infection. Smoking has also been shown to shorten the time span between infection with HIV and the development of AIDS, indicating that smoking does impair immunity. Some street drugs are also known to suppress immunity and other body defenses. Take a moment right now to assess your disease prevention behavior by completing the assessment, In Your Hands: Your Disease-Prevention Behavior.

IMMUNIZATION

Only one disease—smallpox—has ever been completely eradicated. This was accomplished through case-finding and immunization, probably the only way that any disease will ever be eradicated. In the United States, the incidence of many diseases has been drastically reduced through immunization. Some formerly common diseases, such as polio and diphtheria, are now rare because of immunization. This does not mean that you can forget about such diseases. Their pathogens still exist and nonimmunized people are at risk of infection. Immunization is still very important. Each of us is responsible for ensuring that our children are properly immunized (review Table 18.1) and that we obtain certain immunizations for ourselves (review Feature 18.2).

Keeping records of immunizations is another individual responsibility. You need accurate records both for yourself and for your children. With high levels of personal mobility and the changes that are taking place in health care delivery systems, it is easy for records to become lost or difficult to access. When changing physicians, it is important to provide immunization records to your new medical practitioner.

TREATING COMMUNICABLE DISEASES

Treating diseases with drugs is known as chemotherapy. Drugs that control microscopic pathogens are called **antimicrobial agents.** Highly effective drugs are currently available for controlling each group of pathogens, except viruses. As previously mentioned, in their current state of development, antiviral drugs have a more limited usefulness. The progress of some viral diseases, such as AIDS and herpes, can be slowed, but a complete cure is not yet available.

Some of the first really effective antibacterial drugs were the sulfa drugs (sulfonamides), dating back to 1935. Still in use, sulfa drugs prevent the multiplication of bacteria by interfering with their metabolism. Sulfa drugs and many other antibacterial drugs inhibit, but do not kill, bacteria. Their

antimicrobial agents drugs used to treat diseases caused by microorganisms.

effectiveness depends on how well the body defenses can complete the job.

Antibiotics, such as penicillins and tetracyclines, are substances that microorganisms produce in order to inhibit the growth of competing organisms. Antibiotics are made by culturing the producing organisms in large vats of liquid. From the liquid, the antibiotics are then extracted and purified. Many are chemically modified to enhance their effectiveness. Antibiotics, administered orally and by injection, mainly control bacteria and fungi. Antibiotics do not act on viruses. Antibiotics, thus, cannot cure a cold, influenza, AIDS, or any other viral disease. When using antibiotics or any other drugs, be sure to follow the precautions discussed in Feature 18.6.

Drug Resistance

Drug resistance is the ability of a pathogen to remain unharmed by a specific drug. All over the world, drug resistance has become a major health care problem. Some strains of malaria, tuberculosis, staphylococcus, and gonorrhea, to name but a few, have become almost impossible to cure with any of today's drugs.

....

antibiotics drugs produced by microorganisms and administered to fight bacteria and fungi.

drug resistance the ability of a pathogen to remain unharmed by a specific drug.

FEATURE 18.6

USING DRUGS SAFELY

Modern medications can be lifesavers, no doubt about that. Yet when used improperly, the same drugs can be ineffective, dangerous, or even lethal. When you take any medication, be sure to follow these directions.

1. *Follow all instructions exactly,* including proper dosage, number of times per day the medication is taken, whether food is consumed with the medication, and so on.

2. Use a drug only for the illness for which it was prescribed. *Do not save leftover antimicrobial drugs for future use.* Actually, *there should be no leftover antimicrobial drugs* as only the exact amount needed is usually prescribed and all of it should be used. Further, many drugs break down in storage and may become worthless or even harmful.

3. *Avoid borrowing or lending prescriptions.* Entirely different diseases may have very similar symptoms, and a borrowed drug may be very dangerous. (It is also *illegal* to possess a prescription drug without having a prescription.)

4. *Keep all drugs out of the reach of children.*

5. *Avoid unnecessary use of antibiotics.* The indiscriminate use of antibiotics can have two undesirable effects. First, it can lead to severe allergic reactions to the drug, making future use dangerous. Second, it speeds the development of drug-resistant strains of pathogens.

Microbiologists believe that if any drug is used against a pathogen long enough, eventually the pathogen is likely to become resistant to that drug. Some medical microbiologists go so far as to speak of a coming "post-antimicrobial age," in which all major pathogens will have become resistant to all drugs, putting us back where we were in the "pre-antimicrobial age" of long ago. This is a troubling prediction because before antimicrobial drugs (especially the antibiotics) became available, most deaths, even in the United States, were caused by infectious diseases, such as tuberculosis and pneumonia. The average life span was much shorter than it is today, mainly because of such infections. Now tuberculosis is again on the increase, with some strains more virulent and more drug resistant than those of the past.

Drug resistance develops on a global basis. With today's large volume of international travel, a drug-resistant strain of a pathogen that develops anywhere in the world can appear in the United States in a matter of days. How does resistance develop? Three factors are involved: selection, mutations, and recombination.[9]

Selection   Any population of organisms, such as the pathogens causing an infection, has genetic variability. Some of the individual pathogens are inherently more resistant than others to a drug being used against them. Any drug treatment that fails to destroy all of the pathogens present acts to select in favor of the more-resistant individuals, which may survive and continue to multiply. Their offspring will carry the higher level of resistance.

Mutations   Entirely new ways of resisting drugs arise from time to time when pathogens undergo *mutations* (inheritable changes in genes). For example, if a drug affects one specific enzyme of a pathogen, as is often the case, a mutation might result in a new and different enzyme. This new enzyme might perform the same function, but it would not be affected by the drug.

Recombination   Genes producing drug resistance can spread from one pathogen to another through naturally occurring processes of gene **recombination** (any process that produces a new combination of existing genes). These processes include bacterial mating and carrying of bacterial genes from cell to cell by viruses. Recombination can occur within the same species or between two different species of pathogens.

Certain human activities have contributed to the development of drug resistance. Sometimes antimicrobial drugs are used for minor infections that would soon be eliminated by the body's own defenses. Sometimes antibacterial drugs are used when the pathogen is actually a virus. Sometimes drugs are used haphazardly—skipping doses, not taking the full prescription, and so on. This favors selection and the survival of the more-resistant individual pathogens. Finally, antibiotics in animal

....

recombination any process that produces new combinations of existing genes.

feeds have led to some highly resistant strains of pathogens that are now infecting humans.

PUBLIC HEALTH EFFORTS

As emphasized throughout this book, you are largely responsible for keeping yourself healthy. Yet certain disease-preventing measures would be difficult or even impossible for you to carry out alone. The responsibility for some protection, therefore, has been assumed by public health agencies on city, county, state, and federal levels. Some typical public health activities include the following:

- Health education
- Assuring safe water supplies
- Assuring sanitary sewage disposal
- Assuring safety of food offered for sale
- Restaurant inspection
- Dairy inspection and milk testing
- Rodent and insect control
- Immunization clinics
- Sexually transmitted disease clinics
- Investigation of disease outbreaks
- Maintaining birth and death certificates
- Animal control for rabies prevention

CHECKPOINT

1. List as many functions of public health agencies as you can.
2. What aspects of a person's life-style can help prevent communicable diseases?
3. What is the source of antibiotics?

PROFILES OF SOME COMMON DISEASES

The sexually transmitted diseases are of such great importance that they are covered in a chapter of their own (Chapter 19). In the remainder of this chapter, however, we discuss a few other diseases, including Lyme disease, colds, influenza, bacterial pneumonia, measles, mononucleosis, and hepatitis. These diseases are significant in that they are major causes of lost time and productivity due to missed days at work and at school.

LYME DISEASE

Since being identified in Lyme, Connecticut, in 1975, Lyme disease has been found in almost every state. It is most prevalent in the Eastern half of the United States and in California.[10] It is also present in Europe and Australia.

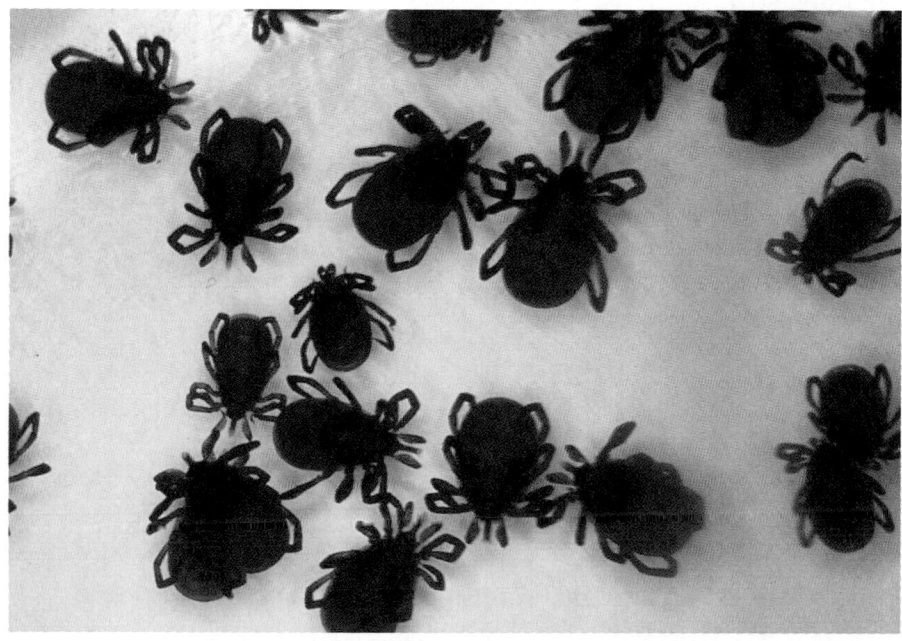

The tick, Ixodes dammini, *one of the vectors of Lyme disease. Actual size is quite small—about the size of a pinhead.*

Lyme disease is caused by a corkscrew-shaped spirochete that is transmitted by the bites of infected ticks. Ticks, in turn, are infected during an immature stage by feeding on infected mice. The complex, two-year life cycle of the tick also includes time spent feeding and mating on deer.

Lyme disease is not fatal, but it can cause crippling, chronic health problems including arthritis, severe headaches, loss of sensation (numbness), and irregularities of the heartbeat. Until Lyme disease became well-known, some people suffered for years from the undiagnosed disease. Now, following diagnosis, often by means of a blood test, Lyme disease can be successfully treated by the use of antibiotics.

The first symptom of Lyme disease is often a "bull's-eye" rash appearing around the site of the tick bite. There may be flulike or mononucleosis-like symptoms such as fever and chills, headache, dizziness, fatigue, and stiff neck. Later, swelling and pain may develop in the joints, especially the knees. This can progress to chronic arthritis.

Lyme disease is prevented by avoiding tick bites through such measures as using effective insect repellents, tucking pants into socks, and wearing long-sleeved, tightly woven shirts (tucked into pants) when working or hiking in tick-infested areas. Try to avoid tall grass and low brush, which are tick havens. Finally, when outdoors, check periodically for ticks attached to your skin and remove them by pulling gently with tweezers. The ticks that transmit Lyme disease are very small and hard to see. Ticks must usually remain attached for 12 hours or longer before the spirochetes are transmitted.

COLDS

The common cold is not a single disease, but a group of over 200 very similar diseases, each caused by its own separate virus[11] (see Feature 18.7). Colds rank at the top among communicable diseases in their nuisance value and the number of days lost from work and school. They also form the basis for a major industry supplying nonprescription remedies, some of which are of dubious value (see Chapter 22).

Colds are highly contagious, with the source of infection being the respiratory discharges of infected people. (Colds are not caused by cold weather.) A cold may be contagious from the day before its symptoms appear until up to five days after their appearance. Transmission is either by the droplet

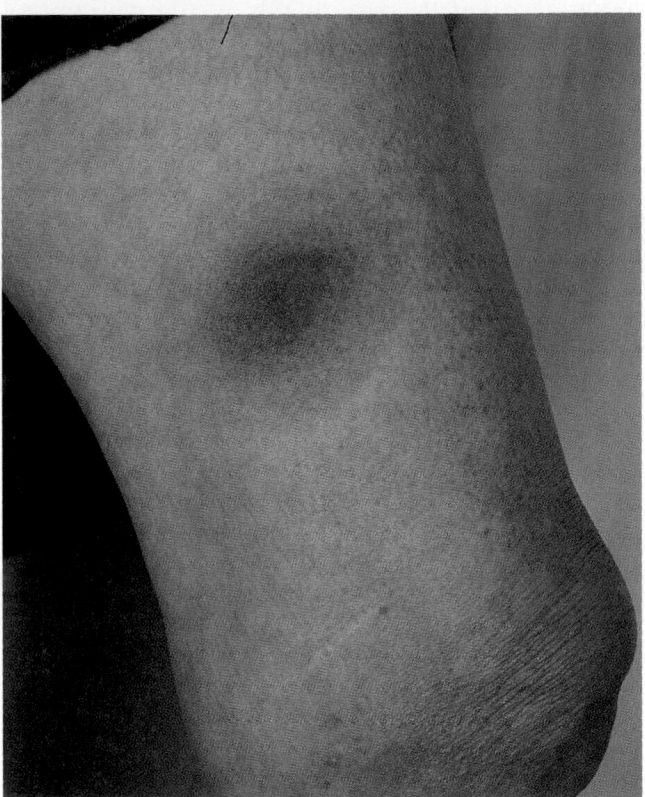

The first symptom of Lyme disease is usually a "bull's-eye rash" that surrounds the area where the tick bite occurred.

infection route or, more often, by rubbing your nose or eyes with virus-contaminated hands.[12] Hand washing is an important preventive measure. The incubation period is short, ranging from about 12–72 hours.

Cold symptoms are quite familiar to most of us: teary eyes, runny nose, sore throat, malaise, aching body, and chills. Even though a room is warm, it may feel icy to you if you have a cold. Your senses of taste and smell are often dulled and, if the cold follows the eustachian tubes into the middle ears, your hearing is affected as well. Although chills typically accompany a fever, there is usually no fever with a cold. If you have coldlike symptoms, but do have a fever, the problem may be influenza or a bacterial infection.

Colds rarely last for more than 7–10 days. This may come as a surprise, because we have all had "colds" that seemed to last much longer than that. Any symptoms that remain beyond a week are very likely the result of a bacterial **secondary infection**

secondary infection one that develops in tissue damaged by a primary infection.

FEATURE 18.7
COLD VIRUSES

The many viruses that cause colds fall into several basic groups:

1. *Rhinoviruses* These are the most frequent causes of colds. Rhinoviruses (*rhino* means nose) mainly infect the cells of the nose and upper respiratory system (rather than the lungs). They produce sneezing, nasal discharges, and teary eyes, but usually no fever (except in young children).

2. *Coronaviruses* These are the second most common causes of colds. Coronavirus colds, like rhinovirus colds, produce mainly sneezing and a runny nose. They are unlike rhinovirus colds in that they are usually transmitted through the air while rhinoviruses spread through hand-to-hand contact. Also, the same coronavirus can infect a person repeatedly, as no immunity develops.

3. *Adenoviruses* Adenovirus colds are more severe than those previously described. They include a dry cough, fever,

red eyes, and a sore throat marked by white or yellowish patches. If the cough becomes productive (sputum is coughed up), a secondary bacterial infection has probably developed in the lungs.

4. *Enteroviruses* Enteroviruses mainly attack the digestive system, but can cause coldlike illness, including coughing, fever, sore throat, and aching muscles.

5. *Respiratory Syncytial Virus (RSV)* Though RSV can infect people of any age, it presents the greatest threat to infants between three weeks and one year of age. With their body defenses not yet well developed, infants sometimes experience very severe infections of RSV, including pneumonia and possible brain damage. After infancy, RSV is usually no worse than any other cold.

(one that develops in tissue damaged by a primary infection) of the membranes that have been disrupted by the viral cold infection. Antibiotics are not useful or recommended for a true viral cold. They are appropriate, though, in treating bacterial infections, which are likely to be the problem when symptoms persist for over a 7–10 days.

What about all of the cough and cold remedies that support your local pharmacy and TV station? There are numerous pros and cons concerning their use (see Feature 18.8 and Chapter 22). One objection to cold-remedy advertising is that it promotes the idea of taking a medication and continuing with normal activities instead of staying home for a day or two, resting, and recovering from the cold. This encourages spreading the virus to others (good for the cold-remedy business) and increases the risk of contracting a secondary bacterial infection.

Even though no medicine available actually cures a cold, you can do some things to alleviate your discomfort and speed your recovery. Foremost is *rest:* Relax, take it easy, and slow down. Your body needs its energy to produce antibodies

FEATURE 18.8
WHAT ABOUT VITAMIN C AND COLDS?

One of the longest-running medical controversies surrounds the value of using Vitamin C to prevent or to treat colds. Dating back to Linus Pauling's 1970 book, *Vitamin C and the Common Cold,* much conflicting information has been published. In one study,[a] male students at the University of Wisconsin were assigned, at random, to receive either Vitamin C (500 mg, four times a day) or identical-looking, inert, placebo tablets. After several weeks of taking the vitamin or placebo tablets, all members of both groups were intentionally exposed to cold viruses through prolonged poker sessions with infected persons. The subjects continued to take their Vitamin C or placebo pills for two additional weeks.

The outcome of this experiment was that Vitamin C *did not prevent* colds. The vitamin recipients were just as likely to

catch a cold as those who received the inert tablets. But the vitamin takers *did experience milder colds* and *recovered more quickly* than placebo takers. Dr. Elliot Dick, who conducted this research, declined to speculate on the significance of the experiment until others have duplicated its results.

In other research, smaller dosages of Vitamin C, ranging from 100 to 200 mg per day, have produced similar results. While some people receiving 2000 mg a day over long periods might experience adverse effects such as development of kidney stones, there is no question about the safety of smaller dosages.

[a]*Medical World News* December 28, 1987, p. 37.

against the cold virus. Try for ten hours of sleep per day. Stay home for a day or two, if possible. Take a good look at your current life-style. What have you been doing—overwork, stress, worry, poor diet, too much alcohol, tobacco, lack of sleep—that has lowered your resistance?

Moisture is very beneficial in keeping nasal passageways and sinuses open and draining. This helps to bring up excess mucus from the lungs. Breathing steam or vapor provides moisture. Take hot showers; breathe the steam from a basin or pan of boiling water; breathe through a warm, damp cloth. Drink plenty of nonalcoholic fluids, especially hot drinks and hot soups. Avoid alcohol. Alcoholic beverages, including beer and wine, actually take more fluid out of your body than they put in. If your throat is sore, *gargle* every hour with a simple solution of one-quarter teaspoon of table salt in eight ounces of warm water.[13]

Cold remedies (see also Chapter 22) may provide some relief of cold symptoms, but do not attack the virus itself.[14] Decongestants contain drugs that shrink the swollen linings of the nose and pharynx, allowing easier breathing. Unfortunately, a rebound response may develop, in which the membranes swell further as the drug begins to wear off, forcing you to continue using the drugs, perpetuating a nonproductive cycle. Also, people with diabetes or hypertension must avoid these drugs as they may raise blood sugar levels and increase blood pressure.

Cough remedies, which suppress the cough reflex, can be of value in several situations. They can help you sleep by controlling dry coughing. They can also help to break a cycle in which coughing acts as an irritant to the lungs, stimulating further coughing. But a cough is usually stimulated by the presence of foreign matter, mucus, or other irritants in the lungs. In this case, the cough reflex *should not be suppressed,* as this material needs to be removed. A cough may also indicate a serious problem such as pneumonia, tuberculosis, congestive heart failure, or lung cancer, which requires prompt medical attention. Cough remedies should not be used for more than a few days.

INFLUENZA ("FLU")

Like colds, influenza (*in"flu-en'za*) is caused by a great number of different viruses. Influenza viruses

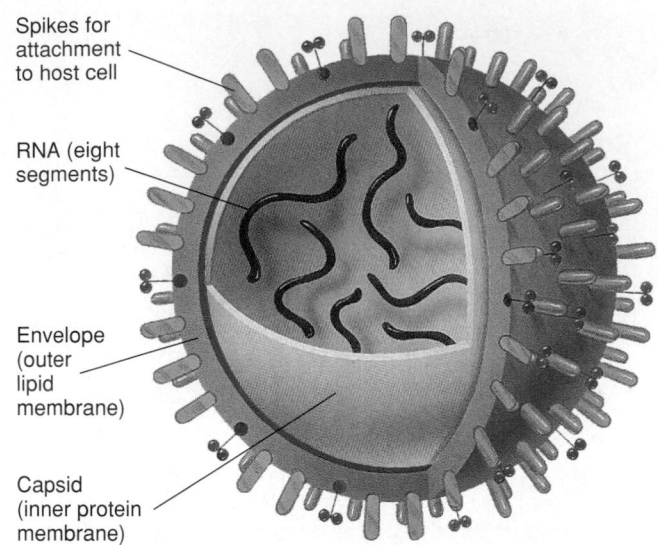

Spikes for attachment to host cell

RNA (eight segments)

Envelope (outer lipid membrane)

Capsid (inner protein membrane)

Figure 18.10
An Influenza Virus

"Flu" viruses are complex in structure and have a high mutation rate.

are grouped into types A, B, and C (see Figure 18.10). Not only are there many viruses in each group, but the mutation rate of these viruses is high, so brand-new forms of influenza appear from time to time. Being infected by a particular influenza virus usually induces a long-term immunity to that specific virus, but not to any other "flu" virus.[15]

Influenza is a respiratory illness, similar in some respects to colds, but more severe. It is especially dangerous to older persons or people with heart or respiratory disorders. Bacterial pneumonia commonly follows the flu in these groups of people. Therefore, the death rate always rises during influenza epidemics.

Like colds, influenza is highly contagious and is transmitted through nose and throat discharges of infected people. Its incubation period is from 24 to 72 hours, leading to a very rapid onset of fever (see Feature 18.9), chills, sore throat, runny nose, headache, muscular aches, and severe coughing. Note that the symptoms do not include digestive disturbances such as diarrhea or vomiting. Many people mistakenly believe that they have the flu when, in fact, they are suffering from food poisoning or a highly contagious viral **gastroenteritis**

gastroenteritis inflammation of the stomach and intestine.

FEATURE 18.9

INFLUENZA AND REYE'S SYNDROME

Reye's (pronounced *rise*) syndrome, first recognized in 1963, includes damage to the brain, liver, and possibly the pancreas, heart, kidneys, spleen, and lymph nodes. It occurs mainly in children under 16 years of age who have taken aspirin to relieve symptoms of influenza or chicken pox. It occurs less commonly in children who have had one of these viral infections and who have not taken aspirin.

Reye's syndrome has also developed in some young adults who have taken aspirin for chicken pox or influenza. Children, adolescents, and young adults are now advised to avoid aspirin if they may have one of those conditions.

Symptoms of Reye's syndrome include nausea and vomiting, disorientation, agitation, seizures, and coma. The cause of Reye's syndrome is not known, but a genetic factor

seems to be involved, as brothers and sisters of victims are also commonly affected. There is no specific cure and about 20 percent of affected children die, sometimes in a matter of hours after the first symptoms appear.

Parents are urged *not* to give aspirin to children who may have influenza or chicken pox. Parents tend to overreact to a child's fever, perhaps not being aware that a fever is part of the body's system of fighting off infections. Only when a child's fever reaches about 101°F should efforts be made to lower the body temperature, unless the child has a history of fever-associated seizures. Even then, if the child has influenza or chicken pox, a physician should be consulted before any medication, including aspirin, is given.

(inflammation of the stomach and intestine). Recovery from the flu should occur within 7–10 days. If symptoms persist beyond 7–10 days, it is likely that secondary bacterial infection has developed and antibiotic therapy may be appropriate.

Annual immunization against influenza is highly recommended for people age 65 or over, those who have chronic circulatory or respiratory disorders, and those whose services are essential to their community. Immunizations are usually given in the fall, as the influenza season usually starts in December, peaks in February or March, and ends in April or May of each year. Each year the vaccine is reformulated in anticipation of the types of flu that seem most likely to become epidemic that year. Some years the vaccine proves highly effective, while other years, it does not. When the vaccine is not effective, it is because of infection by a form of influenza that was not included in the vaccine.

Most of the side effects from influenza vaccine appear in children. They include fever, allergic response to vaccine components, and, in ten of every million vaccinations, *Guillain-Barré* syndrome. Guillain-Barré syndrome is a usually temporary paralysis, although about 5 percent of affected people die (one for every two million immunizations).[16] When this risk is compared with the much higher death rate associated with influenza and its complications, the benefit-to-risk ratio for "flu shots" appears very favorable.

CHECKPOINT

1. How is Lyme disease transmitted to a human?

2. If a person had a runny nose, severe coughing, a sore throat, and a fever, would it more likely be a cold or influenza?

3. If someone has had a "cold" for three weeks, what is likely to be causing the symptoms?

4. What body system does influenza affect?

BACTERIAL PNEUMONIA

Bacterial **pneumonia** (*nu-mō'nē-a;* inflammation of the lungs) can be caused by any of a number of different kinds of bacteria. In the United States, more deaths result from pneumonia than from any other infectious disease.[17] There are over 2 million cases each year, with about 50,000 deaths.[18]

Development of pneumonia is often associated with old age, HIV infection, advanced cancer, chilling, alcoholism and other drug abuse, influenza, and a variety of other disease states. The most common cause of bacterial pneumonia is *Streptococcus pneumoniae,* the pneumococcus. Other bacteria that cause pneumonia include *Staphylococcus*

....

pneumonia inflammation of the lungs.

aureus, Klebsiella pneumoniae, Mycoplasma pneumoniae, Chlamydia pneumoniae, and more.

Pneumonia is usually transmitted by respiratory droplets discharged by healthy asymptomatic carriers. The onset of pneumonia is often sudden. Following a few days of mild respiratory symptoms there may be a high fever (up to 106°F), violent chills, chest pain, and coughing. The **sputum** (substance expelled by coughing) may contain blood, mucus, and pus. With immediate antibiotic therapy the death rate is about 5 percent, but without treatment it is 30 percent.[19]

Pneumonias are classified as lobar or bronchial. **Lobar pneumonia** affects one or more of the five lobes of the lungs. It is usually a **primary infection** (an infection that develops in healthy tissue) as opposed to a secondary infection, and 95 percent of cases are caused by the *pneumococcus.* **Bronchial pneumonia** begins in the bronchi and can spread into the surrounding tissues. Also most often caused by the *pneumococcus,* it is usually a secondary infection following a primary infection such as influenza. It is also common in heart patients.

What is walking pneumonia? **Walking pneumonia,** so named because of its mildness, is usually caused by *Mycoplasma pneumoniae.* Its fatality rate is less than 1 per 1000 cases.[20]

Like many other diseases, pneumonia can be prevented by maintaining good disease resistance through diet and general healthful living habits. A vaccine called Pneumovax will prevent about 80 percent of cases of pneumococcal pneumonia. This vaccine is highly recommended for older people and anyone who has chronic respiratory or circulatory disease.

....

sputum substance expelled by coughing.

lobar pneumonia pneumonia that affects one or more of the five lobes of the lungs, usually a primary infection.

primary infection an infection that develops in healthy tissue.

bronchial pneumonia pneumonia that begins in the bronchi and can spread into the surrounding tissues.

walking pneumonia mild form of pneumonia, usually caused by *Mycoplasma pneumoniae.*

TUBERCULOSIS

Tuberculosis (*tu-ber"ku-lō'sis*) is a bacterial infection caused by the tubercle bacillus, *Mycobacterium tuberculosis.* Similar infections are caused by several other species of Mycobacterium. Most tuberculosis occurs in the lungs, but this bacillus is capable of infecting any part of the body.

Tuberculosis is usually transmitted by inhalation of the bacillus. When inhaled by a healthy person, the bacillus is usually destroyed by phagocytic white blood cells. If the phagocytes fail to destroy all bacillus, the presence of the bacillus stimulates another body defense, in which the bacteria are walled off inside of a small lump of tissue called a **tubercle.** Tubercles, which give the disease its name, contain living bacilli. In less-healthy people, after a period of time the tubercle breaks down to release very large numbers of bacilli that spread destructively throughout the lung and may also spread through the body via the blood and lymphatic system.

Symptoms of advancing tuberculosis include weight loss, coughing, weakness, night sweats, and mild fever. If the spread is not arrested, death results.

Routine testing or screening for tuberculosis involves injecting tuberculin, an antigen obtained from the cells of the tuberculosis organism, into the skin. When checked two days later, a positive test is indicated by the injection site becoming elevated and firm. This indicates that the individual has been infected with tuberculosis at some time, but does not indicate whether the disease is currently active or not. A positive tuberculin test is usually followed up by a chest x-ray. If that shows evidence of tuberculosis, a definitive diagnosis is made by culturing and preparing microscope slides of the sputum (material coughed up from the lungs). The presence of the pathogen in the sputum confirms an active case of tuberculosis.

Tuberculosis is treated by prolonged use of a combination of several drugs. Even when the spread of tuberculosis has been halted, live bacilli

....

tuberculosis an infectious disease caused by the tubercle bacillus.

tubercle the characteristic lesion caused by the tubercle bacillus.

often remain in the lungs and may reactivate at a later date. Reactivation may result from old age, poor nutrition, or any decline in the body defenses, such as in HIV infection. In recent years, drug resistance has made some strains of tuberculosis difficult or even impossible to control.

Tuberculosis has a long history of causing illness and death all over the world. In the past, tuberculosis was the leading cause of death in the United States. At that time, it was called *consumption*. Improved sanitation and diet, along with the introduction of antibiotics, led to a steady decline in the incidence of tuberculosis in the United States until 1985, when it began to increase. Currently, 10–12 million people in the United States are estimated to be infected. Worldwide, at least 3 million people die of tuberculosis every year.[21]

In recent years, tuberculosis has emerged as a special threat to HIV-infected people, as well as those who care for them. In many hospitals, strains of tuberculosis have emerged that are both highly virulent and resistant to many of the important tuberculosis-fighting drugs. Previously, tuberculosis presented little threat to health-care workers, even those with daily contact with infected persons. But newly emerging strains of tuberculosis are highly contagious even to healthy people and are proving more frequently fatal than older strains.

A vaccine, called BCG (bacillus of Calmette and Guerin), is widely used in many countries, but seldom in the United States. Its effectiveness is uncertain and its use causes a positive reaction on the tuberculin skin test that is the main means of screening for cases of tuberculosis in the United States. Here, the emphasis in tuberculosis prevention has been on finding and treating cases to prevent transmission to others. For non-drug-resistant strains, only a short course of treatment is needed to render a person noncontagious to others.

CHECKPOINT

1. What is the most common cause of bacterial pneumonia?

2. Tuberculosis is becoming more of a problem. What groups of people are at greatest risk and what changes in the pathogen are contributing to its increased significance?

MEASLES (RUBEOLA)

Measles (rubeola) (*roo-bē-ō'lǎ*), not to be confused with German measles (rubella), is a dangerous and extremely contagious disease that has been targeted for eradication from the U.S. population. Measles is caused by a virus that is present in the respiratory discharges of infected people and is transmitted through the air, by direct contact with the nose and throat secretions of infected people, or by contact with items contaminated with such secretions. After 8–13 days, fever, headache, conjunctivitis (reddening of the whites of the eyes), and coughing develop, accompanied by the presence of red spots on the lining of the mouth; 3–7 days later, a blotchy red rash appears, beginning on the face and spreading over the body. Measles becomes contagious before any symptoms appear and remains so until about 4 days after appearance of the rash.

Measles. Once viewed as a normal childhood experience, measles is now recognized as a dangerous disease that carries the risk of death or brain damage. Immunization has greatly reduced the incidence of measles in the United States, but cases still occur in nonimmunized or inadequately immunized people.

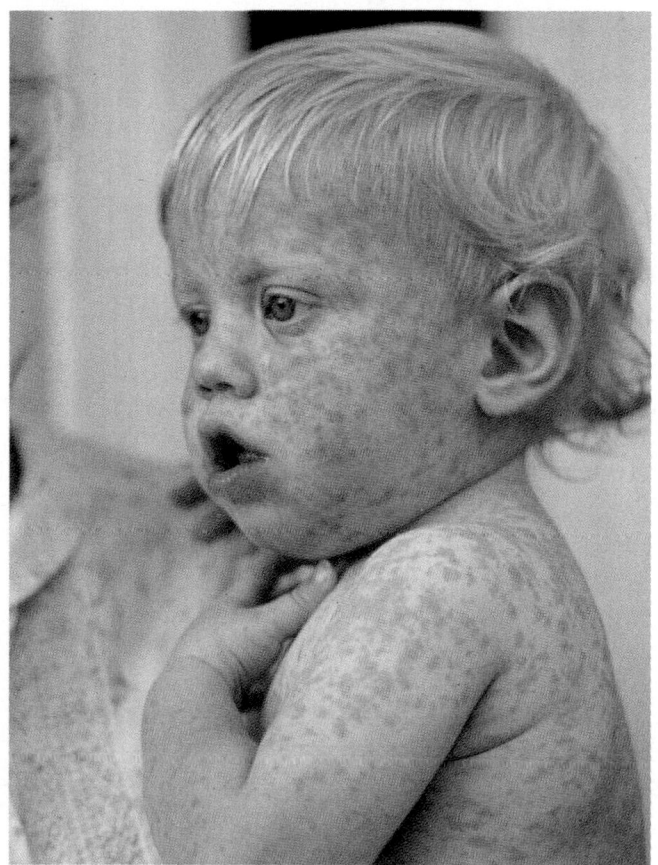

Measles is extremely dangerous, especially for very young or very old people. It is frequently complicated by middle ear infections or pneumonia (inflammation of the lungs) caused by the measles virus itself or by a secondary bacterial infection. In about 1 out of 2000 people with measles, the virus infects the brain, with possible permanent brain damage or death. About 1 in 3000 cases is fatal.[22]

Prior to widespread measles immunization, measles was common in childhood, with over 90 percent of people having had measles by age 20.[23] Since the licensing of a vaccine in 1963, the annual number of cases has declined from over 400,000 to a low of only about 220 cases in 1993. Most cases occur among people who have not been immunized, were immunized too young for a good immune response, or were immunized with an early, less-effective form of vaccine. In addition, although the current vaccine is about 95 percent effective, a few cases occur in people who fail to develop or retain a strong immunity. All parents are urged to ensure that their children are properly immunized against rubeola. This is usually accomplished with MMR (measles-mumps-rubella) vaccine administered at age 15 months.

INFECTIOUS MONONUCLEOSIS ("MONO")

Infectious mononucleosis (*mon-ō-nu"klē-ō'sis*), commonly called "mono," is a viral infection that centers in the lymph nodes. The pathogen is the Epstein-Barr Virus (EBV), a herpes virus that also appears to cause a lymphatic cancer called Burkitt's lymphoma (mainly in Central Africa). It is uncertain why this virus causes cancer in Africa, but seldom causes cancer in the United States.

Mononucleosis is primarily a disease of children and young adults. Recovery from mononucleosis generally confers a high degree of immunity, so most people have it only once. In developing countries, most cases of mononucleosis occur in early childhood and are asymptomatic or produce very mild symptoms, but they still confer immunity. In developed countries, people are infected later, so the disease is most commonly seen in high school and college students.

Transmission of mononucleosis is by contact with the saliva of infected persons through kissing or other close contact. Blood transfusions can also transmit the disease. The incubation period is from four to six weeks.

Symptoms of variable severity include fever, sore throat, fatigue, and enlarged lymph nodes, especially in the neck. The duration of illness is usually from one to several weeks.

The EBV is a herpes virus, which means that it tends to stay with a person for an indefinite period of time, once infection has occurred. In long-term EBV infection, the virus stays in the lymphocytes. An estimated 80 percent of all healthy adults carry the EBV virus in their lymphocytes.[24] Most people who recover from mononucleosis continue to shed the virus in their saliva and may infect others for at least a year after recovery.

VIRAL HEPATITIS

The liver, which performs several hundred important functions, is absolutely essential to human life. **Hepatitis** (*hep-a-tī'tis*), in a general sense, means inflammation of the liver. In addition to viruses, hepatitis can be caused by damage from alcohol or other drugs or exposure to various toxic chemicals. Destruction of liver cells in hepatitis can result in a great loss of liver function, with unpleasant or even fatal effects.

Many different viruses can infect the liver. Table 18.2 compares five forms of viral hepatitis (A through E), each caused by a different virus. It is possible that two different viruses cause what is currently called hepatitis C.[25] Viral hepatitis can be a very severe illness and several forms can lead to long-term consequences such as cirrhosis and liver cancer.

Viral hepatitis is extremely contagious. Hepatitis A and hepatitis E are transmitted primarily through fecal contamination of food or water. Large numbers of cases can result from one infected restaurant employee who fails to wash his or her hands after using the toilet. Hepatitis B, C, and D are transmitted through contaminated blood and blood products, across the placenta during pregnancy, and through semen and other body fluids. Incubation periods (see Table 18.2) range from 2 to 26 weeks for the various types of hepatitis.

Severity of hepatitis can range from asymptomatic (no symptoms at all) to very severe or even

....

hepatitis inflammation of the liver.

Table 18.2
Types of Viral Hepatitis

	Other Names	Usual Means of Transmission	Incubation Period	Severity	Symptoms (See Main Text)	Chronic Infection?	Vaccine?
Hepatitis A	Infectious hepatitis	Fecal contamination of food or water	2–6 weeks	Usually mild, can be severe	Fever and headache present	No	Being tested; temporary protection by injection of immune globulin
Hepatitis B	Serum hepatitis	Blood, semen, other body fluids, can cross placenta	4–26 weeks	Mild to severe; may progress to severe liver damage; most recover completely	Fever and headache absent	Up to 10%; associated with liver cancer	Yes; routine infant immunization; also urged for health care workers and people with multiple sex partners
Hepatitis C	Non-A, non-B hepatitis	Blood and blood products	2–12 weeks (one form is 2–4 weeks, one is 8–12 weeks)	Mild to severe	Similar to hepatitis B	50%; possible association with liver cancer	No
Hepatitis D	Delta hepatitis	Blood; must coinfect with hepatitis B, can cross placenta	2–12 weeks	Severe, with high death rate	Can cause disease only when hepatitis B is also present	Yes	No
Hepatitis E	Non-A, non-B, non-C hepatitis	Fecal contamination of food or water	2–6 weeks	Moderate, but high death rate in pregnant women	Similar to hepatitis A except very severe in pregnant women	No	No

fatal. Typical hepatitis symptoms can include fatigue, loss of appetite, fever and headache for some forms, nausea and vomiting, and several symptoms relating to the orange-colored pigment bilirubin.

Bilirubin comes from the breakdown of the hemoglobin in red blood cells. Normally bilirubin is extracted by the liver and excreted in the bile, where it aids digestion and gives feces its characteristic color. When the hepatitis-damaged liver is unable to extract bilirubin, the pigment builds up in the blood until the skin and whites of the eyes turn yellow. This is **jaundice.** Jaundice is difficult to observe in the skin of darkly pigmented people but is visible in the whites of the eyes. The feces assume a lighter color, while the urine becomes dark when the kidneys take over the job of extracting bilirubin from the blood. Darkened urine is an especially useful sign of hepatitis in darkly pigmented people in whom jaundice is hard to detect.

....

bilirubin pigment from the breakdown of the hemoglobin in red blood cells.

jaundice yellowing of the skin and whites of the eyes.

Hepatitis A and E are prevented by measures such as proper sewage disposal, safe water supplies, and washing of hands by food handlers after using the toilet. Hepatitis B, C, and D are prevented by sterilization of any item that penetrates the skin, careful handling of blood and blood products, avoiding casual sexual partnerships, and applying the safer sex guidelines discussed in the next chapter. An effective vaccine for hepatitis B is routinely administered to infants and is highly recommended for people whose work exposes them to blood or who have multiple sex partners. A vaccine for hepatitis A is being tested; meanwhile exposed people can obtain instant passive immunity through an injection of hepatitis A immune globulin.

CHECKPOINT

1. What are the possible serious complications of measles?

2. Is it unusual for a healthy person to carry the virus that causes mononucleosis?

3. Define the terms *hepatitis* and *jaundice.*

4. How is each form (A–E) of viral hepatitis transmitted?

SUMMARY

Communicable diseases are caused by microscopic parasites, called pathogens, that invade the body. Pathogens are classified into five major categories: viruses, bacteria, fungi, protozoa, and parasitic worms. Of these, viruses are most difficult to control with medications because their simplicity presents few vulnerabilities for drugs to attack.

The source of a pathogen is called its reservoir. For many diseases this is an asymptomatic human carrier. Pathogens leave an infected host by a specific portal of exit and reach a new host by either direct contact, indirect contact, droplets, common vehicle transmission, airborne transmission, or by a vector such as an insect. The portal of entry is where the pathogen enters its new host. It must enter in an infective dosage large enough to overcome body defenses in order to establish infection.

Following infection, the course of a disease progresses through the symptomless incubation period, the prodromal period of early symptoms, the typical illness period, and the convalescence period. Following recovery, some people remain active carriers of the pathogen. Others become carriers without experiencing symptoms. Even in the absence of symptoms, carriers are able to infect other people.

Nonspecific body defenses, collectively called resistance, include unbroken skin and mucous membranes, respiratory cilia, stomach acid, phagocytic white blood cells, inflammation, and interferons. Highly specific body defenses, collectively called immunity, are stimulated by the presence of an antigen, usually a substance that is foreign to the body.

Specific immune responses are carried out by special white blood cells called T lymphocytes and B lymphocytes. T lymphocytes produce cell-mediated immunity, attacking pathogens and abnormal body cells, and also regulate the function of the B lymphocytes. B lymphocytes release antibodies (immunoglobulins) to circulate with the blood. This is humoral immunity.

Active immunity is produced upon exposure to an antigen, either as part of a pathogen or in a vaccine. Active immunity is slow in developing, but it is long term. Passive immunity is produced by passively receiving preformed antibodies from outside of the body. It is instant, but not long term.

Immune deficiency can result from heredity, radiation, chemicals, or viruses, such as HIV (discussed in Chapter 19). Immune deficiency leads to frequent and/or severe infections and increased risk of cancer.

An allergy or hypersensitivity is an immune response against an otherwise harmless substance. Anaphylactic shock is a severe allergic reaction that can be fatal if not treated promptly.

Autoimmune disorders are immune responses against part of your own body. The result is a gradual, progressive degeneration of tissues or organs.

Communicable diseases are prevented through maintaining a healthful life-style, immunization, and public health efforts (education and enforcement of sanitation guidelines). They are treated with antimicrobial drugs such as antibiotics. Drug resistance, however, is reducing the ability of drugs to control many pathogens.

The chapter concluded with a survey of some important communicable diseases. Although communicable diseases are not currently among the top causes of death in the United States, they remain ever-present threats to your health and well-being. Keeping pathogens under control requires ongoing efforts by public health workers and each of us as individuals. *You* must take responsibility for maintaining your own health through practicing healthful living habits and taking advantage of all known precautions, such as getting immunizations, avoiding exposure to contagious pathogens, and obtaining prompt treatment for diseases before serious complications develop.

REFERENCES

1. Stine, G. *Acquired Immune Deficiency Syndrome.* Englewood Cliffs, NJ: Prentice-Hall, 1993.
2. Talaro, K., and Talaro, A. *Foundations in Microbiology.* Dubuque, IA: Wm. C. Brown, 1993.
3. Tortora, G., Funke, B., and Case, C. *Microbiology,* 5th ed. Redwood City, CA: Benjamin/Cummings, 1995.
4. Ibid.
5. Ibid.
6. Benjamini, E., and Leskowitz, S. *Immunology: A Short Course,* 2nd ed. New York: Wiley-Liss, 1991.
7. Ibid.

8. Ibid.
9. Tortora et al., op. cit.
10. U. S. Public Health Service, Centers for Disease Control "Lyme Disease—United States, 1991–1992." *Morbidity and Mortality Weekly Report,* Vol. 42, No. 18 (14 May 1993), 345–348.
11. Tortora et al., op. cit.
12. Anonymous. "Late News on the Cold Front." *University of California at Berkeley Wellness Let.ter* (November 1988), 4–5.
13. Ibid.
14. Ibid.
15. Tortora et al., op. cit.
16. Boyd, R., and Hoerl, B. *Basic Medical Microbiology,* 4th ed. Boston: Little, Brown, 1991.
17. Black, J. *Microbiology,* 2nd ed. Englewood Cliffs, NJ: Prentice-Hall, 1993.
18. Tortora et al., op. cit.
19. Black, op. cit.
20. Black, op. cit.
21. Tortora et al., op. cit.
22. Tortora et al., op. cit.
23. Benenson, A., ed. *Control of Communicable Diseases in Man,* 15th ed. Washington, DC: American Public Health Association, 1990.
24. Tortora et al., op. cit.
25. Black, op. cit.

SUGGESTED READINGS

Benenson, A. (Ed.). *Control of Communicable Diseases in Man,* 15th ed. Washington, DC: American Public Health Association, 1990.

Benjamini, E., and Leskowitz, S. *Immunology: A Short Course,* 2nd ed. New York: Wiley-Liss, 1991.

Black, J. *Microbiology,* 2nd ed. Englewood Cliffs, NJ: Prentice Hall, 1993.

Morbidity and Mortality Weekly Report, published by Centers for Disease Control and Prevention (CDC), Atlanta, Georgia, provides weekly updates on communicable diseases and other public health concerns. Subscriptions available for $56/year through Massachusetts Medical Society, P.O. Box 9120, Waltham, MA 02254-9120.

Morello, J., Mizer, H., Wilson, M., and Granato, P. *Microbiology in Patient Care,* 5th ed. Dubuque, IA: Wm. C. Brown, 1994.

Murray, P., Kobayashi, G., Pfaller, M., and Rosenthal, K. *Medical Microbiology,* 2nd ed. St. Louis: Mosby, 1994.

Talaro, K., and Talaro, A. *Foundations in Microbiology.* Dubuque, IA: Wm. C. Brown, 1993.

Tortora, G., Funke, B., and Case, C. *Microbiology,* 5th ed. Redwood City, CA: Benjamin/Cummings, 1995.

Volk, W. *Microbiology,* 7th ed. New York: HarperCollins, 1992.

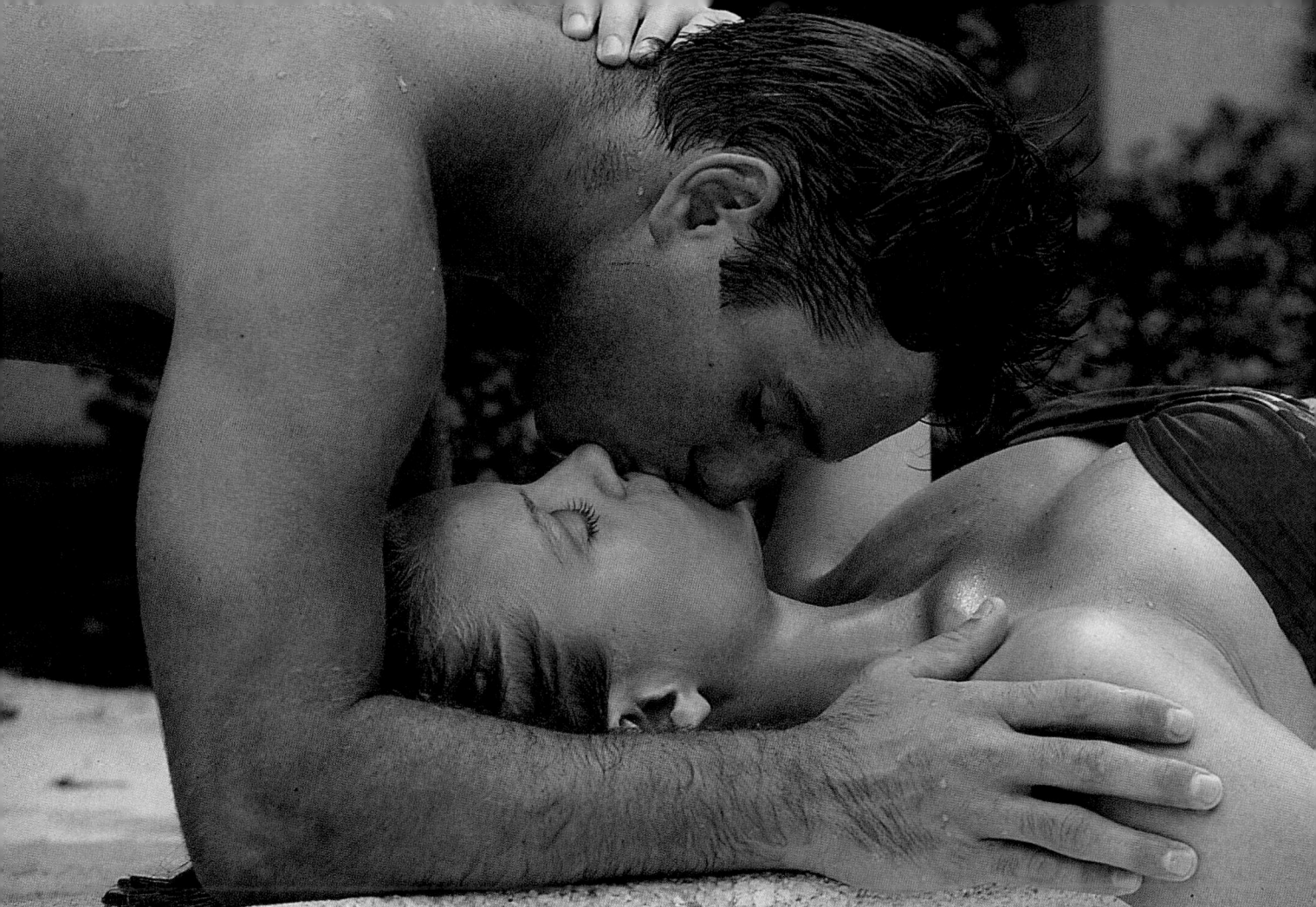

19
SEXUALLY TRANSMITTED DISEASES

Probably few events have caused more people to examine their sexual behaviors than NBA star Magic Johnson's November 1991 announcement that he was infected with HIV. The sexual activity that resulted in his infection had occurred prior to his marriage, but his wife, who was pregnant at the time of the announcement, tested negative for HIV infection. Later, his newborn son also tested negative for infection. His announcement immediately brought attention to heterosexual transmission of HIV. Johnson emphasized prevention of AIDS with safer sex practices. Recently, Johnson has focused more on abstinence in his talks about AIDS prevention. It has become strikingly apparent that no one, regardless of sexual orientation, is immune from HIV infection.

Immediately after his announcement, the interest in information about AIDS increased dramatically. The National AIDS Hotline reported ten times the usual number of inquiries that day. The Centers for Disease Control (CDC) had 10,000 calls per hour in comparison to the usual 200 calls per hour. The number of appointments for HIV testing increased dramatically. In addition, there was an overwhelmingly positive public reaction to Johnson's decision to become a spokesperson for AIDS. With the increased public interest, many of the myths surrounding AIDS were openly dispelled and discussion was stimulated about access to health care, particularly in the African American community. The CDC indicates that the *incidence of heterosexually transmitted AIDS among African American and Hispanic men and women is rising at an alarming rate.*

Whether or not the publicity of Magic Johnson's infection with HIV as a result of heterosexual activity will make a difference in sexual behavior has yet to be determined. His story tells us that AIDS is a disease that crosses all boundaries of sexual orientation, race, and socioeconomic class. Hardly anyone looked healthier than Magic; looks can obviously be deceiving when it comes to taking risks with sexual behavior.

■   ■   ■

In the previous chapter we learned the basic nature of communicable diseases. Now let's examine the most important communicable diseases in the United States today: **sexually transmitted diseases (STDs).**

What do we mean by the "most important communicable diseases"? The number of STD cases exceeds all other communicable diseases combined, with the exception of the common cold. Inherent dangers of STDs include the threat of sterility, diseased or disabled offspring, and even death. In recent years, the sexually transmitted disease AIDS has been unrivaled in its impact on society.

STDs used to be referred to as *venereal diseases,* or VDs. This term, derived from Venus, the goddess of love, is not entirely appropriate, as love often plays no role in the transmission of these diseases.

HISTORY OF STDs

Sexually transmitted diseases are not a new problem (see Feature 19.1). Throughout history, there have been indications of the presence of some of our current STDs. We say "indications" because the early history of all diseases is clouded by confusion and lack of scientific knowledge. Even the idea that diseases are caused by pathogens is a fairly recent development. It was not until 1876 that Robert Koch first proved that bacteria cause disease. Then, in 1879, the German bacteriologist Albert Neisser

proved that syphilis and gonorrhea were separate diseases. Prior to that time, both were thought to be manifestations of the same illness.

Both syphilis and gonorrhea have been known by a variety of names. Gonorrhea has been called *clap, dose, strain,* and *GC,* and syphilis has been called *pox, scab, lues, bad blood,* and *syph.* The word *syphilis* comes from a poem written in 1530 by a physician named Fracastoro about an afflicted Greek shepherd boy named Syphilus who had offended the sun-god.

Genital herpes infection also has a long history. The ancient Greeks knew about herpes and gave herpes its name, derived from the Greek word meaning "to creep," because the lesions (sores) seem to creep over the surface of the skin.

With the introduction of antibiotics in the 1940s, intensive public health efforts, and the prevailing conservative sexual behavior of the 1950s, the incidence of sexually transmitted diseases declined to a low point in the mid-1950s. Then, around 1957, the number of cases started to rise, and this increase continued into the 1980s. While we can only speculate about the cause of this increase, it seems to have coincided with the beginning of a trend toward more casual sexual relationships and a decline in public health emphasis on STDs. Other possible associations are increased use of drugs, bartering of sex for drugs, changing social values, and increased mobility.

STDs gained a new significance in the 1980s when AIDS emerged. For the first time since antibiotics became available in about 1940 there was an STD that was both incurable and likely to prove fatal.

TODAY'S INCIDENCE OF STDs

Accurate figures for incidence of most sexually transmitted diseases are somewhat elusive (see Feature 19.2). Many of the STDs are classified as *reportable diseases;* that is, every diagnosed case is to be reported to public health authorities. This does not mean that the published incidence figures for these diseases are accurate. In the first place, many infected people do not seek treatment, either because they are **asymptomatic** (ā"simp-tō-

....

sexually transmitted diseases (STDs) diseases that are commonly transmitted through sexual contact.

....

asymptomatic having no symptoms.

FEATURE 19.1

HOW DID STDs ORIGINATE?

If we can only catch an STD from another person, not from sheep as was once believed for syphilis or from monkeys as was once believed for AIDS, how did the first person catch an STD?

The human body carries many types of harmless microorganisms; in fact, many are beneficial. But microorganisms have high mutation (genetic change) rates. A virus or bacterium that might have lived on or in some part of the human body for millions of years, but caused little or no problem, could suddenly undergo a genetic change, and as a result, might cause a severe disease, such as an STD.

Several characteristics distinguish the pathogens of STDs from other pathogens. The primary one is that they are present either on the genital membranes or in the genital secre-

tions of infected people, making transmission by sexual contact possible. Another characteristic is that most of them have short lives away from the human body. These "delicate" organisms die when exposed to dryness and/or cold. Therefore, the direct contact of warm, moist membranes is ideal for their transmission.

Exactly how long do STD pathogens survive in the environment? There is no specific answer to this, as there are many variable factors influencing their survival. In general, STD organisms usually survive no more than a few minutes on inanimate objects. Thus, though nonsexual transmission of some STDs is possible, as when a towel is used by one person and then immediately by another, it very rarely occurs.

---

mat'ik; having no symptoms) or because they ignore their symptoms. Further, many cases diagnosed by private physicians are not reported, despite the laws requiring such reporting. Some physicians wish to protect the confidentiality of their patients; some may be too busy to deal with

the paperwork required for reporting cases of STDs.

Some common STDs, such as *Chlamydia,* are reportable in some states, but not in others. Some STDs are not reportable anywhere. For diseases in these categories, we can only guess the number of

---

FEATURE 19.2

INCIDENCE OF SEXUALLY TRANSMITTED DISEASES

Accurate incidence figures for STDs are difficult to obtain. Only some of the STDs are required by law to be reported to public health departments. Even then, the reported number of cases is less than the actual number. Some people fail to seek treatment and some physicians fail to report every case they treat. Here are some reported and estimated numbers of STDs in the United States:

- *AIDS* About 93,000 new cases reported in 1993. Reported cases represent only more advanced cases of HIV infection. The U.S. Centers for Disease Control and Prevention (CDC), in Atlanta, Georgia, estimates that 1.5 million Americans are infected with HIV (AIDS virus). Even those with no symptoms may be a source of virus to other people and almost all will eventually die of AIDS, barring a medical breakthrough.

  AIDS has had a disproportionate impact on several ethnic groups. African Americans, though only 12 percent of the U.S. population, account for 32 percent of AIDS cases. Hispanic Americans, though only 9 percent of the population, account for 19 percent of AIDS cases.[a]

- *Genital herpes* A lifelong infection. Not reportable in most states. An estimated 20–40 million Americans are already infected and about 500,000 new cases occur annually.

- *Papilloma viruses* (genital warts and cervical cancer) The fastest-growing viral STD. Not reportable in most states. Estimates of new cases each year range from 1 to 3 million.

- *Chlamydia* The most common bacteria STD. Not reportable in most states. Estimates range from 3–10 million new cases per year. CDC estimates 4.6 million new cases per year.

- *Gonorrhea* About 392,000 new cases reported in 1993. The actual number of cases is probably several million per year.

- *Syphilis* About 26,000 new cases reported in 1993. True incidence is higher. Many cases are traced to female prostitutes and women who exchange sex for drugs.

Despite the lack of exact figures, it is clear that there are millions of new cases of STDs every year and additional millions of people who are chronically infected and remain contagious to others. Anyone who engages in sex, other than in the context of a mutually monogamous relationship, is at risk of being infected with one or more of the STDs.

[a]United States Public Health Service. *Health United States 1992 and Healthy People 2000 Review.* DHHS Pub. No. (PHS) 93-1232. Hyattsville, MD: Public Health Service, 1993.

cases. Even though our statistics are unreliable, we have enough information to conclude that every year, *millions* of new cases of STDs develop in the United States. This is in addition to the millions of existing untreated cases from previous years. These statistics need to be considered when you make sexual decisions.

WHO GETS STDs?

STDs have permeated American society, crossing all lines of ethnicity, and education and income levels. Risks of STDs significantly increase for those who have multiple partners. For sexually abstinent individuals or **monogamous** couples, assuming neither partner was infected to begin with, the risk of sexually contracting an STD is zero.

In recent years, in response to the increased incidence of herpes and AIDS, many people have modified their sexual habits. Many people have begun to reduce their number of sexual partners, to discuss more openly the risks of disease transmission, and to take greater precautions, such as using condoms to reduce the risk of infection.

WHY ARE STDs SO PREVALENT?

No single explanation accounts for today's high incidence of STDs. Some factors that contribute to the spread of STDs include sexual activity at earlier ages than in past decades, attitudes that discourage obtaining treatment for STDs, and denial by an individual that he or she may be infected with an STD.

Also important are such biological factors as mutations among microorganisms that give rise to entirely new disease agents, and cause drug resistance to develop in existing pathogens. Once new pathogens or newly drug-resistant strains of pathogens develop, world travel becomes a major factor in their spread. A new pathogen or strain of an existing pathogen can arise in any corner of the world and in a very short time be carried to other nations.

According to some authorities, the prevalence of birth control pill use is another factor contribut-

ing to the STD epidemic. By eliminating fear of pregnancy, the pill gives some women a sense of greater sexual freedom. The pill also makes it difficult to motivate people to use condoms and spermicides, both of which help to prevent some STDs, when they are not needed for birth control. Furthermore, the pill reduces the acidity of the vagina, increasing the probability of infection by gonorrhea, *Chlamydia,* and most other STDs when a woman has sex with an infected partner.

TREATMENT OF STDs

If you suspect that you may have an STD or may have been exposed to an STD it is essential to seek professional help. If you are diagnosed as having an STD it is important to inform your partner(s) so that they may also be treated. Treatment can be obtained from a private physician, a public health facility, or a college's student health center. Here, proper diagnosis can be made and appropriate treatment administered or prescribed. If a partner has been treated for an STD the partner's name and where he or she was treated should be mentioned, for confirmation. If the contact has been recent, a person is sometimes treated **prophylactically** (preventively) to kill pathogens before the disease develops.

There is no home remedy, nonprescription drugstore remedy, or folk remedy that can cure any of the STDs. Attempts at self-treatment will only serve to delay effective treatment. During the delay, serious and permanent damage, such as sterility, may result.

Now we will survey some specific STDs, which are arranged by type of pathogen. We will work from the smallest to the largest pathogens: viruses, bacteria, yeast, protozoa, and insect parasites. Table 19.1 summarizes some of these diseases.

CHECKPOINT

1. How recent a problem are the STDs?

2. Which people are most likely to be infected with an STD?

3. What factors are thought to contribute to today's high STD rates?

---

monogamous usually defined as having one sexual partner at a time or as being married to one person at a time. We define a mutually monogamous relationship as one in which, over an extended period of time, two persons engage in sexual activity only with each other.

prophylactically for prevention.

Table 19.1
Summary of Sexually Transmitted Diseases

	HIV/AIDS	Genital Herpes	Hepatitis B	Genital Warts	*Chlamydia*	Gonorrhea	Syphilis	*Candida*	*Trichomonas*
Type of Pathogen	Virus (HIV)	Virus	Virus	Papilloma viruses	Bacterium	Bacterium (coccus)	Bacterium (spirochete)	Yeast	Protozoan
Incubation Period	1–8 weeks to primary illness; can be many years to AIDS	2–12 days	45–160 days	1–20 months	5–7 days or longer	2–8 days or longer	10–90 days	Variable	4–20 days
Initial Symptoms	Enlarged lymph nodes, fever, weight loss, fatigue	Itching, small fluid-filled blisters, fever	Loss of appetite, nause, fatigue, pain in joints, headache, dark urine, jaundice	Warts on penis or labia	Burning during urination, vaginala or urethral discharge	Burning during urination, vaginal or urethral discharge	Chancre(s), then rash and oral and genital lesions	Thick, white vaginal discharge, irritation	Frothy, foul-smelling discharge, irritation, itching
Potential Damages	Severe infections, cancers, death	Infant death or disability	Liver cancer	Cervical cancer is associated with several strains of virus	Sterility, PID, tubal pregnancy, preterm delivery	Sterility, PID, arthritis, heart damage	Permanent damage to central nervous system and other vital organs	Could infect infant	Vaginal bleeding
Treatment	No cure, but drugs prolong the symptomless period and may prolong life	No cure, but acyclovir reduces attack frequency and severity	No cure; vaccine will prevent	Removal by physician or injection of interferon into lesions	Antibiotics	Antibiotics	Antibiotics	Drugs, correct any underlying cause	Drugs

AIDS (ACQUIRED IMMUNE DEFICIENCY SYNDROME)

In 1981 reports began to appear of a new, unnamed disease causing severe illness and death in the United States. Most of the people affected were either homosexual males or intravenous drug abusers. Massive research efforts in France and the United States soon revealed that this disease was a viral infection, which was given the name *acquired immune deficiency syndrome* (AIDS). A **syndrome** is a group of signs and symptoms that characterize a particular disease or condition.

The virus that causes AIDS is **Human Immunodeficiency Virus (HIV)** (see Figure 19.1). Two variants of the virus have been identified and

....

syndrome a group of signs and symptoms that collectively characterize a particular disease or condition.

Human Immunodeficiency Virus (HIV) the virus that causes AIDS.

named HIV-1 and HIV-2. The great majority of AIDS cases in the United States are caused by HIV-1. Both HIV-1 and HIV-2 are unusual pathogens in that they infect the immunity-producing T lymphocytes (refer to Chapter 18). Thus, HIV directly attacks the cells that should be defending the body against viral infection.

Since the emergence of HIV its incidence has continued to climb in most parts of the world. HIV infection is currently spreading most rapidly in developing countries. The World Health Organization says that by the year 2000 at least 30 million people around the world will be infected. Other AIDS experts think the number could reach 110 million by that time.[1] This is especially alarming because no cure for HIV infection has been developed.

Infection with HIV is not synonymous with having AIDS. HIV infection usually requires many years to reach the stage we call AIDS. HIV experts use a six-stage system of classification for the progress of the infection.[2]

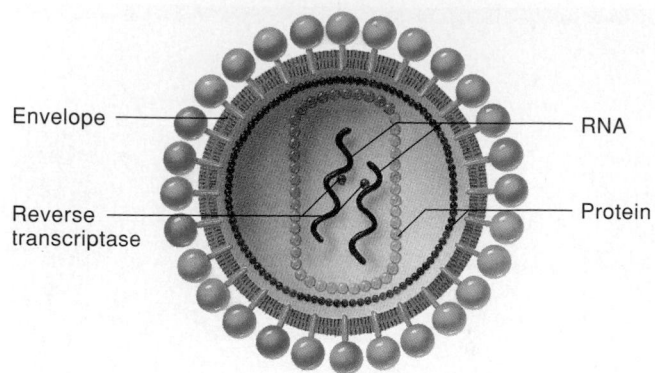

Figure 19.1
The AIDS Virus

Human immunodeficiency virus (HIV), the cause of AIDS. This is a retrovirus, having RNA as its genetic material. It has the ability to produce DNA from RNA, with the DNA then being incorporated into the chromosomes of its human host cells. Actual size is submicroscopic; viruses are visible only with an electron microscope.

Source: Wistreich, G., and Lechtman, M. Microbiology, 5th ed. New York: Macmillan, 1988.

- *Stage 1* begins shortly after infection. Some people experience a mild, mononucleosis-like illness appearing within one to two months after infection. Symptoms may include a mild fever, swollen lymph nodes, and fatigue. These symptoms spontaneously disappear in a few weeks. Most people begin to test positive for HIV antibodies within six months after infection, although some remain negative for a year or more. *We must emphasize that, whether or not a person experiences symptoms of HIV infection, he or she becomes a source of the virus to other people, by all of its methods of transmission, soon after infection, and remains a source of virus for life.*

- *Stage 2* begins after several years and lasts for several additional years. Stage 2 includes chronic swollen lymph nodes and while the individual does not feel especially unwell, the number of viruses in the body is steadily increasing while the number of T4 lymphocytes is declining.

- *Stage 3* begins when the T4 count drops below 400 per milliliter.

- *Stage 4 and Stage 5* are defined in terms of progressive loss of effective immune response, as evidenced by loss of the ability to respond to certain antigens (immune stim-

uli) and by development of infections such as *Candida* (yeast infection). Other symptoms may include swollen lymph nodes, fever, sweating, fatigue, and loss of appetite and weight.

- *Stage 6* is AIDS. In addition to fever, weight loss, diarrhea, and progressive neurological changes, severe opportunistic infections, such as *Pneumocystis* pneumonia, and cancers, such as Kaposi's sarcoma, develop. Even with the best treatments currently available, most people entering this stage will die within about two years.

Beginning in 1993, the definition of AIDS was expanded to include people who test positive for HIV and whose T4 lymphocyte count falls below 200 per cubic millimeter of blood or who suffer from any of about 25 opportunistic infections that are common among HIV-infected people. This had the effect of suddenly increasing the number of reported cases of AIDS, as more HIV-infected people met the definition.[3]

TRANSMISSION OF HIV

One of the greatest public health tasks of all time has been alerting people to the methods of HIV transmission and informing them of appropriate precautions. It has also been necessary to educate the public about how HIV is *not* transmitted, in order to prevent irrational panic (see Feature 19.3).

Although traces of HIV can be detected in most body fluids of infected people, it is present in an infective form and in adequate quantities (an infective dosage) for disease transmission only in blood, vaginal or cervical secretions, breast milk, and semen. Infection almost invariably can be traced to one of the following: sexual contact with an infected person; sharing a needle with an infected person; receiving a blood transfusion or blood product from an infected person; or in some other way, such as being accidentally pricked with an infected needle. Further, in 30–35 percent of the pregnancies of infected women, the virus crosses the placenta into the fetus's blood or the infant is infected during the birth process. *There is no documented case of someone being infected by food prepared or served by an infected person or by working with or simply being around an infected person.*

Any sexual practice that involves exposure to semen or cervical or vaginal secretions can transmit

HOW HIV IS *NOT* TRANSMITTED

A certain amount of hysteria has surrounded the HIV epidemic, just as it has surrounded every disease epidemic in history. The fact that today's scientific knowledge makes the methods of transmission of HIV much better understood than were the transmission of earlier epidemics such as plague, smallpox, and polio has not eliminated myths and misconceptions regarding HIV transmission. We want to clarify some ways that HIV is *not* acquired:

- HIV is *not* acquired through the air. There is no need to fear working with, attending school with, or having other nonsexual contact with infected people.

- HIV is *not* acquired while donating blood. All equipment used to collect blood from donors is perfectly sterile. There is no risk of HIV infection from donating blood.

- HIV is *not* acquired by eating food that has been cooked or served by an HIV-infected person. Even though the virus could theoretically contaminate food if the food handler got cut and bled on the food, the digestive tract is a very poor portal of entry for HIV. There is no known case of someone acquiring HIV in this way.

- HIV is *not* transmitted by mosquito bites. Mosquitoes are effective vectors for some viruses, such as yellow fever, but are not capable of carrying most viruses. For example, there is no mosquito transmission of colds, influenza, polio, rabies, measles, chicken pox, and hepatitis B (which has the same modes of transmission as HIV). Even though some of the places where HIV is most prevalent have plenty of mosquitoes, there has never been a single known case of mosquito-borne HIV.

HIV (see Table 19.2). The most efficient mode of sexual transmission appears to be anal intercourse. The rectal lining is not well suited to withstand the wear and tear of intercourse and abrasions allow entry of HIV. The most likely path of transmission is from the male whose penis is inserted into his sexual partner. Vaginal intercourse has also been documented as a method of transmitting HIV, from either male to female or female to male. The greater risk of transmission, however, is from male to female. Oral sex has not been identified as a major risk factor in studies of either homosexual or heterosexual populations, though there are cases where it has been the method of transmission. It is advisable to avoid oral sex with an infected person or anyone whose HIV status is unknown.[4]

It must be emphasized that not everyone who is infected with HIV will display symptoms. *Even when infected people are not presently experiencing any symptoms, they are capable of infecting others.* Consequently, the potential for the spread of the disease is considerable. One person who is sexually promiscuous or who shares needles could infect many people over a period of years.

FIVE SIGNIFICANT TIME PERIODS

There are five significant time periods related to HIV infection.[5]

They are:

1. The time from when the virus enters the body until it is circulating in the blood in quantities that make the infection *contagious to others.* This takes only one to three weeks, following which the virus remains contagious to others for the remainder of the infected person's life. We want to emphasize that many people who are capable of infecting others with HIV are totally free of symptoms and appear and feel quite healthy.

2. The time from when the virus enters the body until a *short-term illness* (Stage I HIV infection) develops. This period ranges from one to eight weeks. The illness may be mild and mononucleosis-like (fever, fatigue, and enlarged lymph nodes) or more severe.

3. The time from when the virus enters the body until an *HIV antibody test* (the standard blood test for HIV infection) would become positive. This is usually about two to three months, but may be a year or longer.

4. The time from when the virus enters the body until the onset of any *longer-lasting symptoms.* This period may range from one week to many years, but is often about two years.

5. The time from when the virus enters the body until the development of AIDS (Stage 6 HIV infection). This ranges from 6 months to more than 15 years and averages about 10 years.

TYPICAL PROGRESSION OF HIV INFECTION TO AIDS

Symptoms of Stage 2 to Stage 5 HIV infection include enlarged lymph nodes, loss of appetite,

Table 19.2
Relative Risk of HIV Transmission with Various Sexual Activities

No Risk

  Sexual abstinence

  Masturbating alone

  Hugging

  Massage

  Masturbating with another person but not touching each other

  Dry kissing

  Any activity by a mutually monogamous couple as defined on p. 588 if neither is infected when entering the relationship

Slight Risk

  Deep wet kissing

  Mutual masturbation

  "Outercourse" (rubbing penis against external genitals, breasts, etc.) without ejaculation, assuming no contact with preejaculatory fluid

  Cunnilingus

Moderate Risk (in order of increasing risk)

  "Outercourse" with ejaculation (between thighs, on breasts, etc.)

  Fellatio without orgasm

  Fellatio to orgasm with a condom

  Fellatio to orgasm without a condom

  Vaginal intercourse with a latex condom containing nonoxynol-9, withdrawal before ejaculation

  Anal intercourse with a latex condom containing nonoxynol-9, withdrawal before ejaculation

  Vaginal intercourse with a latex condom containing nonoxynol-9, vaginal ejaculation

High Risk (in order of increasing risk)

  Use by more than one person of sex toys exposed to semen or vaginal secretions and not sterilized between uses

  Vaginal intercourse with spermicidal foam, but without a condom, withdrawal before ejaculation

  Anal intercourse with a latex condom containing nonoxynol-9, internal ejaculation

  Vaginal intercourse with spermicidal foam, but without a condom, vaginal ejaculation

  Vaginal intercourse without spermicidal foam or condom, vaginal ejaculation

  Anal intercourse with internal ejaculation and no condom

Note: Relative risks are approximate. Risk increases if any genital lesions such as those of herpes or syphilis are present.

Sources: Modified from Stine, G. Acquired Immune Deficiency Syndrome. Englewood Cliffs, NJ: Prentice-Hall, 1993; Shernoff, M. "Integrating Safer-Sex Counseling into Social Work Practice." Social Casework: The Journal of Contemporary Social Work, Vol. 69, 1988, pp. 334–339.

chronic diarrhea, weight loss, sweating, fever, and fatigue. Neurological symptoms may include slurred speech, loss of peripheral sensation (loss of feeling in hands and feet), memory loss, and general mental deterioration.

In Stage 6 (AIDS) cases, one or both of two conditions usually appear: opportunistic infections (those that the body defenses would normally hold in check) and/or cancer. The opportunistic infection most closely associated with AIDS is pneumonia caused by the fungus *Pneumocystis carinii* (nū-mō-sis'tis kar-i'nē-ī; see Figure 19.2). The form of cancer most closely associated with AIDS is Kaposi's sarcoma (kap'ō-sēz sar-kō'mah), a cancer of the connective tissues (Figure 19.3). Kaposi's sarcoma may occur anywhere on the skin or in the mouth. In its early stages, it may look like a bruise or brownish spot. Both *Pneumocystis* pneumonia and Kaposi's sarcoma are rare in the general population, but common among people with AIDS. Most people who develop AIDS will, in time, die of some type of infection or cancer.

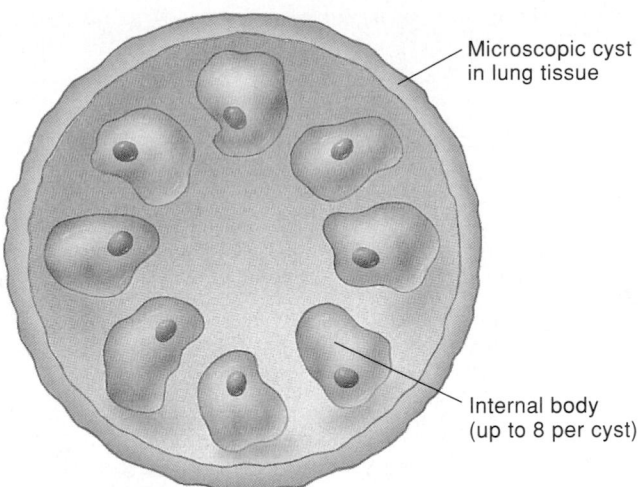

Microscopic cyst in lung tissue

Internal body (up to 8 per cyst)

Figure 19.2
Pneumocystis carinii

This parasitic fungus can be found in the lungs of many healthy people and animals. In people with AIDS it causes an often-fatal pneumonia.

DIAGNOSIS OF HIV INFECTION

Several types of blood tests for detecting HIV infection are available. Actually, these tests detect antibodies against HIV, rather than the virus itself. Initial tests are usually by the ELISA (Enzyme-Linked Immuno-Sorbent Assay) method, which sometimes gives false positive tests. A positive ELISA, therefore, is followed up with the more expensive, but more specific, Western blot test. The fact that current tests detect antibodies, rather than the virus, creates several problems (see also Feature 19.4):

- A newly infected person may continue to test negative on such tests for a period of 1–12 months, yet carry the virus and be able to infect others. Remember that common HIV tests detect antibodies, but HIV reduces a person's ability to produce antibodies, so the most severely affected people may be the slowest to produce enough antibodies to register on the test.

- Current tests are unable to predict whether or not an infected person will, in time, develop AIDS. Over 90 percent will, but some people who are known to have been infected with HIV for 14 years or more remain healthy. These people are being studied to determine what has protected them from severe illness.

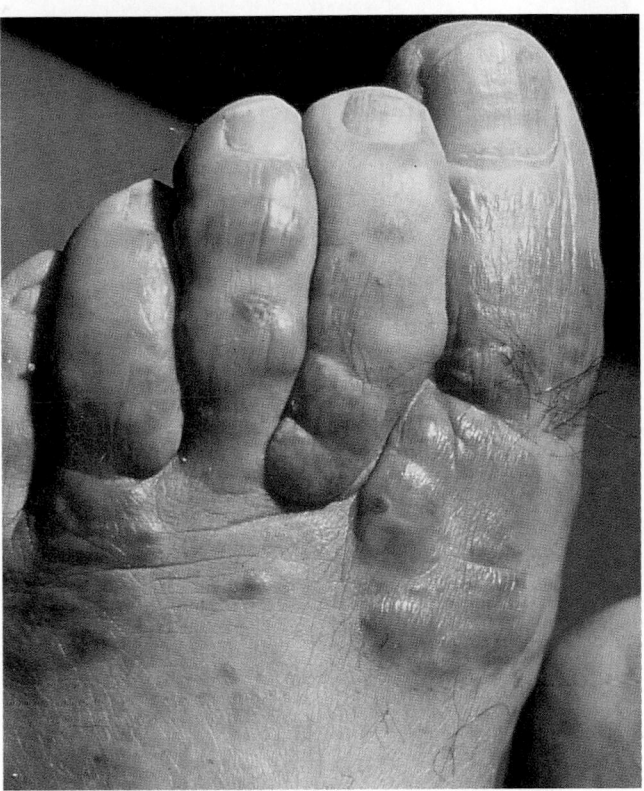

Figure 19.3
Kaposi's Sarcoma

This cancer of the connective tissues is rare among the general population, but common among people with AIDS, for whom it is often a cause of death.

- A positive antibody test in a newborn infant does not reveal whether the infant is HIV infected or just carrying antibodies that have crossed the placenta from the mother.

- The immune mechanisms of some people are so severely impaired by HIV that their blood tests negative for antibodies, even though they are quite ill with AIDS. Their lymphatic tissues do yield an HIV positive test.

Improved tests are being developed. Cost-effective tests that could easily detect the actual virus, rather than antibodies against it, would be ideal.

TREATING HIV INFECTION

Like any viral infection, HIV poses special problems in its treatment. Antibacterial drugs such as antibiotics are of no value against the virus, though

FEATURE 19.4

SOCIAL ISSUES AND AIDS

More than any disease in recent history, AIDS is laden with sensitive social issues. This is because AIDS involves sexuality, and in particular homosexuality, drug abuse, and the risk of death. The complete discussion of all of these issues has filled many books. Any of these issues would make excellent topics for classroom discussion. We will simply list some of them here:

- The overriding issue is the rights of individuals vs. the rights of members of society. To what extent must individual rights be sacrificed to prevent the spread of HIV?

- Do children have the right to a school sexuality education program that teaches about transmission and prevention of AIDS?

- At what age should children receive such education?

- Should drug abusers have legal access to sterile needles?

- Should any specific groups of people—drug users, prostitutes, those having multiple sexual partners, those applying for insurance or marriage licenses, those entering hospitals for any reason, those going to jail—be required to be tested for AIDS? Should everyone be tested? If so, what should happen when someone tests positive?

- Should blood tests be made more accessible to the public, such as through walk-in clinics in shopping malls?

- Who should be informed of the result of HIV blood tests? The individual? His or her spouse? His or her doctor? The health department?

- What are the legal implications if someone with a positive test fails to tell a potential sex partner?

- Should *you* require a potential partner to take a blood test?

- If not, how can you make sure that she or he is not infected?

- Is quarantine of infected people a good idea?

- What are the rights of persons with AIDS relating to employment, housing, and health care?

- Who is going to pay for the enormous health care costs created by AIDS? Does society have a responsibility to the infected?

- What are the rights of infected children?

- Do your answers to any of these questions depend on how a person was infected—whether sexually, through drug abuse, congenitally, or through blood transfusions or other medical procedures?

---

they may be useful for opportunistic infections associated with AIDS. As discussed in Chapter 18, viruses, in general, are difficult to eradicate with drugs as they lack the physiological vulnerabilities characteristic of bacteria. One drug, zidovudine (Retrovir), also known as azidothymidine (AZT), is being widely administered to people with AIDS and is extending the lives of many for an average of about 18 months. AZT inhibits the enzyme (reverse transcriptase) that converts the RNA of HIV to DNA, which is then incorporated into infected cells' chromosomes. Beginning the use of AZT before the illness progresses to advanced symptoms (AIDS) has also proven beneficial. AZT is not an ideal drug because it doesn't eliminate the virus from infected persons, it is very expensive, and it has many side effects. Also, resistant strains of HIV appear in some patients after nine months or more of treatment. Lower doses, earlier treatment, drug-free "rest" periods, and combinations of drugs, such as AZT, ddI (dideoxyinosine), and ddC (dideoyxcytidine) are lengthening survival times

and improving the quality of life for HIV-infected people.[6]

Because of the urgent need for better anti-HIV medications and the near certainty of death for people with advanced AIDS, the FDA allows drugs to be rushed into use in clinical trials more rapidly than it normally allows. Even though the stringent safety tests usually required before clinical testing have not been completed, the risk inherent in partially tested drugs is small compared to the risk of dying of AIDS.

As we have learned, opportunistic infections are characteristic of AIDS and are often the immediate cause of death. In addition to treating the HIV infection itself, intensive treatment for such infections is usually necessary.

PREVENTING HIV TRANSMISSION

Information on the prevention of all sexually transmitted diseases appears later in this chapter, but for now, here is a preview of some of the more important means of preventing transmission of HIV. They include the following:

- Never share needles or any instrument that scratches or penetrates the skin.

- Minimize the number of your sexual partners. Consider abstinence or a long-term monogamous relationship with a noninfected person.

- Avoid sexual activity with people who have many sexual partners or who are or have been intravenous drug abusers.

- Anal intercourse should be reserved for long-term monogamous relationships, and avoided in casual relationships (see Table 19.2).

- In any sexual contact other than in long-term monogamous relationships, *condoms* are a must, even if they are not required for birth control. Latex condoms are necessary, as viruses can pass through the pores of natural "skins" condoms. Condoms that carry the spermicidal chemical nonoxynol-9 are preferred, as this chemical has been shown to destroy HIV. Even though condoms are not 100 percent effective, they *greatly reduce the risk* of HIV transmission.

- Enter into sexual relationships slowly and cautiously. Get to know a person very well before engaging in sexual activity. Insist on mutual HIV testing if either partner might have the slightest chance of being infected.

- Make sure that your health care professionals are wearing gloves and sterilizing instruments. If you have questions about whether adequate precautions are being taken, don't be afraid to ask.

- At the public health level, HIV prevention includes screening blood donors and testing blood and blood products, educating the public about methods of transmission and prevention, and testing sexual contacts of persons known to be infected.

From the public health point of view, there are many obstacles to effective prevention of HIV infection:

1. Some people still do not perceive themselves as vulnerable and are reluctant to change their customary habits and behaviors. There is widespread (erroneous) belief that HIV is very rare among non-drug-abusing, heterosexual people, and that someone who appears to be healthy could not be carrying the virus.

2. Sexual activity may be spontaneous and may take place when judgment is impaired by alcohol or other drugs. Many people will engage in high-risk sexual behaviors or sex with high-risk partners when they have been drinking or using other drugs.

3. Drug-dependent people who are starting to experience withdrawal are likely to use the

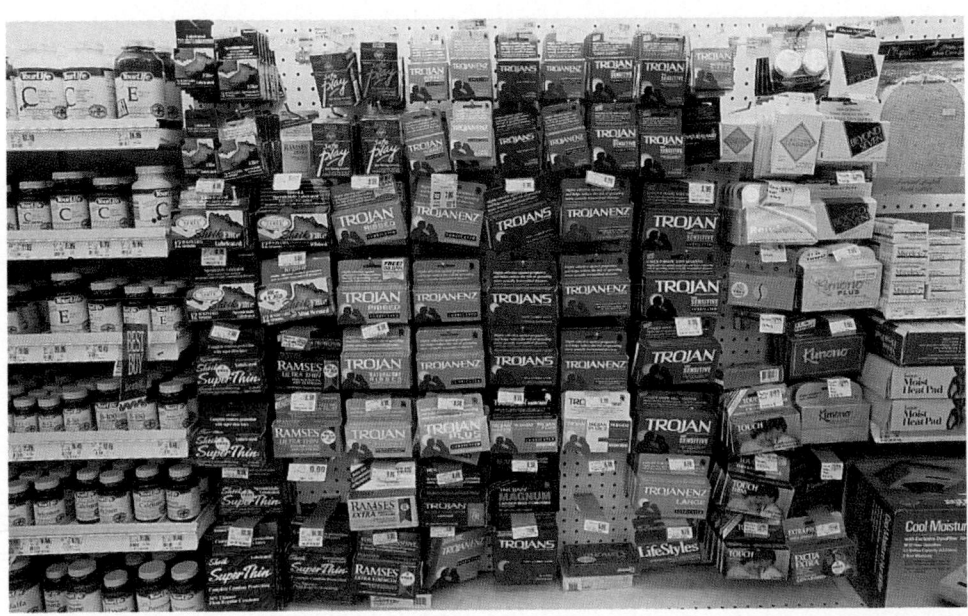

Today, for any sexual contact other than within a mutually monogamous relationship, condoms are a must. Those carrying the spermicide nonoxynol-9 are especially recommended for STD prevention.

first available needle even though they know it is not sterile. Laws in most places make obtaining sterile needles and syringes difficult.

HIV Vaccine Development

The ideal prevention for a disease such as AIDS is an effective vaccine. Many formerly dreaded diseases have been largely controlled through vaccine use. However, development of an effective vaccine against HIV has presented some special challenges:[7]

- Even though an infected person does produce an immune response to HIV (remember, HIV tests detect antibodies to the virus), this immunity does not eradicate the virus from the body or prevent progression of HIV disease.
- HIV integrates its genes into our own chromosomes, creating a very difficult target for an immune response.
- HIV has a high degree of variability and a high mutation rate, making it difficult to produce a vaccine that would be effective against all forms of the virus.
- An effective vaccine would probably be expensive. For example, the vaccine for hepatitis B (the only STD for which we have a vaccine) costs over $120 for the required three injections.

Despite these difficulties, at least eleven potential HIV vaccines are being tested.[8] Should one or more prove to be effective, it will still take years before it becomes available to the public.

C H E C K P O I N T

1. Why is being infected with HIV not synonymous with having AIDS?

2. Which body cells are most directly affected by HIV?

3. How is HIV transmitted and how is it *not* transmitted?

4. What does an HIV screening test actually detect?

GENITAL HERPES VIRUS INFECTIONS

Before the emergence of AIDS, genital herpes was probably the most feared STD in the United States. It still warrants serious concern and precautions. Herpes virus infections are often long-term and *there is currently no cure.* With approximately 20–40 million Americans already infected and 500,000 more becoming infected every year, genital herpes should be influencing the sexual decisions of a great many people. (The above figures are estimates, because herpes is not a reportable disease.)

Two types of herpes viruses (Figure 19.4) are associated with genital infections: herpes simplex virus type 1 (HSV-1) and herpes simplex virus type 2 (HSV-2). HSV-1 more typically attacks the upper parts of the body. About 85 percent of oral herpes infections (commonly called cold sores or fever blisters) are caused by HSV-1; about 15 percent are caused by HSV-2. Genital herpes infections are the opposite: About 85 percent are HSV-2, while about 15 percent are HSV-1. Herpes viruses are transmitted by oral-genital sex as well as by vaginal and anal intercourse, so either virus can attack the oral or genital region. Laboratories can distinguish between the two viruses using viral cultures and blood tests, but because the treatment for both viruses is the same and because these cultures and tests are expensive, they are seldom done.

In addition to causing oral and genital **lesions** (*lē' zhuns;* sores), herpes simplex viruses produce skin lesions, often on the thigh or buttocks, corneal (eye) infection, infection of the membranes covering the brain and spinal cord (meningitis), and brain infection (encephalitis). The meningitis and encephalitis occur primarily in newborns or people with impaired immunity. These two infections are the most dangerous complications of herpes.

Transmission of Herpes

Herpes lesions shed virus from their surface and thus, any contact with a lesion carries the risk of transmission of the disease. Genital herpes is definitely contagious to others whenever an active

---

lesion an area of damaged tissue; a wound or infection.

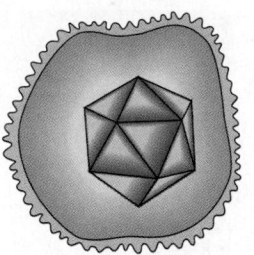

Figure 19.4
Herpes Simplex Virus

Herpes viruses produce long-term infections for which there is currently no cure, though medication such as acyclovir can reduce the frequency and severity of attacks. (Actual size is submicroscopic.)

lesion is present. Further, it is well documented that transmission can occur when no visible lesion is present.[9] This points out the importance of using latex condoms for all sexual activity, even if neither partner shows signs of any infection.

People who have genital herpes have a responsibility to inform potential partners of their infection and let the partners choose whether or not to become involved.[10] Infected people must also refrain from any practices that would expose their partners to virus.

Herpes virus can cross the placenta and infect a fetus. This seems most likely to occur when a woman first acquires genital herpes early in a pregnancy. How frequently this happens is not known. Fetal infection can result in spontaneous abortion or serious damage to the fetus, such as mental retardation and defective sight and/or hearing.[11] As discussed later, infection of an infant can also occur during birth if the mother is shedding virus at that time, with the possibility of serious complications.

LATENT INFECTION

Herpes viruses tend to produce long-term, *latent* (dormant or inactive) infections following a first attack. Infected people carry antibodies against the viruses, but between attacks, herpes viruses reside in the nervous system, where the antibodies cannot reach them.

Herpes viruses can be reactivated by various stimuli, including stress, friction, hormonal changes, and certain foods. Once stimulated, the viruses travel down the nerves, causing a new attack, usually at the same site as previous attacks.

Following the first attack of genital herpes, about 88 percent of those people with HSV-2 virus and about 50 percent of those with HSV-1 virus will have recurrences. If a person is going to have recurrences, the first will usually appear within six months after the primary infection.[12] The frequency of recurrences ranges from once every several years to many times each year.

SYMPTOMS OF GENITAL HERPES

When someone is first infected, herpes symptoms may appear anywhere between 2 and 12 days after contact with the virus. In females, genital herpes lesions may occur on the labia or within the vagina. Lesions occur on the penis or within the urethra in males, or on the thighs or buttocks in either gender.

The first attack of genital herpes is usually the worst. The first sign of a developing herpes attack is tingling, itching, or burning where the lesions are going to appear. Usually within hours after the itching begins, small red marks appear that develop into fluid-filled blisters. There can be from one to many of these blisters. The area around the blisters is red, swollen, hot, and painful. There may also be more general symptoms, including swollen lymph nodes, aching muscles, fever, and malaise.

Over the next two to ten days, the blisters break, leaving open, cratered, painful sores. Scabs form and healing gradually occurs. No scars usually remain. A first attack may require as long as four weeks to completely heal; subsequent attacks usually heal within two weeks. Some people never experience any subsequent attacks. Feature 19.5 (p. 598) discusses how to cope with genital herpes.

DIAGNOSIS OF HERPES

In order to tell if genital sores are caused by herpes simplex, you should visit your physician within three days of the appearance of a lesion. Several diagnostic methods are used. Often the lesions can be diagnosed as herpes on the basis of their appearance alone. Two types of smear tests are used, each of which requires a small amount of cells scraped from an active lesion. One of these tests, the direct fluorescent antibody (DFA) test is immunological, while the other test, the Tzanck (pronounced *zank*) test consists of microscopic

Genital herpes begins as small fluid-filled blisters on a red, swollen background. The blisters soon break, leaving painful, pitted areas.

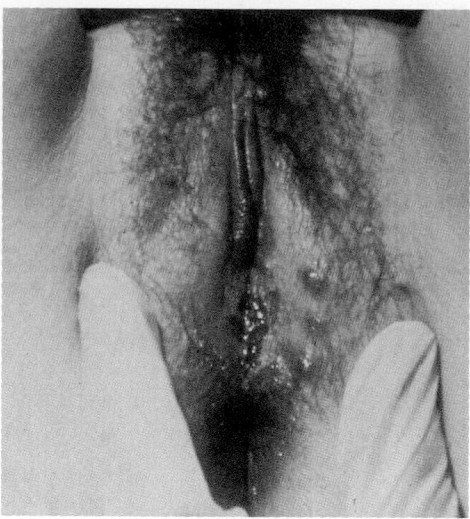 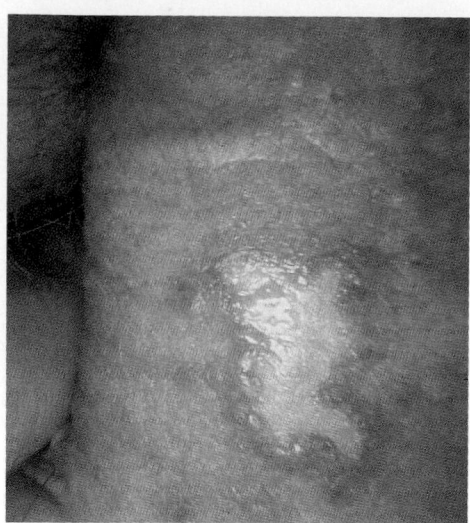

examination of cells scraped from the lesion. Herpes infected cells are unusually large and have multiple nuclei.

Blood tests detect antibodies to herpes viruses. They remain positive even between attacks and do not indicate if a particular sore is or is not herpes; they only indicate that a person has been infected. Viral cultures can also be taken. This is the only way to determine whether or not a person is shedding the virus when lesions are not present.

RELATIONSHIP OF HERPES TO HIV INFECTION

Herpes and HIV are two separate diseases, caused by different viruses, but a disturbing relationship

FEATURE 19.5

COPING WITH GENITAL HERPES

A diagnosis of genital herpes is not the end of the world. Certainly, it causes worry for most infected persons as well as for their sex partners and requires some ongoing precautions. Many people overreact to this situation, however, and come to view themselves as "sexual lepers." Not only do they withdraw from sexual relationships, but some socially isolate themselves, cutting off the support network that is so badly needed.

During an active herpes attack and when symptoms are just beginning to appear, the virus is quite contagious. A few commonsense precautions can reduce the risk of infecting others and can lessen the risks of herpes complications:

1. Discuss your herpes with a potential sexual partner *before* the relationship proceeds to genital contact. This is a moral and legal responsibility (people are being sued by partners whom they have infected).[a] The same standard applies to all other STDs as well. It is also a moral responsibility to tell a potential partner if you have had multiple sexual partners and are thus at increased risk of carrying the AIDS virus or some other STD.

2. Do not have sexual intercourse with anyone during an attack. It is also a good idea to use condoms between attacks if either partner has ever had genital herpes.

3. Discuss with your physician the possibility of obtaining a prescription for acyclovir if your attacks are frequent.

4. Maintain general good health and nutrition. Avoid physical irritation of the genitals as this seems to provoke repeated attacks. Practice effective stress-management techniques, as attacks are often stress related.

5. During attacks, the infected area should be dried well. Be careful not to spread the virus to the eyes by hands, towels, or similar means.

6. Consider joining a herpes support group. There are over a hundred HELP groups in the United States that are affiliated with The Herpes Resource Center, P.O. Box 13827, Research Triangle Park, NC 27709. You can write for membership information.

A diagnosis of genital herpes is no reason to abandon hope. Understanding how herpes infections are transmitted and how symptoms can be successfully treated can help reduce both the pain and the anxiety that accompany the disease.

[a]Davis, M. *Lovers, Doctors, and the Law.* New York: Harper & Row, 1989.

between them has been found.[13, 14] A statistical analysis of 471 heterosexual men and women was made which controlled for the influence of known risk factors for HIV infection, such as having multiple sexual partners. The analysis revealed that men and women who have genital herpes face double the risk of HIV infection of people who do not have genital herpes.

This and other studies suggest that HIV can find its way into the body through the open lesions produced when herpes blisters break. A similar association with HIV is believed to exist for any infection that causes lesions of the skin or mucous membranes.

TREATING GENITAL HERPES

The prescription antiviral medication acyclovir (*a-sī'klō-vir*) (Zovirax; *zō'vir-aks*) is the drug used most frequently for treating genital herpes. When taken orally, it can greatly reduce the frequency of attacks and reduce the severity of those that do occur *but it does not cure the disease.* Acyclovir is most effective if taken within 48 hours of a herpes outbreak. Acyclovir appears to be relatively safe.[15] It should not be used during pregnancy, however. It is also advisable to avoid becoming pregnant or fathering a child until several weeks after use of the drug has been discontinued.

Nonprescription treatments may help relieve pain, itching, and burning, but, like acyclovir, do not cure the disease. Astringent and drying agents, such as Burow's solution or Epsom salts, may also help relieve symptoms. There is little documented evidence that the virus is affected by special diets or vitamins. As with any disease, unproven remedies are best avoided.

Even if an effective cure for herpes is eventually developed, prevention will remain preferable to treatment. What is really needed to prevent herpes, in addition to avoiding exposure, is an effective vaccine. If such a vaccine becomes available, it will prevent new infections, but will not cure existing ones.

HERPES IN INFANTS

The most severe attacks of herpes are those that occur in infants infected before or during birth. The virus can cross the placenta and affect the fetus, causing spontaneous abortion or serious fetal damage, such as mental retardation and defective sight

and hearing. How frequently this happens is not known.

If the fetus of an infected woman remains free of virus until delivery (as confirmed by tests showing the absence of virus in the amniotic fluid), it must be protected from infection during the birth process. If a woman has active herpes lesions as she is giving birth, or if she sheds the virus in the absence of lesions, there is a good chance that the infant will contract the disease during birth. Because an infant's immune system is poorly developed, the infant is unable to fight the virus, which may spread throughout his or her body. Encephalitis (brain infection) may lead to death or permanent disability.

Because of the serious consequences of herpes in infants, many physicians do weekly herpes viral cultures on all infected pregnant women during the final six weeks of pregnancy.[16] If the mother has a positive herpes culture, delivery by cesarean section will protect the infant from infection.

CHECKPOINT

1. About how many Americans are infected with genital herpes?

2. When is someone with herpes contagious to others?

3. What are the symptoms of genital herpes?

HEPATITIS B

Hepatitis B (covered in more depth in the previous chapter) is a serious viral infection of the liver, characterized by jaundice (yellowing of the skin and whites of the eyes), loss of appetite, nausea, and abdominal discomfort. About 10 percent of infected people become chronic carriers of the virus. As is the case with other viral infections, there is no cure for a chronic hepatitis B infection. Chronic carriers, in addition to continuing to be able to infect others, have a greatly increased risk of liver cancer. If they are also infected with the hepatitis D virus, they are at a very high risk of cirrhosis, a potentially fatal degeneration of the liver.[17]

Methods of transmission of hepatitis B are similar to those of HIV, though hepatitis is much more highly contagious. It is transmitted through blood,

Genital warts. Some strains of the papilloma viruses that cause genital warts are believed to also cause cervical cancer.

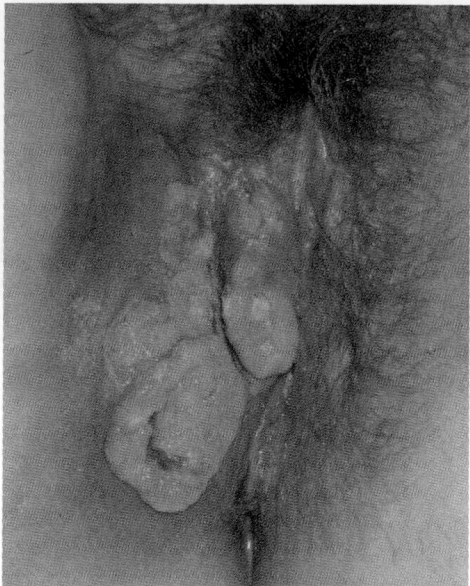 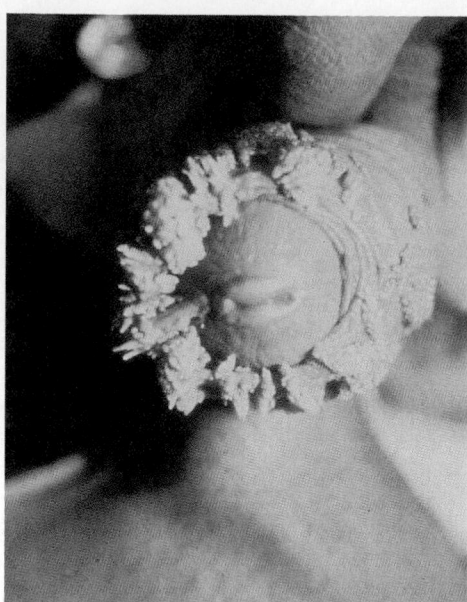

blood products, or penetration of the skin by any item contaminated by blood, such as an injection needle. It is also readily transmitted during sexual contact.

An effective vaccine to prevent hepatitis B is available. It became one of the recommended infant immunizations in 1992. This vaccine is also recommended for people who have occupational exposure to blood or other body fluids and for people who have multiple sex partners.

PAPILLOMA VIRUS INFECTION (GENITAL WARTS)

Evidence suggests that infection by **human papilloma** (*pap-i-lō'ma*) **viruses (HPV)** is today the *fastest-growing* STD in the United States. At least a million new cases are estimated to occur every year. Previously believed to cause only genital warts and similar harmless growths, 3 of the nearly 60 known forms of papilloma virus have now been strongly implicated in cervical cancer. Cervical cancer kills about 6800 women a year in the United States alone. Women with a history of genital warts are four times more likely to develop cervical cancer than women who have never had genital warts.[18] HPV can be found in almost 90 percent of

cervical cancer tissue samples. Further, papilloma virus may play a role in cancers of the vagina, vulva, and penis as well. Fortunately, about 90 percent of cases of genital warts are caused by forms of virus that do not cause cancer.[19]

Researchers have long known that women at greatest risk for cervical cancer are those who have had multiple sexual partners or who first had intercourse at an early age. Since virgin women seldom develop cervical cancer, scientists searched for a sexually transmitted factor in its development. At one time, herpes virus was the prime candidate, but now all the evidence points toward papilloma virus.

In addition to genital warts (which look quite similar to warts on the hands) papilloma viruses cause inconspicuous or even invisible lesions on the vulva, vaginal wall, and penis. Even when these lesions aren't visible, as is often the case, they actively produce and shed viral particles that are easily transmissible through sexual contact.

Physicians traditionally treated genital warts by various methods of physical removal, but they often reoccur following such removal. A newer method of treatment is by injecting interferon (see Chapter 18) directly into the warts. In most cases the warts disappear and do not return.

For now, there is no vaccine to prevent papilloma virus infection. Women are advised to limit the number of their sexual partners, insist that their partners use condoms, and have a Pap smear regularly.

....

human papilloma viruses the viruses that cause genital warts; some forms appear to cause cervical cancer.

CHECKPOINT

1. What are the greatest dangers associated with hepatitis B?

2. What is the most serious outcome of genital papilloma virus infection?

3. Are all papilloma viruses associated with this effect?

CHLAMYDIA INFECTION

Chlamydia trachomatis (kla-mid'ē-ah trah kō'matis) is currently recognized as the *most common* STD in the United States. *Chlamydia* are unusually small bacteria (Figure 19.5), visible only through an electron microscope. They live as intracellular parasites. The same species that causes genital infections also causes the eye infection **trachoma** (*trah-kō'mah*).

Genital *Chlamydia* infection is not a new disease, but has become more prevalent in recent years. Because *Chlamydia* is not reportable in many states, estimates of its prevalence vary but run well into the millions. It is estimated that over 10 percent of sexually active young females and over 5 percent of sexually active young males have genital *Chlamydia*.[20] It is especially prevalent on college campuses. Until recent years, many cases of genital *Chlamydia* were referred to as NSU (nonspecific urethritis) or NGU (nongonococcal urethritis) because testing for *Chlamydia* was difficult and, in some cities, unavailable.

Chlamydia is usually transmitted through vaginal intercourse. In about 70 percent of cases, there are no early symptoms. When symptoms are present, they may include, in males, painful and difficult urination and a thin urethral discharge. In females, symptoms may include painful urination, vaginal discharges, abdominal pain, and bleeding between menstrual periods. Untreated *Chlamydia* in females often progresses to a severe infection called **pelvic inflammatory disease (PID)** (see Feature 19.6, p. 602). About half of all PID (500,000 cases per year) result from *Chlamydia*.[21]

trachoma a severe eye infection that can lead to blindness.

pelvic inflammatory disease (PID) a severe infection of the abdominal cavity which, if left untreated, carries the risk of death.

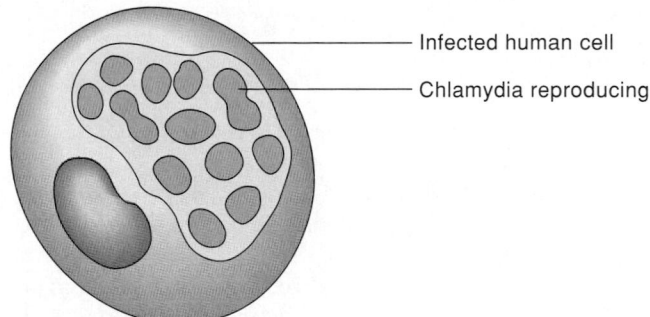

Figure 19.5
Chlamydia trachomatis

These tiny, oval, intracellular parasites cause genital Chlamydia, now recognized as the most common STD in the United States. (Actual size is microscopic.)

It is the long-term effects of untreated *Chlamydia* infection that cause the greatest concern. In either gender, fertility problems are the likely outcome of this genital infection. In males, the vas deferens are blocked by scar tissue, which prevents the movement of sperm from the testes to the urethra. In females, there are numerous effects on childbearing. The fallopian tubes may be blocked, making conception impossible. Seventy-five percent of women with fallopian tube blockage test positive for antibodies indicating *Chlamydia* infection at some time. The risk of ectopic (tubal or abdominal) pregnancy is greatly increased.[22] The risk of premature delivery is tripled.[23] Two-thirds of infants born vaginally to infected mothers are infected during the birth process, developing eye infections or pneumonia.[24]

Physicians can diagnose an active *Chlamydia* infection by culturing the organism from infected areas and can detect a past infection by testing a blood sample for antibodies to the bacteria. Once diagnosed, the organism can be killed by a week-long treatment with a prescribed antibiotic. As both sexes are commonly infected, sex partners need to be simultaneously treated.

CHECKPOINT

1. What are the symptoms of *Chlamydia* infection in each gender?

2. Does *Chlamydia* always produce these symptoms?

3. What long-term effects are associated with untreated *Chlamydia* infection?

FEATURE 19.6

PELVIC INFLAMMATORY DISEASE (PID)

Pelvic inflammatory disease (PID) is a collective term for any extensive bacterial infection of the female pelvic organs, particularly the uterus, cervix, fallopian tubes, and ovaries. Symptoms of PID include severe pain, fever, and sometimes vaginal discharge.

Chlamydia and gonorrhea are the two leading causes of PID; about half of all cases are caused by Chlamydia and about 40 percent by gonorrhea or a combination of gonorrhea and Chlamydia. It is theorized that these bacteria, which have no form of motility (movement) of their own, attach themselves to sperm and are transported by sperm to the fallopian tubes and on into the abdominal cavity.[a] Women using barrier-type contraceptives have lower rates of PID than other sexually active women. Even so, condoms or other barriers are not 100 percent effective in preventing Chlamydia.

The past 20 years have brought a tremendous increase in the number of cases of PID. While in 1970 there were only 17,800 cases of PID, now there are about one million per year and about 150,000 of these require surgery, such as removal of an infected fallopian tube.[a] *Tens of thousands of women have been rendered sterile by PID in recent years.* A woman who has a single case of PID has a 10–15 percent chance of becoming sterile. Among women who have three or more instances of PID, 50–75 percent become sterile. Sterile means *no children ever,* without resorting to difficult, expensive, and uncertainly effective in vitro (test tube) fertilization.

PID is usually treated with the simultaneous administration of two powerful antibiotics—one for Chlamydia and one for gonorrhea. This combination is recommended because many women who are infected with one of these diseases are also infected with the other. Further, to determine which pathogen caused a particular case of PID before treatment started would delay treatment and increase the risk of permanent damage to the reproductive organs.

[a]Tortora, G. Funke, B., and Case, C. *Microbiology*, 5th ed. Redwood City, CA: Benjamin/Cummings, 1995.

GONORRHEA

Gonorrhea (gon-ō-rē'a) is infection by a bacterium (Figure 19.6) called the **gonococcus** (gon" ō-kok' us). Both the pathogen and the disease are called GC in a clinical setting. Gonorrhea is also commonly called *the clap.*

The number of reported cases of gonorrhea has declined from about a million per year in 1980 to about 386,000 in 1993. This is just *reported* cases—the true incidence is much higher. Many infected people do not seek treatment because they are either asymptomatic or experiencing relatively mild symptoms that they choose to ignore. Of cases treated by private physicians, many are not reported, either to protect the patient's confidentiality or to save time for the physician.

TRANSMISSION AND SITES OF INFECTION

Gonorrhea can be transmitted through various kinds of sexual contact—heterosexual or homosexual—including genital, oral-genital, and anal-genital contact. As the gonococcus does not survive for more than a few minutes when exposed to cold or dryness, transmission by contaminated inanimate objects is rare. The incubation period for gonorrhea is usually 2–8 days, but can range up to 30 days.

The gonococcus grows mainly in membranes, including those of the eye, throat, rectum, and sex organs. Gonorrheal infection of the eye is a severe conjunctivitis that, without adequate treatment, can lead to blindness. Gonorrhea in the throat, usually contracted during fellatio, has no symptoms other than a "sore throat." Rectal gonorrhea can be painful or symptomless. If left untreated for a long period of time, gonorrhea may become systemic, attacking the membranes of the heart, brain (meninges), kidneys, blood vessels, and joints, and also causing skin lesions.

Figure 19.6
Neisseria gonorrhoeae

This microscopic bacterium, also called the Gonococcus or GC, causes gonorrhea. It infects several million Americans every year.

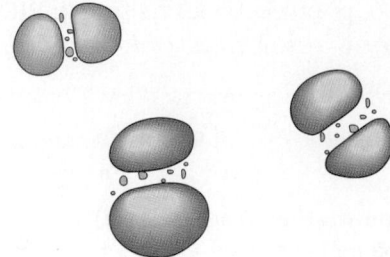

---

gonococcus the bacterium that causes gonorrhea.

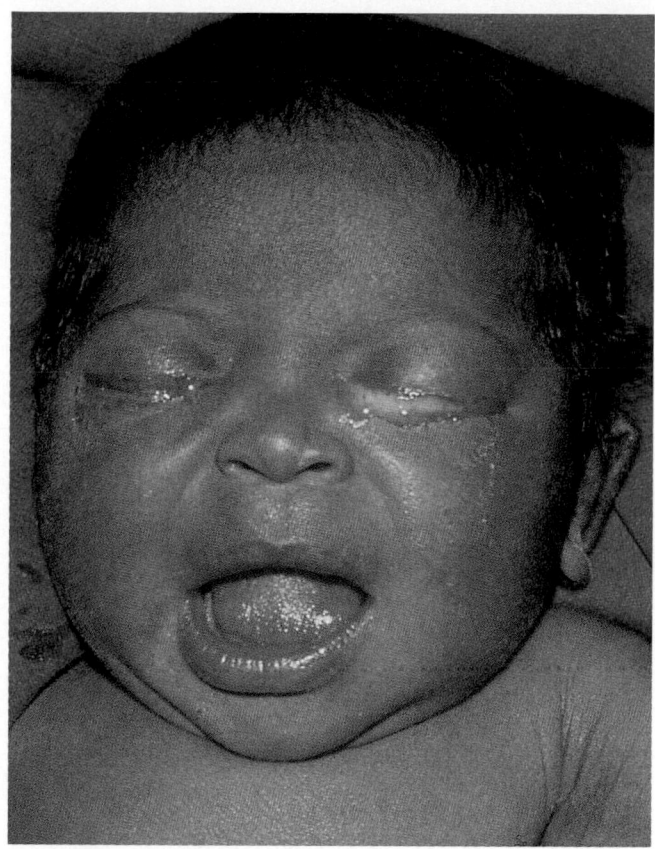

Gonorrheal infection of the eye. Without adequate treatment, this infection can cause blindness.

majority—perhaps 80 percent—of infected women do not realize that they have gonorrhea until their male partners discover their own infections. A female's infection often centers on the cervix, where there are few pain receptors. Chronic female carriers are a major factor in the spread of gonorrhea.

Symptoms among women may include vaginal irritation, pain during intercourse, and vaginal discharge. Untreated, the infection spreads upward through the fallopian tubes, where it causes sterility by blocking the tubes with scar tissue. Like *Chlamydia,* untreated gonorrhea may cause massive infection (pelvic inflammatory disease; see Feature 19.6). It is estimated that 20–30 percent of untreated gonorrhea cases in females progress to PID.[25]

NEONATAL GONORRHEA

When a woman with gonorrhea gives birth, the baby's eyes may be infected during the delivery. Unless promptly treated, this infection may lead to blindness. Laws require that erythromycin or silver nitrate or some other effective antibacterial product be placed in the eyes of every newborn to prevent this infection. Infants may also acquire genital gonorrhea during birth.

SYMPTOMS OF MALE GENITAL GONORRHEA

Male genital gonorrhea usually begins as urethritis, inflammation of the urethra. This typically causes a burning pain during urination and a discharge of pus from the urethra. In early stages of the infection, this discharge tends to be watery or milky. Later, it becomes thick, greenish yellow, and often tinged with blood. At least 10 percent of infected males have no obvious symptoms, and become symptomless carriers.

Without prompt treatment, the infection may spread through the vas deferens, prostate gland, epididymis, testes, bladder, and kidneys. Permanent damage can include urinary obstruction and sterility, as scar tissue blocks the various urogenital ducts.

SYMPTOMS OF FEMALE GENITAL GONORRHEA

Early symptoms of female genital gonorrhea are often so slight that they are ignored. In fact, the

Symptoms of male genital gonorrhea include a thick urethral discharge and a burning sensation while urinating.

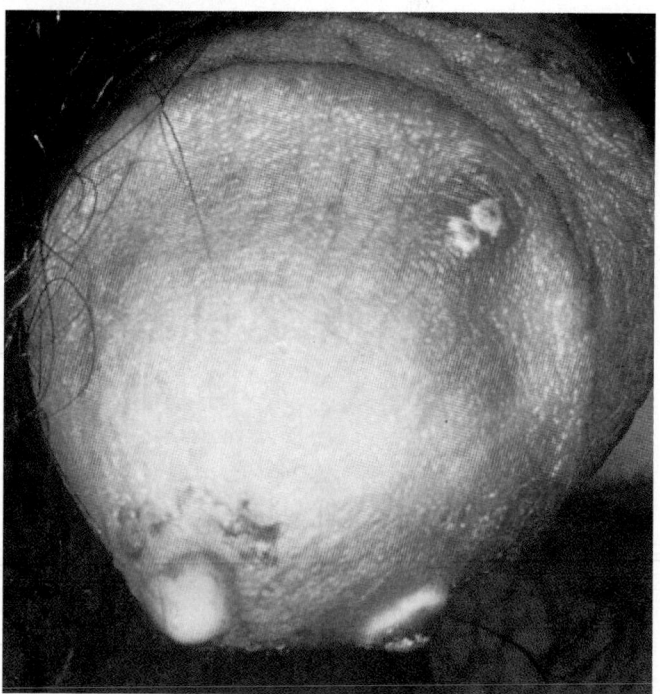

SOME UNCOMMON STDs

Several STDs are currently at low incidence levels in the United States. We will very briefly describe two of them.

CHANCROID

Chancroid (*shang'kroyd*) is a bacterial infection. Its incidence has declined to under 2000 cases per year in the United States. Most cases are traceable to intercourse with prostitutes. The incubation period is 1–14 days. Chancroid produces a deep ulcerlike lesion that spreads laterally, causing tissue destruction, and it may infect other body parts that touch the lesion. Nearby lymph nodes are enlarged. Chancroid is curable with antibiotics.

LYMPHOGRANULOMA VENEREUM

Lymphogranuloma venereum (*lim"fō-gran" ū-lō'mah ve-nē' rē-um*) is caused by specific strains of *Chlamydia trachomatis*, the pathogen of genital *Chlamydia* infection. There are only a few hundred cases per year in the United States, primarily in homosexual males or immigrants from Southeast Asia, Africa, and Central and South America. The incubation period is 3–30 days. Lymphogranuloma venereum may pass through three stages: (1) *the primary lesion:* a painless pimple, blister, or erosion that heals without scarring in two or three days; (2) *the inguinal syndrome:* starts with enlarged, painful lymph nodes. The skin over these nodes breaks down to form multiple cavities that may drain pus for months; and (3) *the genitoanorectal syndrome:* lesions in the rectal wall cause anal discharge. Rectal lymph nodes are enlarged. An opening may develop in the wall between the rectum and vagina. Elephantiasis (enlargement) of the penis, scrotum, or labia may develop. Lymphogranuloma venereum is curable with antibiotics.

DIAGNOSING AND TREATING GONORRHEA

The most reliable tests for gonorrhea are **agar** (a culture medium providing a solid surface for the culture of microorganisms) cultures in which the site of the suspected infection is rubbed with a swab. The swab is then rubbed over the agar, where the gonococcus, if present, will grow. Diagnosis of gonorrhea has been aided by the development of an enzyme-linked antibody (ELISA) test that detects the gonococcus within three hours in material swabbed from the urethra or cervix.[26] A quicker, though less reliable, test is to make a stained microscope slide with pus swabbed from the suspected infected area, such as the urethra, and to examine the slide microscopically for the presence of the gonococcus.

Gonorrhea is treated with antibiotic drugs. Drug resistance is a severe problem with gonorrhea. So far, no totally drug-resistant gonococcus has been identified, though some strains are resistant to many drugs.[27] There is no effective home remedy or nonprescription cure for gonorrhea.

Several other bacterial STDs have been uncommon in recent years. They are described briefly in Feature 19.7.

SYPHILIS

Syphilis is caused by a form of bacteria called a spirochete (*spī'rō-kēt*). Though syphilis is less common than gonorrhea (about 26,000 reported cases in 1993), it is a more dangerous disease because it always enters the bloodstream as a **systemic** infection. In recent years, many cases of syphilis have been traced to chemically dependent female prostitutes. This is a major concern, because prostitutes who are intravenous drug abusers are also likely to be sources of AIDS.

Syphilis, like herpes, is a disease that produces open lesions (sores). These lesions provide an ideal portal of exit for HIV from people who are already infected with HIV and an ideal portal of entry for HIV into people who are not yet infected.[28]

---

agar a culture medium providing a solid surface for the culture of microorganisms.

systemic pertaining to a whole body rather than to one of its parts.

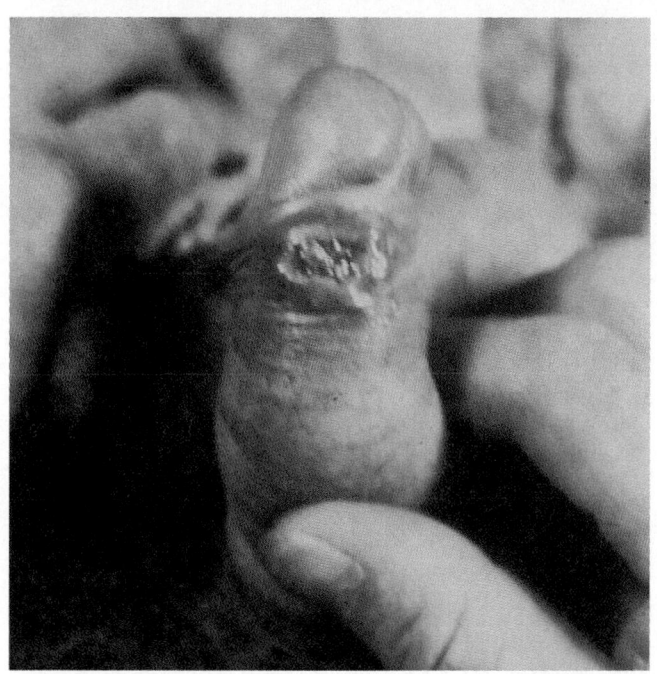

A chancre, the first symptom of syphilis. This lesion, at the point of entry of the spirochetes, can be anywhere on the body, including within the vagina or rectum. It does not hurt, so such hidden chancres might not be noticed.

SOURCE AND TRANSMISSION

Syphilis is transmissible by contact only during those stages (primary and secondary) when lesions are present. Often these lesions, which swarm with spirochetes, are hidden inside the vagina or rectum. Transmission is most often sexual, but kissing and other skin to skin contact with lesions can pass the spirochetes. **Transplacental** (across the placenta) transmission to a fetus occurs at about five months of pregnancy, even in the absence of any lesions. If an infected woman is successfully treated early in her pregnancy, the fetus will be safe.

PRIMARY SYPHILIS

Syphilis is a highly variable disease. Its incubation period ranges from 10 to 90 days. The first symptom to appear is the primary lesion or **chancre** (*shang'ker*). A chancre is a pink or red open sore, which is raised, firm, and painless. It is often the size of a dime, but may be smaller. A chancre appears at the exact spot where spirochetes invad-

....

transplacental across the placenta.

chancre the primary lesion of syphilis; an ulcer swarming with spirochetes.

ed the body, and is often on or near the sex organs, but can be on the lip, tongue, finger, or any part of the body. There may be one or several chancres. In a female, it is often within the vagina, unseen by a male partner, and unfelt by the woman. The chancre's cratered surface is swarming with spirochetes. Any sexual or other direct contact with a chancre is likely to transmit syphilis.

Even without treatment, the chancre disappears in three to six weeks. At about this time, blood tests for syphilis become positive. If the disease has not been treated, it progresses to the secondary stage.

SECONDARY SYPHILIS

Symptoms of secondary syphilis occur throughout the body and appear one to six months after the appearance of the chancre. The most common secondary symptom is a *rash* that does not itch. This rash is variable in appearance and location. It often appears on the palms of the hands and soles of the

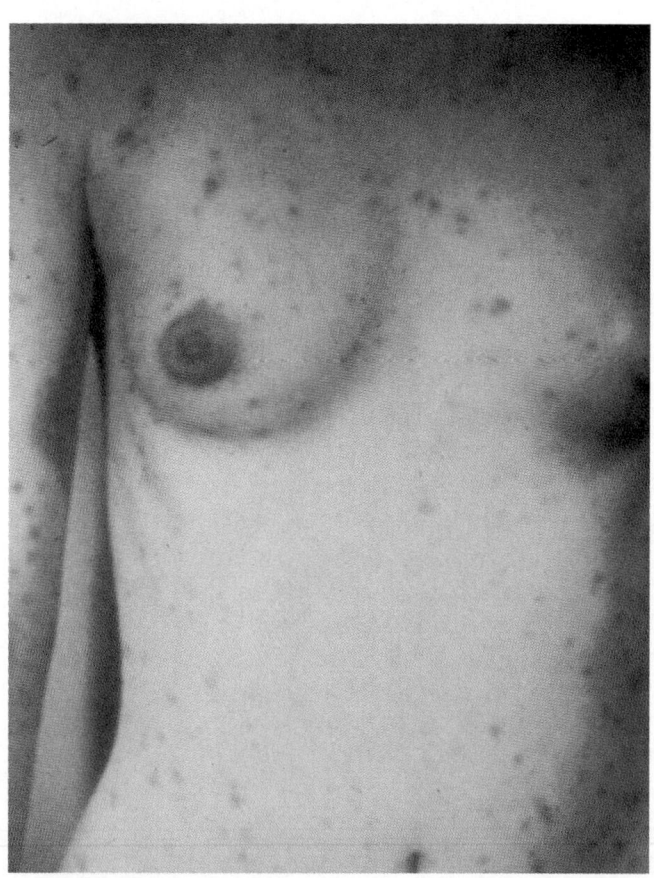

Skin rash characteristic of secondary syphilis. This rash is quite variable and might appear different from this case. It may cover the whole body or any part of it. It often occurs on the palms of the hands or soles of the feet. It does not itch.

feet. Large, moist, *oral and genital lesions* may also be present. Spirochetes are present on their surface and any sexual or other contact, such as kissing, may cause infection. Other secondary symptoms may include a sore throat, headache, fever, red eyes, pain in the joints, and hair loss.

The symptoms of secondary syphilis persist from several weeks to a year. When they disappear, syphilis enters the latent stage. Secondary symptoms can reappear from time to time during the first several years of latent syphilis.

LATENT SYPHILIS

Latent syphilis can last from a few months to a lifetime. Only a blood test can show that the person has syphilis, as there are *no external signs of disease.* Except during recurrences of secondary lesions, syphilis is no longer contagious by person-to-person contact, but it can still be transmitted at any time from a pregnant woman to her fetus.

Some people spontaneously recover from latent syphilis when their body defenses overcome the spirochetes. There are no reliable statistics on the percentage of people who do so.

In other people with latent syphilis, progressive degeneration of the brain, spinal cord, and other organs may occur unnoticed. When these symptoms occur, the last stage of syphilis has begun.

LATE (TERTIARY) SYPHILIS

Tertiary syphilis is characterized by *permanent damage to vital organs.* The most severe damage often occurs in the circulatory and nervous systems.

In the *circulatory system,* arterial walls may weaken, which can cause dangerous **aneurysms** (*an'ū-riz-mz;* bulges in arterial walls) that may rupture, and cause almost instant death due to hemorrhage. Heart valves may also be damaged.

In the *nervous system,* the presence of large numbers of spirochetes causes degeneration of the brain and spinal cord, producing effects collectively called **paresis** (*pah-rē'sis*). Paresis includes per-

....

aneurysm abnormal dilation (bulge) of a blood vessel.

paresis paralysis and mental deterioration caused by degeneration of the brain and spinal cord in late syphilis.

sonality changes, decreased ability to carry out tasks, and impairment of concentration and judgment. Physical symptoms include a progressive loss of muscle control, causing paralysis and loss of reflexes. Progressive loss of vision can also occur. Death eventually results.

CONGENITAL SYPHILIS

Congenital (present at birth) syphilis, resulting from transplacental infection of a fetus, may take various forms. The most extreme outcome of congenital syphilis is stillbirth, in which the fetus dies prior to birth. Among infants surviving with congenital syphilis, many different types of internal and external damage may be present. All pregnant women should be tested for syphilis early in their pregnancies. Treatment in the first few months of pregnancy will prevent fetal infection.

DIAGNOSIS AND TREATMENT OF SYPHILIS

Early syphilis can be diagnosed by examining spirochetes, located in the primary and secondary lesions, microscopically. Around the time the chancre disappears, blood tests become positive and remain so until long after successful treatment. Blood tests may even remain positive for life.

The VDRL (Venereal Disease Research Laboratory) test and the similar RPR (rapid plasma reagin) test are the most common screening tests for syphilis. Both give a significant percentage of false positive reactions for syphilis so a positive test is confirmed with a more specific test such as the FTA (fluorescent treponemal antibody) test.

Some states require a blood test for syphilis in order to issue a marriage license, though this requirement has been challenged as not being cost-effective. Very few cases of syphilis are discovered among people obtaining marriage licenses.

Syphilis is treated with penicillin and other antibiotics in large and prolonged doses. The sooner treatment begins, the smaller the likelihood of permanent organ damage, which cannot be cured. As with other STDs, there is no home remedy that will cure syphilis.

Syphilis is a disease where *preventive* antibiotic use, after a possible exposure to the disease, can

....

congenital present at birth.

be very effective. The long incubation period of syphilis (10–90 days) allows eradication of the spirochetes before the disease symptoms begin.

CHECKPOINT

1. Syphilis progresses in definite stages. Name and describe each of its stages.

2. What are the potential long-term results of untreated syphilis? ✔

BACTERIAL VAGINITIS

Vaginal infections may have various causes, but three pathogens—*Candida (kan'di-da), Trichomonas (trik-ō-mō'nas),* and *Gardnerella (gardner-el' la)*—account for the majority of cases. Table 19.3 compares the three. *Candida* and *Trichomonas* infections are usually referred to as vaginitis (*vaj-in-ī'tis*), inflammation of the vagina. *Gardnerella* infection is sometimes called bacterial vaginosis (*vaj-in-o'sis*), the distinction being the relative lack of inflammation with *Gardnerella.*[29]

The bacterium *Gardnerella vaginalis* accounts for about a third of all vaginal infections, excluding gonorrhea and *Chlamydia.*[30] Bacterial vaginitis is characterized by a frothy vaginal discharge that has a fishy odor. Actually, *Gardnerella* cannot produce vaginitis by itself, but acts in conjunction with other vaginal bacteria. *Gardnerella* usually becomes a problem only when the vagina is less acidic than normal, as might occur when birth control pills are taken or antibiotics or douching have destroyed the vagina's beneficial acid-forming bacteria (see Feature 19.8). Over 90 percent of male partners of women with bacterial vaginitis have asymptomatic urethral colonization by *Gardnerella,* suggesting that sexual transmission of this organism may occur.[31] *Gardnerella* is treated by drugs such as metronidazole, which spare the vagina's acid-forming bacteria.

CHECKPOINT

1. What are the symptoms of bacterial vaginitis?

2. How might douching lead to bacterial vaginitis? ✔

Table 19.3
Characteristics of Three Common Types of Vaginitis

	Candida albicans	Gardnerella vaginalis	Trichomonas vaginalis
Type of organism	Yeast	Bacterium	Protozoan
Amount of discharge	Varies	Abundant	Varies
Consistency of discharge	Curdy	Frothy	Frothy
Color of discharge	White	Gray-white	Greenish-yellow
Odor of discharge	Yeasty	Fishy	Foul
Vaginal lining	Dry, red	Pink	Tender, red

FEATURE 19.8

REDUCE YOUR RISK OF VAGINITIS

Vaginitis (vaginal inflammation) is a common, but often unnecessary, disorder. Since vaginitis is often caused by organisms normally present in the vagina, rather than being a condition that can be "caught" from a partner, there are many things you can do to help prevent this problem.

1. Eat properly. Excessive sugar favors the growth of *Candida* (yeast) and the body's defenses against infection work more effectively with proper nutrition.

2. Keep your vaginal area dry. Wear cotton underwear. Avoid nylon underwear or panty hose. If you buy nylon underwear with a cotton crotch, be sure it is really a cotton inset and not just cotton sewn over the nylon.

3. Wash your vaginal area thoroughly every day and dry the area carefully. Don't use other people's towels or washcloths. Avoid irritating soaps or sprays.

4. Douching (washing out the vagina) is rarely recommended. It may promote vaginitis by eliminating the vagina's protective mucus layer and washing away the beneficial, acid-forming bacteria. If you believe that you must douche, talk to your doctor. Further, a mildly acidic solution, such as one or two tablespoons of vinegar in a quart of warm water, is better than most commercial preparations.

5. Avoid wearing pants that are so tight in the crotch that they "cut" or irritate the genitals.

6. Make sure that your sexual partners are clean. It is a good idea for a man to wash his penis prior to intercourse.

7. Avoid petroleum jellies such as Vaseline for vaginal lubrication. Use water-soluble jellies instead.

8. Avoid any sexual practice that is painful or irritating to your vagina.

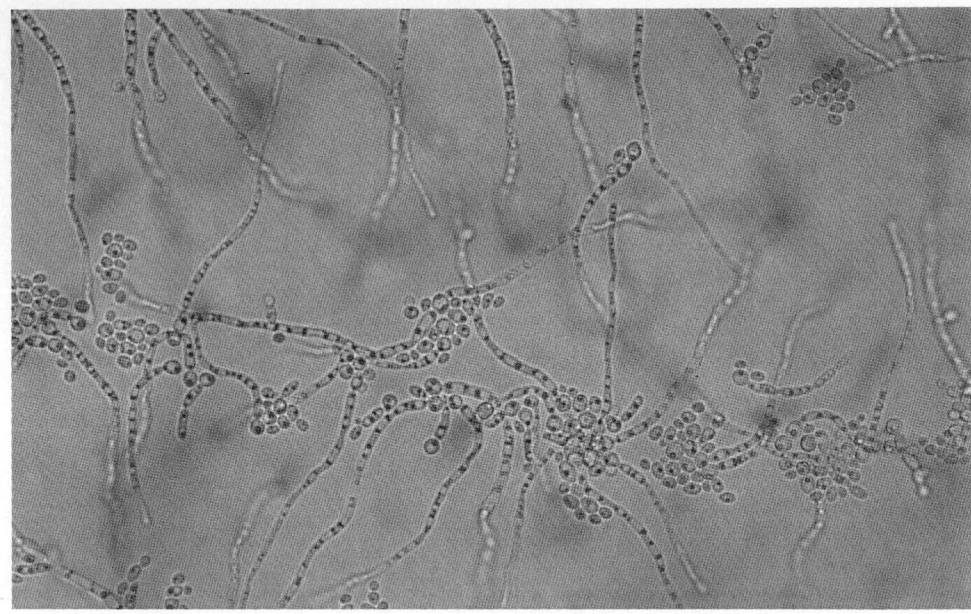

Candida albicans, *the cause of the common vaginal "yeast infection," produces a thick, white discharge. Individual yeast cells are microscopic.*

CANDIDA (YEAST INFECTION)

One of the most common genital infections is caused by the pathogenic yeast, *Candida albicans* (*kan'did-ah al'bi-kans*). *Candida* infection is technically called **candidiasis** (*kan-did-ī'ah-sis*) and is commonly called a "yeast infection." *Candida* is present in the healthy mouth and intestine of most people and in the vagina of most women. The other microorganisms and body defenses usually regulate the amount of yeast that is present. A yeast infection results from any of the following:

- antibiotic use, which may destroy beneficial acid-forming vaginal bacteria
- diabetes, which impairs body defenses and produces high sugar levels in the body, which precipitates the growth of yeast
- pregnancy or oral contraceptives, which may reduce vaginal acidity
- poor diet, especially when it is high in sugar
- moisture buildup, caused by wearing nylon panties, panty hose, or other synthetic fabrics (cotton "breathes" much better)
- douching too often, or with nonacidic solutions

....

candidiasis infection by the yeast *Candida albicans*.

Symptoms of vaginal yeast infections include burning and itching and a thick, whitish discharge. There also may be patches of white membranelike material on the vaginal lining. *Candida* is usually diagnosed by examining a stained microscope slide of the discharge.

A variety of oral and vaginal medications for treating yeast infections are available. To speed the healing process, the vaginal area should be kept dry and any contributing conditions, such as poor nutrition, corrected (see Feature 19.8). Male sexual partners should use condoms while the female has a yeast or other vaginal infection. This avoids the male becoming infected, usually without symptoms, and later reinfecting the female.

CHECKPOINT

1. What symptoms characterize a vaginal yeast infection?

2. What conditions commonly provoke a yeast infection?

TRICHOMONAS

Trichomonas vaginalis (*trik-ō-mō'nas va-jin-al'is*) is a protozoan (one-celled animal-like organism, Figure 19.7) that lives in the vagina of many women without producing any noticeable symptoms. Under some conditions, such as when antibi-

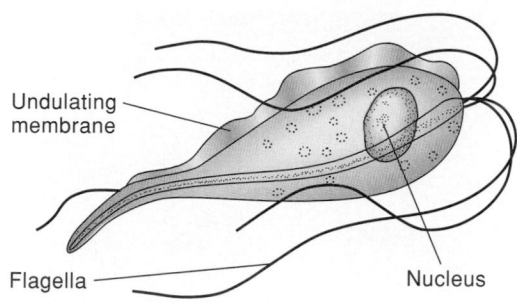

Figure 19.7
Trichomonas vaginalis

This microscopic protozoan causes vaginal infections characterized by a thin, foamy, yellowish discharge.

Undulating membrane

Flagella

Nucleus

otics or birth control pills are being taken, or when a woman is pregnant, *Trichomonas* can multiply enormously in the vagina. Symptoms include intense vaginal itching and burning, rashlike spots on the vaginal lining, and a profuse discharge of a thin, foamy, yellowish substance that may have a foul odor.

In males, symptomless infections of the prostate gland, urethra, and seminal vesicles are common. Symptoms in males, though they rarely occur, include urethritis, or even more rarely, inflammation of the prostate gland or seminal vesicles.

Trichomonas is transmitted sexually, during birth, and possibly through contact with inanimate articles such as towels.[32] Vaginal discharge is examined microscopically so the condition can be diag-

nosed. Prescribed oral or vaginal medications are used to treat *Trichomonas*. Simultaneous treatment of sexual partners is important in preventing reinfection.

One drug used to treat *Trichomonas*—Flagyl (metronidazole)—has several possible side effects. It has been shown to cause cancer in laboratory animals, so any unnecessary use should be avoided. Women in their first trimester of pregnancy should not use this drug because it could cause fetal defects. Also, it should not be used by women who are breastfeeding. Finally, alcohol should be avoided when Flagyl is being taken, since the combination causes dizziness, cramps, vomiting, and headaches.

PUBIC LICE (CRABS)

Pubic lice, called "crabs" or crab lice because of their crablike appearance, are small gray insects, about one-sixteenth of an inch long, that live in the body hair. They prefer pubic hair, but are sometimes found in underarm hair, eyebrows, eyelashes, and beards. They rarely live in scalp hair, because its texture is too fine. Pubic lice suck blood, causing some people intense itching and skin discoloration.

Pubic lice may be transmitted through sexual or other close physical contact. They are also trans-

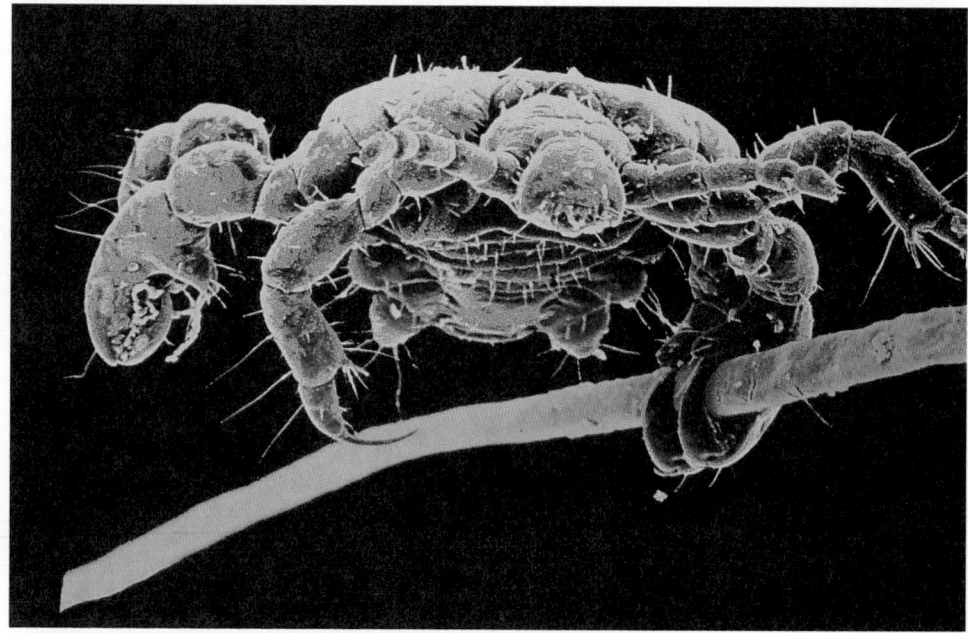

Pubic louse (crab louse), actual size about one-sixteenth inch. These small gray insects live in pubic hair or other body hair and suck blood.

mitted through contaminated clothing, toilet seats, bedding, or towels. They multiply rapidly by attaching eggs, called **nits,** to the hairs.

Crabs can be controlled by special insecticidal shampoos, which are available without prescription at pharmacies. Several applications may be necessary. Infested hair need not be shaved and exposed clothing need not be discarded. Clothing and bedding should be thoroughly washed in hot water before further use, however.

SCABIES (THE ITCH)

Scabies (*skā'bēz*) is parasitism of the skin by tiny, burrowing, spiderlike mites. Scabies is highly contagious, usually by sexual or other direct contact. It is also spread by freshly contaminated clothing or bedding.

Symptoms include burrows that appear as discolored lines on the skin, welts, and water- or pus-filled blisters, which are extremely itchy. In addition to the genital area, scabies may appear under the breasts, in the armpits, between the fingers, and elsewhere. Scabies is diagnosed by recovering the mite from its burrow and identifying it microscopically. Applying ink to the skin and then rinsing it off discloses the burrows. Like crabs, scabies is cured through the use of insecticidal shampoos.

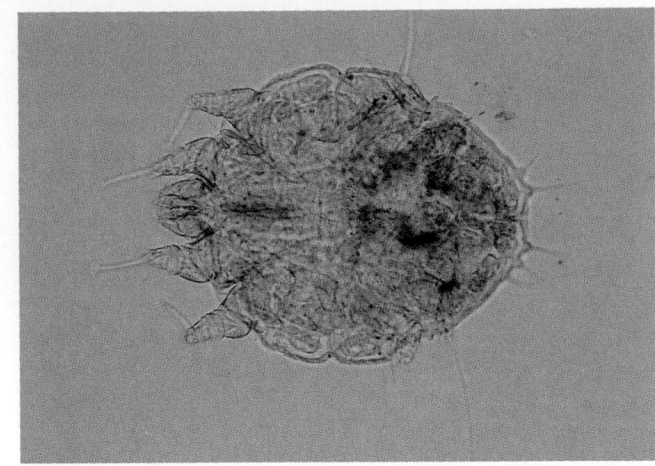

Scabies mite. These tiny mites, spread by sexual or other contact, burrow through the skin and cause intense itching.

CHECKPOINT

1. What type of pathogen is *Trichomonas?*

2. What are the common effects of *Trichomonas* in each gender?

3. How would a person know that he or she had crabs? Scabies?

PREVENTING SEXUALLY TRANSMITTED DISEASES

The best way to avoid contracting sexually transmitted diseases is to practice *abstinence.* The sec-

ond best way is to practice *selective sexual behavior.* In recent years, the threat of AIDS and other STDs has caused many people to reevaluate their sexual habits and place new emphasis on *abstinence* or *long-term, monogamous relationships.* The emergence of AIDS has added a new urgency to the need to control STDs. Preventing STDs involves both personal and public health efforts.

PERSONAL PREVENTION

As with most other diseases, the ultimate responsibility for preventing STDs lies with *you.* The first step is to *minimize the number of your sexual partners* because the more partners you have, the greater the risk of contracting diseases. STDs can be transmitted through heterosexual or homosexual contact, including genital-genital, oral-genital, and anal-genital activity.

Another basic step you must take is to *avoid high-risk activity* or *high-risk sexual partners.* High-risk activities include unprotected (no condom used) vaginal or anal intercourse. The risk increases with the number of partners you have and the less well-known they are to you.

With today's high incidence of STDs, high-risk partners include anyone who has a variety of partners or anyone who has one regular partner who, in turn, has many partners. An example of the latter case is a woman whose bisexual husband has

---

nits eggs of lice.

many male partners. Also, considering the methods of transmission of HIV and hepatitis B, a high-risk partner is anyone who abuses drugs by injection or who has another partner who does. Anyone you don't know very well must be classified as a high-risk partner, even if he or she looks very healthy. Sometimes you think you know someone and you really don't, as when a spouse secretly has other sex partners.

Fearing rejection, people who have histories of a great number of sexual partners or of drug abuse are unlikely to reveal their entire personal histories to potential new partners. Thus, you may not be aware of someone's sexual or drug abuse history after only a few dates. It is best to move into a sexual relationship very slowly, getting to know a potential partner very well before becoming sexually involved. Even then, the following precautions should be taken.

If you insist on coital activity outside of long-term relationships, it is essential to make maximum use of other personal preventive methods to reduce the risk of infection. (We use the word *reduce* rather than *eliminate,* since none of the following methods is totally effective.)

During precoital sex play, *be aware of any signs of possible infection in your partner,* such as urethral discharge or genital lesions of any kind. If such signs are present, immediately discontinue sexual activity with that partner until he or she has been examined by a physician, and if necessary, treated for the condition.

Condoms are highly recommended for disease prevention. Though they aren't 100 percent effective, they *help* prevent transmission of HIV, herpes, gonorrhea, *Chlamydia,* and most other STDs. Research has shown that the risk of HIV transmission is *many* times greater when a condom is not used than when one is used.[33] To be effective, the condom must be applied to the erect penis *before any genital contact is made* (see Chapter 7 for application procedures). Even when condoms are not required for birth-control purposes, a wise person will insist on their use in any situation other than in a long-term, monogamous relationship. Although it has traditionally been a male responsibility to provide condoms, many women now keep a supply available. The female condom, with its greater coverage, appears to be a good choice for disease prevention, although its effectiveness is not yet well documented.

Even when a condom is used, it is still important for both partners to *wash with soap and water* before and after contact because the male condom only covers the penis. The pathogens of diseases such as syphilis and herpes, which can enter the body through the skin, can often be killed or removed with soap and water.

Urinating immediately after sexual contact may help to reduce the chance of urethral infection by diseases such as gonorrhea and *Chlamydia*. It also helps to prevent bladder infection (cystitis), discussed in Chapter 21.

Avoid oral-anal stimulation (anilingus). The incidence of amoebic and other dysenteries is very high among people who practice anilingus.

Antibiotics are occasionally used as a preventive measure after possible exposure to an STD. This might be useful for people who have been sexually involved with someone who has been diagnosed as having a bacterial STD. Antibiotics, however, are not effective against a viral infection such as herpes or HIV. Antibiotics should only be used when prescribed by a physician.

The most effective personal preventive measure, other than abstinence, is a *vaccine* for each disease. Few communicable diseases have ever really been controlled until effective vaccines have been developed against them. *So far, the only STD for which a vaccine is available is hepatitis B.* If you have multiple sexual partners, you should obtain this vaccine. Take a moment right now and complete In Your Hands: Your Behavior and Attitudes Regarding Sexually Transmitted Disease.

PUBLIC HEALTH MEASURES

Even though preventing STDs is mainly an individual responsibility, public health agencies play an important role in STD control. Most public health departments sponsor STD education programs in schools and other locations, and operate clinics for diagnosing and treating STDs at little or no cost to the individual. Laws in most states have been revised to allow for treatment of minors, often as young as 12 years of age, without parental permission or notification. It has been found that when parental permission is required for treatment, many

IN YOUR HANDS

YOUR BEHAVIOR AND ATTITUDES REGARDING SEXUALLY TRANSMITTED DISEASE

In few areas of health-related behavior is the *personal responsibility* greater and the direct cause-and-effect relationship of behavior to health result more obvious than in the prevention of sexually transmitted diseases. How does your behavior in this area rate?

	Almost Always	Sometimes	Almost Never
1. I am sexually abstinent *or* maintain a mutually monogamous relationship.	10	2	0
2. In developing a new sexual partnership, I consider the risk of STD transmission.	4	1	0
3. I avoid sexual relationships with people who have many sexual partners.	4	1	0
4. I avoid sexual relationships with intravenous drug abusers.	4	1	0
5. If a new relationship is becoming sexual, I discuss the topic of STDs with that person before engaging in sexual intercourse.	4	1	0
6. In anything other than a monogamous relationship, I insist on condom use.	4	1	0
7. I avoid anal intercourse in any relationship other than a monogamous one.	4	1	0

8. I know the symptoms (or understand that there may be no symptoms) for:	Yes:	No:	
HIV infection	2	0	
Herpes	2	0	
Gonorrhea	2	0	
Chlamydia	2	0	
Syphilis	2	0	
Genital warts	2	0	

	Almost Always	Sometimes	Almost Never
9. If I suspected I had an STD, I would immediately see a physician or go to a health center.	4	1	0
10. If I learned that I had an STD, I would immediately inform my sex partner(s).	4	1	0

Total points: _____

INTERPRETATION:

50–54 points: Your risk of STD is very low.

46–49 points: Your risk of STD is low.

40–45 points: Your risk of STD is average.

35–39 points: Your risk of STD is higher than average.

Under 35 points: Your risk of STD is very high. These are dangerous diseases that have become very common in our society. Read this chapter very carefully and apply its contents to your own life-style.

young people simply avoid it out of fear of reprisal. In those cases, not only do they then risk permanent damage as a result of their infections, but they serve as a reservoir of infection for others.

Another important public health function in STD control is finding and treating as many active cases of STDs as possible. It is urgent that people being treated for STDs cooperate in naming or personally notifying their sexual contacts because many individuals who have been infected may be asymptomatic, and unless notified, they may suffer severe consequences (see Communication for Wellness: Communicating About STDs). Many people are sterile today because their infected partners

COMMUNICATING ABOUT STDs

Effective communication could greatly reduce the STD problem in the United States. Among the many relationships between STDs and communication are the following:

1. Many young people become sexually active having extremely little factual knowledge of STDs—their symptoms, their dangers, and their prevention. There is an urgent need to include effective STD education in sexuality education programs.

2. Potential sexual partners need to discuss STDs openly and honestly *before* having sex. This discussion needs to include complete disclosure of each person's sexual history—number of and nature of partners, whether any of them had any known STD, and whether each individual has ever been diagnosed with or experienced any symptoms of any STD—and what precautions will be taken to prevent disease transmission. This is not only a moral obligation and good health practice, it is a legal requirement. Anyone who knows or suspects that he or she may have an STD and fails to reveal this

to a potential sex partner is subject to both civil and criminal action. There have been some large judgments made in such cases. You really can't afford not to discuss STDs with a potential sex partner.

3. If you are diagnosed with an STD while you are in a sexual relationship, you need to tell your partner(s) immediately of this development so that he, she, or they can be tested and treated if necessary. Even if this means revealing that you have had sex with someone else, this is something you must do. Failing to tell a partner puts that partner at risk of becoming sterile or experiencing other dangerous complications. It also exposes you to legal risks.

4. When visiting a physician, health department, or college health center with any symptoms that could suggest an STD, it is essential to make a complete disclosure of your sexual activities so an accurate diagnosis can be made. There is no single test that can detect all STDs and knowing your sexual history can help your health care provider to select appropriate tests to perform.

---

failed to inform them of their exposure to an STD. Health departments protect the confidentiality of those who name sexual contacts.

CHECKPOINT

1. Who is primarily responsible for preventing STDs?

2. Outline the personal prevention methods for STDs.

3. What are the roles of public health agencies in STD control?

4. Give several reasons why it is important for recent sexual contacts of people with STDs to be notified.

SUMMARY

Sexually transmitted diseases are the most important communicable diseases in the United States. They are not a new problem, but have assumed a renewed importance in terms of their high total incidence and their effects on our health, reproductive ability, and even our survival.

This chapter surveys major STDs, arranged by their type of pathogen:

1. Viral infections
   - HIV/AIDS
   - Herpes
   - Hepatitis B
   - Papilloma viruses

2. Bacterial infections
   - *Chlamydia*
   - Gonorrhea
   - Syphilis
   - Bacterial vaginitis (*Gardnerella)*

3. Other types of pathogens
   - *Candida* (a yeast)
   - *Trichomonas* (a protozoan)
   - Pubic lice (an insect)
   - Scabies (a mite)

You need to be familiar with the transmission, symptoms, complications, possibility of treatment, and prevention of each of these infections in order to ensure your continuing sexual and physical health and reproductive ability.

While public health departments help to control STDs, the prevention of these diseases requires individual efforts. It is imperative for you to take all possible precautions against infection, to know the symptoms of STDs, to seek prompt treatment if symptoms develop, and to notify recent sexual partners of the possibility of their being infected.

REFERENCES

1. Gorman, C. "Invincible AIDS." *Time* (3 August, 1991), 30–37.
2. Tortora, G. Funke, B., and Case, C. *Microbiology,* 5th ed. Redwood City, CA: Benjamin/Cummings, 1995.
3. Centers for Disease Control. "Impact of the Expanded AIDS Surveillance Case Definition of AIDS Case Reporting—United States, First Quarter, 1993." *Morbidity and Mortality Weekly Report* Vol. 42, No. 16 (30 April 1993), 308–310.
4. Heyward, W., and Curran, J. "The Epidemiology of AIDS in the U.S." *Scientific American* (October 1988), 72–81.
5. Cass, P., and Gallagher, R. *The AIDS Reader.* Dubuque, IA: Kendall/Hunt, 1989.
6. Stine, G. *Acquired Immune Deficiency Syndrome: Biological, Medical, Social, and Legal Issues.* Englewood Cliffs, NJ: Prentice Hall, 1993.
7. Ibid.
8. Ibid.
9. Fackelmann, K. "Herpes, HIV, and the High Risk of Sex." *Science News* (1 February 1992), 68.
10. Davis, M. *Lovers, Doctors, and the Law.* New York: Harper & Row, 1989.
11. Tortora et al., op. cit.
12. Ibid.
13. Fackelmann, op. cit.
14. Stine, op. cit.
15. Straus, S. "Acyclovir: So Far, So Good?" *The Helper* (Fall 1987), 1–6.
16. Tortora et al., op. cit.
17. Black, J. *Microbiology,* 2nd ed. Englewood Cliffs, NJ: Prentice Hall, 1993.
18. Morello, J., Mizer, H., Wilson, M., and Granato, P. *Microbiology in Patient Care,* 5th ed. Dubuque, IA: Wm. C. Brown, 1994.
19. Tortora et al., op. cit.
20. Centers for Disease Control and Prevention. "Recommendations for the Prevention and Management of *Chylamdia trachomatis* infections, 1993." *Morbidity and Mortality Weekly Report* 42, No. RR-12, (6 August 1993), 1–39.
21. Ibid.
22. Gibbons, W. "Clueing in on Chlamydia." *Science News* (20 April, 1991), 250–252.
23. Alger, L. "Chlamydial Infection as a Cause of Preterm Delivery." *Medical Aspects of Human Sexuality* (April 1989), 71.
24. Ibid.
25. Tortora et al., op. cit.
26. Ibid.
27. Higgins, L. "Epidemic of Antibiotic-Resistant Gonorrhea Reshaping Treatment." *Medical World News* (28 November 1988), 12–13.
28. Stine, op. cit.
29. Spiegel, C. "Bacterial Vaginosis." *Clinical Microbiology Reviews* (1991), 485–498.
30. Tortora et al., op. cit.
31. Spiegel, op. cit.
32. Martens, M., and Faro, S. "Update on Trichomonas: Detection and Management." *Medical Aspects of Human Sexuality* (January 1989), 73–79.
33. McGage, E. "The Effectiveness of Latex Condoms: A Barrier to HIV-sized Particles Under Conditions of Simulated Use." *Sexually Transmitted Diseases* (July–August 1992).

SUGGESTED READINGS

Bateson, M., and Goldsby, R. *Thinking AIDS: The Social Response to the Biological Threat.* Reading, MA: Addison-Wesley, 1988.
Cass, P., and Gallagher, R. *The AIDS Reader.* Dubuque, IA: Kendall/Hunt, 1989.
Rathus, S., and Boughn, S. *AIDS: What Every Student Needs to Know.* Fort Worth, TX: Harcourt Brace Jovanovich, 1993.
Schechter, S. *The AIDS Notebooks.* Albany, NY: State University of New York, 1990.
Stine, G. *Acquired Immune Deficiency Syndrome: Biological, Medical, Social, and Legal Issues.* Englewood Cliffs, NJ: Prentice Hall, 1993.
Stine, G. *AIDS Update 1993.* Englewood Cliffs, NJ: Prentice Hall, 1993. (To be updated annually.)
Voeller, B., Reinisch, J., and Gottlieb, M. (eds.). *AIDS and Sex: An Integrated Biomedical and Biobehavioral Approach.* New York: Oxford University Press, 1990.
Wistreich, G. *The Sexually Transmitted Diseases.* Dubuque, IA: Wm. C. Brown, 1992.

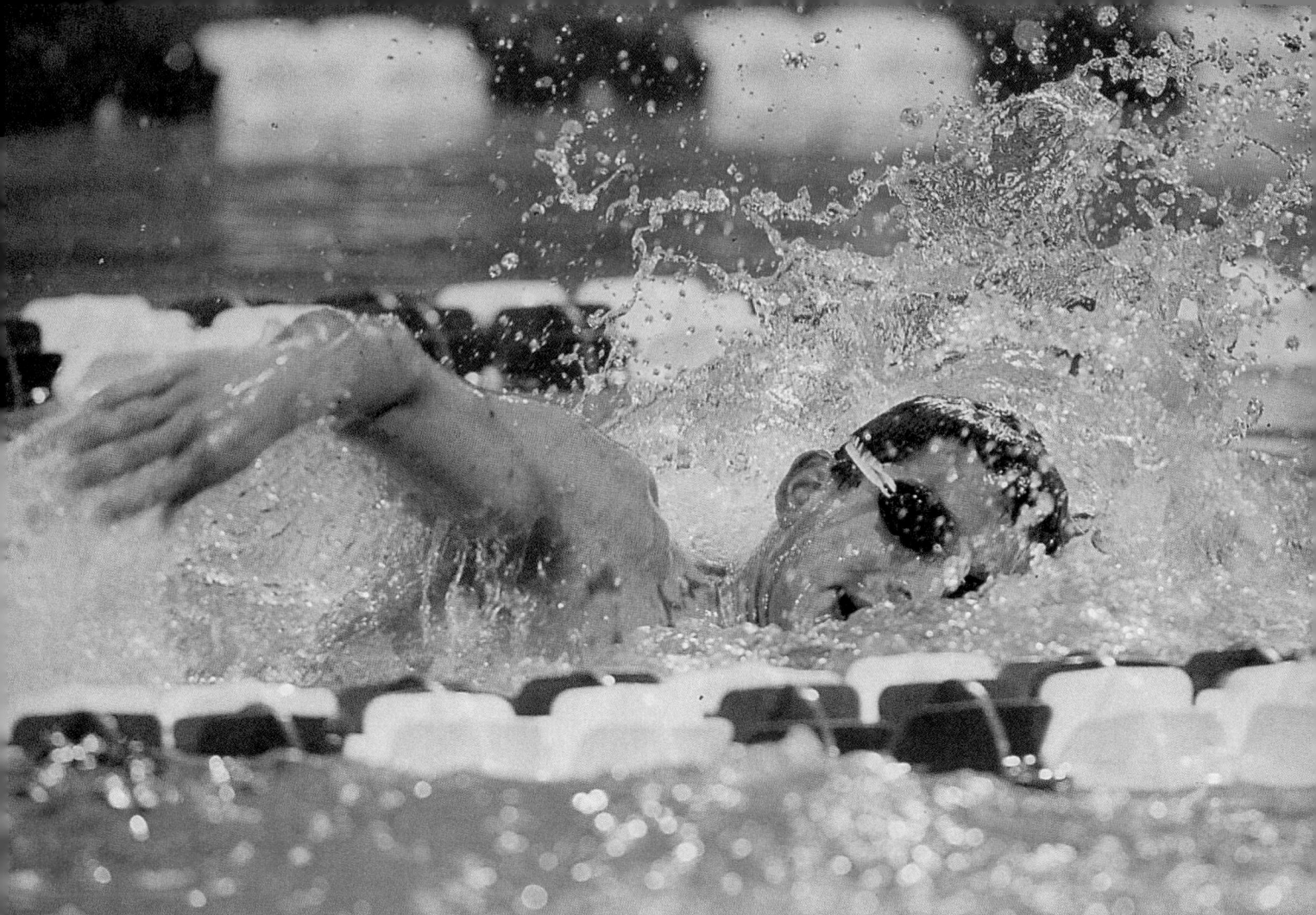

20

CARDIOVASCULAR HEALTH

KNOWLEDGE

- Name the parts of the heart and describe their functions.
- Define the term *atherosclerosis* and explain the changes it brings inside blood vessels.
- Distinguish among a thrombus, an occlusion, and an embolism.
- Identify the incidence of hypertension and contrast primary with secondary hypertension.
- Define the terms *angina pectoris, myocardial infarction,* and *coronary artery disease.*
- Identify those risk factors contributing to cardiovascular diseases that a person can change.
- Identify the sources of the body supply of cholesterol.
- Describe the benefits of regular aerobic exercise to the cardiovascular system.
- List the three kinds of tests used to diagnosis heart diseases.
- Outline the surgical remedies being used to treat damaged hearts.

INSIGHT

- Determine your blood pressure and identify the steps you might take to reduce it if it's too high.
- Explain what you can do to avoid having a stroke.
- Compare, if known, your blood lipid levels to ideal levels.
- Discuss the ways in which cigarette smoking can adversely affect your heart.

DECISION MAKING

- Identify the steps you intend to take if and when you suspect you are having a heart attack.
- Discuss how you plan to go about creating a smoke-free environment if you live or work where you are exposed to cigarette smoke.
- Decide which foods you should eat less of and which you should eat more of to improve your personal cholesterol levels.
- Decide which factors you can alter to reduce your chances of developing heart disease.
- Explain the steps you plan to take to ensure your cardiovascular health.

*C*ardiovascular disease (CVD) remains the number one killer in the United States. Sometimes, CVD is caused by something totally out of our control, such as defective muscle tissue. In other cases, life-style seems to be the reason why CVD may claim a victim. These contrasting causes were vividly seen in the untimely deaths of basketball star Reggie Lewis and actor John Candy.

The death of Reggie Lewis, star of the Boston Celtics professional basketball team, came as a sudden shock. He was shooting some baskets at Brandeis University's Shapiro Gymnasium when he fell to the floor gasping for breath. Less than two hours later, he was pronounced dead at a local hospital emergency room. This was the end of a somewhat bizarre cardiovascular story. Just three months earlier, Reggie Lewis had collapsed during a playoff game with the Charlotte Hornets. Extensive testing followed, *resulting in conflicting diagnoses. One group of cardiologists stated that he had a condition called cardiomyopathy, a potentially fatal condition characterized by defective muscle tissue that causes the heart to pump irregularly and fail to meet the demand for oxygenated blood by other vital organs. Another diagnosis was neurocardiogenic syncope, a nerve condition in which the heart received inappropriate signals from the vagus nerve causing it to beat too slowly during exertion; it can cause fainting, but is not life-threatening. Reggie Lewis obviously decided to believe the less serious diagnosis, and the world lost a respected citizen and basketball player. Some experts indicate that professional athletes may deny possible health problems, as a result of the intense feeling of self-worth they have attached to participation in their sport.*

About seven months after Reggie Lewis's death, another famous person fell victim to cardiovascular disease. John Candy, a 43-year-old comedian and actor, died in his sleep of a massive heart attack while in Mexico filming a movie. John Candy's life-style reflected many of the well-known risks associated with CVD: He weighed about 350 pounds and loved foods rich in fat and cholesterol; he was known for his relentless work schedules; and he was a former smoker. At the time of his death, he was working very long hours while trying hard to lose weight. No doubt all of this was more than his heart could handle.

Cardiovascular disease takes many forms. It is very clear that those who have inherited or congenital heart problems must take precautions to protect themselves against these unpreventable problems. For others, it is essential to maintain a life-style that prevents cardiovascular disease.

Source: Newsweek *9 August 1993, pp. 60–61.*

■ ■ ■

The **cardiovascular** (*kar-dē-ō-vas'kew-ler*) **system** consists of the **heart** and **blood vessels,** the veins,

....

cardiovascular system the circulatory system, consisting of the heart and blood vessels.

heart a muscular contractile organ.

blood vessels a network of tubes that carries blood throughout the body; the veins, arteries, and capillaries.

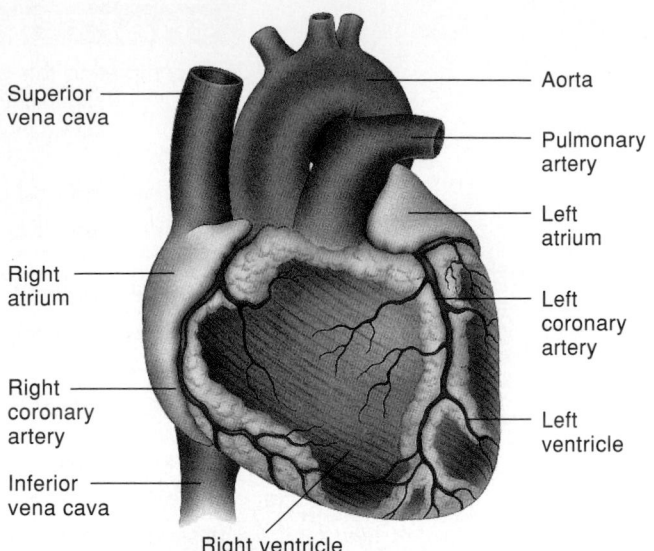

Figure 20.1
Structure of the Heart

The heart with the major branches of the coronary blood vessels shown. These vessels supply the heart with blood and in turn receive their blood from the aorta, just above the aortic valve.

arteries, and capillaries. This system is responsible for the continuous and rapid movement of materials to and from the cells. The body's billions of cells must have a continuous supply of food and oxygen and prompt removal of the waste materials that are produced when the cells turn food into energy.

THE CARDIOVASCULAR SYSTEM

THE HEART

The heart is a muscular organ about the size of a fist (see Figure 20.1), and consists of two separate pumps, one on the right side, and one on the left. These pumps, which move blood by contracting, are separated by a partition called a **septum.** Each side has two chambers (see Figure 20.2). The right and left upper chambers are known as the **atria** (*ā'tri-a*), and fill with blood between heartbeats. The right atrium receives **deoxygenated** (*dē-ox'si-*

....

septum the partition between the right and left sides of the heart.

atria the two upper chambers of the heart.

deoxygenated without oxygen.

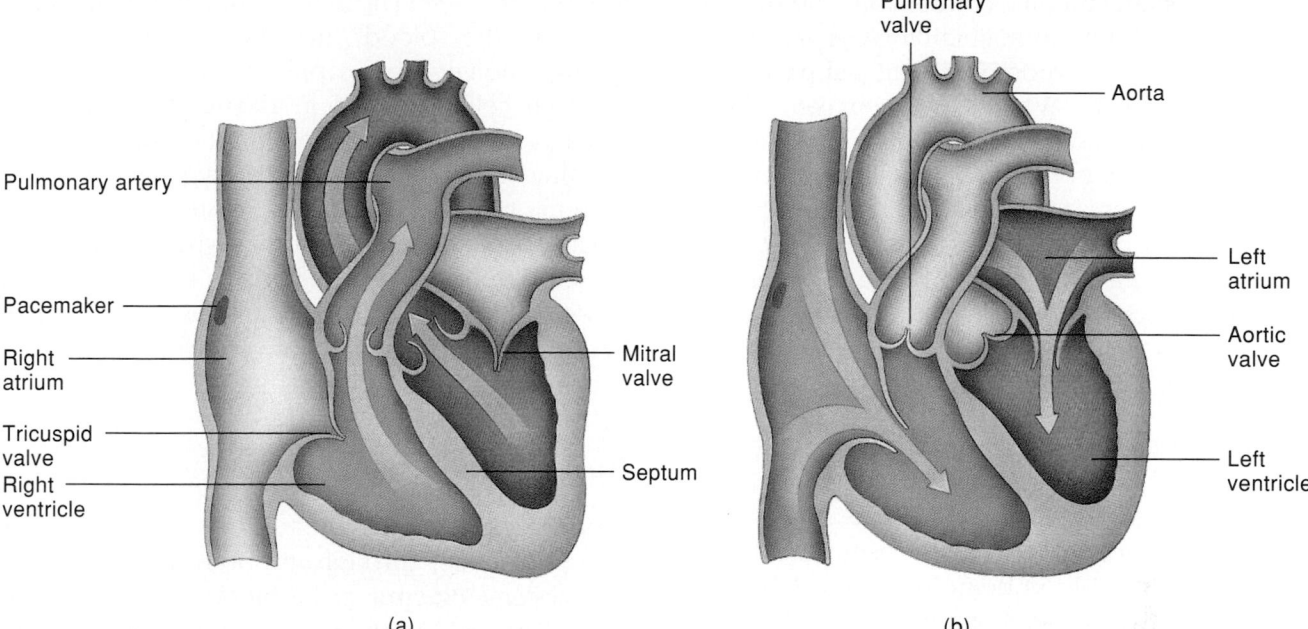

Figure 20.2
Heart Valves and the Cardiac Cycle

(a) Contraction of the ventricles (systole) pumps blood to the lungs and the body.

(b) Relaxation of the ventricles (diastole) allows the ventricles to fill with blood from the lungs and the body.

ji-nā'ted) blood from the body; the left atrium receives oxygenated blood from the lungs. The two atria move blood to the **ventricles** (*ven'tri-kles*), the two lower chambers, which are pumping chambers. The right ventricle pumps blood to the lungs, where carbon dioxide in the blood is exchanged for oxygen. The left ventricle pumps blood to the rest of the body. In the contraction of the heart muscle, both atria contract at the same time, followed by the simultaneous contraction of the two ventricles.

Blood follows a prescribed pathway through the chambers of the heart. Four valves within the heart, one in each chamber, prevent the backflow of blood as it leaves each chamber. The **tricuspid** and **pulmonary valves** are located on the right

ventricles the two lower chambers of the heart.

tricuspid valve the heart valve between the right atrium and right ventricle.

pulmonary valve the valve between the right ventricle and pulmonary artery.

side of the heart; the **bicuspid (mitral)** and **aortic** (*ā-yor'tik*) **valves** are located on the left. If any of the four valves fails to close properly, blood leaks back past the valve, causing an abnormal swishing sound known as a **heart murmur.** Although heart murmurs may have other causes, they most often indicate a valve disorder.[1]

The electrical stimulation needed for the heartbeat originates in a small mass of specialized nerve cells located in the wall of the atrium. Known as the **pacemaker,** this tissue initiates an impulse that causes both atria to contract simultaneously, fol-

bicuspid (mitral) valve the valve between the left atrium and left ventricle.

aortic valve the valve between the left ventricle and aorta.

heart murmur a heart sound that may be caused by a leaking valve.

pacemaker a small mass of nerve tissue in the wall of the right atrium that produces electrical impulses that cause the heart to contract.

lowed by simultaneous contractions of the two ventricles. Difficulty in maintaining cardiac rhythm may call for the insertion of an artificial pacemaker into the chest wall. While the pacemaker initiates the heartbeat, nerves in the brain regulate the speed of the heartbeat. The heart beats approximately 70 times per minute, or approximately 100,000 times per day. With each beat, the heart pumps about three ounces of blood, or over 2000 gallons of blood per day.

Pulse

We can feel the **pulse,** or the rhythmic throbbings of the arterial walls, beating near the surface of the skin in areas such as the wrist, the sides of the neck, and at the temples. What causes the intermittent pulse is the blood being distributed throughout the body. With each contraction of the left ventricle, the blood is pumped into the large artery, or **aorta,** with great force. These contractions cause the blood to spurt rapidly, and the elastic arterial walls to swell. This activity causes a wave, or vibration, from the aorta, through the arteries to the extremities, and thus results in a pulse.

BLOOD VESSELS

There are many different sizes and types of *blood vessels,* which perform different functions while they carry blood throughout the body. **Arteries** carry blood *away* from the heart, and **veins** carry blood *to* the heart. The arteries closest to the heart are large, but divide into smaller vessels called **arterioles** (*ar-tēr'ē-ōlz*), as they move farther away from the heart. The arterioles lead to microscopic vessels called **capillaries** (*cap'i-lar-ēz*), which form an extensive network throughout the body

....

pulse the rhythmic throbbings of the arterial walls.

aorta the large artery that receives blood from the left ventricle and distributes it to the body.

arteries blood vessels that carry blood away from the heart to various parts of the body.

vein any blood vessel that carries blood from various parts of the body back to the heart.

arterioles small branches of arteries.

capillary a microscopic blood vessel between an artery and a vein.

(see Figure 20.3). The actual exchange of materials between the blood and body tissues occurs through the very thin capillary walls.

Each cell is bathed in **tissue fluid,** the fluid that separates from the blood in the capillaries. Tissue fluid is rich in food and oxygen as it comes from the blood, but is rich in waste products, such as carbon dioxide, as it returns to the blood. As tissue fluid from the cells collects in the capillaries, it passes with the blood into small veins called **venules,** which combine into larger veins and lead back to the heart.

BLOOD

Blood is a complex mixture of fluid and cells, which circulates through the body via the circulatory system. **Plasma** is the blood's fluid, and consists of water (90 percent), proteins, blood sugar, lipids (fats), and other chemicals. (Plasma from which the blood-coagulating proteins have been removed is known as **serum.**) The cells within the blood are oxygen-carrying **erythrocytes** (*e-rith'rō-sītz;* red blood cells), protective leukocytes (white blood cells), and **platelets,** which help blood **coagulate** (*cō-ag'ū-lāt*) or clot.

Blood count is the ratio of red cells to white cells in the blood. A healthy ratio is approximately 700 or 800 red cells to every 1 white cell. Since this ratio varies in response to certain illnesses, a blood count is useful for diagnostic purposes.

Blood typing is used to distinguish between major protein differences in the plasma and the red

....

tissue fluid fluid that bathes body cells.

venule a small branch of a vein.

blood a complex mixture of fluid and cells that circulates through the body in the circulatory system.

plasma the liquid portion of the blood.

serum plasma minus its coagulating proteins.

erythrocytes red blood cells.

platelets blood cells that aid in blood clotting.

coagulate to clot.

blood count a count of red blood cells to white blood cells in whole blood.

blood typing the method used to determine the presence of certain proteins in blood.

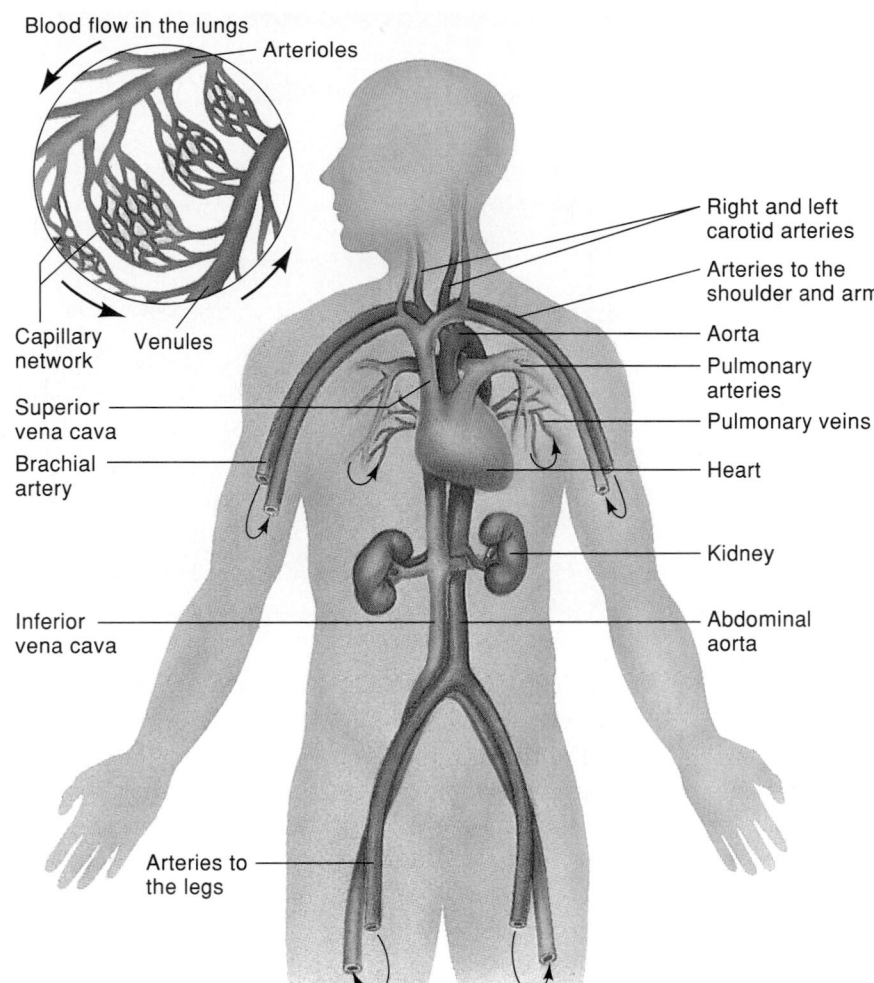

Blood flow in the lungs

Arterioles

Capillary network   Venules

Superior vena cava

Brachial artery

Inferior vena cava

Arteries to the legs

Right and left carotid arteries

Arteries to the shoulder and arm

Aorta

Pulmonary arteries

Pulmonary veins

Heart

Kidney

Abdominal aorta

Figure 20.3
Human Circulatory System

The principal arteries and veins. The insert shows a capillary network.

blood cells. In the most widely used blood-typing system, the ABO System, four types of blood are identified: type A, type B, type O, and type AB. Type O is known as the universal donor and type AB as the universal recipient. In a blood transfusion, if blood types are mismatched, clumping of blood cells can result and seriously impede circulation and result in death.

Another blood protein, the **Rh factor,** is of significance both in transfusions and in childbirth. As with ABO blood types, the Rh factor is inherited. Persons having the Rh factor are said to be Rh positive (Rh⁺), and those without it are Rh negative (Rh⁻). When Rh⁺ blood is injected into an Rh⁻ person, it causes the formation of an antibody. Subsequent transfusions of Rh⁺ blood may result in severe transfusion reactions. Such a reaction may be pronounced in a pregnant Rh⁻ woman who has been sensitized

by blood from an Rh⁺ fetus. Such a reaction in subsequent pregnancies may result in the destruction of red blood cells in the fetus, which may threaten its survival. This is prevented by giving all Rh⁻ mothers an injection of anti-Rh gamma globulin preparation (RhoGAM) soon after a delivery, stillbirth, or abortion. This material prevents the mother's body from producing any antibody, thus protecting the fetus of the next pregnancy.

CHECKPOINT

1. Name the four chambers of the heart. Where does each chamber receive the blood it pumps? Where does each chamber send the blood?

2. Name and identify the location of the four valves within the heart.

3. What are the three kinds of blood vessels in the body? Describe the function of each.

Rh factor a protein found in red blood cells.

4. List the fluid and cellular components of blood.

5. What is your blood type? Why is this important information for you to know?

CARDIOVASCULAR DISEASES

Diseases affecting the heart and blood vessels are called **cardiovascular diseases (CVDs).** The American Heart Association describes the five major CVDs: hypertension, coronary heart disease, stroke, rheumatic (*roo-ma'tik*) heart disease, and congenital heart defects. Each of these diseases, in addition to several others, will be described in the following sections. A person may have more than one of these diseases at the same time.

INCIDENCE AND COST

Cardiovascular diseases are the number one killer in the United States (see Table 20.1).[2, 3] In 1992, nearly 1 million Americans died from CVDs. This is almost as many deaths as those caused by a combination of cancer, AIDS, accidents, pneumonia, and influenza. Looking at this statistic from yet another perspective:

- 54,246 Americans died in the Korean War
- 58,012 Americans died in Vietnam
- 116,708 Americans died in World War I
- 407,316 Americans died in World War II, but
- 930,500 Americans died from cardiovascular disease in a recent year.[4]

The significance of cardiovascular diseases is sometimes underestimated, perhaps because they are often diseases attributed to the elderly. Nearly 43.8 percent of all deaths in the United States are due to CVDs. Five percent of all heart attacks strike people under age 40, and 45 percent strike people under 65. Heart attacks are the leading cause of death in the United States today.[5]

Cardiovascular diseases do not affect everyone equally. Based on 1990 data, the death rate from

....

cardiovascular diseases (CVDs) diseases of the heart and blood vessels.

Table 20.1
Prevalence of the Major Cardiovascular Diseases in the United States, 1993

CVD Type	Prevalence (in millions)
Hypertensive Disease	63.64
Coronary Heart Disease	6.23
Stroke	3.02
Rheumatic Heart Disease	1.32

- One in nine women ages 45–64 has some form of heart disease or stroke; this ratio rises to one in three at age 65 and beyond.

- One in six men ages 45–64 has some form of heart or blood vessel disease; in men of age 65 and over the ratio is one in eight.

Source: American Heart Association. 1993 Heart and Stroke Facts Statistics, Dallas, TX: American Heart Association, 1993.

heart disease for men ages 45–74 was greater than for women in the same age group. Among white men the death rate was 2.2 times the rate for white women; the rate for African American men was 1.7 times the rate for African American women. When compared to the white population, the death rate was greater for African Americans. Among African American women, the death rate from heart disease was 1.8 times greater than for white women; the rate for African American men was 1.4 times the rate for white men. Among African American women heart diseases were the leading cause of death, but the second leading cause of death for white women; among both African American men and white men, heart diseases were the leading cause of death.[6]

The American Heart Association estimates the cost of cardiovascular diseases in 1993 at $117.7 billion. Included in this are the costs of physician and nursing services, hospital and nursing home services, medications, and lost productivity due to disability.[7]

ATHEROSCLEROSIS

Arteriosclerosis, or hardening of the arteries, is a disease that causes the arteries to become narrower and to lose their elasticity. The most common form of this disease is *atherosclerosis.* Arteries become narrower when deposits of cholesterol and other fatty substances, called *plaque,* accumulate on the inner walls of the arteries (see Figure

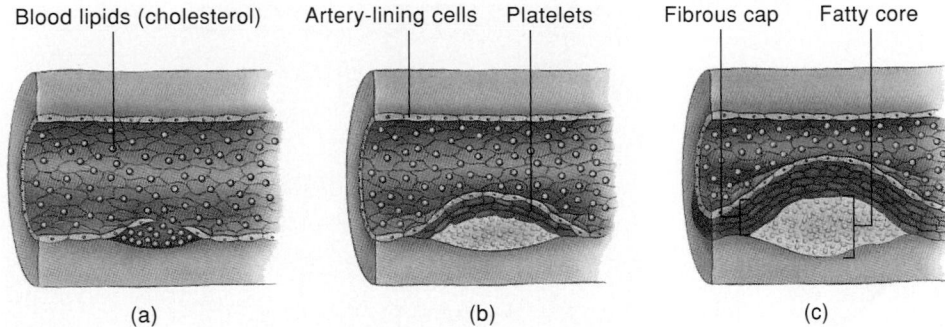

Blood lipids (cholesterol)   Artery-lining cells   Platelets   Fibrous cap   Fatty core

(a)   (b)   (c)

Figure 20.4
Stages of Plaque Buildup

(a) Plaque formation begins when excess cholesterol and fat particles collect beneath cells lining an artery that has been damaged by high blood pressure, smoking, or other causes.

(b) Blood platelets collects over the damaged area, isolating the plaque within the artery wall.

(c) The narrowed artery is now subject to blockage by clots that form over the damaged area.

20.4). Plaque may partially or completely block the flow of blood through the artery. Where the plaque forms there are two things that can happen: Bleeding into the plaque can occur, or a blood clot, a **thrombus,** can occur on the surface of the plaque. Either of these can lead to a complete blockage, or *occlusion,* of the artery, causing a heart attack or stroke. Usually large- and medium-sized arteries are affected.

The cause of atherosclerosis is not fully understood. For some reason the innermost lining of the artery, the *endothelium,* becomes damaged. Whatever triggers the damage, two events follow: The smooth muscle fibers proliferate and lipids build up both within the cells and between them. The accumulating cholesterol, triglycerides, and cells form a lesion called an *atherosclerotic plaque* (Figure 20.5).[8]

The plaque then provides a rough surface on which blood platelets release a substance that promotes the further proliferation of endothelial cells, causing the lesion to grow larger. The platelets also release clot-forming substances, enhancing the growth of clots. As these materials build up they gradually narrow and block the artery. Sometimes these clots break loose from the diseased artery and are carried to another point in the circulatory system, where they become lodged and form an

obstruction, or **embolism.** While this can occur in any blood vessel, it is most serious when it occurs in the heart or the brain.

The factors seen as significant risks leading to plaque buildup are: elevated blood lipids (cholesterol and triglycerides), high blood pressure, and cigarette smoking. Smoking is believed to accelerate the development of atherosclerosis in the coronary arteries, aorta, and arteries of the legs.[9]

HYPERTENSION

Blood pressure is the force blood exerts against the walls of the arteries and arterioles as the heart contracts and relaxes. The walls of these vessels can contract and expand, altering the resistance to blood flow. Each contraction, or **systole** (*sis'tō-lē*), creates pressure in the artery. Between beats when the heart relaxes, called **diastole** (*dī-as'tō-lē*), the pressure falls. Regulation of the size (inner diameter) of the arterioles is significant in controlling

thrombus a blood clot that forms inside a blood vessel.

embolism a blood clot that has moved and lodged in a blood vessel.

blood pressure the force exerted by the blood against the artery walls.

systole the part of the heart cycle when the heart is in contraction.

diastole the part of the heart cycle when the heart is relaxed.

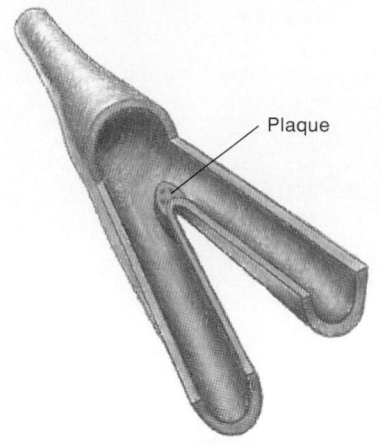

(a) An artery (section) with plaque just beginning to form. Plaques can easily appear in a person as young as 15.

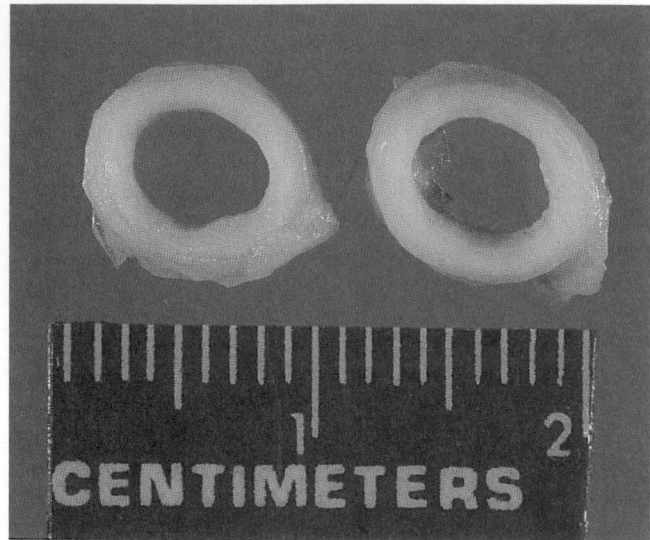

Plaque

Outer layer
(supportive tissues)

Middle layer
(smooth muscle)

Inner layer
(artery lining)

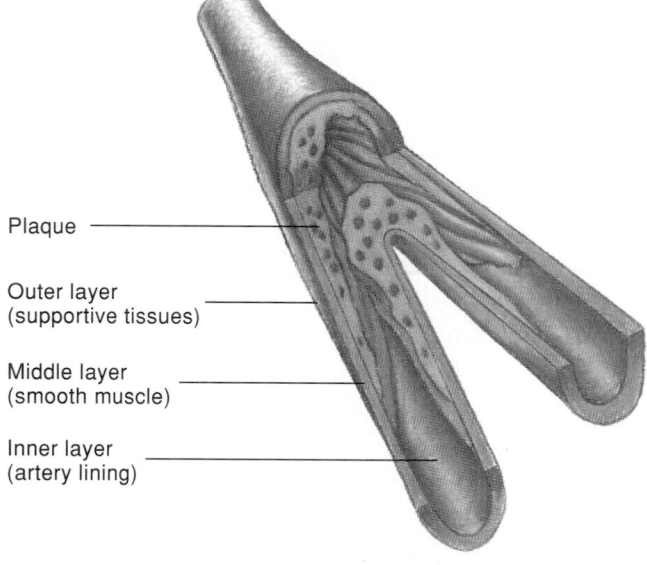

(b) The same artery (section) years later, half blocked by plaque.

Figure 20.5
The Formation of Plaques in Atherosclerosis

(a) An artery (section) with plaque just beginning to form. Plaques can easily appear in a person as young as a teenager.

A healthy artery provides an open passage for the flow of blood.

(b) The same artery, years later, half-blocked by plaque.

Plaques along an artery narrow its diameter and obstruct blood flow. Clots can form, aggravating the problem.

Source: Whitney, E., and Rolfes, S. Understanding Nutrition, 6th ed. St. Paul, MN: West, 1993, p. 557.

blood flow and determining blood pressure. The harder it is for the blood to flow the higher the pressure will be. If the vessels remain constricted, a condition called *hypertension,* or high blood pressure, can occur.

Measuring Blood Pressure

Blood pressure is measured using an instrument (see Figure 20.6) called a **sphygmomanometer** (*sfig-mō-man-om'et-er*). A common type of sphygomomanometer consists of a rubber cuff which is wrapped around the arm above the elbow. Using the pump, the cuff is inflated until it stops the blood flow in the artery in the arm. Then, as the air is released, the person measuring the blood pressure listens with a stethoscope. When the blood begins to flow through the artery, it makes a sound, which continues until the pressure in the artery exceeds the pressure in the cuff. The blood pressure is reflected in a column of mercury marked off in millimeters of mercury (mm Hg). Standard readings are obtained with mercury-type instruments. Some instruments use an analog dial or digital readout convenience. When the heart contracts, the blood pressure should raise the mercury about 120 millimeters (mm). When the heart relaxes, the pressure should raise the mercury about 80 mm. Blood pressure readings are presented as systolic pressure over diastolic pressure, for example 120/80.

Systolic pressures of 110 to 139 and diastolic pressures of 70 to 89 are considered within a normal range. Most people's blood pressure varies from time to time. Sleeping and sitting cause blood pressure to drop, while exercising causes it to rise. A persistent reading of 140/90, or higher, indicates a problem. Because blood pressures vary, and because of possible errors, a single blood pressure reading is not sufficient. Several readings should be taken at different times for a more accurate indication of a person's true blood pressure.

The Effects of Hypertension

Hypertension is the most common disease affecting blood vessels and the heart. An estimated 27 percent of women and 32 percent of men 18 years

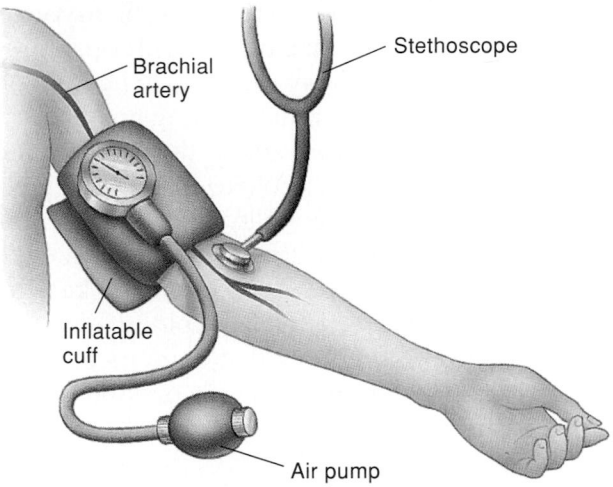

Figure 20.6
Measuring Blood Pressure

Blood pressure is measured with an instrument called a sphygmomanometer. A quick, simple, painless procedure, a measurement is made of how much pressure in the inflatable cuff is required to stop the flow of blood through the artery in the arm. The pressure is commonly measured by a column of mercury calibrated in millimeters; other times (as shown here), the pressure is measured with other instruments based on the mercury column. The presence or absence of blood flow is monitored with a stethoscope.

of age and over have high blood pressure.[10] African Americans, Puerto Ricans, and Cuban and Mexican Americans are more likely to suffer from high blood pressure than Anglo Americans. In 1989 the death rates per 100,000 persons were 6.2 for white men, 28.7 for African American men, 4.6 for white women, and 21.4 for African American women.[11]

Primary (essential) hypertension is persistently high blood pressure that cannot be related to any particular organic cause. Ninety to ninety-five percent of all hypertension is primary. The remaining 5–10 percent of high blood pressure, or *secondary hypertension,* has some known cause, such as kidney disease, adrenal (referring to a gland atop each kidney) oversecretion, or congenital defect of the aorta. Hypertension puts strain on the brain and kidneys, but especially on the heart. Due to the extra work required to pump the blood, the heart muscle becomes thickened, and the heart enlarges. Working harder, the heart muscle needs more oxygen. If unable to meet the demands put upon it, **angina pectoris,** chest pains due to an oxygen

---

sphygmomanometer an instrument for measuring blood pressure.

angina pectoris chest pain resulting from the heart muscle receiving insufficient blood supply.

insufficiency to the heart, may occur, or **myocardial infarction,** the damaging or death of an area of the heart muscle, may develop. High blood pressure leads to the eventual scarring and hardening of the arterioles. Arterioles of the kidneys and brain are especially susceptible to high blood pressure. Even though the mortality figures from high blood pressure seem low, the numbers are seen to be deceptive. Many of the deaths from strokes and heart attacks are caused by high blood pressure. Because of this and the fact that many people are unaware they have high blood pressure, it is known as the "silent killer."

Causes of Hypertension

There are several mechanisms that cause high blood pressure. One cause relates to the arterioles, the tiny vessels that feed into the capillaries. Normally, the muscles in the walls of the arterioles contract as needed, allowing less blood to enter the capillaries. When more blood is required, such as for digestion, the arterioles in the intestines open up. In some people, however, the arteriole muscle cells tighten up and stay tightened, causing the heart to pump harder, raising blood pressure. Why arterioles constrict abnormally is not known.[12]

Atherosclerosis, as discussed earlier, inhibits the blood flow. This also causes the heart to work harder because it has to push the blood through the narrowed arteries. The resulting high blood pressure further injures the arterial walls and induces further atherosclerosis.

Sodium Excessive sodium in the diet increases blood pressure in some people. The main source of sodium is table salt (sodium chloride), which is about 40 percent sodium. Although sodium is essential for normal body functions, the average healthy adult requires only 500 mg of sodium (1250 mg, or ¼ teaspoon salt) per day.

The National Academy of Sciences advises limiting the daily sodium intake to less than 2.4 g (6 g salt).[13] Yet, the average person daily takes in 3.3 g of sodium (8.25 g salt), or 1½–2 teaspoons daily.

This is one-and-a-half to two times more than recommended.[14]

The kidneys usually filter excess sodium out of the blood into the urine. After eating salted foods, thirst follows, ensuring consumption of more water. Then the kidneys excrete the extra fluid along with extra sodium. Most people can safely consume more salt than needed. Some people, however, are "sodium sensitive," and experience high blood pressure from excess sodium intake. Their blood retains more sodium, increasing water retention and affecting blood pressure. If high blood pressure is not sodium-related, restricting salt intake will not help lower it.

Control of Hypertension

Although primary hypertension is based on an organic cause, certain steps can significantly reduce it. An increase in physical activity, weight reduction, stopping smoking, decrease in or stopping the use of alcohol, a decrease in salt consumption, stress management, and an increase in calcium and potassium intake, if not adequate, may help reduce high blood pressure. Since secondary hypertension has known causes, any successful treatment of the underlying causes may lead to the control of the hypertension.

Medication

Various types of medications are being used to control hypertension. *Diuretics* can be taken to reduce blood volume, and thus pressure, by increasing urine production and ridding the body of excess fluids and sodium. *Beta blockers* are used to reduce heart rate and thus blood output by the heart. The nerves that stimulate the arterioles to contract can be blocked by *sympathetic nerve inhibitors. Vasodilators* relax the smooth muscles in arterial walls. *Calcium antagonists* and *angiotension converting enzyme inhibitors* help the blood vessels to relax. The effectiveness of any of these medications must be determined on an individual basis by a qualified health professional.

HEART ATTACK

Heart attack is the largest single cause of death in the United States, accounting for over 22 percent of

---

myocardial infarction (MI) the damaging or death of an area of the heart muscle.

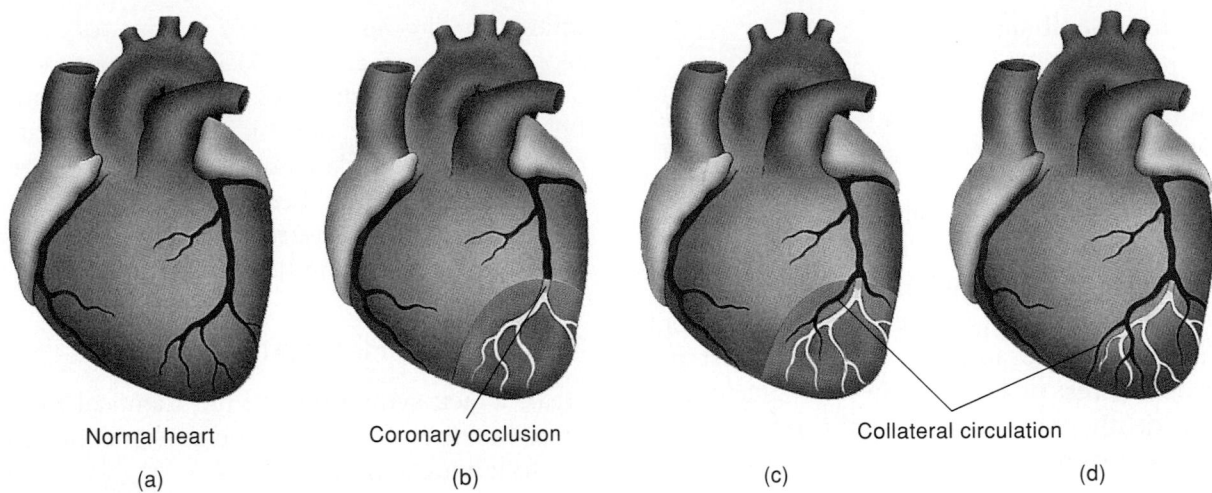

Normal heart
(a)

Coronary occlusion
(b)

Collateral circulation
(c)   (d)

Figure 20.7
Development of a Heart Obstruction and Repair

(a) A normal heart; (b) a coronary occlusion occurs; (c) collateral circulation reroutes circulation; (d) restoration of coronary circulation repairs the heart muscle tissue.

all deaths each year, and 36 percent of all deaths among males ages 35–64. One-quarter of heart attack victims die very quickly; in most cases, a heart attack victim dies within two hours. Other heart attack victims may suffer severe impairments.[15] Unfortunately, about half of all heart attack victims wait two or more hours before deciding to get help.[16]

Heart attacks most commonly result from one or more diseases of the coronary arteries that supply blood to the heart muscle, or the **myocardium** (*mī-ō-car'dē-um*). When there is diminished blood flow to tissue, known as **ischemia** (*is-kē'mi-a*), the tissue is deprived of oxygen and nutrients, and it begins to die (an **infarct**; *in'farkt*). Such damage to the heart is known as a myocardial infarction (MI), or a heart attack (see Figure 20.7). Blood vessel disease of the heart is commonly referred to as **coronary artery disease (CAD)** or **coronary heart disease (CHD).**

....

myocardium the muscular wall of the heart.

ischemia a diminished flow of blood to a tissue.

infarct the dying of tissue.

coronary artery disease (CAD) an impeding of coronary blood flow to the heart; also known as **coronary heart disease (CHD)**

Angina Pectoris

Angina pectoris is severe pain in the chest, which indicates that the coronary arteries are unable to supply enough oxygen-rich blood to the heart muscle. The pain is most intense in the center of the chest and may radiate to the neck and jaw, shoulders, and down the left or both arms. Literally meaning "strangled chest," the pain of angina is described by some as a tight or squeezing sensation, as though the chest were in a vise. Labored breathing, dizziness, and sweating are other reported symptoms. Angina usually flares up during physical exertion, emotional excitement or stress, or other times when the heart demands an increased supply of oxygen.

Angina pectoris discomfort should not be ignored. Although it may disappear on its own, it is a sign of severe coronary artery disease, and indicates a high risk of heart attack. Anyone experiencing these pains should consult a physician promptly. The discomfort of angina can be controlled in many coronary heart disease patients with one of a variety of drugs, such as nitroglycerine.

Some people experience myocardial ischemia, but without prior warning, such as pain. People with angina may experience episodes of such "silent ischemia" which can be dangerous since a heart attack is a likely result of lack of treatment. Such symptomless angina can sometimes be diagnosed with the help of exercise tests or 24-hour portable monitors.

Coronary Occlusion

A complete blockage of a coronary artery, or **coronary occlusion,** often is the result of a clot, or **coronary thrombosis.** Obstruction within a coronary artery can also be caused by intermittent coronary artery spasm, in which the smooth muscle of a coronary artery undergoes a sudden contraction, causing a narrowing of the blood vessel. Coronary artery spasm usually occurs in people with atherosclerosis and may result in chest pain either during rest or exertion, in heart attack, or in sudden death. Although unconfirmed, smoking and stress are strongly suspected to be factors.

When the blockage takes place in a large coronary artery, this affects a large area of the heart, and may be referred to as a *massive* coronary. The term *massive heart attack* is sometimes used in the media to indicate that the person being referred to has died, or died suddenly. If used to refer to sudden death (see Sudden Cardiac Death in this chapter), the term is being used incorrectly. Massive coronaries are often, but not always, fatal.

If the attack is not fatal the heart muscle begins to repair itself over time by developing new blood vessels into the damaged area. Unfortunately, the tissue beyond the obstruction dies and is replaced by noncontractile scar tissue. As a result the heart muscle loses some of its strength. In addition to killing tissue, the infarction may disrupt the heart's conduction network and may trigger **fibrillation,** a rapid and uncontrolled contraction of individual heart muscle fibers, which may result in sudden death.

Supplemental, or **collateral circulation,** involves new or different arteries to provide blood flow around the damaged area of the heart. Although everyone has potential collateral vessels, they may not develop and open. Collateral circulation may begin forming prior to a myocardial

coronary occlusion an obstruction in a coronary artery.

coronary thrombosis formation of a blood clot in a coronary artery.

fibrillation rapid and uncontrolled contractions of individual heart muscle fibers.

collateral circulation a system of smaller arteries that may open up and start to carry blood to a part of the heart when a coronary artery is blocked; also develops as a result of engaging in regular aerobic exercise.

infarction during the early stages of coronary blockage (see Figure 20.7). A heart attack stimulates the development of collateral circulation. A benefit of regular aerobic exercise is that such exercise also stimulates the development of collateral circulation in the heart, and may, if a blockage occurs, provide an alternate route for blood, which prevents a devastating heart attack.

Symptoms of Heart Attack

Heart attack symptoms are not identical in all victims, but they frequently include one or more of the following sensations:

- uncomfortable pressure, fullness, squeezing, or pain in the center of the chest that lasts more than two minutes, or goes away and comes back
- pain spreading to the shoulders, neck, jaw, arms, or back
- chest discomfort with lightheadedness, fainting, sweating, nausea, or shortness of breath

Not everyone experiencing chest pain is having a heart attack. Nor do all of these warning signs occur in every heart attack. If some start to occur, however, don't wait. Get help immediately (see Feature 20.1). Many people die each year because they fail to recognize the symptoms of an attack. Delay can be deadly!

Cardiac Arrest

Cardiac arrest occurs when the heart stops beating. Cardiac arrest results from a heart attack, but can also result from arrhythmia, suffocation, a *near* drowning, a drug overdose, stroke, or an electrocution. During cardiac arrest the tissues of the brain and other organs begin dying within minutes. Sixty percent of cardiac arrest victims die before they reach the hospital.

Until emergency help arrives, it is essential that **cardiopulmonary resuscitation (CPR)** be performed. CPR is a method of combining closed

cardiac arrest when the heart stops beating.

cardiopulmonary resuscitation (CPR) a combination of closed chest massage and mouth-to-mouth breathing used during a cardiac arrest to keep blood flowing to the heart muscle and brain.

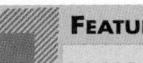

FEATURE 20.1

WHAT TO DO IF YOU SUSPECT A HEART ATTACK

KNOW WHAT TO DO IN AN EMERGENCY:

- Find out which area hospitals have 24-hour emergency cardiac care.

- Know (in advance) which hospital or medical facility is nearest to your home and office, and tell your family and friends to call this facility in an emergency.

- Keep a list of emergency rescue service numbers next to the telephone and in your pocket, wallet, or purse.

- If you have chest discomfort that lasts more than a few minutes, call the emergency rescue service.

- If you can get to a hospital faster by going yourself and not waiting for an ambulance, have someone drive you there. Do not attempt to drive if you think you may be having a heart attack!

BE A HEART SAVER

- If you're with someone experiencing the signs of a heart attack—and the warning signs last more than a few minutes—act immediately.

- Expect "denial." It's normal for someone with chest discomfort to deny the possibility of something as serious as a heart attack. But don't take no for an answer. Insist on taking prompt action.

- Call the emergency service, or get to the nearest hospital emergency room that offers 24-hour emergency cardiac care.

- Give CPR (mouth to mouth breathing and chest compression) if it's necessary and you're properly trained.

Source: Heart and Stroke Facts. Dallas, TX: American Heart Association, 1992.

chest massage with mouth-to-mouth resuscitation in an effort to restore breathing and circulation. CPR must be administered within minutes of cardiac arrest. Most medical, police, and fire personnel are trained in CPR.

Training is required before a person is prepared to perform CPR. It is a very significant lifesaving tool that everyone should be encouraged to learn how to administer. If you are interested in learning CPR, contact your nearest branch of the American Red Cross, American Heart Association, or your local hospital.

Heart Attack Recovery

When a heart attack victim receives prompt treatment, the damage to the heart can be significantly reduced. This is part of the reason 80 percent of heart attack survivors can return to work within three months. After a coronary artery blockage, the

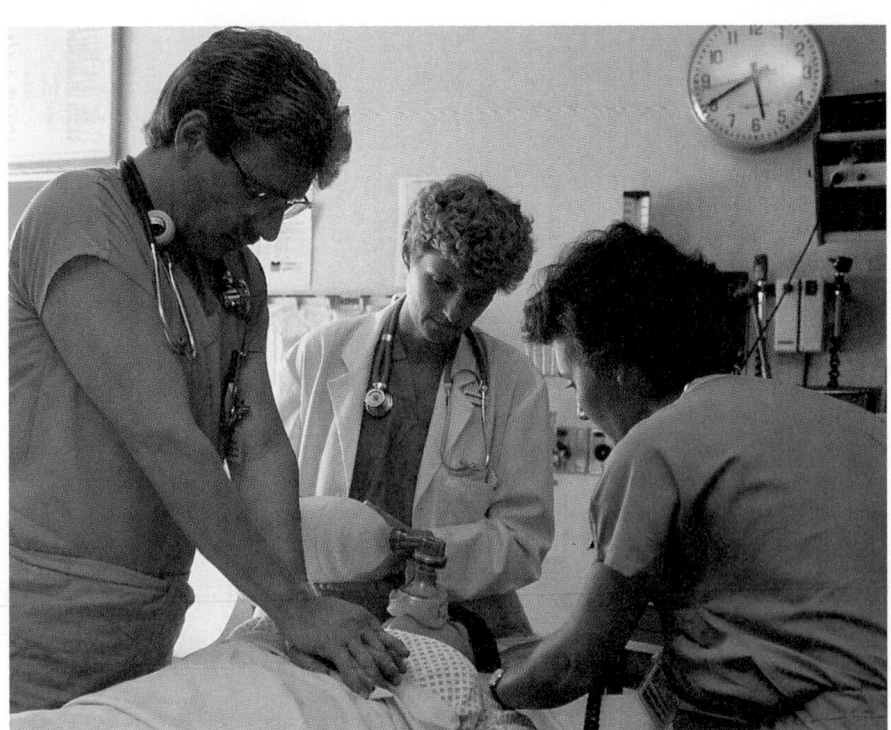

Heart attacks usually strike when a person least expects them. While many victims die before reaching a hospital, the use of lifesaving emergency care, provided immediately, can save many victims.

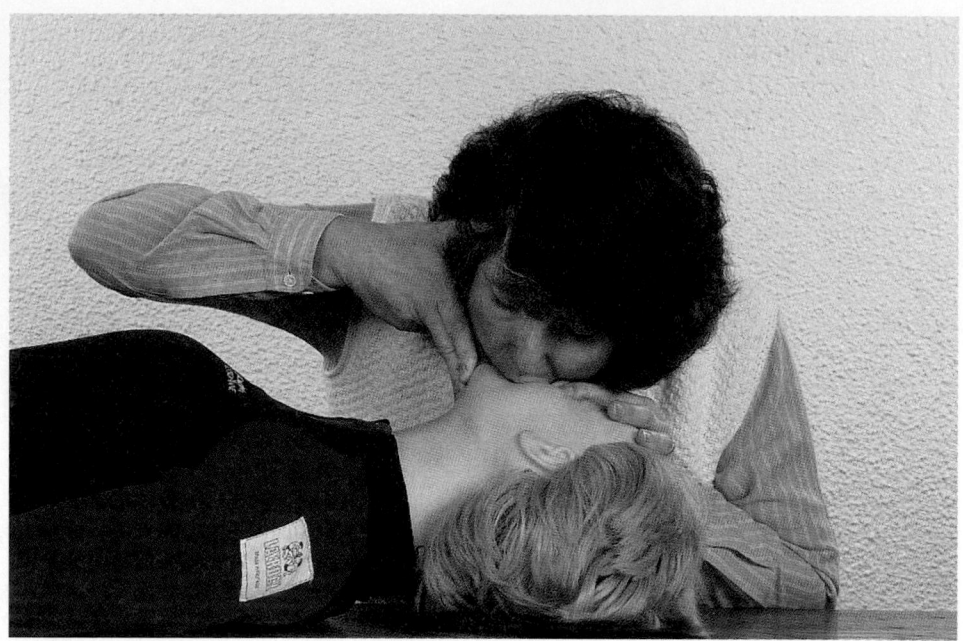

Cardiopulmonary resuscitation (CPR) can be a lifesaver for a heart attack victim. If heartbeat is arrested, the person will die unless heart action is quickly restored. Until emergency care arrives, the most important help is CPR. Many lives have been saved because of lay people who have been trained in giving CPR.

affected heart tissues do not die immediately. Damage increases, however, the longer the artery remains blocked. Emergency treatment allows the application of various tissue-saving therapies. One such treatment is called *reperfusion therapy* or *thrombolysis,* which involves the injection of a thrombolytic (clot-dissolving) agent to dissolve the coronary artery clot and restore partial blood flow before all of the affected heart tissue dies. The sooner the drug is used, the more effective it is; best effects occur if the drug is used within one to three hours of the attack.

Once heart muscle dies, its contracting function cannot be restored. However, function can be restored to areas suffering decreased blood flow. Such restoration may be aided by coronary artery bypass surgery, or angioplasty, discussed later in the chapter.

STROKE

A **stroke,** or **cerebrovascular accident (CVA),** occurs when the blood supply to the brain is cut off. The brain receives about 15 percent of the

stroke or **cerebrovascular accident (CVA)** in which the blood supply to part of the brain is interrupted through rupture or blockage of a blood vessel supplying the brain.

blood pumped from the heart, and it needs a continuous supply of oxygen-rich and glucose-rich blood in order to function properly. While the brain represents only about 2 percent of the body's weight, it uses about 25 percent of the body's oxygen supply and about 70 percent of the glucose. Brain cells, unlike cells in other organs, are unable to store the energy they make from oxygen and glucose. Therefore, when the brain cells lack oxygen, for example, when a person stops breathing or when a person's heart stops beating, that person can survive for only a few minutes. Once dead, brain tissue can not be regenerated.[17]

Kinds of Strokes

There are four main kinds of strokes: Two are caused by clots and two by hemorrhages. About 70–80 percent of all strokes are caused by clots that block an artery: a cerebral thrombosis or a cerebral embolus.

The most common type of stroke, the **cerebral thrombosis,** is caused by a blood clot (thrombus) that forms and blocks a cerebral artery (Figure 20.8). This most often happens in arteries previously damaged by atherosclerosis. This kind of

cerebral thrombosis formation of a blood clot in an artery that supplies part of the brain.

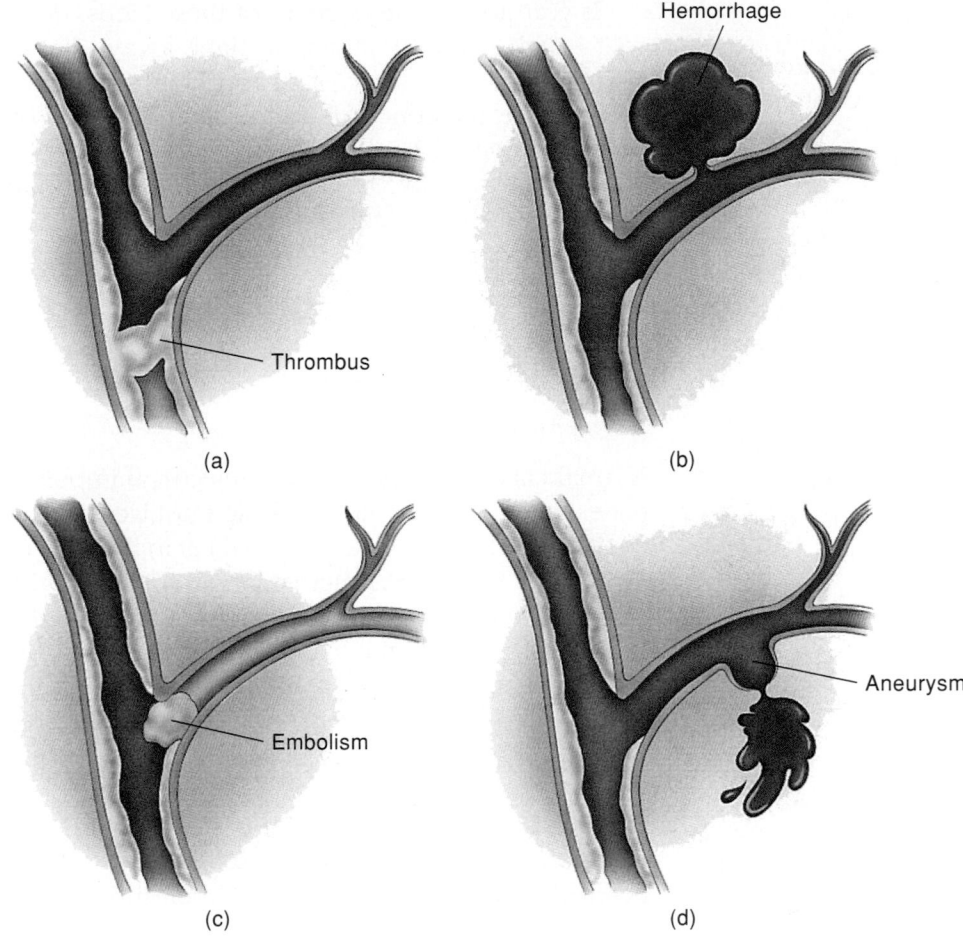

Hemorrhage

Thrombus

(a)

(b)

Embolism

(c)

Aneurysm

(d)

Figure 20.8
A Cerebrovascular Accident, or Stroke

Blood supply to the brain may be interrupted by one of several cases: (a) thrombus, (b) hemorrhage, (c) embolism, and (d) aneurysm (rupture).

stroke usually occurs at night or first thing in the morning when blood pressure is low. It is frequently preceded by a "mini-stroke" known as **transient ischemic attack (TIA).** TIAs are very important warning signs of a potential stroke.

Cerebral emboli are traveling blood clots, or some other particles, that lodge in a smaller artery. Emboli usually occur in an artery leading to the brain (see Figure 20.8). The most common cause of emboli are clots formed by a malfunctioning heart in which the atria do not empty completely, allowing blood to pool and clot.

A hemorrhage can occur when a blood vessel in or on the surface of the brain bursts. A *sub-*

arachnoid hemorrhage occurs on the surface of the brain, with bleeding into the space between the brain and the skull. If it occurs in the wall of a blood vessel in the brain, a **cerebral hemorrhage** floods the surrounding tissue with blood. Hemorrhage of an artery can be caused by a head injury, or by an *aneurysm* (a weakened spot in an artery wall). Aneurysms may burst due to high blood pressure. In a hemorrhage, blood accumulates, putting pressure on surrounding brain tissue. Hemorrhagic strokes account for 15–20 percent of all strokes. Although they are fatal in about 50 percent of all cases, the survivors tend to recover much more often than victims of strokes caused by clots. Persons suffering from both atherosclerosis and hypertension are more likely to suffer cerebral hemorrhage than persons suffering from just one of these conditions.

....

transient ischemic attack (TIA) a temporary stroke-like event that lasts for only a short time and is caused by a temporarily blocked blood vessel.

cerebral emboli blood clots formed in one part of the body and then carried by the bloodstream to the brain, where it blocks an artery.

....

cerebral hemorrhage the rupture of a diseased blood vessel in the brain.

Likely Victims of Stroke

Older people more commonly have strokes. Men have strokes about 30 percent more often than females. African Americans have strokes 60 percent more often than whites, perhaps due to their having a greater incidence of high blood pressure. Diabetics are much more likely to suffer stroke than nondiabetics. Heart disease increases the risk of stroke. Atherosclerosis and other heart diseases double the risk of stroke as compared to normal functioning hearts. Some factors cannot be changed. Others are caused by life-style and environmental factors that may be changed (see Major Risk Factors That You Can Modify, p. 636).

Higher-than-average rates of death from stroke occur in the southeastern United States, an area known as the "Stroke Belt." In 11 states from Virginia to Georgia, and Louisiana to Indiana, the stroke deaths are 10 percent higher than the national average of 40 per 100,000 population, according to the National Heart, Lung, and Blood Institute. South Carolina leads the list with 58.6 stroke deaths per 100,000. This area also has a higher percentage of smokers, a higher percentage of overweight persons, a higher tendency toward a high-fat high-salt diet, and many residents who are poor and have little access to health care.[18]

Warning Symptoms of a Stroke

There is an advance warning in about 10 percent of all impending strokes. A TIA may occur, causing blindness in one eye, speaking or writing difficulty, or numbness to one side of the body. Such ministrokes usually last less than 30 minutes, and are followed by a return to normal.

When a clot-caused stroke occurs, symptoms commonly last from a few minutes to several hours. The warning signals of stroke are:

- sudden weakness or numbness of the face, arm or leg on one side of the body
- sudden dimness or loss of vision, particularly in only one eye
- loss of speech, or trouble talking or understanding speech
- sudden severe, unexplained headaches
- unexplained dizziness, unsteadiness or sudden falls, especially along with any of the previous symptoms

If you notice one or more of these signs, don't wait—seek medical attention right away! Today fewer people are dying of stroke. During the past decade, the incidence of strokes has declined by approximately 50 percent. While the reason for this is uncertain, it may be due to increased attention by Americans to weight control, exercise, diet, and blood cholesterol levels, which all affect the alterable risk factors discussed earlier.[19]

OTHER CARDIOVASCULAR DISORDERS

Arrhythmias

Normal cardiac rhythm is set by electrical impulses generated within the heart. These impulses start in the sinoatrial (S-A) node (pacemaker) in the wall of the atrium, then spread across the atria, then to the atrioventricular (A-V) node near the center of the heart, and finally to the walls of the ventricles. This allows an orderly series of contractions in the various chambers of the heart, resulting in an effective pumping of blood through and away from the heart.

An **arrhythmia** (*a-rith'mē-a*) is any change in this normal sequence, resulting in an abnormal heartbeat. Some arrhythmias are brief and temporary; others are sustained. When the heartbeat is less than 60 beats per minute, the abnormal beat is known as **bradycardia** (*brad-i-kar'di-a*); when more than 100 beats per minute, it is termed **tachycardia** (*tak-i-kar'di-a*).

An arrhythmia may be caused by a **heart block,** in which impulses may not be conducted through all parts of the heart. This results in dropped beats, with decreased cardiac output and blood flow as a result of which, patients may experience dizziness, unconsciousness, and convulsions.

....

arrhythmia an abnormal heartbeat.

bradycardia a slow heartbeat characterized by a pulse rate under 60 beats per minute.

tachycardia an abnormally rapid heartbeat characterized by a pulse rate over 100 beats per minute.

heart block condition in which the conducting tissues of the heart fails to conduct impulses normally from the atrium to the ventricles. This causes altered rhythm of the heartbeat.

Another arrhythmia is **flutter,** in which there are many atrial beats per minute, often from 240 to 360. These may be accompanied by a blockage of ventricular contractions. This may be caused by rheumatic heart disease, coronary artery disease, or certain congenital heart defects.

In *fibrillation* there are rapid, uncoordinated contractions of individual heart muscle fibers. These chaotic contractions may affect the atria or the ventricles. *Atrial fibrillation* can reduce the pumping action of the heart by 20–30 percent. *Ventricular fibrillation* is far more serious and almost always indicates imminent death unless corrected quickly. The rate of beat may be rapid or slow, ventricular pumping becomes ineffective, blood flow is halted, and circulatory failure and death occur. The application of a strong electric current across the chest for a short interval, called **defibrillation,** can stop ventricular fibrillation. Some patients with repeated episodes of fibrillation can have a defibrillator device implanted in their chest that monitors heartbeat and automatically delivers lifesaving defibrillation when necessary.

Yet another arrhythmia is **ventricular premature contractions,** in which nerve cells outside the pacemaker deliver an occasional, abnormal impulse between the normal impulses. Relatively nonthreatening, premature contractions may be caused by emotional stress, use of substances containing caffeine and nicotine, and lack of sleep. Such contractions may also relate to an underlying heart disease.

Sudden Cardiac Death (SCD)

Almost half of all deaths from heart diseases are due to **sudden cardiac death (SCD).** A sudden and unexpected cardiac arrest, SCD is usually the result of a rapid and chaotic heartbeat. Occurring at an average age of about 60 years, the unexpectedness of SCD, often during a person's most productive years, leaves families devastated. SCD is *not* synonymous with a heart attack, in which death of the heart muscle tissue is due to loss of blood supply.

Behind most cases of SCD is an underlying heart disease. Atherosclerosis is typically responsible, with a narrowing of coronary arteries or scarring of heart muscle from a prior heart attack. Thus, risk factors for SCD are similar to those for atherosclerosis, including cigarette smoking and high blood pressure. Hearts that are diseased, scarred, or enlarged are subject to life-threatening arrhythmias. Significant changes in blood levels of potassium and magnesium, as often happens with the use of *diuretics* (taken in some weight-loss programs) can cause life-threatening arrhythmias. In young people, recreational drug abuse is a common cause of SCD.

Cardiac arrest is reversible in most victims if treated within a few minutes. With the advent of coronary care units and electrical shock devices, in-hospital survival rates have improved significantly. Now, adequately trained and staffed emergency rescue teams, using CPR and defibrillators, can save many lives as long as they reach the victim in time.

Congestive Heart Failure

When the heart is unable to pump adequately all of the blood that it receives, the blood backs up in the veins leading to the heart. **Edema,** or the build-up of fluid in the body tissues occurs, especially in the lungs and extremities, and may eventually lead to **congestive heart failure.** The accumulation of fluid in the lungs causes pulmonary congestion, which makes breathing difficult. Symptoms of this condition may include swelling in the ankles and legs. Due to insufficient blood pressure, the kidneys are unable to excrete sufficient water and sodium, which adds to the edema.

Congestive heart failure may ensue when the heart is damaged from a heart attack, atherosclerosis, hypertension, rheumatic fever, or birth defects.

....

flutter a tremulous, rapid movement of the heart.

defibrillation use of electric currents to reestablish normal heart contraction rhythms.

ventricular premature contractions an occasional abnormal impulse between normal impulses delivered by nerve cells outside the pacemaker.

sudden cardiac death death that occurs unexpectedly and instantaneously, or shortly after the onset of symptoms.

....

edema swelling due to an abnormally large amount of fluid in body tissues.

congestive heart failure the inability of the heart to pump out all the blood that returns to it.

Treatment for congestive heart failure involves rest, proper diet, reduced physical activity, and medications, such as *diuretics* to help the body excrete excess fluid, *digitalis* to improve the heart's pumping action, and *vasodilators* to expand blood vessels and decrease resistance to blood flow.

Rheumatic Heart Disease

Rheumatic heart disease, which develops in response to **rheumatic fever,** is a disease in which there is permanent damage to the valves of the heart. An inflammatory disease, rheumatic fever starts with a streptococcal infection ("strep throat") that affects the body's connective tissues, especially those of the heart, joints, brain, and skin. Usually occurring in children 5–15 years of age, rheumatic fever may be recognized by fever, swelling and pain in the joints, poor appetite, fatigue, and an inability to gain weight. Treating strep throat with antibiotics can often prevent acute rheumatic fever from developing.

Due to inflammation of the inner lining of the heart, the valves may scar and thicken to the degree that they may fail to open completely or close properly. Such heart valve leakage can, by the use of a stethoscope, be heard as a "swishing" sound called a *heart murmur.* An insufficiently opening valve forces the heart to work harder to pump enough blood through the openings. A valve not closing properly allows blood to "leak" back into the chamber from which it was pumped, again causing the heart to work harder.

Damaged heart valves may go unnoticed, but if serious enough, will eventually cause problems. Mitral valve problems can prevent the heart from pumping properly, and allow blood to back up into the lungs; this can cause shortness of breath and even fluid retention, or *edema,* in the body tissues.

Treatment for rheumatic heart disease may include the surgical replacement of one or more valves of the heart, with an artificial valve made of metal or plastic. Parents can help prevent rheumatic heart disease by paying attention to severe sore

rheumatic heart disease damage done to the heart, particularly the heart valves, by one or more attacks of rheumatic fever.

rheumatic fever an infectious disease that inflames the inner lining of the heart and causes rheumatic heart disease.

throats and fevers. A physician should be seen when a fever reaches 101 degrees in a child.

Congenital Heart Defects

Infants born with a malformation of the heart or of a major blood vessel of the heart have a **congenital heart defect.** Such defects, which occur in about 1 percent of all newborns, are the most common congenital malformation.[20]

Congenital heart defects most often obstruct blood flow in the heart or vessels near it, or cause blood to flow through the heart in an abnormal pattern. Some defects are holes in the septum between the ventricles and the atria (Figure. 20.9). These openings allow deoxygenated blood from the right side of the heart to mix with oxygenated blood from the left side of the heart. Since blood flowing to the body cannot carry enough oxygen, it gives the skin a bluish tone. Babies born with this condition are **cyanotic** (*sī-an-ot'ik*) and are called "blue babies."

Another congenital defect obstructs the flow of blood in or near the heart. The three most common obstructions are pulmonary valve stenosis, aortic valve **stenosis,** and coarctation of the aorta. In a stenosis there is a narrowing of the valves that results in an impeding of the flow of blood through the valves. Another defect is a narrowing, or **coarctation** (*kō-ark-tā'shun*) of the aorta, constricting the flow of blood to the body. Sometimes the arteries delivering blood to the lungs and to the body are switched so they attach to the wrong ventricles. As a result, oxygen-rich blood is delivered to the lungs and oxygen-poor blood to the body. Yet another defect, **patent ductus arteriosus,** is a persistent passageway between the pulmonary artery and aorta following birth, allowing oxygen-poor blood in the pulmonary artery to mix with the oxygen-rich blood in the aorta. The ductus arteriosis is a normal passageway between the two vessels

congenital heart defect malformation of the heart or of its major blood vessels.

cyanotic having a blueness of skin caused by insufficient oxygen in the blood.

stenosis constricting or narrowing of a heart valve or blood vessel.

coarctation compression of the walls of a blood vessel.

patent ductus arteriosus a persistent pathway between the main pulmonary artery and the aorta of the fetus.

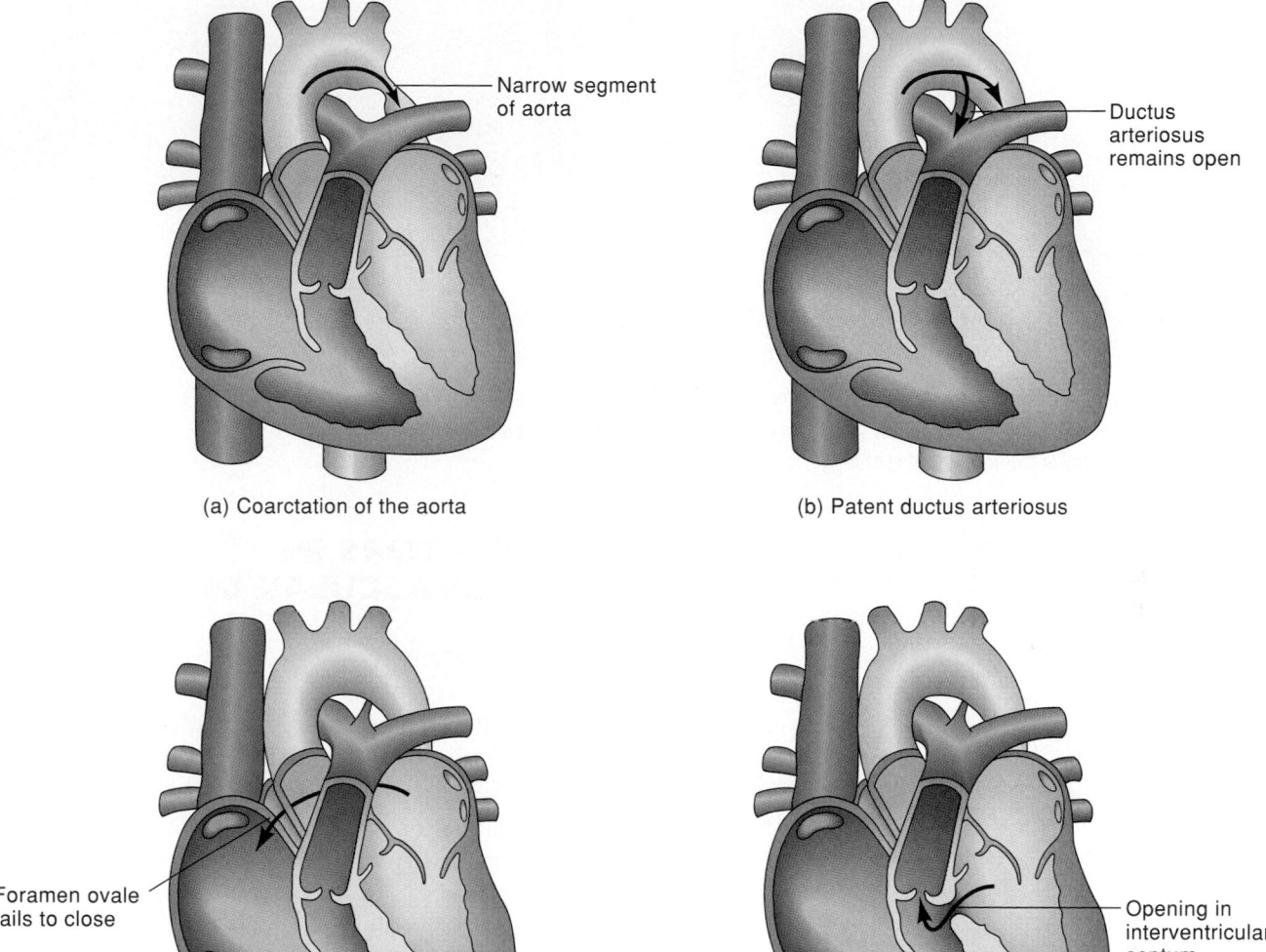

(a) Coarctation of the aorta

(b) Patent ductus arteriosus

(c) Interatrial septal defect

(d) Interventricular septal defect

Figure 20.9

Some Common Heart Defects That Exist at Birth

(a) Coarctation, or narrowing, of the aorta; (b) patent ductus arteriosus, or a passageway between the aorta and pulmonary artery that exists after birth; (c) interatrial septal defect, or a hole in the septum between the two atria; and (d) interventricular septal defect, or a hole in the septum between the two ventricles.

Source: Tortora, G., and Grabowski, S. Principles of Anatomy and Physiology, 7th ed. New York: HarperCollins, 1993.

before birth, but should close at or near the time of birth. Prior to birth, before the child must use his or her own lungs, the mother's body is processing oxygen-poor blood for the unborn child. Because all blood going through the unborn child's heart is oxygen-rich, prior to birth both of these major vessels carry oxygen-rich blood.

A serious congenital heart defect is usually diagnosed at birth or during infancy. The physician may detect an abnormal heart sound or the child may be cyanotic. Causes of congenital heart defects are not fully understood. One known cause, however, is rubella, or German measles. Children of mothers who contract this virus during the first three months of pregnancy are at greater risk of heart defects, as well as deafness, cataracts, and mental retardation. Contact with other viral diseases is also thought to be a cause. All women of childbearing age should

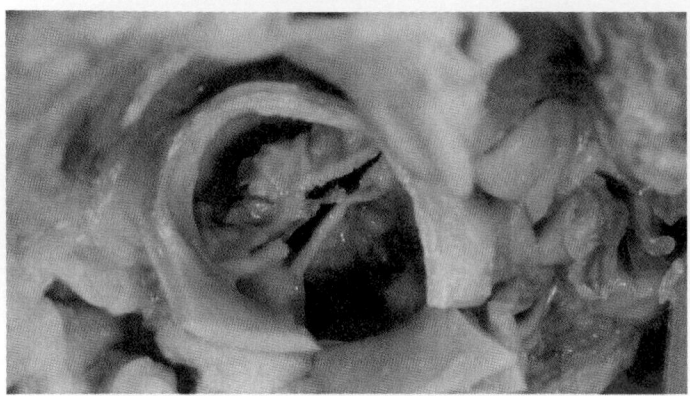
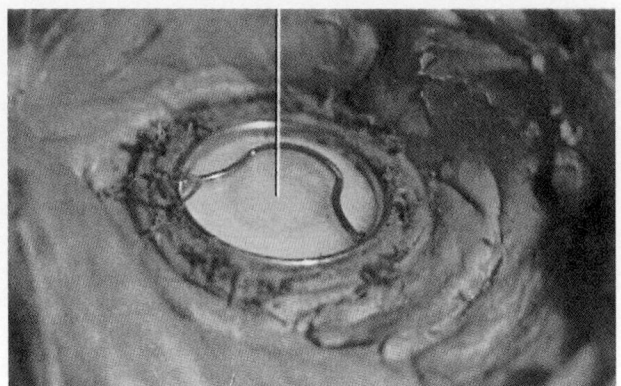

Heart valves which have been damaged by disease (left) may interfere with the flow of blood because they fail to open or close properly. In such cases, valve replacement surgery, in which the diseased valve is replaced with an artificial valve (right) made of metal or plastic, is recommended.

be vaccinated against rubella. Rubella antibodies in the blood, either from vaccination or contact with the disease, indicates an immunity to the disease. Congenital defects can also be caused by a mother drinking alcohol or using drugs such as cocaine during pregnancy.

Congenital heart defects can be treated with medicine or surgery. The surgery is designed to repair the defect as completely as possible. Some congenital heart conditions do not require surgery, but respond to medical treatment. Many congenital heart defects are correctable, and treatment can restore the child to a normal life.

CHECKPOINT

1. List the five major cardiovascular diseases described by the American Heart Association.

2. How do cardiovascular diseases rank as a cause of death in the United States?

3. Describe atherosclerosis and explain what happens to the arteries in this disease.

4. What are the causes and effects of hypertension?

5. Define the terms *myocardial infarction, ischemia, angina pectoris,* and *coronary thrombosis.*

6. List the symptoms of a heart attack.

7. What is a stroke? What is its major cause?

8. Describe arrhythmia, congestive heart failure, and rheumatic heart disease.

RISK FACTORS IN CARDIOVASCULAR DISEASES

The United States Public Health Service has, since 1948, been following the cardiac history of more than 10,000 residents of Framingham, Massachusetts. An intent of the Framingham Heart Study has been to identify risk factors in the incidence of cardiovascular diseases. The study has documented that a person's overall risk of cardiovascular disease is increased as the severity of these factors increases, and that the risk also increases as the number of factors present increases.

Risk factors are grouped into two categories: major risk factors and contributing risk factors. Major risk factors are those definitely associated with a significant increase in the risk of cardiovascular diseases. Contributing factors are those associated with increased risk of cardiovascular disease, but whose significance and prevalence have not yet been precisely determined. Some major risk factors can be changed, others cannot.[21]

MAJOR RISK FACTORS THAT YOU CAN MODIFY

Major risk factors that result from life-style habits that can be modified are cigarette smoking, high blood pressure, high blood lipid levels, and physical inactivity.

Cigarette Smoking

The Surgeon General has identified smoking as the most dangerous cardiovascular disease risk factor

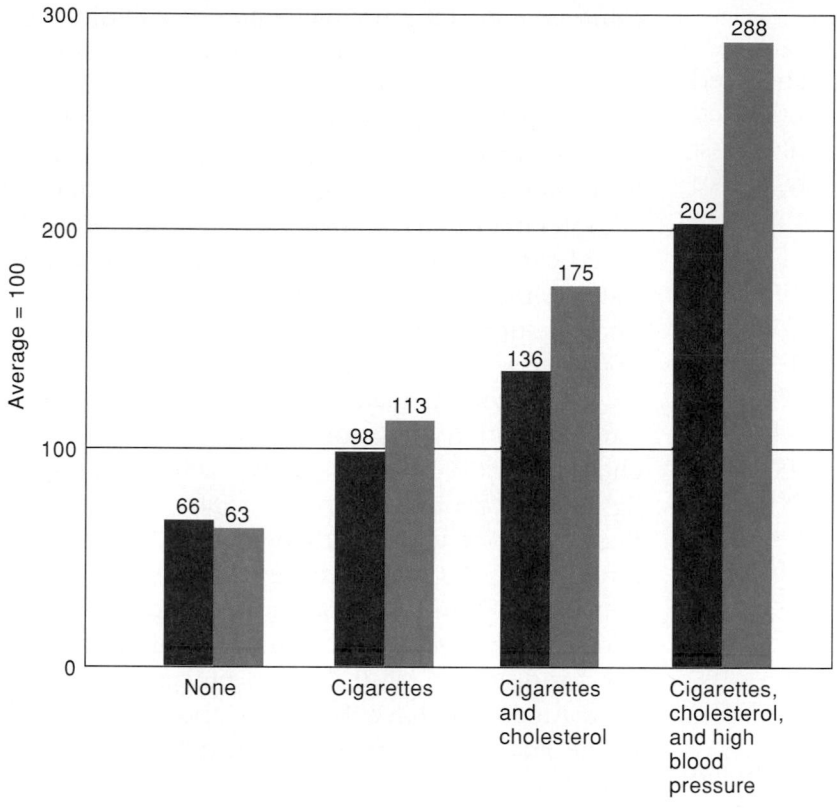

Figure 20.10

The Danger of Heart Attack Increases with the Number of Risk Factors Present

This chart shows how a combination of three major risk factors can increase the likelihood of heart attack. For purposes of illustration, this chart uses an abnormal blood pressure level of 150 systolic and a cholesterol level of 260 in a 55-year-old male and female.

Source: Framingham Heart Study, Section 37: "The Probability of Developing Certain CV Diseases in Eight Years at Specified Values of Some Characteristics," August 1987.

(Figure 20.10). The more a person smokes, the greater the risk of cardiovascular disease. Smokers face two to four times more risk of sudden cardiac death than nonsmokers. When combined with other risk factors, such as hypertension and high blood cholesterol levels, the danger is *synergistic,* or increases by more than the combined effects of the single risk factors. Smoking is the biggest risk factor for *peripheral vascular disease* (narrowing of blood vessels carrying blood to leg and arm muscles); in fact, this condition is found almost exclusively among smokers. Persons with peripheral vascular disease run a greater risk of developing gangrene and requiring leg amputation due to poor circulation.[22]

There are several possible explanations for the heart damage caused by smoking:

1. Nicotine stimulates a rise in heart rate and blood pressure. It causes heart muscle irritability, which can lead to cardiac arrhythmias.

2. Carbon monoxide (CO) from cigarette smoke displaces oxygen (O_2) in the blood, be-cause the hemoglobin of red blood cells has a greater affinity for CO than for O_2; thus the heart works harder to supply the body tissues with oxygen.

3. Smoking damages the lining (endothelium) of the coronary arteries, which leads to plaque buildup and increase in clot (thrombus) formation.[23] Smoking produces a three-fold increase in the risk of sudden death following a myocardial infarction.[24]

4. Smoking causes a lowering of the levels of high-density lipoprotein (HDL) cholesterol in the blood.

Second-hand smoke also increases the risk of heart disease. The risk of death is increased by 30 percent in nonsmokers exposed to environmental smoke at home, and it can be even higher among people exposed to second-hand smoke at work.[25] When people stop smoking, the risk of heart disease is rapidly reduced. Within a few years, the risk of heart disease drops and becomes equal to that of a nonsmoker.

Hypertension

Affecting almost one-third of people in the United States, hypertension is one of the most overlooked causes of CVD. Hypertension is the single most important risk factor for stroke. Fortunately, stroke from high blood pressure has been dropping in incidence in recent years.

The higher a person's blood pressure, the greater the risk of CVD. High blood pressure means the heart must work harder to pump blood, and over a period of time the heart becomes enlarged and weakened. High blood pressure increases the risk of congestive heart failure, heart attack, and kidney failure. When combined with cigarette smoking, obesity, high blood cholesterol levels, or diabetes, hypertension increases the risk of heart attack and stroke several times over. Men have a greater risk of high blood pressure than women until age 55, when the risk becomes the same until age 65; after age 65 women face a greater risk than men.[26]

A person with high blood pressure should monitor blood pressure regularly, exercise consistently, reduce salt (sodium) intake, control fat and calorie intake, and take medication if recommended by a physician. A diet lower in saturated fats and cholesterol and higher in fibers is recommended. High blood pressure can also be reduced by stopping smoking and limiting alcohol intake.[27, 28] Hypertension is rarely cured. Any course prescribed to reduce and control it will need to be followed for life.

Blood Lipid Levels

Lipids (fats), such as cholesterol and triglycerides, are transported in the blood (see Chapter 8). To be carried in the blood they must combine with protein, forming lipoproteins. Each lipoprotein molecule consists of protein, triglycerides, and cholesterol. The term *blood lipid* is frequently used when referring to the presence of cholesterol and triglycerides in the blood.

Many Americans have undesirably high levels of cholesterol and triglycerides. We have already discussed how blood lipids infiltrate the walls of the blood vessels in the formation of atherosclerotic plaques. A poor blood lipid profile is believed to be the most significant factor in the development of CHD.

Cholesterol Of particular interest is cholesterol; many researchers see a link between high levels of cholesterol in the blood and cardiovascular disease, especially CHD. Cholesterol is introduced into the body in two ways. The body, primarily the liver, produces about 1000 mg a day. An additional 400–500 mg per day comes directly from foods. As stated earlier, certain animal products contain cholesterol; plants do not contain it. The body's production supplies most or all of the cholesterol the body needs.

The recommendations of the National Cholesterol Education Program (NCEP) is to keep total cholesterol (TC) levels below 200 mg/dl (milligrams of cholesterol per deciliter of blood; a deciliter is one-tenth of a liter, or the equivalent of three ounces). Cholesterol levels (see Table 20.2) between 200 and 239 mg/dl are borderline high, and levels of 240 mg/dl and above indicate high risk for disease.[29] More than 50 percent of middle-aged Americans have TC levels above 200 mg/dl. In the Framingham Heart Study, not a single individual with a TC level of 150 mg/dl or lower has had a heart attack.[30] As the TC level increases above 150 mg/dl, the risk of coronary artery disease slowly begins to rise. Above 200 mg/dl the risk rises more rapidly. The chance of a heart attack doubles with every 50 mg/dl increase in TC once the level goes over 200 mg/dl.[31]

You have it within your power to help your blood vessels retain their original level of wellness longer. Communication for Wellness: How to Make Your Arteries Younger (or Older) Than They Are is a message of what you can do to speed up or slow down the clock of arterial aging. The time to begin affecting your arterial clock is now.

Total cholesterol is found distributed in three kinds of lipoproteins: low-density lipoproteins (LDLs), high-density lipoproteins (HDLs), and very-low-density lipoproteins (VLDLs). LDLs contain 25 percent protein, 20 percent triglycerides, and *55 percent cholesterol*. LDLs deliver cholesterol to cells that need it, but with too high a level of LDL cholesterol being deposited in the lining of blood vessels, speeding up the process of atherosclerosis. Thus LDLs are called "bad cholesterol." HDLs contain 50 percent protein, 37 percent triglycerides, and *only 13 percent cholesterol*. Their low levels of cholesterol allows HDLs to remove cholesterol from body cells and deliver it to the liver for elimination, reducing the buildup of cholesterol in the

Table 20.2
Standards for Blood Lipids

	Level	Risk
Total cholesterol	< 200 mg/dl	Desirable
(TC)	200–239 mg/dl	Borderline high
	> 239 mg/dl	High
Low Density Lipoprotein	< 130 mg/dl	Desirable
(LDL)	130–159 mg/dl	Borderline high
	> 159 mg/dl	High
High Density Lipoprotein	> 40 mg/dl	Desirable
(HDL)	35–40 mg/dl	Borderline low
	< 35 mg/dl	Low
Triglycerides	< 190 mg/dl	Desirable
	190–500 mg/dl	Borderline high
	> 500 mg/dl	High

Source: Tortora, G., and Grabowski, S. Principles of Anatomy and Physiology, 7th ed. New York: HarperCollins, 1993, p. 614.

blood and preventing plaque from forming in the arteries. VLDLs contain about 10 percent proteins, 65 percent triglycerides, and 25 percent cholesterol, and carry triglycerides from liver cells to adipose cells (see Triglycerides, this page).[32] Thus, a high level of HDL indicates a lowered risk of heart disease from plaque formation. Accordingly, HDLs are called "good cholesterol." Both high levels of HDL and low levels of LDL are associated with a decreased risk of heart disease.

In adults, desirable levels of blood cholesterol are: TC less than 200 mg/dl, LDL under 131 mg/dl, HDL over 40 mg/dl, and triglycerides (VLDLs) less than 190 mg/dl (see Table 20.2). The risk of developing CHD can be predicted by determining the ratio of TC to HDL. For instance, a TC of 180 and

an HDL of 60 gives a ratio of 3. Ratios above 4 are viewed as undesirable. The higher the ratio the higher the risk of developing CHD.[33]

Triglycerides   The most plentiful lipids in a person's body are triglycerides (fats and oils). As discussed in Chapter 8, they are either saturated or unsaturated, depending on whether the molecules contain the maximum number of hydrogen atoms. Carried in the blood mainly by VLDLs, triglycerides are transported from liver cells to fat (adipose) tissue for storage. The higher the fat diet, the greater the number of VLDLs. After their transport duties are complete, *VLDLs are converted to LDLs*. In this way a high-fat diet contributes to the formation of fatty plaques. Normally, triglycerides in the blood are in the range of 10 to 190 mg/dl (see Table 20.2).

Three important therapies in reducing blood cholesterol are exercise (see Chapter 10), diet (see Chapter 8), and medications. Regular physical exercise at or near aerobic levels tends to raise the number of HDLs. Dietary practices should lower the intake of fat in any form, especially saturated fats and cholesterol, and raise fiber intake (Table 20.3). In a study, people who lowered their fat-calorie diet to 10 percent of intake and did regular aerobic exercise (mostly walking) reduced their blood cholesterol by an average of 23 percent.[34] Medications used to treat high cholesterol levels include Questran and Colestid, which promote bile excretion in the feces, and Lipo-nicin (nicotinic acid) and Mcvacor, which blocks synthesis of cholesterol by liver cells. (For more regarding medications used to treat heart disease, see p. 645.)

COMMUNICATION FOR WELLNESS

HOW TO MAKE YOUR ARTERIES YOUNGER (OR OLDER) THAN THEY ARE

Although the rate of fatty cholesterol deposit varies from person to person, the average person with a blood cholesterol level of 200 milligrams per deciliter (mg/dl) and no other risk factors will probably develop a significant amount of plaque formation by the age of 70. If, however, a person's blood cholesterol level is 250 mg/dl, a comparable amount of arterial plaque will accumulate by age 60. At 300 mg/dl, a 50-year-old's arteries will be similar to those of a 70-year-old.

Add other risk factors to high cholesterol, such as smoking and hypertension, and the clock speeds up. A person

with a cholesterol level of 250 mg/dl and who smokes, may reach a critical degree of plaque formation at age 50, rather than at age 60.

You have the power to change these progressions. You can slow down the clock. Keep your cholesterol levels well below 200, and at age 70 you may have the arteries of a 50-year-old. (Note: A deciliter is one-tenth of a liter, or the equivalent of 3 ounces.)

Source: Berkeley Wellness Letter, June 1987, p. 5.

Table 20.3
Food for a Healthy Heart

There is no longer any doubt that diet affects blood cholesterol levels which, in turn, can cause atherosclerosis, leading to heart attacks and strokes. As a result, many people today are choosing their foods more carefully.

The first table contains some foods to consume in moderation, since they are high in cholesterol and saturated fats. The second contains foods that can be eaten more often, since they are low in cholesterol and saturated fats.

Consume in Moderation	Cholesterol (milligrams)	Saturated Fat (grams)
Beef liver, fried (3 oz)	408	2.3
One egg	212	1.5
Shrimp, raw, large (14)	152	0.3
Ice cream, hardened, 16% fat (1 cup)	90	14.8
Ground beef patty, broiled, lean (3 oz)	87	6.0
Prime rib of beef, lean and fat (3 oz)	72	10.8
Beef hot dog, large (1)	35	6.9
Whole milk (1 cup)	33	5.1
Butter (1 tbsp)	31	7.1
Donut, cake type, plain (1)	18	1.9
Milk, chocolate, 2% fat (1 cup)	17	3.1

Preferred Types of Foods	Cholesterol (milligrams)	Saturated Fat (grams)
Most fruits and vegetables	0	trace
Popcorn, popped in vegetable oil (1 cup)	0	0.5
Angel food cake (1/12 of cake)	0	0.1
Peanut butter (1 tbsp)	0	2.4
Margarine, hard (1 tbsp)	0	2.2
Skim milk (nonfat, 1 cup)	4	0.3
Parmesan cheese (1 tbsp)	4	0.9
Cottage cheese, dry curd (1 cup)	10	0.4
Ice milk (1 cup)	18	3.5
Yogurt (1 cup)	14	2.3
Tuna, light, water pack (3 oz)	25	0.2
Turkey, white meat (3 oz)	59	0.9
Steak, lean (3 oz)	76	2.6
Chicken, breast, without skin, lean (3 oz)	78	1.1

Source: Whitney, E., and Rolfe, S. Understanding Nutrition, 6th ed. St. Paul: West, 1993.

Physical Inactivity

A primary benefit of regular physical activity is protection against coronary heart disease, which is consistently higher in people who have inactive or sedentary occupations than in those who have active occupations. Coronary heart disease is almost two times more likely to develop in physically inactive people than in active ones. Yet, in spite of well-publicized benefits of physical activity, there are only slightly more than one in ten people in the United States who report daily physical activity of 30 minutes or more.[35]

Regular aerobic exercise that works large body muscles for at least 20 minutes, 3–5 times a week, improves the health of the cardiovascular system. Such activities include brisk walking, jogging, running, bicycling, aerobics, swimming, cross-country skiing, and sports such as basketball, soccer, tennis, and racquetball.

Low-intensity physical activity, even at modest levels, is helpful in reducing risk if done regularly and for extended periods. In a study of people bicycling at 65 percent of maximum capacity for 30 minutes, three times a week, there was a reduction of systolic pressure by 4 mm Hg, and of diastolic pressure by 5 mm Hg.[36]

Actually, there is scientific evidence that regular, moderate-intensity physical activity promotes significant health benefits. The U.S. Centers for Disease Control and Prevention and the American College of Sports Medicine, in cooperation with the President's Council on Physical Fitness and Sports, now recommends that *every American adult should accumulate 30 minutes of more than moderate-intensity physical activity over the course of most days of the week.* Such activities include walking up stairs, gardening, raking leaves, dancing, and walking part or all of the way to and from work. It may come from planned exercise or recreation, such as jogging, playing tennis, swimming, and cycling, or from walking two miles briskly each day.[37]

The benefits of physical activities include an increase in HDLs, a decrease in triglyceride levels, and improved lung function. It helps reduce blood pressure, anxiety, and depression; controls weight; and increases the body's ability to dissolve blood clots.[38]

MAJOR RISK FACTORS THAT YOU CANNOT CHANGE

There are some risk factors in cardiovascular diseases that cannot be changed voluntarily.

Heredity

Some risk of heart disease appears to be inherited. People whose parents have had atherosclerosis have a greater tendency toward developing it themselves. Among African Americans the incidence of severe hypertension is reported three times as often as among whites, and moderate hypertension twice as often.[39] Some contest these findings. In a study of 457 African Americans, high blood pressure was found only among those who had low socioeconomic status or who had not graduated from high school. A combination of socioeconomic disadvantages and a behavior of repressing hostility and anger may be more significant than any genetic predisposition.[40, 41]

Sex

Cardiovascular disease may also relate to a person's sex. Traditional wisdom has stated that heart attacks are a man's disease. Before menopause, when a woman has the protection of estrogen, the incidence of heart attacks is higher in men, but after menopause the heart attack rate in women increases, until by age 65, incidence is almost equal (Feature 20.2).

Age

As a person ages, the risk of heart attack increases. More than half of all heart attack victims are age 65 or older. Five out of six deaths due to stroke occur in people over 65 years of age.[42]

CONTRIBUTING RISK FACTORS

Factors associated with increased risk of CVD, but whose significance and prevalence have not yet been precisely determined, are called *contributing risk factors*. Such factors include diabetes, stress, and obesity.

Diabetes

Diabetes is a generalized term for diseases characterized by excessive loss of urine. The term is most often used for diabetes mellitus, a disorder in which

---

diabetes a general term for diseases characterized by excessive urination; commonly refers to diabetes mellitus, a chronic disorder of carbohydrate processing in the body due to inadequate insulin production or utilization.

there is an inability of the body to metabolize or use glucose properly. As a result, the body cells rely upon fats to produce energy. But as the lipids are transported around the body, they are deposited in the walls of blood vessels. This leads to the formation of atherosclerotic plaques and a host of cardiovascular problems. Small blood vessels, especially in the eyes and extremities, tend to deteriorate.

Occurring most often in middle-aged and overweight persons, diabetes may go unnoticed for many years if its effects are mild. People with diabetes face increased risks of kidney disease, blindness, nerve and blood vessel damage, as well as increased risks of developing CVD.

Diabetes can be controlled. By changing eating habits, controlling weight, exercising regularly, and taking prescribed drugs (if necessary), people with diabetes can control their disease and reduce the risk of CVD. (For further discussion of diabetes, see Chapter 21.)

Stress

Defining and measuring a person's stress level is difficult, if not impossible. People feel and react to stressors in very different ways. Stress in and of itself may not be harmful. Some stress, such as moderate levels, increases performance and achievement. Chronic, or excessive stress, however, has the potential for being harmful. Work-related stress may be especially harmful. In a study of 215 men ages 30–60, job-related stress was found to cause both high blood pressure and potentially hazardous changes in the heart. Loss of control over day-to-day decisions, especially in jobs with high psychological demands, seems to create the greatest stress. People working under these conditions had three times greater risk of high blood pressure. Younger men in the study who were in high-stress jobs showed measurable thickening in parts of the heart muscle, a condition that commonly precedes heart disease and heart attack.[43] A person's life stress, behavioral habits, and socioeconomic status have been shown to relate to CHD. These factors may affect established risk factors. For instance, a person in a stressful situation may start to smoke or may smoke more than he or she otherwise would.[44]

The idea that excess stress may be the single most important personality factor in the development of heart disease among middle-aged adults developed in the 1950s. People were divided into

FEATURE 20.2

WOMEN AND HEART DISEASE

Long-neglected in the media and the medical profession is the fact that heart disease is a killer of women. Early findings by the Framingham Heart Study indicated that heart disease was a middle-aged-man's disease. Underlying this gender-based point of view was belief that women are immune to heart disease due to estrogen (which raises the level of HDL in women). Although estrogen offers protection during the first half of life, with menopause, estrogen production declines and heart attack rates soar in women.

Pointing to the need for better diagnosis and treatment for women, studies show the following:

1. Women over age 70 are more likely to suffer heart attacks than men.

2. Women heart victims with chest pains are less likely to be treated with clot-busting drugs within the critical first four hours after chest pains start.

3. Women who undergo angioplasty, the tiny balloon therapy, are more than ten times as likely to die in the hospital.

4. Women who suffer the symptoms of a heart attack are likely to have a vague, lingering chest discomfort and nausea (in contrast to crushing chest pains in men).

5. Women have a 1-in-11 chance of developing breast cancer, but a 1-in-2 chance of a cardiovascular disease.

6. Women who take estrogen pills after menopause have 50 percent fewer heart attack deaths.

7. Women are rarely given treadmill tests, in contrast to men.

8. Women are 2–8 times as likely to die shortly after surgery from a coronary bypass operation than are men.

9. Women under stress sleep less, exercise less, weigh more, feel more anger, and smoke more.

Ways for a woman to cut down the risk of heart disease include the following:

• Stop smoking!

• Keep your blood pressure below 140/90.

• Keep the TC to HDL ratio at 4.5 or less.

• Keep HDL levels up to at least 40 mg/dl, and LDL levels under 160 (130 if you smoke).

• Keep triglyceride levels under 150 mg.

Source: Diethrich, E. *Women and Heart Disease: What You Can Do to Stop the #1 Killer of Women.* New York: Random House, 1992.

two general behavioral, stress-related categories: Type A and Type B. Type A personalities were hard-driving, competitive, impatient, compulsive, and hostile. Type B personalities were more relaxed and placid. After more than 40 years of study, this concept is still hotly debated. Of all of the traits associated with Type A behavior, hostility is the only trait that now appears to correspond directly to heart disease.[45, 46] Others, disagreeing with this, contend that a critical factor of Type A behavior is inappropriate competitiveness.

Obesity

Obesity relates to CVD largely because it has an influence on blood pressure and blood lipid levels and often leads to diabetes. People whose body weight is more than 30 percent above their ideal body weight often develop heart disease and stroke, even if they have no other risk factors.[47] Recent evidence suggests that *where* fat is deposited may affect the risk of CHD. For men, a waist/hip ratio of more than 1.0 (waist measurement exceeding hip mea-

surement) indicates increased risk. For a woman to avoid increased CHD risk, her waist/hip ratio should not exceed 0.8 (her waist measurement should not be more than 80 percent of her hip measurement).[48]

Now that you have finished reading the major and contributing risk factors in cardiovascular diseases, you can determine your own risk of heart disease by completing the assessment, In Your Hands: Taking Your Measure of Heart Disease Risk.

CHECKPOINT

1. List the four most modifiable factors that contribute to the development of heart disease.

2. Explain how cigarette smoking damages the heart.

3. Identify the steps you can take to reduce and control high blood pressure.

4. What are major risk factors of heart disease that you cannot change?

IN YOUR HANDS

TAKING YOUR MEASURE OF HEART DISEASE RISK

In each of the following categories pick your answer, then add up the corresponding points from each category to calculate your score. To find the correct answer in some categories, you may need medical information.

PERSONAL
Your sex and age is:
   0   Woman younger than 55
  +1   Man younger than 55
  +2   Woman 55 or older
  +3   Man 55 to 65
  +4   Man 65 or older

Among your close blood relatives, there have been heart attacks:
   0   In no parent, grandparent, aunt, or uncle before age 60
  +1   In one or more parents, grandparents, aunts, or uncles after age 60
  +2   In one parent, grandparent, aunt, or uncle before age 60
  +3   In two of the above relatives before age 60
  +4   In more than two of the above relatives before age 60

Among your close relatives, the following medical conditions have existed:
   0   No serious high blood pressure, diabetes, or high cholesterol level
  +1   Serious high blood pressure, diabetes, or high cholesterol level in only one close relative
  +2   Serious high blood pressure, diabetes, or high cholesterol levels in two close relatives
  +3   Serious high blood pressure, diabetes, or high cholesterol levels in more than two close relatives

STRESS
You feel overstressed:
   0   Rarely at work or at home
  +3   Somewhat at home but not at work
  +5   Somewhat at work but not at home
  +7   Somewhat at work and at home
  +9   Usually, at work or at home
  +12 Usually, at work and at home

DIABETES
Your diabetes history is:
   0   Blood sugar always normal
  +2   Blood glucose slightly high (prediabetic) or slightly low (hypoglycemic)
  +4   Diabetes beginning after age 40 requiring strict dietary or insulin control
  +5   Diabetes beginning before age 30 requiring strict dietary or insulin control

ALCOHOL
You drink alcoholic beverages:
   0   Never or only socially, about once or twice a month, or only one 5-ounce glass of wine or 12-ounce glass of beer or 1½ ounces of hard liquor about five times a week

  +2   Two to three 5-ounce glasses of wine or 12-ounce glasses of beer or 1½-ounce cocktails about five times a week
  +4   More than three 1½-ounce cocktails or more than three 5-ounce glasses of wine or 12-ounce glasses of beer almost every day

CHOLESTEROL
Your serum cholesterol level is:
   0   190 or below
  +2   191 to 230
  +6   231 to 289
  +12 290 to 319
  +16 320 or over

Your HDL cholesterol is:
  −2   Over 60
   0   45–60
  +2   35–44
  +6   29–34
  +12 23–28
  +16 Below 23

SMOKING
You smoke now or have in the past:
   0   Never smoked, or quit more than 5 years ago
  +1   Quit 2 to 4 years ago
  +3   Quit about 1 year ago
  +6   Quit during the past year

You now smoke:
  +9   ½ to 1 pack a day
  +12 1 to 2 packs a day
  +15 More than 2 packs a day

The quality of the air you breathe is:
   0   Unpolluted by smoke, exhaust, or industry at home and at work
  +2   Live or work with smokers in unpolluted area
  +4   Live and work with smokers in unpolluted area
  +6   Live or work with smokers and live or work in air-polluted area
  +8   Live and work with smokers and live and work in air-polluted area

BLOOD PRESSURE
Your blood pressure is:
   0   below 120/75
  +2   120/75 to 140/85
  +6   140/85 to 150/90
  +8   150/90 to 175/100
  +10 175/100 to 190/110
  +12 190/110 or above

EXERCISE
Your exercise habits are:
   0   Exercise vigorously 4–5 times a week
  +2   Exercise moderately 4–5 times a week
  +4   Exercise only on weekends
  +6   Exercise occasionally
  +8   Little or no exercise

(continues)

WEAPONS AGAINST HEART DISEASE

There is reason for continuing optimism in the fight against CVD. The death rate from heart disease has declined by about 45 percent since 1970. Credit for the decline is due to several factors. People are increasingly health conscious and concerned with personal health—quitting smoking, controlling high blood pressure, lowering cholesterol and triglyceride levels, and maintaining physical fitness. During the last several decades, there have been dramatic breakthroughs in discovering some of the causes of heart disease and in developing techniques for treating these conditions. At the same time cardiac-intensive-care units have come into widespread use in hospitals and heart surgery has become commonplace. In addition, continuing research has provided the basis for improved diagnosis and treatment of CVD. The role played by national organizations, such as the American Heart Association, in helping raise money for research and educating the public on ways to reduce the risks of heart disease has been one of the major reasons for the progress made against CVD.

DIAGNOSTIC TESTS

A physician may be able to diagnose the presence of heart disease before an attack by examining the results of one of a number of different diagnostic tests. Tests are of three types.[49]

A. *Tests that make picture images, resembling x-rays, of the brain, heart, and larger blood vessels:*

   1. *Radionuclide Imaging* Injected radioactive compounds follow the blood into the heart, then computer-generated pictures are taken, indicating the supply of blood to the heart muscle, functioning of the chambers, and extent of any damage to the heart by an attack.

   2. *Magnetic Resonance Imaging (MRI)* The atoms in the human body are made to resonate by the action of radio waves on a strong magnet. Each type of body tissue gives off a unique signal, allowing a computer to generate two dimensional images. The pictures image the heart muscle and identify heart damage, congenital heart defects, and diseased blood vessels.

   3. *Computed Tomography (CT) Scanning* Previously known as computerized axial tomographic (CAT) scanning, this is the most well-known imaging test. A beam moves through an arc around the body, producing a cross-sectioned, three-dimensional image (CT scan) used in diagnosing tumors and aneurysms.

B. *Tests that measure the electrical activity of the brain, heart, and larger blood vessels and that give useful information about normal or abnormal functioning:*

   1. *Electrocardiogram (EKG)* Variously located electrodes on the body's surface detect normal and abnormal electrical currents generated by the heart that are recorded as tracings on long strips of paper.

   2. *Electroencephalogram (EEG)* Electrodes placed on the scalp pick up normal and abnormal electrical impulses from brain cells that are recorded as tracings on long strips of paper.

C. *Tests that measure blood flow, detect blockages in blood vessels, and reveal areas of significant atherosclerosis in carotid arteries:*

1. *Digital Cardiac Angiography (DCA) or Digital Subtraction Angiography (DSA)* A computer compares an x-ray of a region of the body before and after a contrast dye has been injected into a blood vessel. This form of imaging is used primarily to study blood vessels in the brain and heart.

2. *Doppler Ultrasound Test* A gel, through which a technician listens with a probe, is put on the neck to allow monitoring of blood flowing in an artery (carotid in neck). Careful analysis can detect occlusions.

MEDICATIONS

The Food and Drug Administration has approved a new class of drugs, known as "clotbusters." These drugs dissolve blood clots that form on the fatty plaques in the coronary arteries and cut off blood flow. Such drugs are administered through a **catheter,** which is a flexible tube inserted through an arm or leg artery into the heart. The drugs can dissolve clots and restore blood flow to the oxygen-deprived heart muscle. In order to be effective, treatment must be started promptly after heart attack symptoms begin. One of these drugs, TPA (tissue plasminogen activator) can be injected directly into a vein by the victims themselves when they first detect heart attack symptoms. The drug dissolves a clot within 30–60 minutes.

There are also many drugs that help reduce blood cholesterol levels. Lovastatin reduces the production of cholesterol-raising LDLs by as much as 40 percent, and raises the level of heart-protecting HDLs (also see Chapter 8). Nicotinic acid, part of the B-complex vitamin family, inhibits the production of fats, decreases blood cholesterol, and raises HDL levels. (See the earlier discussion in this chapter on medications to lower cholesterol levels, p. 639.) Probucol is another drug that reduces cholesterol levels.

Calcium blockers lower blood pressure, increase cardiac output during heart failure, relieve angina, and control arrhythmias. By controlling the flow of calcium ions, which cause muscle cells to contract, heart vessel spasms that can close an artery may be prevented. *Beta blockers* are able to slow the heart rate, and thus by requiring less blood flow help patients with partially blocked coronary arteries and high blood pressure. All of these medications require a prescription and must be used under supervision of a qualified physician.

Aspirin

A nonsurgical therapy to lower the risk of heart attack and prevent recurrence of heart attack is the regular use of aspirin. Aspirin has an anticlotting effect and it prevents the platelets in the blood from sticking to arterial plaques and forming clots. However, aspirin should be used with caution. First, you should discuss the matter with your personal physician, since people with certain medical problems, such as peptic ulcer, gastrointestinal bleeding, and liver or kidney disease, may be advised against taking aspirin. The frequent use of aspirin can lead to ulcers, and aspirin use has been shown to relate to certain types of stroke. When used, aspirin should be adjunct therapy, not used as a substitute for reducing other CVD risk factors, such as smoking, hypertension, diabetes, high cholesterol levels, and obesity.

SURGICAL REMEDIES

Some of the most recognized breakthroughs in treating heart disease have been surgical improvements.

Bypass Surgery

The surgical procedure most commonly performed on heart patients is **coronary artery bypass graft (CABG) surgery.** This surgical technique bypasses clogged arteries and maintains flow to the heart. A segment of blood vessel, usually taken from the leg or from inside the chest wall, is used to create a detour around the obstruction (see Figure 20.11).

---

catheter a tube passed through the body, often through a blood vessel, for injecting fluids into a body structure, such as the heart.

coronary artery bypass graft surgery surgery to improve the blood supply to the heart muscle.

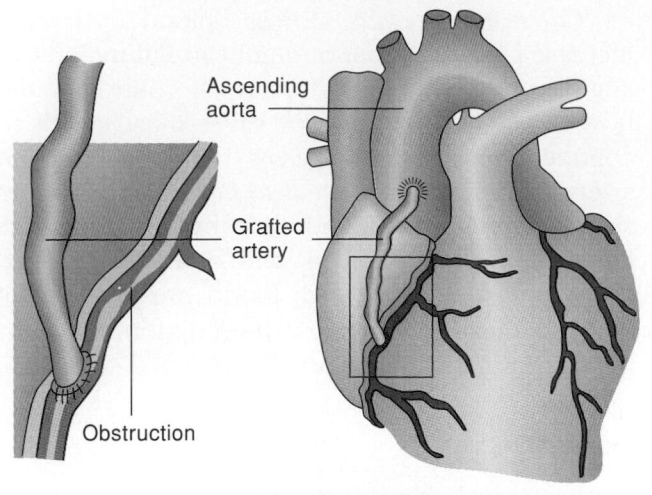

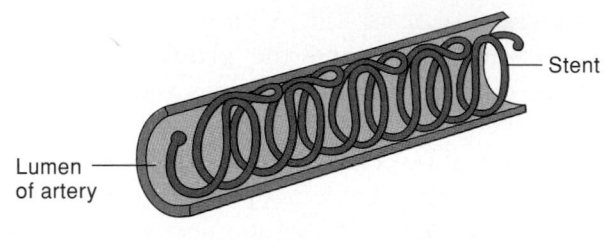

(a) Coronary artery bypass grafting (CABG)

(c) Stent in an artery

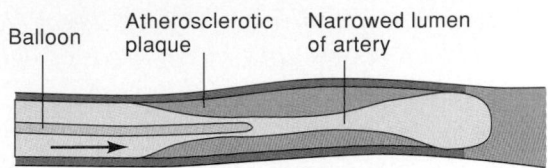

Balloon catheter with uninflated balloon approaches obstructed area in artery

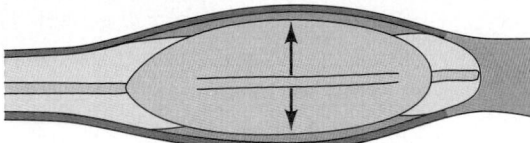

When balloon is inflated, it breaks up atherosclerotic plaque

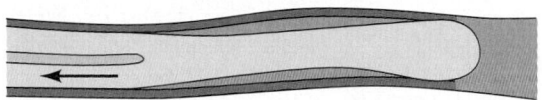

After lumen is widened, balloon catheter with uninflated balloon is withdrawn

(b) Percutaneous transluminal coronary angioplasty (PTCA)

Figure 20.11

Several Procedures for Reestablishing Blood Flow in Occluded Coronary Arteries.

(a) In coronary artery bypass grafting (CABG), the internal mammary artery is removed from the patient's chest, and grafted at one end to the aorta and at the other end to the coronary artery at some point beyond the obstruction; (b) percutaneous transluminal coronary angioplasty (PTCA), is a nonsurgical procedure in which a balloon is inserted by catheter into the blocked vessel, inflated with air to squash the plaque against the blood vessel wall, then withdrawn; (c) a stent is inserted into the artery to avoid a renarrowing of the opened blood vessel.

Source: Tortora, G., and Grabowski, S. Principles of Anatomy and Physiology, 7th ed. New York: HarperCollins, 1993.

One end of the vessel is attached above the blockage and the other end to the coronary artery below the blocked area. During the surgery, circulation is maintained by a heart-lung machine. One or more bypasses may be done at the same time.

Angioplasty

Also known as balloon angioplasty or *percutaneous transluminal coronary angioplasty* (PTCA), **angioplasty** (*an'jē-ō-plas-tē*) is an alternative to bypass surgery. PTCA is a nonsurgical procedure designed to widen or expand coronary arteries and

angioplasty a procedure used to widen narrowed arteries.

increase the blood supply to the heart muscle. A balloon catheter (plastic tube) is inserted into the artery of an arm or leg and guided through the arterial system to the obstructed coronary artery under x-ray observation (Figure 20.11). Then, while a liquid dye visible in x-ray is released through the catheter, angiograms (x-ray movies of blood vessels) record the course of the dye and identify obstructed areas. Next, the balloon is inflated with air at the arterial blockage to compress the plaque against the arterial wall and widen the channel so that blood can flow more easily. Then the balloon is deflated and the catheters are withdrawn. PTCA is most often used after angina pectoris.

In about 25–30 percent of cases, the PTCA-opened arteries renarrow. This usually occurs with-

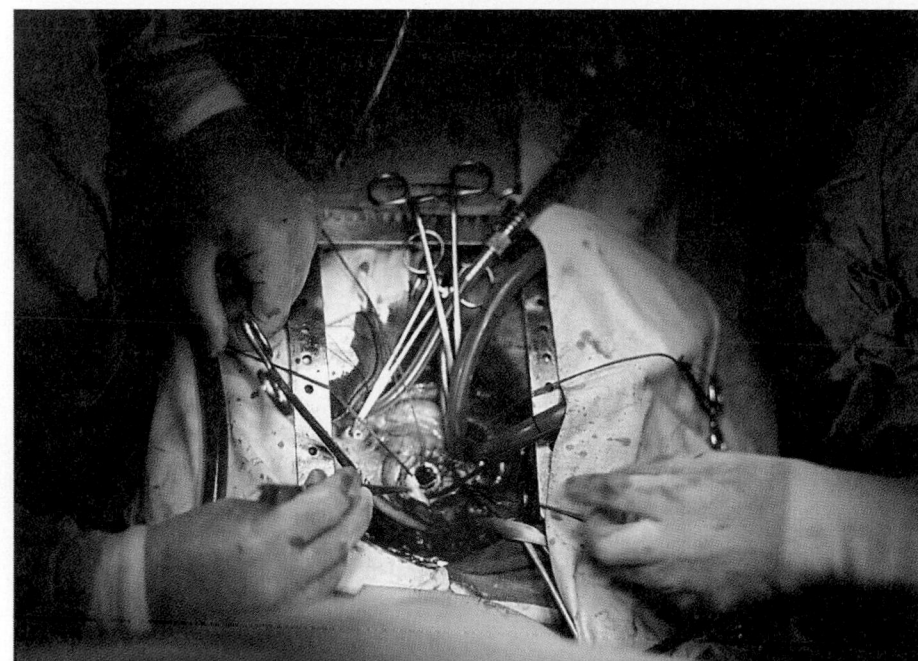

Heart transplant is a procedure in which a donor heart is used to replace a diseased heart in the recipient. Unfortunately, the procedure has not been as successful as hoped.

in the first six months. If this is the case, there are several options. The PTCA may be repeated. A *stent,* which is a stainless steel device resembling a spring coil, may be inserted through the catheter and permanently placed in the artery to keep the artery open.

Laser

Another technique for cleaning clogged arteries is **laser angioplasty.** The laser, an instrument that emits an intense, highly focused beam of light and energy, is attached to the tip of the catheter. Once in place, short bursts are fired at the obstruction, vaporizing the plaque and opening the channel. The debris is sucked up through a vacuum tube.

Two recently developed techniques are **balloon-laser welding** and **catheter artherectomy.** In balloon-laser welding, the affected artery is widened by PTCA, then a laser heats the surround-

....

laser angioplasty surgery using a device that emits intense heat and power at close range by converting light into one small and extremely intense beam.

balloon-laser welding heating by laser of an artery, which has been widened by angioplasty, in order to stretch and weld the artery wall into a smooth surface.

catheter artherectomy the use of a catheter rotating drill to shave off a plaque.

ing tissue to stretch and weld the wall into a smooth surface. In catheter artherectomy, a rotating drill shaves off the plaque, then the debris is trapped and removed.

Heart Transplant

Millions of people suffer from the effects of diseased or damaged hearts. Heart disease is the number one cause of premature death in the industrialized world. One of every five persons who reaches age 60 will have a myocardial infarction. Although various drugs and therapies are available and helpful, at some point they are no longer adequate because too much functional cardiac muscle has been lost.[50]

One recourse for a failing heart is a **heart transplant,** a procedure in which the heart and, on occasion, the lungs, are transplanted from a donor's body. People whose heart failure does not respond to other available treatment may be candidates for heart transplants.

Before a transplant can be considered, it must be determined that the donor's tissue *antigens* are sufficiently similar to those of the recipient in order to avert tissue rejection. The drug cyclosporine has helped suppress transplant rejection, though such

....

heart transplant the transfer of a heart from one person to another.

suppression weakens the patient's immune system and leaves him or her open to severe infection.

Unfortunately, the availability of donor hearts is very limited. In 1991, with 50,000–100,000 candidates needing donor hearts, only 1,935 heart transplants were performed. Of these, the five-year survival rate, when using a three-drug regimen, is 71 percent. Another alternative not currently in use is the artificial heart. During the 1980s several patients received artificial heart transplants. Due to problems with blood clotting, strokes, and infection, the Food and Drug Administration in 1990 banned further use of the devices. Research into other possible types of artificial hearts continues.[51, 52]

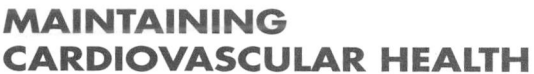

CHECKPOINT

1. How are drugs used to combat heart disease?

2. What are some of the surgical techniques used to treat heart disease?

MAINTAINING CARDIOVASCULAR HEALTH

The fight in the United States against cardiovascular diseases, particularly coronary heart disease, is looking better. In fact, the death rate from coronary heart disease has fallen by over 30 percent since 1972.[53] Apparently we as a country are learning how to better protect ourselves from these diseases. But more remains to be done. The National Heart, Lung, and Blood Institute estimates that if no one had high blood cholesterol or high blood pressure, and no one smoked, the number of heart attacks in the United States would only be 20–25 percent of what it is now.[54] Premature coronary heart disease can be prevented.

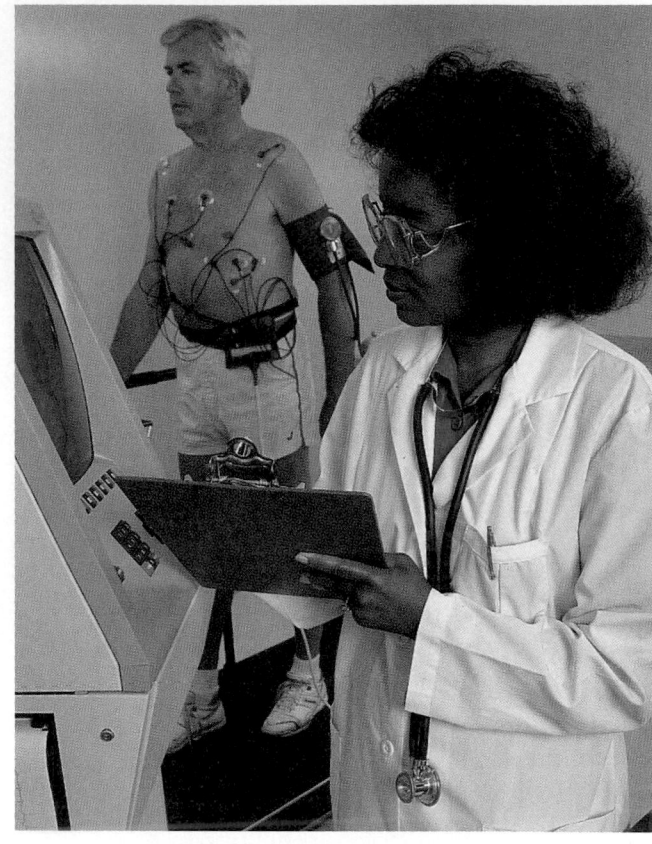

An exercise test—running on a treadmill as an electrocardiograph monitors the flow of the blood to the heart—is recommended for persons who are about to start on an exercise program or who are at risk of heart disease.

Following are some steps that can be taken to maintain cardiovascular health, some of which were already documented in this chapter:

1. If you smoke, stop smoking. If exposed to passive, or second-hand, smoke, eliminate or reduce the amount of exposure.

2. Have regular medical checkups, which include checking your blood pressure and blood cholesterol (see Feature 20.3); also take a treadmill

FEATURE 20.3

WHAT DOES THE BLOOD SAY?

If you have never had a blood chemistry test taken you need one. The first test establishes a baseline for further reference. In having a blood test, be certain that it includes the HDL component, since this factor is not regularly included in routine blood workups. Observe any dietary and exercise guidelines given by your physician as a result of the test, and if there are

no unusual blood lipid levels, such as high cholesterol or triglycerides, or low HDL, a blood analysis every 3–5 years up to age 35 should be adequate. After that, a yearly blood lipid test should be conducted, along with a yearly preventive physical examination.

test (stress electrocardiogram) while heart performance is monitored.

3. Have your cholesterol level tested. If it is high (over 200 mg/dl in the average adult) talk to your physician about changing your diet.

4. Have your HDL levels and the ratio of total cholesterol to HDL cholesterol checked. Your goal is a ratio of four or less (see Chapter 8).

5. Limit your saturated fat intake and replace it with foods that are low in saturated fats; also, use polyunsaturated and monounsaturated fats for cooking (see Chapter 8).

6. Accumulate at least 30 minutes or more of moderate-intensity physical activity over the course of most days of the week.

7. Control diabetes by changing eating habits, controlling weight, exercising regularly, and taking prescribed medication as instructed.

8. Reduce your chronic or excessive stress by practicing stress-management techniques such as

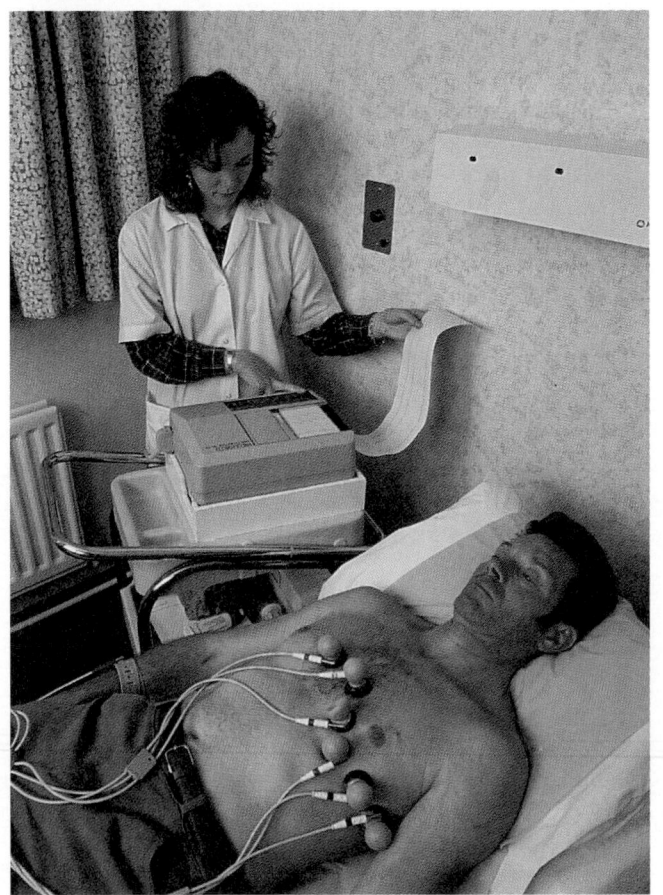

An electrocardiograph (EKG), an instrument used to measure the electrical activity of the heart, is used to aid in the diagnosis of certain heart diseases and abnormalities.

physical exercise, progressive muscle relaxation, and breathing techniques.

9. Control obesity by losing fat if obese and by making permanent dietary changes, by balancing food intake against energy output, and by engaging in a lifelong exercise program.

CHECKPOINT

1. What has been the percentage change in the death rate from coronary heart disease in the United States since 1972?

2. List the steps you can take to maintain cardiovascular health.

SUMMARY

The cardiovascular system, the heart and blood vessels, supplies the body with food and oxygen and helps remove wastes. The heart is a double pump—the right side supplies the lungs, the left the rest of the body. The blood vessels consist of the arteries, which carry blood from the heart, and the veins, which carry blood to it. Between the arteries and veins are the arterioles, venules, and the capillaries where tissue fluids leave the blood. Blood is a mixture of fluid (plasma) and blood cells.

Cardiovascular diseases (CVD) are the number one killer in the United States. They include coronary heart disease (CHD), hypertension, stroke, congenital heart defect, and rheumatic heart disease. The blood vessels of the heart, the coronaries, may become diseased and thickened due to fat deposits, allowing blood clots to form. Such damage can lead to heart attack. Hypertension, or high blood pressure, results from narrowed vessels, and is a major contributor to CHD. Stroke is a cerebrovascular accident, which may occur from a clot or a hemorrhage, and often results in some degree of paralysis. Other CV disorders include arrhythmia (abnormal heartbeat), congestive heart failure (heart weakness), rheumatic heart disease resulting from rheumatic fever, and congenital heart defects.

There are many risk factors that encourage the development of CVD. Factors you can modify include cigarette smoking, hypertension, high cholesterol and saturated fat levels in the blood, diabetes, obesity, chronic or excessive stress, and too little exercise. Factors such as heredity, age, race, and sex are beyond your control.

Heart disease is treatable with surgery and medications. New drugs dissolve clots, reduce cholesterol, and slow the heart rate. Surgical procedures include bypass surgery, angioplasty, laser therapy, and heart transplants.

Exercising regularly, having regular medical checkups, quitting smoking, eating a healthy diet, and reducing chronic or excessive stress are all steps you can take to reduce your risk of heart disease.

REFERENCES

1. Tortora, G., and Grabowski, S. *Principles of Anatomy and Physiology,* 7th ed. New York: Harper-Collins, 1993.
2. American Heart Association. News Release 1992, Greater Los Angeles Affiliate, Inc.
3. American Heart Association. *1993 Heart and Stroke Facts Statistics.* Dallas, TX: American Heart Association, 1993.
4. Ibid.
5. National Center for Health Statistics. "Births, Marriages, Divorces, and Deaths for May 1993." *Monthly Vital Statistics Report* Vol. 42, No. 5 (21 October 1993).
6. Ibid.
7. American Heart Association. *1993 Heart and Stroke Facts Statistics,* op. cit.
8. Tortora, op. cit.
9. American Heart Association. *Heart and Stroke Facts.* Dallas, TX: American Heart Association, 1992.
10. Ibid.
11. American Heart Association. *1993 Heart and Stroke Facts Statistics,* op. cit.
12. Zamala, E. "A Primer on High Blood Pressure." *FDA Consumer* (September 1986), 24–27.
13. National Academy of Sciences. *Diet and Health: Implications for Reducing Chronic Disease Risk.* Washington, DC: National Academy Press, 1989.
14. Wright, H. et. al. "The 1987–88 Nationwide Food Survey: An Update on the Nutrient Intake for Respondents." *Nutrition Today* (May/June 1991) 21–27.
15. Zamala, op. cit.
16. American Heart Association. *Heart and Stroke Facts,* op. cit.
17. Zamala, E. "Stroke: Fighting Back Against America's No. 3 Killer." *FDA Consumer* (July–August 1986), 6–11.
18. Skerrett, P. "The Southeast Leads the Way in Stroke Prevention." *Medical World News* (February 1992), 29.
19. Zamala, *A Primer,* op. cit.
20. American Heart Association. *Heart and Stroke Facts,* op. cit.
21. Ibid.
22. Ibid.
23. Tortora, op. cit.
24. Hoeger, W., and Hoeger, S. *Fitness and Wellness,* 2nd ed. Englewood, CO: Morton, 1993.
25. American Heart Association. *Heart and Stroke Facts,* op. cit.
26. Ibid.
27. Yetiv, J. *Popular Nutritional Practices: A Scientific Appraisal.* Toledo, OH: Popular Medicine Press, 1986.
28. Zamala, op. cit.
29. National Cholesterol Education Program. "Report of the Expert Panel on Detection, Evaluation, and Treatment of High Blood Cholesterol in Adults." *Annals of Internal Medicine* (December 1987).
30. Hoeger, op. cit.
31. Tortora, op. cit.
32. Ibid.
33. Ibid.
34. Barnard, J. "Effects of Life-style Modification on Serum Lipids." *Archives of Internal Medicine* 151 (1991), 1389–1394.
35. American Heart Association. *1993 Heart and Stroke Facts Statistics.* op. cit.
36. Zoler, M. "Low-level Exercise Can Reduce BP." *Medical World News* (October 1991), 9.
37. American College of Sports Medicine. "Summary Statement, Workshop in Physical Activity and Public Health; Sponsored by the U.S. Centers for Communicable Diseases and Prevention and the American College of Sports Mecicine, in cooperation with the President's Council on Physical Fitness and Sports." *Sports Medicine Bulletin* 4 (1993), 7.
38. Tortora, op. cit.
39. American Heart Association. *Heart and Stroke Facts,* op. cit.
40. Murray, R. "Skin Color and Blood Pressure." *JAMA* 5 (1991), 639–640.
41. American Heart Association. *1993 Heart and Stroke Facts Statistics,* op. cit.
42. American Heart Association. *Heart and Stroke Facts,* op. cit.
43. Schnall, P. et al. "The Relationship Between 'Job Strain,' Workplace Diastolic Blood Pressure, and Left Ventricular Mass Index." *JAMA* 14 (1990), 1929–1935.
44. American Heart Association. *Heart and Stroke Facts,* op. cit.
45. "Type A Minus." *Time* (26 May 1986), 60.

46. Higgins, L. 'Hostility Theory Rekindles Debate Over Type A Behavior." *Medical World News* (27 February 1989), 21.

47. American Heart Association. *Heart and Stroke Facts,* op. cit.

48. Ibid.

49. Ibid.

50. Tortora, op. cit.

51. Ibid.

52. American Heart Association. *1993 Heart and Stroke Facts Statistics,* op. cit.

53. Carey, J., and Selberner, J. "Fending Off the Leading Killers." *U.S. News and World Report* (17 August 1987), 56–64.

54. Ibid.

SUGGESTED READINGS

American Heart Association. *The American Heart Association Cookbook,* 5th ed. New York: Random House, 1991.

Consumer's Guide. *Cholesterol: Your Guide to a Healthy Heart.* Lincolnwood, IL: Publications International, 1989.

Cooper, K. *Overcoming Hypertension.* New York: Bantam, 1990.

Goldman, M. *The Handbook of Heart Drugs.* New York: Holt, 1992.

Griffin, G., and Castell, W. *How to Lower Your Cholesterol and Beat the Odds of a Heart Attack.* Tucson, AZ: Fisher, 1989.

Hoffman, G., and Birkner, B. *The Blood Handbook.* Vancouver, BC: Hartley and Marks, 1991.

Kraus, B. *The Dictionary of Sodium, Fats, and Cholesterol,* 2nd ed. New York: Perigee, 1990.

Kwiterovich, P. *The Johns Hopkins Complete Guide for Preventing and Reversing Heart Disease.* New York: Prima, 1993.

Kunz, J., and Finkel, A. (eds.). *The American Medical Association Family Medical Guide.* New York: Random House, 1987.

Legato, M., and Colman, C. *The Female Heart.* New York: Avon, 1991.

McGoon, M. (ed.) *Mayo Clinic Heart Book.* New York: Morrow, 1993.

Mogadam, M. *Choosing for a Healthy Heart.* Yonkers, NY: Consumer Reports Books, 1993.

Moser, M. *Lower Your Blood Pressure and Live Longer.* Toronto: Berkley, 1989.

Moser, M. *Week by Week to a Strong Heart.* Emmaus, PA: Rodale, 1992.

Ornish, D. *Dr. Dean Ornish's Program for Reversing Heart Disease.* New York: Ballantine, 1990.

Pashkow, K., and Libov, C. *The Woman's Heart Book.* New York: Dutton, 1993.

Stark, R., and Winston, M. *The AHA Low-salt Cookbook.* New York: Random, 1990.

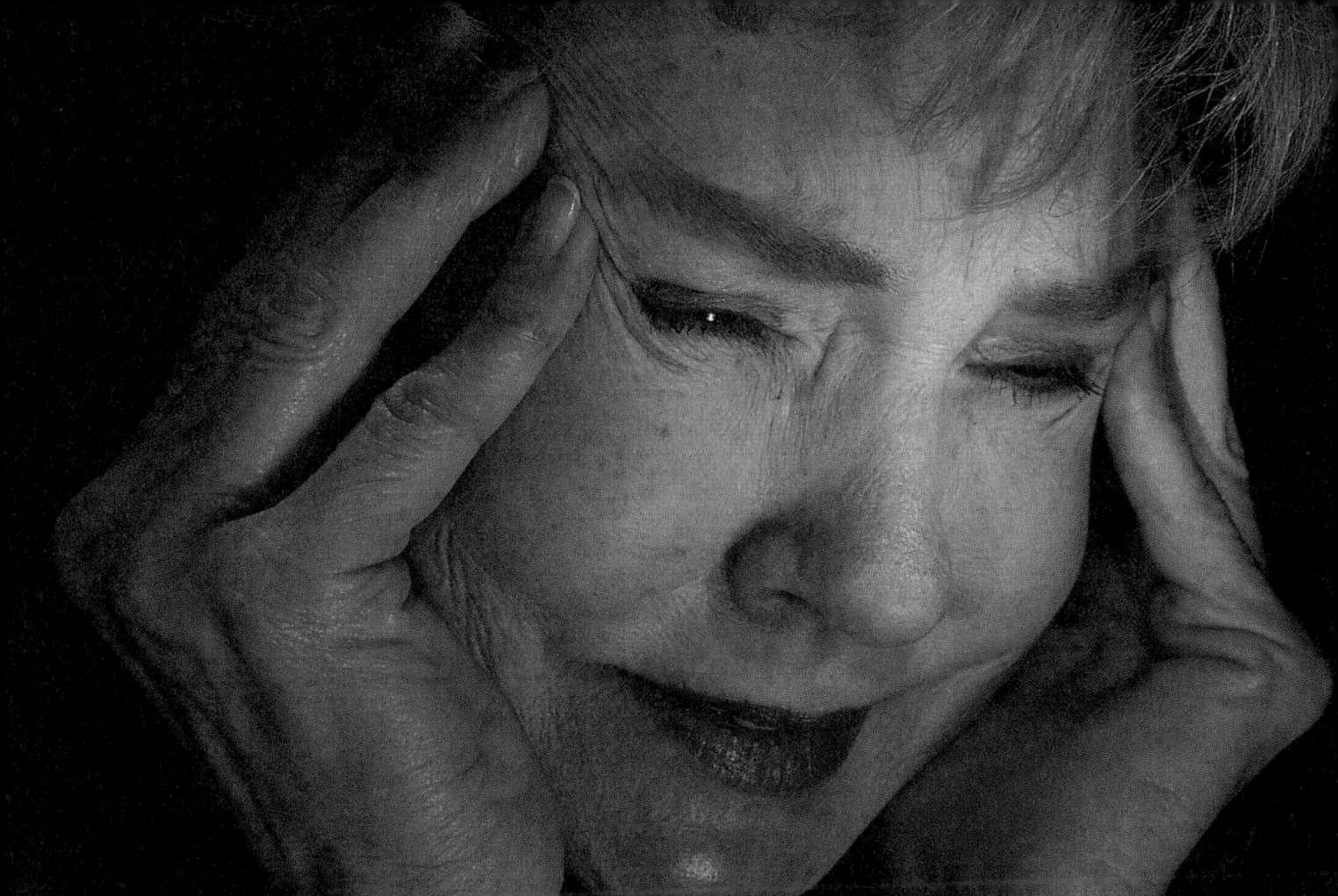

21
CANCER AND OTHER CHRONIC DISORDERS

CHAPTER OBJECTIVES

Upon completing this chapter, you will be able to:

KNOWLEDGE

- Distinguish between malignant tumors and benign tumors.
- Describe the relationship between tobacco smoke and lung cancer, both for smokers and nonsmokers.
- Identify the risk factors for breast cancer.
- Identify the early warning signals of cancer.
- Distinguish between Type I and Type II diabetes.
- Define arthritis; explain who and how many it affects.
- Describe the three most common types of seizure disorders.
- Define the symptoms of Alzheimer's disease and the persons who are most affected by it.
- Identify the number of people in the United States who have lower back problems.

INSIGHT

- Describe the steps you can take to avoid cancer.
- Outline the steps you could take to treat arthritis.
- List steps you can take to maintain kidney health.
- Identify the steps you can take to prevent low back pain.

DECISION MAKING

- Discuss how you intend to reduce your chances and those of older men in your family of developing prostate cancer.
- Decide on the steps you can take to check yourself for possible cancers.
- Identify the ways in which you can reduce your chances of developing diabetes.
- Decide the ways in which you intend to avoid developing chronic obstructive pulmonary disease.
- Explain what you are doing now and what you intend to do to reduce your having low back pain.

Cancer is a disease that strikes people of all races, religions, and social classes. No amount of wealth, dedication to religion, degree of personal goodness, or worth to society can stop cancer from taking its toll. A person's economic position may make a difference in how early this disease is detected and how it is treated; however, as you can see from the following list of well-known and respected people who fell victim to cancer, this is an equal opportunity disease.

- Steve McQueen, actor, died of lung cancer in 1980 at the age of 50.
- Ingrid Bergman, actress, died of breast cancer in 1982 at the age of 67.
- James Baldwin, playwright and poet, died of stomach cancer in 1987 at the age of 63.
- Gilda Radner, actress and comedienne, died of ovarian cancer in 1989 at the age of 43.
- Jill Ireland, actress and writer, died of breast cancer in 1990 at the age of 54.
- Sammy Davis, Jr., actor, died of throat cancer in 1990 at the age of 64.

- *Michael Landon, actor and director, died of pancreatic cancer in 1991 at the age of 54.*
- *Jim Valvano, basketball coach and sports announcer, died of liver cancer in 1993 at the age of 47.*
- *Frank Zappa, singer and songwriter, died of prostate cancer in 1993 at the age of 52.*

There are many others, famous and not so famous, who have survived cancer and are able to live full and enjoyable lives. Ronald Reagan has survived several bouts with cancer, including prostate, skin, and colon cancer. Betty Ford was diagnosed with breast cancer while in the White House. Ann Jillian, a popular actress, was only 40 years old when she was diagnosed with breast cancer. She had a double mastectomy, and was soon back to work. In 1988, she won a Golden Globe award for portraying her own struggle with breast cancer in a made-for-TV movie. Dave Dravecky, a professional baseball player, was diagnosed with a cancerous tumor in his pitching arm. The cancer forced him out of baseball, but it did not force him out of living.

Most of those who survive have the cancer detected early and treated aggressively. The most important step you can take is to make cancer prevention a part of day-to-day behavior. A healthy life-style in combination with recommended regular checkups is the best way to minimize your risk of cancer.

■　　■　　■

This chapter examines cancer and some other important chronic disorders, and completes our four-chapter sequence on diseases. Throughout the chapter, individual responsibility for your health and wellness is emphasized. The impact of all of the conditions discussed in this chapter can be reduced if you assume responsibility for prevention and for recovery, should illness occur.

CANCER

Cancer is second only to cardiovascular disorders as a leading cause of death in the developed countries. Cancer affects people of every age and ethnic group. Cancer is not always random, however. Its incidence often relates to environmental factors determined by occupation, place of residence, diet, and other elements of life-style.

Even though our knowledge of cancer is incomplete, many of today's cancer deaths could be avoided simply by applying existing knowledge of prevention, detection, and early treatment. The best way to reduce the risk of dying of cancer is to maintain a healthy life-style, and obtain prompt medical attention for any cancerlike symptom that may develop.

NATURE OF CANCER

Cancer is a group of more than 100 diseases characterized by uncontrolled growth and spread of abnormal body cells.[1] Cancer cells differ from normal cells in many ways.[2] For example:

- Cancer cells lack the constraints that regulate proliferation (cell division) in normal cells.
- Cancer cells live longer than many types of normal cells.
- Cancer cells are undifferentiated (they lack the specialized structure and ability to perform useful functions that characterize normal cells).
- The metabolic rate of cancer cells is higher than that of normal cells (they are able to compete aggressively with normal cells for the available nutrient supply).

Generally a cancer cell can be distinguished from a normal cell by its appearance. The nucleus of a cancer cell is usually larger than that of a normal cell and differs in the number and appearance of its chromosomes.

Many forms of cancer produce **tumors**, also called **neoplasms**, which are masses of new tissue that grow without serving any useful function. The study of tumors is called **oncology** (*on-kal'ō-jē*). Not all of these tumors are cancerous. Cancerous tumors are referred to as **malignant** (*ma-lig'nant*);

....

cancer a group of diseases characterized by uncontrolled growth and spread of abnormal body cells.

tumor or **neoplasm** a mass of new tissue that grows without serving any useful function.

oncology the branch of medicine dealing with tumors.

malignant cancerous.

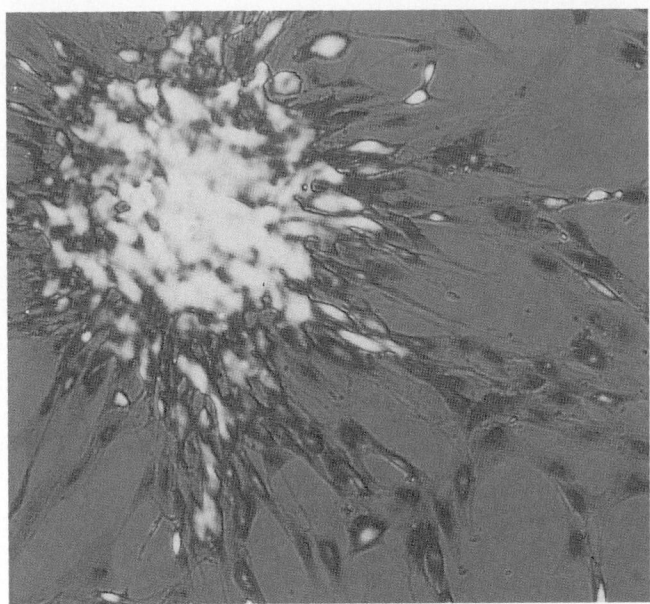 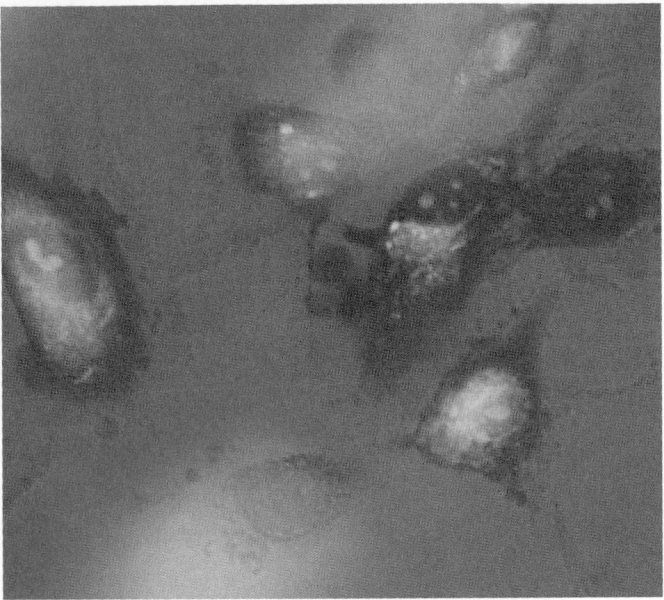

Cancer Cells. A microphotograph of cancer cells (left), compared with normal cells (right). The cancer cells are jumbled masses, with no orderly arrangement of cells; cancer cells are detached; with no cohesiveness to a cellular mass, cells are often carried away.

noncancerous tumors are **benign** (*bē-nīn'*). Benign tumors do not spread to other parts of the body and are seldom a threat to life. The cells of malignant tumors reproduce continuously, quickly, and without control. This excessive proliferation of normal cells is called **hyperplasia** (*hī-per-plā'zē-a*). Other cancers, such as **leukemias,** in which the number of white blood cells increases abnormally, do not produce any tumor mass.

Invasiveness

Cancer is **invasive.** In normal cells, division is slowed or stopped by close contact with surrounding cells. In contrast, cancer cells continue to divide and push into and invade the surrounding normal tissues, much like the roots of a tree push through soil. Healthy tissues become infiltrated with destructive cancerous growth. Early detection and treatment are important in reducing the damage caused by this invasiveness.

benign not cancerous.

leukemia uncontrolled growth of white blood cells.

hyperplasia excessive proliferation of blood cells.

invasive tending to spread into healthy tissue.

Metastasis

Cancerous growths tend to shed living cancer cells. These can be picked up by the blood or lymph vessels (see Figure 21.1) and carried to parts of the body far-removed from the original tumor. Likely secondary tumor sites can be predicted from the direction of the lymph flow from the original site. Wherever these cells happen to lodge, they begin to grow, divide, and invade. This process of spreading disease to a distant part of the body is called **metastasis** (*me-tas'ta-sis*). For example, if a person's cancer originated in his or her lungs, it might *metastasize* (*me-tas'ta-sīz*) to the liver, brain, and other body parts. Cancer experts can usually tell where the cancer originated by the appearance of the cells. Early detection and treatment of cancer reduces the risk of metastasis.

Remission

Remission (*rē-mish'un*) occurs when the symptoms of a disease decrease or disappear. It can be

metastasis the spread of disease from one organ or body part to another.

remission a decrease in or abatement of the symptoms of a disease.

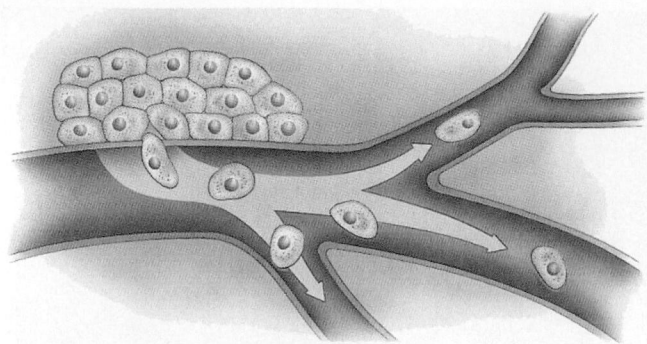

Figure 21.1
Metastasis

The process of metastasis. Cancer cells entering a blood vessel can be carried to remote parts of the body.

temporary or permanent and is common with cancer. Remission can result from one's own body defenses or from treatment. It is not always clear which of these is the case. A patient may be receiving a treatment that is not effective; however, the body's defenses may be working simultaneously to fight the disease. The resulting spontaneous remission may be erroneously attributed to the treatment. This sometimes give credibility to worthless treatments and complicates research on cancer therapy.

How Cancer Kills

Cancer cells do not directly "kill" normal cells, but do so indirectly through their competition for space and vital nutrients. Actively dividing, undifferentiated cancer cells can "crowd out" the normal, differentiated (specialized) cells of the body. Cancer cells aggressively compete for vital nutrients and "starve" the normal cells. As a result, normal tissues, organs, and body systems eventually fail to perform their vital functions. In addition, malignant tumors can also obstruct blood vessels, the digestive tract, urinary tract, or other body structures. Eating and absorption of nutrients may become difficult or impossible, causing wasting of the body. The lungs may fill with tumors, reducing their ability to oxygenate blood. Finally, the body's ability to fight pathogens decreases due to a weakening of the immune system and death results from infection.

Before proceeding further, stop and assess your knowledge of and attitudes toward cancer by completing the assessment, In Your Hands: Assessing Your Cancer-related Attitudes, Knowledge, and Behavior. After completing your reading of the entire section on cancers, you may wish to retake this test and compare the improved results as indication of your improved knowledge of cancers.

CLASSIFICATION AND TYPES OF CANCER

Cancer can affect almost any part of the human body and is classified according to the type of tissue in which it originates. The names of most human cancers are derived from the type of tissue in which they develop. There are several general categories of cancers: carcinomas, sarcomas, leukemias, and lymphomas.

Carcinoma

Carcinoma (*kar-si-nō'ma*) is cancer arising from epithelial, or membranous, tissue. It is estimated that 90 percent of all human cancers are of this type. Most of these cancers begin on surfaces that come into contact with elements from the external environment (skin, linings of airways, and linings of the stomach and intestines). Carcinomas include unpigmented skin cancer, cervical cancer, endometrial cancer, and most lung cancers. Examples include *melanoma* and *adenocarcinoma*.

Sarcoma

A **sarcoma** (*sar-kō'ma*) arises from connective tissues, such as bone and cartilage, or muscle cells. One example is *osteogenic sarcoma*, bone cancer (*osteo* = bone; *genic* = origin).

Leukemia

Leukemias are cancers of blood-forming organs, characterized by the rapid growth and abnormal development of white blood cells, or leukocytes.

....

carcinoma a malignant tumor occurring in epithelial tissue.

sarcoma a malignant tumor occurring in connective tissue.

IN YOUR HANDS

ASSESSING YOUR CANCER-RELATED ATTITUDES, KNOWLEDGE, AND BEHAVIOR

Cancer is the second leading cause of death in the United States, yet many of these deaths are avoidable, either by preventing the cancer in the first place or through prompt detection and treatment of cancer that does develop. Preventing cancer deaths involves healthful attitudes, knowledge, and behavior.

Attitudes and Knowledge	Strongly Agree	Somewhat Agree	Strongly disagree
1. Cancer is a matter of luck; either I'm going to get it or I'm not.	0	2	4
2. If I do get cancer, I'm going to die from it.	0	2	4
3. I believe that I can reduce my chances of getting cancer.	4	2	0
4. Most cancers can be cured if treated early enough.	4	2	0
5. List as many warning signals of cancer as you know.	_____ (write 0–7)		

Behaviors	Almost Always	Sometimes	Almost Never
6. I avoid using tobacco in any form.	4	1	0
7. I avoid unnecessary exposure to x-rays.	4	2	0
8. I choose my foods carefully to minimize exposure to possible cancer-causing chemicals *and* to obtain plenty of vitamins.	4	2	0
9. I follow an effective stress-management program.	4	2	0
10. I discourage other people from smoking in my presence.	4	2	0
11. I avoid overexposing my skin to the sun; I use high-SPF sunscreens during exposure.	4	2	0
12a. *Females only:* I examine my breasts for signs of cancer every month *and* I get annual Pap smears.	4	2	0
12b. *Males only:* I perform testicular self-examination every month.	4	2	0

Total points: _____

INTERPRETATION:

45–51 points: Your knowledge, attitudes, and behavior are highly favorable toward cancer control. You appear to be taking most of the known precautions.

35–44 points: You are taking some unnecessary risks with cancer. A more cautious attitude about cancer might be helpful.

34 points or less: You are definitely placing yourself at risk of cancer through your attitudes and/or behavior.

Lymphoma

A **lymphoma** is a malignant disease of lymphatic tissue, such as lymph nodes. *Hodgkin's disease* is a lymphoma.

....

lymphoma a malignant tumor occurring in the lymphatic system.

INCIDENCE OF CANCERS

Since there is no national office that records every new case of cancer, there is no way to know exactly how many new cases occur each year. All incidence figures in this chapter are estimates by the American Cancer Society of cases in the United States.[3] These statistics are based on extrapolations of data from reliable data bases, such as the U.S. Centers for Disease Control.

FEATURE 21.1

CANCER SURVIVAL

Being diagnosed as having cancer is not a death sentence. Today's treatment methods have increased the five-year survival rate (which in most cases represents a "cure"). In 1900, the long-term hope of survival from cancer was virtually nil. In the 1930s, the five-year survival rate (or survival of five years after treatment) was less than 20 percent. By the 1940s the five-year survival rate was 1 in 4, and by the 1960s it had climbed to 1 in 3. Today, about 4 out of 10 patients will be alive five years after diagnosis. This rise in five-year survival represents more than 80,000 persons saved from death by cancer each year. This "observed" survival rate, when adjusted for normal life expectancy factors (such as dying of heart disease, accidents, and disease common in old age), becomes a "relative" survival rate of 52 percent for all cancers. This relative survival rate is often used to measure progress in early detection and treatment.

Cancers of the breast, tongue, mouth, colon, rectum, cervix, prostate, testis, and skin can be detected, by regular screening and self-examination, at an early stage when treatment is more likely to be successful. Of these cancers, about two-thirds of all patients now survive for five years, although about 90 percent would survive with early detection. This comes to about 100,000 more potential survivals if these cancers are detected early and treated promptly.

Of the approximately 526,000 annual cancer deaths, about 100,000 could be prevented by earlier diagnosis and prompt treatment. This means that anyone who assumes responsibility for his or her health, heeds the warning signs of cancer, and seeks prompt medical attention stands an excellent chance of a cure. Some survival rates for specific cancers can be found in Table 21.2.

Source: Cancer Facts and Figures, 1993. New York: American Cancer Society.

About 1.17 million people are diagnosed each year as having cancer of some form other than nonmelanoma skin cancer or cervical carcinoma **in situ** (*in-sī'tū*), a tiny spot of localized cancer that has not begun to spread. These two cancers are excluded because they are common and easily cured with prompt treatment. Incidence figures and other information for specific cancers are presented in Table 21.1.

Each year, about 526,000 people die from cancer. Yet, equally as or more important is the hope of long-term survival for cancer patients (see Feature 21.1).

CAUSES OF CANCER

A number of factors are involved in the onset of cancer. For any specific case of cancer, it is likely that more than one of these factors will be involved.

Environment Factors

Chemicals or other environmental agents producing cancer are called **carcinogens** (*car-sin'ō-jens;* cancer-causing *agents*), and can be found in the substances in the air we breathe, the water we drink, and the food we eat. The World Health Organization (WHO) estimates that 60–90 percent of all human cancers are associated with carcinogens. Avoiding environmental carcinogens and adopting a cancer-prevention life-style can help reduce your chances of getting cancer. Environmental agents include chemicals, radiation, and viruses.

Chemicals Many drugs, pesticides, and other environmental chemicals have been identified as carcinogens. Table 21.3 (p. 660) is a partial listing of chemical carcinogens. Chemical carcinogens, researchers believe, cause cancer by activating **oncogenes** (*ong'kō-jēnz*), genes that have the ability to transform a normal cell into a cancerous one.

Cigarette smoke is a leading source of chemical carcinogens for both smokers and the nonsmokers who are exposed to it. The transformation of normal cells to cancerous cells by the chemicals in tobacco smoke is well known. The blood receives the carcinogens from smoke via the lungs and carries them throughout the body, where they contribute to cancers of the lungs, mouth cavity, larynx, esophagus, stomach, pancreas, breast, kidney,

in situ in position, localized.

carcinogens cancer-causing agents.

oncogene a gene that has the ability to transform a normal cell into a cancerous one.

Table 21.1
Information on Some Major Cancers

Site	Number of New Cases Per Year		Number of deaths per Year		Warning Signals
	Male	Female	Male	Female	
Lung	100,000	70,000	93,000	56,000	Persistent cough
Breast (invasive)	1,000	182,000	300	46,000	Lump or thickening in breast
Colon and rectum	77,000	75,000	28,800	28,200	Change in bowel habits; bleeding from the rectum; blood in the stool
Prostate	165,000		35,000		Difficulty in urinating
Cervix (invasive)		13,500		4,400	Unusual vaginal bleeding or discharge
Endometrium and body of uterus		31,000		5,700	Unusual vaginal bleeding or discharge
Pancreas	13,500	14,200	12,000	13,000	Nausea, "fullness," abdominal discomfort
Lymphomas	28,500	22,400	11,500	10,500	Painless enlargement of lymph nodes; pain in abdomen and back; persistent sore; throat, trouble swallowing
Ovary		22,000		13,300	Abdominal pain
Stomach	14,800	9,200	8,200	5,400	Chronic indigestion; aversion to rich food; decreasing appetite, tarry stool
Leukemia	16,700	12,600	10,100	8,500	Weakness; weight loss; fatigue; bleeding from mucous membranes; enlarged liver or spleen
Bladder and Kidney	55,800	23,700	20,800	13,000	Blood in urine; frequent, painful urination
Mouth and throat	20,300	9,500	4,975	2,725	Sore that does not heal; difficulty in swallowing; hoarseness
Skin (melanoma only)	17,000	15,000	4,200	2,600	Sore that does not heal; change in wart or mole

Site	Safeguards	Additional Information
Lung	Do not smoke	Leading cause of cancer deaths in both sexes
Breast (invasive)	Periodic checkup; monthly self-examination	Develops most frequently in females who have not breastfed infants; does occur in males
Colon and rectum	Periodic proctoscopy and tests for blood in feces	Highly curable with early detection
Prostate	Periodic checkup by physician	Usually develops in males past age 60
Cervix (invasive)	Periodic pelvic exam and Pap smear; avoid casual sexual contacts; use condoms	Cervical cancer linked to sexually transmitted papilloma viruses; Pap smears save thousands of lives annually
Endometrium and body of uterus	Periodic pelvic exam	
Pancreas	Periodic checkup by physician	High fatality rate
Lymphomas	Avoid exposure to radiation and carcinogenic chemicals	Affected people often lead normal lives; these cancers are found throughout the body in the lymphatic system
Ovary	Period checkup	Tumor may become quite large before producing pain
Stomach	Bring chronic indigestion to attention of a physician	Often mistaken for a stomach ulcer
Leukemia		Some forms are being very successfully treated with drugs
Bladder and Kidney	Do not use tobacco; report bloody urine to physician	Most cases occur in tobacco users
Mouth and throat	Do not use tobacco	Often detected in dental examinations
Skin (melanoma only)	Periodic checkup; avoid overexposure to sun or tanning machines; use high-SPF sunscreen	Skin cancer is increasing; over 550,000 nonmelanoma skin cancer cases each year

Source: Cancer Facts and Figures, 1993. *New York: American Cancer Society, 1993.*

Table 21.2
Cancer Survival Rates

| | Percent Surviving Five Years | | | |
| | White Americans | | African Americans | |
Cancer	1960	1988	1960	1988
All Sites	39	54	27	38
Mouth and pharynx	45	54	—	32
Stomach	11	16	8	17
Colon	43	59	34	48
Larynx	53	67	—	53
Lung	8	13	5	11
Liver	2	6	—	5
Melanoma of skin	60	83	—	68
Breast (females)	63	79	46	62
Cervix of uterus (invasive)	58	68	47	55
Body of uterus	73	84	31	54
Ovary	32	39	32	37
Testis	63	93	—	84
Prostate	50	78	35	63
Thyroid	83	94	—	93
Hodgkin's disease	40	78	—	74
Leukemia	14	38	—	29

Source: Cancer Facts and Figures, 1993. New York: American Cancer Society, 1993.

Table 21.3
Some Cancer-Causing Chemicals (Carcinogens)

These chemicals (and many others) may cause cancer when absorbed through the skin, ingested with food, or inhaled:

Aflatoxin (in moldy peanuts)

Arsenic (in old house paints and old wallpaper)

Asbestos (in building materials and some auto brake linings)

Benzene

Benzidine (in some dyes)

Benzopyrene (produced in charcoal broiling of meats)

Cadmium (in some paints)

Carbon tetrachloride (solvent and in some old fire extinguishers)

Chlorinated hydrocarbons (some insecticides, polluted water)

Chromium (in paints, dyes, and auto trim)

Cigarette smoke (carries many different carcinogens)

Coal tar

Coke oven (where coal is converted to coke) fumes

Creosote (in paints, fabrics, and building materials)

Dioxin (contaminant in herbicides)

Ethylene dibromide (fumigant)

Food colorings (red dyes No. 2, 3, and 4)

Lead (in paints)

Marijuana smoke (all smoke contains carcinogens)

Nickel

Nitrosamines

Pesticides (chlordane, dieldrin, lindane, parathion, etc.)

Petroleum products

Saccharin (low level of risk)

Sodium nitrite (meat preservative that produces nitrosamines)

Soot

Tars

Vinyl chloride

bladder, and cervix. Use of smokeless tobacco is also associated with increased risk of many of these cancers, especially cancer of the cheek and gums. There has been an increase in the use of all forms of smokeless tobacco (snuff, plug, and leaf), especially snuff. When smokeless tobacco is placed between the cheek and gum, both nicotine and carcinogens are readily absorbed by the membranes of the mouth. Because of this direct contact, the use of snuff is associated with a greatly increased risk of oral cancer. Thirty percent of all cancer deaths overall are directly related to the use of tobacco in any form.

Radiation Radiation is a powerful carcinogen. Many cancer experts believe that, as with viruses and chemicals, radiation produces cancer by activating oncogenes.

Radiation exposure at any level causes genetic changes in cells. There is no safe radiation dose. While natural background radiation, such as radon and cosmic rays, has always been present, some people also receive large doses of radiation from artificial sources, including x-rays and industrial and medical uses of radioisotopes. The benefits obtained from x-rays usually outweigh the risks; however, any unnecessary use of x-rays should be avoided.

Ultraviolet (UV) radiation, sometimes called "black light," is the element in the sun's rays that tans—or burns—skin. It also prematurely ages the skin and causes skin cancer. Ultraviolet exposure that results in sunburn is believed to carry an especially high risk of cancer. People who tan easily

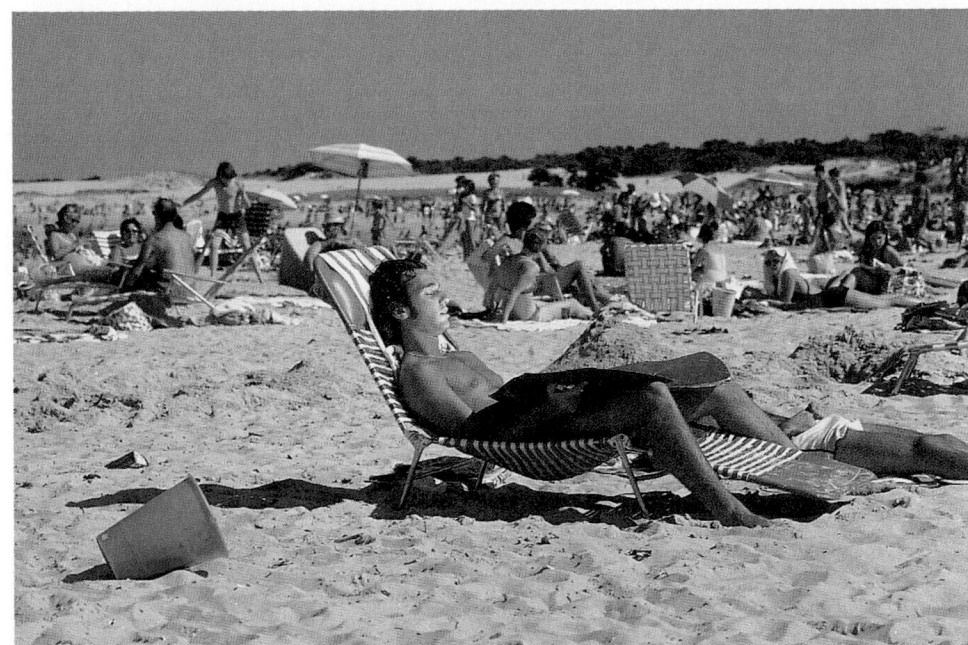

Tan with care! In addition to causing painful sunburns, the sun's ultraviolet rays cause premature aging of skin and skin cancer.

and burn rarely are less likely to develop skin cancer than are people who tan with difficulty and burn easily.

Tanning-machine manufacturers like to make a distinction between the safety of the "UV-A" wavelengths produced by their machines and the "UV-B" that is more abundant in sunlight. The longer-wavelength UV-A rays penetrate the skin more deeply and cause slower tanning or burning, but, because of this deeper penetration, also carry greater risk of suppressing the immune system, damaging the eyes, prematurely aging the skin, and causing skin cancer. According to medical authorities, UV-A is just as harmful as UV-B wavelengths.[4] The Food and Drug Administration (FDA) and most skin experts caution against excessive exposure to any form of UV radiation.

Viruses   Viruses are tiny units of nucleic acids, either DNA or RNA, that can infect cells and convert them into virus-producers. Years ago, experiments proved that many cancers in animals are caused by communicable viruses. Similar experiments in humans would, of course, be illegal and unethical. In recent years, however, a number of viruses have been isolated from human cancers. When these viruses are transferred to laboratory cultures of human body cells, the human cells become cancerous. This is very strong evidence that at least some human cancers are caused by viruses. Some examples of human cancers and the viruses associated with them are indicated in Table 21.4.

Heredity

Though few forms of cancer are directly linked to heredity, it does play a definite, though little understood, role. One of the most intensely studied aspects of cancer in recent years has been the role of oncogenes, which are cancer-causing genes. Found in tumor cells, these genes have the ability to transform a normal cell into a cancerous cell when activated inappropriately. Oncogenes develop from normal genes controlling growth and development.

Table 21.4
Viruses Causing Human Cancers

Viruses	Type of Cancer
Human immunodeficiency virus (HIV-1)	Kaposi's sarcoma (a cancer of the inner lining of some blood vessels; often seen in those who have AIDS)
Human T-cell leukemia-lymphoma (HTLV-1; HTLV-2)	Leukemias (cancers of blood-forming tissues); lymphoma (cancer of lymphoid tissue)
Epstein-Barr Virus (EBV)	Burkitt's lymphoma (cancer of white blood cells); Hodgkin's disease (lymphatic system cancer)
Papilloma virus	Some strains are associated with cancer of the cervix, vagina, penis, and colon

As these genes undergo some type of change, the growth pattern of the cell containing them becomes abnormal, making them reproduce new cells in excessive amounts or at the wrong time.

Over 40 different oncogenes have been identified, but how these genes cause cancer is still uncertain.[5] It is clear that the presence of a particular form of cancer, such as breast cancer, in a family is associated with an increased risk of that form of cancer for other family members. Methods are being developed to screen family members for oncogenes. Until such tests become available, if a certain form of cancer is present in your family, it is wise to take any special precautions and be checked for signs on a regular basis.

Immune Deficiency

Cancer researchers believe that cancer cells arise in all of us from time to time. Usually the body's immune system recognizes these cells as abnormal and destroys them. Thus, a tumor can begin to form only when the immune system is weak. Once a rapidly growing malignancy develops, it may be beyond the ability of even a healthy immune system to destroy it.

Several forms of evidence support this view of cancer as an immune deficiency disorder. The incidence of certain kinds of cancer sharply increases in people whose immunity has been intentionally suppressed. This is often done to prevent the rejection of transplanted organs or tissue. People with AIDS have a very high incidence of an otherwise rare cancer—Kaposi's sarcoma—apparently because their immune systems are no longer able to destroy cancer cells.

Anything you do to help maintain a strong immune system contributes to cancer prevention. Since stress can impair immunity, stress management is an important prevention measure. Avoiding exposure to immunity-suppressing agents, such as radiation and certain drugs, including steroid hormones, is another. The relationship of diet to cancer will be explored later in this chapter.

LUNG CANCER

Lung cancer, or **bronchial carcinoma,** is the leading cause of cancer deaths in both sexes. Human

....

bronchial carcinoma lung cancer.

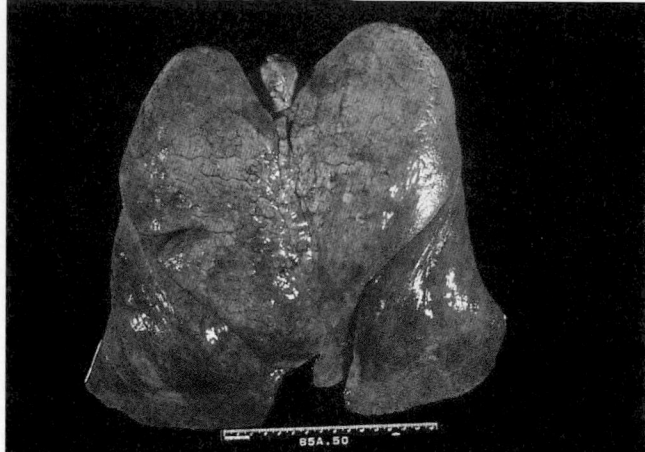

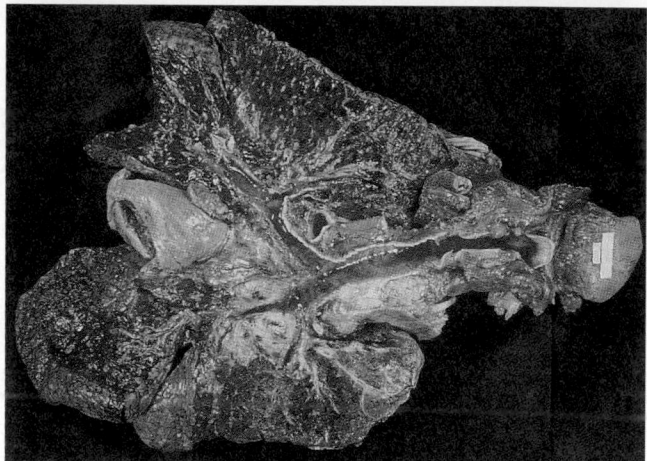

Cancer and Emphysema. (top) Normal lung; (bottom) Cancerous and emphysematous lung. Normal cells disappear as they are replaced by cancer cells. As this happens, the malignant growth spreads throughout the lung, eventually blocking the bronchial tubes.

Source: Tortora, G. & Grabowski, S. Principles of Anatomy & Physiology, 7th ed., Harper-Collins, New York, 1993, p. 758.

life is totally dependent upon the ability of the lungs to oxygenate the blood. In lung cancer, the lungs fill with tumorous growths, and oxygenation of the blood is progressively reduced. Unless lung cancer is treated very early, death, after a long, painful illness, is almost always the end result. Lung cancer has one of the lowest survival rates of the major cancers. Only about 13 percent of those people diagnosed as having lung cancer survive for five years or more after diagnosis. Only 16 percent of all lung cancers are discovered while the cancer is localized and most treatable.[6]

The average person inhales and exhales over 12,000 liters (over 13,000 quarts) of air every day. If this air contains any cancer-causing substance, some of that substance will remain in the lungs and possibly trigger the development of cancer in one or more of the lung cells. If even one cell becomes cancerous and is not quickly destroyed by the immune system, cancer will begin to spread throughout the lungs.

One of the richest known sources of cancer-causing substances is tobacco smoke. Inhaled smoke and pollutants cause damage to the cells in the tissues lining the bronchial tubes within the lungs. Cells enlarge, give off excessive mucus, undergo rapid cell division, and eventually become cancerous. The American Cancer Society estimates that 87 percent of lung cancer cases are due to smoking.[7] Many studies have shown that the risk of developing lung cancer increases with the number of cigarettes smoked (both the number per day and the number over a period of years). In smokers who stop smoking before the cancerous tissue has started forming, the damaged bronchial lining tissues often return to normal.

People who do not smoke, but are exposed to tobacco smoke, are also exposed to increased risk. Known as *environmental tobacco smoke (ETS)*, such second-hand, or "passive," smoke is a known carcinogen and contains a higher concentration of the toxic carcinogenic substances than found in mainstream smoke. In addition to carrying cancers, such smoke impairs blood circulation; increases the severity and frequency of pneumonia, bronchitis, and asthma in children; worsens asthmatic conditions in general; and creates significant health hazards for unborn and young children.[8]

Air pollution also plays a role in lung cancer. The cancer-causing effect of asbestos particles in the air has been well publicized. Even here, tobacco smoke plays a role. Among asbestos workers, the risk of lung cancer is 60 times greater for smokers than for nonsmokers.[9]

Radon, a radioactive gas released from disintegrating uranium and other radioactive materials, is a suspected cause of lung cancer in some non-smokers (smoking raises the risk of radon-related cancer to a level 15 times higher than that for non-smokers).[10] The soil in many parts of the nation emits radon. As homes and workplaces have been made increasingly airtight in order to save heating and cooling energy, radon levels have sometimes risen to hazardous levels. Refer to Table 24.3 (p. 770) for more on this problem.

Depending on the type and stage of lung cancer, the therapy options include surgery, radiation therapy, and chemotherapy. If the cancer is localized, surgery is the preferred treatment. Yet by the time lung cancer is discovered, it has usually metastasized, or spread, mandating radiation therapy, and/or chemotherapy, as well as surgical removal of part or all of the lung. Once the cancer has spread, none of these therapies may be effective.

Even though some exposure to airborne carcinogens is unavoidable for most of us, each of us does have control over the single most important cause of cancer. By not using tobacco in any form, we can reduce our risk of all cancers collectively by about 30 percent and of lung cancer by about 87 percent.

BREAST CANCER

There are 2.8 million victims of breast cancer in the United States, and 46,000 women die from it every year.[11] Breast cancer has become the leading cause of death for women between the ages of 32 and 52 and is second only to lung cancer among cancers causing deaths of women.[12] The incidence rate that had been increasing gradually for many years has leveled off since 1987.[13]

The risk of getting breast cancer is related largely to age. The average risk of developing breast cancer, for the woman who lives to age 95, in other words over a woman's entire lifetime, is 1 in 8. Yet, the younger the woman, the lower the likelihood of developing breast cancer (see Table 21.5). There are, however, some ethnic differences in risk. African American woman run a higher risk of developing breast cancer until age 40, after which the risk, relative to white women, begins to drop.[14] Other risks factors include the following[15]:

- Previous cancer in one breast
- Having a mother, grandmother, or sister who has had breast cancer
- Exposure to ionizing radiation (such as x-rays)
- Early age at menarche (first menstrual period)
- Late age at menopause
- Excessive fat and alcohol intake
- Obesity
- Cigarette smoking

Of the risk factors for breast cancer you can control, cutting down on the fat in your diet is the single most important step. Diets high in fat appear to relate to a high incidence of breast cancer. The

Table 21.5
Odds of Developing Breast Cancer

Age:	Odds:
25	1 in 19,608
30	2,525
35	622
40	217
45	93
50	50
55	33
60	24
65	17
70	14
75	11
80	10
85	9
95 or older	8

Source: Lifetime Probability of Breast Cancer in American Women, *National Cancer Institute: Bethesda, MD, 1993.*

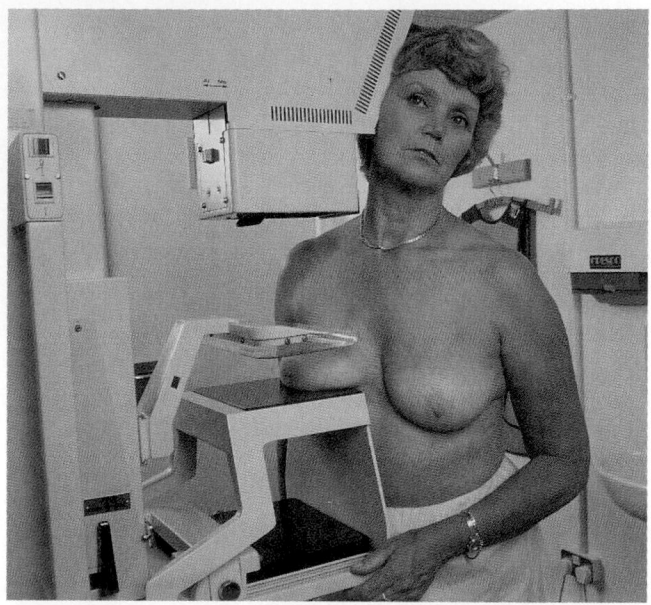

Mammography can detect breast cancers in their earliest and most curable stages, long before a woman or her physician can feel a lump or other change in the breast. The risk from the low dose of x-ray is about the same as being in a fatal car accident while driving fifteen miles in a car.

National Cancer Institute, the National Academy of Sciences, and the American Cancer Society have all issued guidelines regarding high-fat diets and cancer. The breast is also vulnerable to x-rays at younger ages. If possible, avoid unnecessary x-rays, especially during puberty and pregnancy.[16] Although there is some disagreement, most studies show that women who take the birth control pill are not as likely to develop cancer as are women who do not take it. At the same time, such information should not become a deciding factor for going on the pill, as there are other effects of pill use (see Chapter 6).[17]

Most deaths from breast cancer are unnecessary. Breast cancer can be survived if it is detected early through monthly breast self-examination and periodic breast x-ray, or **mammogram** (*mam'ō-gram*). Self-examination, as described in Feature 21.2, should be performed every menstrual cycle or month, beginning no later than age 20 and continuing for life. This should be augmented by a physician's examination every three years from age 20 through age 40, and then every year after that. The American Cancer Society recommends that a mammogram should be performed every one to two years between ages 40 and 49 and every year

thereafter. One "baseline" mammogram is recommended between the ages of 35 and 39 which can serve as a basis for comparison for later mammograms.[18] The National Cancer Institute recommends routine mammography screening be started for all women age 50 and older, and only for those women ages 40–49 who have a family history of breast cancer or who are otherwise at high risk for breast cancer.[19]

Once a breast lump is detected, mammography can identify any other possible lesions too small to be felt. Mammograms only indicate *possible* cancerous areas, and may incorrectly identify the presence (false positives) or absence (false negatives) of cancer. Sometimes *ultrasound* is used to determine whether a lump is benign, a fluid-filled cyst, or a solid (and possibly malignant) tumor. Most breast lumps are *not* malignant, but a subjective diagnosis of lumps must be made by a physician. Cancers are usually more irregular, harder, and less freely moving than benign growths. For a definitive diagnosis of all suspicious lumps, a **biopsy** (*bī'op-sē*), or microscopic examination of tissue, should

mammogram x-ray of the breast.

biopsy removal of a small piece of living tissue for microscopic examination.

FEATURE 21.2

BREAST SELF-EXAMINATION

Breast cancer, *if it is detected and treated early,* can be cured. Most breast cancers are detected by the woman herself, rather than by her physician. With regular breast self-examinations, a woman is very likely to detect any cancer that may develop while it is still in an early stage.

What do you look for in breast self-examination? It's very simple: *look for something that was not there before.* It might be a lump, thickening of skin or deeper tissue, dimpling, or a discharge.

BREAST FAMILIARIZATION

All women have minor lumps or irregularities in their breasts. How do you know that something was not there before? Become very familiar with your breasts through a series of 30–40 complete self-examinations, one each day, before beginning monthly self-examination.

WHEN TO EXAMINE BREASTS

If you haven't already started, start now. The best time is about a week after each menstrual period ends, since lumps are easiest to detect at this time. Those women whose periods are irregular or who have already been through menopause should perform a self-examination once each calendar month.

THE PROCEDURE

Examine your breasts in three stages:

1. Start the examination in the shower or bath, with plenty of soap on your hands and breasts. (Hands slide easi-ly over soapy skin.) Lift your left arm over your head and use your right hand to examine the left breast. Keep your fingers flat and move them over every part of each breast (illustration a). Switch arms and examine the right breast. Check for any *new* lump or thickening.

2. Standing before a mirror, visually inspect your breasts for any changes in shape, swelling, dimpling of the skin, or changes in the nipple. First check with your arms at your sides, then check with your arms high over your head (illustration b).

3. Lie down with a pillow under your right shoulder and your right hand behind your head. With your left hand, starting at the top of your right breast, press fingers gently in small circular motions around the breast. When you get back around to the top, move your fingers in about an inch and make another circle. Keep making circles until you reach the nipple (illustrations c and d). Then squeeze each nipple gently, checking for a discharge (illustration e). Repeat this for your left breast, moving the pillow to your left shoulder and raising your left hand behind your head.

Any discharge from the nipple or any new lump or thickening or other irregularity should be reported to your physician immediately. Most lumps will be benign; should a lump be cancerous, early detection will often mean less extensive forms of surgery and can save your life.

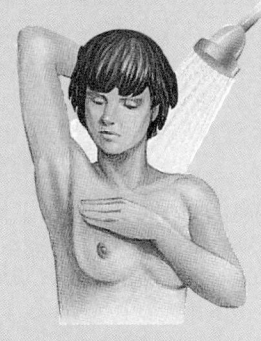

(a)

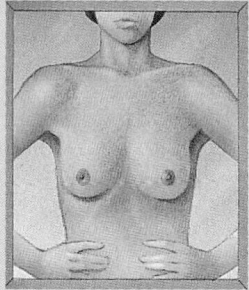
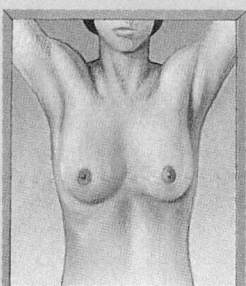

(b)

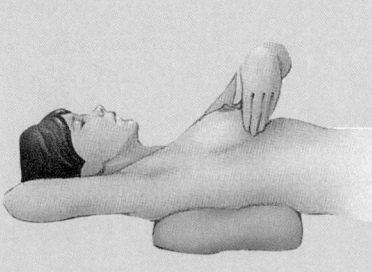

(c)

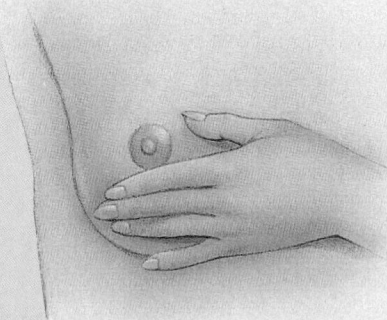

(d)

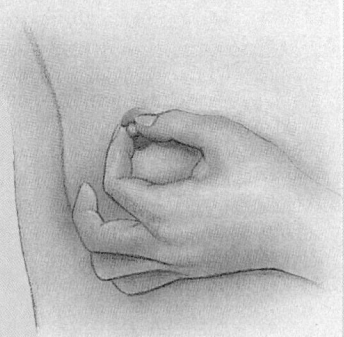

(e)

be done even though the findings from the mammography may be described as normal.

Breast cancer treatment is one of the most controversial areas in medicine. Debate centers on how much surgery is necessary, and on the kinds of nonsurgical therapies that are necessary. Surgical treatment is the usual treatment if the cancer is small and localized. The question is how much of the breast to remove. In **lumpectomy** only the lump and nearby tissue is removed. **Mastectomy,** or removal of the breast itself, may be partial or total. A total mastectomy may be removal of the breast only (*simple mastectomy*), or additional removal of chest muscles and lymph nodes (*radical mastectomy*).

Most women receive a combination of surgical and nonsurgical therapies to treat the breast cancer, which may involve hormone therapy, chemotherapy, and radiation therapy. Since most invasive malignancies such as breast cancer can be associated with the spread of the cancer to other parts of the body, therapy to eliminate any distant cancer sites is appropriate. Chemotherapy can reduce mortality from breast cancer by 25 percent.[20] Most often, radiation therapy is used along with lumpectomy or mastectomy.

The key in breast cancer diagnosis is *early*. According to National Cancer Institute data, the five-year survival rate (generally considered equal to a total cure) of breast cancers detected by mammograms before they have spread beyond an individual milk duct or gland, is 92 percent. For tumors that have spread slightly, but are under two centimeters (about four-fifths of an inch) in diameter, the survival rate is as much as 71 percent. But when diagnosis is delayed until cancer has metastasized to other parts of the body, the survival rate drops to 14 percent. Further, breast cancers detected early generally require less-extensive surgery than those that have been allowed to spread.

Given the associations of breasts to body image and feelings of femininity and sexual adequacy, mastectomy carries powerful emotional implications. When mastectomy is necessary, breast reconstruction by a skilled plastic surgeon can be a boon to the emotional healing process. In some cases, reconstruction can be started at the same time as the mastectomy. Surgical reconstruction involves using either an artificial implant or moving fat and skin tissue from the woman's back, abdomen, or buttocks.[21]

Whether breast cancer is treated by mastectomy or lumpectomy, another emotional concern characteristic of most forms of cancer is the ongoing fear of a recurrence. In most communities, support groups are available for people who have had breast or other forms of cancer. A local office of the American Cancer Society, regional office of the National Cancer Institute, your local hospital, or YWCA can often provide information on such support groups.

Men are not immune to breast cancer. Though the incidence in males is much lower than in females, a man should bring any sign of possible breast cancer to the attention of his physician.

SKIN CANCER

Excessive exposure to the sun can result in skin cancer. Everyone, regardless of the darkness of skin pigmentation or coloration, can be affected if the exposure is sufficiently prolonged and intense. Of all forms of skin cancer, the fastest-growing form and by far the most fatal is **melanoma,** a form of skin cancer in which there is a darkening of the skin. Over three-quarters of all skin cancer deaths (6800 out of 9100) each year are from melanoma.[22]

There is a simple ABCD rule to help identify a possible melanoma (see Figure 21.2). **A** is for asymmetry—melanoma looks like a mole in which one half does not match the other. **B** is for border irregularity—the edges are ragged, notched, or blurred. **C** is for color—the growth is darkly, but irregularly pigmented. **D** is for diameter—any growth that is more than 6 mm (about ¼ inch) in diameter or is increasing in diameter. A skin spot with any of these features should be examined by a physician. Adults should practice skin self-examination once a month, and any suspicious spots should be brought to the attention of a physician.

....

lumpectomy removing only a tumor and nearby tissue.

mastectomy removal of a breast.

....

melanoma a form of skin cancer in which there is a darkening of the skin.

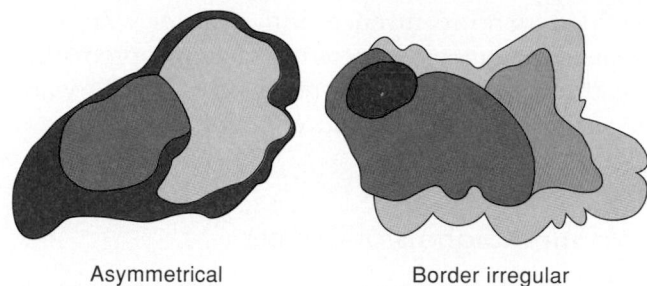

Asymmetrical   Border irregular

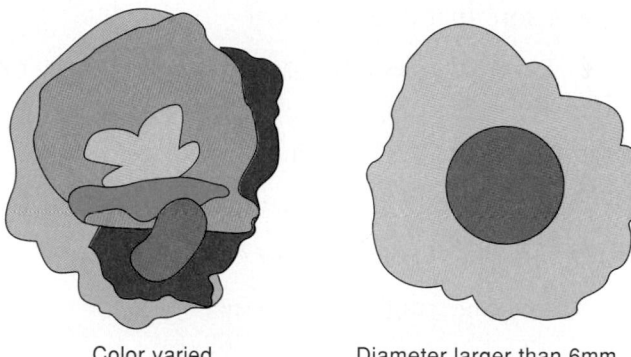

Color varied   Diameter larger than 6mm

Figure 21.2
Skin Cancer Danger Signs

The American Academy of Dermatology advises: Know your spots and do a spot check. Also, have your skin checked by a physician for any changes once a year. If you notice one of the following changes in your skin, see your family physician or dermatologist immediately.

- **Melanoma** *Remember your ABCDs. A. Symmetry: One-half of a mole or lesion doesn't look like the other half. B. Border. A mole has an irregular, scalloped, or not clearly defined border. C. Color: The color varies or is not uniform from one area of a mole or lesion to another, whether the color is tan, brown, black, white, red, or blue. D. Diameter: The lesion is larger than 6 millimeters or larger than a pencil eraser.*

- **Basal-cell or squamous-cell carcinoma:** *any lesion that is new, that starts growing, that starts changing, that bleeds, that is scabby, or that doesn't heal.*

- **Actinic ketatosis:** *a precancerous skin lesion that is dry, scaly, reddish, and slightly raised.*

Source: Greeley, A. "Skin Cancer Danger Signs." FDA Consumer, May 1991, pp. 20–21.

Most cases of malignant melanoma stem from excessive sun exposure. Malignant melanoma can be prevented by using a sunscreen with a sun protection factor of 15 during sun exposure, wearing protective clothing, and avoiding the midday sun, when ultraviolet rays are strongest. Some research has shown that severe sunburn in childhood carries with it an excessive risk of melanoma in adult life, so children, in particular, should be protected.

PROSTATE CANCER

In men, prostate cancer is the second most common cancer and the second leading cause of death from cancer. Both benign and malignant growths in the prostate are common in older men. An enlarged prostate, two to four times the normal size, occurs in about half of all males over age 60. Because the prostate surrounds the urethra, both types of growths put pressure on it, making urination painful and difficult. Even if the tumor is benign, treatment and/or surgery may be required to alleviate difficulty in eliminating urine.

Prostate cancer may be detected by a combination of tests. Digital rectal examination, performed by a physician inserting a gloved finger into the rectum, can indicate prostate enlargement. Two blood tests can also help confirm prostate cancer. One test is *prostatic acid phosphatase (PAP);* elevated levels of this acid in the blood usually indicate prostate cancer and the spread of the cancer to other parts of the body, especially to the bone. A second blood test is used to measure the level of *prostate-specific antigen (PSA)* in the blood. The level of PSA rises in cases of cancer of the prostate gland. Another diagnostic test used along with the two blood tests is transrectal ultrasonography. In this test a rectal probe, inserted into the rectum, is used to bounce waves off the prostate gland and locate cancers as small as a grain of rice. The sonographic waves are used to create an image that can be viewed and printed. Suspected tissue can then be biopsied with a fine needle and examined to determine the presence of malignant cells.

Treatment for prostate cancer consists of surgery, alone or in combination with radiation and/or hormones and anticancer drugs. The use of hormones and anticancer drugs can shrink the size of the tumor, relieving pain and controlling the cancer for long periods of time.

The incidence of prostate cancer increases with age; over 80 percent of prostate cancers are diagnosed in men over age 65. African American men have the highest incidence of prostate cancer in the world. The cause of prostate cancer remains unknown. It is unclear whether prostate cancer is due to genetic or environmental factors. Dietary fat may be a factor.[23]

Sixty percent of all cases of prostate cancer are discovered before the cancer has spread, and among these the five-year survival rate is 88 percent. In fact, the survival rates for all stages is 74 percent.[24] Men over 40 years of age should have a digital rectal exam as a part of any regular physical checkup, and all men 50 and older should have a rectal exam, along with a PAP and PSA test, at least once a year.

CANCER IN ETHNIC GROUPS

In 1993, according to the American Cancer Society, the incidence of cancer and mortality rates was higher for African Americans than for white Americans.[25] In 1989, the incidence rates were 380 per 100,000 for whites and 401 for African Americans. In the same year, the mortality rates were 227 for African Americans and 169 for whites.

Cancer incidence and mortality for African Americans was significantly higher in cancer of the esophagus, cervix, stomach, liver, prostate, larynx, and bone marrow. Esophageal cancer rates are over three times higher among African Americans than whites. The five-year survival rates for cancers in African Americans are also lower than among whites. Survival rates for cancers diagnosed from 1983 through 1988 were about 38 percent for African Americans compared with 54 percent for whites. These differences may be due, in part, to cancers for which early diagnosis is possible, but which were not detected and treated when in a localized stage.

By contrast, cancer incidence and mortality rates for other ethnic groups, such as Hispanics, are often lower than for black or white Americans. Such ethnic and cultural differences can be due to life-style and behavioral differences, such as dietary patterns, use of alcohol, sexual and reproductive behaviors, frequencies of seeking medical care, and to economic limitations, such as lack of health insurance.

DETECTING AND DIAGNOSING CANCER

Early detection and treatment of cancer can mean the difference between a complete cure (usually defined as no recurrence of the cancer within five years) and an unexpectedly early, or premature, death. Early detection involves knowing the warning signals of cancer and conducting certain routine examinations.

Warning Signals of Cancer

It is extremely important to be able to recognize the early warning signals of cancer. The following acronym will help you to remember them:

C Changes in bowel or bladder habits

A A sore that does not heal

U Unusual bleeding or other discharge or weight loss

T Thickening or lump in breast or elsewhere

I Indigestion or difficulty in swallowing

O Obvious change in wart or mole

N Nagging cough or hoarseness

If any of these warning signs persist, see your physician immediately. Any of these symptoms can result from some condition other than cancer, but prompt cancer treatment is so essential that it is foolish to take a "wait and see" attitude. If cancer is discovered, it can be promptly treated; if cancer is not present, needless worry can be avoided.

Receiving the diagnosis of cancer is emotionally difficult for both the patient and his or her family. Although most cases are now curable with early detection and treatment, the fear of the five D's remains: fear of death, disfigurement, disability, dependence, and disruption of important relationships.

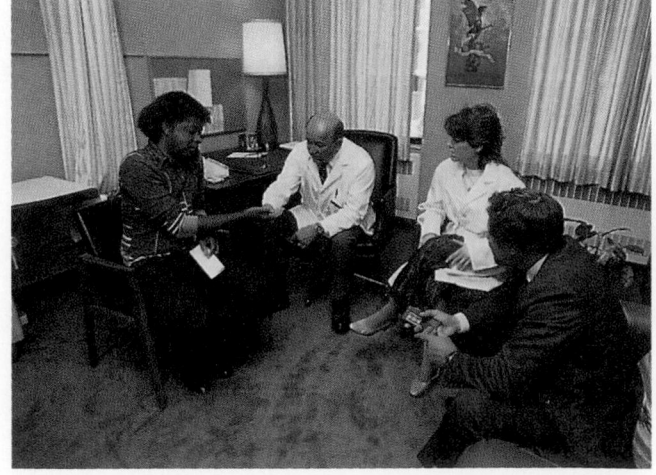

Routine Examinations

Routine examinations may detect many forms of cancer at an early stage. The chance of successful treatment is excellent when cancer is found early. Recommended examinations are outlined in the following sections.

Breast Cancer Detection   Monthly breast self-examinations (see Feature 21.2, p. 665) and yearly mammograms for women 50 years of age and older, and a clinical breast examination every three years for women ages 20–40 are recommended. All suspicious breast lumps should be biopsied.

Testicular Cancer Detection   Testicular cancer accounts for only 1–2 percent of all cancer in men, but it is the most common cancer in men between the ages of 15 and 35. It is four times as common in white males as in African American males.[26] No single cause of testicular cancer has been identified, although a major risk factor is having an un-

descended testicle (cryptorchidism), which carries a risk of cancer five times that of men who do not have this condition. Monthly self-examination for signs of testicular cancer is recommended for men from age 15 (see Feature 21.3).

Cervical Cancer Detection   All women who are or have been sexually active *or* who have reached 18 years of age should have annual Pap (Papanicolaou) tests and pelvic examinations to detect early cervical cancer. In a Pap test, the cervix and its opening are swabbed (see Figure 21.3) and a microscope slide is prepared from the swab, stained, and examined for abnormal cells. This allows detection of cervical cancer while it is still a tiny spot on the cervix that can be removed easily.

Colon and Rectal Cancer Detection   The American Cancer Society recommends three different tests for early detection of cancer of the colon and rectum.[27] A digital (by finger) rectal examination, performed by a physician, should be per-

---

FEATURE 21.3

TESTICULAR SELF-EXAMINATION

The leading cause of cancer deaths for college-age males is testicular cancer. With early detection and treatment, testicular cancer has one of the highest survival rates of all cancers (97 percent). The most common symptom of this cancer is a scrotal lump that gradually increases in size, but usually produces no pain or other symptoms. Men under age 30, in particular, should perform testicular self-examination (TSE) monthly.

TSE should be performed when the scrotum is relaxed, such as after a warm shower or bath. A normal testis is egg-

shaped, smooth, and firm, with the epididymis felt as a raised area at the rear of each testis (illustration a). Using the thumb and fingertips, feel the entire surface of the testis for any lump, hardening, or enlargement (illustration b). Do not confuse the epididymis with a tumor. The epididymis will feel about the same on both testes, while a tumor will be on one testis only. Any suspicious hard lumps should be reported to a physician immediately.

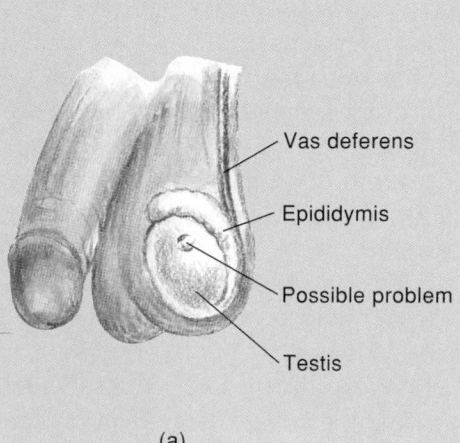

Vas deferens

Epididymis

Possible problem

Testis

(a)

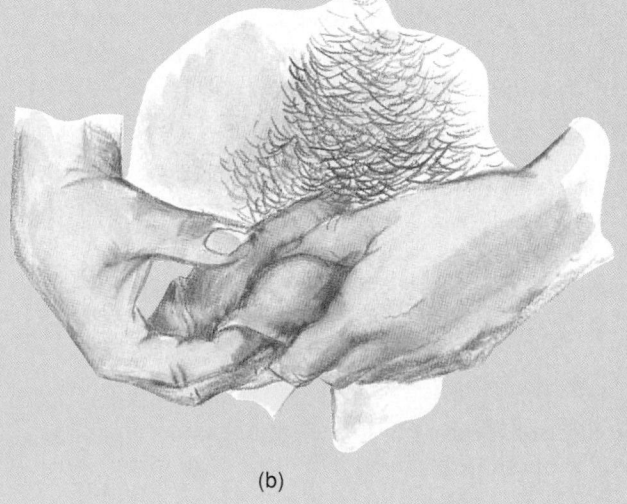

(b)

Figure 21.3
Procedure for the Pap Smear

In a Pap smear, the cervix is swabbed, then a microscope slide is smeared with the material on the swab, stained, and examined for abnormal cells.

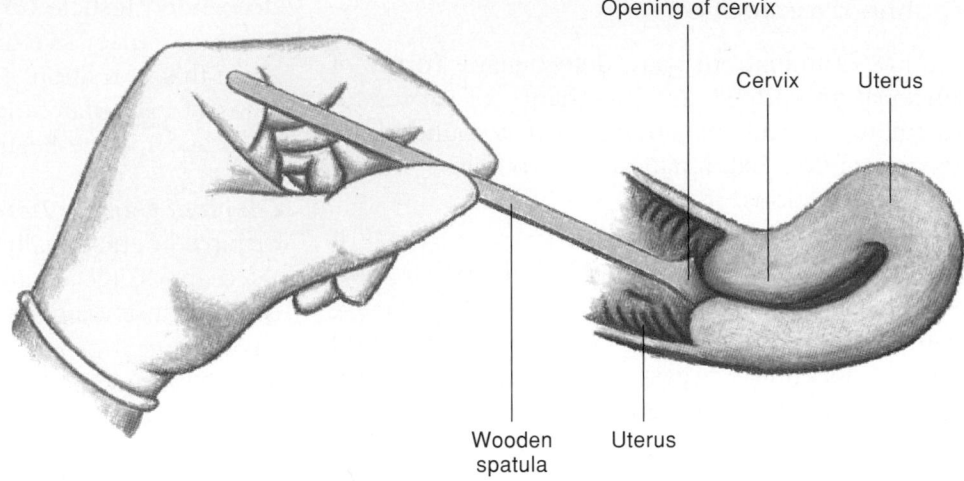

formed every year for individuals age 40 and over. The feces should be tested for blood every year after age 50. And the lower colon should be visually examined using an instrument that allows the physician to see the lining of the colon. Called **proctosigmoidoscopy** (*proktō-sig-moyd-os'kō-pē*), this examination is recommended every three to five years after age 50, following two annual exams with negative results. Anyone of any age experiencing rectal bleeding, abdominal pain, or a change in bowel habits, however, should see a physician immediately.

The Cancer-Related Checkup The American Cancer Society recommends that people ages 20–39 who have no cancer symptoms should be checked for signs of cancer every three years. Individuals 40 and over should be checked every year, and more often if at some particular risk. During these checkups, a physician looks for cancer of the thyroid gland, testes, prostate, mouth, ovaries, breasts, cervix, skin, and lymph nodes.[28] Table 21.6 summarizes the tests the American Cancer Society recommends that people undergo for the early detection of cancer.

TREATING CANCER

Great strides have been made in cancer treatment in recent years. Survival rates (see Table 21.2) have

....

proctosigmoidoscopy visual examination of the rectum and sigmoid (lower) colon by use of an instrument (sigmoidoscope).

increased while treatment side effects have lessened.[29] Because of the following medical advances there is less and less reason for dismay upon hearing a diagnosis of cancer.

Modern Surgical Procedures

Over one-fifth of all cases of cancer diagnosed each year can be cured by surgery alone. This form of treatment is usually successful for cases that have been diagnosed before extensive invasion of surrounding tissues (metastasis) has occurred. Surgery is also used to reduce the size of a tumor to make it more vulnerable to radiation and chemotherapy, or to reconstruct certain areas of the body, such as breasts, that have been damaged by cancer.

Radiation

It may seem surprising that radiation is used to treat cancer when it is also a cause of cancer. Both x-rays and radioisotopes (radioactive chemicals) are used in cancer therapy. The doses used in treating cancer are very intensive—much greater than in dental or other x-rays—and are focused into the cancerous tissue.

About a tenth of all cancer cases may be cured with radiation alone or in conjunction with surgery. Radiation is effective due to the increased speed of cancer cell divisions and the increased vascularization (development of new blood vessels) of tumorous growths. Therapy works by ionizing (breaking up) cell chemicals, including genes. Radiation is selective in that it has a greater effect on cancerous cells because they are dividing much more rapidly

Table 21.6
Tests for Early Detection of Cancer

Test or Procedure	Population		
	Sex	Age	Frequency
Sigmoidoscopy, preferably flexible	M and F	50 and over	Every 3–5 years
Fecal occult blood test	M and F	50 and over	Every year
Digital rectal examination	M and F	40 and over	Every year
Prostate exam[a]	M	50 and over	Every year
Pap test	F	All women who are, or who have been, sexually active, or have reached age 18, should have an annual Pap test and pelvic examination. After a woman has had three or more consecutive satisfactory normal annual examinations, the Pap test may be performed less frequently at the discretion of her physician.	
Pelvic examination	F	18–40	Every 1–3 years with Pap test
		Over 40	Every year
Endometrial tissue sample	F	At menopause, if at high risk[b]	At menopause and thereafter at the discretion of the physician
Breast self-examination	F	20 and over	Every month
Breast clinical examination	F	20–40	Every 3 years
		Over 40	Every year
Mammography[c]	F	40–49	Every 1–2 years
		50 and over	Every year
Health counseling and cancer checkup[d]	M and F	Over 20	Every 3 years
	M and F	Over 40	Every year

[a]Annual digital rectal examination and prostate-specific antigen test should be performed on men 50 years and older. If either is abnormal, further evaluation should be considered.
[b]History of infertility, obesity, failure to ovulate, abnormal uterine bleeding, or unopposed estrogen or tamoxifen therapy
[c]Screening mammography should begin by age 40.
[d]To include examination for cancers of the thyroid, testicles, ovaries, lymph nodes, anal region, and skin.

Source: "Tests for Early Detection of Cancer" from Cancer Facts and Figures, *1993.*

than noncancerous cells. Many of the adverse effects formerly associated with radiation therapy, such as digestive disorders and impaired immunity, have been eliminated or reduced by recent technical advances. Total dosages are now divided into multiple small daily doses and focused very accurately at the cancerous tissue.

Chemotherapy

Chemotherapy is a very general term, describing the use of any form of drug to treat any physical or mental disorder. In cancer chemotherapy, drugs are used that are selectively more toxic to cancer cells than to healthy body cells.

The majority of today's cancer cases are treated with anticancer drugs, either alone or in combination with surgery, and/or radiation. Using anticancer drugs in combination with surgery and radiation therapy increases the chances of success. Anticancer drugs are taken either orally or by injection. Because these drugs are distributed throughout the entire body, they can kill cancer cells that have metastasized to distant sites. When drugs are used in conjunction with surgery, the surgery can often be less extensive and therefore less debilitating.

Chemotherapy for cancer has improved vastly in recent years. Many cases of cancer that only a few years ago would have been viewed as "incurable" are now successfully cured. Usually, several anticancer drugs are used together, increasing the chance of killing every single cancer cell to produce a complete cure.[30]

Immunotherapy

In almost every type of cancer, the body's natural defenses attempt to control the malignant cells.[31, 32] **Immunotherapy** strengthens the body's ability to control, reject, and kill the malignant cells without affecting the normal ones. Several forms of immunotherapy are being tested; all are still experimental and may or may not prove effective.

Vaccines Cancer cells carry specific antigens (see Chapter 18) on their surfaces, raising the possibility that anticancer vaccines might someday be available, either to prevent cancer from developing or to stimulate the immune system to attack existing cancer cells.

Interferons As described in Chapter 18, interferons are naturally occurring proteins that enable cells to resist being infected by viruses by killing the cancer cells or stopping their growth. Interferons are normally produced by cells that are infected by viruses. In addition to their antiviral effects, interferons also suppress the growth of cells. Experiments are currently assessing the ability of interferons to suppress cancer.

Monoclonal Antibodies **Monoclonal antibodies** are highly specific antibodies made outside the body by cultures of antibody-forming cells (see Figure 21.4). Monoclonal antibodies can be produced in great quantities. They are being used as experimental cancer therapy in several ways, including the following:[33]

- By directly attacking cancer cells.
- By delivering anticancer drugs or radiation directly to specific target cells, thereby increasing their effectiveness of the drugs while reducing damage to healthy cells.

....

immunotherapy the production or enhancement of immunity in treating disease.

monoclonal antibodies antibodies made outside the body by cultures of antibody-forming cells.

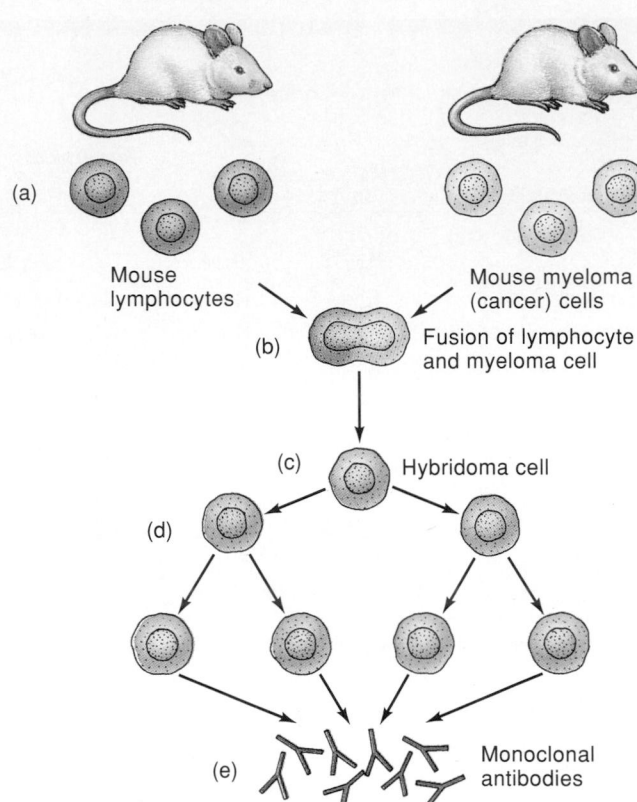

(a)
Mouse lymphocytes

Mouse myeloma (cancer) cells

(b) Fusion of lymphocyte and myeloma cell

(c) Hybridoma cell

(d)

(e) Monoclonal antibodies

Figure 21.4
Monoclonal Antibody Production

Antibody-producing mouse lymphocytes (a) and mouse myeloma (cancer) cells are fused together (b) by mixing them in the presence of the chemical, polyethylene glycol. The resulting hybridoma cell (c) undergoes cell division (d) to produce a large number of antibody-producing hybridoma cells. Culture of hybridoma cells is grown commercially to produce the desired monoclonal antibodies (e).

- By attacking "tumor growth factors," which are chemicals produced by cancer cells that stimulate the growth of other cancer cells of the same type.

Before immunotherapy becomes a standard approach to cancer treatment, much research and testing will be required. Its potential, however, looks promising (see also Feature 18.3 on p. 567).

Directions of Current and Future Research

New developments in the early detection and diagnosis and treatment of cancer are bringing cures to various forms of cancer once thought incurable, including Hodgkin's disease, children's leukemia,

Burkitt's lymphoma, and testicular cancer. Research continues on many fronts.

A sampling of some current cancer research follows:

- *Bone marrow transplantation* has been used with some leukemia patients. *Autologous bone marrow transplants* involve a person's own marrow which is removed, treated, saved, and later restored, avoiding problems of tissue matching.

- *Diagnostic imaging techniques* have replaced exploratory surgery. *Magnetic resonance imaging (MRI)* and *computerized tomography (CT)* scanning, used to detect hidden tumors, are painless noninvasive procedures sparing normal tissue during radiation therapy.

- *Neoadjuvant chemotherapy* is being used to shrink cancers, which can then be removed surgically.

- *Hyperthermia*—or temperatures of 108°–109°F—makes cells more susceptible to the effects of chemotherapy and radiation. A temperature of 113°F kills cancer cells.

- *Suppressor genes* exist in normal cells to control growth. When altered, these genes may cause cancers, including breast and lung cancer. Members of families in which there is known genetic transmission of some suppression genes can now be screened for genetic abnormality before the cancer develops.

- *Genetic engineering* is the correction of impaired immune systems by transplanting normal copies of genes into cells that have mutated forms of these genes.

Cancer Quackery

Every year people spend billions of dollars on unproven, faddist cancer "cures" and other worthless remedies. In addition to the dollar cost of cancer **quackery,** the more tragic cost is that people often lose precious time trying ineffective remedies instead of pursuing effective therapies that could save their lives.

....

quackery the practice of pretending to have knowledge or skill in medicine.

People try unproven cancer remedies for several reasons:[34]

- They are *desperate* and quacks promise a cure, whereas ethical physicians are reluctant to make promises

- They are *afraid* of surgery, radiation, and anticancer drugs and are looking for less-frightening alternatives

- They are *uninformed* and simply do not realize the difference between proven and unproven cures

- They are *gullible* and are taken in by the testimonials of those who claim to have been "cured" but who never actually had cancer in the first place or those who went into remissions that were spontaneous, not caused by the "cure."

There are too many ineffective cancer cures to mention all of them, but some of the more common categories include the following:

- *Special diets* that may be severely deficient in many important nutrients, thereby causing more harm than good.

- *Megadoses* (extremely large doses) of vitamins such as Vitamin C or Vitamin E or of minerals such as zinc. Megadoses may cause toxic effects and in some cases may impair, rather than enhance, the body's defenses against cancer.

- *Secret or exclusive drugs* or other cures available nowhere else. This claim is almost always a sign of quackery, because if a treatment is effective, it usually becomes available to all physicians.

- *Unusual remedies* such as coffee enemas or sitting under lights of special colors or types. Repeated enemas can deplete the body of important minerals.

Obtaining the Best Treatment

Cancer treatment is highly specialized and is constantly making rapid advances. Only a physician who is a specialist can stay up-to-the-minute on the latest cancer treatments. When cancer is diagnosed by a nonspecialist, such as a family physician, a referral to a cancer specialist is appropriate. Communication for Wellness: Coping with Cancer sug-

---

COPING WITH CANCER

A diagnosis of cancer is laden with implications that are extremely difficult emotionally for both the person with cancer and his or her family. Common fears associated with cancer are referred to as the five D's: fear of *Death, Disfigurement, Disability, Dependence,* and *Disruption* of important relationships.[a] These concerns, although very difficult to deal with, can be managed by the person with cancer and his or her family by recognizing them as normal and by using techniques to deal with them directly.

Research[a] suggests that the kind of people who best manage the stresses of cancer are those who:

- feel personally responsible for maintaining their health

- learn as much as possible about their disease

- follow their physician's advice

- have an optimistic outlook and will fight the disease without giving up

- maintain close contact with family and friends, talk about the illness, and express both their positive and negative feelings

- have a sense of humor, particularly about things that cannot be changed

- continue with activities that have been important, such as work, socializing, religion, and recreational activities

It is important that each day provides pleasure. Positive thinking and optimism, expressed by receiving and giving affection, hope, love, joy, and laughter all contribute to a better psychological outlook and, according to some research, to a higher rate of recovery.

When a family member has cancer, it affects every member of that family, individually and in their relationship to one another. Many physicians like to include their patient's family members in all conversations with the patient about his or her condition, if the patient will agree to this. This encourages open communication and discourages secrets and misconceptions.

Healthy individuals must be sensitive to the needs of someone with cancer. When visiting a friend or family member who has cancer, it is important to act naturally. Try not to be self-conscious—if a kiss, hug, or handshake was how you greeted the person before his or her illness, don't change your behavior; he or she may be sensitive to any signs of possible rejection. Don't pretend that the person is not ill, however. Allow him or her to lead the conversation and be prepared to follow his or her lead, even if it leads to painful thoughts. It is important, psychologically, for someone with cancer to be able to share worries and feelings with others. Don't feel obligated to solve problems or cheer up the person. Listening and trying to understand is what is important.

Above all, it is important to recognize that people can and do recover from cancer. An optimistic outlook, good coping strategies, support from family and friends, and competent medical care are all parts of the formula for successfully living with cancer.

Most cancers are assumed to be cured when symptoms disappear for five years. For years beyond that point, however, it is normal for anyone who has had cancer to experience fear or panic when any ache or pain occurs.

[a]Holland, J., and Cullen, L. "Living with Cancer." In Holleb, A. (ed.). *The American Cancer Society Cancer Book.* Garden City, NJ: Doubleday, 1986.

---

gests ways in which you can cope with a cancer diagnosis.

AVOIDING CANCER

Not every case of cancer can be prevented. By applying what we do know of cancer prevention, however, many cancer cases can be prevented.

Tobacco

As we have already discussed, at least 30 percent of all cancer deaths are directly attributable to the use of tobacco. Cancers of the mouth, throat, larynx, trachea, lung, kidney, and bladder are all associated with smoking or the use of smokeless tobacco (snuff and chewing tobacco). Avoiding tobacco use is the single most important way of preventing cancer. Those who smoke two or more packs of cigarettes a day have lung cancer mortality rates 15–25 times greater than nonsmokers.[35]

Alcohol

Excessive alcohol consumption is associated with cancers of the mouth, throat, larynx, esophagus, and liver. The combination of alcohol and tobacco use is especially hazardous as the two drugs are synergistic in producing cancer.[36, 37]

Sunlight

Ultraviolet radiation from sunshine is a major cause of skin cancer. Avoid excessive ultraviolet by using a sunscreen product with a high sun protection factor (SPF, see Chapter 22) during outdoor activities.

Ionizing Radiation

Avoid unnecessary x-rays and other radiation exposure. Before a physician or dentist takes x-rays, ask how important they are to your diagnosis and treatment. Minimize exposure to chemical carcinogens (Table 21.3) by not smoking, by reducing the radon level in your home if necessary, by eating pure foods, and by taking precautions to reduce occupational chemical exposure. If an x-ray is necessary, the lowest possible dosage should be used.

Occupational Hazards

Many cases of cancer in the United States are related to personal habits, life-styles, and physical surroundings. Various industrial agents, such as asbestos, vinyl chloride, and tars, have been shown to be carcinogenic. Asbestos, when combined with cigarette smoking, increases the risk of cancer nearly 60 times. Workers exposed to radiation and who smoke have an increased rate of lung cancer.

Diet

Perhaps the most controversial area of cancer prevention has been the role of diet. There are two basic issues: Do certain foods increase one's risk of cancer and can certain foods reduce one's risk of cancer? These questions have generated a lot of conflicting research data. On the basis of the accumulation of a considerable body of research, the American Cancer Society offers the following guidelines to reduce cancer risks.[38] This report was directed at foods, and specifically stated that additives legally allowed in foods were not implicated as causes of cancer.

1. *Control total food energy intake.* Persons who are 40 percent or more overweight increase their risks of developing cancers of the breast, colon, gallbladder, ovary, prostate, and uterus. The control of total food intake helps control obesity. Obesity is associated with marked increases in cancers of the ovary, uterus, gallbladder, prostate, colon, and breast.

2. *Cut down on total fat intake—both saturated and unsaturated fats.* Of all dietary components, the intake of fat is uniquely correlated with cancer. The fats do not appear to initiate cancers, but seem to promote its development once a person has been exposed to a known carcinogen. A high-fat diet is unique as a cancer promoter in several ways:

- By causing the body to secrete more hormones, including certain ones (such as estrogen) favorable to the development of certain cancers (such as breast cancer).

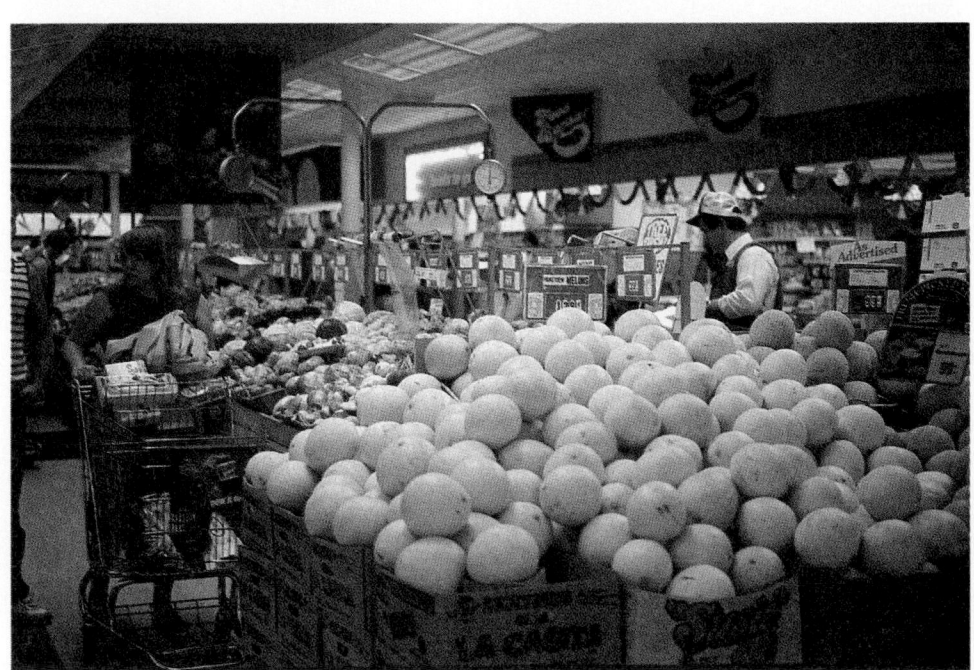

A "cancer-prevention diet" centers around the produce section of the store. It is high in fiber (abundant in most fruits and vegetables), high in Vitamin A (dark green and deep yellow vegetables and some fruits, see text) and Vitamin C (citrus, tomatoes, peppers, broccoli), contains crucifiers (cabbage, broccoli), and is low in fat and calories.

- By promoting bile secretion into the intestine, bile is converted in the colon into cancer-producing compounds.
- By being incorporated into the cell membrane and there attached so they provide a reduced defense against cancer.

Certain forms of fat in particular seem to be implicated in promoting cancer. The polyunsaturated fatty acids from vegetable oils are more likely to promote cancer than *omega-3 fatty acids* from fish and fish oils and *monounsaturated fatty acids* from olive oil. This means cutting down on certain fats— salad dressings, mayonnaise, margarine, butter, and relying on fish oils and olive oils.[39]

3. *Eat more high-fiber foods, such as whole grain cereals, breads, pasta, and more fruits and vegetables.* It is thought that fibers may help by protecting against some cancers by speeding up the movement of all materials through the colon. The more quickly food wastes move through the intestine, the less the time of exposure to any carcinogens that may be present. The carcinogens may also bind to the fiber, so that they are carried through the intestine rather than being absorbed. Studies have indicated that people with colon cancer have a diet of more meat, less fiber, and more saturated fat than others without cancer.[40, 41] Although dietary fats act as promoters of cancers, fibers appear to act as antipromoters. The frequent intake of vegetables relates to a reduced incidence of cancer of the stomach and colon.

4. *Include foods rich in Vitamin A and Vitamin C in the daily diet.* Vitamin A regulates cellular differentiation. Vitamin A also helps maintain the immune system, which works against cancer even after a tumor has begun to form. Getting Vitamin A, Vitamin C and fiber from green vegetables and fruits has a greater effect than getting the same vitamins from pills because of the fibers.[42] Members of the cabbage family of plants, the so-called **crucifers** (cabbage, broccoli, brussels sprouts, turnips, cauliflower, and rutabagas), contain compounds that activate enzymes that destroy carcinogens.[43]

5. *Use moderation in consuming salt-cured, nitrate-cured, and smoked foods.* This food catego-

ry includes salted or smoked fish, ham, bacon, salami, wieners, and similar cured meats. In populations that consume these foods frequently, such as in parts of Asia and Africa, there is a high incidence of cancer of the esophagus and stomach.[44]

6. *Cut down on alcohol consumption, if you drink at all.* The excessive use of alcohol, especially when combined with cigarette smoking or smokeless tobacco use, increases risk of cancers of the mouth, throat, larynx, esophagus, and liver.

The "bottom line" on cancer is that by applying what you know about its prevention, detection, and treatment, you can greatly reduce your chance of a premature death from cancer.

CHECKPOINT

1. In what ways do cancer cells differ from normal cells?
2. What is the difference between malignant and benign tumors?
3. What are the known causes of cancer?
4. List the seven warning signs of cancer.
5. What are the recognized treatments for cancer?
6. How can a person reduce his or her chances of getting cancer?

DIABETES

Diabetes is a generalized term for a group of diseases in which there is excessive urination. Unless otherwise indicated, use of the term diabetes usually refers to diabetes mellitus. **Diabetes mellitus** (*dī-a-bē'tez mel-ī'tis*) is a disorder of carbohydrate metabolism and results in excessive sugar in the

crucifers edible vegetables from the mustard plant family (Cruciferae).

diabetes a general term for diseases characterized by excessive urination.

diabetes mellitus a disorder of carbohydrate metabolism resulting in excessive sugar in the blood and sugar in the urine.

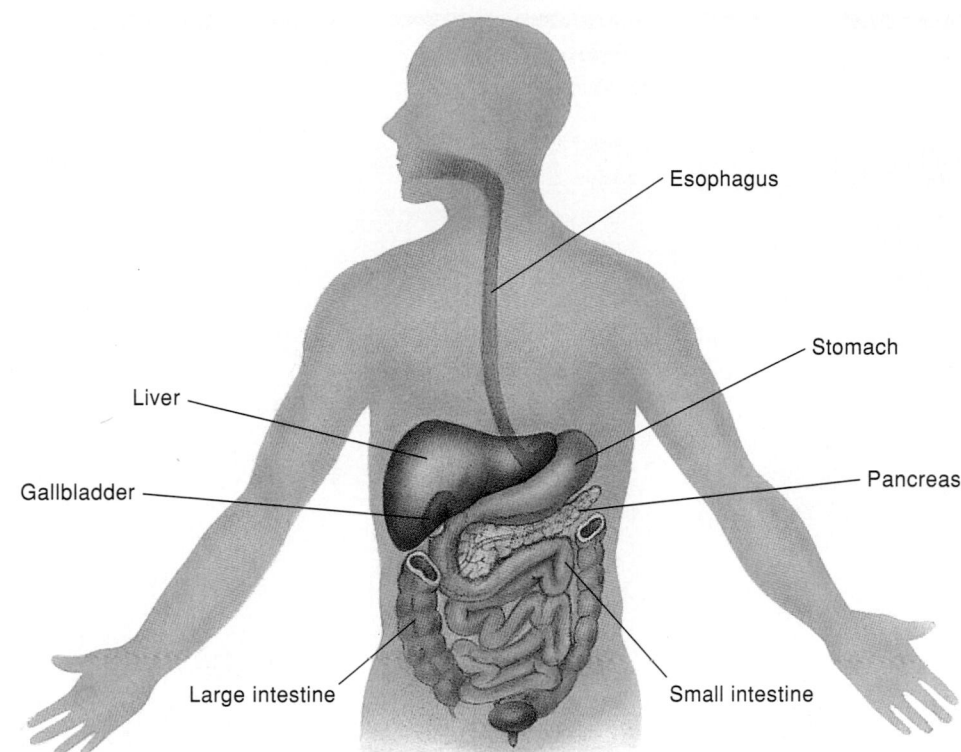

Figure 21.5
The Pancreas

Scattered within the pancreas are small clusters of insulin-producing cells. The pancreas is also an important source of digestive enzymes.

blood (*hyperglycemia*) and sugar in the urine (*glycosuria*) due to an inadequate production or use of insulin. People with diabetes also display excessive urine production (*polyuria*), excessive thirst (*polydipsia*), and excessive eating (*polyphagia*). **Insulin** is a hormone produced by specific cells within the **pancreas,** an organ located just under the stomach (see Figure 21.5). The function of insulin is to transport sugar (glucose) from the blood into each body cell. People with diabetes may have a blood sugar level several times higher than normal, but the body cells are unable to absorb sugar, which is normally the main energy source for all human cells. As a result, the cells starve, despite the high level of sugar in the blood. To compensate for the lack of sugar, the cells break down their own fats and proteins for energy and thus damage them-

selves. Also, toxic by-products (ketones) from the breakdown of fatty acids accumulate in the body, increasing the acidity of the blood and impairing many body functions.[45]

About 12 million people in the United States have diabetes.[46] The incidence of diabetes increases with age and for unknown reasons, is higher among African Americans than in other ethnic groups (see Table 21.7).

Unfortunately, only about half of the people who have diabetes are aware of their condition. Inadequately treated, diabetes has very severe consequences, including blindness, atherosclerotic disease leading to amputation of limbs, heart attacks, and early death. Symptoms of diabetes are listed in Table 21.8. Some people experience none of these symptoms and the disease progresses silently. Thus, periodic testing for diabetes is recommended for everyone.

The tendency toward diabetes is often inherited. Not everyone who inherits the tendency actually develops the disease, however. In other instances, people develop diabetes even though there is no family history of the problem. There are two major types of diabetes mellitus: Type I and Type II.

insulin a hormone produced by the pancreas and necessary for movement of sugar from the blood into the body cells.

pancreas a gland located behind the stomach and connected by a duct to the small intestine. The gland produces both pancreatic juice to assist in food digestion and insulin to assist cells in blood sugar absorption.

Table 21.7
Comparative Incidence of Diabetes, in Cases per 1000 People

	Cases per 1000 People	
Group	Male	Female
Age		
Under 17	0.7	1.1
17–44	7.7	10.4
45–64	55.0	55.1
65–74	87.9	87.7
Ethnic Group		
African American	33.7	46.2
Hispanic	25.6	35.9
White	22.7	23.4
Other	32.6	43.9
Education		
Under 12 years	36.9	50.6
12 years	30.4	26.2
Over 12 years	28.4	20.2

Source: Drury, T., and Powell, A. Prevalence, Impact, and Demography of Known Diabetes in the United States. Advance data from Vital and Health Statistics, U. S. Public Health Service, No. 114, 12 February 1986.

Table 21.8
Symptoms of Diabetes

Frequent urination (polyuria)

Excessive thirst (polydipsia)

Craving for sweets and starches; increased food intake (polyphagia)

Weight loss

General weakness

Fatigue

Visual disturbances—blurred vision

Personality changes—moodiness, difficulty in coping

Impaired sexual response—male or female

Increased number of infections—skin, mouth, vagina, and so on

Itching, often around the genitals

Nausea and vomiting

Drowsiness

Tingling or numbness in feet

Note: Children usually exhibit dramatic and sudden symptoms, requiring prompt medical attention, but adults can have diabetes with none of these symptoms. Periodic blood or urine tests are important for everyone.

TYPE I DIABETES

Type I diabetes, called **insulin-dependent diabetes mellitus (IDDM),** was formerly known as juvenile-onset diabetes because it commonly develops in children and adolescents. In IDDM, which is the more severe form of diabetes, there is an absolute deficiency of insulin. IDDM occurs when a person's immune system produces antibodies that destroy the insulin-producing cells within his or her own pancreas. (Review Chapter 18 for discussion of such autoimmune disorders.) The cause of this autoimmune destruction is unknown, but it appears to occur in genetically susceptible people, and may involve, in at least some cases, infection of the insulin-producing cells with viruses.[47, 48] There is

....

insulin-dependent diabetes mellitus (IDDM) a form of diabetes mellitus in which regular injections of insulin are required to prevent death. Also known as Type I diabetes. Previously known as juvenile-onset diabetes.

some evidence that a peptide in cow's milk may trigger the onset of IDDM. Investigations are being conducted to see whether withholding cow's milk from an infant's diet during the first three months of life will protect against IDDM.[49]

Since blood glucose is unable to enter the cells, the cells must rely on fats and proteins for energy. As blood lipids are transported to the cells, lipid particles are deposited in the walls of blood vessels, leading to atherosclerosis and other cardiovascular problems (cerebrovascular insufficiency, coronary heart disease, peripheral vascular disease, and gangrene). Loss of vision and kidney problems are common.[50] Cyclosporine, a drug that suppresses the immune system, shows some indication of being able to interrupt the destruction of the insulin-producing cells.

Most people with Type I diabetes must inject insulin (insulin does not work if taken orally as it is broken down by digestive enzymes). Some Type I diabetics receive their insulin from small, implanted insulin pumps. Research continues on an artificial pancreas that monitors blood glucose level and administers insulin automatically. Transplantation has been tried in several ways. Whole pancreas transplants face possible rejection by the recipient's body, and thus require immunosuppressant drugs.

Another approach includes implanting clusters of insulin-producing cells into the pancreas.[51]

TYPE II DIABETES

Type II diabetes is much more common than Type I, and occurs in more than 90 percent of all cases. Typically found in people who are over age 40 and overweight, it was once called adult (maturity-onset) diabetes. Many people with Type II diabetes have sufficient insulin in the blood, but if additional insulin is needed, drugs to stimulate the insulin-producing cells of the pancreas can be taken. For this reason, Type II diabetes is called **non-insulin-dependent diabetes mellitus (NIDDM).** In persons with NIDDM, the problem is an increased resistance by cells to insulin. Possible causes include the following:[52]

- Inadequate amounts of insulin are produced in relation to the body's need.
- Insulin is destroyed before it can take effect, perhaps by antibodies.
- Insulin release is out of phase with food intake and blood-sugar levels.
- The number of available insulin receptors (specific places where insulin attaches) on the body cells is decreased. In an autoimmune process, antibodies bind to the insulin receptor sites and diminish the effectiveness of insulin, since few sites remain free for the hormone to bind.[53]

Obesity is a common characteristic of individuals who develop Type II diabetes. Eighty percent of people who develop Type II diabetes are obese at the time of its onset. Many of these persons have a sufficient amount or even surplus of insulin in the blood, but their cells become less sensitive to it, possibly due to the reduced sensitivity of the insulin receptors. As fat cells in a person enlarge, the cells become increasingly resistant to the effects of insulin. The greater the insulin resistance,

....

non-insulin-dependent diabetes mellitus (NIDDM) a form of diabetes mellitus in which there is sufficient insulin present, but cells become less sensitive to it. Also known as Type II diabetes. Previously known as adult (mature)-onset diabetes.

the more the person overeats, setting up an unfortunate cycle.[54] Type II diabetes can usually be controlled with weight loss, oral medications, a proper diet, and exercise.

HYPOGLYCEMIA

Hypoglycemia (*hī-pō-glī-sē'mē-a*), or low blood sugar, can arise in a person after going without food longer than usual, or can indicate one of various disease conditions. It may be accompanied by symptoms similar to those of an anxiety attack: weakness, rapid heartbeat, sweating, anxiety, hunger, and trembling—all symptoms caused by *epinephrine* (adrenalin, the "emergency hormone"). Epinephrine works to stimulate release of glycogen from the liver cells. Released when you are under stress, it acts quickly to ensure that your body cells have enough energy fuel.

After eating, a person's blood glucose level rises, followed by a decline while glucose is primarily stored. Once no more glucose is available from digestion, the liver starts releasing the glucose it has stored as glycogen for use by the body (fasting state). Through all this the blood glucose remains within its normal range.

In some people the transition from the fed state to the fasting stage is not smooth, causing the release of epinephrine. These people must compensate by eating or drinking something sweet every two to three hours. In other people, the fasting state lasts too long, and a drop in blood glucose occurs.

If you have a tendency toward hypoglycemia, it may help for you to eat normal mixed meals rather than sugar snacks. Eating balanced meals including complex carbohydrates (starches and whole grains), on a regular basis, may alleviate the condition.[55]

CHECKPOINT

1. What are the differences between Type I and Type II diabetes?
2. How can your chances of getting diabetes or hypoglycemia be reduced?

....

hypoglycemia low blood-sugar level.

ARTHRITIS

Arthritis is inflammation in one or more of a person's joints, usually accompanied by pain and, frequently, changes in structure. This painful and often disabling condition affects over 36 million Americans. An astounding 97 percent of people over the age of 60 show some degree of arthritis.

There are more than a hundred different forms of arthritis; general symptoms typically include pain, swelling, deformity, and difficulty moving the affected joint. We will briefly describe some of the most common forms of arthritis.

In healthy joints, bone never touches bone, as each articulating surface is covered with a layer of cartilage. **Cartilage** is a dense, firm tissue capable of resisting considerable pressure or tension. It occurs in many parts of the body. **Osteoarthritis** (*os'tē-ō-ar-thrī'tis*) is characterized by gradual degeneration of the cartilage of the joint along with overgrowth of bone tissue. It usually develops in people over the age of 40 and affects joints in the fingers, hips, knees, and spinal column. Because the normally flexible cartilage degenerates, it is called the "wear and tear" arthritis. New bone replaces the cartilage and forms at the margins of the joint. Small burrs, or spurs, develop at the ends of bones, decreasing the space in the joints between the bones, further restricting movement. Symptoms include swelling, deformity, pain, and restricted movement of the affected joints. Possible causes of osteoarthritis include metabolic disorders, physical injury, obesity, and excessive use (wear and tear) of specific joints, as may occur in certain occupations. Treatments include weight loss, reduced use of the affected joints, heat applications, and medications such as aspirin or ibuprofen.

Rheumatoid (*roo'ma-toyd*) **arthritis** is an autoimmune process in which the joints are attacked by one's own immune mechanism. Rheumatoid arthritis often affects young adults, as well as older persons, and is more prevalent in females than in males. Early symptoms include stiffness and joint pain. More advanced cases include severe pain, swelling, redness, limited movement, and severe joint deformity. In addition to the joints, the lungs, eyes, skin, and nervous system may be involved. Acute attacks sometimes alternate with periods of remission. Possible causes include stress and genetic predisposition. There is no cure at this time, but treatments include anti-inflammatory agents and in severe cases only, suppression of the immune system.[56]

Systemic lupus erythematosus (*lū'pus er-i-thē-ma-tō'sus*) **(SLE)** is another autoimmune disease in which the skin and internal organs, as well as the joints, are attacked. The disease mainly affects women aged 20–40 and is characterized by alternating attacks and remissions.[57] In addition to arthritic joint pain, symptoms commonly include skin rashes, pleurisy (inflammation of the membrane surrounding the lungs), and kidney damage. Most treatments of SLE, like those for rheumatoid arthritis, either reduce inflammation or suppress the immune system. There is, at this time, no way to suppress the specific, harmful, autoimmune response in either of these diseases.

Gout is a hereditary metabolic disease producing acute attacks of arthritis caused by deposits of **urate** crystals in the joints. Urates come from the breakdown of several nitrogen-rich body chemicals and are normally excreted with the urine in the form of uric acid. In people with gout, this excretion is reduced. Urates thus accumulate in the blood, and deposit as crystals in and around one or more joints. This condition is extremely painful. Gout affects men seven times as frequently as women and is the most common form of inflammatory joint disease in men over 40. Treatment of gout includes long-term use of medications, main-

---

arthritis inflammation in one or more of a person's joints, usually accompanied by pain and, frequently, changes in structure.

cartilage a dense, firm tissue capable of resisting considerable pressure or tension.

osteoarthritis gradual destruction of the cartilage of a joint and overgrowth of bone in the joint.

rheumatoid arthritis an autoimmune disorder marked by severe inflammation of the joints and sometimes other organs.

---

systemic lupus erythematosus (SLE) an autoimmune disease affecting the joints, skin, kidneys, and other body systems.

gout hereditary metabolic disease characterized by acute attacks of arthritis caused by deposits of urate crystals in the joints.

urates salts of uric acid, normally present in the urine.

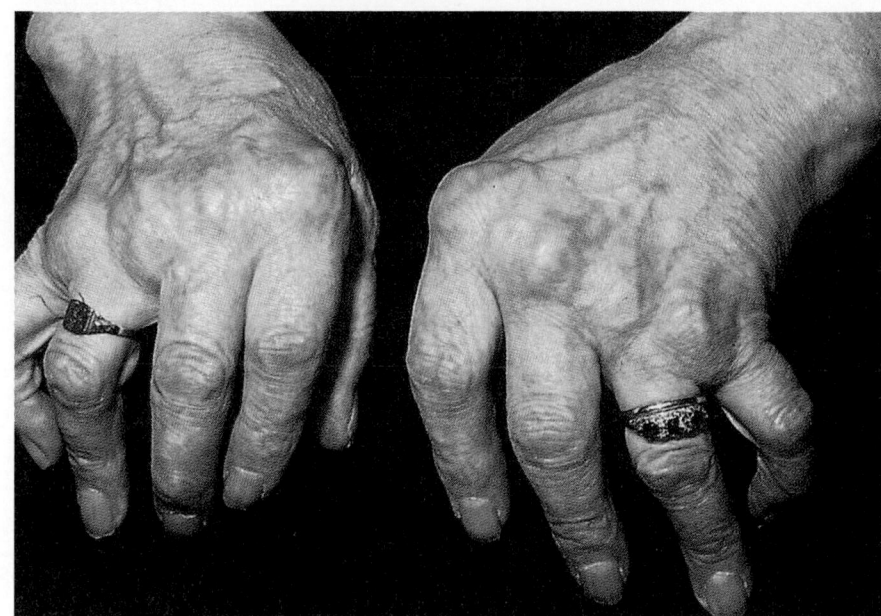

In addition to pain, arthritis often produces swelling and crippling deformity of joints.

taining ideal weight, and moderation in alcohol consumption.[58]

Infection of a joint by a pathogen can also cause arthritis. Many types of bacteria can enter the blood and settle into the joints, causing arthritis. Examples include Lyme disease (a spirochete transmitted by tick bites), gonorrhea, tuberculosis, and syphilis. Such bacterial infections are curable using antibacterial drugs.

Severe arthritic joint damage can often be prevented if arthritis is diagnosed and if treatment begins while the disease is still at an early stage. Consult a physician if any of the following signs appear:

- recurring pain or tenderness in one or more joints
- swelling or deformity in one or more joints
- stiffness in one or more joints
- redness and heat in one or more joints
- inability to move a joint through its normal range of motion
- fever, weight loss, or weakness in association with joint pain.

Most types of arthritis, other than those caused by bacterial infection, are not yet actually curable, but their symptoms can often be relieved by anti-inflammatory and pain relieving drugs. A total joint can be replaced surgically with one of plastic and/or metal if damage is severe enough. Other treatments include the following:

- *Exercise* Under the supervision of a physician or physical therapist, gentle exercise may be very beneficial in relief of stiffness or soreness.
- *Heat* Hot baths or showers or direct application of heat to a painful joint is often recommended to relieve pain and facilitate movement.
- *Rest* Rest periods scheduled throughout the day may help relieve pain.
- *Diet* Although there are no specific diets recommended for most forms of arthritis, a well-balanced, nutritious diet is recommended for maintaining a strong immune system and restricting weight gain. Excess weight places a greater burden on the joints.

As with cancers, millions of people are victimized every year by fads and quackery in arthritis treatment. Not only are quack remedies a waste of money, using these methods may delay arthritis victims from obtaining effective treatments. Severe and irreversible joint damage may take place during this delay.

CHECKPOINT

1. What is believed to cause both rheumatoid arthritis and systemic lupus erythematosus?

2. Why is prompt treatment for arthritis essential?

FEATURE 21.4

THE PRICE OF HEADACHES

People who don't suffer from headaches may have little concept of how disabling they can be. Consider these facts:

- Headaches are a severe problem for approximately 45 million Americans.

- Headaches cause over 50 million visits to doctors each year.

- Over $400 million is spent on nonprescription pain relievers each year, a large portion of which are taken because of headaches.

- Students in grades 1–12 lose 1.3 million days of school each year because of headaches.

- Job absenteeism because of headaches costs at least $55 million each year.

- More than 64 million work days are lost each year due to headaches.

Source: Clark, M. "Headaches." *Newsweek,* 7 December 1987, pp. 76–82.

NEUROLOGICAL DISORDERS

Neurological (*nū-rō-loj'i-kal*) disorders are organic or biological disorders of the nervous system. They can range from minor headaches to fatal brain deterioration.

HEADACHES

Headaches are among the most common of all health problems (see Feature 21.4). Let's briefly examine some of the more common types of headaches.

Stress or Tension Headaches

Tension often causes muscles located in the neck, shoulders, and back to contract, producing pain that feels as if it is inside of the head. This pain is typically a dull, constricting headache on both sides of the head and may run into the neck and shoulders.

Stress management (see Chapter 4) can often prevent these headaches. When tension headaches do develop, vigorous massage will often help contracted muscles to relax. Physical exercise can be very helpful. A good workout of the offending neck or shoulder muscles frequently causes them to relax and the headache to disappear. Relaxation techniques, sleep, meditation, yoga, stretching, and hot baths may help. Nonnarcotic pain relievers may also alleviate the distress.

neurological pertaining to the nervous system.

Migraine (Vascular) Headaches

Migraine (*mī'grān*) headaches are characterized by severe, throbbing pain, often on one side of the head. Attacks may be preceded by an **aura,** such as glowing spots before the eyes. Nausea, aversion to light and sound, and temporary loss of vision may accompany these headaches. Migraine headaches may last from four hours to two days or longer and may be entirely disabling.

Migraine headaches are caused by excessive dilation of blood vessels within the head. The tendency toward migraines is often hereditary; however, specific attacks are often triggered by stress, menstruation, or chemicals in certain foods or beverages (see Feature 21.5).

Prescribed medications can help prevent or relieve migraine attacks. Medication does not always work; resting in a quiet, dark place often offers the best relief.

Cluster Headaches

Cluster headaches produce severe pain, nearly always on one side of the head. As they recur, they are almost always on the same side of the head. The eye on that side often becomes teary and the nose clogged. Cluster headaches last from 20 minutes to 2 hours and occur at least once a day (and up to 14 times a day) for weeks or months; they

migraine periodic headache attacks often accompanied by visual disturbances and nausea.

aura a subjective sensation preceding an attack of some condition.

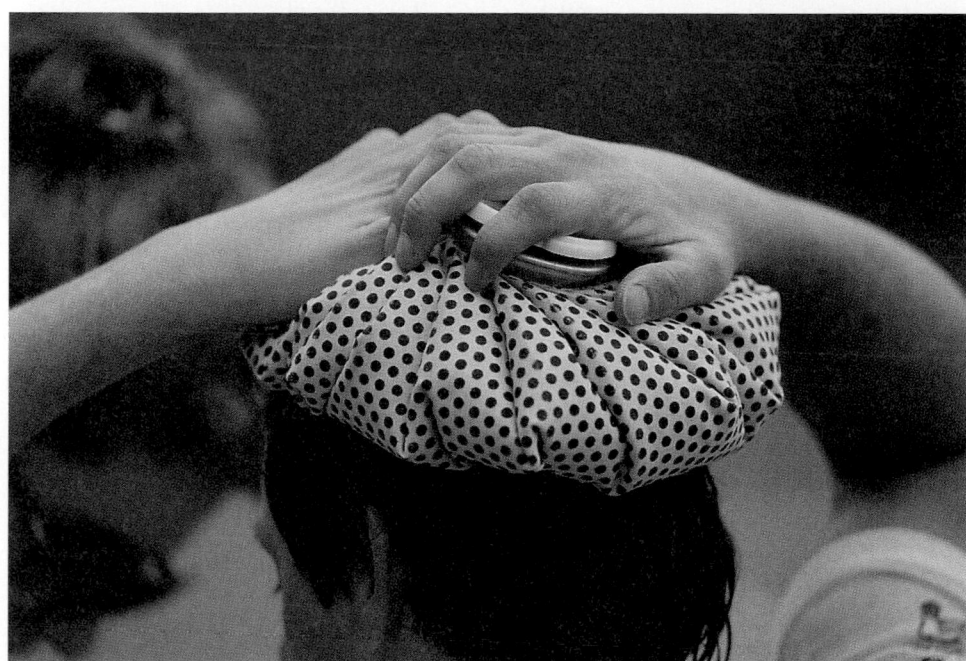

Headaches are among the most common health problems. The headache of an alcoholic hangover comes from the toxic effects of alcohol and its breakdown products such as acetaldehyde.

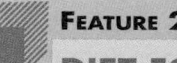
FEATURE 21.5

DIET FOR HEADACHE PREVENTION

Some people find that certain foods, beverages, or environmental changes may cause their migraine headaches. All of the following items have been reported to cause migraines in some people. Many people are able to determine their own "headache foods" by keeping a diary of food and beverages consumed on days that their headaches occur. Problem foods, drinks, and physical and environmental causes for some people include the following:

- Alcoholic beverages (especially tequila, beer, and red wine)

- Altitude changes

- Anchovies

- Avocados

- Bananas (in excessive amounts)

- Caffeine

- Chicken livers

- Chocolate

- Citrus fruits (in excessive amounts)

- Cultured milk products (yogurt, sour cream, etc.)

- Cured meats (bologna, salami, sausage, pepperoni, hot dogs)

- Fermented, pickled, or marinated foods

- Figs (excessive amounts)

- Guacamole

- Herring (pickled)

- Hot fresh breads, coffee cakes, and donuts

- Hunger

- Menstruation

- Monosodium glutamate (MSG; a flavor enhancer used in some Asian foods and in many processed American food products)

- Nuts, peanut butter, sunflower seeds, pumpkin seeds

- Onions

- Pizza

- Pods of broad beans (lima beans or pea pods)

- Pork

- Sleep (lack of, excessive amounts)

- Smog

- Stress and anxiety

- Sunlight glare

- Vinegar (except white vinegar)

- Yeasty foods (excessive amounts)

may stop for months before recurring. These headaches are more common in men. Treatment includes various prescription medications such as ergotamine tartrate.

Toxic Headaches

Many poisonous chemicals produce headaches. Alcohol and its breakdown products, such as acetaldehyde, produce the "hangover" headache. Other chemicals that may provoke headaches include engine exhaust fumes, industrial chemicals, toxins from bacterial infections such as sinus or tooth infections, and various types of drugs, such as quinine or morphine. Toxic headaches can be prevented by avoiding their chemical causes and treating infections promptly. Their treatment includes aspirin and abundant nonalcoholic fluids to counteract dehydration and in some cases, to help flush the chemicals from the body.

Other Headaches

Some people develop a dull or intense headache during or after sexual activity. These headaches usually last up to two hours. They can often be relieved with aspirin or a prescribed medication.

More common is the hunger headache, caused by low blood-sugar levels occurring when a person goes without food for a long period. These headaches can be prevented by eating regular, low-sugar meals to prevent periods of low blood sugar. As discussed previously in the section on hypoglycemia, a high-sugar meal produces a high insulin level which, in turn, causes the blood-sugar level to drop rapidly.

When someone who usually does not get headaches suddenly develops severe headaches, they may be symptoms of a serious organic disorder. In such cases, consult a physician immediately.

MULTIPLE SCLEROSIS

Multiple sclerosis (MS) is a progressive degeneration of the **myelin sheaths** surrounding the neuron fibers in the brain and spinal cord (see Figure

....

multiple sclerosis progressive degeneration of the myelin sheaths.

myelin sheath a fatlike covering over the fibers of some of the neurons of the brain and spinal cord.

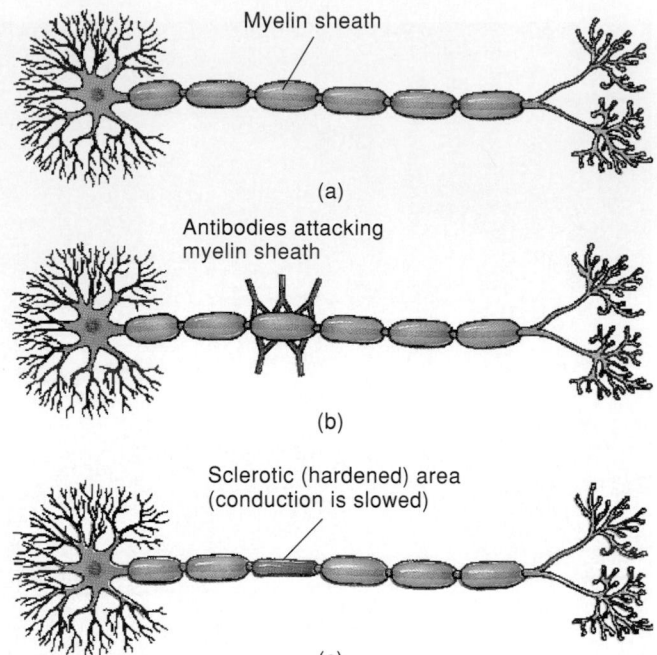

Figure 21.6
Development of Multiple Sclerosis

Development of multiple sclerosis, an autoimmune process. (a) Neuron with normal myelin sheath; (b) antibodies attacking the myelin sheath; (c) sclerotic (hardened) area caused by destruction of myelin sheath. Conduction of nerve impulses through the damaged area is slowed.

21.6). The sheaths deteriorate to *scleroses,* or hardened plaques or scars, in multiple regions. The loss of myelin sheaths leads to a slowing down of nerve impulses in the affected neurons. Since interactions among neurons are complex, slowing the impulses in even a few neurons can lead to severe neurological impairment.

The first symptoms occur at an average age of 33 years. Flare-ups are greatest during the first 3–4 years of the disease. In some people the first attack is so mild it escapes medical attention. In others, the first attack is not followed by another attack for 10–20 years. The cause of MS is unknown and there is no satisfactory treatment.[59]

First symptoms of MS may include muscular weakness in one or more extremity; pricking or burning sensations in the arms or legs; changes in the manner of walking; visual impairment, including double vision, and problems with color perception; constant involuntary movements of the eyeballs; speech impediment; incoordination, dizziness; and feelings of urinary urgency. As the disease progresses movement becomes increasingly impaired and mental function may also deteriorate. One attack follows another, usually every year or two. The result is a progressive loss of function interspersed with remission periods during which undamaged neurons again function normally.

As already stated, the cause of MS is unknown. It is currently believed to be an autoimmune process, possibly induced by prior exposure of the myelin sheath to some yet unidentified virus.[60] As with other autoimmune disorders, treatment often includes anti-inflammatory and immunosuppressive drugs given during acute attacks.

SEIZURE DISORDERS (EPILEPSIES)

Commonly called epilepsies, seizure disorders are a group of brain disorders, that can take the form of recurring sudden attacks of loss of consciousness, involuntary muscle contractions, or both. Seizure disorders are the second most common neurological disorder after stroke; about 1 percent of the population suffers from some form of seizure disorder. There are many types of seizure disorders; we will describe the three most common.

Absence (Petit Mal) Seizures

Absence seizures, formerly called *petit mal* epilepsy, are brief seizures in which a person loses contact with the environment for a few seconds, his or her eyes or muscles flutter, and sometimes he or she loses muscle tone. Absence seizures are believed to be hereditary, occur mainly in children, and rarely occur after 20 years of age. Persons having absence seizures usually do not fall down and after the attack may not even realize that it has occurred.

Complex Partial (Psychomotor) Seizures

Complex partial seizures, formerly called **psychomotor** seizures, are characterized by a one- to two-minute loss of contact with one's surroundings. Someone experiencing this attack is mentally confused, may stagger, perform purposeless move-

ments, and utter unintelligible sounds. He or she will not understand what others say and may refuse aid. Psychomotor attacks may begin at any age and are caused by physical injury to the brain.

Tonic-Clonic (Grand Mal) Seizures

Tonic-clonic seizures, formerly called *grand mal* seizures, include loss of consciousness, falling, and **convulsions,** which are sudden, repeated, and involuntary contractions of all of the body's muscles. There may be loss of bladder and bowel control. *Grand mal* seizures usually last two to five minutes. Sleep or confusion often follows these attacks. First aid for tonic-clonic attacks is described in Feature 21.6.

Causes of Seizure Disorders

The tendency toward some seizure disorders is inherited. When either parent has a personal or family history of seizures, their child has an increased risk of developing seizures. If both members of a couple have a history of seizures, the risk is quite high; in such cases, some physicians advise against having children.

Many seizures have no identifiable cause; others appear to be due to brain damage at birth, metabolic disturbances, infection, toxins, vascular disturbances, head injuries, or brain tumors and abscesses. In any case, random dispersed firings of neurons in the brain stimulate the muscles to contract. Many cases of seizure disorders result from head injuries; in these cases, heredity plays little or no role.[61] The relationship between head injuries and seizures is strong enough that many physicians automatically begin antiseizure medication following head injuries, without waiting to see if seizures occur.

Treating Seizure Disorders

Seizure disorders are effectively treated with medications, such as carbamazepine (Tegretol), pheny-

----

absence seizures seizures characterized by brief loss of contact with the environment, eye and muscle fluttering, and sometimes, loss of muscle tone.

complex partial seizures seizures characterized by a brief loss of contact with one's surroundings, mental confusion, staggering, and/or unintelligible sounds.

psychomotor physical activity associated with mental processes.

tonic-clonic convulsive episodes, accompanied by loss of consciousness and falling.

convulsion sudden and repeated involuntary contraction of all of the body's muscles.

FIRST AID FOR TONIC-CLONIC (GRAND MAL) SEIZURES

Tonic-clonic (grand mal) seizures are not uncommon and most of us will, at some time, be present when someone is experiencing one. What should be done?

1. *Do* move the person to a safe place (out of a street, for example) if necessary.

2. *Don't* try to restrain the convulsions.

3. *Do* place a sweater or folded jacket under the person's head.

4. *Do* loosen tight collars, ties, and so on.

5. *Do* turn the person on his or her side to help keep the airway clear.

6. *Don't* put anything in the person's mouth or between his or her teeth.

7. *Don't* try to give liquids during or just after the seizure.

8. *Don't* try to hold the person's tongue; it can't be swallowed.

9. *Do* look for a medical identification bracelet.

10. *Do* reassure the person when consciousness returns.

11. *Do*, after a single seizure that has lasted less than ten minutes, ask if the person wants medical assistance.

12. *Do*, if seizures are multiple or if one seizure lasts more than ten minutes, call for assistance or take the person to an emergency room.

toin (Dilantin), and valproic acid (Depkene). Once the correct dosage of the proper drug or combination of drugs is established, seizures can be completely controlled in the majority of cases.

People whose seizures are adequately controlled should be able to live active, full lives. Most can work, participate in sports, go to school, drive a car (if seizure control is complete), and have healthy children. For many, a major obstacle is lingering public misunderstanding of seizure disorders. The Epilepsy Foundation of America (see the *Study Guide* for address) and other organizations are actively working to overcome public prejudice against people who have had seizures.

ALZHEIMER'S DISEASE

Alzheimer's (*Alts'hī-merz*) **disease** is a degenerative brain disorder afflicting about 11 percent of the population over age 65. It affects over 4 million people and claims over 100,000 lives per year, and is the fourth leading cause of death among the elderly, after heart disease, cancer, and stroke. Its causes are unknown, and it has no cure.

Victims progressively lose their ability to read, write, talk, eat, and walk. The ability to reason and

....

Alzheimer's disease a degenerative brain disorder in which persons progressively lose the ability to read, write, talk, eat, and walk.

ability for self-care are lost. Bedridden and requiring total care, the person may die of pneumonia or some similar terminating complication.

Alzheimer's disease usually begins to develop between the ages of 40 and 60, and more often occurs in women than in men. Victims initially have trouble remembering recent events. Confusion, repeating of questions, and getting lost while traveling to familiar places are early symptoms. Gradually, over a period of time of several months to four or five years, past memories fade, and disorientation grows. Some experience paranoia, hallucinations, and violent mood changes.

Alzheimer's disease is difficult to diagnose, especially in its early stages, because of the lack of definitive tests. Only when well-advanced, and other possible causes have been ruled out, can probable diagnosis be made. Autopsied brains of victims show the presence of abnormal protein plaques deposited outside of neurons, loss of neurons, especially in brain regions important in memory and learning, and tangled protein filaments within neurons. The plaques consist of the accumulation of an abnormal protein called *beta amyloid*. These amyloid plaques are thought to be toxic to neurons and responsible for the loss of those neurons responsible for learning and memory.[62]

Researchers studying the disease are focusing on genetic factors that appear to be involved, on possible viral links, and how these two factors may interact with each other.[63] Other factors, such as toxic environmental chemicals, are also being examined.[64] So far, no suggestions for prevention or cures have emerged from this research.

KIDNEY DISORDERS

The excretory system consists of two *kidneys,* two *ureters* that carry urine from the kidneys to the *bladder,* and the *urethra,* which carries urine from the bladder to the exterior of the body (see Figure 21.7). The kidneys lie in the back of the abdominal cavity, just below the bottom rib. Because of the kidneys' location, pain from a kidney problem can be mistaken for a backache.

Kidneys remove not only excess water, but also many toxic waste products and surplus chemicals from the body. Although the total loss of kidney function no longer carries the certainty of death that it did in the past, kidney disorders are still considered very serious and are responsible for many physical restrictions.

People who lose kidney function must either receive kidney transplants or undergo frequent dialysis. Transplants require suppression of the immune mechanism to prevent rejection and still, some transplant attempts fail.

Dialysis is inconvenient, carries risk of infection, and is not as selective as a living kidney. It is either performed by circulating one's blood through a dialysis machine or by performing a fluid wash of the abdominal cavity several times a day. People who depend on dialysis are never quite as healthy as people who have normal kidney func-

tion. Taking care of your kidneys is essential as there is no regeneration of a damaged kidney—*kidney damage is permanent.*

SYMPTOMS OF URINARY DISORDERS

If a developing urinary problem is detected early enough, it may be corrected before serious loss of kidney function occurs. Thus, it is important to recognize when a problem arises and promptly consult with a physician for any of the symptoms of urinary problems:

1. *Increased urinary frequency.* This can be a symptom of an infection of the bladder or urethra. If not treated, these infections can spread into the kidneys, causing severe and permanent damage. In men, frequent urination can also result from prostate disorders (see next item).

2. *Difficulty in starting urine flow or weak flow of urine.* These problems, in males, are often associated with disorders of the prostate gland. Swelling of the prostate may pinch the urethra as it passes through the prostate. The bladder then fails to empty completely, causing frequent urination and contributing to the development of **cystitis** (*sis-tī´tis*), an inflammation of the bladder usually associated with infection. Cystitis is also very common in women due to the more moist condition of the opening to the urinary duct and the shorter length of the duct than in men.

3. *Burning or stinging during urination.* In either sex, painful urination is often caused by bacterial infection of the urethra or bladder. These infections may spread on up into the kidneys.

4. *Urethral discharge or unusual appearance of urine.* These symptoms may indicate bacterial infection and a physician should be consulted promptly.

5. *Pain in the lower back or side.* This could indicate an infection or a "stone," technically called a **calculus** (*kal´kū-lus*), in the kidney or ureter (see Feature 21.7).

dialysis the process of circulating the blood through a machine to remove toxic materials, or by performing a fluid wash of the abdominal cavity, in cases of impaired kidney function.

cystitis inflammation of the urinary bladder, usually associated with infection.

calculus an abnormal stonelike deposit, usually of mineral salts, somewhere in the body.

Figure 21.7
The Human Urinary System

Each kidney receives blood and returns it to circulation after excess water and wastes are removed. The ureters carry urine from the kidneys to the bladder, while the urethra carries urine from the bladder to the exterior of the body.

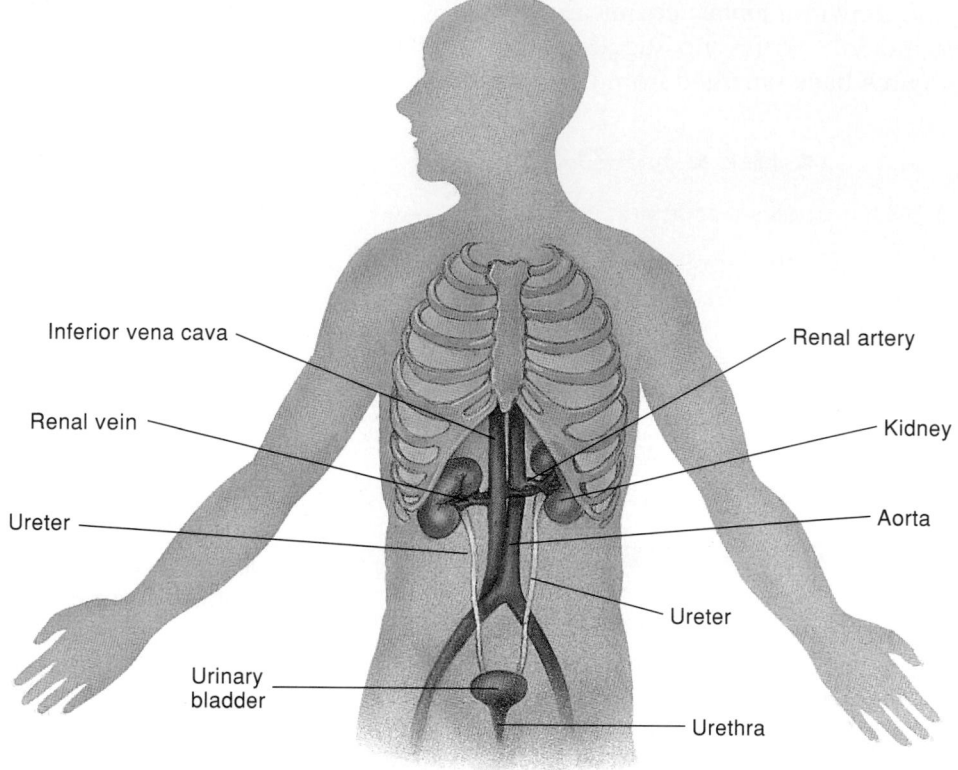

Inferior vena cava
Renal vein
Ureter
Urinary bladder
Renal artery
Kidney
Aorta
Ureter
Urethra

6. *Edema (swelling of tissues).* Edema of the hands, face, feet, ankles, or other body parts indicates an excess accumulation of fluid in the tissues. Edema can be caused by severe loss of kidney function, heart problems, too much salt in the diet, high blood pressure, or other conditions. Edema should always receive the prompt attention of a physician.

7. *High blood pressure.* High blood pressure can be either a cause or a symptom of kidney damage. Like the other symptoms listed here, it must receive prompt medical attention.

MAINTAINING KIDNEY HEALTH

Much kidney disease can be prevented by taking the following precautions:

- *Drink plenty of nonalcoholic fluids.* This can help prevent formation of kidney and bladder stones (see Feature 21.7) and the flushing effect of abundant dilute urine can help prevent infections of the kidney, bladder, or urethra. It is uncertain whether fruit juices, such as cranberry juice, have any value to

the urinary system beyond the liquid they provide.

- *Urinate as soon as practical when the need is felt.* Holding urine for long periods of time stretches the bladder, and promotes infection.

- *Urinate after sexual intercourse.* Vigorous intercourse can force bacteria up into the urethra; urination may flush them away before they can establish infection.

- *Promptly treat high blood pressure.* High blood pressure can result in serious kidney damage, causing thickening and hardening of microscopic blood vessels within the kidneys, which reduces the kidneys' ability to concentrate waste products in the urine.[65]

- *Avoid toxic chemicals.* Some chemicals, such as mercury and lead, are quite destructive to the kidneys. Mercury exposure is usually occupational, while the main sources of lead include old house paint and the glazes on some imported dinnerware items (see Chapter 24, p. 775).

FEATURE 21.7

URINARY STONES

Occasionally crystals of salts present in urine solidify into insoluble "stones," or calculi. Calculi may be formed in any part of the urinary tract. They may occur in the kidney (renal calculi), ureters, bladder, or urethra (see Figure 21.7). (Stones may also occur in the pancreas, gallbladder, and prostate gland.) Once formed, the stones may block the flow of urine from the kidney or bladder, causing infection and excruciating pain.

The stones are composed of various chemicals, but commonly consist of calcium oxalate, uric acid, and calcium phosphate crystals. Stones have many causes, including inherited metabolic disorders, inadequate fluid intake, immobility (which causes resorption of calcium from the bones into the blood and urine), and excessive intake of Vitamin D.

The method of treating urinary stones depends upon the type of stone and its underlying causes. Sometimes medicines can relax the smooth muscle of the urinary system and allow passage. Sometimes surgical removal is required. A newer and less-expensive therapy requiring no incision is **shock wave lithotripsy** (*lith'ō-trip-sē*). High-intensity sound waves bombard the stones, breaking them up into tiny fragments that can pass with the urine. Lithotripsy requires minimal recovery time.

Prevention of further stones almost always involves increased fluid intake. Specific drugs may be prescribed depending on the type of stones that have been a problem. Also, depending on the type of stones, the urine may either be acidified or alkalinized through dietary adjustments.

CHECKPOINT

1. What are the symptoms of a possible disorder in the urinary system?

2. What things can you do to maintain a healthy urinary system?

RESPIRATORY DISORDERS

Physical stamina, endurance, and the overall health of your body depends on the ability of the lungs to provide the blood with enough oxygen. Respiratory disorders rank high on the list of causes for disability and death. Fortunately, the incidence of many respiratory problems can be reduced by healthful behaviors such as not smoking and by seeking prompt treatment for respiratory infections. Some of these diseases cause some degree of obstruction of the flow of air into and/or out of the lungs. The term *chronic obstructive pulmonary disease (COPD)* is used in reference to asthma, bronchitis, and emphysema. Such obstruction is indicated by symptoms such as coughing, wheezing, and dyspnea (painful or labored breathing). We will discuss four major obstructive lung disorders, in which the flow of air into and/or out of the lungs is in some way restricted. The first of these disorders, asthma, is usually episodical—it occurs in definite episodes or attacks, with symptomless periods in between the episodes. The other

three—chronic bronchitis, emphysema, and cystic fibrosis—are all forms in which the flow of air is restricted all or much of the time.

ASTHMA

Asthma attacks make breathing very difficult by narrowing the bronchioles, which are the many small tubes inside the lungs (see Figure 21.8). Between 8 and 10 million people in the United States suffer from asthma. The disease affects people of all ages and is the most common cause of chronic illness in children under age 17.[66]

Asthma is characterized by a temporary spasm (constriction) of the bronchioles, swelling of the mucous membrane that lines the bronchioles, and increased production of mucus. When an asthma attack occurs, breathing becomes labored, and the victim wheezes and experiences shortness of breath. An attack can be mild or so severe that immediate medical treatment is required. Asthma attacks can be precipitated by one or more of the following:

- allergic reactions (the most common cause), such as to dust, pollen, and animal hair
- bacterial infections

shock wave lithotripsy crushing of a calculus in the bladder or urethra by the use of high-intensity sound waves.

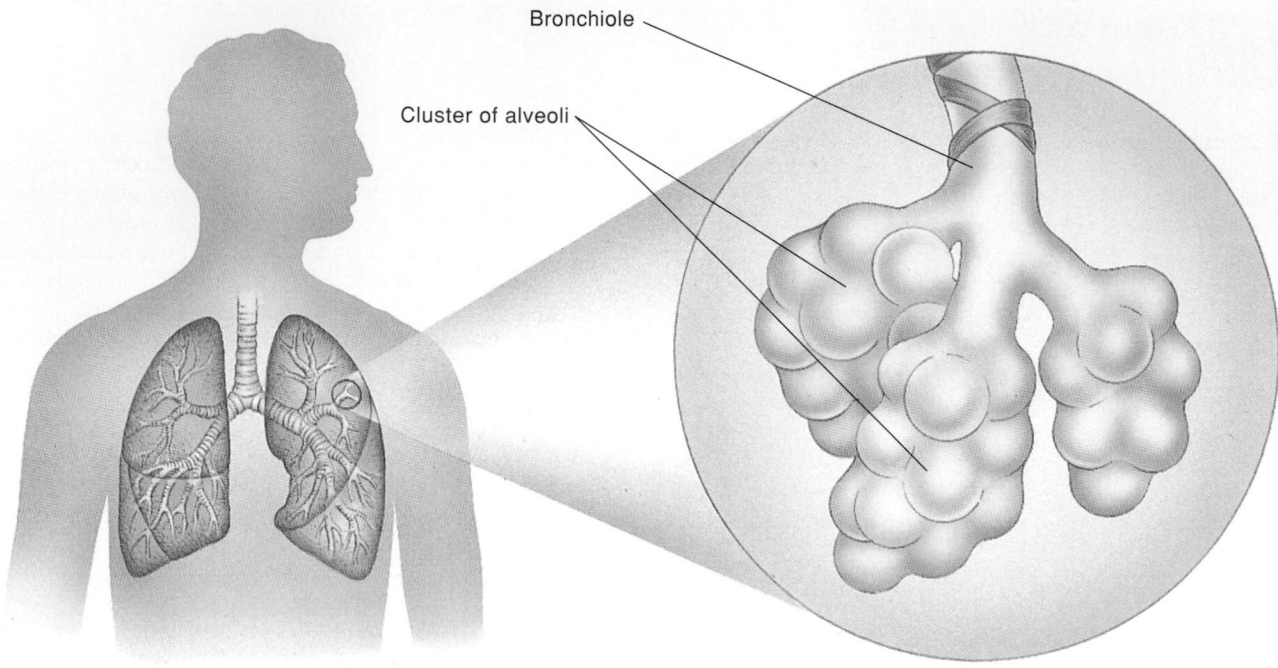

Bronchiole

Cluster of alveoli

Figure 21.8

Microscopic Structure of the Lungs

Each spongelike lung consists of millions of microscopic air sacs (alveoli) supplied with air by tiny tubes (bronchioles). Asthma consists of temporary episodes of obstruction of airflow through the bronchioles. In chronic bronchitis, such obstruction is an ongoing problem.

- vigorous exercise, especially in cold air
- weather changes
- fatigue
- various drugs, including aspirin and ibuprofen
- exposure to fumes, such as cigarette smoke
- emotional conflict or stressful situations

Asthma should receive adequate medical treatment under supervision of a physician. Treatment may include inhaling bronchodilators such as *corticosteroids*. Prolonged or repeated asthma attacks can cause permanent damage to the lungs and heart.

CHRONIC BRONCHITIS

Chronic bronchitis is caused by an inflammation of the bronchi, and characterized by the enlargement and increased activity of the mucus-secreting glands lining the airways. This is a chronic condition in which a considerable amount of greenish-yellowish *sputum* may be coughed up every day.

The raising of sputum, defined as a productive cough, is the most prominent feature of chronic bronchitis. The disease is characterized by inflammation and swelling of the bronchioles and overproduction of mucus. Viral and bacterial infections are common and are often a result, rather than a cause, of the problem.

As the disease progresses, shortness of breath develops, due to airway obstruction. Breathing becomes increasingly labored, at first during exertion and eventually when the person is at rest. The skin may take on a blue tone, indicating poor oxygenation of the blood. In advanced cases, the fingertips become clubbed (see Figure 21.9), also a result of insufficient oxygen. In contrast with people with emphysema, those with chronic bronchitis usually maintain a normal or elevated body weight. Chronic bronchitis places a great burden on the heart and often leads to death from heart failure.

Chronic bronchitis is caused by chronic irritation from inhaled substances and fumes, and from recurrent infections. In the United States, smoking is the most frequent cause of chronic bronchitis.[67] Other causes include the following:

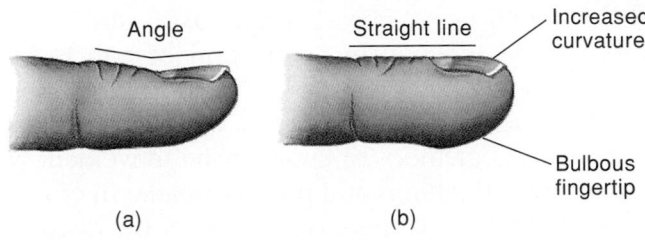

Angle   Straight line   Increased curvature

Bulbous fingertip

(a)   (b)

Figure 21.9
Clubbed Fingers in Bronchitis

Clubbing of the fingers is common in chronic bronchitis and is a result of inadequate oxygen supply. (a) Normal fingertip—note angle formed by nail and finger; (b) clubbed finger—note relatively straight line formed by nail and finger, also increased curvature of nail.

- breathing "secondhand" smoke
- occupational exposure to irritating chemicals

Whatever the cause, chronic bronchitis should be promptly treated under direction of a physician. Treatments include:

- avoidance of cigarette smoking and environmental irritants
- prompt antibiotic treatment of respiratory infections
- maintenance of optimal nutrition and adequate fluid intake
- medications such as epinephrine or theophylline

- physical therapy
- oxygen in advanced cases

EMPHYSEMA

Emphysema (em-fi-sē'ma) is characterized by a breakdown of the walls of the microscopic alveoli (air sacs) at the ends of the bronchioles, producing large air spaces that remain filled with air during expiration (see Figure 21.10). Several tiny sacs break down to form one larger sac. Air becomes trapped within the lungs because they have lost their elastic fiber. This larger sac offers less surface area for absorption of oxygen than did the combined walls of the former smaller air sacs. Further, the lungs lose their elasticity, limiting the amount of air that can be exhaled (see the section of this chapter on lung cancer, p. 662). Any small degree of exertion causes shortness of breath. The key symptom is a reduced forced expiratory volume. The person has to work voluntarily to exhale. Over a period of time the added exertion increases the size of the chest cage, resulting in a "barrel chest" typical of the emphysema sufferer.

With less surface area within the lungs for gas exchange, less oxygen is absorbed. Blood oxygen levels are lowered, and any mild exercise that increases the oxygen needs of the cells leaves the person breathless. All of this places an added burden on the heart, because the heart must attempt to pump enough blood through the lungs to meet the

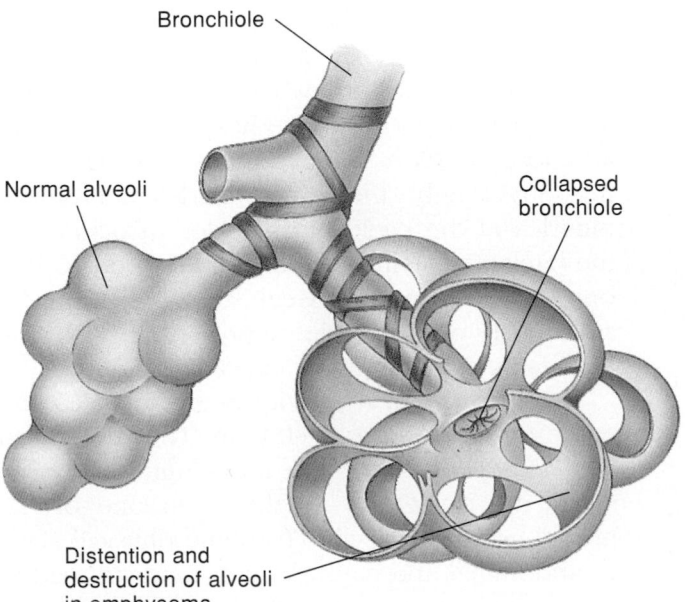

Bronchiole

Normal alveoli

Collapsed bronchiole

Distention and destruction of alveoli in emphysema

Figure 21.10
Emphysema

The bronchiole and alveoli to the left are normal while the bronchiole and alveoli to the right are typical of emphysema. The ability to move air into and out of the lungs is reduced by loss of elasticity of lung tissue, while the capacity for absorption of oxygen into the blood is reduced by loss of alveolar surface area.

body's oxygen needs. As in chronic bronchitis, the risk of heart failure is increased.

Blood circulates with difficulty through lungs damaged by emphysema. This creates a great burden on the heart, because the heart must pump all of the blood through the lungs before it can circulate to the body. As in chronic bronchitis, death often results from heart failure.

There are several known or suspected causes of emphysema, the most important of which is smoking. The risk of emphysema increases with the number of cigarettes smoked. A second cause is an inherited deficiency of a body chemical (alpha$_1$-antitrypsin) that blocks the action of protein-dissolving enzymes. Without alpha$_1$-antitrypsin, these enzymes destroy the alveolar walls. There is also evidence that smoking, over time, reduces the level of alpha$_1$-antitrypsin.[68]

There is no way to restore alveoli destroyed by emphysema; the most one can hope to do is to arrest its further development. Emphysema is treated in the same ways as chronic bronchitis.

CYSTIC FIBROSIS

Cystic fibrosis, a hereditary disease affecting 30,000 newborns each year, is a hereditary disease transmitted as a recessive gene.[69] The disease accordingly only affects children who have received this gene from both parents. Cystic fibrosis causes the production and accumulation of sticky mucus in the pancreas, lungs, and sweat glands. Usually beginning in infancy, cystic fibrosis causes severe obstruction of the airflow in the bronchioles. The secretion inflames the passageways, which respond by producing connective tissue that blocks the passageways. The pancreatic ducts also become blocked, reducing the amount of pancreatic fluid reaching the intestine. This fluid helps in the digestion of fats; consequently, the person absorbs fewer fat molecules and the fat-soluble vitamins carried by them. Thus Vitamin A, Vitamin D, and Vitamin K deficiency is common. Other aspects of the disease include very salty sweat

---

cystic fibrosis a hereditary disease causing production and accumulation of sticky mucus in the pancreas, lungs, and sweat glands.

(babies with cystic fibrosis often taste salty when kissed) and inadequate production of pancreatic digestive enzymes.

Treatment of cystic fibrosis includes medical and physical methods to improve the movement of mucus from the lungs and prompt treatment of respiratory infections. There is no cure for the disease, but the use of effective antibiotics has prolonged the life of many patients.

CHECKPOINT

1. What is the difference between asthma and COPD?

2. What is actually taking place in asthma, chronic bronchitis, emphysema, and cystic fibrosis?

3. What is the most important cause of chronic bronchitis and emphysema?

BACK PROBLEMS

One of the most common physical complaints has to do with low back pain. About 192 million, or 80 percent, of people in this country have trouble with lower back pain at some time.[70] Seventy-five million people in the United States suffer from chronic low back pain, of which about 80 percent is preventable. Few people are able to totally avoid low back pain.[71]

People may say their "back is out," or that they have a "slipped disc." Most likely, a muscle has been strained or torn while the spine is out of alignment, or poor posture has been practiced. In addition, the term "back muscles" can be misleading. Structurally, the term includes not only the muscles of the back, but muscles *associated* with the back; they fall into four muscle groups. If any one of these groups is weak, the alignment of the spine will be affected, putting strain on it and increasing the chances of backache.

Lack of physical activity is the most common cause of chronic low back pain. The strength of a muscle depends on its size and length. Many backaches are caused by weakness in one or more groups of back muscles. Too little physical activity of abdominal and back muscles tends to lead to a

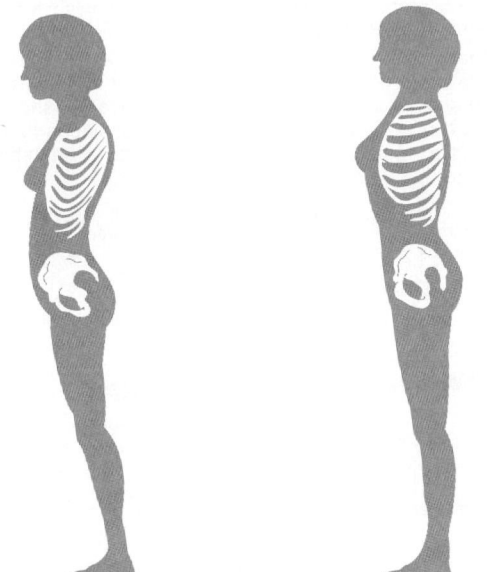

Figure 21.11
Back Alignment

Incorrect (left) and correct (right) pelvic alignment.

Source: Hoeger, W., and Hoeger, S. Fitness & Wellness, Englewood, CO: Morton, 1993, p. 51.

forward tilt of the pelvis (Figure 21.11), which puts pressure on the spinal vertebrae, producing pain in the lower back. Some people have tight hamstring muscles, which pull on the pelvis, causing pelvic tilt. The accumulative storage of fat around the midsection of the body can also contribute to the forward tilt of the pelvis, adding to the pain. Low back pain is often related to faulty posture and improper bodily positions when sleeping, sitting, standing, walking, driving, and exercising. Incorrect posture not only puts unnecessary strain on back muscles, but on joints, ligaments, and various bones as well (Figure 21.12). Back pain may also be due to herniated disks, an increasingly common cause among younger people. Some research is linking stress levels to back pain.

Specific stretching and strengthening exercises can reduce the frequency and severity of low back pains. But, if the back pains are serious or persistent, you should first see your physician, who can determine if there is any other cause for the pain. The physician might also prescribe some physical therapy, muscle relaxant, or anti-inflammatory medication. Once pain-free, the patient can start a back muscle strengthening program. The incidence

of low back pain can be greatly reduced, or even prevented, by using specific stretching and strengthening exercises as a part of any program of physical exercise. Specific exercises for rehabilitating the back may be prescribed by a physical fitness instructor, physical therapist, or physician.

SUMMARY

Cancer is second only to cardiovascular disorders as a leading cause of death in developed countries. Cancer affects people of every age and ethnic group, and often is the result of environmental factors. Cancer can affect almost any body part and is classified by the type of tissue in which it originates. Of particular concern are cancers of the lung, breast, skin, prostate, testes, cervix, colon, and rectum. Cancer therapies include surgery, radiation, and chemotherapy.

Diabetes is a group of diseases causing excessive urination. Most commonly the term is used in reference to diabetes mellitus, a disorder of carbohydrate metabolism. Two forms of diabetes mellitus occur: insulin-dependent diabetes mellitus (IDDM) normally develops in children and adolescents, and non-insulin-dependent diabetes mellitus (NIDDM) commonly develops in people over age 40.

Arthritis is a painful inflammation of the joints. It occurs in more than a hundred forms. A common form of arthritis is rheumatoid arthritis, in which a person's joints are attacked by his or her own immune system. Neurological disorders that commonly occur include headaches, multiple sclerosis, epilepsy, and Alzheimer's disease.

Kidney disorders may lead to an inability to rid the body of excess water, toxic wastes, and surplus chemicals. Respiratory disorders impede the ability of the body to obtain sufficient oxygen. Chronic obstructive pulmonary disease (COPD) includes asthma, bronchitis, and emphysema. Back problems, which affect about 80 percent of all people in this country, are often preventable through proper exercising.

Many degenerative health problems threaten your well-being. Though it may seem that luck dictates who is affected by these conditions, the reality is that many of the disorders described in this chapter can be entirely prevented by healthful living habits. For those diseases that cannot be avoid-

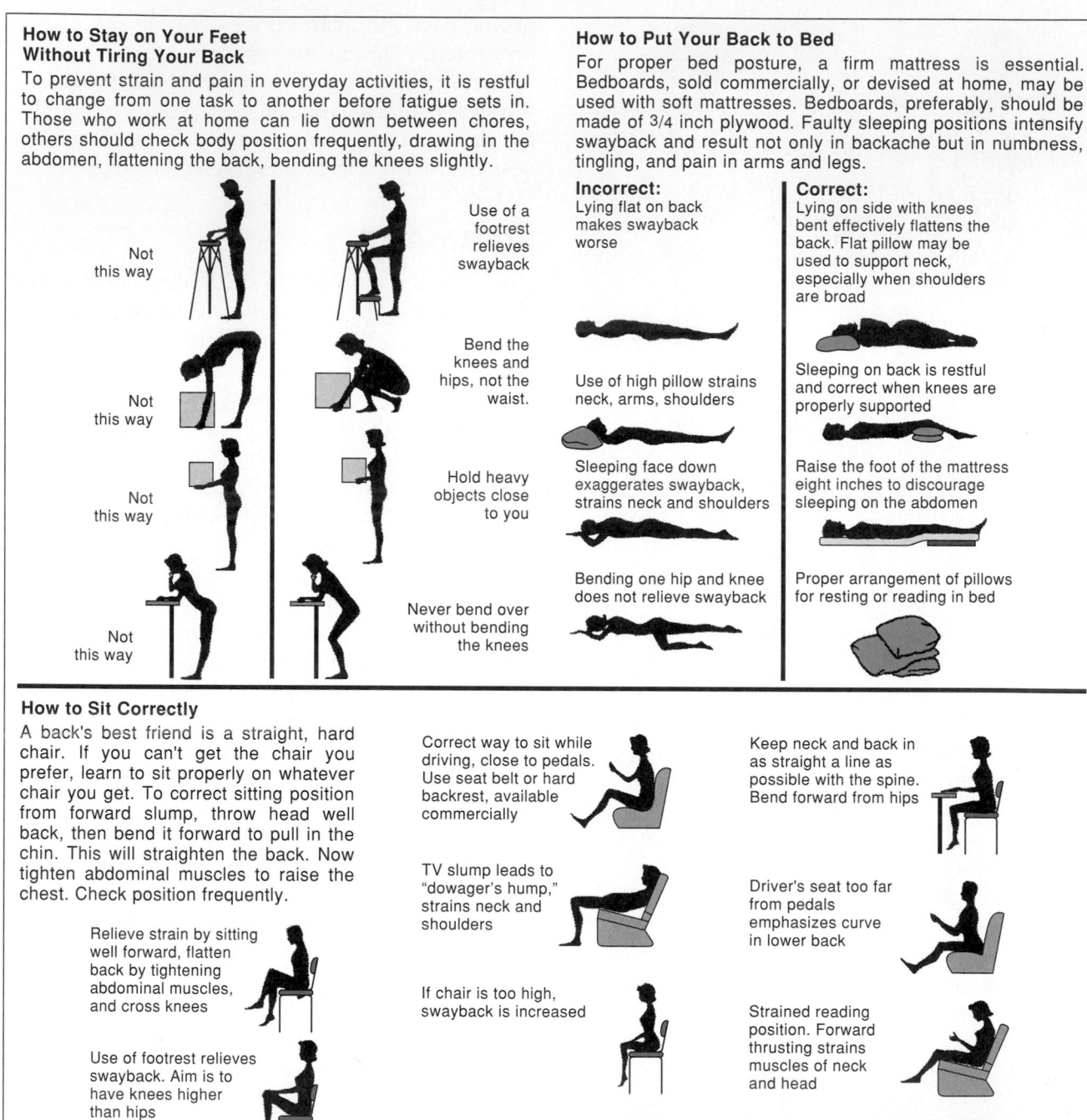

How to Stay on Your Feet Without Tiring Your Back

To prevent strain and pain in everyday activities, it is restful to change from one task to another before fatigue sets in. Those who work at home can lie down between chores, others should check body position frequently, drawing in the abdomen, flattening the back, bending the knees slightly.

Not this way

Use of a footrest relieves swayback

Not this way

Bend the knees and hips, not the waist.

Not this way

Hold heavy objects close to you

Not this way

Never bend over without bending the knees

How to Put Your Back to Bed

For proper bed posture, a firm mattress is essential. Bedboards, sold commercially, or devised at home, may be used with soft mattresses. Bedboards, preferably, should be made of 3/4 inch plywood. Faulty sleeping positions intensify swayback and result not only in backache but in numbness, tingling, and pain in arms and legs.

Incorrect:
Lying flat on back makes swayback worse

Correct:
Lying on side with knees bent effectively flattens the back. Flat pillow may be used to support neck, especially when shoulders are broad

Use of high pillow strains neck, arms, shoulders

Sleeping on back is restful and correct when knees are properly supported

Sleeping face down exaggerates swayback, strains neck and shoulders

Raise the foot of the mattress eight inches to discourage sleeping on the abdomen

Bending one hip and knee does not relieve swayback

Proper arrangement of pillows for resting or reading in bed

How to Sit Correctly

A back's best friend is a straight, hard chair. If you can't get the chair you prefer, learn to sit properly on whatever chair you get. To correct sitting position from forward slump, throw head well back, then bend it forward to pull in the chin. This will straighten the back. Now tighten abdominal muscles to raise the chest. Check position frequently.

Relieve strain by sitting well forward, flatten back by tightening abdominal muscles, and cross knees

Use of footrest relieves swayback. Aim is to have knees higher than hips

Correct way to sit while driving, close to pedals. Use seat belt or hard backrest, available commercially

TV slump leads to "dowager's hump," strains neck and shoulders

If chair is too high, swayback is increased

Keep neck and back in as straight a line as possible with the spine. Bend forward from hips

Driver's seat too far from pedals emphasizes curve in lower back

Strained reading position. Forward thrusting strains muscles of neck and head

Reproduced with permission of Schering Corporation. Copyright Schering Corporation, Kenilworth, NJ.

Figure 21.12
Your Back and How to Care for It

ed, their impact on your life can be minimized by early detection and prompt, effective treatment. Assuming responsibility for your own health is essential for disease prevention, early detection, and effective treatment. In essence, you can and must participate in your own personal wellness.

REFERENCES

1. National Cancer Institute. *What You Need to Know About Prostate Cancer.* National Institutes of Health Publ. No. 90-1576, 1990.
2. Coleman, R., et al. *Fundamental Immunology,* 2nd ed. Dubuque, IA: Brown, 1992.

3. American Cancer Society. *Cancer Facts and Figures, 1993.* New York: American Cancer Society, 1993.

4. Tortora, G., and Grabowski, S. *Principles of Anatomy and Physiology,* 7th ed. New York: HarperCollins, 1993.

5. Thomas, P. "Oncogenes: Redirecting the Clinical Attack on Cancer." *Medical World News* (23 February 1987), 28–36.

6. American Cancer Society, op. cit.

7. Ibid.

8. Ibid.

9. Ibid.

10. Tortora, op. cit.

11. American Cancer Society, op. cit.

12. Zuckerman, M. "Battling Breast Cancer." *U.S. News and World Report* 23 (November 1992), 104.

13. American Cancer Society, op. cit.

14. Rubin, R. "The Breast Cancer Scare." *U.S. News and World Report* (15 March 1993), 68–72.

15. Cowley, G. "In Pursuit of a Terrible Killer." *Newsweek* (10 December 1990), 66–68.

16. Boston Women's Health Book Collective. *The New Our Bodies, Ourselves.* New York: Touchstone, 1992.

17. National Women's Health Network. "The Latest Studies in Breast Cancer and OC." *The Network News* 2 (1989), p. 4.

18. American Cancer Society, op. cit.

19. Rubin, op. cit.

20. Boston Women's Health Book Collective, op. cit.

21. Ibid.

22. American Cancer Society, op. cit.

23. Ibid.

24. Ibid.

25. Ibid.

26. Murphy, G. "Cancer of the Male Reproductive System." In Holleb, A. (ed.), *The American Cancer Society Cancer Book.* Garden City, NY: Doubleday, 1986.

27. American Cancer Society, op. cit.

28. Ibid.

29. DiVita, V., et al. "Modern Cancer Therapy." In Holleb, A. (ed.), *The American Cancer Society Cancer Book.* Garden City, NY: Doubleday, 1986.

30. Skolnick, A. "Opinions Vary, But Some Recommend Hitting Certain Cancers 'Harder and Earlier'." *JAMA* 17 (1991), 2165–2171.

31. Freireich, E. "Experimental Treatments and Research." In Holleb, A. (ed.), *The American Cancer Society Cancer Book.* Garden City, NY: Doubleday, 1986.

32. Coleman, op. cit.

33. Ibid.

34. Herbert, V. "Questionable Cancer Remedies." In Holleb, A. (ed.), *The American Cancer Society Cancer Book.* Garden City, NY: Doubleday, 1986.

35. American Cancer Society, op. cit.

36. Ibid.

37. Crowley, op. cit.

38. American Cancer Society, op. cit.

39. Whitney, E., and Rolfes, S. *Understanding Nutrition,* 6th ed. St. Paul: West, 1993.

40. Grosvenor, M. "Diet and Colon Cancer." *Nutrition and the M.D.* 4 (1989).

41. Bingham, S. "Meat, Starch, and Nonstarch Polysaccharides and Large Bowel Cancer." *American Journal of Clinical Nutrition* 48 (1988), 762–776.

42. Coleman, op. cit.

43. Whitney, op. cit.

44. Ibid.

45. Tortora, op. cit.

46. Porth, C. *Pathophysiology,* 3rd ed. Philadelphia: Lippincott, 1990.

47. Tortora, op. cit.

48. Coleman, op. cit.

49. Hurley, D. "On the Trail of a Diabetes Cure." *Medical World News* (September 1992), 16–17.

50. Whitney, op. cit.

51. Tortora, op. cit.

52. Porth, op. cit.

53. Coleman, op. cit.

54. Lillioja, S., et al. "Impaired Glucose Tolerance as a Disorder of Insulin Action." *New England Journal of Medicine* 318 (1988), 1217–1225.

55. Whitney, op. cit.

56. Coleman, op. cit.

57. Ibid.

58. Porth, op. cit.

59. Tortora, op. cit.

60. Ibid.

61. Ibid.

62. Ibid.

63. Ibid.

64. "Update: Alzheimer's/Aluminum." *University of California at Berkeley Wellness Letter* (April 1993).

65. Porth, op. cit.

66. Ibid.

67. Ibid.

68. Ibid.

69. Glick, D. and Hager, M. "When DNA Isn't Destiny." *Newsweek* (6 December 1993), 53–54.

70. Althoff, S., et al. *Choices in Health and Fitness for Life,* 2nd ed. Scottsdale, AZ: Gorsick Scarisbrick, 1992.

71. Hoeger, W., and Hoeger, S., *Fitness and Wellness,* 2nd ed. Englewood, CO: Morton, 1993.

SUGGESTED READINGS

American Cancer Society. *Cancer Facts and Figures, 1993.* New York: American Cancer Society, 1993.

Arthritis Foundation. *Understanding Arthritis.* New York: Scribner's, 1984.

Brackenridge, B., and Dolinar, R. *Diabetes 101,* 2nd ed. Minneapolis: Chronimed, 1993.

Dollinger, M., et. al. *Everyone's Guide to Cancer Therapy.* Toronto: Somerville, 1991.

Edelwick, J., and Brodsky, A. *Diabetes: Caring for Your Emotions as Well as Your Health.* Reading, MA: Addison-Wesley, 1986.

Fries, J. *Arthritis.* Reading, MA: Addison-Wesley, 1990.

Hoeger, W., and Hoeger, S. *Fitness and Wellness,* 2nd ed. Englewood, CO: Morton, 1993.

Holleb, A. (ed.). *The American Cancer Society Cancer Book.* Garden City, NY: Doubleday, 1986.

Kunz, J., and Finkel, A. *The American Medical Association Family Medical Guide,* rev. ed. New York: Random, 1987.

Morra, M., and Potts, E. *Choices, Realistic Alternatives in Cancer Treatment,* rev. ed. New York: Avon, 1987.

Rosenbloom, A., and Tonnessen, D. *Living with Diabetes.* New York: Plume, 1993.

Thygerson, A. *Fitness and Health: Life-Style Strategies.* Boston: Jones and Bartlett, 1989.

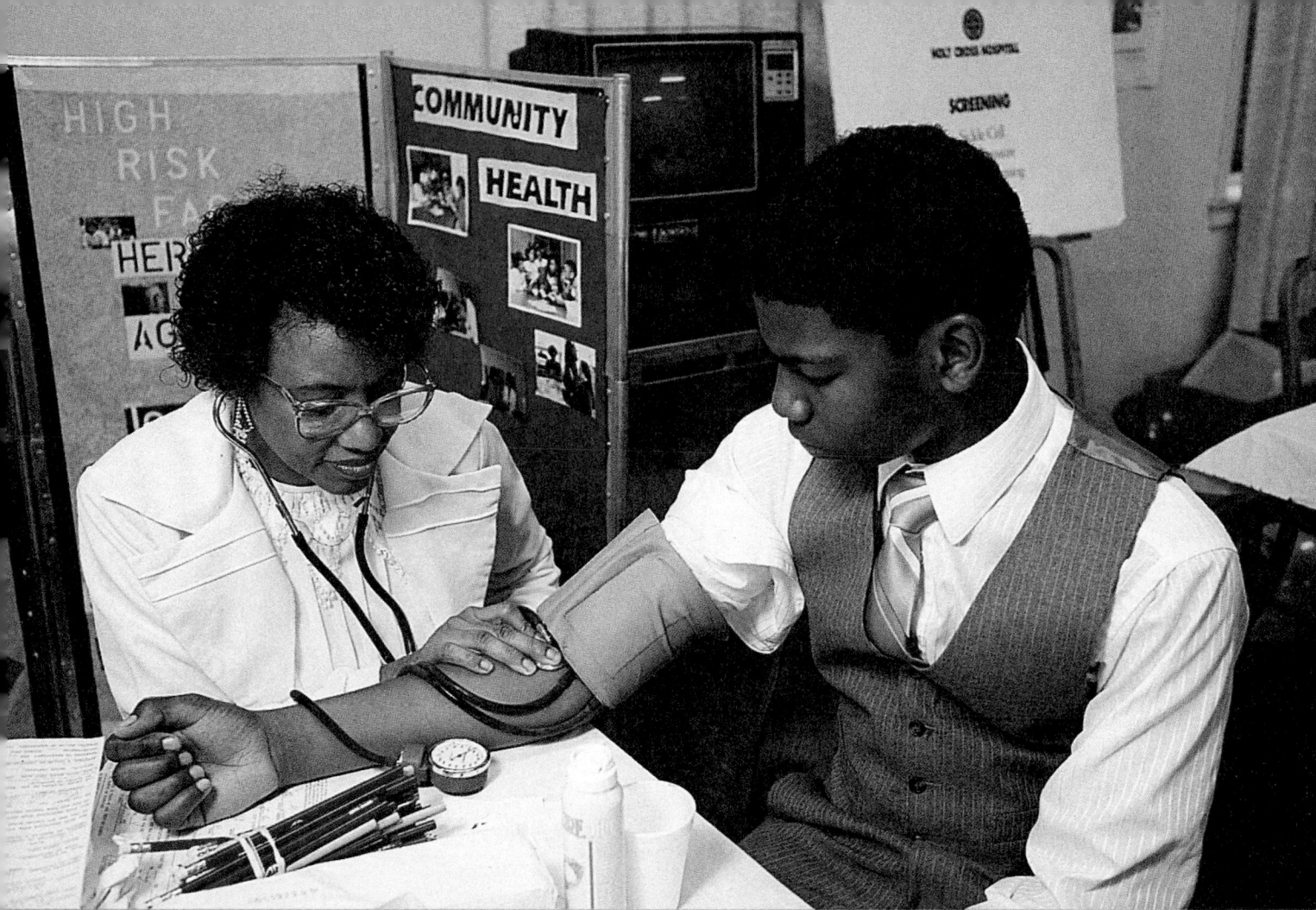

EIGHT

CONSUMER ACTION AND ENVIRONMENTAL HEALTH

We usually think of ourselves as consumers only when we are purchasing a product or a service. Often we attach value to something only when money changes hands.

When we buy cough medicine or a pair of sunglasses, we are buying a product that relates to our well-being. If for no other reason than we are contributing to the profit of the manufacturer, we have the responsibility to demand drugs and cosmetics that are both safe and effective. We also pay for the expertise of physicians and dentists, and of hospitals and nursing homes. Since our well-being is at stake, we have the right to expect qualified and affordable health care. The availability of health services to all should be an absolute right.

While it may be easy not to place environmental concerns into the same perspective as goods and services we exchange money for, there is no mistaking the ultimate costs to each of us of polluted water and air, and of noise and radiation pollution. All of our efforts to achieve internal well-being mean little if our external world is unusable. This unit concludes this text by placing all of our collective health concerns into a global perspective.

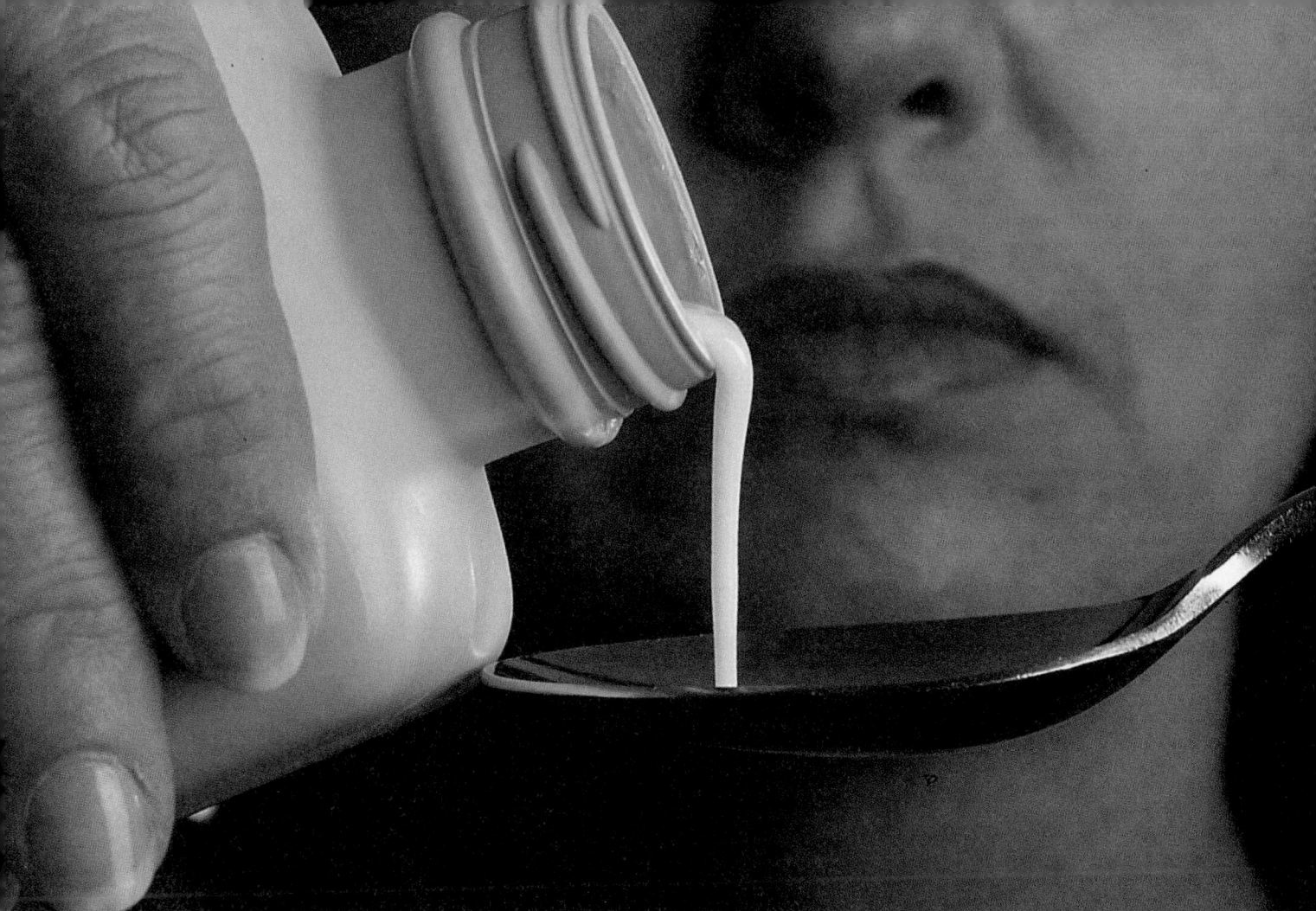

22

HEALTH FOR THE SMART CONSUMER

CHAPTER OBJECTIVES

Upon completing this chapter, you will be able to:

KNOWLEDGE

- List the benefits of taking charge of your health.
- Identify the amount of training required to become a pharmacist.
- Explain the risks of multiple drug use.
- Contrast the actions of an expectorant with those of a cough suppressant.
- Define a cosmetic.
- Discuss the risks of ultraviolet radiation.
- Distinguish between the functions of an ophthalmologist and an optometrist.
- Identify the conditions under which cavities in teeth occur.
- Classify the available home test kits.
- List the top ten health frauds.

INSIGHT

- Identify the ways in which you can gain assistance from your pharmacist in your drug choices.
- Explain all of the possible benefits of aspirin use versus all of the hazards.
- Explain which type of sunglasses you should select based on UV-A/UV-B radiation protection.
- Outline the tips to observe when using home health tests.

DECISION MAKING

- Decide which factors are important to you when deciding between a brand name vs. a generic form of a drug.
- Identify ways in which you intend to become more selective when purchasing OTC medications.
- Decide the criteria you intend to use in choosing pain-relief medication in the future.
- Identify the criteria you might use in deciding which SPF to look for when selecting a sunscreen.
- Decide how you intend to protect yourself against quack health products and procedures.

The tonics and snake oils that were once sold by salesmen from wagons that traveled across the country still exist. Gone are the wagons, but all too prevalent are the individuals and companies selling their wonder drugs and fountains of youth capitalizing on trusting, hopeful people. At particular risk are groups such as those with terminal illnesses and older persons. However, one recent federal investigation led to a 198-count indictment that will, we can only hope, send a message to these modern-day snake oil salesmen.

A federal grand jury in San Diego returned that indictment in response to charges against five individuals and five corporations that have been smuggling into the country tons of substances purported to enhance sexual vitality and reverse the aging process. Those who were indicted only represent a small portion of the health fraud problem in the United States. The anti-aging-drug market alone is estimated to be worth $2 billion per year.

These products were primarily of three types. Zumba Forte is billed as a "sexual tonic." Procaine hydrochloride derivatives known as Gerovital are advertised as rejuvenation products and as treatment for Parkinson's disease, hypertension, and neuralgia. Cell therapy products isolate ribonucleic acid from the organs and tissues of young sheep or cattle and are promoted to cure over a hundred medical conditions, including sterility.

Among the 15 tons of anti-aging drugs found during this investigation, many can cause very serious health problems, even death. For example, one of the primary ingredients in these "fountain of youth" drugs is yohimbine, which is considered dangerous to those who have renal (kidney) disease. Kidney disease is common among those who would be most likely to buy an anti-aging drug.

This type of drug therapy is not only bogus, it is dangerous. In almost all cases, the Food and Drug Administration has no idea how these drugs are manufactured or what their ingredients are. Indictments such as the one in San Diego should send a message to modern-day "snake oil salesmen." The public must be educated as well, so they will be less vulnerable to these potentially deadly treatments.

Source: Drug Topics 4 *May 1992, p. 59 (2).*

■   ■   ■

Over the last decade, we have witnessed a continuing interest by people in taking personal responsibility for health matters, thus the focus on personal responsibility of this text. This is due partly to a growing awareness that treating sickness is more expensive than it used to be and that the cost of health care continues to spiral upward. Also, evidence continues to mount that how long we live relates in some degree to how well we take care of ourselves. About 70 percent of all deaths in this country are due to cardiovascular diseases and cancer. Of these deaths, it is estimated that about 80 percent could be delayed by a healthy life-style.[1,2]

As a consequence, many people are taking an increased degree of control over their own personal health. Surveys show that although Americans have many everyday aches and pains, in nine out of ten cases they take care of them without professional help.[3] People either use home remedies or drugs they can purchase **over-the-counter (OTC)** without a prescription, or simply wait for the discomfort to pass.

TAKING CHARGE OF YOUR HEALTH

You can do more for our own health and well-being than any physician, clinic, or hospital. You can lower your health risks by not smoking, by maintaining a regular exercise program, by eating healthy foods and balanced meals, and by learning to recognize and deal with stress.

Benefits of taking charge of your health include fewer serious health problems, reduced absenteeism, considerable monetary savings, and positive mental aspects, such as an improved sense of well-being. Savings come not only in the actual out-of-pocket costs for medicines and care, but in reduced costs for health insurance, which rise in direct proportion to how much care we need and use.

CONSUMER VULNERABILITY

Taking greater control of your personal health is not always easy, and it takes time and understanding. The vast increase in medical research has led to a proliferation of reports about new drugs and medical devices. Because the fields of medicine and biotechnology are advancing so rapidly, consumers' expectations are high, and they believe that there must be a cure for everything. Unfortunately, this is not always the case. Because people conclude that everything can be treated or cured, consumers can become an easy target for promoters of fraudulent cures. These promoters play on people's fears and levels of despair. The more vulnerable consumers are, the greater the success of these promoters of newfangled cures.

With the help of medical specialists and sophisticated drugs, the care of the body is increasingly specialized and precise. To be an intelligent consumer, you need to know something of the complexity of the body and how it works, and to understand the nature of illnesses and how they can be relieved by medications. Some of these medications are under the control of pharmacists

over-the-counter (OTC) drugs nonprescription drugs.

and others are available to consumers over the counter. You also need to know how to read labels and follow directions. All of these issues will be addressed in the following pages.

CHECKPOINT

1. Approximately what proportion of people take care of their own aches and pains?

2. List the benefits of taking charge of your own health.

3. Describe why today's health consumer may be more vulnerable than ever before.

PRESCRIPTION DRUGS

Prescription drugs are medicines that must be obtained through a prescription written by a licensed practitioner (physician, dentist, or podiatrist). Each year more than 1.6 billion prescriptions are written. Although few of us can understand the abbreviated language of a written prescription (Table 22.1), and even fewer from physicians with sloppy handwriting, we must trust that it has been prescribed and written properly and interpreted correctly by a pharmacist. This isn't always the case. In a study at one teaching hospital, 290,000 prescriptions were written in one year, of which only 905, or 0.3 percent, were incorrect. About half of these errors were serious enough to pose a health risk. Errors involved overdosing, underdosing, omitting information from the prescription, and not recognizing the patient's allergy to a drug.[4]

Once in the patient's hands, a medication is effective only if taken as directed. But patient compliance is not guaranteed. Only about 75 percent of medications are taken exactly as prescribed.[5] Patients take them at the wrong times, do not take all of the pills, take too many, or don't take them at all. This is drug misuse. As a result, infections may not be completely wiped out, recovery may not be as expected, and sometimes medical emergencies may occur. It is estimated that failure to take drugs properly costs people in the United States about $22 billion in physician visits, diagnostic tests, and additional medications.[6]

A part of taking medications properly is patient instruction. Often patients fail to ask questions,

Table 22.1
Prescription Abbreviations

aa	Equal amounts of each
aq	Water (*aqua*)
b.i.d.	Twice a day
coch or cochl	Spoonful
dim	One-half
ea	Each
g	Gram
gr	Grain
gt	Drop (plural: gtt)
l.a.s.	Label as such, i.e., label with the name of the drug. The AMA recommends this practice unless there is a reason to leave the patient in ignorance.
p.o.	By mouth
p.r.n.	As needed
q.2 h.	Every 2 hours; similarly, q.3 h., etc.
q.d.	Every day
q.i.d.	Four times a day
ss.	A half
t.i.d.	Three times a day
ut dict	As directed. The AMA counsels against this abbreviation on prescriptions, and recommends that instructions for taking medicine be written on the label.

Source: Taber's Cyclopedic Medical Dictionary, *17th ed. Davis: Philadelphia, 1993.*

especially when a new medication is being prescribed. It's important for physicians and/or pharmacists to explain to the patient any necessary precautions and possible side effects. Whether to take drugs with or without food, whether the drug interacts adversely with some other prescribed or over-the-counter drug, or alcohol, the patient is taking, or whether the drug should be taken at a particular time are all matters about which the patient should be informed. Patient compliance is important to help guarantee that the infection or condition is being taken care of properly. Some people stop taking their pills as soon as they think they feel better, saving the leftover pills until the next time they feel sick. Others take too many pills if they think the medication is not working or is not working quickly enough, running the risk of drug overdose. Some people use friends' prescriptions left over from a previous illness. As a result there is a good likelihood they may be taking the wrong drug at the wrong dosage. Effective medical care may be delayed or unnecessary adverse reactions may occur if you use medication that was prescribed for someone else.

GENERIC VS. BRAND NAMES

In an effort to help contain costs, many health insurance providers are requiring their insurees to insist on lower-priced **generic** versions of brand-name drugs when having their prescriptions filled. Generic versions of brand-name drugs are prescription drugs that contain the same active ingredients in the same amounts as a brand-name drug; there are also generic versions of nonprescription drugs. The cost savings could stretch the health care dollar to cover other necessary, or helpful, therapies. The result has been the mushrooming of generic drug sales, especially since 1984, when Congress passed a law eliminating the need for duplicate safety and efficacy testing for generic drugs whose brand-name versions have already been approved, helping pharmaceutical companies save both time and money.[7]

At the same time, the **Food and Drug Administration (FDA),** the federal agency responsible for consumer protection, issued guidelines on the **bioequivalency** of generic drugs. To be the bioequivalent of a brand-name drug, the generic must be identical to it in active ingredients. Ingredients other than the active ingredients are similar, but are not identical in *bioavailability* (absorption, distribution within the body, and elimination). Although generic drugs do not need to repeat the extensive clinical trials required of brand-name drugs, the manufacturers must show that the generic drug is the bioequivalent of the brand-name drug. The original version, or pioneer drug, is marketed under a brand name. For instance, the generic drug diazepam (an antianxiety drug) was first marketed

under the brand-name Valium. The brand name has patent protection for 17 years, with market exclusivity. This protects the drug firm's investment in developing the drug. Once this protection expires, other drug companies may apply to the FDA for generic licensing to produce and market their generic version of that drug. Almost 80 percent of generic drugs are produced by brand-name drug firms.[8]

When being prescribed a new medication, there are steps you should take in consultation with your physician. Before walking out of the office:

- Make sure the physician is aware of any allergies or other conditions you may have, or other medications you are taking.

- Ask the physician if there are any side effects so you know what to anticipate as a normal response to the drug.

- Decide, with your physician, whether a generic drug is available and acceptable, then stick with that decision. If a switch between a brand-name and generic drug is made, be sure the physician is aware of the switch so he or she can accurately monitor the drug's effect on you.

THE PHARMACIST AS A HEALTH ADVISOR

The one health care professional with whom you do not need an appointment is the **pharmacist,** the professional trained to formulate and dispense drugs. Pharmacists are not only the most accessible health care professionals, they are drug experts who receive four or more years of training in *pharmacology,* or the study of drugs. Much of a pharmacist's time is taken up filling prescriptions; in fact, other than a physician, the pharmacist is the only professional who can fill a prescription. A particularly valuable service provided by the pharmacist is calling the customer's attention to labeling, directions for use, and warnings. An FDA survey

generic drug a prescription drug that has the same active ingredients as a brand-name drug; there may also be generic versions of nonprescription drugs.

Food and Drug Administration (FDA) the U.S. Department of Health and Human Services agency responsible for consumer protection.

bioequivalency fact that the active ingredient(s) in a generic drug are identical to those in its comparable brand-name drug.

pharmacist a professional trained to formulate and dispense drugs; a druggist.

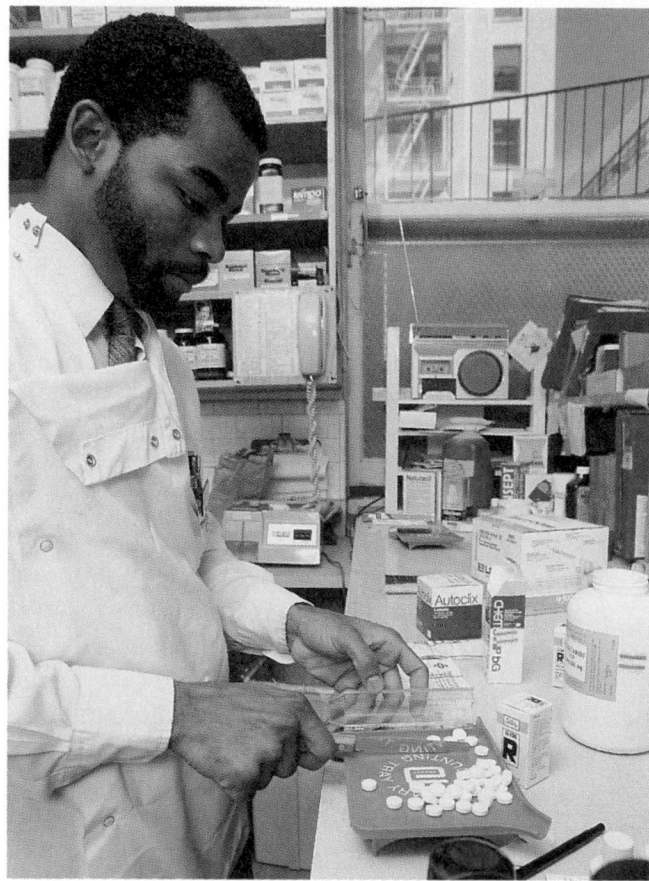

Pharmacists are the most accessible health care professionals. Their specialized training in drug composition and effect enables them to assess all medications better than anyone else.

using more than one pharmacy could easily hide such a problem. Some pharmacies now have records on computer to print out potentially conflicting drugs, and some maintain complete profiles of the patient. Patients who are taking multiple drugs and need to avoid drug interaction, who have trouble complying with directions or scheduling, or who have trouble reading and/or understanding the labels need to have a reliable pharmacist. A 1990 Gallup poll showed that Americans rated pharmacists as the most trusted of 25 different professionals.[10]

The consumer should deal with a pharmacy where he or she feels comfortable asking health questions. Pharmacists do not charge for their advice.

CHECKPOINT

1. In what ways can a pharmacist help you as a drug consumer?

2. Why is the pharmacist such a valuable resource in drug matters?

3. Define the term *bioequivalency*.

showed that about 23 percent of pharmacist's time is spent counseling customers.[9] Customers have questions on how and when to take medications, drug side effects, dangers of extended use, drug use with alcohol, drug use during pregnancy, and proper storage. Pharmacists are equally valuable in answering questions about OTC drugs located on the open shelves of the drug store. Their specialized training in drug composition and effects enables them to assess all medications better than anyone else.

To help build a relationship with a pharmacist, customers are encouraged to choose a single pharmacy for filling all prescriptions. This way people can find a pharmacy where they feel comfortable in asking for counsel and pharmacists can learn to know their customers and help them avert problems. Some customers see more than one physician, and get overlapping or incompatible drugs. An alert pharmacist can detect such problems, but

NONPRESCRIPTION (OVER-THE-COUNTER) DRUGS

Several thousand drugs designed for minor ailments can be purchased without a physician's prescription in drug stores, supermarkets, and convenience stores. These nonprescription, or over-the-counter (OTC) drugs are used to treat a wide range of conditions such as acne, allergies, hemorrhoids, headaches, and warts. Unlike prescription drugs, most OTC medications simply relieve the symptoms of a disease or condition, with some capable of curing minor conditions. Yet, all OTC drugs should be taken with caution. Many of them have the potential for adverse side effects.

Where once OTC drugs carried the reputation of "patent medicines" that were chemically trivial, the presence of useless drugs in OTC is now the exception rather than the rule. During the past two decades the FDA has banned some 400 of the 700 drug ingredients used in the 300,000 OTC products they started looking into in 1972.[11] Yet, as the incidence of self-care has grown, OTC drugs have

Table 22.2
Crossover Drugs

Selected drugs that were once available only by prescription but have become available over the counter in recent years.

Drug	Ailment	Brand	Year
Clemastine	Allergies	Tavist-D	1992
Miconazole	Antifungal	Monistat-7	1991
Clotrimazole	Yeast infection	Gyne-Lotrimin	1990
Permethrin	Lice	Nix	1990
Loperamide	Diarrhea	Imodium A-D	1988
Doxylamine succinate	Sinus or cold	Vicks Nyquil	1987
Pseudoephedrine hydrochloride and triprolidine hydrochloride	Sinus or cold	Actifed	1985
Diphenhydramine hydrochloride	Cough	Benadryl	1985

been accounting for an increasingly large market share of drugs sold in this country. In 1960 OTC drugs accounted for less than 20 percent of the total legitimate drug market, but now they represent about 40 percent of that market. OTC drugs account for 60 percent of the drugs people buy.[12]

The OTC market is growing partly due to the FDA giving OTC status to "crossover" drugs that it deems safe enough for use without a physician's prescription and partly due to the expiration of licensing patents for some "best-selling" prescrip-

tion drugs. During the last decade more than 200 drug products were "switched" from prescription to OTC status, including such products as Actifed, Coricidin Nasal Mist, Dimetapp, Sominex, Bactine, Motrin, and OcuClear.[13] (See Table 22.2.) The growth of OTC drugs is also the result of drug manufacturers developing new drug combinations, new ways of dispensing them, and new packaging ideas. Tylenol, for instance, is marketed in over 230 different package sizes, forms, and strengths.

Self-diagnosing and subsequent OTC drug use has risks. The early symptoms of a vaginal, bladder, or kidney infection could be the same. Treating an apparent vaginal yeast infection which is actually a bladder infection could postpone effective treatment.

Labeling prescription drugs is very different from labeling OTC drugs. Prescription drug labels provide information such as the name and address of the dispenser, the serial number, the date of the prescription, the name of the patient, directions for use, and any necessary warnings. Consumers using OTC drugs are not provided with instructions specific to the customer and must read all the information provided to determine proper dosage (Figure 22.1). (For example, children's dosages vary widely by age and weight.) See Communication for Wellness: Reading Drug Labels (p. 706) for instructions in interpreting labels.

The FDA is responsible for making sure that OTC drugs are safe and effective. The agency has the authority to require the clearance of new drugs

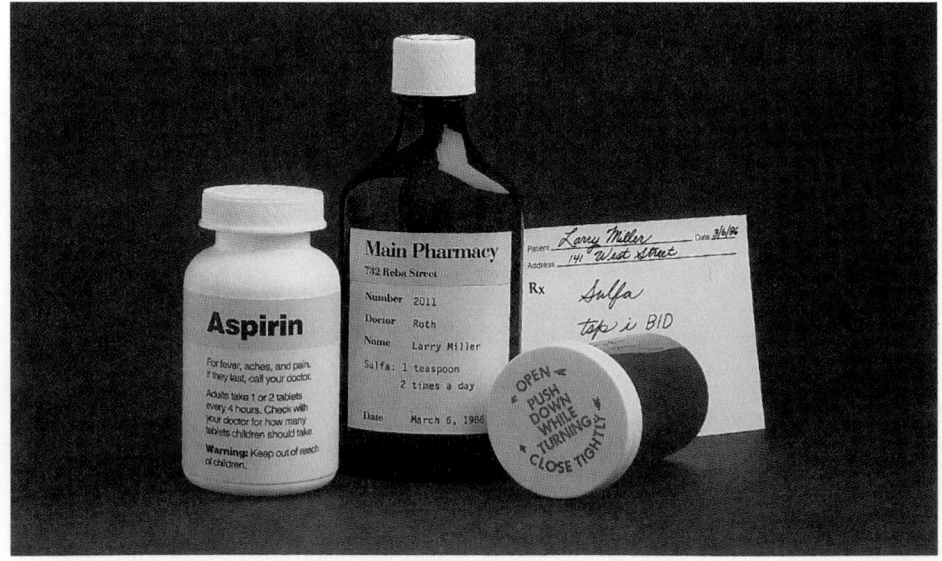

The labeling of a prescription drug is different from the labeling of an over-the-counter (OTC) drug. Prescription drug labeling provides information on the name and address of the dispenser, the serial number, the name of the physician and the patient, directions for use, and the data. Since OTC drug labeling does not include such specific information, manufacturers of OTC drugs must provide enough information for the safe use of the drug.

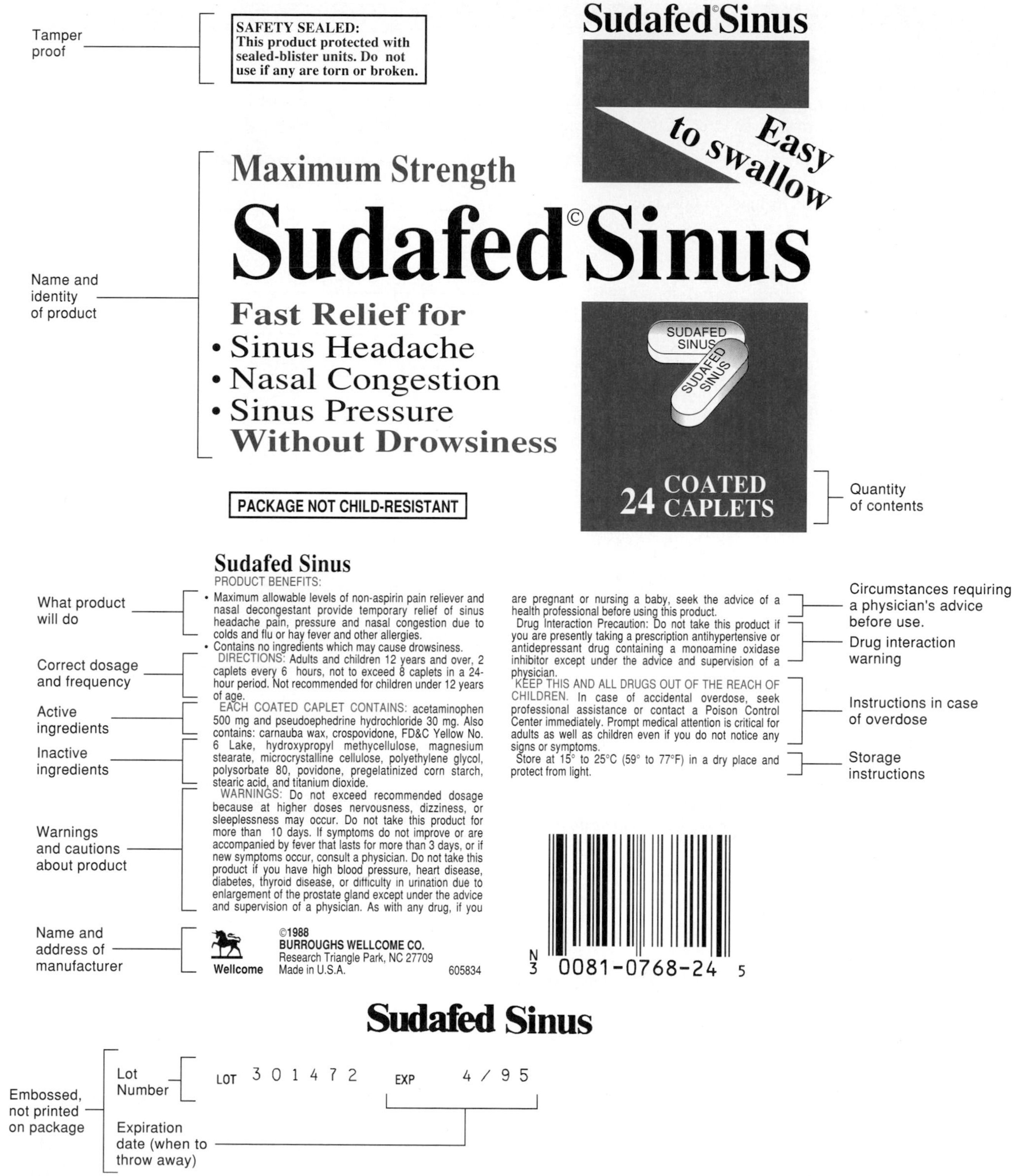

Tamper proof

SAFETY SEALED:
This product protected with
sealed-blister units. Do not
use if any are torn or broken.

Sudafed©Sinus

to swallow *Easy*

Name and identity of product

Maximum Strength

Sudafed©Sinus

Fast Relief for
• Sinus Headache
• Nasal Congestion
• Sinus Pressure
Without Drowsiness

PACKAGE NOT CHILD-RESISTANT

SUDAFED SINUS
SUDAFED SINUS

24 COATED CAPLETS

Quantity of contents

Sudafed Sinus
PRODUCT BENEFITS:

What product will do

• Maximum allowable levels of non-aspirin pain reliever and nasal decongestant provide temporary relief of sinus headache pain, pressure and nasal congestion due to colds and flu or hay fever and other allergies.
• Contains no ingredients which may cause drowsiness.

Correct dosage and frequency

DIRECTIONS: Adults and children 12 years and over, 2 caplets every 6 hours, not to exceed 8 caplets in a 24-hour period. Not recommended for children under 12 years of age.

Active ingredients

EACH COATED CAPLET CONTAINS: acetaminophen 500 mg and pseudoephedrine hydrochloride 30 mg. Also contains: carnauba wax, crospovidone, FD&C Yellow No.

Inactive ingredients

6 Lake, hydroxypropyl methycellulose, magnesium stearate, microcrystalline cellulose, polyethylene glycol, polysorbate 80, povidone, pregelatinized corn starch, stearic acid, and titanium dioxide.

Warnings and cautions about product

WARNINGS: Do not exceed recommended dosage because at higher doses nervousness, dizziness, or sleeplessness may occur. Do not take this product for more than 10 days. If symptoms do not improve or are accompanied by fever that lasts for more than 3 days, or if new symptoms occur, consult a physician. Do not take this product if you have high blood pressure, heart disease, diabetes, thyroid disease, or difficulty in urination due to enlargement of the prostate gland except under the advice and supervision of a physician. As with any drug, if you

are pregnant or nursing a baby, seek the advice of a health professional before using this product.
Drug Interaction Precaution: Do not take this product if you are presently taking a prescription antihypertensive or antidepressant drug containing a monoamine oxidase inhibitor except under the advice and supervision of a physician.

Circumstances requiring a physician's advice before use.

Drug interaction warning

KEEP THIS AND ALL DRUGS OUT OF THE REACH OF CHILDREN. In case of accidental overdose, seek professional assistance or contact a Poison Control Center immediately. Prompt medical attention is critical for adults as well as children even if you do not notice any signs or symptoms.

Instructions in case of overdose

Store at 15° to 25°C (59° to 77°F) in a dry place and protect from light.

Storage instructions

Name and address of manufacturer

©1988
BURROUGHS WELLCOME CO.
Research Triangle Park, NC 27709
Wellcome   Made in U.S.A.   605834

N3 0081-0768-24 5

Sudafed Sinus

Embossed, not printed on package

Lot Number   LOT 3 0 1 4 7 2   EXP   4 / 9 5

Expiration date (when to throw away)

Figure 22.1
Looking at Labels: OTCs

COMMUNICATION FOR WELLNESS

READING DRUG LABELS

Manufacturers of OTC drugs must provide sufficient information for the safe use of any given drug. OTC drugs must include the following information.

Label Items

- name of the drug and its function (identity)
- active ingredients
- inactive ingredients
- quantity of contents
- batch number
- expiration date (when to discard)
- what the drug will do
- warnings and cautions about the drug
- limits to duration of use
- circumstances that may require a physician's advice before use (when the drug should not be taken and who should not take it)
- correct dosage and frequency
- name and address of the manufacturer
- tamper-proofing

Your information

_____

_____

_____

_____

_____

_____

_____

_____

_____

_____

_____

_____

_____

Now, locate and review the label of an OTC product in your home. Look for each of these items on the label and write this information in the proper spaces above. If you need an example of an OTC product, refer to that in Figure 22.1.

---

before they reach the market. Beyond this, consumers must make sure that they use OTCs as instructed. You must keep in mind the following:

- Use an OTC drug properly; improper use may aggravate symptoms or cover up serious conditions.
- Read the label on the drug container carefully _before_ using it.
- Reread the label each time you buy the product, as directions may change slightly.
- Read warnings carefully and check with a physician or pharmacist regarding questions about certain drugs in relation to allergies or chronic health problems.

- Check expiration dates and discard outdated drugs.
- Check with a physician or pharmacist before using a drug if you are pregnant, nursing, or taking other drugs (prescription or OTC).

MULTIPLE DRUG USE (POLYPHARMACY)

One of the problems with the use of OTC drugs and self-medication is the risk of people using several drugs together without supervision, and without awareness of the potential for adverse interactions between different drugs. Very young and older patients are especially at risk. In 1989, the U.S. Inspector General's Office reported that

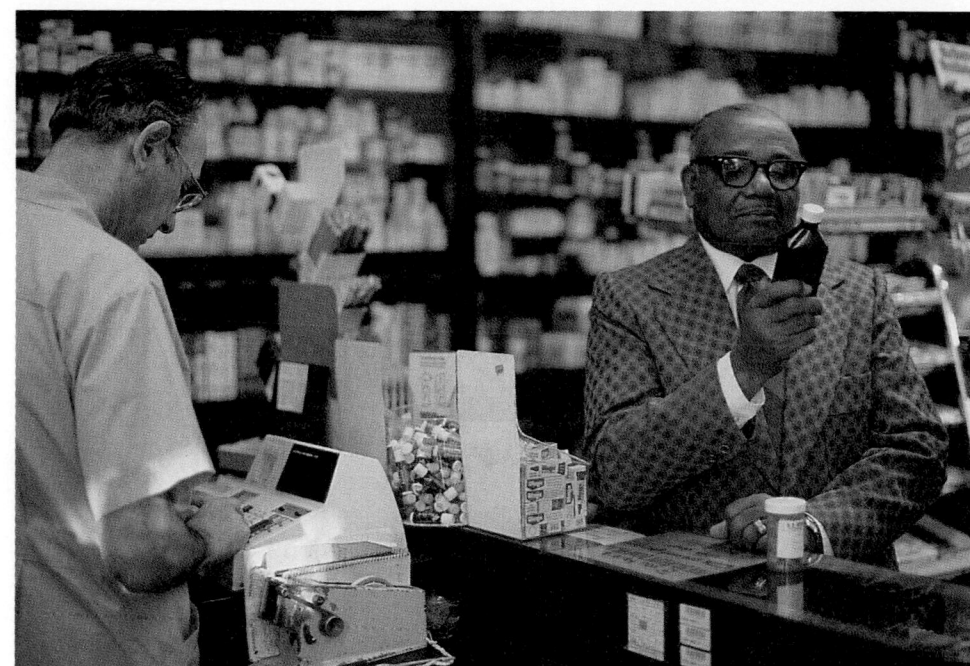

Consumers of an OTC drug are responsible for reading the label on the drug container carefully before using it and for using the drug only as instructed.

people over age 60 make up 17 percent of the U.S. population, yet consume 25 percent of all prescription medications and 40 percent of all OTC drugs.[14] Many older people take several different kinds of medication daily. There have been cases where a person may be taking a prescription drug, such as Motrin, yet at the same time be self-medicating on an OTC drug, such as Advil, two drugs whose action may essentially be the same, thus inadvertently doubling the dosage. In other cases, an OTC drug a person is taking may actually interfere with a prescription drug and negate its intended effect. Although multiple drug taking may be more common among the elderly (see Feature 12.3 Overmedication: A Problem for Some Older People, on p. 386), it is a risk for people of any age.

Physicians who are giving their patients prescriptions for drugs must question them regarding all of the drugs they may be taking, including vitamins. This is especially important as the range of OTC choices broadens. You as a patient also have the responsibility to share with your physician information about any drugs you may be taking, whether an illegal street drug or a prescribed one. You should feel free to consult with your pharmacist, not only when you have a prescription filled, but when you are purchasing OTC drugs, especially ones you are not accustomed to taking.

CHECKPOINT

1. Distinguish a nonprescription drug from a prescription drug.

2. What agency approves drugs for OTC status?

3. List the items of information that must be included on an OTC drug label.

4. What things should a responsible consumer do when using an OTC drug?

5. Explain the potential risks involved in multiple drug use.

OTC PRODUCTS: GOOD AND BAD

In this section, we discuss some of the better known types of OTCs in the vast array of products available. This discussion will help you make safer, more intelligent decisions when purchasing and using these products. Before looking at the types of OTC products, it would be useful to stop and assess why you buy certain brands (In Your Hands: Reasons I Buy Certain Brands, p. 708). As you read the content of each of the following kinds of OTC products, compare that information against the brand choices you have selected in the past.

PAIN RELIEVERS

Pain is a protective mechanism that warns us when tissue is damaged. OTC pain relievers, or **analgesics,** are the most widely sold of all nonprescription drugs. Pain relievers are most effective when used to treat musculoskeletal pain. OTC analgesics are also commonly used for headaches or for pain associated with **peripheral nerves,** nerves supplying the outside, or periphery, of the body, or supplying muscles or joints. Three types of analgesics used for pain relief are **aspirin, acetaminophen** (o-set"a-min'ō-fen), and **ibuprofen** (ībū-prō'phen).

....

analgesic a drug that relieves pain.

peripheral nerve any nerve supplying the outer part of the body.

aspirin acetylsalicylic acid; one of the most widely used analgesics and antipyretics.

acetaminophen a synthetic drug with analgesic actions similar to those of aspirin.

ibuprofen a synthetic drug with analgesic actions similar to those of aspirin.

Aspirin

Aspirin belongs to a group of drugs called **salicylates** (sal-i-sil'āts). The active ingredient, salicylic acid, is found in the bark of willow trees. Synthesized as acetylsalicylic (a-sē-til-sal-i-sil'ik) acid, aspirin is the most popular nonprescription drug on the market.[15] Acetylsalicylic acid is the principal active ingredient in hundreds of OTC drugs; in many, it is the only effective ingredient. The cost of these drugs, however, is much greater than that of plain aspirin tablets.

In addition to its pain-relieving qualities, aspirin has several other benefits. As an **antipyretic** (an-ti-pī-ret'ik), it helps reduce fevers by increasing sweating and blood flow to the skin. As an **anti-inflammatory** drug, aspirin reduces inflammation in body tissue, such as that caused by arthritis. Aspirin is also used under supervision to

....

salicylate any form of salicylic acid, the active ingredient in aspirin.

antipyretic a drug that reduces fever.

anti-inflammatory a drug that reduces inflammation.

prevent heart attacks and strokes by reducing blood clotting that may lead to blood vessel obstruction, to reduce pregnancy-induced hypertension, and can cut down on the occurrence of migraine and other disabling headaches.[16]

Aspirin is available in tablets, capsules, and in chewing gum. Because aspirin is an acid, it may irritate the stomach. Taking aspirin with water or milk, or using a buffered aspirin, which contains an **antacid** to neutralize acidity, is less irritating to the stomach. Tablets and capsules may be time-released, which means they are gradually dissolved in the body. Tablets may also be **enteric-coated;** these tablets do not dissolve until they reach the small intestine, and are less likely to cause ulcers and stomach erosion than plain or buffered aspirin. "Extra strength" or "maximum strength" aspirins contain more than the usual adult dosage of 325 mg of aspirin per pill, or combine aspirin with another analgesic.[17] Other aspirin products contain caffeine, which is a mild stimulant, or **antihistamines,** which reduce mucus secretions, relieving **rhinorrhea** (*rī-nō-rē'a;* a runny nose). These aspirin products may cost more, but are no more effective in relieving pain than plain aspirin.

Aspirin is widely available by its generic name, as well as under familiar brand names such as Bayer, St. Joseph, Anacin, A.S.A. Compound, and Empirin. While some brands of aspirin are advertised as being more effective than others, the active ingredient remains the same. The only difference between generic and brand names, or among brand names, would be any additive present.

Aspirin is considered safe for most people, but it does have side effects. The most common of these are nausea or vomiting and other stomach irritation. Stomach pain experienced when using aspirin should be reported to a physician. Recommended dosages should not be exceeded. Dosages above

....

antacid an agent that neutralizes acidity.

enteric-coated any drug tablet or capsule that is coated with a special substance that will not dissolve until it reaches the small intestine.

antihistamine any drug that reduces mucus secretions by opposing the action of histamine, a body substance released from injured cells and that causes flushing of the skin, headaches, and lower blood pressure.

rhinorrhea thin watery discharge from the nose.

the recommended level are *not* more effective and may be harmful. Every drug has a maximum dosage, above which no therapeutic gain is realized, yet side effects are increased. Possible signs of aspirin overdose or **salicylism** *(sal'i-sil-izm),* include bloody urine, diarrhea, dizziness, severe drowsiness, and ringing or buzzing in the ears.[18]

Aspirin should only be used for long periods of time under a physician's supervision and on a physician's recommendation. Pregnant and lactating women, patients anticipating surgery, people who regularly consume alcoholic beverages, patients on anticoagulants, people with diabetes, people with asthma, and children under the age of 16 who have chicken pox or the flu (and who may be subject to the rare, but sometimes fatal disease called **Reye's** (*rīz*) **Syndrome,** an acute condition affecting the brain and liver, and seen in children after a serious virus infection, should consult a physician before taking aspirin.[19, 20] Prior to administering OTC products, parents need to read labels thoroughly to see if they contain aspirin. Aspirin is one of the leading causes of accidental poisoning of young children, because they may think it is candy. Childproof caps on drugs have greatly reduced accidental poisonings, but aspirin, like other medications, should be kept out of the reach of children.

Acetaminophen

One of the most widely prescribed drugs is the pain-relieving drug *acetaminophen.* Although it is as effective in relieving pain and reducing fever as aspirin, an advantage for some users, such as people who are already on a blood-thinning agent or patients on an anti-inflammatory agent such as Naprosyn, is that it has no effect on inflammation or blood clotting. Acetaminophen has fewer side effects than aspirin, and is often recommended for people who cannot take aspirin. Since it does not irritate the stomach and rarely causes allergic reactions, it can be used successfully by people who have ulcers or aspirin allergies. The greatest danger

....

salicylism toxic condition caused by an overdose of salicylic acid.

Reye's Syndrome an acute condition affecting the brain and liver; seen in children after a serious virus infection.

from acetaminophen comes from its effect on the liver. Single massive dosages (30–50 extra-extra-strength tablets) or chronic excessive use for several weeks can cause liver problems. Since drinking alcohol makes side effects of acetaminophen on the liver more likely, do not use alcohol with this drug. Because of its possible adverse effects on the liver, acetaminophen should not be taken by people who have liver disease or a viral infection.

Acetaminophen products include Tylenol, Datril, Bromo-Seltzer, Allerest, Tempra, and Anacin-3. When combined with aspirin in products such as Excedrin, it is often difficult to assess which active ingredient is achieving the desired response. The most widely used prescription pain reliever in the United States is acetaminophen-codeine, a combination of two medicines: *acetaminophen,* the pain-reliever, and *codeine,* the pain-killer. This combination of drugs is commonly prescribed for such diverse conditions as migraine headaches, broken bones, and dental and postsurgical pain. The combination may be sold under brand names such as Tylenol with Codeine, Empracet with Codeine, Proval, Acetaco, and Ty-Tab with Codeine.

Ibuprofen

Ibuprofen is a relatively new OTC drug that offers pain relief and reduces fever, inflammation, and blood clotting. Ibuprofen has fewer side effects than aspirin, such as less irritation on the stomach lining, but it has more side effects than acetaminophen. Common side effects include heartburn, nausea, stomach pain, and abdominal pain. It is an excellent choice for people who have stomach problems. Large doses of ibuprofen are less toxic than either aspirin or acetaminophen. If you are allergic to aspirin, however, you should not take ibuprofen. Since ibuprofen is part of the same family of drugs as aspirin, it must still be taken with food or milk to prevent stomach distress. As with aspirin, any stomach pain should be reported to a physician. Ibuprofen is more expensive than either aspirin or acetaminophen. Common ibuprofen products include Advil, Nuprin, Motrin, and Mediprin.

COLD AND COUGH REMEDIES

Every year new cold remedies are introduced to the public through massive advertising campaigns,

only to drop quietly off the market when a new remedy is discovered. No matter how many cold remedies are introduced and no matter how many medical advances are made, there is still no cure for the common cold.

To understand the function of cold and cough remedies, one needs to understand that a cold is caused by a virus and that, to date, only limited progress has been made toward producing drugs that will cure viral infections (see Chapter 18). The role of cold medicine, then, is to alleviate the symptoms of a cold in order to relieve overall discomfort.

Most cold remedies contain an analgesic to relieve aches and pain, although they are available without analgesics. The active analgesic agents are aspirin, acetaminophen, and ibuprofen. Before taking a cold remedy containing an analgesic, check the label for instructions and precautions.

Decongestants

Decongestants, drug agents that ease congestion or swelling, are also known as **sympathomimetics** *(sim-pa-thō-mim-et'iks)* and are drugs that mimic the effects of the sympathetic nervous system. They ease a stuffy nose by constricting inflamed blood vessels in the nasal tissues, resulting in shrinkage of the mucus membranes, thus helping prevent a mucus buildup that might lead to sinus infection. Decongestants tend to produce stimulation.

Antihistamines

Antihistamines are drugs that oppose the action of *histamines,* those substances produced by injured cells, and which cause flushing of the skin, headache, and lowered blood pressure. Antihistamines are common in cough remedy products, although the FDA has found antihistamines ineffective for treating colds. OTC antihistamines tend to produce drowsiness. Effective for treating allergies and hay fever, the active agents of antihista-

....

decongestant drug agents that reduce congestion or swelling.

sympathomimetic a drug that mimics the effects of the sympathetic nervous system.

mines may be tripolidine, diphenhydramine, chlorpheniramine maleate, or promethazine.

Cough remedies may contain a cough suppressant and/or an expectorant. **Cough suppressants** work on the brain to inhibit the cough reflex and are useful when you have a dry, nonproductive cough; they may contain the active ingredients codeine, or dextromethorphan. **Expectorants** are useful for the productive phase of a cough when you "bring up" phlegm. They increase the secretions in the lungs to make the phlegm loose and less sticky; the active ingredient is guaifenesin. Although some medications combine a cough suppressant and an expectorant, it is better to use one or the other, depending upon your needs at the time. A popular form of cold remedy contains a combination of products. Called "shotgun" remedies, some contain as many as five active ingredients for five different actions. Although convenient to buy and take, some dosage levels may be too low, or they may target actions that are not needed. For these reasons, some physicians recommend using only single-action products, or at most, three-action products.

Precautions are called for when purchasing cough remedies, especially for children. Cough remedies containing aspirin should not be given to children due to its link to Reye's syndrome. Reading the labels will also tell the amount of sugar and alcohol in the product. *Syrups* are water- and sugar-based, and *elixirs* contain alcohol. Products containing alcohol are often labeled for nighttime use.

By eliminating the symptoms of a cold, but not the cause, cough and cold remedies may, in the long run, prove harmful. For example, when symptoms are relieved, people with colds are tempted to continue their normal activities when they should go to bed and rest. If you rest at the onset of a cold, it can often hasten recovery and prevent secondary infections and other complications. The result of fighting a cold by disguising the symptoms is often a secondary bacterial infection in the middle ear, sinus cavities, or lungs; these complications may lead to more severe illnesses.

....

cough suppressant a drug that inhibits coughing.

expectorant a drug that leads to the expulsion of mucus or phlegm from the throat or lungs.

RELIEF FOR GASTROINTESTINAL DISORDERS

Most people take in food every day as their source of energy, and their bodies must process that food and excrete the wastes. Their bodies are engaged in a constant process of **gastrointestinal (GI)** activity. Often this process runs smoothly, but it's not uncommon for parts of the process to malfunction. Some of the common forms of distress with GI activity such as indigestion and heartburn, occur when food enters the system, and when wastes leave the system, such as diarrhea, constipation, and hemorrhoids.

Heartburn and Indigestion

After having eaten a big meal—multiple courses, a helping or two of dessert, along with one or more drinks—it is not uncommon for a person to pay for it a second time, but now with a "burning sensation" in the stomach.

Indigestion is a catch-all term for any kind of stomach distress caused by conditions such as too much stomach acid, inflammation of the stomach lining, or by an ulcer. **Heartburn** occurs when the stomach's contents, including foods and gastric juices, shoot back up into the *esophagus* (the food tube leading into the stomach) causing a "burning" sensation. A small circular muscle between the esophagus and stomach, which prevents such backup, fails to function properly in this condition.

To relieve the distress, many persons go for their favorite *antacid*. Used to counter heartburn and indigestion, antacids are OTC drugs used to neutralize stomach acidity. But frequent and prolonged use can damage the heart, kidneys, and bones, and some people with special medical conditions should never use them.[21] The names of antacids commonly available reads like a Who's Who of TV advertising—Alka-Seltzer, Bromo Seltzer, Tums, Maalox, Mylanta, Rolaids, and Simethicone. Although antacids may bring temporary

....

gastrointestinal (GI) pertaining to the stomach and intestines.

indigestion incomplete or imperfect digestion, usually accompanied by feelings of physical distress.

heartburn return of the stomach's acid contents into the esophagus, causing a burning sensation.

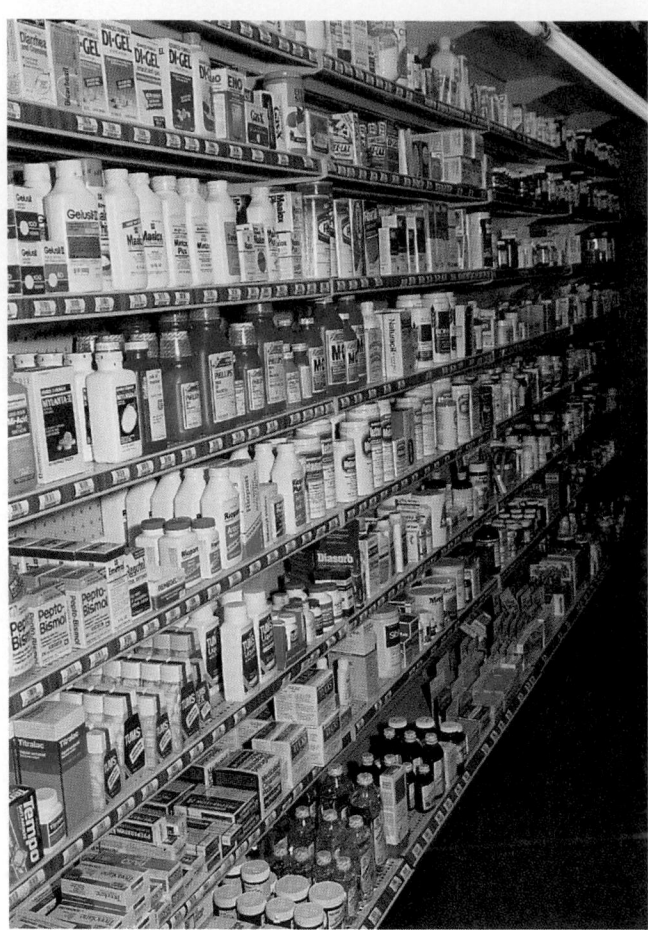

The shelves of drug stores contain many brands of many different kinds of OTC drugs from which you must make the most appropriate selections.

relief, eating less, eating more slowly, cutting down on the caffeine, alcohol, and tobacco, and not eating large amounts of food close to bedtime will prevent the problem.

Diarrhea

Diarrhea is the frequent passage of abnormally watery stools, or bowel movements. Excess water that is normally absorbed from the intestine is excreted through the rectum during diarrhea. If too much water is lost, it may lead to dehydration, a condition especially serious in small children. Diarrhea is usually a symptom of food poisoning or an intestinal infection. The most commonly used antidiarrheal agents are absorbents in products such as Kaopectate, Pepto-Bismol, Imodium AD,

....

diarrhea frequent passage of abnormally watery bowel movements.

and Donnagel PG, which slow intestinal motility, reducing the amount of diarrhea and the loss of fluid from the GI tract.

Constipation

Some people believe that a good state of health entails a daily bowel movement, or evacuation, and that anything less than this is health endangering. Actually, infrequent bowel movements may not be unusual; in fact, the normal range varies from as many as three movements a day to as few as three per week.[22] If bowel movements become difficult and the fecal material is unduly dry and hard, the person may be suffering from **constipation.** This condition can be alleviated in most cases by increased exercise, increased fluid intake, and eating a well-balanced diet, including unprocessed bran, whole wheat bread, and plenty of fruits and vegetables.

When a well-balanced diet does not relieve constipation, OTC **laxatives** are available to loosen the bowels. They come in various liquid and solid forms and work in different ways to promote stool evacuation. Laxatives should be used only on a short-term basis, or the body may become dependent on them, especially if they are stimulants (i.e., Dulcolax, Senokot, or Correctol). If use of laxatives does not lead to relief after one week, or if rectal bleeding occurs, the laxative should be discontinued and a physician consulted.[23] Overuse of laxatives can lead to reduced neurological and muscular control of the large intestine, as well as depletion of body fluids, salts, vitamins, and minerals. If taken in the presence of abdominal pain, nausea, or vomiting, the laxative could mask an attack of appendicitis.

Hemorrhoids

Hemorrhoids and other anal-rectal disorders are some of the most annoying and uncomfortable GI disorders. A hemorrhoid is a mass of enlarged, exposed veins in the **rectum,** or lower part of the

....

constipation infrequent and difficult bowel movements.

laxative a substance that acts to loosen the bowels.

rectum lower part of the large intestine.

intestine near the opening of the anus. Hemorrhoids may be caused by extreme and prolonged rectal straining, such as in forced bowel movements and in childbirth.

Hemorrhoids may be treated with stool softeners or improved anal hygiene. Severe cases of hemorrhoids may require surgery. OTC products, such as Preparation H and Anusol HC, are available for relief of the minor symptoms such as burning, pain, itching, swelling, inflammation, and general discomfort. Severe symptoms, such as bleeding or severe persistent pain, should be attended by a physician.

SLEEP AIDS, SEDATIVES, AND STIMULANTS

Insomnia, or the inability to sleep, affects an estimated one-half of the American population. About 33 percent of people with insomnia view it as an ongoing problem.[24] Some people have trouble falling asleep; others awaken in the middle of the night, or too early in the morning. For those seeking relief from insomnia, OTC sleeping aids are available. For those who need to stay awake, OTC stimulants are available.

Sleep Aids and Sedatives

Many OTC products are advertised as providing "safe and restful sleep" or relief from "simple nervous tension." Such claims are unsubstantiated.[25] For instance, some products contain low dosages of antihistamines. While **sedation,** or calming, is a drug side effect of antihistamines, at low dosages they produce minimal or no sedation. To obtain the desired sedation, some people may exceed recommended dosages and suffer toxic effects of the drug. OTC sleep aids may also contain salicylates and salicylamides to relieve mild pain. Common sleep aid products include Alva Tranquil, Sominex, Quiet Tabs, and Somnicaps.

In 1979, the FDA determined that all OTC drugs used for daytime sedation were unsafe, and directed that they not be marketed for that purpose. People should never drive a car or operate hazardous machinery after taking a sleep aid or any drugs containing antihistamines.

Insomnia is caused by a wide variety of factors. Stress, anxiety, depression, pain or discomfort, changes in work hours, jet lag, growing older, drug use, hormonal disorders, and epilepsy are some contributing factors. While some of these are temporary problems, a physician should be consulted if insomnia persists.

Insomnia may be relieved without drugs in several ways. Try the following:

- Drink warm milk at bedtime.
- Do not drink any beverages containing caffeine before bedtime.
- Relax before going to bed by engaging in activities such as reading, watching television, or listening to soothing music.
- Go to bed at around the same time each night.

A glass of warm milk and a good novel are but two ways to prepare for a good night's sleep.

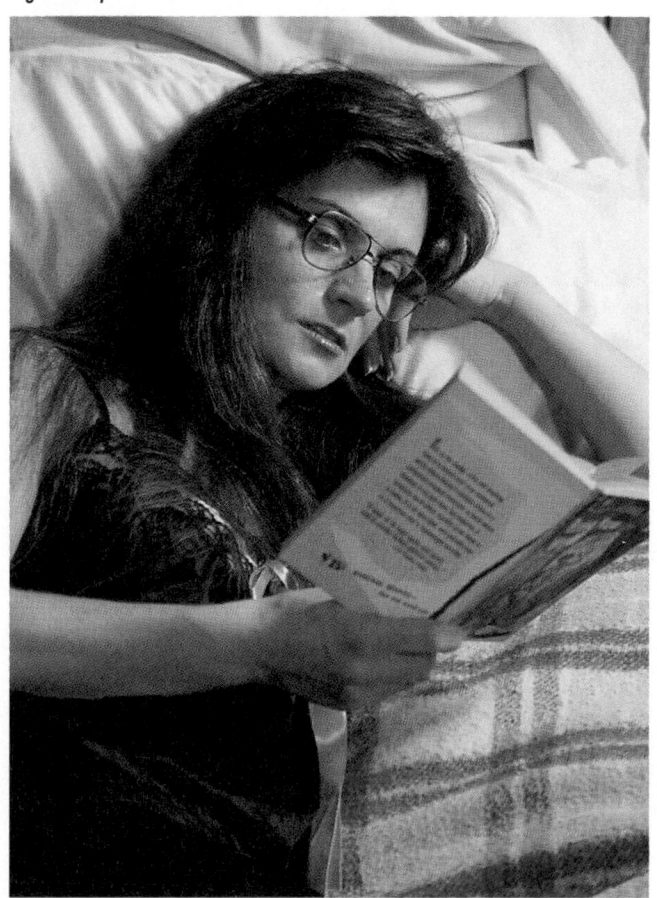

insomnia inability to sleep.

sedation state of being calmed.

- Don't worry if you can't sleep. Anxiety can contribute to insomnia.
- Wake up at the same time each morning regardless of how well you slept the previous night. After a few nights of poor sleep, your sleeping may become more regular.
- Avoid daytime naps.
- Participate in stimulating daytime activities.
- Exercise regularly, but not within two to three hours of bedtime.

Stimulants

Monotonous activity, such as highway driving, fatigue, or boredom may induce sleepiness. To maintain alertness, people sometimes resort to using nonprescription **stimulants.** OTC stimulants that are advertised as helping people stay awake usually contain caffeine. Common OTC stimulant products include Nodoz Tablets, Amostat Tablets, Pep-Back, and Tirend Tablets. Many beverages and foods also contain caffeine, as do many OTC drugs (see Table 22.3).

Small doses of caffeine (50–200 mg) stimulate brain functions associated with conscious mental processes; ideas become clearer, thoughts flow more easily and rapidly, and feelings of fatigue and drowsiness decrease, although manual dexterity may not be improved. Not everyone reacts to caffeine in the same way, but usually doses larger than 250 mg prevent sleep and often cause restlessness, irritability, nervousness ("coffee nerves"), tremors, or headaches. Caffeine also causes the heart to beat faster.

Caffeine-containing pills taken to prevent sleep will have the same affect on a person as coffee does. One tablet of a caffeine product is about equal to one cup of strong coffee. Regular use of these pills can be quite unhealthy because they cause the person's body to ignore its fatigue without replenishing depleted energy with adequate rest.

Students sometimes take caffeine pills so they can study an extra hour or two, but after that, the ability to absorb information drops considerably. When driving long distances, it is better to combat fatigue by stopping frequently, or if possible, by

---

Table 22.3
Caffeine in Some Common Drinks and Drugs

This table gives the average caffeine content of several drinks and drugs. The chart will help you to calculate your daily caffeine intake. Remember, caffeine content varies widely, depending on the product you use and how it is prepared.

Beverages	Serving Size	Caffeine (mg)
Coffee, drip	5 oz	110–150
Coffee, perk	5 oz	60–125
Coffee, instant	5 oz	40–105
Coffee, decaffeinated	5 oz	2–5
Tea, 5-minute steep	5 oz	40–100
Tea, 3-minute steep	5 oz	20–50
Hot cocoa	5 oz	2–10
Coca-Cola	12 oz	45
Mountain Dew	12 oz	50
Over-the-Counter Drugs	**Dose**	**Caffeine (mg)**
Anacin, Empirin, or Midol	2 tablets	64
Excedrin	2 tablets	130
Aspirin, plain	2 tablets	0

Source: University of California at Berkeley Wellness Letter, *February 1985, p. 5 and July 1988, p. 4.*

---

driving with the windows down to allow fresh air to keep the driver awake.

OTC stimulants should be used with caution. It is not a good idea to fight fatigue by taking stimulants. For simple fatigue, rest is the best remedy. For chronic fatigue, a physician should be consulted.

EYE CARE

Many OTC products are available to treat eye discomfort, such as dry eyes, inflammation and irritation, and the effects of air pollutants, wind, and sunlight. Because our eyes are such important sense organs, care must be taken when selecting eye products to treat any eye irritation.

Decongestants, Artificial Tears, and Eyewashes

Many physicians warn against self-prescribing any OTC eye preparations. Some of these contain ingredients that raise eye pressure or raise blood

---

stimulant any drug that increases functional activity.

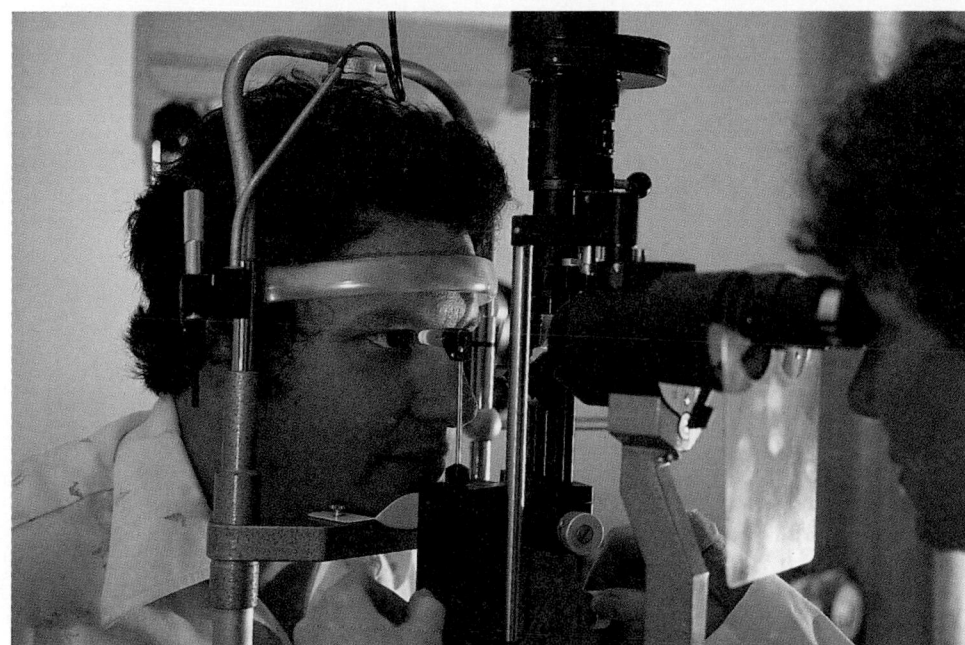

An examination of the eyes is necessary to test them for refractory disorders and for diseases. Such an examination needs to be made before a prescription for lenses can be given.

pressure, cause allergies, and affect eye fluid pH; they may also be easily contaminated.

Various eye preparations are intended to do different things. Decongestants are used primarily for allergic symptoms that leave the eye tissues red and swollen, and are not to be considered as eyewashes. Some common decongestants are Murine Plus, Visine, VasoClear, and Phenylzin. Artificial tears are used for dry eyes or artificial tear production, although many physicians believe that the natural flow of tears in the eyes constitutes the best means of cleansing the eye of dust, foreign objects, and pollutants. Some common artificial tear preparations are Hypotears, Lacril, Refresh, and Tears Plus. Eyewashes are used to remove loose foreign materials, such as dust. Common OTC eyewashes include Dacriose and Collyrium.

As with many kinds of self-treatment, eye preparations may relieve and disguise the symptoms of serious eye disorders that need the immediate attention of a physician. If any redness or irritation lasts longer than a day or two, a physician should take a look.

EYEGLASSES

Some types of eyeglasses, especially reading glasses, are available over-the-counter. Most commonly, however, eyeglasses are prescribed by a physician who specializes in the eye, an **ophthalmologist (oculist),** after a complete eye examination. He or she is qualified to examine the eyes for diseases, test vision, prescribe lenses, prescribe medications, and perform surgery. An **optometrist** (O.D.) is a nonmedical eye specialist who can test the eyes for inability to focus properly, or **refractory disorders,** and prescribe lenses, but may not administer or prescribe medication or perform surgery. An **optician** is a technician who prepares lenses for eyeglasses.

To reduce the risk of injury from shattering eyeglass lenses, the FDA regulations, as cited in the FDA Impact-Resistance Standards, require that eyeglass and sunglass lenses be resistant to breakage upon impact. Goggles and face masks, such as those used when swimming and skiing, are not so regulated.

....

ophthalmologist a physician who specializes in the treatment of refractory disorders and diseases of the eye; also called an oculist.

optometrist a nonphysician who is trained to examine the eyes for refractory disorders.

refractory disorder inability to focus the eyes or to perceive images correctly.

optician a person who makes optical appliances.

CONTACT LENSES

Contact lenses, an alternative to eyeglasses, are small plastic disks that ride on a thin layer of tears directly over the clear, front portion of the eye, or the **cornea,** and under the eyelids. Tears lubricate the cornea and eyelid, keep the surface of the cornea clean of dust, and nourish it. All contact lenses must be disinfected when not in the eye and all lenses must be kept wet in storage. As with eyeglasses, contact lenses are fitted by an ophthalmologist, or optometrist. There are several types of contact lenses on the market, including hard lenses, soft lenses, disposable lenses, extended-wear soft lenses, and gas-permeable lenses.

Hard contact lenses are made of rigid plastic and are intended for daily wear only; they must be removed before going to sleep. Not everyone adapts well to hard lenses. Unlike other types of lenses, hard contacts require a break-in period. Hard contact lenses are the least expensive on the market. They correct most refractory problems and are the easiest to care for. Due to a decrease in popularity, fewer companies are making them, and they are becoming more difficult to get.

Soft contact lenses are made of soft plastic; most are intended for daily wear. They are popular because they are usually comfortable from the first day and require little break-in period. Soft lenses cover more of the eye surface than hard lenses and are less likely to pop out of the eye because they are more flexible. Soft lenses are costlier than hard lenses, are more easily damaged, and must be replaced every year. As with hard contacts, most soft lenses must be removed before sleeping. Soft lenses worn on a daily basis are generally considered to be safer than soft lenses worn as extended wear lenses. Those left in longer are associated with a higher risk of corneal infection.

Disposable lenses are soft lenses meant to be discarded after a week of use and are typically purchased a year's worth at a time. Being disposable, the lenses do not require the care and cleaning required of most contact lenses. Disposable lens users do not encounter the discomfort that can accompany protein buildup on soft lenses. Protein,

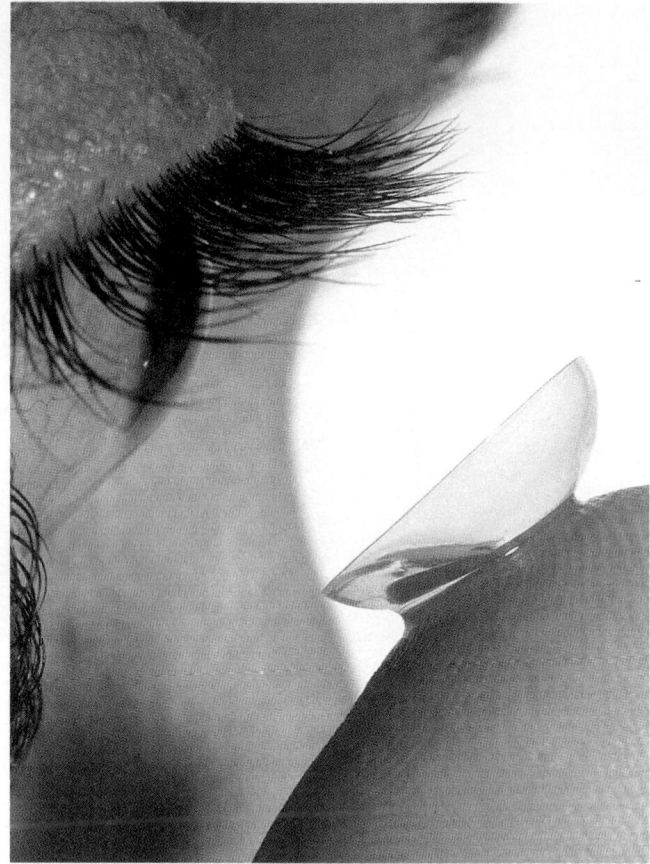

There are several types of contact lenses on the market including soft, disposable, extended-wear, gas-permeable, and hard lenses.

found in human tears, builds up on contact lenses like plaque on teeth. Use of disposables is referred to by some as a planned replacement program.

Extended-wear soft lenses are designed to be worn for up to 30 days. Yet, recent studies have shown that extended-wear lenses can increase the risk of eye infections. The FDA has asked the makers of extended-wear lenses to recommend that they be worn for no more than three days at a time. Other medical consultants recommend that extended-wear contacts be taken out every night, or at least every other night.[26] Extended-wear lenses may also be prescribed for daily wear for those whose eyes are over-sensitive or damaged. These lenses allow more oxygen to reach the eye and are less irritating than other types of contact lenses.[27]

Gas-permeable extended-wear lenses are rigid. These lenses cover less of the cornea than soft lenses, so there is more oxygen flow. Easier to wear, these lenses are in the hard lens category in that they must be taken out nightly. While some believe these lenses may be easier on the eyes, no

....

contact lenses a small lens that fits over the cornea of the eye.

cornea the clear, transparent front portion of the eye.

conclusive evidence has been found to substantiate this claim.

Contact lens wearers may be bothered by dry air, tobacco smoke, aerosol sprays, and other airborne irritants. All contact lens wearers should have a pair of properly fitted eyeglasses they can wear when their eyes become fatigued or irritated.

SUNGLASSES

Some people wear a pair of sunglasses to add an air of mystery to the face; but sunglasses are more than a fashion statement. Their main function is to protect the eye by reducing the amount of light and nonvisual radiation reaching the eye. Invisible **ultraviolet radiation (UV)** can damage the unprotected refracting **lens** and nerve-containing **retina,** and lead to possible loss of transparency of the lens, or *cataract.* It's important to protect your eyes not only in summer, but all year long. Although these claims have not been substantiated, much sunglass technology has, nevertheless, been directed at improving UV blockage. (For a further discussion on UV radiation see p. 720.)

Most sunglasses reduce glare and block much of the visible light. Studies show that the makers of sunglasses have improved their ability to block UV light considerably in recent years. Many eye specialists now recommend that everyone wear UV-absorbing sunglasses whenever exposed to the sun. As yet, the only industry standard for UV absorption was established by the American National Standards Institute (ANSI) in New York. Glasses conforming to ANSI standards have "Z-80.3" printed on the frame.[28] When buying sunglasses, look at the labeling. Most sunglass manufacturers label sunglasses according to standards established by the ANSI.

Sunglasses fall into three categories.[29]

- *Cosmetic-use sunglasses* are lightly tinted, may be worn in mild sunlight, and should block at least 70 percent of the UV-B and 60 percent of the UV-A radiation.

- *General-use sunglasses* are medium- to dark-tinted, are for outdoor use, and should block at least 95 percent of UV-B and at least 60 percent of UV-A.

- *Special-use sunglasses* are dark tinted, are used for intense sunlight, and should block at least 99 percent of UV-B and 98 percent of UV-A.

For greatest protection, you should wear sunglasses that block 95–100 percent of both UV-A and UV-B radiation. A wide frame that wraps around is better than small glasses that allow a lot of light into the eyes. Plastic sunglass lenses, if properly coated, can provide greater UV protection than glass lenses. Cost is not the only factor; even some inexpensive glasses offer good protection. Polarized lenses are designed to cut down glare and, though dark in color, may not do a good job of blocking out UV light.

Other considerations in the purchasing and use of sunglasses include the following:

- Lenses that distort images will not hurt your eyes, but may give you a headache. To check nonprescription sunglasses, hold them at an arm's length and look at straight lines in the distance. Move the lenses back and forth; if the line bends or sways, the lenses are imperfect and might bother your eyes (see Figure 22.2, p. 718).

- Lenses should be large enough to protect against light reaching the eye from the sides, top, or bottom. They should fit snugly so they don't slip down your nose.

- "Fashion" tints of lenses, giving a range of hues, may not be dark enough to block out the sun's rays. Dark gray gives the least distortion of natural color, followed by green.

- All sunglasses must pass the FDA's safety test for breakage.

- If there is no label giving an ANSI standard, the glasses should be dark enough so that you cannot see your eyes in the mirror.

- Sunglasses should never be worn at night, in tunnels, or in other dim environments.

By law, sunglass lenses must meet FDA impact-resistance standards. Plastic lenses are lighter weight and, if handled properly, last as long and perform as well as glass lenses.

---

ultraviolet radiation (UV) rays beyond visible light at the violet end of the spectrum.

lens the transparent refracting body within the eye.

retina the nerve-containing innermost layer of the eye, which receives the images formed by the lens.

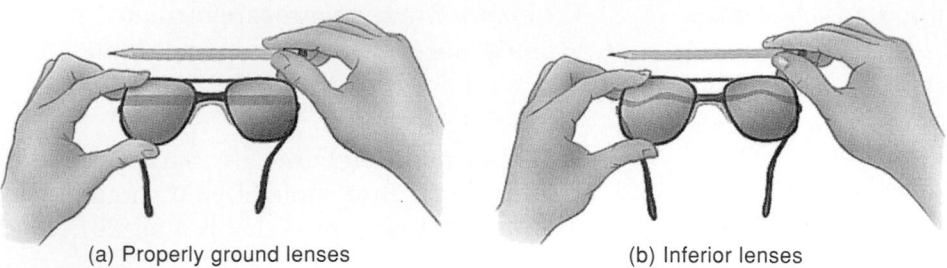

(a) Properly ground lenses   (b) Inferior lenses

Figure 22.2
A Simple Optical Quality Test for Sunglasses

To check if nonprescription sunglasses distort, hold the glasses at arm's length and slowly move a pencil up and down in front of the lenses. (a) Properly ground lenses reflect without distorting. (b) Inferiorly ground lenses transmit a distorted image to the eye.

CHECKPOINT

1. Why is aspirin considered such a valuable drug?

2. Why is it impossible for a cold remedy to cure the common cold?

3. List several ways in which insomnia can be relieved without the use of drugs.

4. Describe how a person's body reacts to caffeine.

5. Compare the different types of contact lenses.

6. List the features to look for when shopping for sunglasses. ✓

COSMETICS

Cosmetics may bring to mind images of eye shadow, lipstick, and blush. There are many types of cosmetics. The FDA defines cosmetics as "articles other than soap which are applied to the human body for cleansing, beautifying, promoting attractiveness, or altering the appearance."[30] The FDA has classified more than 80 types of products as cosmetics. We will discuss several of these in the following pages.

Items that one would consider to be cosmetics may actually be classified as drugs by the FDA if they alter a body function. For example, **deodorant** is regulated as a cosmetic, because it is *intended* to prevent odor. An **antiperspirant,** however, is regulated as a drug because it is *intended* to reduce perspiration, which is a normal body function. Toothpaste is classified as a cosmetic to clean and brighten teeth; if it contains fluoride it is considered a drug because it prevents tooth decay. Tooth decay is considered a disease, and therefore needs to be treated, or altered. Determining whether a product is a drug, a cosmetic, or both is the obligation of the manufacturer.

If a product is classified as a drug, its working, or **active ingredients** must be listed ahead of all other ingredients. For example, this is done on the labels of dandruff shampoos, antiperspirants, and medicated cosmetics.

DEODORIZERS

Controlling body odors is a concern of most socially aware people and many products are available to destroy these odors. For body odor, antiperspirants and deodorants are available; for bad breath, mouthwashes and sprays may be purchased.

Deodorants and antiperspirants have evolved to eliminate body or underarm odor. While deodorants fight body odor, antiperspirants fight

deodorant a substance that masks or absorbs body odors.

antiperspirant a substance that inhibits perspiration.

active ingredient an ingredient responsible for the primary purpose of a drug preparation.

cosmetics preparations for cleansing, beautifying, promoting attractiveness, or altering the appearance.

both wetness and body odor. Today, combination antiperspirants/deodorants, which come in the form of creams, roll-ons, sticks, or aerosols are available.

Most brands of antiperspirants contain an aluminum compound, which is a safe and effective active ingredient. No antiperspirant can stop sweating completely; although it can reduce sweating by 20–70 percent. Antiperspirants work best when applied to dry skin. Those that are applied directly to the skin and are rubbed on, such as sticks, roll-ons, and creams, provide the best protection and are more environmentally friendly than sprays.

Deodorants work either by inhibiting or removing the number of odor-causing bacteria; some mask the odor with another scent, such as a perfume.

The best way to control body odor is with a combination of methods. Regular use of an antibacterial soap or use of a deodorant will keep most people free of natural body odor for up to 24 hours; but deodorants by themselves only kill or inhibit the bacteria. If you are allergic to a certain brand of antiperspirant or deodorant, switch to a different brand with different ingredients.

Mouthwashes are another kind of deodorizer. Most commercially available mouthwashes are cosmetic in that they freshen breath or help clean out mouth debris. Contrary to advertised claims of mouthwashes being medicated to "kill germs," there is no conclusive evidence that mouthwashes can effectively kill microorganisms or treat oral infections.[31] The American Dental Association sees mouthwash use as having the potential to cover up disease conditions in the mouth, as well as in the gastrointestinal tract, and delay treatment. They suggest that if bad breath persists after proper tooth brushing, the cause should be investigated rather than masked with a mouthwash.[32]

SHAMPOOS

The hair and scalp need to be washed regularly to eliminate the normal buildup of dandruff, oil, bacteria, and dirt. While any ordinary bath soap will cleanse hair in soft water, detergents work better in hard waters. Today most shampoos contain detergents. The amount of foam a shampoo produces is no indication of its cleansing ability. Low-foam shampoos cleanse as well as high-foam shampoos. The stronger the detergent in a shampoo, the more likely it will strip off hair dyes and tints, remove natural oils in the hair, and neutralize the effects of conditioning agents.[33]

Hair conditioners have also been added to some shampoos. Conditioners make the hair appear soft, smooth, and lustrous. Conditioners also get rid of snarls, making hair easier to comb, brush, and style.

Medicated shampoos, whether prescribed or OTC, contain ingredients for relieving excessive dandruff (small flakes of dead skin shed from the scalp), psoriasis, and eczema. While some flaking skin on the scalp is normal it may be twice as great in a dandruff sufferer. Since dandruff shampoo treats dandruff and cleanses the hair, the FDA treats it both as a drug and a cosmetic.

HAIR DYES

It's estimated that 40 percent of women and a smaller percentage of men dye their hair to enhance or change their natural color. There are four types of coloring agents used: temporary, semi-permanent, permanent, and gradual or progressive.[34]

The degree of safety in the use of hair dyes is unclear. Most hair dyes are legally exempt from premarket safety testing that is required of other cosmetic color additives. Recent studies have linked an increased risk of certain cancers with the use of hair dyes. At the same time, other studies provide conflicting results that question these risks.[35] Of special concern are the coal-tar hair dyes and the ability of such dyes to produce cancers in test animals. Only the gradual dyes do not contain such compounds.

The FDA recommends that hair dyes be used in moderation and with the use of good judgment. Using less dye and waiting to use dyes until your hair turns gray is recommended. The FDA makes the following additional recommendations:[36]

- Don't leave dye on your head any longer than necessary.
- Rinse the scalp thoroughly with water after use.
- Wear gloves when applying hair dye.
- Carefully follow the directions on the package.
- Never mix hair dye products.
- Do a patch test for allergic reactions before applying the dye to your hair.
- Never dye your eyebrows or eyelashes.

REMEDIES FOR OVEREXPOSURE TO THE SUN

Many lightly pigmented people believe that a suntan enhances their physical appearance. Almost everyone has a feeling of well-being when warmed by the sun. In reality, however, the adverse effects of the sun far outweigh any beneficial effects.

Those who like to tan deeply should be aware of several possible effects. Sunbathing ages the skin, giving it wrinkles and a leathery texture, and can leave it mottled or discolored. Overexposure to the sun eventually makes you look older than you are. Sunbathing also increases your risk of skin cancer. Basking in the sun is not healthy.[37]

Sunburns are caused by certain wavelengths of *ultraviolet radiation (UV)* (Figure 22.3). UV alters the layers of the skin, causing reactions such as redness, blistering, tanning, and skin cancer (see Chapter 21). UV radiation includes two bands: UV-A radiation and UV-B radiation.

- UV-B radiation turns the skin red rather quickly, causing sunburn, and can cause damage to genetic material in cells and tissues which, if not repaired correctly, can lead to skin cancer. Most of the damage to genetic material in cells comes from UV-B. Although people of all backgrounds are vulnerable to skin cancer, African Americans show a very low incidence of skin cancer because their skin contains a greater amount of the pigment melanin.[38, 39] UV-B also impairs the body's immune system.[40, 41] UV-B rays are more intense in summer months, especially between the hours of 10 AM and 2 PM, at high altitudes, and near the equator.

- UV-A radiation is the largest component of UV radiation. Thought by many to be harmless "tanning rays," UV-A penetrates to the *dermis,* or second layer of skin, causing changes in blood vessels and creating sags and bags associated with premature aging of the skin (Figure 22.3). UV-A rays, present year-round, are especially strong in the early morning and late afternoon.

Most sunburns are first-degree burns that damage only the outer layer of skin and cause redness and slight swelling. For the pain of mild burns, topical analgesics containing benzocaine, lidocaine, camphor, or phenol will temporarily soothe the pain.[42] When the skin begins to peel, moisturizers such as cocoa butter and petrolatum can work to relieve the dryness. Blisters, swelling, and/or oozing are signs of a second-degree burn, which should be treated by a physician. Creams or lotions, when applied to second-degree burns, may do more damage than good because of the danger of infection.[43]

Sunscreens and Other Suntan Preparations

If you must get a tan, you should take several safety precautions to protect your skin. You can start by using lotions, creams, or oils that contain chemicals called **sunscreens,** which absorb and block UV-B radiation to some degree. Sunscreens are used to prevent sunburn and help achieve a tan.

The FDA regulates sunscreen products as OTC drugs and categorizes them as:[44]

To relieve the burn of sunburns, apply cold compresses or soak in cold water to carry the heat away from the skin.

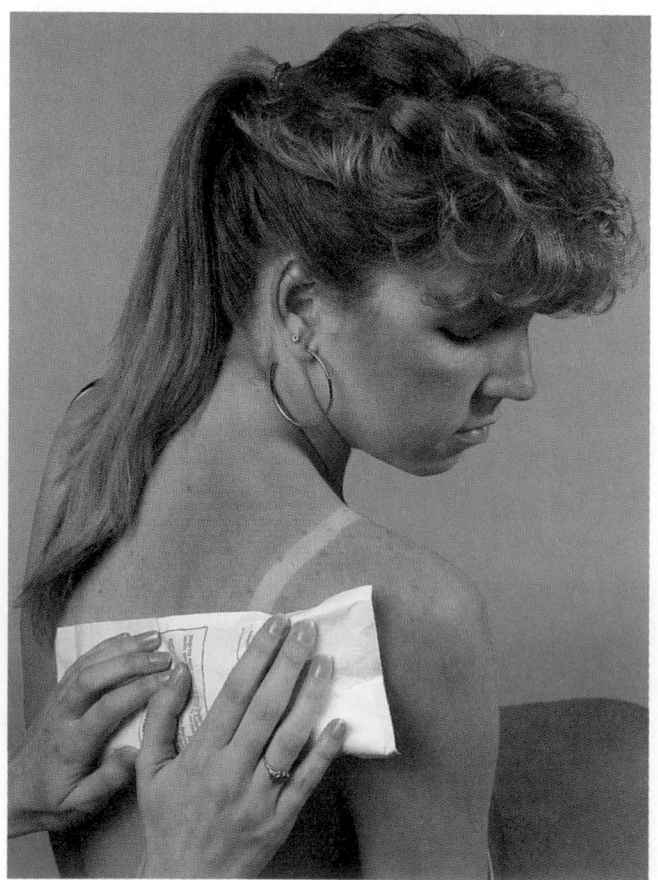

sunscreen a substance used to protect the skin from UV rays.

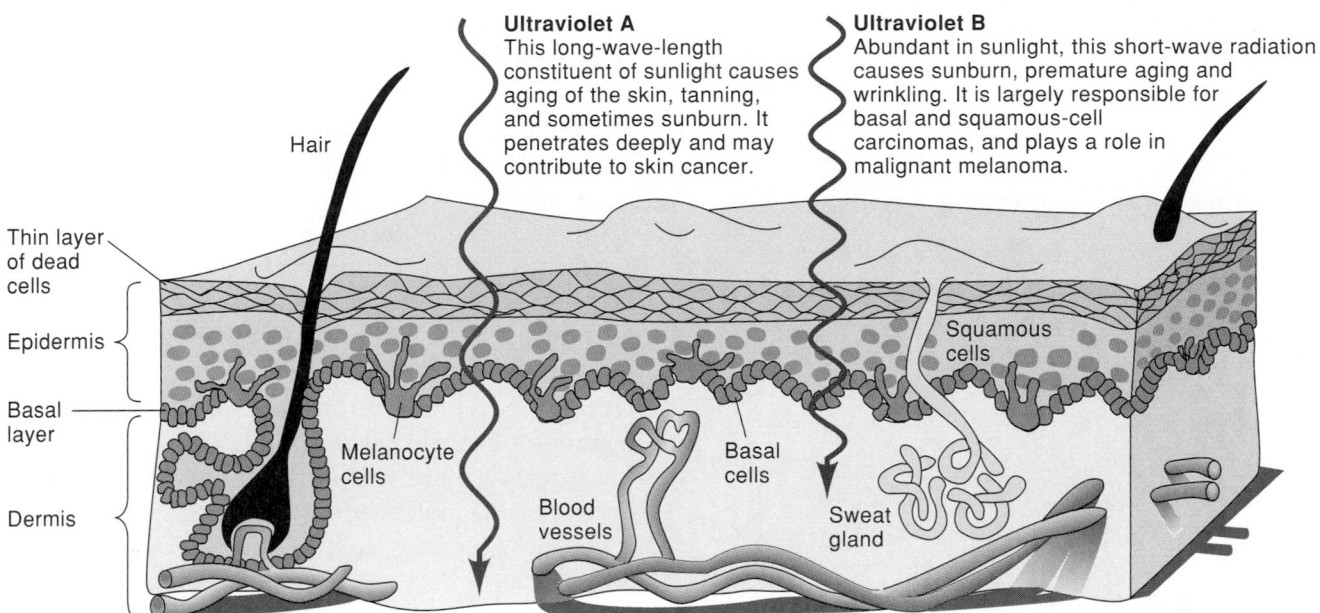

Ultraviolet A
This long-wave-length constituent of sunlight causes aging of the skin, tanning, and sometimes sunburn. It penetrates deeply and may contribute to skin cancer.

Ultraviolet B
Abundant in sunlight, this short-wave radiation causes sunburn, premature aging and wrinkling. It is largely responsible for basal and squamous-cell carcinomas, and plays a role in malignant melanoma.

Hair

Thin layer of dead cells

Epidermis

Basal layer

Dermis

Melanocyte cells

Blood vessels

Basal cells

Squamous cells

Sweat gland

Figure 22.3
Assault on the Skin

1. *Sunscreen-sunburn prevention products* contain an active ingredient that absorbs 95 percent of the UV-B rays.

2. *Sunscreen-suntanning products* contain an active ingredient that absorbs at least 85 percent of the UV-B rays and part of the UV-A rays and transmits the rest.

3. *Sunscreen-opaque sunblock products* contain an opaque substance, such as zinc oxide, that reflects all ultraviolet radiation.

Many products contain a combination of the first two types of ingredients. The basic difference between a suntanning product and a sunburn-prevention product is the amount of the active ingredient. Suntan products are not able to "promote" a tan. The FDA warns that any product claiming otherwise is making unsubstantiated claims.

Sunscreens are rated by their ability to prevent sunburn. The rating is expressed as a number called the **sun protection factor (SPF)** and pertains only to UV-B rays. The higher the SPF, the more effectively the product prevents sunburn. An SPF of 6, for instance, means that you can stay in the sun six times longer before burning than if you were wearing no sunscreen. The American Acade-

my of Dermatology and the National Institutes of Health agree that everyone should use a product with an SPF of at least 15. Although the FDA has proposed an upper limit of SPF 30, manufacturers market products with SPFs as high as 50.[45, 46]

The FDA is constantly evaluating the amount of UV-A rays that sunscreen products need to screen out. Some sunscreen ingredients filter out only part of UV-A radiation and others all of it. In screening out all UV-A, those rays that permit tanning will also be curtailed.

If using sunscreen, apply it at least 30–45 minutes before exposure, then reapply it periodically, especially after you swim or sweat. It is especially important to protect children. One or more severe sunburns with blisters in childhood or adolescence can double the risk of the skin cancer melanoma later in life.[47] Additional protection can be provided by a wide-brimmed hat to protect your head and face, and opaque clothing to cover those body areas you wish to protect. Any fabric or material you can see through, including some beach umbrellas, does not give full protection. You should stay out of the sun between 10 AM and 2 PM when the rays are strongest.

Sun exposure while on certain medications can decrease the time necessary to promote sunburn, premature skin aging, cataracts, skin damage, allergic reactions, and reduced immunity. Drugs causing increasing light sensitivity include antihista-

....

sun protection factor (SPF) a measurement of the ability of a sunscreen product to prevent sunburn.

mines, dandruff shampoos, oral contraceptives, ibuprofen, antinausea drugs, sulfa drugs, water pills, oral anti-diabetic agents, tetracyclines, and antidepressants.[48]

Sunlamps and Pigmenting Agents

For those wanting the bronzing effects of a tan without sun exposure, there are two other options: tanning lamps and skin dyes.

Sunlamps Sunlamps are often used in health club tanning booths. They give off UV radiation, concentrated more intensely than that in sunlight; and it thus takes less time to affect the skin. To give people more color, these lamps commonly provide over 95 percent UV-A and less than 5 percent UV-B radiation, a different mix than found in sunlight. Yet, dermatologists warn that UV-A radiation can still adversely affect the eyes and the skin of the recipient, including causing skin cancer melanoma. Research also shows that people who use tanning devices often show signs of suppressed immunity, as shown by more colds and outbreaks of cold sores (oral herpes).[49] Although the FDA has set standards for tanning salons, studies have shown that many salon operators have not posted the mandatory warning signs, and many do not follow safety standards. Such warnings give instructions on how long to stay under the lights, the use of protective eye cover, who should seek a physician's advice before using a tanning bed, and the dangers of using tanning beds.[50] Dermatologists take sharp exception to claims by salon operators that salon tanning is safe and healthy. According to the FDA, the risks associated with tanning salons include the following:[51]

- allergic reactions from the lights
- herpes rash and warts from unsanitary tanning beds
- eye damage, including corneal burns, retina damage, and cataracts, from not wearing protective eye covers
- weakened connective tissue in the skin, leading to wrinkling or sagging
- increased risk of skin cancer.

Skin Dyes There are four different types of skin dyes that can give an "artificial" tan without sunlight. *Bronzers* are color additives that interact with protein on the skin's surface. They stain the skin without damaging it, yet give the skin no protection against the sun. Difficult to apply evenly, the intensity of the tan also corresponds to the thickness and dryness of the skin. Dry elbows and kneecaps can "overtan," as can palms and fingers if the dye is not promptly washed off them after application. Some bronzers are synthetic in origin, and others come from natural sources such as walnut juice. With soap and water these can be washed off. Under any circumstance, after several weeks the dye fades and needs to be reapplied if continued bronzing is desired.[52, 53]

Extenders are color additives that cause a chemical reaction with the protein of the skin. Presently only one such product is available for cosmetic use. *Tanning pills* contain additives from substances similar to beta carotene, which gives carrots their orange color. When taken, these additives are distributed throughout the body, especially in the skin, making it orange. Since oral tanning pills containing these color additives may be harmful, they may not be marketed legally for use in the cosmetic coloring of the skin. *Tanning accelerators* containing amino acids are promoted as substances to hasten development of melanin in sunlight. At this time these drugs are not approved by the FDA as being safe and effective.[54]

PRODUCTS FOR THE TEETH

About two-thirds of all 9-year-old Americans have never had decay in their permanent teeth. According to the Public Health Service, this is more than twice the number of 9-year-olds that were cavity-free a mere decade earlier.[55]

Cavities (caries), or gradual decay in teeth, occurs when three requirements are present: teeth, bacteria, and sugar. Tooth enamel, the hard outer covering on teeth, is vulnerable to certain acids that are produced by bacteria in the mouth. The bacteria feed on carbohydrates, especially sucrose (table sugar). Dental research has shown that approximately 96 percent of all harmful bacteria in the mouth live in the tiny crevices between the tooth and the gum. An age-old technique to protect the teeth we have all been taught is to brush the teeth to remove the sugars the bacteria feed on.

....

cavities (caries) gradual decay of a tooth.

Best done immediately after meals, brushing has always been difficult to practice. Another technique is to remove food particles from between the teeth by using dental floss after eating. Dental floss is a waxed or unwaxed thread that is pulled between the teeth to remove any food lodging there.

Another technique is to strengthen the teeth structurally to resist the acid attack on the enamel. Infants and children who receive **fluoride** from the time the teeth are forming until the baby teeth are lost, have permanent teeth that are stronger and more resistant to bacterial decay. The trick is that the fluoride must be taken internally in drinking water or in food supplements before the permanent teeth have erupted. Once the child's permanent teeth appear, ingested fluoride is of no help. From then on, fluoride applied to the surface of the teeth through fluoride-containing toothpaste and mouth washes can add some protection to the outer layers of the teeth.

Fluoride concentrations are measured in parts per million (ppm). The ideal level is about 1 ppm; less than 0.7 ppm is ineffective, and more than 1.5 to 2.0 ppm can cause mild dental *fluorosis,* a cosmetic effect in which a mottling, or small white contrasting areas on the teeth, occurs. Between 2 ppm and 4 ppm, the effect of excess fluoride is cosmetic only, but above 4 ppm there may be a health effect. The federal Environmental Protection Agency (EPA) can legally require states to defluoride water with a fluoride content in excess of 4 ppm because of the possibility of adverse health effects.[56] Such water can cause an actual pitting of the enamel, making the teeth more susceptible to decay.

When water is artificially fluoridated, the EPA calls for an optimal range in fluoride of 0.7–1.2 ppm. The practice of fluoridating water supplies is endorsed by the American Medical Association, the American Dental Association, the U.S. Public Health Service, and the National Research Council.[57]

Dentifrices (toothpastes and toothpowders for tooth cleaning) do not kill bacteria, nor do they neutralize any acids produced. Unless these dental products also contain fluorides, they are classified as cosmetics, not drugs. The ingredients in dentifrices include abrasives, detergents, flavoring, and in many cases, fluorides. Fluorides are now a major ingredient in 95 percent of the toothpaste we purchase.[58]

In addition to brushing your teeth after each meal and flossing daily, it is essential that you visit a dentist or dental hygienist once or twice each year to have your teeth examined and cleaned. Such attention is an important way of preventing the expense and inconvenience of tooth loss and replacement.

USING COSMETICS SAFELY

Although there are no government or industry regulations that protect the consumer, according to the FDA, today's cosmetics are among the safest products available. As with prescription and over-the-counter products, it is very important that consumers follow label directions and warnings.

Some rules for preventing adverse reactions to cosmetics include the following:

1. Follow all directions and warnings on products.

2. Wash your hands before applying a cosmetic. Also, remember to close containers after each use; dust and microorganisms can easily settle into any product left uncovered.

3. Never borrow another person's cosmetics.

4. When water must be added to a cosmetic before it can be used, do not substitute saliva, which could transfer the bacteria from the mouth to any skin openings.

5. If you develop any adverse reaction to a cosmetic that does not disappear within a day or two, see your physician.

Your welfare depends on how well you watch out for your health and safety, so be smart and choose and use your products wisely.

CHECKPOINT

1. Define the term *cosmetic*. What is the difference between a cosmetic and a drug?

2. Distinguish between the action of a deodorant and an antiperspirant.

3. Distinguish between UV-A and UV-B radiation.

---

fluoride a chemical element that is present in, or added to, water that helps reduce the rate of tooth decay.

dentifrice a powder or other substance for cleaning teeth.

4. Name the precautions a person should observe when using a sunlamp.

5. Identify the factors that have helped reduce the incidence of dental cavities in the United States. ✔

DO-IT-YOURSELF TESTS

An element in people taking charge of their own health is the use of *do-it-yourself* health tests—simple diagnostic tests that people can give themselves to get some indication of their state of health in some given respect. There are an increasing number of these tests available. See Feature 23.2, on p. 735 for a list of home medical tests.

The expanding number of home medical tests makes it easier for people to monitor and maintain their own health. The benefits of home testing are clear. Early pregnancy detection can mean better prenatal care, closer monitoring of glucose can translate into fewer complications from diabetes, and heart disease can be prevented by early discovery of high cholesterol levels.

The home tests approved by the FDA are cheaper than the same tests conducted in laboratories and can be performed without a visit to a physician. Besides being far cheaper, they may also be more accurate. Glucose monitoring kits that allow people with diabetes to monitor blood sugar levels one or more times a day give more accurate results than a once-a-month visit to a physician. Some people with diabetes using home glucose testing have been able to reduce their doctor visits from once a month to once every several months.

The use of in-home testing not only allows for early detection, but can give you more knowledge of and control over your own health. The use of such tests by the general public can reduce days lost to illness and help save lives. The FDA is currently investigating many other tests now available only in physician's offices that might safely be done at home.[59]

There are also problems with home medical tests that need to be reckoned with (Feature 22.1). One is that medical diagnostics is not an exact science. Not all tests are definitive, and the possibility exists for "false" results that might lull a person into unnecessarily delaying a visit to a physician for a more thorough and detailed diagnosis. Not all people are reliable testers and observers. Unless they have technical ability, they can perform the test incorrectly, sometimes even with simple tests, and the results can be misread and misinterpreted. Misread test results can adversely affect the patient if they lead to delays in treatment of serious conditions.

Home tests are no substitute for an initial diagnosis or development of treatment plans. Some medical tests, such as testing for the detection of HIV/AIDS, carry emotional implications and subjects may require psychological counseling. This is one of the reasons the FDA has not approved home tests for the detection of HIV/AIDS.

Some wonder whether home testing will threaten the existence of medical laboratories. Medical observers note that even if a home test screening picks up some conditions, a lab would still need to do the followup; consequently the labs receive more business than if the condition had not been spotted.

Home medical testing increases consumer awareness of their health. With an aging, as well as

FEATURE 22.1

HOME TESTING TIPS

The FDA warns that home medical tests are never 100 percent accurate. They recommend that you consider the following before taking one of these tests:

- Note the expiration date of test kits that contain chemicals.

- Pay attention to whether the product needs protection from heat or cold while in storage.

- If the directions are not clear, do not guess at what they mean. Consult a pharmacist or health professional or check the package insert for information about who to call for assistance.

- Review what the test is intended to do and its limitations.

- Note any special precautions, such as avoiding exercise or food or drugs before taking the test.

- Follow the sequence of instructions exactly. Do not skip any steps.

- Wash urine specimen containers with distilled water, which is usually purer than tap or bottled water.

- When a step is timed, be precise. Use a stopwatch or a watch with a second hand.

FEATURE 22.2

TOP TEN HEALTH FRAUDS

When you entrust your health care to unqualified individuals and buy unproven remedies from them, you are involved in the world of health quackery. Health fraud is big business that has invaded many health practices. According to the FDA, the top ten health frauds include the following:

1. *Fraudulent arthritis products.* Copper bracelets, Chinese herbal remedies, large vitamin doses, and snake or bee venom are used. Symptoms of arthritis go into remission periodically, leading people who use unproven remedies to associate them with the remission.

2. *Spurious cancer clinics.* Use of Laetrile, vitamins, and minerals in questionable clinics, often outside the United States, may cause people to abandon or bypass legitimate cancer treatments.

3. *Bogus HIV/AIDS cures.* Underground or "guerrilla clinics" offering the latest cure for HIV/AIDS have sprung up in the United States, the Caribbean, and Europe. Victims of this so-far incurable disease are further victimized by unproven "cures" of massive doses of antibiotics, typhus vaccine, and herbal tea.

4. *Instant weight loss schemes.* Since weight loss is a concern of many people, weight-loss frauds promising rapid, dramatic, and easy weight loss are widespread and promoted through newspaper and magazine ads and on TV and radio. *There is no quick, painless way to lose weight.*

5. *Fraudulent sexual aids.* No nonprescription drug agents have been shown to serve as safe or effective aphrodisiacs, and use of some involves serious health risks. The FDA thus bans the use of nonprescription aphrodisiacs. Sexual problems should not be treated with OTC products.

6. *Quack baldness remedies and other appearance modifiers.* Aside from one prescription product that has been approved for growing hair on some bald men, there are no effective nonprescription substances for treating baldness or wrinkles, or for increasing breast size.

7. *False nutritional schemes.* So-called "perfect" foods or products, such as bee pollen, wheat germ capsules, and OTC herbal remedies are promoted as surefire cures for various diseases and nutritional shortcomings.

8. *Chelation therapy.* Promoters claim that injection or tablets of certain chemical substances taken with vitamins and minerals cleans out arteries by breaking down arterial plaques, thereby preventing circulatory disease, heart attacks, chest pains, and strokes as an alternative to heart bypass surgery.

9. *Unproven use of muscle stimulators.* Although muscle stimulators have been used legitimately to relax muscle spasms, rehabilitate muscle functions after a stroke, and prevent blood clots, health spas and figure salons have been promoting muscle stimulators to remove wrinkles, perform facelifts, reduce breast size and remove cellulite, uses which the FDA views as fraudulent.

10. *Candidiasis hypersensitivity. Candida* is a fungus found naturally in small amounts in warm parts of the body, but with weakened body resistance, the fungus can multiply and severe infections occur. Some promoters claim that people can suffer from a *Candida* hypersensitivity that triggers fatigue, constipation, diarrhea, depression, impotence, and infertility. By taking antifungal drugs, and vitamin and mineral supplements, promoters claim the problem can be corrected.

Source: "Top 10 Health Frauds." *FDA Consumer* October 1989, pp. 28–31.

---

better-informed, U.S. population, the issue of home testing and diagnosis will inevitably become more focused.

QUACKERY

As discussed in Chapter 20, *quackery* is the commercialization of unproven, worthless, and sometimes dangerous health products and procedures. The promotion and sale of these "health" services is alive and thriving, even among the educated public. Quacks play on people's fear and desperation, and that accounts for much of their success.

The FDA estimates that more than $27 billion a year is spent on fraudulent health practices; more than $1 billion a year is spent on fraudulent HIV/AIDS therapies alone (Feature 22.2). The FDA estimates that at least 38 million people use fraudulent health products each year. Not without risk, it is believed that 1 out of every 10 people who use quack remedies are harmed by their side effects.[60, 61]

WHO ARE THE QUACKS?

Most commonly, quacks have little or no scientific training and pretend to be experts in chemistry and the human body. "Dr. Sebi," a Brooklyn herbalist who posed as a physician, was arrested for treating HIV/AIDS with his herbal compounds for a fee of $500 per treatment.[62] Some quacks operate in respected medical clinics; however, they use unorthodox remedies. This was the case for the antiviral drug HPA-23, developed by the Pasteur Institute. Before knowing much about the drug, physicians at Pasteur prescribed it for Rock Hudson. As studies of the drug were completed, findings showed that the drug had excessive toxicity and was of little, if any, benefit to the HIV/AIDS patient.[63]

Other forms of quackery are practiced by corporations that falsely promote their products. One example is Lubraseptic, an FDA-approved drug promoted as a condom lubricant/spermicide. When studies showed that the chemical would kill the HIV/AIDS virus in the test tube, the manufacturer promoted the drug as an HIV/AIDS preventive in the body without further studies. No drug, to date, is able to prevent HIV/AIDS.

WHO ARE THE QUACKS' CUSTOMERS?

According to a national health fraud survey by Louis Harris, more than one out of four Americans said they had used health care treatments of questionable safety or effectiveness. Surprisingly, the survey found that college graduates were more likely to use questionable treatments than those with less formal education, and that most of those using these products had at least some college education.[64]

Health frauds are often targeted at vulnerable groups of people, such as:

- Teenagers concerned with self-image (undersized breasts, underdeveloped muscles, weight and complexion problems)[65]

- The elderly, who may become depressed over chronic health problems

- Recent immigrants whose language and cultural differences limit their access to information about health fraud

- Victims of life-threatening diseases, such as HIV/AIDS, arthritis, and some cancers. More than one-third of arthritis sufferers and about one-sixth of cancer victims have used questionable therapies for their conditions.[66]

- The very rich, because they have the money to pay for miracle cures.

- The poor, who lack access to affordable and ethical care.

Because so many people fear rejection if they don't measure up to a specific image, they'll go to almost any length to change. To accommodate these people, fraudulent products cover a spectrum that includes weight-loss products, hair-restoration schemes, wrinkle removers, and products to cure hemorrhoids, varicose veins, and gray hair. Many people accept almost any information they hear as reliable and anything they read as gospel. See Feature 22.3 for some signs of quackery.

CONSUMER PROTECTION AGAINST QUACKERY

Consumers have a right to safe cosmetic products, as well as responsible, honest, high-quality medical care. Federal and state governments and private organizations are helping to provide such protection.

Food and Drug Administration (FDA)

The FDA is a federal agency responsible for protecting the consumer against the dangers of contaminated food and hazardous and worthless drugs and health devices. It has the authority to require that new products meet a set of criteria for safety *before* they reach the marketplace and to ensure that products offered for sale are both effective *and* safe.

Federal Trade Commission (FTC)

The **Federal Trade Commission (FTC)** is an agency responsible for protecting the consumer by acting against false and misleading advertising and selling practices for products that could adversely affect the health and safety of consumers. It also protects the consumer against products that just do not work.

U.S. Postal Service

The postal Service, through its postal inspection process, works to prevent the mails from being used in schemes to defraud the public. Postal laws prohibit the use of mail to obtain money or property by means of false or fraudulent representations, pretenses, or promises.

....

Federal Trade Commission (FTC) the federal agency responsible for regulating false and misleading advertising and the selling of dangerous and ineffectual products.

FEATURE 22.3

SIGNS OF QUACKERY

It is important for you to be aware of signs of quackery. Following are some red flags to watch for.

A "secret formula" available only from this one company. Legitimate scientists share their knowledge so other scientists can review their data. Once proven effective, all qualified medical pracititioners are free to use it, not one person or company.

A computer-scored questionnaire for diagnosing "nutrient deficiencies." Computers used for such tests are programmed to recommend supplements for virtually everyone, regardless of symptoms or medical conditions.

The treatment is promoted only in back pages of magazines, over the phone, by mail-order newspaper ads in the format of news stories, or 30-minute infomercials. Bona fide medical studies are reported first in medical journals. Information appearing only via these other means probably does not pass scientific scrutiny.

Products that claim an easy way to lose weight. Beware. There is no magic pill or magic device to lose weight easily. Products that promise to trim you down and tone you up effortlessly are false. Losing weight requires the self-discipline to eat less and exercise more.

Testimonials and anecdotes from satisfied customers to support claims. There is no way of knowing whether the "satisfied" users ever had the disease the product was supposed to cure, whether they are paid spokespersons, or whether they even exist. Many chronic ailments have symptom-free periods that may be mistaken for a cure, and many single episodes of disease disappear over a period of time. Remem-

ber that 50–75 percent of all doctors' office visits are the result of psychosomatic complaints that often disappear due to the power of suggestion.

Claims that most doctors are "butchers," that the medical community is against them, and that the government will not accept this wonderful discovery. Actually, as with other notable discoveries, anyone finding a cure for HIV/AIDS or other serious conditions would be appropriately honored with grant money and scientific honors, such as the Nobel Prize. Legitimate doctors do not conspire to suppress cures.

"Limited supply—act now." "Don't miss this once-in-a-lifetime opportunity." This sales approach, so commonly used in all lines of business, is intended to scare the customer into acting without taking time to think about the offer and to check its validity.

"Recommended by doctors and nurses." This advertisement seldom states who these doctors and nurses are, or what type, for that matter.

Guarantee of cure or satisfaction. Ethical physicians never guarantee a cure. They do the best they can, but medical science has not progressed to the point where results are that certain. Even with a "guarantee," a quack is seldom known to refund any money.

"Approved by independent research laboratories." It is not difficult for the patent medicine producer to find some chemist who is willing to set up an "independent research laboratory," perhaps in a garage, and for a fee, to approve almost any product.

Source: "How to Spot a Quack." FDA Consumer October 1989, p. 30.

State Departments

Some states now have a separate Department of Consumer Affairs, and they all have Attorney Generals offices that initiate the prosecution of consumer violations. In order to establish complete accountability in the marketplace, the departments and offices ask that consumers take a greater part in policing for misleading advertising. Check your local telephone listings for the addresses and phone numbers of such offices in your area.

Private Agencies

Many privately funded groups actively participate in consumer protection efforts. These include the Bureau of Investigation of the American Medical Association, the Better Business Bureau, the Consumer's Union, and Ralph Nader and Associates. Although these organizations have no legal regulatory powers, they can bring cases of fraud to the

attention of the public and the proper regulatory authorities. Check your local telephone listings for the location of such agencies in your area.

As consumers, we all must share the responsibility for protecting ourselves against health frauds. We should heed warnings about quackery and be wary whenever we encounter products that seem "too good to be true." They probably are.

C H E C K P O I N T

1. Define the term *quackery.* What are some of the characteristics of a quack?

2. List some examples of HIV/AIDS quackery.

3. Who are the common targets of health frauds?

4. Name several agencies that help protect consumers against health frauds.

SUMMARY

Ours is a consumer-oriented society. Many people are well read and well educated, and everyone has access to a wide array of health products. While we can do much for our own well-being, we need product protection and counsel in understanding the content and proper use of these products. The success you find in the use of these and other such products will in no small way have a bearing on your peace of mind and bring a sense of confidence in taking care of that most precious of endowments—your physical body.

Drug products that can be used safely and effectively without a physician's supervision are nonprescription, or over-the-counter (OTC), products. The FDA decides which drugs are to be placed in this category. Since consumers select and administer such drugs, they include more labeling. Pharmacists are a helpful resource for the consumer in the use of both prescription and OTC products.

The most widely sold of all OTC drugs are pain-relievers, or analgesics. Aspirin, the most popular analgesic, reduces inflammation and reduces fever. Two other common analgesics are acetaminophen and ibuprofen.

There is no cure for the common cold. Many drugs are available for treating cold symptoms—relieve pain, dry up mucous membranes, and reduce nasal congestion. Other cold remedies suppress coughing and phlegm production.

Another category of OTC drugs is intended to treat gastrointestinal disorders, such as diarrhea, constipation, and hemorrhoids. Sleep aides and sedatives, which are intended to promote sleep and quiet a person, often contain antihistamines, while stimulants often contain caffeine. Eye products include eyewashes and eyedrops.

Eyeglasses are available both OTC and as a prescription product from an ophthalmologist or optometrist. An alternative to eyeglasses are contact lenses, which may be hard or soft. Some soft contacts are designed as extended-wear lenses and some as disposable lenses.

Substances that are intended to beautify, yet not alter body function, are called cosmetics. Deodorants, mouthwashes, shampoos, sunscreens, pigmenting agents, and dentifrices fall in this category. Some products, such as antiperspirants, may be both a drug and a cosmetic.

Quackery is the commercialization of unproven, often worthless, health products or procedures. Nowhere is quackery more glaring than with those promoting HIV/AIDS remedies. Quacks often, though not always, lack scientific training. Their clients are the young, old, sick, rich, and poor. Respected corporations and medical clinics sometimes traffic in quackery. Many agencies have been created to protect the consumer from quackery, such as the FDA, FTC, Department of Consumer Affairs, and various private agencies.

REFERENCES

1. *Heart and Stroke Facts.* Dallas, TX: American Heart Association, 1992.
2. *Cancer Facts and Figures, 1992.* Atlanta, GA: American Cancer Society, 1992.
3. Hecht, A. "OTC Drug Labels: 'Must' Reading." *FDA Consumer* (October 1985), 33–35.
4. Lesar, T., et al. "Medication Teaching Error in a Teaching Hospital." *JAMA* 17 (1990), 2329–2334.
5. Cramer, J., et al. "How Often Is Medication Taken as Prescribed?" *JAMA* 22 (1989), 3273–3277.
6. Ibid.
7. Yorke, J. "FDA Ensures Equivalency of Generic Drugs." *FDA Consumer* (September 1992), 11–15.
8. Ibid.
9. Blumenthal, D. "Pharmacists Help Solve Medication Mysteries." *FDA Consumer* (January–February 1991), 27–30.
10. Ibid.
11. Thomas, P. "OTC Drugs." *Medical World News* (December 1990), 32–42.
12. Ibid.
13. Segal, M. "Rx to OTC: The Switch Is On." *FDA Consumer* (March 1991), 8–11.
14. Thomas, op. cit.
15. Hecht, A. "Aspirin vs. Acetaminophen." *FDA Consumer* (February 1983), 6–9.
16. American Pharmaceutical Association. *Handbook of Non-prescription Drugs,* 9th ed. Washington, DC: American Pharmaceutical Association, 1990.
17. Hecht, 1983, op. cit.
18. Ibid.
19. Ibid.
20. American Pharmaceutical Association, op. cit.
21. Cramer, T. "When Do You Need an Antacid?" *FDA Consumer* (January–February 1992), 119–122.
22. Cumings, M. "Overuse Hazardous: Laxatives Rarely Needed." *FDA Consumer* (April 1991), 33–35.
23. American Pharmaceutical Association, op. cit.

24. Ibid.

25. Ibid.

26. "Buying Glasses." *Consumer Reports* (August 1993), 459–503.

27. "Wrapup: Contact Lenses." *University of California at Berkeley Wellness Letter* (July 1986), 4–5.

28. "Buying Sunglasses: The Eight Key Questions." *University of California at Berkeley Wellness Letter* (June 1988), 3.

29. Greeley, A. "Dodging the Rays." *FDA Consumer* (July–August 1993), 30–33.

30. Stehlin, D. "Cosmetic Safety More Complex Than First Blush." *FDA Consumer* (November 1991), 18–23.

31. American Pharmaceutical Association, op. cit.

32. American Dental Association. *Accepted Dental Therapeutics,* 40th ed. Chicago, IL: American Dental Association, 1984.

33. Hopkins, H. "What Does Shampoo Do?" *FDA Consumer* (June 1984), 8–11.

34. Patlak, M. "Hair Dye Dilemmas." *FDA Consumer* (April 1993), 31–34.

35. Ibid.

36. Ibid.

37. Pine, D. "The Right Shades." *FDA Consumer* (June 1992), 20–25.

38. Greeley, 1993, op. cit.

39. Ibid.

40. Greeley, A. "No Safe Tan." *FDA Consumer* (May 1991), 16–21.

41. Greeley, 1993, op. cit.

42. Pine, op. cit.

43. "A Soothing Look at Sunburn." *University of California at Berkeley Wellness Letter* (August 1985), 7.

44. Greeley, 1993, op. cit.

45. Greeley, 1991, op. cit.

46. Greeley, 1993, op. cit.

47. Pine, op. cit.

48. Ibid.

49. Greeley, 1993, op. cit.

50. Roan, S. "Burning Issue for Tanning Salons." *Los Angeles Times* (14 May 1991), E-1, 12.

51. Ibid.

52. Pine, op. cit.

53. Greeley, 1993, op. cit.

54. Ibid.

55. Schultz, D. "Fluoride: Cavity Fighter on Tap." *FDA Consumer* (January–February 1991), 34–38.

56. Ibid.

57. Ibid.

58. Ibid.

59. Schrage, M. "Do-It-Yourself Health Tests: Over Time, Costs Will Soar." *Los Angeles Times* (11 March 1993), A-1, 5.

60. "Top 10 Health Frauds." *FDA Consumer* (October 1989), 28–31.

61. Segal, M. "Defrauding the Desperate: Quackery and AIDS." *FDA Consumer* (October 1987), 17–19.

62. Ibid.

63. Ibid.

64. Young, F. "Allies in the War Against Health Fraud." *FDA Consumer* (March 1988), 6–7.

65. Food and Drug Administration and Council of Better Business Bureaus, "Quackery Targets Teens." *FDA Consumer* (February 1988), 24–27.

66. Young, op. cit.

SUGGESTED READINGS

Arnot, R. *The Best Medicine.* Reading, MA: Addison Wesley, 1992.

Consumer Reports Books. *Complete Drug Reference,* 1993 ed. Mt. Vernon, NY: Consumer's Union, 1992.

Consumer Reports Books. *U.S. Pharmacopeia: Drug Information for the Consumer,* 1989 ed. Mt. Vernon, NY: Consumer's Union, 1989.

FDA Consumer. A periodical, published monthly, except for two issues, at $15 per year. For information, write: the Superintendent of Documents, P.O. Box 371954, Pittsburgh, PA 15250-7954.

Griffith, H. W. *Complete Guide to Prescription and Nonprescription Drugs,* 7th ed. Los Angeles: The Body Press, 1992.

Long, J. *The Essential Guide to Prescription Drugs,* 1989 ed. New York: Perennial Library, 1989.

Margolis, S. (ed.). *The Johns Hopkins Handbook of Drugs.* New York: Rebus, 1993.

Sherman, H., and Simon, G. *The Pill Book,* 5th ed. New York: Bantam, 1992.

University of California at Berkeley Wellness Letter. A periodical that is published in association with the School of Public Health. Published monthly at $24 per year. For information, write: Health Letter Associates, 5 Water Oak, Fernandina Beach, FL 32034.

Wolfe, S., and Hope, R. *Worst Pills, Best Pills II.* Washington, DC: Public Citizen Health Research Group, 1993.

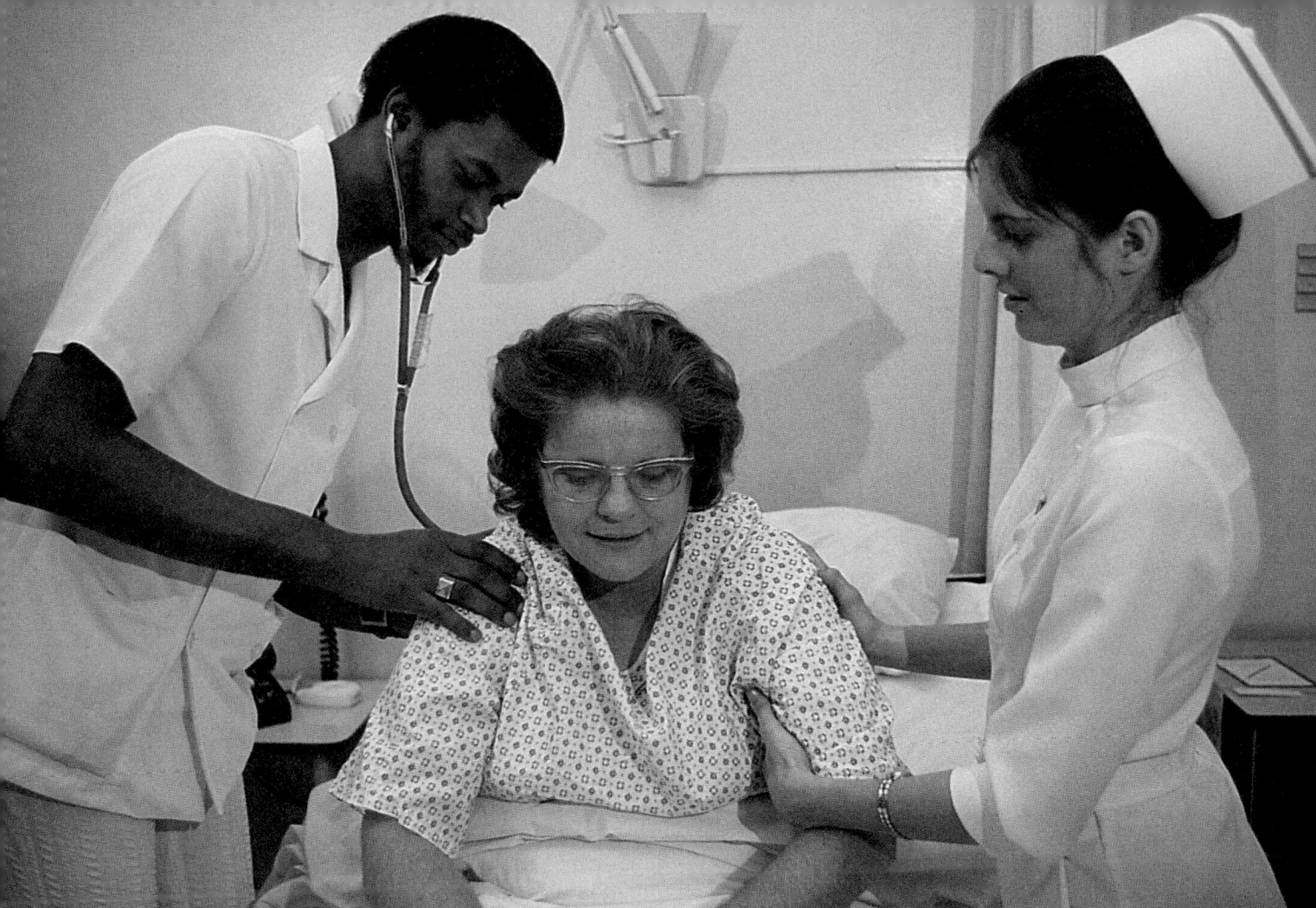

23

HEALTH CARE SYSTEMS

CHAPTER OBJECTIVES

Upon completing this chapter, you will be able to:

KNOWLEDGE

- Explain the basis for the great interest people have in self-care.
- Describe the average amount of money spent yearly by people in the United States on health care.
- Outline the kind and amount of training a physician must have and the requirements he or she must meet in order to become a general practitioner.
- Name several of the more common medical specialties.
- List the common kinds of health care facilities.
- Define *fee-for-care* medical care.
- Explain the meaning of HMO and PPO.
- Explain the meaning of *managed competition* in the proposed national health care reforms.
- In what ways has the government gotten involved in tax-supported public insurance?
- Give some of the reasons some people feel there is need for health care reform in the United States.

INSIGHT

- Explain why you would or would not choose alternative health care over traditional medicine for the treatment of an illness you might have.
- Outline some home medical tests you can carry out for yourself without seeing a physician.
- Understand your own health insurance coverage.

DECISION MAKING

- Decide on the type of physician that would best suit your needs of primary care.
- Explain the criteria most important to you in selecting a primary physician.
- Identify whether health insurance through an HMO or a PPO would better serve your health needs.
- Decide how you feel about the proposed national health plan.

Most residents of the United States enjoy the benefits of one of the world's most advanced health care systems. However, we are experiencing significant problems with this system. The cost of health care has been increasing dramatically each year, far exceeding the overall inflation rate. The spiraling cost of health care represents only one of the many problems with the current health care system. An alarming number of Americans, children as well as adults, have no insurance coverage. As a result, they may not attend to health-related problems until they reach a crisis point, or they may have difficulty receiving appropriate care when they require it.

The state of medical practice has changed a great deal over the past 50 years. Fewer physicians practice alone or are self-employed; more practice in groups or organizations. Physicians now depend a great deal on payment for services by public and private third parties, such as Medicare, Medicaid, and private insurance companies. Also, there has been an increasing emphasis on outside review and control of *medical practice, resulting in physicians being more obligated to follow standardized rules of clinical procedure. Health care professionals complain of overregulation and duplication of administrative tasks that take them away from time with patients. The way these changes have been addressed is directly related to the problems of rising health care costs, lack of insurance for many, and the administrative overload faced by most physicians today.*

Most experts believe that changes in our current system of health care are not only important, but essential. Most likely, our political process will prevent or at least slow any truly sweeping changes in the health care system. There is no doubt, however, that changes must occur to improve the administration of health care in the United States.

■ ■ ■

HEALTH CARE AND YOU

We in the United States have a great deal of interest in health care. We are the benefactors of the greatest advances ever in medical technology, medications, hospital services, and insurance programs. Each of these elements has become so technical and sophisticated that the system has become unwieldy and very costly. In fact, major deficiencies in the system have caused the delivery of health care to become a major issue on the national agenda. Not everyone in this country has easy and affordable access to these services. In this chapter we will examine the nature of health care, how it is provided, and by whom. We will also be looking at some of the troublesome areas and what is being proposed to fix them.

Before proceeding further into the chapter, stop and check your knowledge as a health care consumer by completing the assessment, In Your Hands: Rating Your Own Health Consumer Skills. As you read the chapter, look for ways to improve your health care consumer skills.

HEALTH CARE IN THE UNITED STATES

Satisfaction with the delivery of health care in the United States can be measured by public opinion.

According to surveys, 94 percent of the people in the country believe their own physician does a good job, and 53 percent say they would be willing to pay more to keep their own physician, yet 81 percent feel that physicians charge too much.[1] There is no question that each of us spends a great amount of money on health care. As a nation we spend a yearly average of about $3000 per person on health care.[2] The effect of this has been that almost one in four of us put off health treatment for fear we can not afford it, and nearly half of us believe we could not afford good care if we were to become critically ill.[3] Further complicating the picture is the fact that 37 million, or 14 percent of people in the United States, have no health insurance coverage whatsoever. All of this has happened in a country that spends more per person on health care than any other country in the world, 12.2 percent of the nation's gross national product.

A possible cure for health care problems in the United States must take several issues into account. One is that everyone must take responsibility for as much self-care as possible. A second is that we need an adequate supply of health care professionals. A third is that health care must be easily available and affordable.

SELF-CARE

Most Americans are interested in taking an active role in promoting their own health. Many of us can be trained to do a good deal to care for ourselves. In taking more responsibility for our health, we are a part of the movement toward **self-care.**

There are many reasons for engaging in self-care. We have more interest in exercising control over our own health practices. As a result, we are learning about preventive measures to ward off illnesses and injuries (see Feature 23.1, p. 734). We are also learning to monitor and assess our activities in ways that had once been left up to our physicians.

Self-care helps lower health care costs, provides more effective care for certain conditions, reduces physicians' patient loads, and frees physicians to spend more time with more critically ill

....

self-care health care we can provide to ourselves.

IN YOUR HANDS
RATING YOUR OWN HEALTH CONSUMER SKILLS

Circle the selection that best describes your behavior. Then total your points for an interpretation of your health consumer skills.

	Lowest			Highest
1. I understand the services that a general practitioner provides.	1	2	3	4
2. I have a family physician who has accepted me as a patient.	1	2	3	4
3. I have investigated the credentials of my family physician.	1	2	3	4
4. I have a family physician with whom I can openly discuss any physical condition I might face.	1	2	3	4
5. I have checked out the hospital in which my physician practices; It is accredited by the Joint Commission on Accreditation of Healthcare Organizations.	1	2	3	4
6. When I visit my physician, I make it a point to ask about his/her diagnosis and why he/she is recommending the particular treatment.	1	2	3	4
7. When I have a physical condition that persists for more than several days, I don't hesitate to see my physician.	1	2	3	4
8. I know the basis for my physician's fees and I am satisfied with them.	1	2	3	4
9. I have sought a second opinion when my physician's diagnosis of a condition seemed questionable.	1	2	3	4
10. I practice preventive health care.	1	2	3	4
11. I have my teeth examined at least twice a year.	1	2	3	4
12. I have a tuberculosis test every two years.	1	2	3	4
13. I know how to practice breast (females) or testicular (males) self-examination and perform it regularly.	1	2	3	4
14. I have checked into whether I am covered by a health insurance plan.	1	2	3	4
15. I have recently read my health insurance policy and understand its benefits.	1	2	3	4
16. I am acquainted with the annual deductible in my health insurance policy.	1	2	3	4

Total points: _____

INTERPRETATION:

57–64 points: A highly skilled health consumer

41–56 points: An adequately skilled health consumer

25–40 points: An inadequately skilled health consumer

16–24 points: A very poorly skilled health consumer

---

patients. This philosophy has also been responsible for the increased interest in health-related activities. Self-care is preferable to professional care in at least three areas. *First,* self-care is often appropriate for certain acute conditions that occur frequently and are self-limiting, such as common colds, first-aid for common injuries, and headaches. *Second,* self-care can be used for therapy. For example, people with diabetes can test blood sugar levels and administer their own insulin shots, and patients with hypertension can monitor their own blood pressure. *Third,* self-care can be used for health promotion. Breast and testicular self-examination, exercise programs, stress management, weight-loss programs, and first-aid classes all lend themselves to self-care. Various community organizations specialize in health promotion, such as fitness clubs and Weight Watchers.

More can be done in the area of self-care once people know what to look for (see Feature 23.2, p. 735). People interested in performing self-care must be alert consumers. Books, self-care equipment, and self-help groups are increasingly available. It is important to learn how to buy reliable equipment (pregnancy test kits, blood pressure measuring devices, stethoscopes) and to learn how to use it accurately. Self-care demands time, money, and a willingness to become a smart consumer.

FEATURE 23.1

PREVENTIVE CARE

The object of preventive care is to prevent illness and disease. If disease should occur, good care will lessen the chances of long-term effects. Preventive measures may include:

- Immunizations: a physician can recommend an appropriate schedule.

- Periodic physical examinations: your physician may recommend a schedule that is appropriate for your age and condition.

- Blood pressure readings: take your own or have it done inexpensively at a screening center.

- Pap smears: should be performed by a physician once every six months to three years for the early detection of cervical cancer.

- Breast self-examination: every woman should learn how to examine her breasts, and then examine herself monthly.

- Testicular self-examination: every man should learn how to examine his testicles, and then examine himself monthly.

- Glaucoma: many physicians recommend annual tests after age 40, especially if there is a family history of the disease.

- Tuberculosis: many employers require a TB test once every two years, especially if exposed to TB; and

- Dental checkups: annual or semiannual checkups and teeth cleaning.

Multiphasic screenings, or a series of tests for multiple conditions, are available from wellness clinics, or centers for health promotion. Multiple health tests may include treadmill and resting electrocardiograms, blood pressure measurement, blood cell and blood chemistry profile, lung function tests, colon cancer screening, health risk profile, health analysis, and body fat analysis. Some hospitals and medical schools conduct health- and risk-evaluation programs for a package price, which may be much less than conducting the same tests separately in a hospital. Many of these tests may be available at your college or university student health center.

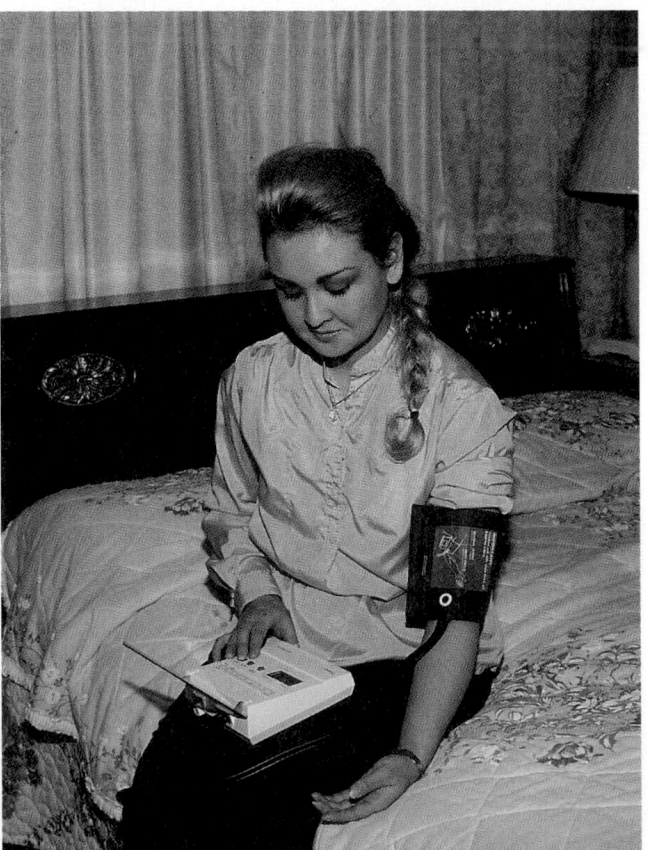

Providing self-care. Home blood pressure readings can be self-administered to detect the presence of hypertension.

CHECKPOINT

1. List the advantages of self-care.

2. Name steps you can take in the direction of preventive care.

3. List several home medical tests and the reasons you would use them.

HEALTH CARE PROFESSIONALS

Health care services are provided by a cadre of health care workers, both professional and non-professional, whose expertise spans every facet of the health care system. These workers run the gamut from the highly trained physician specialists to orderlies and security personnel. Their training ranges from extended postgraduate programs to on-the-job training.

Due to the fact that the delivery of health care is so complex, knowing to whom to turn for help requires knowledge of the system. As a health care consumer, you need to be informed about the different types of health care providers and what they have to offer.

FEATURE 23.2

HOME MEDICAL TESTS

Following are some simple medical tests and procedures that can be part of a self-care assessment.

Procedure	*Purpose*
Blood glucose test	To detect the level of glucose in the blood
Blood pressure measurement	To detect the presence of hypertension
Body fat measurement	To determine the percentage of body fat
Breast examination	To detect lumps or fluid-filled cysts in the tissue of the breasts
Gonorrhea test	To detect the bacterium that causes gonorrhea in a specimen of pus from the penis
Hidden fecal blood test	To detect hidden blood in stools
Impotence test	To detect and measure the rigidity of the penis during sleep
Ovulation monitoring	To measure the amount of the hormone LH, the hormone which triggers ovulation, in urine
Pregnancy test	To detect the hormone HCG, the hormone which is produced by a developing placenta (see Chapter 8), in urine
Testicular examination	To detect the presence of tumors in the tissue of the testicles
Urinary tract test	To detect nitrites in the urine; the presence of nitrites indicates a urinary tract infection
Vision test	To screen for visual acuity, problems with retinal degeneration, and glaucoma

PHYSICIANS

There are many ideas as to the best way to treat persons who are sick and injured. Orthodox medicine, which uses drugs or other remedies, is represented by two traditional approaches. Medical doctors, or **medical physicians,** stress the use of agents, often drugs or medicines, such as antibiotics, and combine this emphasis with surgical methods and various therapies. **Osteopathic physicians** focus on the musculoskeletal system and how it interacts with body organs in both health and disease, and combine this emphasis with medical and surgical methods of treatment. We will discuss both approaches.

Training

Earning a *doctor of medicine* (M.D.) degree or a *doctor of osteopathy* (D.O.) degree requires four years of training in an accredited college of medicine or a college of osteopathic medicine. To prac-

....

medical physician a trained and licensed practitioner of medical arts.

osteopathic physician a trained and licensed practitioner of osteopathic medicine.

tice with either degree, most states require an additional one-year hospital internship in order to gain experience, and require that the physician candidate pass a licensing examination given by either the state or by the national board of medical or osteopathic examiners.

A physician who completes these requirements is known as a **general practitioner (G.P.).** If the physician wishes to specialize in a specific field of medicine, two to five years of additional training and hospital practice, called a *residency,* is required. In order to become a *board-certified,* or fully qualified, specialist, a physician must complete a residency, and pass an examination in his or her specialization. After completing these requirements, the physician receives a certificate designating him or her as a diplomate or fellow of the board of that specialty. For example, an M.D. might become a *Diplomate of the American Board of Pediatrics,* while a D.O. might become a *Fellow of the American College of Osteopathic Pediatricians.* To confirm whether a physician is certified by a board, consult *The Directory of Medical Spe-*

....

general practitioner (G.P.) a physician who has met the professional and legal requirements to provide general health care.

The health care system in the United States includes many kinds of personnel. Surrounding this patient are the various kinds of professional and nonprofessional persons whose services are needed to provide him with care.

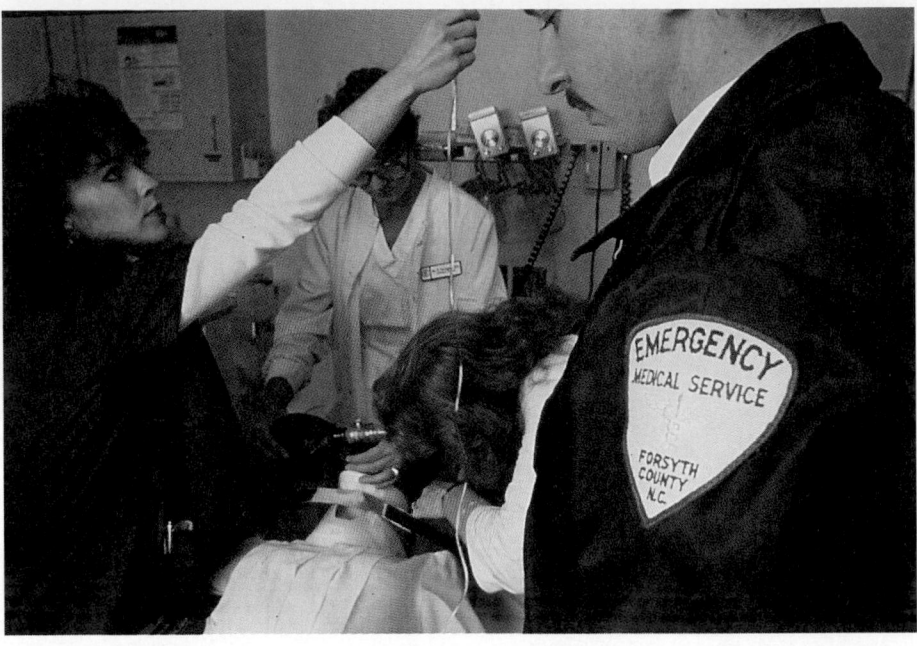

cialists or *The AOA Yearbook and Directory of Osteopathic Physicians,* national publications that list information on all physician diplomates or fellows. Some specialties are sufficiently complex that they are subdivided into subspecialties, such as cardiology being a subspecialty of internal medicine. See Table 23.1 for descriptions of some of the more common specialties and subspecialties.

It is important to know that if a physician claims to specialize in a certain area, he or she has earned board certification in that particular specialty. Studies show that significant numbers of physicians advertise themselves as specialists, implying that they in some way confine their practice to certain areas of medical care rather than their having earned board certification in a particular specialty.[4] Physicians can legally practice any form of medicine they wish regardless of their training.

THE FAMILY PHYSICIAN

Everyone should have a physician they can call upon for basic, or general, health care. The care you receive on your first contact with the health care system is **primary care** (see Feature 23.3, p. 738). One of several types of physicians should be able to meet this criteria. Except for those specialists who also serve as primary care physicians,

most specialists provide **secondary care** upon referral from a person's primary care physician. Your physicians will develop and keep confidential medical records of your condition, illnesses, injuries, treatments, and tests. In the event you change physicians, it is important to your best medical care that your medical record move with you. Feature 23.4 (p. 739) explains how you can share in the proper handling of your own medical records.

Various kinds of physicians can provide primary care, and include the following:

- *General practitioners (G.P.s)* are physicians who have met the professional and legal requirements to provide general health care, but who have not earned advanced certification in a medical specialty. G.P.s most commonly provide basic, or primary, medical care for a wide range of physical conditions.

- **Family practitioners** are diplomates or fellows whose specialty is Family Practice. In many places family practitioners have replaced general practitioners as the first choice

....

primary care basic, or general, care given at the person's first contact with the health care system.

secondary care medical care provided by another physician upon referral by a patient's primary care physician.

family practitioner a specialist in providing comprehensive medical care to the family unit.

Table 23.1
Medical and Osteopathic Specialties and Subspecialties

Specialty	*Description*
Allergy and Immunology	A subspecialty of internal medicine that diagnoses and treats allergic reactions
Anesthesiology	Administration of drugs to block pain or induce unconsciousness during surgical operations or diagnostic procedures
Cardiology	A subspecialty of internal medicine that diagnoses and treats disorders of the heart and blood vessels
Dermatology	Diagnosis and treatment of skin diseases
Family Practice	Comprehensive medical care with emphasis on the family unit
Gastroenterology	A subspecialty of internal medicine that diagnoses and treats disorders of the stomach and intestinal tract
Geneticist	Diagnosis and treatment of genetic diseases
Hematology	Diagnosis and treatment of blood-related disorders
Internal Medicine	Diagnosis and treatment of disorders of organs and organ systems of the body that do not require surgery
Neurology	Diagnoses and treats nonsurgical disorders of the brain, spinal cord, and nerves
Neurological Surgery	Diagnosis and surgical treatment of nervous system disorders
Nuclear Medicine	Use of radioactive substances to diagnose and treat disease
Obstetrics and Gynecology	Care for pregnant women and treatment of disorders of the female reproductive system
Oncology	Diagnosis and treatment of new and abnormal growths or tumors
Ophthalmology	Medical and surgical eye care, including prescription of corrective lenses
Orthopedic Surgery	Diagnosis and treatment of diseases of the muscles, fractures, and deformities of the bones and joints
Otolaryngology	Diagnosis and treatment of ear, nose, and throat disorders
Pathology	Examination of body organs, tissues, body fluids, and excrement to detect disease
Pediatrics	Provision of care for children from birth through adolescence
Rehabilitation Medicine	Treatment of convalescing and physically handicapped individuals
Plastic and Reconstructive Surgery	Correction and repair of body or facial structures through surgery
Psychiatry	Diagnosis, treatment, and prevention of mental illness
Pulmonary Medicine	A subspecialty of internal medicine concerned with lung diseases
Radiology	Use of radiation for diagnosis and treatment of disease
Urology	Diagnosis and treatment of urinary tract disorders in males and females, and the reproductive system in males

for a family physician. Family practitioners are able to provide primary care.

- **Pediatricians** specialize in providing primary care to children from birth to adolescence. At some point in childhood or adolescence, families transfer from a pediatrician to some other type of physician for continuing primary care.

pediatrician a specialist in the treatment of children's diseases.

- **General internists** specialize in **internal medicine,** that branch of medicine that treats, by nonsurgical means, diseases of the internal organs. General internists often provide primary care to adults.

general internist a physician who practices internal medicine.

internal medicine the branch of medicine that treats diseases of the internal organs by nonsurgical means.

FEATURE 23.3

SHOPPING FOR A PHYSICIAN

Whether you choose a physician by picking a name out of the yellow pages, by talking to your pharmacist, or by following the recommendation of a friend, make sure that the physician you choose is someone with whom you are comfortable. As health insurance and medical technology become more complex, finding the right physician who can diagnose, treat, and/or advise you becomes more challenging. What you need is a primary care physician who will serve as your personal physician and provide referrals when specialists are needed.

Take the following steps when choosing a physician:

1. Decide on your requirements for a primary care physician. Do you want a physician who can treat all members of your family? Do you want a male or a female physician? Do you want him or her to have special training? Do you want a specialist or a general practitioner? Must he or she be located in a given area, town, or on the staff of a given hospital?

2. Assemble names of physicians in your vicinity who meet your requirements. Sources for names include pharmacists, nurses, local medical or osteopathic societies, accredited hospitals, and friends.

3. Check a physician's basic credentials. These can be found through a local or state medical or osteopathic society.

(These resources, however, will tell you little about his or her competency, personality, or philosophy.)

4. Make sure that the hospital in which the physician practices is accredited by the Joint Commission on Accreditation of Healthcare Organizations. The hospital can provide you with this information. When hospitalized, you will have to go where your physician has hospital staff privileges.

5. Check the medical or osteopathic societies or organizations to which the physician belongs. The *American Medical Directory* or the *AOA Yearbook and Directory of Osteopathic Physicians* will list these.

6. From your list, select names of several physicians who are conveniently located and who meet your requirements.

7. Make an appointment with the leading candidate. Ask about fees, office hours, and coverage when he or she is unavailable or in case of emergency. Find out if advice is given by phone, the types of health insurance the office accepts, and who submits the claim for the insurance payment. You may wish to schedule a physical exam with the physician before you make up your mind.

8. If your candidate appears to be a person you can trust, and if your questions are answered satisfactorily, your investment of time and money will have paid off.

The medical needs of children often are provided by a pediatrician, a physician specialist trained in providing care of children.

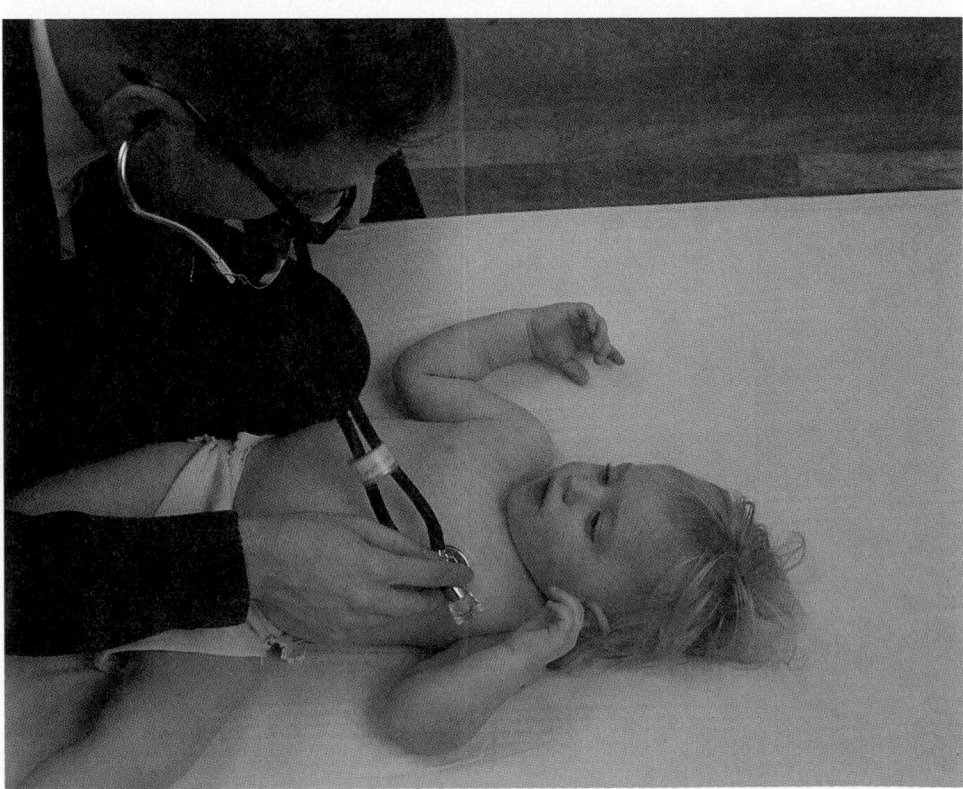

FEATURE 23.4

YOUR MEDICAL RECORDS

Your medical records are confidential. These records are on file in your physician's office and in any hospital where you have been a patient. Medical information that you supply when you apply for health, disability, or life insurance may, however, become a part of a control data base called the Medical Information Bureau, and be shared among health insurance companies and, with your permission, be made available to employers, schools, and government agencies.

It may be useful for you to have a complete, up-to-date, set of your medical records. In the event your physician retires and your records are not transferred to another physician or you wish to provide them to a new physician, you have a copy of your records. Such records provide continuity of care and may help avoid the unnecessary repetition of tests. About half of the states now guarantee you access to your medical records; in those that do not, many physicians and hospitals honor requests for copies. Expect to pay a charge for photocopying and mailing.

For information on accessing your medical records, you may purchase a booklet entitled "Medical Records: Getting Yours" for $10 from Public Citizen, 2000 P Street, NW, Suite 600, Washington DC 20036. To obtain a free copy of your records on file with the Medical Information Bureau, write to: P.O. Box 105, Essex Station, Boston, Massachusetts 02112.

Source: "Take Charge of Your Medical Records." University of California at Berkeley Wellness Letter November 1993, p. 1.

OTHER HEALTH CARE PROFESSIONS

Health care professionals who are not medical doctors are limited by law in the procedures they can perform. Some of the more common examples are dentists, registered nurses, podiatrists, optometrists, and pharmacists.

Dentistry

Dentists diagnose and treat conditions of the gums and teeth. Dentists hold either a *Doctor of Dental Surgery (D.D.S.),* or a *Doctor of Dental Medicine (D.D.M.)* degree. Most dentists are general practitioners and provide a wide range of care. Some dentists specialize in providing basic dental care to children (pedodontists), realigning teeth (orthodontists), root-canal therapy (endodontists), conditions of the gums and underlying bone (periodontists), and extraction of teeth and surgical procedures (oral surgeons).

Nursing

Nurses provide patient care ranging from simple health care tasks to the most expert professional

....

dentist a medical practitioner specializing in the care of the teeth and gums.

nurse a medical professional who provides patient care ranging from simple health care tasks to expert professional techniques.

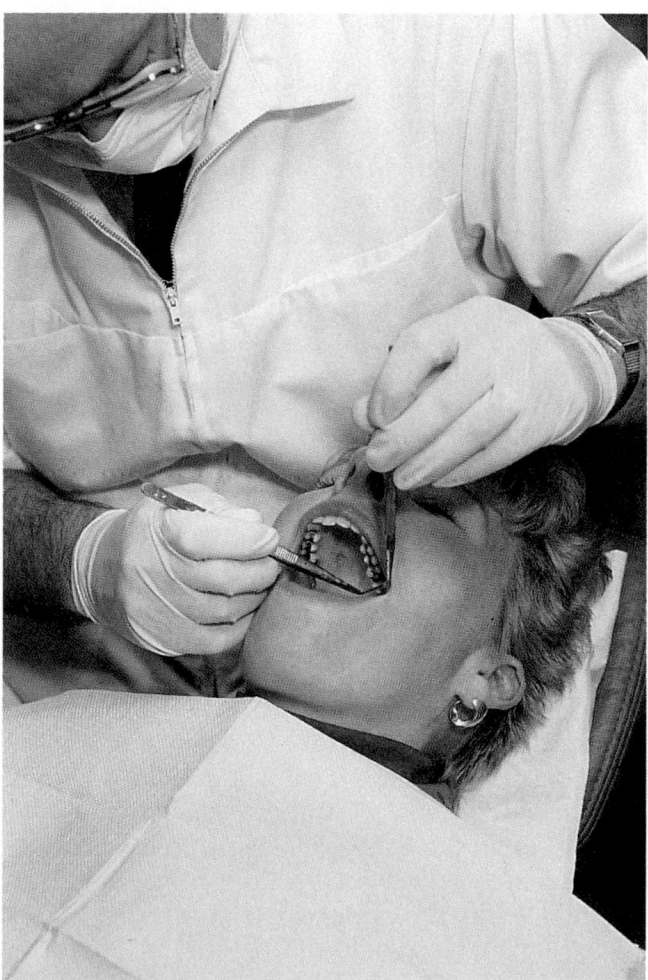

Regular dental check-ups and cleanings are essential to help prevent tooth decay and gum disease.

techniques. The health care team includes the registered nurse (R.N.), nurse-practitioner (N.P.), and licensed practical (vocational) nurse (L.P.N. or L.V.N.).

- *Registered Nurse (R.N.)* A person may enter one of three state-approved types of training for registered nursing. Associate degree programs, often found in community colleges, usually require two years of training. Diploma programs are conducted by hospitals and independent schools and require three years of training. Bachelor degree programs usually require four years of education at a college or university. Nurses must pass a state board examination in order to become licensed.

  Some registered nurses take specialty training in fields such as nurse practitioner, nurse midwifery, psychiatric nursing, health education, obstetrics, pediatrics, medical/surgical, family health, oncology, critical care, and life support. Upon passing a certification examination, these nurse specialists receive certification in their area of training.

- *Licensed Practical Nurse (L.P.N.)* or *Licensed Vocational Nurse (L.V.N.)* These nurses undergo a shorter period of training than registered nurses and work under the supervision of physicians or R.N.s.

Podiatry

The *Doctor of Podiatric Medicine (D.P.M.),* or the *Doctor of Podiatry (D.P.),* is a medical specialist who treats foot disorders by performing surgery, prescribing drugs, and/or fitting braces. **Podiatrists** are sometimes also known as chiropodists.

Optometry

As discussed in Chapter 22, the *Doctor of Optometry (O.D.)* is a professional who is trained and licensed to diagnose refractory disorders and to prescribe and fit corrective lenses. The *optometrist* is not to be confused with the *ophthalmologist,* a physician specializing in eye conditions, who is also qualified to dispense drugs and perform eye surgery.

------

podiatrist a medical practitioner who treats foot conditions.

Pharmacy

Also, as discussed in Chapter 22, the *pharmacists* are medical professionals who specialize in pharmaceutics. The role of the pharmacist is to formulate drugs, fill drug prescriptions, and provide information about using different drugs. Many pharmacists now hold *Doctor of Pharmacy (Pharm. D.)* degrees.

ALLIED HEALTH CARE PROFESSIONS

There are many other health care workers in fields often referred to as the **allied health professions,** whose disciplines are seen as professions and whose members are essential to the health care team (Table 23.2). Trained in a specialty area, their services are auxiliary to the work of physicians and other primary health care workers. The amount of training allied health care professionals receive varies from graduate or bachelor degree programs to associate programs.

ALTERNATIVE HEALTH CARE THERAPIES

There are alternative health care systems of healing that are nontraditional and that have not been tested according to the same standards as have orthodox health care methods. Such systems are gaining an increasing foothold in the United States. A *Time*/CNN poll found that 30 percent of those questioned had tried some form of alternative therapy, half of them within the last year.[5] Some of these patients are dissatisfied with conventional medicine, which may be pathology-oriented, and with too great a focus on crisis intervention rather than on staying healthy. Other people feel that traditional medicine places an undue reliance on the use of drugs as a therapy tool.

There is support for some of the claims of alternative health care therapies. For example, there are research findings that an acupuncturist's needles inserted into the skin stimulate nerve cells to release *endorphins,* opiate-like substance that relieve pain.[6] Critics answer that there is no objective evidence as to the usefulness of such uncon-

------

allied health professionals health care professionals whose specialty areas are auxiliary to physicians and other health care professionals.

Table 23.2
Some of the Allied Health Care Professionals

Health Worker	Description
Dental hygienists	Provide services for the maintenance of oral health, including cleaning and scaling of teeth
Medical records personnel	Responsible for keeping patients' records complete, accurate, up-to-date, and confidential
Medical technologists	Perform laboratory tests to help in the diagnosis of disease and to determine its extent and possible causes
Occupational therapists	Work with disabled patients to help them adapt to their disabilities; this may involve relearning skills needed for daily activities and modifying the physical environment
Orthotists and prosthetists	Prepare and fit braces and artificial limbs
Physical therapists	Provide services designed to prevent loss of function and to restore function in the disabled; exercise, heat, cold, and water are among the agents they use
Physician assistants	Perform physical examinations, provide counseling, and prescribe certain medications under a physician's supervision
Radiologic technicians	Prepare patients for x-ray and take and develop x-rays
Recreational therapists	Provide services to improve patients' well-being through music, dance, and other artistic activities
Registered dietitians	Licensed to apply dietary principles to the maintenance of health and the treatment of disease
Respiratory therapists	Treat breathing disorders, according to the physician's directions; assist in postoperative rehabilitation
Speech pathologists and audiologists	Measure hearing ability and treat disorders of verbal communications

Source: Columbia University College of Physicians and Surgeons. Complete Home Medical Guide, rev. ed. New York: Crown Publishers, 1989.

sionals should be prepared to demonstrate proof of adequate training as indicated by a degree, credential or accreditation, and by licensing and regulation within the state in which they practice.

Chiropractic

Chiropractic treatment is based on the belief that many human diseases are due to the misalignment, or **subluxation,** of vertebrae of the spinal column, which leads to pressure on the nerves. **Chiropractors** often diagnose conditions by using x-rays, and then treat conditions by manipulating the bones, especially the vertebrae. Chiropractors are not allowed to use surgery or to prescribe drugs. They hold the degree of *Doctor of Chiropractic (D.C.),* which is granted after four years of training in chiropractic.

Homeopathy

Homeopathy is based on Hippocrates' law of similar conditions, the tenet that "like cures like." By administering a large dose of a drug to a healthy person, a set of drug-caused reactions, or symptoms, result. The drug, diluted to microdoses and given to patients with similar disease-caused reactions, or symptoms, stimulates the body's healing processes.

Naturopathy

Naturopathy is treatment based on the belief that disease occurs when natural principles relating to the body have been abused. Diseases are seen as the body's effort to repel impurities and substances harmful to it. Naturopathic treatment involves

ventional techniques. They insist that there is a risk in a person relying on alternative therapies for conditions, such as some cancers, that may have been treatable with traditional medicine, but which have now gotten out of hand due to inordinate delay and/or reliance on some unproven therapy. They make the point that unconventional therapies, when unregulated, are subject to quackery and fads (see Chapter 22). There is also the unnecessary cost of any ineffectual therapy.

Some of the alternative health care fields are commonly recognized professions, although others are nonprofessional fields. All health care profes-

subluxation a partial or incomplete dislocation of the vertebrae.

chiropractor the professional who treats health conditions by methods that include musculoskeletal manipulation.

homeopathy a system of disease treatment in which minute doses of a drug or remedy are administered, a large dose of which would in healthy persons produce symptoms of the disease; the theory that "like cures like."

naturopathy a therapeutic system that does not use drugs or therapy, but employs natural forces such as light, heat, air, water, and massage.

Acupuncture is based on the theory that illness results from an imbalance of vital energy flowing through the body along twelve meridians, each of which corresponds to a vital organ. The acupuncturist inserts needles at specific points. The free ends of the needles may be twirled or used to conduct a weak electric current.

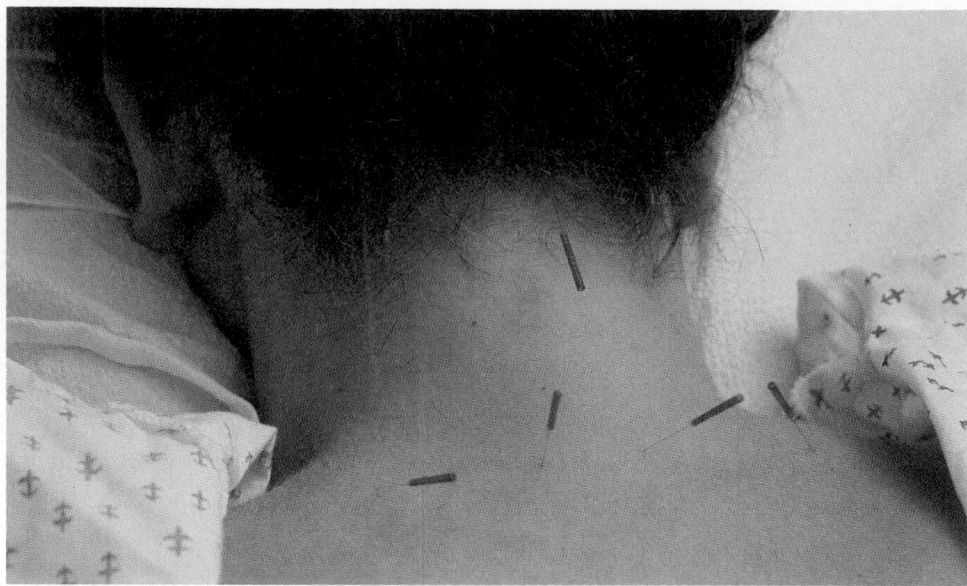

using natural forces such as light, heat, air, water, sunlight, "natural" foods, vitamins, herbs, minerals, and salts. Surgery and drugs (other than naturally occurring ones) are not used. The practice of naturopathy is licensed in only certain states.

Naturopathy does not satisfactorily allow for the presence of disease-producing organisms, or the need for drugs or surgery.

Faith Healing

Today there is a revival of spiritual, or **faith healing** in the United States. This practice is based on the belief that a divine being or higher power can heal, and that there is no need for medical or chemical treatment. Some faith healers also advocate traditional medicine.

Acupuncture

Acupuncture is a method of treatment based on a centuries-old Chinese technique of inserting special needles into the skin or muscles at one or more meridians, which are invisible points that represent various internal organs. Acupuncture practitioners

....

faith healing healing accomplished by supplication to a divine being or power without medical or chemical treatment.

acupuncture a technique for treating certain painful conditions by passing long thin needles through the skin to specific points representing specific organs.

believe that this method balances the flow of the body's life force, or *Chi.*

Acupuncture is reported to relieve pain in those who believe in its efficacy. An anesthetic effect sufficient to permit abdominal, thoracic, and head and neck surgery has been produced by acupuncture alone. Some dentists regularly use acupuncture in place of conventional anesthetics and some insurance companies cover such therapy if it is shown to be medically necessary.[7, 8]

Many forms of alternative health care have long been practiced worldwide. An increasing number of such therapies have found their way into the practice of health care in the United States, especially among the great numbers of foreign-born persons entering the United States in recent years. Some other forms of alternative health care are described in Table 23.3.

CHECKPOINT

1. Discuss the training required to become a medical doctor or doctor of osteopathy.

2. How can a person know whether a physician is a certified specialist?

3. Name the types of physicians an individual or family would look to for primary health care.

4. Explain why a person should not seek a chiropractor, homeopath, or naturopath to provide them with primary health care.

Table 23.3
Other Forms of Alternative Health Care

Practice	Description
Acupressure	Like acupuncture, except using fingers to replace needles
Alexander technique	Training in improved posture to alleviate pain
Aromatherapy	Use of essential plant oils for skin massage and inhaling
Ayurvedic medicine	Use of herbs and massage, depending on body type
Bioenergetics	Exchange of "energy" between patient and therapist
Biofeedback	Use of machines to train people to control involuntary functions
Color healing	Use of colored light on body to alter its "vibrations" or aura
Crystal healing	Healing by deriving energy from quartz and other minerals
Guided imagery	Envisioning your own immune systems to battle disease
Holistic medicine	Treatment of whole person emphasizing life-style and psychological factors
Hypnotherapy	Using therapeutic suggestions while patient is in a semi-conscious trance to relieve pain and induce healing
Macrobiotics	Dietary and health discipline based on balancing yin (passive energy) and yang (active energy)
Medicinal herbalism	Use of plant-derived potions to promote healing
Reflexology	Manipulating areas on the feet to affect the rest of the body
Rolfing	Deep, perhaps painful, massage to realign body
Shiatsu	Japanese therapeutic massage using pressure points

HEALTH CARE FACILITIES

One important health care issue is knowing where to go when you need medical care. For some people this becomes a matter of whether they will be accepted for treatment; for some, where they will receive the best care, especially if a person's life is in question; for many it's a matter of whether they will be able to cover the costs. Yet for others it is a question of where the facility is located, whether it's open, and how much time it will take. All of these matters can become magnified if there are children or elderly persons in the family. Before committing yourself to any kind of medical care, it's important to review the kinds of facilities available and the pros and cons of the different kinds of facilities.

COLLEGE HEALTH SERVICES

Colleges and universities provide campus-based student health services. A major resource to college students, such facilities commonly provide medical services, psychological services, nursing services, emergency service and first aid, and health education and consultation. Additional services may include laboratory tests, medications, vision screening tests, tuberculin skin tests, and immunizations.

Costs for college health services are often covered by fees that are included as a part of the total payments made at the time of registration. Some are covered by supplementary insurance policies.

PRIVATE PHYSICIANS' OFFICES

Many physicians have their own solo practices, or are part of a group partnership with one or more other physicians. Some physicians are family physicians and provide primary care such as routine office visits, immunizations, and physical exams. Other physicians are specialists who provide secondary care, often upon referral from a patient's primary-care physician.

CLINICS

Clinics are medical treatment centers that generally provide more equipment and/or personnel than a private physician's office. Some clinics provide primary care, secondary care, or both. Clinics may be private or public. County or city health departments often operate public, low-cost diagnostic and treatment clinics for family planning, sexually transmitted diseases, and immunizations for persons not otherwise able to obtain such services. Some clinics are large and have established reputations, such as the Mayo Clinic in Rochester, Minnesota; others are staffed by a small number of professional and clerical people. While some clinics provide comprehensive ambulatory care, others specialize in x-rays, headache and pain control, orthopedic and back treatment, physical therapy, or birth-control counseling. There is a growing trend toward organizing free-standing 24-hour emergency-care clinics that provide greater convenience and lower cost than those found in many traditional hospitals. Clinics may or may not have facilities for performing minor surgery.

HOSPITALS

Hospitals are health centers providing an array of clinical and surgical services on both an inpatient

Hospitals provide a wide array of clinical and surgical services. As a health facility hospitals usually offer the most comprehensive level of medical care.

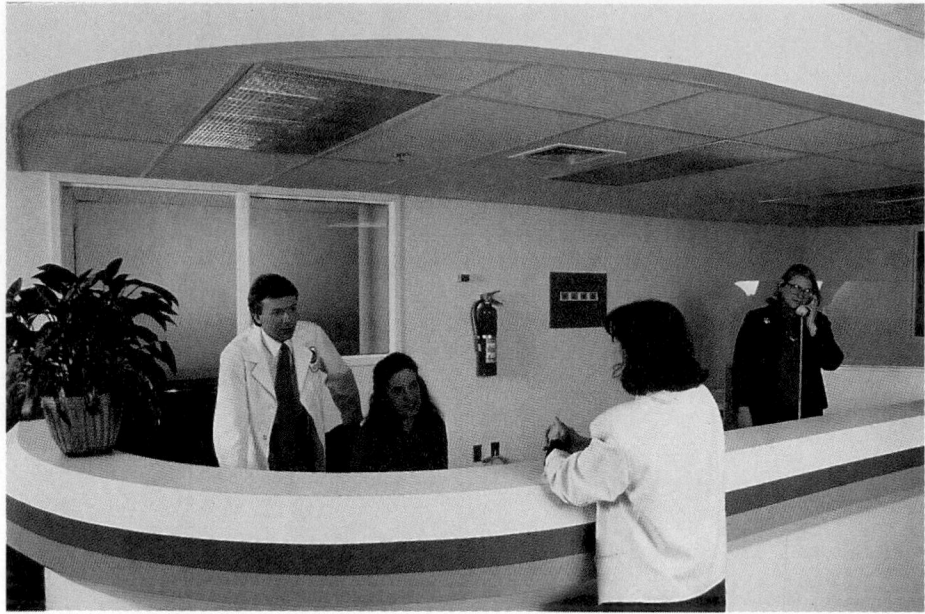

and outpatient basis. They generally offer the most comprehensive level of care of any health facility. Hospitals vary considerably in size, type of services offered, and ownership.

To help guarantee that it maintains a certain quality of care, a hospital should seek accreditation by JCAHO. Once accredited, the hospital may seek reaccreditation every two to three years. Accreditation is based on a hospital's staff physicians, records, laboratory operations, food handling, and cleanliness. If a hospital is denied accreditation, it is not eligible to train interns, residents, or nurses, and may be denied some government funding. Today, more than 89 percent of all hospitals in the United States are accredited.

Hospitals are commonly categorized by type of ownership. The three major types of hospitals are those privately owned and operated to make a profit, those privately owned and operated as nonprofit institutions, and those publicly owned.

Proprietary Hospitals

Proprietary hospitals are often owned and operated by individuals or corporations, and are intended to make a profit. There has been a rapid growth of investor-owned multihospital chains. These hospitals often emphasize such cost-reduction meth-

ods as labor-saving measures, group purchasing and management, and shorter patient stays. Proprietary hospitals are generally medium-sized (100–250 beds) facilities.

Nonprofit Hospitals

Nonprofit, or **voluntary, hospitals** are maintained as public institutions. Because their goals are not monetary, these hospitals often provide for patients who cannot pay for their treatment. Often referred to as community hospitals, they are frequently owned by the community and operated under a governing board of community leaders. Voluntary hospitals usually offer a wide range of comprehensive therapeutic services, and many of them are developing wellness clinics, which provide preventive and rehabilitative services.

Public Hospitals

Public hospitals are supported mostly by tax dollars and fees for available services. They are often large facilities that contain from 500 to 1000 patient beds. Many of these hospitals are known as gov-

proprietary hospitals hospitals whose operations are intended to make a profit.

nonprofit or voluntary hospitals hospitals that are publicly owned and are operated as nonprofit institutions.

public hospitals hospitals that are owned and operated by some level of federal, state, county, or local government.

ernment hospitals, because they are operated by county, state, or federal agencies, such as the Veterans Administration, the Public Health Service, or the military. On the local level, public hospitals may be operated by the county or city.

Specialized Care Centers

Specialized care is often needed on a short-term to long-term basis. Common types of such centers are nursing homes, rehabilitation centers, and convalescent centers.

- *Nursing homes* are usually used as long-term care facilities for the elderly or chronically ill. They may be categorized by the level of care they offer.
  - *Sheltered care* is for residents who need some assistance in daily living, but who need little attention.
  - *Intermediate care* is for residents who need help with activities of daily living on a regular basis.
  - *Skilled-nursing care* is for residents who need intensive, personalized, and professional health supervision on a 24-hour basis. Some homes also provide specialized care for those afflicted with conditions such as Alzheimer's disease.
- *Rehabilitative centers* serve burn victims, orthopedically injured people, or the handicapped or chronically ill.
- *Convalescent centers* provide care to people recovering from an illness, injury, or surgery who need extended care, but at a lower cost than in a hospital.

EMERGENCY CARE

Life-threatening emergencies rarely occur to most people. But when they do happen, you must get help immediately. If your community does not have a 911 emergency number, keep the numbers of an ambulance service, police, fire department, and your physician handy. In desperate situations, call the operator. If you are with someone whose heartbeat or breathing has stopped, or if severe bleeding or unconsciousness occurs, seek immediate attention.

Hospital emergency rooms should be used only for life-threatening emergencies. Some physi-

cians direct their patients to a hospital emergency room if a crisis occurs after regular office hours. Some people who do not have a primary care physician use emergency rooms for routine care. Such misuse of emergency rooms reduces their efficiency and increases their operating costs. If there is a non-life-threatening emergency, such as a bone fracture, animal bite, or laceration, find out where the nearest independent 24-hour emergency care, or urgent care, center is located.

WOMEN AND HEALTH CARE

Women have a unique interest in the health care system. Whether for themselves, their children, mates, or parents, they are part of the health care system more than twice as often as are men. Women are the bearers of children and the nurturers of infants. Much of the flow of health care communication among physician's offices, hospitals, and families comes through women. So involved are women in health care that some health care analysts refer to women as the "primary health care workers."

Beyond their crucial role in communicating medical information, women have particular health care needs themselves. These needs are heavily influenced by the woman's role as a mother or potential mother. Her lifetime phases of adolescence and menarche, of young adulthood and childbearing, and of older years and menopause require medical attention that is quite different from that of the man. As a childbearer, her body is heavily influenced by the reproductive hormones estrogens and progesterone. As childbearing passes, she must adjust to significant shifts in hormone levels.

Among older women estrogen replacement therapy (ERT) is now recognized as playing a significant role in affecting the incidence of heart disease and the incidence of bone fracture due to osteoporosis.[9] This is important, in part, because it is now known that one of the biggest health risks women face is cardiovascular disease (particularly stroke and coronary disease), a mortality risk that is more than two times greater than that of cancers of the breast, ovary, and uterus combined.[10] The causes of morbidity (sickness) and mortality (death) differ between women and men, and women tend to live longer (by about seven years on average).

The quality of a woman's health is pivotal in the home, in the support of her children's education, and in her adult relationships. The health care of women deserves attention since the poor are disproportionately women and children, some of whom do not have access to survivable levels of income or to adequate insurance coverage. This is especially important since 14 million women of childbearing age have no health care coverage, and the health insurance of 5 million more women excludes coverage for prenatal care and delivery.[11]

Even for those women who have access to the full range of medical services, it is appropriate to identify health care services that are directed at women's needs. A good model of such care specializing in women's needs is women's health centers and clinics, some of which are run by women. Such clinics provide services in well-woman care, gynecological exams, and birth control and abortion services. Here patients can talk with female health workers and other female patients, and can be referred to appropriate specialists. While much quality health care is available to both genders, any shortcomings in the care of women needs to be addressed especially promptly and effectively because of their high rate of use of the health care system.

CHECKPOINT

1. Distinguish between private physicians' offices and clinics with regard to the type of care each can provide.

2. How is the quality of health care that is provided by hospitals measured?

3. On what basis is a hospital classified as proprietary, nonprofit, or governmental? Compare the kinds of services that can be provided by each.

4. Under what conditions might a person seek out emergency health care?

5. List the types of preventive care a person might practice in order to avert illness.

THE COST OF HEALTH CARE IN THE UNITED STATES

Each year, the cost of medical care in the United States increases. Reasons for the rise in costs include a greater demand for health services, costlier medical techniques and procedures, greater availability of health insurance to foot the bills,

and the rising proportion of older persons in the population.

In 1991, national health care spending increased 9.1 percent over the previous year. This amounted to $738.2 billion dollars, or 13 percent of the gross national product (see Figure 23.1). On an individual basis, personal health care expenses reached an average of $2817 per person (see Figure 23.2, p. 748).

FINANCING HEALTH CARE

Health care in the United States is financed by a combination of patient payments, private and public insurance plans, and public assistance. Unfortunately, this system of financing doesn't cover everyone and the system contains some large gaps. Many low-income persons go without health care because they are unable to afford health insurance or adequate care. An estimated 14 million poor people in this country do not go to physicians because they cannot afford medical services. Thirty-seven million, or 14 percent of Americans have no health insurance. Two-thirds of the uninsured are in families of full-year steadily employed workers. Nearly half of uninsured workers are self-employed or employed in firms with fewer than 25 workers.[12]

Children are most in need of health care. For them, many health conditions are preventable at a relatively low cost per child, but lack of such care can become very costly in terms of a child's life expectancy. The American Academy of Pediatrics now advises that children receive 14–15 immunizations by age 2 as protection against 9 diseases; yet, nationally only 63 percent of 2-year-olds have had their immunizations and the rate is as low as 10 percent in some areas of the country.[13]

Many employers do not provide any health care coverage. Self-employed people often go without insurance because it is too expensive. Some payment options for health care insurance are available, and will be discussed in following sections.

PAY-AS-YOU-GO

Some Americans pay for their health care on a pay-as-you-go, or **fee-for-service,** basis. Less than 23

fee-for-service a payment as the service is rendered; also called pay-as-you-go.

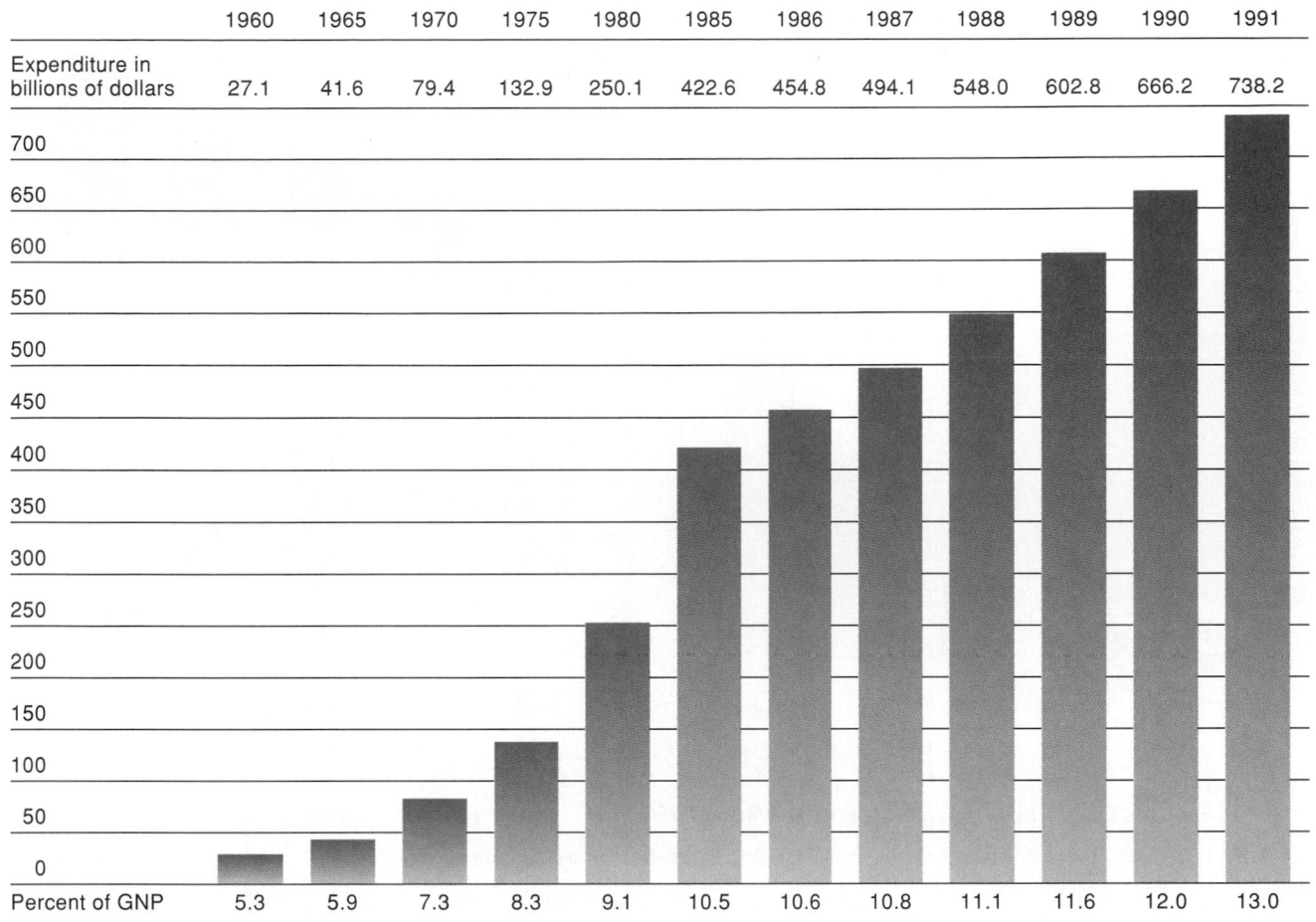

	1960	1965	1970	1975	1980	1985	1986	1987	1988	1989	1990	1991
Expenditure in billions of dollars	27.1	41.6	79.4	132.9	250.1	422.6	454.8	494.1	548.0	602.8	666.2	738.2
Percent of GNP	5.3	5.9	7.3	8.3	9.1	10.5	10.6	10.8	11.1	11.6	12.0	13.0

Figure 23.1

National Health Expenditures and Percent of Gross National Product

Source: Health Insurance Association, 1992 Source Book of Health Insurance Data. Washington, DC: Health Insurance Association of America, 1992.

percent of the total health care payments in the United States are direct payments to a health care person or facility. Fee-for-service means that the patient either pays the physician, another health care professional, or pays the facility for services rendered.

Many people are covered by some form of insurance, but their policies carry a deductible portion that they must pay before the insurance will cover the remaining costs. Other people run the risk of carrying no insurance, either because the premiums are more than they can afford or they decide to forego such costs. These people pay their own medical costs as they arise, hoping they stay well.

HEALTH INSURANCE

In the United States we take it for granted that everyone is entitled to an education—the nurturing

of the mind; and yet not everyone has access to health care—the nurturing of the body. The United States is the only industrialized country in the Western world that does not guarantee basic health insurance coverage for all of its citizens.

Health insurance is a contract agreement between an insurance company or insurer, and the person being insured, or policyholder, for the payment of health care costs (see Feature 23.5, p. 749). The policyholder pays a premium to an insurance company, which covers him or her for specific health costs. The coverage for injury and illness differs with each policy. Most insurance policies provide for a part of the medical costs; but usually do not cover the entire cost.

health insurance a contract between an insurance company and a policyholder for the payment of health care costs.

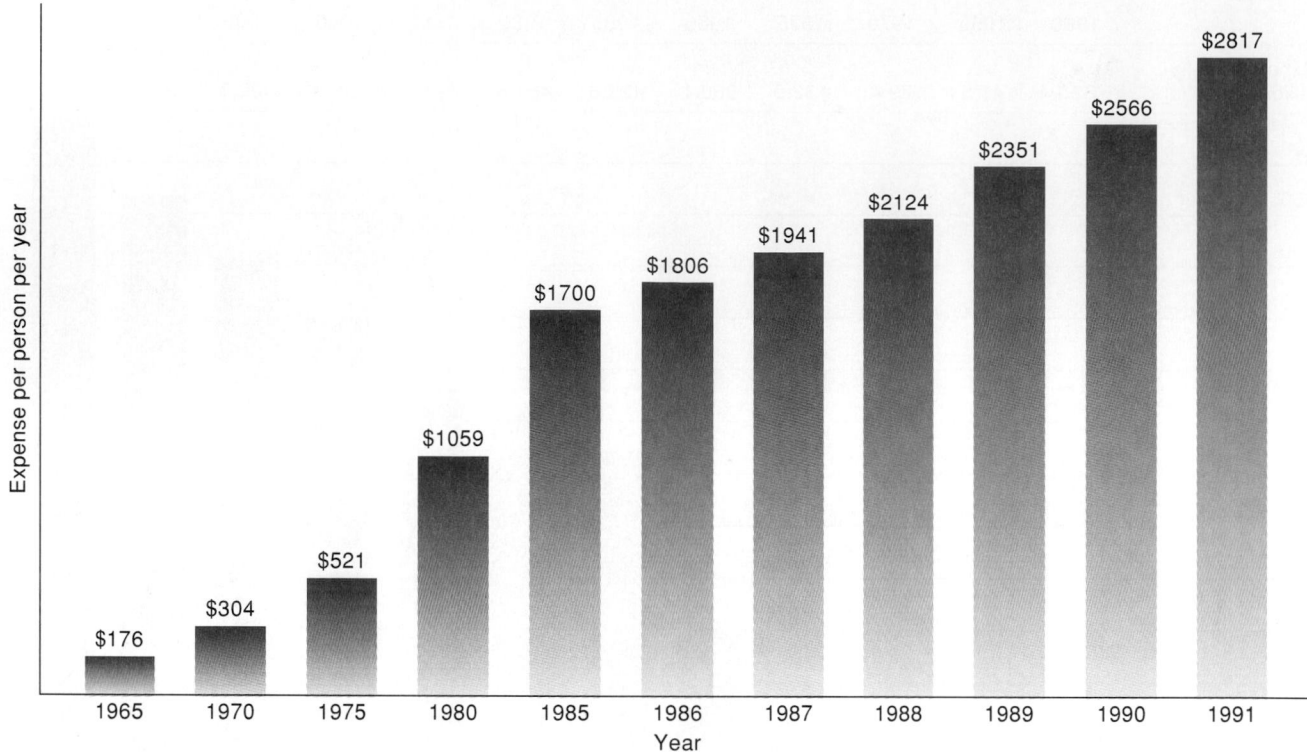

Figure 23.2
Personal Health Care Expenses per Person, 1965–1991

Source: Health Insurance Association. 1992 Source Book of Health Insurance Data. Washington, DC: Health Insurance Association of America, 1992.

Health insurance is usually obtained through either a **group health insurance plan** or an **individual (family) health insurance plan.** The most favorable rates, and the more inclusive coverages, are usually available when a policy is written for a group of individuals, often through an employer. If a person changes employment, he or she may lose eligibility for membership in the group. Individual, or family, policies are usually written for an individual policyholder and/or his or her family.

Students often take health insurance for granted. After being covered on their parents' policies while living at home, they may lose that coverage without being aware of it. Some policies stop coverage of dependents when they turn 18 or 21 years

of age, when they are no longer full-time students, or when they move away from home. Some colleges provide limited health insurance for every student enrolled. If you do not know whether or not you are covered, check immediately. If you are not, look into purchasing an individual, low-cost policy from a private insurance company. Also, if a period of time lapses between the time you graduate from college and the time of your first full-time job, check to see if you are still covered. At minimum, be sure you are always protected against catastrophic medical expenses.

Private Health Insurance

To protect individuals from unexpected health care costs, insurance companies pool the subscribers' risks. The company assesses the risks of illness or injury of that group, then determines a premium based on those risks. The premium may be paid by the individual directly, but more likely by an employer as a salary benefit, providing specified insurance benefits.

group health insurance plan a policy that is written for a group of individuals at a uniform cost.

individual (family) health insurance plan a policy that is written for an individual or family at a particular cost.

Health care coverage is provided either through private health insurance by a commercial insurance company, group self-insurance, Blue Cross-Blue Shield plans, or prepayment plans such as HMOs. Some health care is provided through public health care coverage under federal, state, and local programs.

Commercial Insurance Companies The insurer may be a profit-making commercial insurance company, such as Prudential, Aetna, or one of hundreds of similar companies. Most commercial health insurance companies provide two basic

categories of coverage: *medical expense insurance* providing broad benefits for hospital and medical care, and related service, and *disability income insurance* providing periodic payments as a result of sickness or injury.

Group Self-insurance Today many large companies and unions representing sizable work forces, have acted to provide *self-insurance*. Rather than providing health care coverage for their workers through a profit-making commercial company, the employer or union sets aside money to pay health care claims of their employees and

FEATURE 23.5

GLOSSARY OF HEALTH INSURANCE TERMS

Because health insurance policies are legal contracts, they use precise legal language. Some of these terms appear in all policies, while others appear just in some. Understanding them will help you figure out how a policy works and what it actually covers. Following are terms not defined elsewhere in this chapter.

Assignment of Benefits By signing a form (usually the insurance claim form), you authorize the insurance company to pay the physician or other provider directly. Otherwise payment must be made directly to you. Most providers will ask you to sign the form if you don't want to pay your bill before the insurance company pays its share.

Co-insurance An arrangement whereby you and the insurance company share, in a specific ratio, payment for costs covered by the policy after the deductible is met. Typically, the insurer pays 75–85 percent of covered costs and you pay the rest. Some policies set an upper limit to coinsurance expense, after which the company pays all additional charges.

Conversion Privilege A provision that enables those insured by group contracts to, under various circumstances, such as leaving the job that provided the group coverage, obtain an individual policy without evidence of medical insurability.

Coordination of Benefits A provision that prohibits you from collecting identical benefits from two or more policies, thereby exceeding 100 percent of the medical costs. After the primary company pays, other companies will calculate their coverage of the remainder. All group policies contain a coordination clause, but most individual policies do not.

Deductible The amount you must pay before the insurance company starts paying.

Exclusions (Exceptions) Specified conditions or circumstances for which the policy does not provide benefits.

Grace Period The number of days that you may without penalty delay payment of your premium without losing your insurance.

Guaranteed Renewability A policy under which the company agrees to continue insuring you up to a certain age (or for life) as long as you pay the premium. Under this provision, the premium structure cannot be raised unless it is raised for all members of a group or class of insured, such as all people living in your state with the same kind of policy.

Inpatient Services Services received at a hospital, clinic, or dispensary while being hospitalized.

Notice of Claim Written notice the insurance company must receive for the payment of benefits after services have been rendered. Typically it must be received within 20 days or as soon thereafter as reasonably possible.

Outpatient Services Services obtained at a hospital, clinic, or dispensary, without being hospitalized.

Participating Physician A physician who agrees to abide by the rules of a plan in return for direct payment by the insurance company. The agreement includes acceptance of a fixed fee schedule, a monthly fee per eligible patient, or other fee limitation.

Preexisting Condition A health problem you had before becoming insured. Some policies exclude these conditions, while others do not.

Provider Any source of health care services, such as a hospital, physician, pharmacist, or laboratory.

Reasonable and Customary Charges The amount a company will pay for a given service based on what most providers charge for it.

Rider An attachment to the basic insurance policy that changes its coverage.

Waiting Period A specified time between issuance of a policy and coverage of certain conditions. Typically there are waiting periods for preexisting conditions and maternity benefits.

assumes all or part of the responsibility for paying claims. Not only does the firm save the extra costs charged by a profit-making company, they also retain control over their funds until a medical bill needs to be paid. Self-insurance plans may be administered by the employer or union, or by some outside firm. Many companies are convinced that it pays to spend money to help their employees stay well. See Communication for Wellness: Promoting Wellness for examples of what some companies are doing.

Blue Cross-Blue Shield Plans Health care coverage is also provided by nonprofit membership plans, such as Blue Cross-Blue Shield plans serving state and regional areas. These plans structure the premium charged to equal the costs of benefits paid. Because they do not need to make a profit, such plans are often able to compete successfully with commercial companies for subscribers.

Prepaid Health Insurance **Prepaid health insurance** plans meet all of the medical needs of their members for a predetermined amount of premium. The most common form of prepaid health care is the **health maintenance organization (HMO).** HMOs provide a wide range of comprehensive health care services to subscribers enrolled within a specified geographical area. The care is provided by physicians and other therapists who are hired by, and who contract with, the HMO. There are various models of HMOs. In the "staff model," the HMO employs its own physicians, who commonly practice under one roof.

Almost any organization can sponsor an HMO, including the government, medical schools, hospital, employers, labor unions, and insurance companies. According to the federal HMO Act of 1973, any company with more than 25 employees must offer its employees one of several HMO options.

·····

prepaid health insurance health insurance, which for a predetermined amount of money, meets all of the medical needs of members.

health maintenance organization (HMO) an organization that provides a wide range of comprehensive health care services for a specified group at a fixed premium.

Over 556 HMOs now serve more than 38 million, or 15 percent of, people in this country.

MANAGED CARE

Containing the ever-rising cost of health care has become one of the most pressing concerns in the United States. During the 1980s, management of the provision and finances of health care, or *managed care,* evolved at a pace few anticipated. To contain costs, networks of physicians and hospitals were organized to give patients access to care at greatly reduced cost. With managed care the members are restricted to physicians and selected hospitals at a lower than usual cost. The best examples of managed care are the HMOs and preferred provider organizations.

HMOs

Cost containment is one of the most important features of HMOs. Medical services are centralized, reducing unnecessary duplication and record-keeping for equipment, facilities, and staff. HMOs routinely promote preventive practices for their patients, which is in keeping with their philosophy that the fewer services required, the greater the cost savings. HMOs also emphasize care provided on an outpatient, or ambulatory basis rather than in an inpatient hospital setting. One objection to some HMOs is that the patient has a limited choice of physician or that the patient does not have a single primary care physician. In many organizations, however, the member may select his or her primary practitioner by scheduling appointments in advance.

Preferred Provider Organizations

Preferred provider organizations (PPOs) are another form of managed care that provides more freedom in choice of physician and hospital than an HMO. In a PPO, physicians and hospitals agree

·····

preferred provider organization (PPO) an arrangement whereby a third-party payer contracts with a group of physicians who furnish services at lower than usual fees in return for prompt payment and a certain volume of patients.

PROMOTING WELLNESS

Illness is expensive. It results in loss of productivity and income, costs for medical care and medications, feelings of sickness and despair, work overload for other people, and sometimes, higher insurance rates. Wellness implies a variety of activities that help you implement positive behavior to improve your quality of life and well-being (see Chapter 11). Realizing that it is cheaper to invest in ways to keep their employees well, many companies have developed Wellness Plans.

Quaker Oats, in their Chicago headquarters, has modeled one such plan. They installed a fitness center, which includes activities such as stress-management, proper nutrition, substance-abuse control and smoking cessation, and health education programs. They set up classes to teach employees ways to get the most for their health care dollars, such as ways to avoid unnecessary surgery and how to cut down on hospital stays. Over several years Quaker saw the average number of hospital days per every 1000 employees cut by more than half. As a dividend, Quaker reimbursed employees with refunds from the amount of money allocated for each employee for medical expenses. Any employee who does not use the full allocation gets a refund.

Other companies, as a part of their health plans, offer the employees incentives, including cash bonuses, for staying well. Although no wellness plan can keep all employees from getting sick, the payback comes in fitter employees and trimmer corporate insurance budgets.

Source: Schwartz, J. "'Wellness' Plans: An Ounce of Prevention." *Newsweek* 30 January 1989, p. 51.

---

to provide medical services to an insurance company or employer with discounts for their services in return for prompt payment and a certain volume of patients. Patients can choose from a number of PPO physicians in the network or can receive treatment outside the system. Patients get 80–100 percent reimbursement for treatment in a PPO versus 60–70 percent outside it; thus there is incentive to use PPO providers as much as possible. Often, a given procedure must be reviewed and authorized by the insurer to minimize unnecessary tests and treatments. EPOs (exclusive provider organizations) are PPOs in which subscribers are only reimbursed if they receive care from within the network.

GOVERNMENT INSURANCE PLANS

Tax-supported public insurance is sponsored by the government in two major programs: Medicare and Medicaid.

Medicare

Medicare, in effect since 1966, is a federally administered program providing hospital and medical protection to persons 65 years of age and older, and to disabled persons who are entitled to Social Security benefits. Medicare consists of two parts. *Medicare Plan A* is a compulsory hospital insurance providing coverage for hospital-related expenses. *Medicare Plan B* is an optional supplemental medical insurance that pays for physicians' services, medical services, and supplies not covered under Part A. Part B is voluntary and is paid for by monthly premiums of those who enroll and by the federal government. Both Part A and Part B include an annual deductible that the subscriber must pay, and which is subject to annual adjustments. The deductible amounts for both Part A and Part B, and the premium for Part B, are subject to annual changes. Since Medicare pays only a portion of health care costs for the elderly, some people subscribe to supplemental private insurance plans to help pay for the costs not covered by Medicare.

Medicaid

Medicaid is a state government health insurance program for low-income people or medically needy people who are receiving public welfare assistance. Medicaid is designed to cover hospital, physician, and nursing home expenses, and it has

---

Medicare the hospital insurance system and the supplemental medical insurance for the elderly under Social Security.

Medicaid state programs of public health care assistance provided to people who are unable to afford medical expenses.

no age requirements. It is financed and administered cooperatively among the federal government and most of the 50 states.

Limiting Public Health Care Costs Cost containment has been a persistent problem for government health care programs. In 1972, professional standards review organizations (PSROs) were established to encourage physicians in each state to review hospital admission and costs under Medicare and Medicaid. However, this attempt proved ineffective in controlling costs.

In 1984, the federal government ordered hospitals to accept Medicare payments based on what Medicare estimated the treatment should cost, rather than on what individual physicians and hospitals estimated the actual cost to be. Medicare's estimates are referred to as diagnostic-related groups (DRG). Under this system, hospitals receive only a fixed fee for treatment of all Medicare or Medicaid patients with a given condition. The result is that hospitals have begun to control costs more closely and cut down on expenses. In addition, the length of a patient's hospital stay tends to be shorter under DRGs.

NATIONAL HEALTH CARE REFORM

The need for health care reform in the United States has long been apparent; too few people are covered and costs are too high. The price for a modified radical mastectomy can run $7,900; coronary bypass surgery, $49,000; delivery of a baby by Cesarean section, $7,500; and a psychotherapist's time, $160 an hour.[14] The consequence is that as many as 25 percent of Americans put off medical treatment for fear they cannot afford it.[15]

With the election of President Bill Clinton in 1993 came the promise to overhaul the U.S. health care system. According to the plan, which has not yet been enacted by the Congress, it would guarantee coverage for an estimated 37 million Americans who are currently without health care insurance and would significantly alter the way many Americans approach health care.

At the center of the proposal is managed competition, in which the federal government would be the top manager and set the terms for coverage. Regardless of employer or type of health care

provider selected, everyone would be guaranteed a package of benefits including reimbursement for physician and hospital bills, prescription drugs, and preventive care.

TYPES OF PLANS

States may be required to set up insurance buying cooperatives known as *health alliances*. Each cooperative would offer a menu of plans, including several HMOs, a traditional fee-for-service plan, and a combination plan:[16]

- The *HMO plans* offer the lowest costs for individuals and employers. All medical care is provided under one roof or from an approved network of physicians and costs from $10–$15. In return, you lose the privilege of choosing your own physician. This is similar to the managed-care plans familiar to people who now belong to an HMO or PPO.

- The *fee-for-service plan* allows you to choose your own physician, but is the most expensive health plan. After reaching a $400 deductible, the typical family pays about 20 percent of medical bills up to an annual $3000 out-of-pocket maximum. Rural areas beyond the reach of an HMO need to rely on conventional fee-for-service plans.

- With the *combination plan,* you choose a physician from the plan's network and pay a small copayment of $10–$25. If you wish to choose some physician outside the network, it costs extra.

BENEFITS PROVIDED

The plan would guarantee a broad range of benefits. A sampling of some of these benefits follows:[17]

- *Professional Services*—physicians' office visits, emergency-room care, laboratory and ambulance fees.

- *Hospitalization*—a semiprivate room unless a private room is medically necessary; otherwise private rooms would cost extra.

- *Long-term care*—nursing homes and residential treatments would be covered when they can be justified as an alternative to hospitalization; a 100-day maximum per calendar year would be allowed.

- *Dental care*—preventive care for children is covered; adult care would be phased in by year 2000.
- *Prescription drugs*—$5 per prescription or a $250 yearly maximum depending on the plan you choose.
- *Preventive care*—immunizations, prenatal and infant checkups, cholesterol screening, physicals with increasing frequency as patient ages; mammograms for women older than 50.
- *Psychotherapy*—would be phased in. Until year 2000, limited psychotherapy sessions, inpatient care, and psychiatry would be covered; after 2000, comprehensive mental-health care would be provided.

HOW PEOPLE ARE COVERED

One of the biggest questions is "How will National Health Care be paid for, and who would do the paying?" According to the blueprints of the plan, the costs would be borne in the following way:[18]

- *Corporations* with more than 5000 employees can set up their own private health alliances, offering the same three basic health plans as their government counterparts. In any case, big business would pay 80 percent of the employees' insurance, and the employee 20 percent.
- *Midsize companies* with more than 50, but fewer than 5000 workers would pay 80 percent of the workers' insurance premiums, and the worker would pay 20 percent.
- *Small business* owners would pay 80 percent of the employees' insurance premiums, and the worker would pay 20 percent. But for companies with fewer than 50 workers, government subsidies would keep health care costs at 3.5 percent of payroll for all workers making less than $24,000.
- *Self-employed workers* would pay for their own health insurance premiums, which could be $1,800 for individuals and $4,200 for a family. However, the worker could deduct the entire amount from taxes.
- *Unemployed workers* would be expected to pay something toward their health plan, since everyone is expected to pay something. If income was a percent below the poverty line, the government would help pay the premium.
- *College students* would be covered for health costs under the family policy if the college is located close to home. If located far from home, college students would join the local health alliance.
- *Retirees* under age 65 would get government subsidies for premium payments, if necessary. Over age 65, Medicare pays for the premium, for prescriptions, and for in-home health care.
- *Poor people* under Medicaid would join health alliances just like everyone else and pick the health plan of their choice. Federal and state governments would pay the premiums, but only for plans priced at or below the average of all those offered.
- *Undocumented workers* would not be able to join a health alliance unless they have working papers. In no case would emergency care be denied.

The cost of the whole new health package is assumed to require some significant new taxes. Which taxes to raise or create would be contested. There appears to be broad support among the people in this country for some health care reform that guarantees health care for all.

Some states are not waiting for the enactment of a national health care reform, but are setting up their own programs. States such as Massachusetts, Minnesota, Oregon, Washington, Maryland, Hawaii, and Florida have passed legislation providing basic coverage for all residents, affordable insurance for low-income people, or new insurance purchasing arrangements. Some physicians' groups and hospitals are beginning to structure set fees and standardized procedures for certain kinds of surgeries and treatments, and some companies are instituting new cost-efficient health contracts with hospitals and physician groups. Some national health insurance groups, both commercial and nonprofit, are moving to evaluate the quality of managed health plans.[19]

Whatever the process, the road to congressional approval and implementation of a national health care plan is bound to be tedious and may require a span of years to accomplish. Nonetheless, there is wide evidence of a movement to solve a decades-old problem.

CHECKPOINT

1. What categories of citizens are often not covered by health insurance or have no ability to pay?

2. How many people in the United States do not go to physicians because of cost? Who are these people?

3. Describe the advantages of being covered by health insurance.

4. Compare the advantages of an individual health insurance plan with the advantages of a group health insurance plan.

5. Describe the differences between an HMO and a PPO.

6. What steps is the government taking to contain health care costs?

SUMMARY

The U.S. health care system is the most costly of any country in the world. Yet 15 percent of all Americans go without health insurance, and 1 in every 100 infants dies before his or her first birthday. This is one indication that the most costly health care is not equal to the best health care.

There are many different approaches to health care. Self-care is increasingly used by those who desire to take an active role in their own wellness. For those who need help from physicians, the two traditional approaches are medicine and osteopathy. Medical doctors rely on drugs and surgery to treat patients, whereas osteopathy combines musculoskeletal manipulation with drugs and therapy. Primary health care is usually provided by general practitioners, family practitioners, pediatricians, or general internists. Other health professionals include dentists, nurses, podiatrists, optometrists, and pharmacists. Alternative health care is available from chiropractors, homeopaths, naturopaths, faith healers, and acupuncturists.

Health care is provided through various types of facilities. For college and university students, health care is usually available through campus-based student health services. For many people,

primary care is provided through private physicians or at clinics; other facilities include hospitals, emergency care offices, and nursing homes. As health care centers, hospitals may be organized as proprietary, voluntary, or governmental.

Unfortunately, health care costs in the United States continue to climb. By the early 1990s health care costs had exceeded an average $2500 per person. Financing of health care is usually done through fee-for-service and health insurance. Insurance may be purchased through private insurance companies, through prepaid health plans such as HMOs, or provided by the government through Medicare and Medicaid. Cost containment is an ongoing need in all health care programs. The need for a national health insurance program continues to be hotly debated.

Currently, adequate health care is not available to or affordable enough for everyone in the United States. Lack of access is most often a problem for infants, the elderly, pregnant women, and accident victims. Access to quality care should be the right of all citizens in this country.

REFERENCES

1. Beck, M. et al. "Doctors Under the Knife." *Newsweek* (5 April 1993), 28–33.
2. Health Insurance Association of America. *Source Book of Health Insurance Data, 1992.* Washington, DC: Health Insurance Association of America, 1992.
3. Scott, J. "Many Believe They Can't Afford Good Health Care." *Los Angeles Times* (5 February 1990), A-1, 23.
4. Parachini, A. "When Looking for a Specialist, Patient Beware." *Los Angeles Times* (26 March 1987), Part 5-1, 2.
5. Wallis, C. "Why New Age Medicine Is Catching On." *Time* (4 November 1991), 68–76.
6. Ibid.
7. Flanagan, W. "Me and Dr. Gong." *Forbes* (9 December 1991), 320–321.
8. Stix, D. "Stick It in Your Ear." *Forbes* (9 December 1991), 321.
9. Shaffer, M. "Roundtable: Women's Health Comes to the Forefront of Medicine." *Medical World News* (November 1992), 18–24.
10. Ibid.
11. Zittel, N. "Medicine: The War Between the Sexes." *Medical World News* (November 1992), 2.
12. Health Insurance Association of America, op. cit.
13. Brink, S. et al. "Top 10 Health Stories to Watch." *U.S. News and World Report* (10 May 1993), 81–82.

14. Castro, op. cit.

15. Scott, op. cit.

16. Murr, A., et al. "The Clinton Cure." *Newsweek* (4 October 1993), 36–43.

17. Ibid.

18. Rogers, P. "Healthtown, U.S.A." *Newsweek* (4 October 1993), 44–45.

19. Brink, op. cit.

SUGGESTED READINGS

Boston's Women's Health Book Collective. *The New Our Bodies, Ourselves*. New York: Simon and Schuster, 1992.

Breyfogle, N. *The Common Sense Medical Guide and Outdoor Reference*. New York: McGraw-Hill, 1988.

Carlson, R., and Shield, B. *Healers on Healing*. Los Angeles: Tarcher, 1989.

Consumer Guide. *The Home Remedies Handbook*. Lincolnwood, IL: Publications International, 1993.

Drury, N., and Drury, S. *Illustrated Dictionary of Natural Health*. New York: Sterling, 1989.

Fein, R. *Medical Care, Medical Costs*. Cambridge, MA: Harvard University Press, 1989.

Harrison, L. *Helping Yourself with Natural Healing*. Englewood Cliffs, NJ: Prentice-Hall, 1988.

Horowitz, D., and Shilling, D. *The Fight Back Guide to Health Insurance*. New York: Dell, 1993.

Islander, C., and Weiner, E. *Take This Book to the Hospital with You*. Allentown, PA: People's Medical Society, 1993.

Kunz, J., and Finkel, A. (eds.). *American Medical Association Family Medical Guide,* rev. New York: Random House, 1987.

Lockie, A. *The Family Guide to Homeopathy*. New York: Simon and Schuster, 1993.

Mole, P. *Acupuncture*. Rockport, MA: Element, 1992.

Rossman, M. *Healing Yourself*. New York: Pocket Books, 1987.

Simons, A. et al. *Before You Call the Doctor*. Boston: Ballantine, 1992.

Stewart, F., et al. *Understanding Your Body: Every Woman's Guide to Gynecology and Health*. New York: Bantam, 1987.

Vickery, D., and Fries, J. *Take Care of Yourself,* 5th ed. Reading, MA: Addison Wesley, 1993.

Weil, A. *Natural Health, Natural Medicine*. Boston: Houghton Mifflin, 1990.

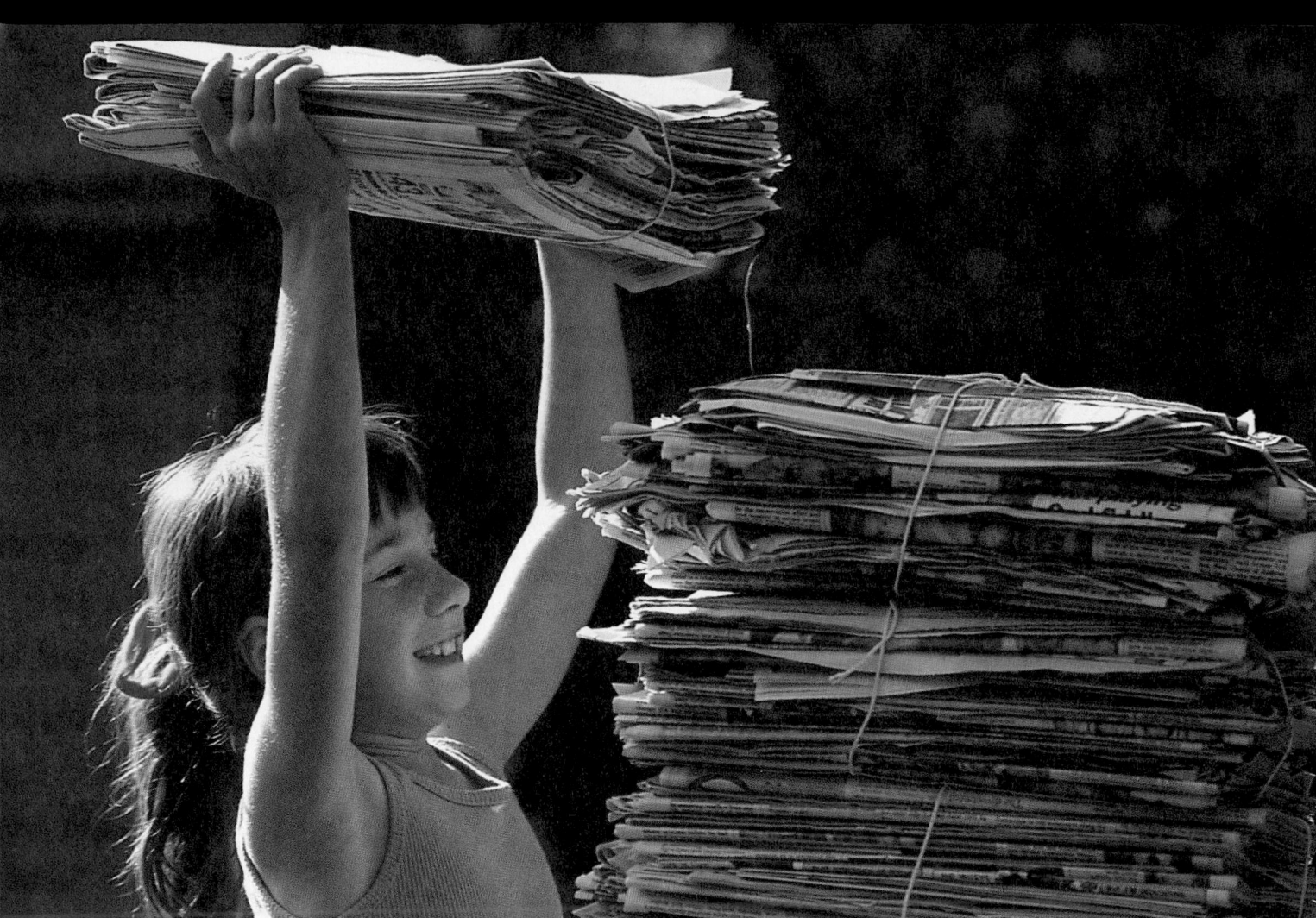

24
ENVIRONMENTAL HEALTH

KNOWLEDGE

- Define the terms *ecology, ecosystem,* and *biosphere.*
- List the interrelationships that govern us humans as members of the global community.
- List the six most common kinds of pollutants.
- Define the term *air pollution.*
- Discuss the stratospheric ozone layer and how human activities are affecting it.
- Define the term *solid waste.*
- Name some hazardous wastes.
- Contrast sound and noise.
- Give the present United States and world population totals.
- List five slow-growth countries and five rapid-growth countries.

INSIGHT

- Identify the principles that you might include in an Environmental Bill of Rights.
- Describe ways in which you might be inadvertently affected by lead poisoning.
- Discuss your feelings on the use of nuclear power plants as an energy source.
- Identify your expectations on the number of children you anticipate having and why.
- List some ways in which you can respond responsibly to environmental problems.

DECISION MAKING

- Decide if your community is the ideal place for you to live.
- Identify what you are going to do to improve the quality of the air in the house in which you live.
- Outline steps you plan to take to reduce the amount of urban garbage that is being hauled to landfills.
- Outline ways in which you are going to increase the amount of recycling you do.
- Decide how you intend to commit yourself to protecting the health of the environment.

I n 1989, the Exxon Valdez *oil spill in Alaska's Prince William Sound created great concern among those who value the health of the environment. This oil spill devastated the wildlife in the area and their habitats. In 1993, Exxon's reports were released and company officials made the statement that the Sound had "almost fully recovered" from this oil spill. Some environmentalists were suspicious about this statement and the results of the Exxon studies.*

Scientists are still learning from this event, the most scrutinized disaster of its kind. On the fifth anniversary of the spill, in March 1994, two conferences were held in Anchorage. Reports from the state of Alaska detail damage to wildlife. Harbor seals, sea otters, pink salmon, Pacific herring and several kinds of birds show "little or no sign" of recovery in the Prince William Sound. However, other species, such as killer whales, proved resilient; state scientists say that the group of whales is growing again after losing 13 between 1988 and 1990.

Close inspection revealed that oil remnants could be found in the Sound's deep sediments and its shallow tidal sediments. There were three possible sources of this oil: (1) natural crude-oil seeps dating back over 160 years that would affect the deeper sediments; (2) diesel oil, perhaps spilled when a ship was refueling, and/or (3) oil from the Exxon Valdez oil spill.

Scientists from Exxon and the environmental scientists determined that the oil from the deep sediment samples was from natural crude-oil seepage. Determining the source of the oil from the shallow sediment samples was more difficult and complex. Exxon scientists argued that this oil was from a combination of sources, including possibly the Exxon Valdez. Therefore, they concluded, Exxon was only partially responsible. Other scientists claimed that the primary source of this oil must be the spill.

Other controversies in this case included the overall harmful impact of the spill on fish and birds that inhabit the Sound area. Exxon maintains that the impact has been minimal, while the state has argued that the long-term consequences to the wildlife are substantial, and some of them as-yet unrecognized.

This controversy represents the public's healthy concern about the state of the environment. The quality of the overall environment, including the air we breathe, the water we drink, and the land we inhabit, is very important to personal health.

Source: Science News May, 1993, pp. 294–295.

■ ■ ■

The Exxon Valdez incident is a frightening case that illustrates how human interests can intrude into the natural environment and affect a scenic treasure and wildlife habitat. Although environmental changes don't always have such immediate and devastating effects, the environment plays a very important role in all of our lives.

WHAT IS A HEALTHFUL ENVIRONMENT?

From the beginning of recorded history, humans have sought to dominate nature. While paying tribute to natural wonders, industrial societies have also developed a throwaway ethic, by which we assume that humans are apart from and above nature, and that the role of humans is to conquer and subdue nature.

Yet, all parts of nature are interconnected and interdependent. We must acknowledge that humans are *part* of nature, and that in order for the earth to survive, humans must protect the earth's limited resources and care for all living things—human and nonhuman. We are entitled to interfere with nature only to provide for vital human needs.

Our quality of life depends on the quality of our environment. Clean water, pure air, and productive soil are all essential for healthy living. Without clean air the human respiratory defenses against air pollutants can be overwhelmed. The water essential to our existence, if polluted, can become a carrier of disease-producing organisms and toxic compounds. Contaminated soil pollutes groundwater and reduces or destroys the productivity of the land. The contamination of these resources poses health hazards and limits the supply of these necessary resources.

There has been an increasing call to guarantee environmental-quality rights through a constitutional process. Many states have already adopted statements in their constitutions that guarantee certain environmental rights. In 1987, the National Wildlife Federation passed a resolution calling for the amending of the U.S. Constitution to include an Environmental Bill of Rights. An Environmental Quality Amendment, as outlined by the National Wildlife Federation, would embody the following principles:

The people have a right to clean air, pure water, productive soils, and to the conservation of the natural, scenic, historic, recreational, esthetic, and economic values of the environment. America's natural resources are the common property of all people, including generations yet to come. As trustee of these resources, the United States Government should conserve and maintain them for the benefit of all the people.

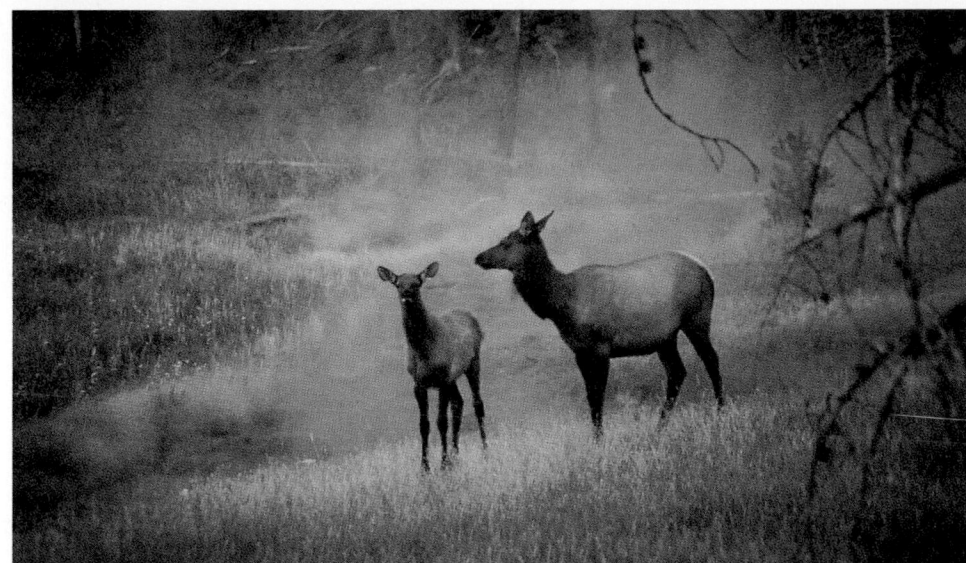

The natural world is the common property of all creatures—both animals and people. Maintaining the well-being of the natural environment is the task of all people.

The environment is vast, and is governed by age-old forces of natural progression. Yet, on an individual level each one of us lives somewhere and belongs to some community. As an individual, what are your expectations for your community that can help you realize your dreams as a person? Before continuing, assess what you would like to see in your community that would make it an ideal place to live by completing In Your Hands: Your Community—An Ideal Place to Live? on p. 760. If you live in or near a college or university campus, you may wish to use that area for your evaluation.

CHECKPOINT

1. On what things does our quality of life depend?

2. Describe the throwaway ethic, and explain how humans have excused themselves in their abuse of nature.

ECOSYSTEMS

Nature consists of an array of living organisms in their natural habitats. The study of **ecology** looks at how these plants and animals interact with each other within their physical environments, and how these interactions affect nature.

Living organisms tend to reproduce naturally in groups or **populations.** Plant and animal populations live in an environment that includes nonliving components, such as air, water, light, and soil. The various combinations of components are known as **ecosystems.** A forest is an ecosystem; it is a collection of trees, smaller plants, and animals, living with nonliving factors. Deserts, prairies, ponds, and oceans are other ecosystems. All of the ecosystems of the world collectively are known as the **biosphere.** To us the most important living organisms in the biosphere are humans. Since this text examines the human condition, our focus will be on human organisms and their interactions with the environment.

The nonliving substances of the earth consist of simple chemicals, the most essential of which are carbon, oxygen, hydrogen, nitrogen, phosphorus, and sulfur. Plants and animals have only a small portion of the earth's chemicals available to them.

ecology the study of the interactions of living things with their environments.

populations groups of individuals of the same species living in the same geographical area.

ecosystem plants and animals and their nonliving environmental factors in a defined area.

biosphere all of the earth's ecosystems, collectively.

IN YOUR HANDS

YOUR COMMUNITY—AN IDEAL PLACE TO LIVE?

The following list contains statements describing certain living conditions. Respond to each statement by relating to what degree it helps you fulfill your health needs or helps you to grow as a person. Circle the number for each statement that best describes the status in your community.

DOES YOUR COMMUNITY HELP YOU TO:

	Usually	Often	Sometimes	Never
1. Feel mentally relaxed?	5	3	1	0
2. Feel content and happy?	10	7	2	0
3. Find relief from tensions?	5	3	1	0
4. Grow as a person?	10	6	2	0
5. Be productive?	5	3	1	0

DOES YOUR COMMUNITY HAVE:

	Very Many	Many	Some	None
6. Good roads?	5	3	1	0
7. Bikeways?	5	3	1	0
8. Camping sites?	5	3	1	0
9. Wooded areas (open spaces)?	5	3	1	0
10. Playgrounds?	5	3	1	0
11. Gardens, green grass, and parks?	5	3	1	0
12. Walkways?	5	3	1	0
13. Quiet neighborhoods?	5	3	1	0
14. Clean beaches or swimming pools?	5	3	1	0

	Usually	Often	Sometimes	Never
15. Clean, fresh air (outdoors)	10	7	3	0
16. Bright sunshine (year round)	5	3	1	0

DOES YOUR COMMUNITY ENFORCE LAWS REGARDING:

	Usually	Often	Sometimes	Never
17. Noise ordinances?	5	3	1	0
18. Litter?	5	3	1	0
19. Sewage dumping?	5	3	1	0
20. Dogs on the beach?	5	3	1	0
21. Industrial wastes dumping?	5	3	1	0
22. Pesticide spraying?	5	3	1	0
23. Automobile air pollution?	10	8	3	0
24. Industrial air pollution?	10	7	3	0
25. Smoking in the workplace?	30	20	5	0

Total Points: _____

INTERPRETATIONS:

175–139 points: Very satisfactory place to live

138–108 points: Desirable place to live

107–75 points: Acceptable place to live

74–42 points: Tolerable place to live

41–0 points: Intolerable place to live

Source: Adapted from Sorochan, W. *Promoting Your Health.* New York: Wiley, 1981.

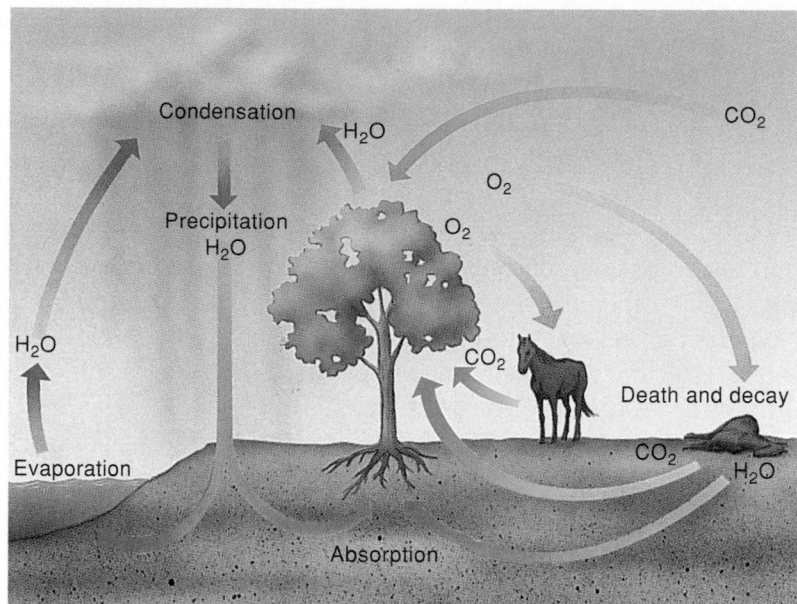

Figure 24.1

The Three Cycles—Oxygen, Carbon Dioxide, and Water

These three cycles are intimately connected through the action of biological, chemical, and geological processes.

Because a fixed supply of essential chemicals is continuously cycled through the air, water, and soil, these needs are easily met. For example, as a chemical travels through a cycle, it may be a part of you now and at some other time a part of the non-living environment. Oxygen, for instance, at various times may be a part of water, carbon dioxide, and food (see Figure 24.1). There are also cycles for carbon, oxygen, and nitrogen.

As members of the global community, we as humans must be reminded that we are ultimately and absolutely governed by the laws that control all other life on this planet. Four ecological laws, or principles, spell out the basis of this interrelationship:

1. In nature we can never do just one thing; everything we do creates effects, some of which are unexpected.

2. Everything is interconnected with everything else; we are all in this together.

3. Nature knows best. It is not only more complex than we think, but more complex than we can ever think.

4. No chemical that we produce should interfere with the earth's natural chemical cycles in ways that adversely affect, or pollute, earth's life support systems for us or other species.

Humans often violate these laws and interfere with natural cycles of the biosphere. By altering chemical cycles for our own use, such as by cultivating land using commercial fertilizers, or by flattening lands to construct housing developments, we are affecting the environment. The result of our efforts is that we often produce waste that can not continue through the natural cycle. These wastes interfere with nature's cycles by changing the physical, chemical, and biological characteristics of the air, soil, and water. Such changes, which are identified as **pollution,** may take many forms.

CHECKPOINT

1. Define the term *ecology*.

2. Explain the difference among a population, the ecosystem, and the biosphere.

3. Name some chemical substances that are continuously cycled.

4. Define the term *pollution*.

pollution a change in the physical, chemical, or biological characteristics of the air, water, or soil that can affect the health, survival, or activities of humans or other living organisms in a harmful way.

PERSONAL RESPONSIBILITY— A GLOBAL PERSPECTIVE

In this chapter, you will examine many factors that are wreaking havoc on the environment. Many of these factors are hazards, such as air and water pollution, and hazardous waste and radiation contamination. You live with some of these hazards daily; others you only encounter on occasion. You can ask: How did this happen? Who can I blame? But in the end, what you need to investigate is what you can do to protect yourself and your environment for the future. To help you assess your commitment to environmental stewardship, complete the assessment, In Your Hands: Environmental Ethics.

G. Tyler Miller, in *Living in the Environment* (7th edition), states some universal principles on resources, pollution, and environmental degrada-

tion that we will address in this chapter. These principles are as follows:

1. *Principle of Limits*—Resources are limited and we must not waste them; there is not always more.

2. *Principle That "Band-aids" Are Temporary*—Although pollution control and waste management are better than nothing, these are merely bandages and do not cure the basic problem. Once the environment is polluted, it is difficult and expensive to "undo" it.

3. *Principle of Pollution Prevention*—The prevention of pollution and the reduction of wastes are the best and cheapest ways to sustain the earth.

4. *Principle of the "3 Rs"*—Reducing our consumption and use of natural resources is the most important priority. If we use these resources, then we should reuse them, if possible, or recycle them.

IN YOUR HANDS

ENVIRONMENTAL ETHICS

Indicate your level of agreement with each of the following statements. Total your points and check the interpretation following the quiz.

1 Disagree
2 Undecided
3 Agree

1. Humans have the right to accumulate personal luxuries and conveniences even though the environment is fouled.	1	2	3
2. An individual is entitled to consume as much of the world's resources as he or she can pay for.	1	2	3
3. Corporate profit margins are more important than the control of waste generated by corporations.	1	2	3
4. It is acceptable for an industry to dump wastes into a river if it costs too much to install waste water-treatment facilities.	1	2	3
5. Private property rights take precedence over social and environmental concerns.	1	2	3
6. Success is measured by the production and consumption of material goods.	1	2	3
7. As a citizen, I am guaranteed the right to own goods I desire even though it is at the expense of others in the world or those in the future.	1	2	3
8. As a member of a developed country I have the right to look upon conveniences as necessities.	1	2	3

Total points: _____

INTERPRETATION:

8–12 points: Reflects an ethic of responsible environmental stewardship

13–20 points: Reflects an undecided ethical standard

21–24 points: Reflects an exploitive or unresponsible environmental ethic

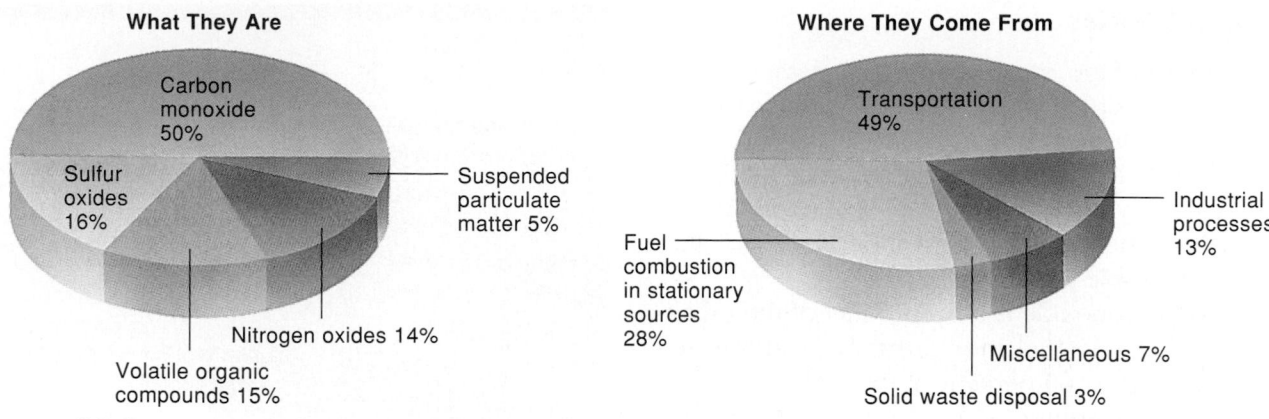

What They Are

Carbon monoxide 50%

Sulfur oxides 16%

Suspended particulate matter 5%

Nitrogen oxides 14%

Volatile organic compounds 15%

Where They Come From

Transportation 49%

Industrial processes 13%

Fuel combustion in stationary sources 28%

Miscellaneous 7%

Solid waste disposal 3%

Figure 24.2

Emissions of Major Air Pollutants in the United States

Source: EPA. In Miller, G. Living in the Environment, 7th ed. Belmont, CA: Wadsworth, 1992.

Reduce, reuse, and *recycle* are the "3 Rs" of earth care.

5. *Principle That Wastes Are Potential Resources*—Wastes are potential resources that we should be reusing and recycling. Humans are the only beings that deliberately waste resources.

6. *Principle of Sustainable Yield*—We should use locally available and renewable resources, and use these no faster than they are replenished by natural processes.

7. *Principle of Global Commons*—Everyone is affected by everyone else; we are all dependent upon everyone else.

Sometimes tragedy and fear bring people together. Perhaps fear of destruction has alerted us to the danger of apathy and has created a determination to clean up our environment. As the president of the National Wildlife Federation stated, "the greatest accomplishment of the environmental movement since Earth Day (1970) in the United States has been putting our strong desire for environmental protection at the heart of the quality of life in our society."[1]

AIR POLLUTION

Most living things need clean air to survive. Humans need oxygen from the air to carry out the processes within body cells. Once oxygen enters the lungs, it is released into the blood and carried to each body cell. In the lungs, the oxygen is exchanged for carbon dioxide, which then leaves the body. When chemical substances in the atmosphere build up in concentrations to the point of harming humans, other animals, vegetation, or materials it is known as **air pollution.** Of special concern is the effect of air pollution in interfering with oxygen entering the lungs, and reducing cell functions throughout the body. Pregnant women are especially affected by air pollution because oxygen is critical to the fetal development.

Estimates reveal that each year in the United States, air pollution causes more than 50,000 deaths and respiratory problems for tens of millions of people.[2] Some air pollutants are gaseous; others are particles that stay suspended in the air for varying periods of time (see Figure 24.2).

OUTDOOR AIR POLLUTION

Most of the recognized outdoor air pollution in the United States comes from six groups of pollutants: carbon monoxide (CO), nitrogen oxides, sulfur oxides, hydrocarbons (and other volatile organic compounds), ozone, and suspended particulate matter. Many of these pollutants come from the burning of fossil fuels (coal, oils, gasoline, natural gas) in power and industrial plants, and in automobiles.

....

air pollution the buildup of chemical concentrations in the atmosphere to the point of causing harm to humans, other animals, vegetation, and materials such as metals and stone.

Carbon Oxides

Carbon monoxide is a colorless, odorless, tasteless gas that is absorbed by the lungs and enters the red blood cells. When carbon monoxide bonds with the red blood cells, it reduces the cells' ability to transport oxygen. The results of exposure to increasing amounts of carbon monoxide are summarized in Table 24.1.

Carbon monoxide is a by-product of the breakdown of burning fuel into carbon dioxide, water, and heat. Almost 60 percent of the carbon monoxide in the atmosphere is from automobile exhaust emissions. Another common source of carbon monoxide is tobacco smoke. Both smokers and nonsmokers who breath passive smoke inhale amounts of carbon monoxide that exceed levels considered to be safe (see Chapter 16).

Carbon dioxide is a gas naturally present in the atmosphere. Because of its basic role in photosynthesis, the synthesis of food by plants, and in respiration, carbon dioxide is not always regarded as an air pollutant. But since the beginning of the industrial revolution, the increasing use of coal, oil, and gas for combustion has released great amounts of carbon dioxide into the atmosphere.

The innermost layer of the atmosphere is the **troposphere,** which extends 11 miles above sea level, and contains about 95 percent of the earth's air. The carbon dioxide level in the troposphere is now the highest it has been in the last 130,000 years, and it is rising. The greatest carbon dioxide emission comes from the United States, which is responsible for 20 percent of the world's total carbon dioxide emission.[3]

Carbon dioxide in the atmosphere, along with water vapor and other gases, allows visible sunlight to reach the earth. Upon striking the earth, some of the visible radiation is transformed into heat. This heat, rather than flowing back toward space from the earth's surface, is absorbed by carbon dioxide, and other gases in the lower atmosphere, and builds up, causing a gradual warming trend on the surface of the earth. Global warming produced in this manner is known as the *greenhouse effect.* From the data presently available, it appears there could be a global warming of 2–5 degrees fahrenheit before the end of the twenty-first century. Such global warming could pose a

Table 24.1 Carbon Monoxide in the Air	
Prolonged Exposure to Harmful Levels	**Some Actual Levels Reached**
50–100 parts per million (ppm) causes headaches, fatigue	10–75 ppm on freeways and expressways at rush hours.
250 ppm causes severe headaches, dizziness, eventually coma	25–115 ppm on downtown streets with peaks to 400 ppm in traffic jams
750 ppm causes death	200–400 ppm in cigarette smoke (ties up 5%–15% of the smoker's oxygen-carrying hemoglobin)

Source: Data from the Environmental Protection Agency.

threat of massive polar ice cap melting, with resultant flooding of low-lying coastal areas worldwide.[4]

Warmer temperatures may also contribute to a drop in the agricultural productivity of range- and cropland. A decrease in productivity of 10 percent or more is known as *desertification.* Eventually, desertification leads to a loss of the ability of people in affected areas to feed themselves. Significantly large areas of the world are becoming desertified.

Hydrocarbons

Hydrocarbons are compounds that contain carbon and hydrogen. Various forms of hydrocarbons in the air are methane, propane, ethylene, benzene, and toluene. Methane, which can be used as a fuel, is produced by bacteria in landfills and water-logged soils. This gas is about 25 times more efficient in producing global warming than each molecule of carbon dioxide.[5] More than half of the hydrocarbons in the atmosphere are produced by internal combustion engines. Hydrocarbons evaporate into the atmosphere from spilled and partially burned gasoline and industrial solvents. Hydrocarbons are a part of the mixture of atmospheric pollutants known as **smog.**

Nitrogen Oxides

About 78 percent of the air we breathe is nitrogen gas. Nitrogen oxides include nitrous oxide, nitric

....

troposphere the innermost layer of the atmosphere.

hydrocarbons compounds containing carbon and hydrogen.

smog see photochemical smog, p. 765.

FEATURE 24.1

THERMAL INVERSIONS

During the daytime the sun warms the earth's surface, causing air to expand and rise. As it expands and rises, pollutants in the air are diluted and carried into the upper atmosphere. Generally air temperature drops at a constant rate as it rises, but sometimes this is not the case. At times, air temperature drops steadily as it rises to 1500–3000 feet, then the temperature rises for the next few thousand feet, and then it resumes a steady decrease. Such a temperature reversal is called a *thermal* or *temperature inversion*. As shown in Figure 24.3, such a "lid" of warm, high-pressure air prevents the dissipation of pollutants generated from below. Pollutants spread out below the inversion layer and accumulate in the surface air.

Inversion layers are warm and dry, and remain cloudless most of the time. They allow the energy of sunlight to interact with the trapped pollutants, producing new pollutants, known as *photochemical smog*. The occurrence of photochemical smog realizes its peak during summer months, during midday hours, when the surface temperature is 75–90°F and the humidity is low. Such thermal inversions usually last only a few hours. However, they may last for several days when a high-pressure air mass stalls over a geographical area. The photochemical smog created is a brownish-yellow haze, and is most commonly found in sunny, warm, dry cities such as Los Angeles, Salt Lake City, and Denver, which have large numbers of motor vehicles.

---

oxide, and nitrogen dioxide. These gases are a by-product of high-temperature **combustion** (or burning) from motor vehicles, power plants, and from industries. When nitrogen oxides in the air combine with water to form nitric acid, it may fall to the earth as **acid precipitation.**

People exposed to nitrogen oxides experience eye and respiratory irritations. Extended exposure may cause permanent respiratory damage and lung diseases, such as emphysema (see Chapter 15). Cigarette smoke also contains nitrogen oxides; therefore cigarette smokers living in cities where there is a high level of air pollution have a higher incidence of chronic lung disorders than smokers living in less-polluted areas (see Chapter 15).

Photochemical smog is a complex mixture of air pollutants trapped under a **thermal inversion layer** (see Feature 24.1). Occurring during certain atmospheric conditions, such as on a dry, warm, cloudless day, the inversion layer traps hydrocarbons and nitrogen oxides near the ground, and

under the influence of sunlight allows them to react, producing a second generation of new photochemical pollutants (see Figure 24.3). This mixture includes **ozone,** a three-atom type of oxygen found in the lower atmosphere, and other chemicals similar to tear gas. (Ozone also occurs in the upper atmosphere, as is discussed on p. 766.)

A recent study showed that a few hours of exposure to ozone levels as low as 0.12 ppm, which is the maximum allowable level according to standards of the EPA, can cause chest pains, coughing, and nausea. This level of ozone is less than the peak concentration of ozone in many cities on a day of bad pollution (see Table 24.2, p. 766). Ozone damages lung tissue, causing tiny scars to form, which makes the tissue less elastic than normal. In plants, high ozone levels are responsible for decreased food crop yield, and for slow growth and dying of trees in affected areas.[6]

Sulfur Oxides

Sulfur oxides are produced from the combustion of sulfur-containing coal and fuel oils by homes, industries, and power plants. The principal offenders are sulfur dioxide and sulfur trioxide. Sulfur oxides, as well as nitrogen oxides, react with water vapor in the air to produce sulfuric acid and nitric acid, which may fall to the earth as acid precipita-

---

combustion burning.

acid precipitation rain, snow, sleet, fog, or dew that contains higher than normal levels of sulfuric or nitric acid.

photochemical smog a complex mixture of air pollutants produced in the atmosphere by the reaction of hydrocarbons and nitrogen oxides under the influence of sunlight.

thermal inversion layer a layer of air trapped under a layer of less-dense warm air, thus reversing the usual situation.

---

ozone a three-atom type of oxygen formed when an atom of oxygen reacts with oxygen already in the atmosphere.

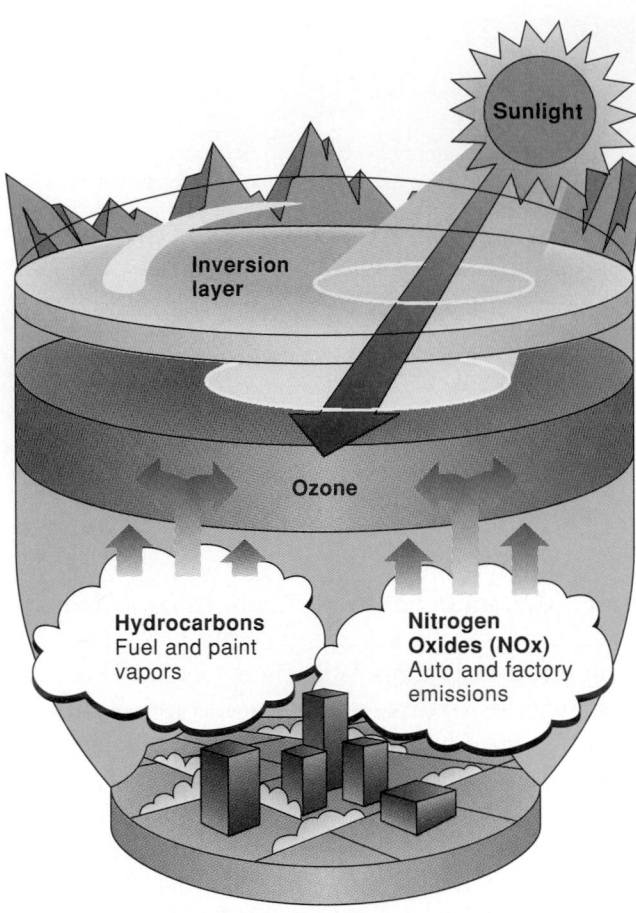

Figure 24.3

Ozone

Ozone is a colorless, pungent, highly reactive gas that is the main component of smog. It is formed by a chemical reaction of two principal air pollutants—nitrogen oxides and reactive organic gases—in the presence of sunlight. The pollutant reaches peak levels in mid-afternoon. In coastal areas it may be carried inland by sea breezes, and may become trapped in natural topographical basins. An inversion layer of warm air traps ozone near the ground.

Source: "What Is Ozone?" Los Angeles Times 23 April 1991, p. A-44.

Table 24.2
Living in a Fog of Ozone

Many cities in the United States have failed to meet federal EPA ozone standards of 0.12 ppm. Many cities and counties are regularly exposed to air that is dangerously high in ozone.

Metropolitan Area	Peak Ozone Level[a]
Los Angeles	0.36
Houston-Galveston-Brazoria	0.25
Greater Connecticut	0.23
New York City	0.22
San Diego	0.21
Chicago-Gary-Lake County	0.20
Atlantic City, New Jersey	0.19
Providence-Pawtucket-Fall River	0.18
Philadelphia	0.18
Sacramento	0.18
Baltimore	0.17
Cincinnati-Hamilton	0.17
Fresno, California	0.17
Milwaukee-Racine	0.17
San Francisco	0.17
Atlanta	0.16
Baton Rouge, Louisiana	0.16
Boston-Lawrence-Salem	0.16
Dallas-Fort Worth	0.16
Phoenix	0.16
Portland, Maine	0.16
St. Louis	0.16
Washington, D.C.	0.16
Louisville	0.15
Salt Lake City-Ogden	0.15
Seaford, Delaware	0.15

[a]Peak ozone level for any given day.

Source: Uehling, M. "Missing the Deadline on Ozone." National Wildlife October/November 1987, pp. 34–37.

tion. Sulfuric acid is corrosive to metals and harmful to vegetation and wildlife (see Feature 24.2).

Sulfur oxides irritate the respiratory system and impair breathing. They also cause reduced mucus secretion, which reduces the lungs' ability to trap and remove foreign particles. People with asthma are particularly susceptible to developing complications.

Ozone

The ozone that is created in photochemical smog is a pollutant that can damage plants and human health. This undesirable ozone in the lower atmosphere should not be confused with the highly beneficial layer of ozone that is found in the upper atmosphere about 20–50 kilometers, or 12–31 miles, above us. The upper atmosphere, also known as the stratosphere, contains a few parts of ozone per million parts of air. This is not really very much. If purified and held under ordinary sea-level

FEATURE 24.2

ACID PRECIPITATION

When fossil fuels are burned, large amounts of sulfur oxides and nitrogen oxides are carried into the air, where they combine with water to form sulfuric acid and nitric acid. In the air, they may fall to earth as acid rain, snow, sleet, fog, and dew.

Natural precipitation is slightly acidic, with an average *pH value* of 5.6 due to carbon dioxide and traces of sulfur and nitrogen compounds. The pH value is a numerical value that indicates the relative acidity or alkalinity of a substance on a scale of 0–14, with the neutral point at 7.0 (see illustration a). Acid solutions have pH values lower than 7.0, and alkaline solutions have pH values greater than 7.0. Acid rain is any rain below a pH of 5.6. In the Adirondack Mountains of New York State, once renowned for its unspoiled wilderness, acid deposition originating in Pennsylvania and the upper midwest has affected all forms of wildlife. In the lakes, fish migration and reproduction has been prevented by levels of acid as low as pH 5.0–5.5. As acid levels increase, no

form of life can survive in a lake. Approximately two hundred lakes in the Adirondacks are unable to support fish populations.

Acid precipitation kills fish, aquatic plants, and microorganisms in lakes and streams. It can also damage wood, metal and concrete buildings, forests, and crops. Acid precipitation is a serious problem throughout the northeastern United States, southeast Canada, Eastern Europe, and Scandinavia. Acid precipitation often originates in one country or state and then falls in another; some of the acid rain that falls in Canada originates in the United States. This becomes an international political issue in which one country must try to exert diplomatic pressure on the other country to control gaseous pollutants.

Power-generating plants that burn high-sulfur coal and oil produce some of the acid rain. This can be prevented by installing "scrubbers," devices that remove the sulfur from combustion fumes by passing them through a chemical bath.

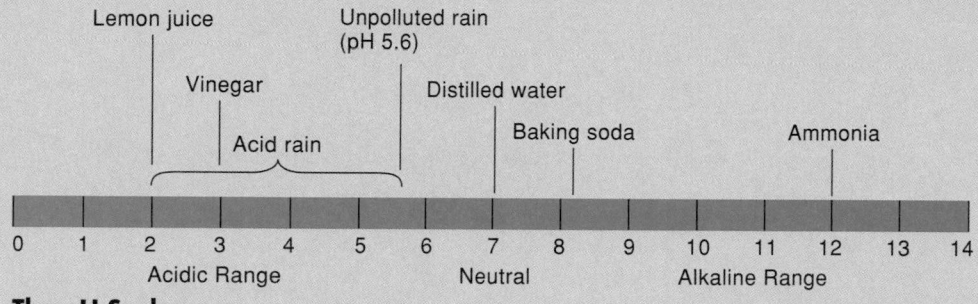

The pH Scale.

A pH of 7 is neutral. Smaller numbers indicate acidity, larger numbers alkalinity. Each point to the right or left on the scale represents a ten-fold increase in strength; therefore a pH of 2 is 1000 times as acidic as a pH of 5.

Source: Kaufman, D., and Franz, C. *Biosphere 2000.* New York: HarperCollins, 1993.

atmospheric pressure, it would form a layer only about as thick as a dime.

Without the lower stratospheric ozone, we could not survive. Ozone screens out about 99 percent of the harmful high-energy ultraviolet radiation from sunlight (see Figure 24.4, p. 768). After only a brief exposure to the full intensity of this UV we would be severely burned. Even a slight depletion of this ozone layer increases the incidence of skin cancer, eye cataracts, and weakened immunity. There is already evidence that increased UV radiation is penetrating surface waters around Antarctic, adversely affecting ocean life and damaging land crops.[7]

Researchers have discovered that the ozone layer is already being depleted. They are currently

examining a "hole," or thinning, in the ozone layer over the South Pole, where there is up to a 50 percent depletion in the ozone layer, and a smaller "hole" over the North Pole where there is a 15–25 percent depletion in the ozone layer.

The average concentration of ozone in the atmosphere is being decreased by **chlorofluorocarbons (CFCs),** which are propellants in aerosol spray cans, refrigerator and air conditioning coolants, industrial solvents, styrofoam and other plastic foams for insulating houses, hot food con-

....

chlorofluorocarbons (CFCs) propellants found in aerosol spray cans, industrial solvents, and styrofoam-type containers.

Figure 24.4

Effects of Chlorofluorocarbons (CFCs)

Allowing more UV rays through could have catastrophic health effects: Incidences of skin cancer could increase dramatically, agriculture could suffer losses, and increased heat could melt polar ice caps and cause flooding.

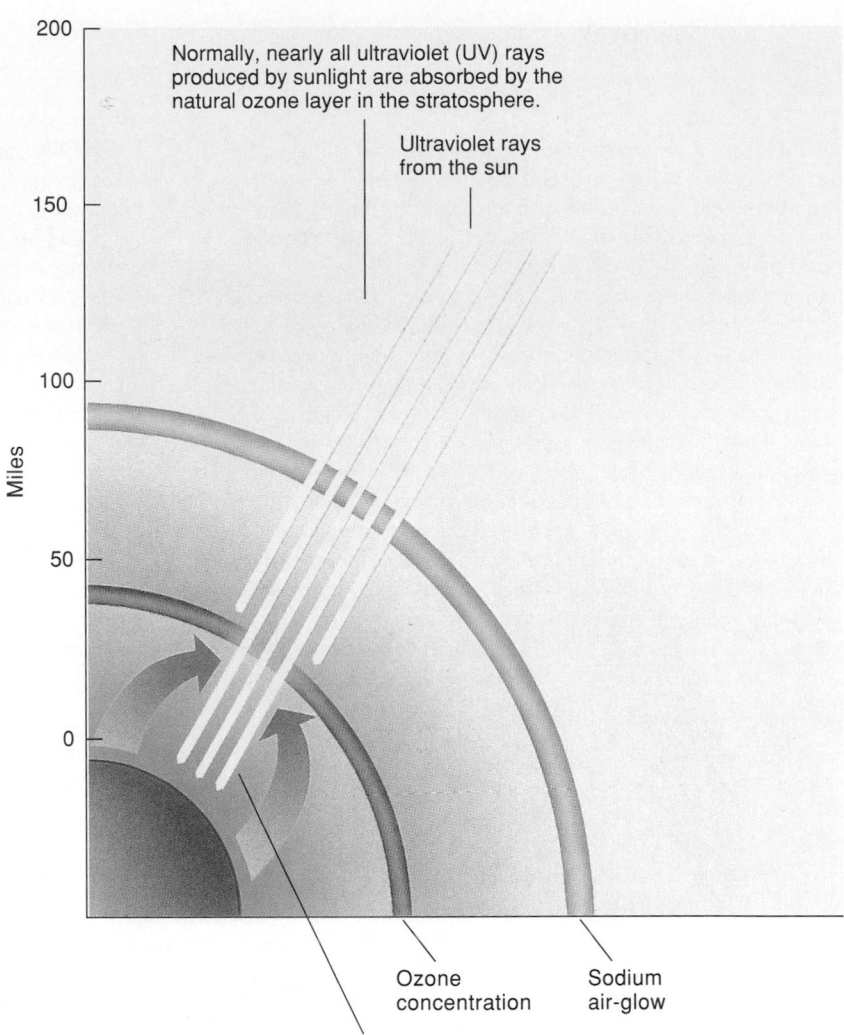

Normally, nearly all ultraviolet (UV) rays produced by sunlight are absorbed by the natural ozone layer in the stratosphere.

Ultraviolet rays from the sun

Ozone concentration

Sodium air-glow

CFCs, a manufactured substance used in refrigerators, destroys ozone, weakening Earth's protective shield and allowing UV rays through.

tainers, and packing for shipping. Since 1978, most uses of CFCs in aerosol spray cans has been banned in the United States, Canada, and most Scandinavian countries, but worldwide nonaerosol CFC use has risen sharply.

Suspended Particulate Matter

Particulate matter includes nongaseous air pollutants, such as soot, dust particles, dirt, and ash. Some forms of particulate matter are toxic to humans, such as asbestos, soot, lead, beryllium, and fluoride compounds. Asbestos is a mineral

....

particulate matter solid particles or liquid droplets suspended or carried in the air.

once widely used in cement, insulation, plaster, and in ceiling and floor tiles. Asbestos fibers, which are easily inhaled, lodge themselves in the lungs and become chronic irritants to lung tissue. Inhalation of asbestos fibers may lead to lung cancer. Soot is produced from the burning of oil, diesel fuel, wood, and other combustibles. Soot often forms as a dirty film on windows and walls and may settle in the lungs, reducing their function.

INDOOR AIR POLLUTION

It's estimated that Americans spend 70–98 percent of their time indoors. For this reason the EPA has called indoor air quality "the most significant environmental issue we have to face."[8] Unfortunately, the insides of buildings are heavily exposed to hazardous chemicals, of which as many as 20–150 are found in concentrations 10–40 times greater than those in the outdoors.[9] Especially vulnerable to this pollution are the elderly, young children, sick persons, pregnant women, those with respiratory and heart problems, and others who spend a good deal of time indoors. The consequences of exposure to indoor pollutants include premature deaths, cancer, headaches, dizziness, nausea, coughing, respiratory problems, and flulike symptoms. The four worst offenders are formaldehyde, asbestos, radioactive radon-222 gas, and cigarette smoke.

Formaldehyde

A colorless, pungent, irritating gas emitted from building materials, pressed wood products, particle board and paneling, insulation, and fiber board is **formaldehyde.** These materials end up in countertops, furniture, kitchen cabinets, and subflooring. Formaldehyde is also found in draperies, permanent-press clothing, and upholstery. Many mobile homes contain an especially large amount of formaldehyde because many of the materials used to build them contain formaldehyde. Exposure to formaldehyde can cause chronic respiratory problems, sore throat, eye irritation, and cancer.

Asbestos

Asbestos is a group of natural minerals that are made up of tiny fibers; these fibers crumble into dust-sized particles that are easily suspended in the air and inhaled into the lungs. Prolonged exposure to these fibers can lead to lung cancer and **asbestosis** (a chronic lung condition). People exposed to high levels of asbestos in the air include auto mechanics, pipe fitters, and insulators. Such people's chances of dying from lung cancer are increased if they also smoke. Until 1974, when it was banned for the following uses, asbestos was sprayed on ceilings for fire-proofing and sound-deadening, and used for insulating pipes and for

....

formaldehyde a colorless, pungent, irritating gas commonly made by the oxidation of methyl alcohol.

asbestos a fibrous, incombustible natural mineral used in insulation material.

asbestosis a chronic lung condition resulting from prolonged exposure to asbestos particles.

decorating walls. A further ban by the FDA was placed on other uses in 1989.

Asbestos is of danger to people only if the fibers can escape into the air. In some products it is sealed into the product, such as with vinyl flooring and roof shingles, and is not fragmented unless the products are sanded or cut. In other products, such as spray-on ceiling coverings, the asbestos can be easily crumbled by hand, or is *friable*, and can release asbestos fibers. In 1989, the EPA estimated that one in seven commercial-public buildings in the United States contained friable asbestos. In 1986, the U.S. Congress passed a law requiring all schools to be checked for friable asbestos, and have any removed. In some cases, the subsequent removal has been done improperly, increasing asbestos risks to workers doing the removal and to children and employees who return to the buildings.

Radioactive Radon-222

Radon-222 is a naturally occurring radioactive gas produced by the normal decay of uranium-238 in soil and rock. Usually such radon gas seeps upward in soil and is released into the air, where it quickly and harmlessly decays. Sometimes, however, the gas seeps in through cracks into buildings and collects in basements, or into water in underground wells, where the gas can build up to high levels. Radon is measured in units called *picocuries* per liter of air (see Table 24.3, p. 770). Prolonged exposure to high levels of radon over a lifetime causes increased risk of lung cancer. The risk is increased by a combination of high radon levels and smoking.

In 1988, the EPA and U.S. Surgeon General's Office recommended that everyone living in separate houses, or on the lower floors of apartment buildings, test for radon. Although radon gas can be easily tested for, very few homes have been tested.

When unsafe levels of radon are found, methods are available to reduce it. Detection kits to test your own home are available and easy to use.[10] If unsafe levels are found, such levels can often be reduced by proper ventilation, or installation of air-exchange devices. Methods are also available for removal of radon from contaminated well water. At present, there are no laws in the United States mandating new construction procedures that ensure against radon contamination. Environmentalists recommend such enactment, as well as the testing

Table 24.3
Possible Risks from Radon

Exposure (Picocuries[a] per Liter of Air)	Lung-Cancer Deaths Per 1000 People Exposed (for a lifetime of 70 years)	Comparable Lifetime Risk (70 years)	Recommended Action
200	440–470	Smoking 4 packs cigarettes a day	**20–200 picocuries** Lower levels within several months; if
100	270–630	2000 chest x-rays a year	higher than 200, remedy within a few
40	120–380	Smoking 2 packs of cigarettes a day	weeks or move out until lower levels are reached.
20	60–210	Smoking 1 pack of cigarettes a day	**4–20 picocuries** You've got a few years to make
10	30–120	5 times the lung-cancer risk of a nonsmoker	changes, but do it sooner if you're at the top of the scale
4	13–50		
2	7–30	200 chest x-rays a year	**Below 4 picocuries** Once you get around 4, it's nearly
1	3–13	Same lung-cancer risk as a nonsmoker	impossible to bring levels lower
0.2	1–3	20 chest x-rays a year	

[a]A picocurie is a trillionth of a curie, a standard measure of ionizing radiation.

Source: Miller, G. Living in the Environment, 7th ed. Belmont, CA: Wadsworth, 1992.

of soil and well water by individuals before building or the testing of indoor air before buying a house.

Cigarette Smoke More deaths are caused by tobacco smoking than by any other environmental factor. Worldwide, at least 2.5 million people die prematurely each year from heart disease, lung cancer, other cancers, bronchitis, emphysema, and stroke—all related to smoking. In 1989, smoking in the United States killed about 434,000 Americans or an average of 1,190 per day (see Figure 24.5).[11] Passive smoke inhaled by nonsmokers causes a significant increase in the incidence of lung cancer. Fortunately, the percentage of the adult population in the United States that smokes has dropped from 42 percent in 1966 to 27 percent in 1990. The longer an ex-smoker has not smoked, the lower the risks of dying from heart disease and lung cancer.

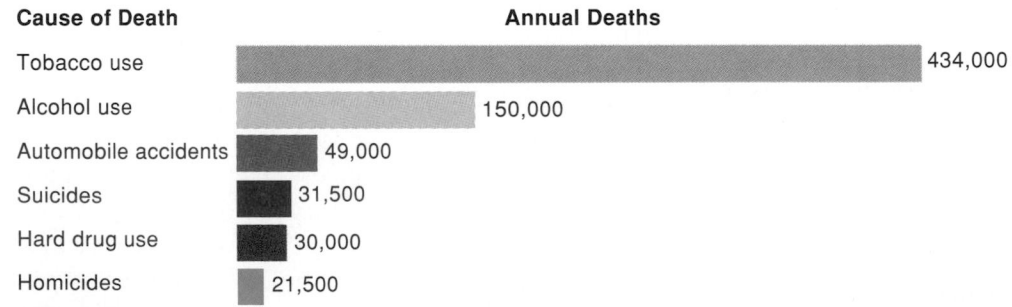

Cause of Death	Annual Deaths
Tobacco use	434,000
Alcohol use	150,000
Automobile accidents	49,000
Suicides	31,500
Hard drug use	30,000
Homicides	21,500

Figure 24.5

Annual Deaths in the United States in 1989 Related to Tobacco Use and Other Causes

Smoking is by far the leading cause of preventable death in the United States. It causes almost twice as many premature deaths each year as all of the other categories shown in this figure combined.

Source: Miller, G. Living in the Environment: 7th ed. Belmont, CA: Wadsworth, 1992.

HOW YOU CAN REDUCE AIR POLLUTION

The human body has built-in defenses that protect it from air pollution. Most of the small ducts of the respiratory tract are lined with millions of tiny hair-like processes called cilia. These hairs continuously wave back and forth, moving mucus and pollutants to the throat where they are swallowed or expelled. If the lungs are irritated, a greater amount of mucus is produced and released in order to help remove the irritants and stimulate coughing, which discharges the dirty mucus and air.

Pollutants and particles may paralyze the cilia for minutes to hours. During these periods, the cilia cannot remove the pollutants. The respiratory system then becomes vulnerable to viral, bacterial, and fungal attacks. When the body's natural defenses are overloaded with contaminants, the system may become impaired, leading to chronic bronchitis, emphysema, or lung cancer.

As individuals, we can help control air pollution. Walk or bicycle where possible instead of driving. Many localities have been encouraging ride-sharing to reduce the number of automobiles on freeways; some employers have switched employee schedules from five 8-hour days to four 10-hour days per week to reduce automobile usage. Gasoline vapors are more volatile during hotter daytime hours than cooler nighttime hours; in those states where gasoline-fume-retrieval devices are not mandated for gasoline pump hoses, hydrocarbon fumes from exposed or spilled gasoline can be reduced by nighttime refueling of vehicles.

State and federal governments have taken steps to control air pollution. Many states now require vehicle inspections for emissions and require the use of antipollution devices on vehicles. The United States passed Clean Air Acts in 1970, 1977, and again in 1990 (see Feature 24.3). The 1990 Act requires that each state develop and enforce a plan of implementation for attaining these standards.

CHECKPOINT

1. Define the term *air pollution*.

2. What is the *greenhouse effect?*

3. Describe the origin and nature of photochemical smog.

4. Explain the relationship between CFCs and the ozone "holes" over the North and South poles.

5. Discuss the ways in which you can combat air pollution.

FEATURE 24.3

PROVISIONS OF THE 1990 FEDERAL CLEAN AIR ACT

1. Reduce the mass of 1988 CFC emissions 20 percent by 1993 and 50 percent by mid-1999.

2. Require industries to use the best available technology to reduce the mass of industrial emissions of 1890 toxic chemicals by 90 percent between 1995 and 2003.

3. Require 87 cities not meeting federal emissions standards for ozone to meet such standards between 1993 and 1999; give 8 severely polluted cities until between 2005 and 2007 to meet those standards (Los Angeles has until 2010, although it must meet even tougher state standards).

4. Reduce auto emission of hydrocarbons 35 percent and nitrogen oxide 60 percent for all new cars by 1994. By 1998, all new cars must have emission-control systems good for 10 years or 100,000 miles, instead of the current 5 years or 50,000 miles.

5. Require all diesel trucks to cut emissions of particulate matter 90 percent by 1998 compared to uncontrolled levels. Buses in urban areas must do better than trucks in controlling harmful emissions.

6. Require oil companies to sell cleaner-burning gasoline and other fuels in the 9 dirtiest cities (Los Angeles, Baltimore, Chicago, Houston, Milwaukee, Muskegon, New York, Philadelphia, and San Diego) by 1995, and to sell at least 150,000 electric or other clean-fuel vehicles in California by 1996.

7. Require coal-burning power plants to cut their annual sulfur dioxide emissions by 10 million tons (about half the current levels) by year 2000, or by 2005 if they switch to low-sulfur coal or other clean-coal technologies, and to cut the emissions of nitrogen oxides to 2 million tons below 1980 levels. In year 2003, stricter emission standards to go into effect.

8. Establish an emissions trading policy by allowing companies to buy and sell pollution rights for sulfur dioxide emissions from one another. Companies that reduce emissions below their limit will receive credit in the form of permits that they can use for new facilities, or sell to other companies (thus creating a financial incentive to reduce emissions).

WATER POLLUTION

All chemical reactions in the body occur in water. Water is the most abundant compound on the earth's surface and is essential to the survival of all living creatures. It is also the most abundant substance in all living cells.

Maintaining an adequate and usable water supply has become increasingly more difficult because of **water pollution,** or physical or chemical changes to surface or groundwater that can adversely affect living organisms. Pollutants enter water supplies from a variety of sources. The nation's fresh waterways—rivers and lakes—have historically been used as handy dumping sites for both solid and liquid wastes. Many of these wastes have been identified as hazardous; some as toxic. In recent years the dumping has been extended out into our oceans. Fish, shellfish, mammals, and birds are affected along our coastlines. The tides have washed up dangerous hospital debris, including vials of disease-laden fluids, onto heavily used recreational beaches.

About 97 percent of the earth's water is found in oceans and salt lakes, and is too salty for drinking. Over three-fourths of the 3 percent of the earth's water that is fresh water is locked in glaciers or polar ice caps.

Only about 0.5 percent of all water is recoverable fresh water, yet much of this water is either polluted or too expensive to recover. Only about 0.003 percent of the world's water is available for all human, agricultural, and industrial use. Put another way, out of 26 gallons, only one-half teaspoon is usable.[12]

SURFACE WATER

The fresh water people use comes from two sources: surface water and groundwater. **Surface water** is precipitation that does not filter into the

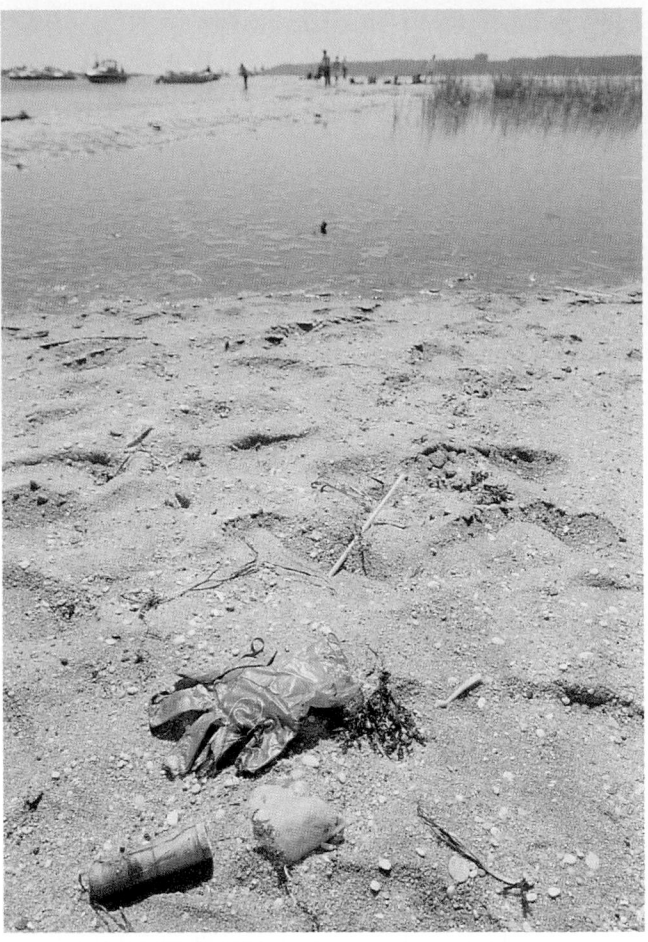

The oceans are prized as places of solitude, recreation, and industry. Yet, the ocean has become a place to dump wastes. A pandora's box of discarded items may be washed ashore by the relentless tides. Alarmingly, this debris has included hazardous and pathogenic medical throw-aways.

ground or evaporate; instead it runs off into streams, rivers, lakes, or reservoirs. Areas of land that drain runoff water into bodies of surface water are called *drainage basins,* or watersheds. Almost 70 percent of the water reaching the world's rivers comes from rain and melted snow, or *surface runoff;* the rest comes up from groundwater. Surface runoff, collecting in rivers, flows into the ocean as *river runoff.* These river basins occupy 60 percent of the earth's total land area and support 90 percent of the world's population.[13] There has been noticeable improvement in many streams and lakes. Today, surface runoff in the United States is affected largely by farmland runoff containing fertilizers and pesticides. The watersheds can be improved by reforestation to control runoff, and by the reduction of agricultural pollutants.

---

water pollution any physical or chemical change in surface or groundwater that can adversely affect living organisms.

surface water precipitation that does not filter into the ground, but becomes runoff into rivers, streams, and lakes.

GROUNDWATER

Groundwater is precipitation that seeps into the ground. This groundwater is confined in layers of sand, gravel, and porous rock in the earth's crust, forming saturated zones in which the water may be stored for long periods. The upper surface of these underground water zones is the *water table.* There is 40 times as much groundwater below the earth's surface as there is surface water. The pooling of ground water in porous soil and rock forms an **aquifer,** a large underground area of water, or "lake." Much of our drinking water comes from these aquifers.

Groundwater does not cleanse itself as surface water does. The water is cold and cut off from the oxygen of the atmosphere; thus contaminants are not effectively diluted and dispersed. All of this means that hundreds of years may be required for groundwater to cleanse itself of degradable wastes.

Groundwater is easily contaminated by *pesticides* (chemicals used to kill pests), by leaks from underground storage tanks, and by seepage of hazardous organic chemicals and *toxic* (poisonous synthetic chemicals) heavy metal compounds from landfills, abandoned hazardous-waste dumps, and industrial-waste storage lagoons situated near aquifers (Figure 24.6, p. 773).[14] Several hundred different chemicals are found in groundwater, yet only 38 are presently included in federal water quality standards and routinely tested for.[15]

While only an estimated 2 percent of the volume of all U.S. groundwater is contaminated, up to 25 percent by volume of the usable groundwater is contaminated; in some localities, up to 75 percent of the water is contaminated. In the state of New Jersey every major aquifer is contaminated.

HOW YOU CAN REDUCE WATER POLLUTION

Since 1972 the United States has passed laws requiring cities and industries to install facilities for the treatment of household and industrial wastewater and the purification of drinking water. In 1987 a federal Clean Water Act was passed. A small, but important part of that act was allocating money to help states starting the control of "nonpoint" pollution, or rainwater runoff from sources such as farms, streets, and mines containing residues from fertilizers, herbicides, acids, and petroleum products. Prior federal clean-water legislation focused almost entirely on "point source" pollution, such as wastewater from industrial plants and sewage treatment plants.[16]

As individuals, we can take steps to reduce water pollution. Never pour harmful chemicals down house or street drains or flush them down toilets. Waste crankcase oil and radiator fluid drained from automobiles should be contained and taken to a nearby recycling center. Radiators should be drained away from water supplies. Insecticides, herbicides, paints, lacquers, thinners, and household cleaners should be disposed of according to instructions from local health or water departments. Reduced use of commercial fertilizers, detergents, and of water itself can help reduce water pollution. What steps are you taking to help reduce water pollution?

CHECKPOINT

1. Define the term *water pollution*.
2. Distinguish between surface water and groundwater.
3. Explain the meaning of the word *aquifer*.
4. Discuss the ways in which you can combat water pollution. ✔

PESTICIDES AND TOXIC METALS

Both pesticides and toxic metals can be hazardous to your health. They are especially widespread because they get into surface or groundwater and thus can be transported great distances. They both may also get into the food supply.

PESTICIDES

Pesticides, also known as biocides, are used to kill organisms that are considered undesirable. The

---

groundwater water that sinks into the soil, where it may be stored for long periods.

aquifer a layer of the earth's crust that contains groundwater.

pesticide any chemical used to kill plant or animal pests.

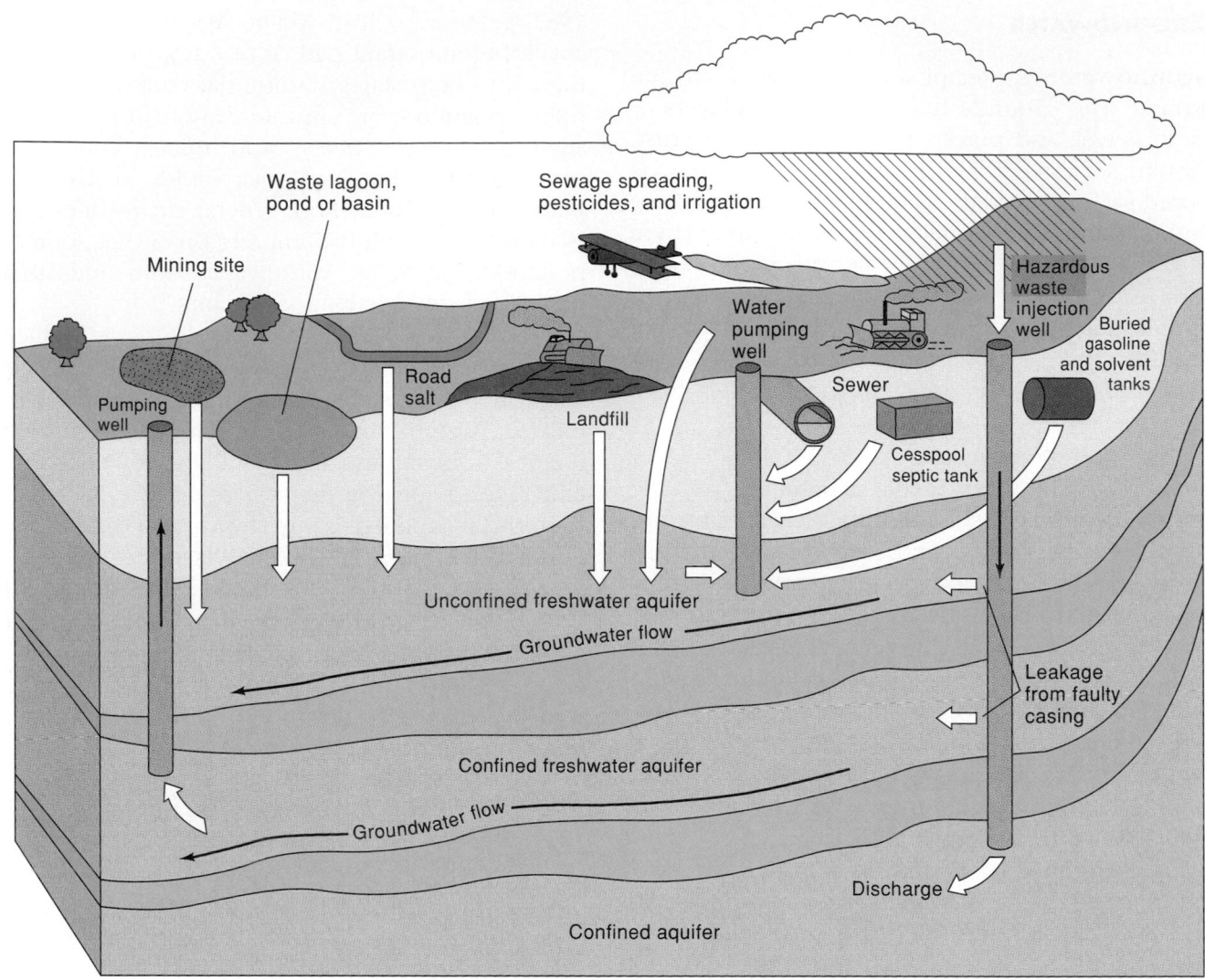

Figure 24.6
Principal Sources of Groundwater Contamination in the United States

Source: Miller, G. Living in the Environment, 7th ed. Belmont, CA: Wadsworth, 1992.

most common forms are *insecticides* (insect killers), *herbicides* (weed killers), *fungicides* (fungus-killers), *nematocides* (nematode killers), and *rodenticides* (rodent killers). Although pesticides are used to protect food crops from pest destruction, pests still succeed in destroying about one-third of the world's food crops each year.[17]

In 1939 DDT, the first on a long list of synthetic organic pesticides, was developed. Since then, annual pesticide use has increased worldwide to an average of one pound of pesticide for each person on the earth. While many of these products are used on crops, 92 percent of all U.S. households use one or more types of pesticides. In fact, according to a study by the EPA, homeowners

apply about five times more pesticides per unit of land than do farmers.[18]

Since 1972, DDT use has been officially banned in the United States. Yet, a 1983 study showed that it is present in many fruits and vegetables. Some of this is due to illegal smuggling of DDT from Mexico; some due to U.S.-produced DDT being shipped to other countries where it is used legally in the production of food that is imported by the United States. Although banned, a 1988 amendment to the 1972 law by Congress allows other insecticide products sold in the United States to contain up to 15 percent DDT.[19]

Of special concern are the long-term effects of pesticides on human health. According to the

National Academy of Sciences,[20] the active ingredients in 90 percent of all fungicides, 60 percent of all herbicides, and 30 percent of all insecticides in use in the United States may cause anywhere from 4,000 to 20,000 cases of cancer per year in the United States. In terms of cancer risk, the EPA ranked pesticide residues the third most serious environmental health threat in the United States.[21] Aside from cancer, some scientists are seriously concerned about possible genetic mutations, birth defects, nervous system disorders, and effects on the immune and endocrine systems caused by exposure to low levels of pesticides over a long period of time.

Some say that pesticides are greatly overused. Although the use of pesticides has increased by 33 times since 1940, U.S. crop losses to pests has increased from 31 percent in 1940 to 37 percent today.[22] Unfortunately, only 1–5 percent of pesticides reach the target pests. The rest ends up in the soil, surface water, groundwater, food, and other nontarget organisms, including people.[23] Slowly degradable insecticides, such as DDT and PCBs (polychlorinated biphenyls) can be biologically amplified thousands to millions of times in the **food chains** and webs in which food energy moves from green plants to humans.

Ways to Combat the Use of Pesticides

You can combat pesticides through your handling of foods that have been exposed to them, as well as by replacing the use of pesticides with alternative forms of pest control.

Although no amount of peeling or washing can remove all pesticides from fruits and vegetables you eat, some ways to reduce your exposure to them include the following:

- Wash all produce thoroughly. A few drops of mild dishwashing detergent in some water will remove more pesticides than water alone. When finished, rinse well.
- Use a vegetable scrub brush on hard produce, such as carrots, potatoes, and sweet potatoes.

- Chop rough-surfaced produce, such as broccoli and cauliflower, before you wash it.
- Peel any fruit or vegetable that has a wax coating, such as apples, eggplants, and cucumbers.
- Discard the outer leaves of cabbage and iceberg lettuce.
- Trim off the leaves of celery.

Opponents of pesticide proliferation insist there are safer and more effective alternatives to pesticide use by homeowners and farmers. A few of these alternatives include the following:

- Remove diseased or infested plants and stalks and other plant residues that harbor pests.
- Mow weeds around crops and shrubs, instead of using herbicides.
- Use vacuum machines that gently remove bugs from plants.
- Use photodegradable plastic between shrubs and rows of some crops to prevent the growth of weeds.
- Use crop rotation (crops are changed from year to year), so that populations of pests do not have time to multiply to uncontrollable levels.

TOXIC METALS

Various metallic elements or their compounds have been found to be hazardous to our health. Of particular concern to people in the United States has been lead.

Lead

We are exposed to lead every day in our food, water, and air. According to a 1986 EPA study, 88 percent of all children and 77 percent of adults have 10 or more micrograms of lead per deciliter (mcg/dl) of blood in their systems. A level of 25 mcg/dl, the currently accepted danger level, is believed by some to be too high. The Center for Disease Control (CDC) and Department of Health and Human Services (DHHS) favor lowering the danger level to 10 mcg/dl.[24] The body of the average person contains 5–6 mcg/dl of lead.

Lead serves no known function or health benefit in humans. Once inside the body, it is handled

food chain the sequential transfer of food energy from green plants to humans and other animals.

like calcium, because the body cannot distinguish between the two. After several weeks in the blood, lead is absorbed by bone and accumulates there over a lifetime. When lead enters the blood, about 90 percent is stored in the bones, and the rest is excreted. Lead interferes with many body systems, especially the nervous, reproductive, cardiovascular, immune, and gastrointestinal, as well as damaging the kidneys and liver. Intellectual development and red blood cell formation are especially affected.

The most profound effect of lead poisoning is seen in children. Continuous low levels of lead exposure can cause a range of physical and mental problems (including learning disabilities) and is especially dangerous for fetuses and small children. The activities and behavior of children—playing in dirt, putting hands in the mouth, and ingesting nonfoods—increase their exposure. Lead poisoning is more likely among poor children who live near sources of lead, such as older housing with old and peeling paints. In addition, children naturally absorb more minerals than adults do, especially during periods of rapid growth. Infants and young children absorb 5–10 percent more lead than adults do.[25] Lead toxicity is found primarily in children younger than 6 years old. Malnourished children are especially vulnerable to lead poisoning. More lead is absorbed if the stomach is empty, if there is an iron deficiency, or if calcium and zinc intake is low.[26] The American Academy of Pediatrics and the CDC recommend screening all children for lead.[27] If your child has not received the blood test, ask your physician or health department for advice.

Mild lead poisoning can result in general symptoms such as diarrhea, irritability, and lethargy. At higher levels of poisoning there is effect on balance; verbal, perceptual, and cognitive abilities; and the development of learning disabilities. One year of exposure can permanently impair the brain, nervous system, and psychological functioning.[28] Each year 12,000–16,000 children are treated for acute lead poisoning; 200 of these children die. Survivors of lead poisoning may suffer from palsy, partial paralysis, blindness, and mental retardation.[29]

All foods contain some lead, although most lead is the result of industrial pollution. People are exposed to lead from gasoline, paint, newspaper ink, batteries, shotgun ammunition, pesticides, and industrial processes. Lead gets into food from tin cans sealed with lead solder, and old or imported pottery decorated with lead glazes, especially from lead-glazed pottery not fired at sufficiently high temperatures to keep the lead from leaching into the food.

A number of measures have been taken to eliminate lead from our environment. In 1973, all new cars were required to use only unleaded gasoline. In 1986, that law was amended to make the requirement more rigid, reducing the amount of lead in unleaded gasoline from 2.5 grams per gallon to 0.1 gram per gallon. In 1976, a measure was enacted requiring paint manufacturers to reduce the amount of lead used in their products. Since 1987 the use of pipes and solder containing lead for public water systems has been banned. Yet many older houses, buildings, and drinking fountains have pipes and solder joints containing lead. Even some home water-filtering systems and bottled spring water may contain lead. Levels of lead in food and drinks today are the lowest in history—90 percent lower than 12 years ago.[30]

Protecting Yourself Against Lead Poisoning

The following are some measures you can take to protect yourself and your family against lead poisoning:

1. Make sure children's hands are clean before they eat.

2. If using leaded crystal for drinking, do not use it on a daily basis, or store liquids in it, or let children use it, or use it while pregnant.

3. Test tap and bottled water for lead content.

4. Be cautious about using foods from imported lead-soldered cans, especially acidic foods such as tomatoes and citrus juices, coffee, tea, apple juice, and cola soft drinks.

5. If using older or imported ceramic products, avoid storing acid foods in them, or have them tested to determine if they are safe for food use; limit use of antique or collectible dishware for food or beverage use to special occasions.

6. Keep painted surfaces in good repair to avoid chipping or peeling of older paint layers; never allow children to eat paint chips; take special precautions when remodeling older houses.

7. Never use lead solder to repair plumbing.

8. Follow label directions on any ornamental product with wording such as "Not for Food Use—Plate May Poison Food. For Decorative Purposes Only."

9. If wine is sealed with a foil capsule, wipe the rim of the bottle with a cloth dampened with water or lemon juice before removing the cork.

CHECKPOINT

1. List the most common forms of pesticides.

2. When was DDT developed, how has it been used, and why has it been banned from use in the United States?

3. What are the effects of lead poisoning on a person?

4. List some measures you can take to protect yourself from lead poisoning.

WASTE DISPOSAL

SOLID WASTES

The United States generates enormous amounts of solid wastes. With only 4.5 percent of the world's population, the United States produces 33 percent of the world's solid waste. **Solid waste** is any unwanted or discarded material that is not a liquid or a gas. This includes our everyday garbage, such as cans, bottles, and newspapers, as well as worn-out furniture, old appliances, animal manure, and any other cast-off materials.

Approximately 11 billion tons of solid waste are produced annually in the United States. This represents an annual per-person production of 44 tons, two to four times that of any other developed country.[31] About 75 percent of this comes from mining, natural gas and oil production, and industrial and agricultural activities. Thirteen percent of this waste is produced on farms; most farm-generated waste, such as manure, is recycled. Nine-and-

a-half percent is generated by industrial operations, homes, and businesses. One percent is sewage sludge. The remaining 1.5 percent of solid waste is municipal solid waste from homes and businesses, or garbage. It has been estimated that each of us produces almost four pounds of garbage, waste paper, and rubbish each day, or 51 tons over a 70-year lifetime.[32]

Many of us throw away most of our solid wastes, then set it out for garbage collectors to pick up. Of the garbage and rubbish Americans throw away, about 59 percent is paper, cardboard, and yard wastes (Figure 24.7). Of this, only 13 percent is being recycled or composted, the other 87 percent is hauled away and dumped or burned at a cost of $6 billion per year.[33] Trash collectors take urban trash to garbage dumps. As garbage dumps fill up, however, everyday waste is carted farther away at increased cost. At present, about 73 percent of all urban garbage is hauled to landfills, where garbage is compacted and covered with dirt each day. The location of these landfills is chosen to minimize water pollution. Landfills may fill in canyons, quarries, or form new hills. Once these sites are filled, they may be allowed to settle or compact. Due to the many years required for settling, landfills are not suitable locations for buildings; they are often used instead as parks, golf courses, baseball fields, or wildlife areas.

WHAT WE CAN DO TO COMBAT WASTE POLLUTION

Because many existing landfills are full and sites for new landfills are becoming harder to find, alternatives are being considered. Some dumps are burning wastes instead of burying them. Although incineration is currently a more expensive option and has the drawback of causing air pollution, it is increasingly feasible. At other dumping sites, **composting** is used to dispose of biodegradable wastes, which can then be used as soil conditioners and fertilizers (see Feature 24.4, p. 779).

An alternative to landfill disposal of wastes is recycling. Recycling involves collecting used mate-

---

solid wastes any unwanted or discarded material that is not a liquid or a gas.

composting the accelerated breakdown of grass clippings and other organic solid wastes in the presence of bacteria to produce a humuslike product used as a soil conditioner.

Figure 24.7

Composition of municipal solid waste thrown away in the United States. The proportions of the types of solid waste in the total mixture change over time. Today's solid waste contains more paper and plastics than in the past, whereas the amounts of glass and steel have declined.

Source: Raven, P. et al. Environment. New York: Saunders, 1993.

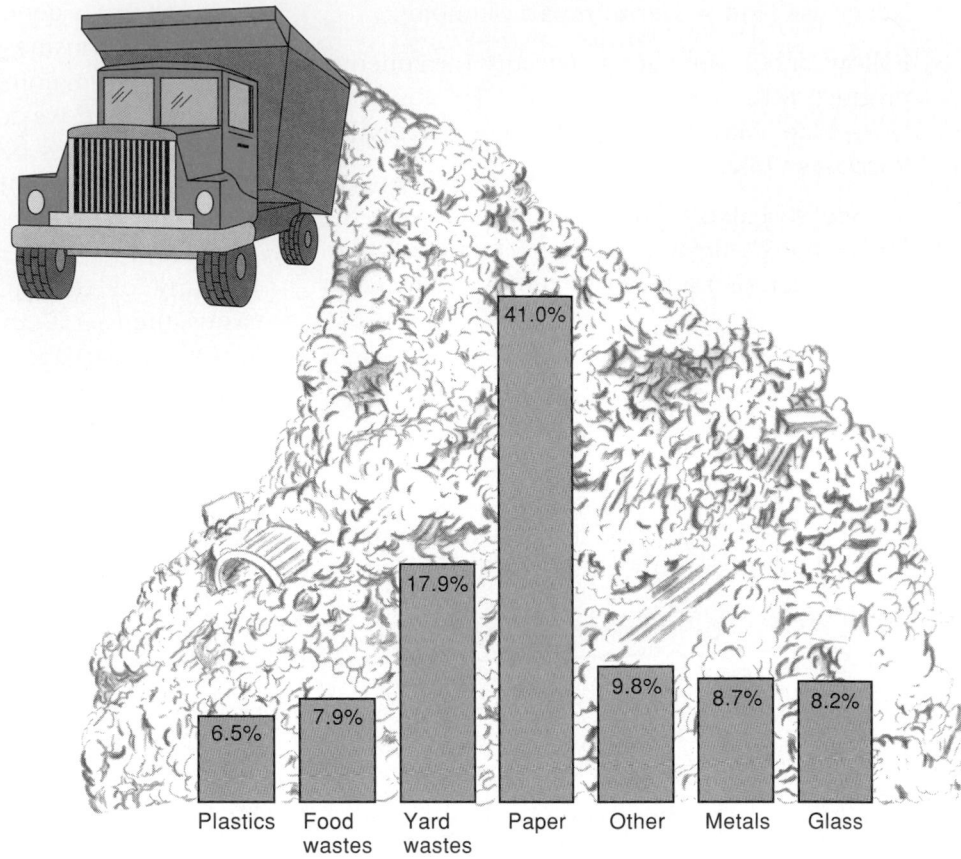

Plastics	Food wastes	Yard wastes	Paper	Other	Metals	Glass
6.5%	7.9%	17.9%	41.0%	9.8%	8.7%	8.2%

rials, such as paper (see Feature 24.5, p. 780), glass, aluminum, and iron, and reprocessing them to make new products. Recycling extends the life of resources and reduces the use of virgin resources, as well as cuts down on waste disposal costs. Only ten states, affecting about one-quarter of the U.S. population, have beverage-container deposit laws that reduce litter and encourage recycling of glass and metal containers. A significant commitment you can make toward protecting the environment and saving it from unnecessary destruction is to become a recycler. Feature 24.6 (p. 781) gives you

As landfills reach capacity and new sites become scarcer and more expensive, North Americans will need to develop and pay for more innovative options for the handling of solid wastes.

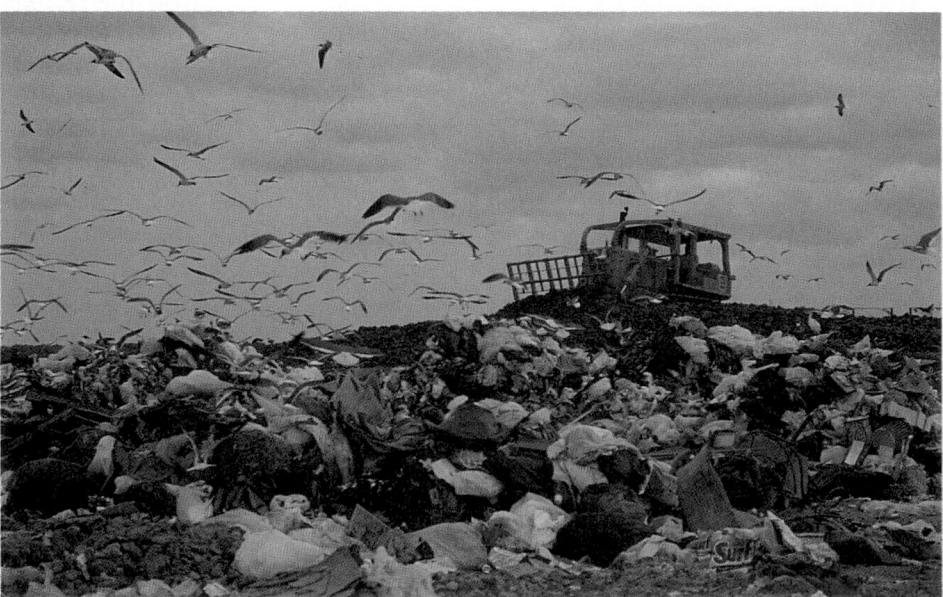

FEATURE 24.4

COMPOSTING AROUND YOUR HOME

Compost is a rich natural soil conditioner and fertilizer. It is produced by making alternating layers of kitchen and yard wastes, cuttings and leaves, animal manure, and topsoil. This makes a home for microorganisms that aid the decomposition of the wastes, and produces a sweet-smelling, dark humus material rich in organic material and soil nutrients. It can be used as a soil conditioner, topsoil, or soil dressing around plants.

You can begin your own composting by constructing a home compost bin as shown in the illustration. Once the lay-ers have been constructed, you can either allow the pile to collect rainwater, or if necessary moisten the pile occasionally. The pile should be turned once a month. During winter months in cold areas the pile should be covered with a tarp. Small compost bins have been developed for use in apartments or condominiums. If necessary, one or more layers of cat litter can help reduce any odors.

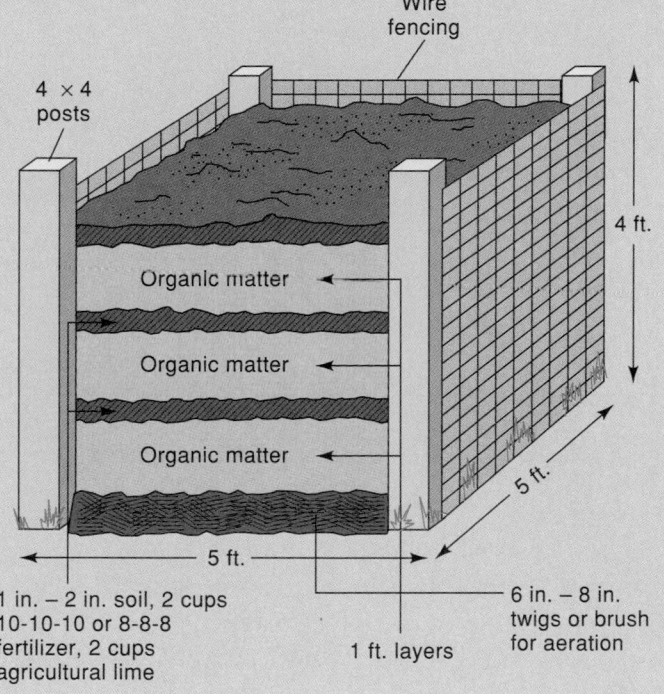

A simple home compost bin can be used to produce mulch for garden and yard plants.

Source: Miller, G. Living in the Environment, 7th ed. Belmont, CA: Wadsworth, 1992.

a number of ideas on how you can begin or expand your practice of recycling, thereby extending the life and health of the earth.

An even better strategy than recycling is to use the same packaging, such as beverage bottles, over and over again in its original form. This used to be a common practice with milk bottles. Reuse extends the supply of the resource, reduces the use of energy, and lessens pollution even more than recycling. It takes three times as much energy to crush and remelt a glass bottle to make a new one than it does to refill it.[34]

Other options include trying to produce less waste by reducing consumption, reducing the amount of material used in packaging, and repairing products to keep them working longer. Although some replacement strategies are being used today, many more are needed for the future.

HAZARDOUS WASTES

Discarded materials that pose a threat to human health or to the environment are called **hazardous wastes.** These wastes may be solid, liquid, or gaseous, and include many toxic, corrosive, and ignitable substances. Until a little more than a decade ago, an estimated 6 billion tons of hazardous wastes were being dumped in 26,000 des-

....

hazardous waste discarded solid, liquid, or gaseous wastes that threaten human health or the environment.

FEATURE 24.5

RECYCLING PAPER

Even though paper is highly recyclable, only about 25 percent of the world's wastepaper is now recycled. While The Netherlands recycles 53 percent of its paper, the United States recycles only 25 percent of its paper. Some countries, such as Sweden, have enacted laws requiring paper recycling. The United States could be doing better than it now is. During World War II, as a part of all civil defense efforts, the nation recycled about 45 percent of its wastepaper.

Recycling paper in the United States makes good sense. Every American uses an average of 699 pounds of paper each year, or about eight times the world average per person. One Sunday edition of the *New York Times* alone requires the weekly consumption of 150 acres of forest to produce the needed paper. About three-quarters of U.S. paper products end up as trash. This is more significant since paper also makes up over 40 percent of the volume of urban solid waste produced each year. Americans spend about 10 percent of their grocery dollars on paper packaging, which they throw out.

Recycling paper is energy efficient. Paper recycling requires about 30–64 percent less energy than that needed to produce paper from virgin pulpwood. The U.S. paper industry is the country's third-largest consumer of energy and the largest user of fuel oil. Not only does recycling save on energy, it also saves on pollution. Recycling paper cuts down on air pollution from pulp mills from 74 to 95 percent, and reduces water pollution by 35 percent. At the same time, recycling paper conserves large volumes of water and saves landfill space. Half of the trash the government discards is paper. The state of Florida now adds a tax to every ton of virgin newsprint used, a model that could be followed by other states. If half of the discarded paper were recycled, the United States would save enough energy to provide 10 million people with electric power each year. An increasing number of cities are now requiring residences and businesses to sort newspapers and cardboard for pickup and recycling.

Unfortunately, since 1988 the supply of recycled newspapers has exceeded the capacity of U.S. paper mills to use it, causing the price of recycled paper to plunge. A strategy of increasing demand for recycled paper is needed. One place to begin using recycled paper products is with the federal and state governments, which are large consumers of paper. The state of New Jersey has now passed a law requiring that a given percentage of government purchases of paper be recycled paper. Conservationists seek public, national, state, and local policies that could result in recycling of half of wastepaper in the United States by the year 2000.

Source: Data from Organization for Economic Cooperation and Development. In Miller, G. *Living in the Environment,* 7th ed. Belmont, CA: Wadsworth, 1992.

---

ignated sites around the country. These sites included municipal landfills, farm fields, and chemical dump sites from which chemicals leaked into surrounding water supplies. Love Canal in Niagara Falls, New York, a neighborhood of almost a thousand homes, was affected by toxic and carcinogenic chemicals from an abandoned chemical dump nearby. The government declared the area a federal disaster area and was forced to relocate people, demolish homes, and pay settlements to many of the families affected by the disaster.[35]

In 1987, the EPA compiled a list of the worst hazardous waste sites among the thousands of sites in the United States, and began to clean them up. The EPA has estimated that eventually, as many as 10,000 sites may need to be cleaned up over the next 50 years, at a cost of as much as $100 billion.[36]

The United States generates 264 million tons of hazardous wastes annually, for an average of 1 ton per person. Yet, the American Chemical Society believes the true amount is two to ten times greater than the EPA estimate.[37] Sewage sludge, radioactive waste, and toxic household waste are not included in that statistic because these wastes are not EPA regulated. Approximately 93 percent of all hazardous waste in the United States comes from the chemical-, petroleum-, and metal-related industries.

In 1980, Congress passed what was to become the Superfund program, a five-year, $1.6 billion crash program to clean up the 500 worst toxic dumps across the country. It has twice been extended, once in 1986 and again in 1990, and immensely expanded. Now more than 13 years and $13 billion in public funding later, the end of its job appears little closer, and further extensions are certain. It was to be financed jointly by federal and state governments, supplemented by taxes on the chemical and petrochemical industries. A prompt cleanup seemed a reasonable goal. Unfortunately, taxes on industry-generated wastes have amounted to only about $1 billion per year.

In 1989 the EPA estimated that there are more than 32,000 sites containing potentially hazardous wastes. The General Accounting Office estimates

FEATURE 24.6

WAYS YOU CAN RECYCLE

Environmentalists are helping us understand that all of us need to be shifting from a dumping, burying, burning mentality to a recycling, reusing, composting one. Trash cans need to be seen as *resource containers,* used to collect trash for separating into useful materials for recycling. In some areas, families have achieved a recycling rate as high as 84 percent. Environmentalists insist that a recycling rate of 60 percent is an attainable goal in all communities. Although more than half of the states recycle less than 5 percent of their municipal solid waste, some states have set the goal of recycling 50 percent of their municipal solid waste by the year 2000; the state of New Jersey is aiming for 60 percent.

Salvaging usable metals, paper, plastics, and glass from municipal solid waste and selling them to industries for recycling and reuse is called **resource recovery.** In special resource-recovery plants, mixed municipal wastes are separated and then sold to manufacturing industries as raw materials for recycling. The remaining combustible wastes can then be incinerated. Less expensive yet is letting consumers separate trash into recyclable categories before it is picked up.

Steps you can take to reduce, reuse, or recycle include the following:

- Use refillable glass containers for beverages, rather than cans or throwaway bottles.

- Make a conscious effort to produce less waste by not using disposable paper, plastic, and metal products when alternatives are available, and by deciding whether you really need a product before you buy it.

- Use a plastic or metal lunch box or reusable paper lunch bags; use biodegradable wax paper for wrapping sandwiches or put them in reusable plastic containers. Store refrigerated food in reusable containers rather than in plastic wrap or aluminum foil.

- Reuse cardboard and computer paper boxes as storage files.

- Use rechargeable batteries. Manufacturing a standard disposable battery requires 50 times more electricity than the battery generates; plus disposable batteries are a source of toxic metals in landfills.

- Lobby for the use of washable, reusable dishes and flatware in school and business cafeterias.

- Lobby schools and companies to switch their paper stock to recycled products.

- Use both sides of paper you write on.

- Push for the setting up of ways to recycle computer and other office paper.

- Select products that do not have excessive packaging; buy fresh fruit and vegetables that are loose, rather than wrapped in plastic and on trays.

- Reduce the amount of junk mail you receive by writing to Mail Preference Services, Direct Marketing Association, 11 W. 42nd Street, P.O. Box 3681, New York, NY 10163-3861, asking that your name not be sold to mailing list companies.

- Use junk mail at home as scrap paper for writing phone messages, notes, and shopping lists.

- Use washable cloth napkins, dish towels, and sponges rather than paper ones.

- Use as few plastic or paper bags as possible when purchasing groceries and other products; take your own cloth or reusable bags with you when shopping.

- When purchasing appliances insist on repairable items and ones that last longer.

Source: Miller, G. *Living in the Environment,* 7th ed. Belmont, CA: Wadsworth, 1992.

that the number of such sites could reach well over 100,000. In 1991, the EPA placed 1,211 of these sites on a National Priorities List. Not included in these numbers are Defense and Energy Department sites. Of these, only 64 have been declared cleaned up and removed from the priority list. The EPA now projects a cost of $77 billion to clean up all of the sites on the list.[38]

resource recovery salvaging usable metals, paper, and glass from solid waste and selling them to manufacturing industries for recycling or reuse.

Running up the cost of cleanup have been issues of liability. In one example, Glenwood Landing, New York, petroleum was stored and wastes were dumped for four decades. Put on the National Priorities List in 1984, the EPA identified 257 parties, ranging from multinational corporations to a local film-developing lab, which it saw as potentially liable for cleanup costs. By 1991, 136 law firms had been engaged to defend the litigants, and 4 of the parties had sued 442 insurance companies for cleanup reimbursement. Due to the mass of litigation that accompanies cleanup efforts, the typical site cleanup takes more than a decade.

How You Can Reduce Hazardous Waste

As with other types of pollutants, hazardous waste exposure can be reduced both by individual and industrial commitment to action.

A first option in combating hazardous waste would be to redesign manufacturing processes to eliminate as much as possible the need for materials that may become hazardous wastes. Some wastes that are generated can be reused or recycled, as already discussed regarding paper.

Hazardous organic compounds containing little or no toxic compounds or volatile materials can be detoxified biologically by applying them to forest and farm lands. If unfit for spreading on the land, hazardous wastes can be handled by incineration. While incineration is used to dispose of the bulk of hazardous wastes in some Western European countries, only a small amount of such wastes are incinerated in this country.

Industry can reduce the adverse effects of hazardous waste by disposing of it in secured landfills for long-term storage. Figure 24.8 illustrates a suggested method for constructing a secured landfill.

Individuals can act to combat hazardous wastes by monitoring the enforcement of laws governing such waste and by helping lobby for adequate funding of responsible agencies. Individuals can also help by replacing hazardous household cleaning products with less-hazardous ones (see Table 24.4).

Figure 24.8
Secure Landfill

A secure landfill is designed to contain hazardous wastes, preventing hazardous water seepage from contaminating groundwater, nearby surface waters, and soils.

Source: Kaufman, D., and Franz. C. Biosphere 2000. New York: HarperCollins, 1993.

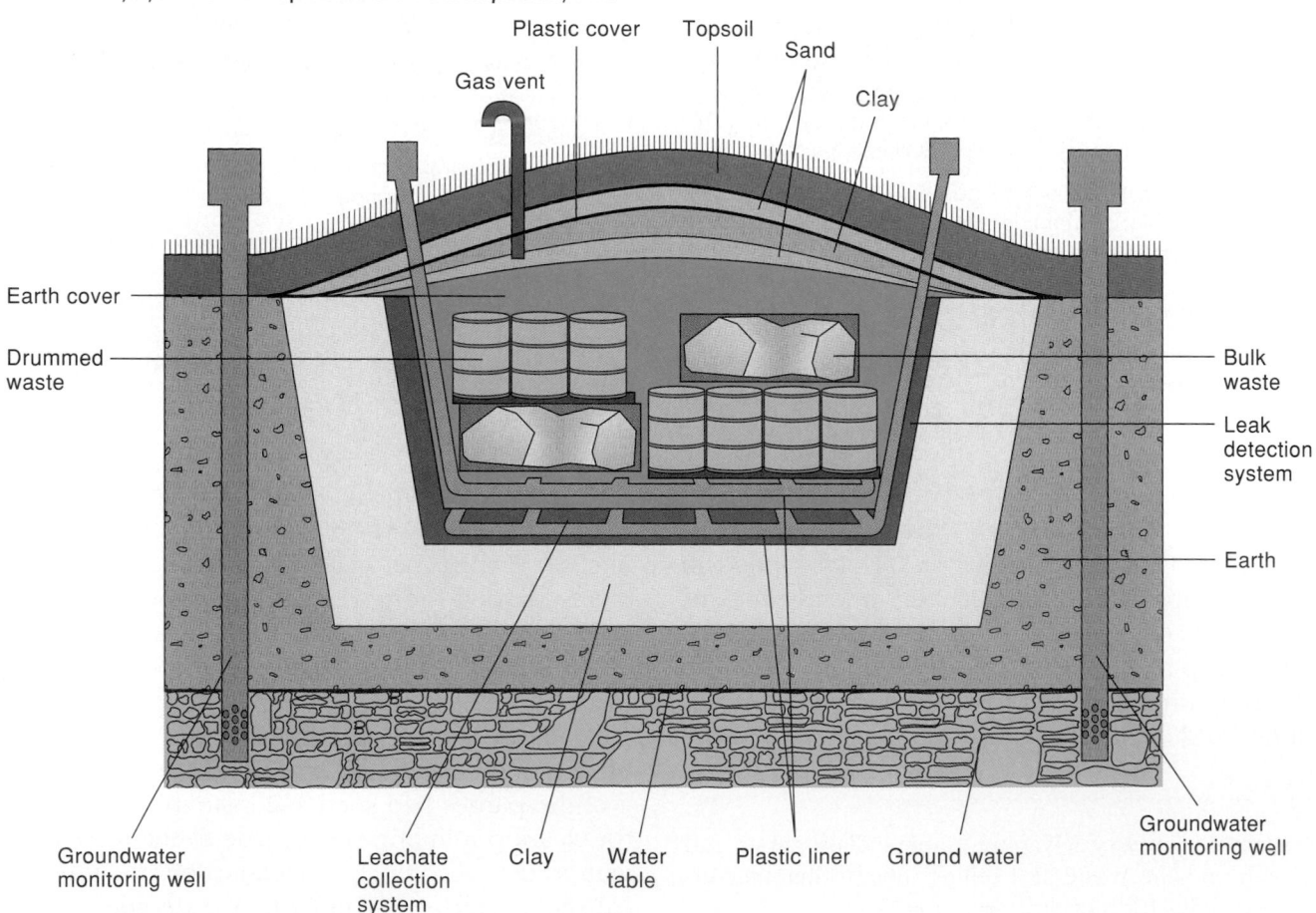

Table 24.4
Replacements for Some Hazardous Household Chemicals

Chemical	Alternative
Oven cleaner	Use baking soda for scouring; for baked-on grease, apply ¼ cup of ammonia in oven overnight to loosen; scrub the next day with baking soda.
Drain cleaner	Pour ½ cup salt down drain, followed by boiling water; flush with hot tap water
Glass polish	Use ammonia and soap
Wall and floor cleaners containing organic solvents	Use detergents to clean large areas and then rinse with water
Toilet bowl, tub, and tile cleaner	Mix borax and lemon juice in a paste; rub on paste and let set two hours before scrubbing
Mildew stain remover and disinfectant cleaner	Chlorine bleach
Furniture polish	Melt 1 pound carnauba wax into 2 cups of mineral oil; for lemon oil polish, dissolve 1 teaspoon of lemon oil into 1 pint of mineral oil
Shoe polish	Use polishes that do not contain methylene chloride, trichloroethylene, or nitrobenzene
Spot removers	Launder fabrics when possible to remove stains; also try cornstarch or vinegar
Carpet and rug shampoos	Cornstarch
Detergents and detergent boosters	Washing soda and soap powder
Water softeners	Washing soda
Pesticides (indoor and outdoor)	Use natural biological controls; use boric acid for roaches
Mothballs	Soak dried lavender, equal parts of rosemary and mint, dried tobacco, whole peppercorns, and cedar chips in real cedar oil and place in a cotton bag

Source: Miller, G. Living in the Environment, 6th ed. Belmont, CA: Wadsworth, 1988.

OTHER TOXIC SUBSTANCES

A number of other common metallic substances are hazardous. Arsenic, beryllium, and cadmium are all released when fossil fuel is burned. Cadmium is inhaled with smoke from cigarettes, and plants absorb it from commercial fertilizers. Arsenic is released when ores are refined.

Each of these toxic substances is a known carcinogen, and in sufficient concentrations, can be hazardous to our bodies. As these substances accumulate in the body they can cause liver, kidney, and respiratory damage as well as heart disease.

They have also been found to cause birth defects and cancer.

CHECKPOINT

1. Define the term *solid waste*.
2. How much solid waste do people in this country produce daily per person?
3. Explain composting.
4. Define the term *hazardous waste*.
5. Explain the Superfund program.

RADIATION

Radiation is the emission of radiant energy in the form of fast-moving particles from certain naturally occurring elements, such as uranium, thorium, and radium. Those elements capable of giving off radiation are said to be **radioactive.** Radium gives off three kinds of radiation, *alpha, beta,* and *gamma.* When radium gives off alpha particles, a radioactive gas called **radon** is formed (see Air Pollution earlier in this chapter). Alpha and beta particles are barely able to penetrate the skin, although when either kind of particle is inhaled or ingested, significant damage may result. Gamma radiation, which is similar to x-rays, can penetrate the human body and most other substances with ease.

Many elements are made up of atoms that vary in weight, but are otherwise identical. Such atoms are called **isotopes.** Radioactive isotopes are known as **radioisotopes,** and the radiation they emit is called **ionizing radiation.** Ionizing radiation can damage living tissue. Radio waves, infrared light, and ordinary visible light are exam-

....

radiation transmission of energy through matter and space in the form of fast-moving particles.

radioactive capable of giving off radiation.

radon a radioactive gas.

isotopes atoms that vary only in weight.

radioisotopes radioactive isotopes.

ionizing radiation radiation emitted by radioisotopes.

Table 24.5
Half-lives of Some Representative Radioactive Materials

Isotope	Half-life[a]
Uranium-238	4,510,000,000 years
Uranium-235	700,000,000 years
Plutonium-239	25,000 years
Radium-226	1,600 years
Strontium-90	28 years
Iodine-131	8 days

[a]Half-life is the length of time required for one-half of a quantity of a radioactive isotope to decay (break down) to nonradioactive materials. After two half-lives, one-fourth of the original radioactivity remains; after three half-lives, one-eighth remains, and so forth.

Table 24.6
Health Effects of Exposure to Radiation

Sudden, whole-body exposure to radiation can cause the following general effects.

Dose (rems)	Effects
0–100	Nausea, vomiting
100–200	Moderately depressed white blood cell count; not immediately fatal but long-term cancer risk
200–600	Heavily depressed white blood count; blotched skin in 4–6 weeks; 80–100 percent possibility of death
600–1000	Diarrhea, fever, blood-chemical imbalance in 1 to 14 days; almost 100 percent probability of death

Source: Kaufman, D., and Franz, C. Biosphere 2000. New York: HarperCollins, 1993.

ples of *nonionizing radiation,* which do not damage living tissue. Radioisotopes vary not only in the kind of radiation emitted, but in their longevity. Longevity of radioisotopes is expressed in the time it takes for one-half of their radioactivity to dissipate, or *half-life* (see Table 24.5).

There are various units, such as the curie, roentgen, rem, and millirem, used to describe the forms of radiation. Of interest to us is the **rem,** and the **millirem (mrem),** which are measures of radiation dosage in human tissues. The probable effects of various dosages of radiation are given in Table 24.6.[39]

Radiation is one of the most hazardous of all environmental pollutants. It is tasteless, odorless, and invisible, and the day-to-day exposure to ionizing radiation may have serious health effects. While a massive dose of radiation may result in rapid death, smaller, nonlethal doses may produce permanent genetic alterations and certain types of cancers.

SOURCES OF RADIATION

No one is able to avoid all exposure to ionizing radiation. Some radiation is **natural,** or **background, radiation,** arising in the natural environment. About one-fourth of such radiation is found in cosmic rays, which bombard us from outer space; another one-fourth comes from radioactive elements in our bodies, which have been deposited there through the air we breathe, the water we drink, and the food we eat. The rest of the natural radiation comes from soil and rocks, such as the radioactive gas radon.[40]

We are exposed to additional radiation as the result of **artificial,** or **human-related,** activities, such as dental and medical x-rays, diagnostic tests involving the injection or ingestion of radioisotopes, and myriad other sources such as computer display screens, microwave ovens, television sets, and luminous watch dials (see Table 24.7). A small amount of radiation arises from the normal operation of nuclear power plants.

Americans are exposed to an annual average of 230 millirems (or 0.23 rem) of ionizing radiation. Natural sources supply an average of 130 mrem, and artificial sources add another 100 mrem. There is no agreement by scientists as to a "safe" level of radiation exposure. The recommended maximum "safe" dosage ranges from 0.5 to 5 rem per year.[41] Current federal and international standards set the maximum allowable occupational exposure at 5000 mrem, or 5 rem, per year.

FOOD IRRADIATION

Ionizing radiation is being used as an alternative to chemical additives for some FDA-approved foods.

rem roentgen equivalent in humans.

millirem (mrem) one one-thousandth of a rem.

natural, or **background, radiation** radiation arising in the natural environment.

artificial, or **human-related, radiation** radiation arising as a result of human activities.

Table 24.7

Major Sources of Artificial Radiation in the United States (Per Person per Year)

Source	Amount of Radiation (mrem)
Medical x-rays	72.0
Nuclear weapons fallout	4.0
TV, consumer products, and air travel	2.7
Radioactive isotopes used to diagnose and treat disease	2.0
On-the-job exposure	0.8
Nuclear power plants, fuel-processing plants, and nuclear research facilities	0.3

It is being used to kill insects and prevent them from reproducing in certain foods after harvest, to destroy certain parasitic worms (*trichinae*) and bacteria (*salmonella*), to extend shelf life of some perishable foods, to inhibit the growth of sprouts on potatoes and onions, and to delay ripening in certain fruits. Treatment with radiation does not change flavor, color, or texture.[42]

Irradiation never makes foods radioactive, just as being exposed to airport scanners does not leave the body radioactive. Yet it is known that the irradiation creates small chemical changes in the food, the exact nature of which is the subject of ongoing research.[43] Although the doses of radiation needed to achieve these effects varies, the levels are low. In 1986, the FDA gave approval for the use of low doses of ionizing radiation on fruits, vegetables, wheat and wheat flour, pork, nuts, seeds, teas, and spices. In 1990, FDA approval was given for use of radiation on poultry, followed by final clearance by the U.S. Department of Agriculture in 1992.[44] Approval for the use of radiation on seafood is expected. In the United States, irradiated foods carry a characteristic logo along with a label stating that the food has been treated by or with irradiation (Figure 24.9). The use of this term is due to the belief that some consumers may react negatively to the use of the term *radiation* and associate it with the radiation particles that persist after a nuclear accident.

RADIATION POLLUTION

There is profound public concern over the effects of radiation pollution. Of particular concern are radioactive fallout, commercial nuclear power plants, disposal of radioactive wastes, and radiation in medicine and therapy.

Radioactive Fallout

Radioactive fallout consists of the dirt and debris, sucked up and made radioactive by a nuclear blast, which falls back to earth near the site of an explosion or on downwind areas hundreds and thousands of miles away. The history of the two small nuclear bomb blasts in Japan in 1945 tells a morbid story of over 100,000 people dead from radioactive fallout, and of many more who developed cataracts, and leukemia and other lethal cancers years later. While the United States, the USSR, and Great Britain agreed in 1963 to stop atmospheric testing of nuclear weapons, the testing of nuclear devices has continued, many of them underground. While nuclear testing has added only about 1 percent to natural background radiation, this percentage could increase significantly as more countries develop nuclear capability.

Nuclear Power Plants

Nuclear power was initially seen as a clean, cheap, and safe source of energy. Only a fraction of the projected plants were built. Currently in the United States only 111 licensed commercial nuclear power plants are functioning, generating about 20 percent of the country's electricity. This percentage is expected to decline as old plants are decommissioned and no new plants are built.

The entire issue of the appropriateness of using nuclear power as an energy source has been very debatable. Proponents insist that nuclear fission is

Figure 24.9
Radiation Logo

The international symbol identifies retail foods that have been irradiated. The words "Treated by irradiation" or "Treated with irradiation" must accompany the symbol.

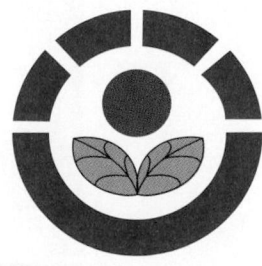

The safety of nuclear power plants continues to be of high public concern. While no new plants are being built, the fate of operating and decommissioned plants requires the greatest public surveillance.

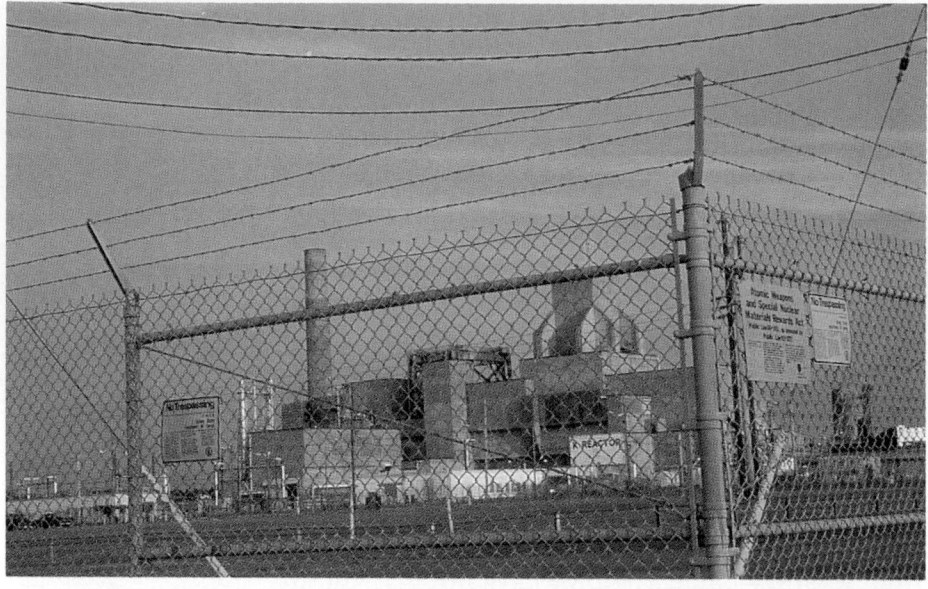

the cheapest, most nonpolluting, and most efficient method of generating electricity, and that it does not depend upon coal and oil. Opponents reply that plant malfunctions, billion-dollar construction cost overruns, the risk of nuclear accident, and unresolved disposal of radioactive wastes make it a price too high for the public to pay.[45]

Thirty years after the first nuclear power plant began operating in the United States, there is still no officially accepted study of how safe these plants are.[46] There are fears over nuclear accidents, such as the ones at Three Mile Island in Pennsylva-

nia and at Chernobyl in the USSR. A reactor core meltdown or reactor building explosion could kill or injure thousands and could contaminate large areas for hundreds of years.

Radiation in Medicine

Radiation that is used in the health sciences for diagnostic and therapeutic purposes accounts for our greatest exposure to artificial radiation. X-rays and radioactive isotopes have been used to treat diseases and extend many lives. While radiation is

Radioactivity properly used is an important tool in the diagnosis and therapy of certain health conditions. While such radiation may be beneficial, it is essential that unnecessary exposure to it be minimized.

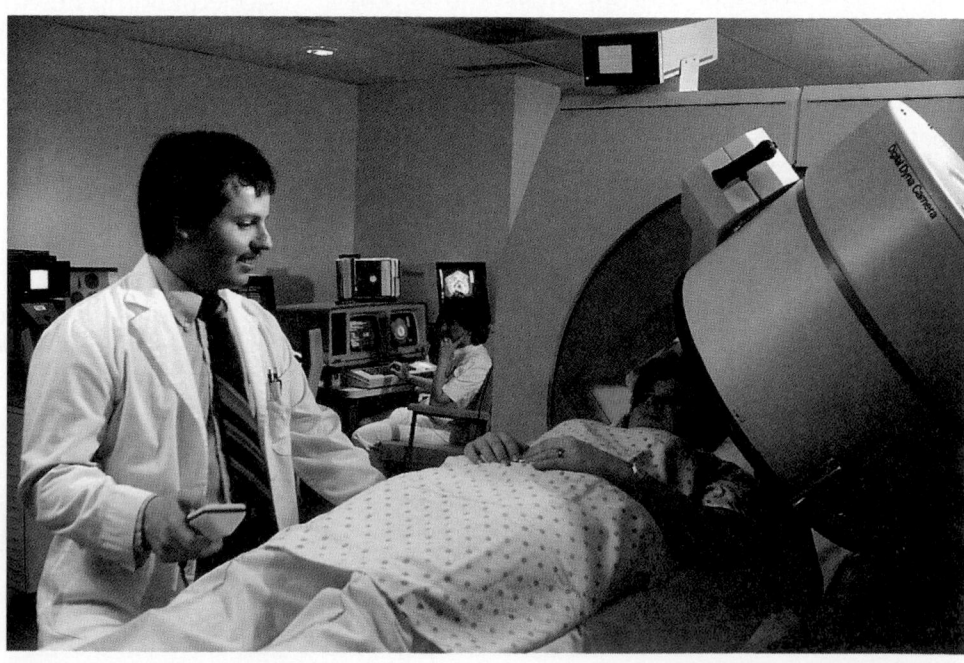

beneficial in these instances, it is essential to minimize unnecessary exposure to radiation. X-rays should be ordered only when no other methods of diagnosis are sufficient, and precautions must always be taken to minimize the emission of stray radiation.

Radioactive Wastes

The disposal of radioactive waste produced by nuclear power plants, hospitals, universities, and industry is a grave problem, and one that seriously threatens our environment. At the heart of the problem is the fact that the only way to destroy radioactivity is to allow time for it to decay. Some radioactive waste is low-level and has a short half-life. But the spent fuel rods from commercial nuclear power plants are high-level, with half-lives of thousands of years. According to the EPA, spent fuel rods require 10,000 years before they decay to acceptable levels of radioactivity.[47]

There is still no widely agreed upon way to store high-level radiation wastes safely. Most citizens strongly object to locating nuclear waste disposal sites anywhere close to them. Almost half of the states have enacted laws banning radiation waste disposal within their boundaries because of possible geological and water contamination.

CHECKPOINT

1. Distinguish among radioactivity, radioactive isotopes, and ionizing radiation.

2. What is the difference between a rem and a millirem?

3. Contrast natural background radiation with artificial radiation.

4. Name the major sources of radiation pollution.

NOISE POLLUTION

Sound, defined as any identifiable noise, is perceived by tiny hair cells in the fluid-filled inner ear. Sound produces reaction in these hair cells that produces electrical impulses, which travel via the auditory nerve to the brain, where the impulses are interpreted as sound.

People with normal hearing can perceive sounds with frequencies ranging from 16 to 20,000 cycles per second, or *Hertz (Hz)*. If sounds are too loud, hair cells are flattened, leading to a sense of fullness or pressure in the ears, or for some, a buzzing. Unrelenting noisy assaults sooner or later cause the hair cells to lose their resilience and die. They do not regenerate and the result is a gradual loss of hearing. About 28 million Americans, or 11 percent, suffer serious hearing loss, and more than one-third of these cases result from too much exposure to loud noise.[48]

Noise, defined as unwanted sound, is a part of our everyday lives. Many of us begin our day to the sounds of flushing toilets, clanking pipes, and voices. Suburbanites head for work on trains, buses, and freeways, and listen to the constant noise of cars, buses, sirens, and radios. At work, there is noise from ringing telephones, computer printers, and more voices. In some places people come home to residences located near or under the flight paths of jet planes. Our days are so filled with a steady stream of noise that the absence of noise almost leaves us bewildered. Whether a sound is noise is a matter of personal opinion. One person's noise is another person's music.

The intensity, or loudness, of a sound is measured in terms of a reference sound that is so soft it is almost inaudible to the human ear. The relative loudness of a sound is expressed by a numbered **decibel (db)** scale or a modified **decibel-A (dbA)** scale. As shown in Table 24.8, for every rise of 10 decibels (dbA), there is a ten-fold increase in volume intensity.

Industrial workers commonly suffer hearing loss. It is estimated that of an industrial work force of 75 million people, 19 million suffer hearing damage.[49] Hearing damage is also common among people who listen to loud music on home stereos, car stereos, with earphones, or who are exposed to jet plane engine roar, revved up motorcycles, pneumatic drills, and leaf blowers. Sound pres-

sound any identifiable noise.

noise unwanted sound.

decibel (db) unit used to measure the intensity, or loudness, of a sound.

decibel-A (dbA) a modified decibel scale.

Table 24.8

The Intensity of Some Common Sound

Sound Source Exposure	Decibels (dbA)	Relative Sound Intensity	Effect on Hearing (Prolonged Exposure)
	0[a]	1	Audibility threshold
Breathing	10	10	
Whisper, rustling leaves	20	100	Very quiet
Quiet rural nighttime	30	1000	
Library, soft music	40	10,000	
Normal conversation	50	100,000	Quiet
Average office	60	1,000,000	
Vacuum cleaner	70	10,000,000	Annoying
Garbage disposal	80	100,000,000	Possible hearing damage
City traffic, diesel truck	90	1,000,000,000	Hearing damage (8 hours or more exposure)
Garbage truck, chain saw	100	10,000,000,000	Serious hearing damage (8 hours or more exposure)
Live rock band; portable stereo held close to ear	110	100,000,000,000	
Siren (close range); jet takeoff (200 yds)	120	1,000,000,000,000	Hearing pain threshold
Crack of gunfire	130	10,000,000,000,000	
Aircraft carrier deck	140	100,000,000,000,000	
Jet takeoff (close range)	150	1,000,000,000,000,000	Eardrum ruptures

[a]The threshold of hearing is 0 decibels because the scale is logarithmic, and the logarithm of 1 is 0.

Source: Miller, G. Living in the Environment, 7th ed., Belmont, CA: Wadsworth, 1992.

sures can damage a person's hearing at 75 dbA, and be painful at 120 dbA. Continued exposure to high-intensity sounds can permanently damage the hair cells in the inner ear. Deafness usually begins with loss of sensitivity to high-pitched sounds, but may not be noticed until the destruction is extensive. For this reason, ear protectors should be worn by persons exposed to high-intensity noises. Today, employers in the United States must require ear protectors for workers when occupational noise levels exceed 90 dbA.[50] Above 120 dbA, the sound level of loud rock bands, the nerve damage can lead to a persistent ringing in the ears, a condition called *tinnitus,* for which there is no treatment.

Notice that according to Table 24.8, the dbA sound pressure scales are logarithmic. With every 10 dbA rise, there is a 10-fold increase in sound pressure. A rise of 30 db amounts to a 1000-fold increase in sound pressure on the ear.

One study has shown that 60 percent of incoming freshmen at the University of Tennessee have significant hearing loss in the high-frequency range. Their hearing capability is the equivalent of a person 60–69 years old. Studies have also shown that by age 30, most people can hear nothing above 16,000 Hz; by age 65, most people are unable to hear sounds above 8,000 Hz.[51]

Loud noises not only affect hearing, but the person's whole body. Noise causes automatic stress reactions, including constricted blood vessels, dilated pupils, muscle tension, elevated heart rate and blood pressure, holding of the breath, and stomach spasms. Constriction of blood vessels may become permanent, increasing blood pressure and contributing to heart disease.

HOW YOU CAN REDUCE NOISE POLLUTION

Noise can be combated; it is one of the easiest types of pollution to control. You can keep your stereo and television turned down, wear ear protectors, limit exposure to damaging sounds such as rock bands, and buy quieter household equipment and appliances. At work people can wear ear plugs, factory machines can be totally or partially enclosed, and buildings can be insulated. You can also work for the enactment and enforcement of stricter noise standards where you work and in the community where you live. Unfortunately, the control of noise pollution in the United States has been crippled by budgetary cutbacks and by the virtual elimination of the portion of the EPA's budget for noise-pollution control.

CHECKPOINT

1. Define the term *noise*.

2. Discuss the meaning of *decibel* and how volume relates to a rise in decibels.

3. Describe the ways in which noise can be combated.

POPULATION DYNAMICS

Population growth is the single most important factor contributing to environmental problems. The world population continues to increase at astounding rates (see Figure 24.10, p. 790). By this time tomorrow, there will be about 245,986 more people on earth; 194,663 in *less-developed countries (LDC)*, and 51,123 in *more-developed countries (MDC)*.

Birth rates in less developed nations are more than twice what they are in developed nations (see Figure 24.11, p. 791). Overall, the *natural increase,* which is the birth rate minus the death rate, in the LDCs is four times what it is in the MDCs. The greatest amount of population change is occurring in Africa, Latin America, and Asia (Table 24.9). The rate of population increase worldwide is 1.6 percent per year, which, if sustained, will lead to a doubling of the population in 43 years. The U.S. population is currently increasing at a rate of 0.7 percent per year, which means that it will double in about ninety-eight years.

The best indication of the potential for growth of a population is its *total fertility rate (TFR),* or the average number of live births a woman will have throughout her childbearing years (usually considered to be ages 15–49). In 1994, the TFR was 3.2 per woman for the world as a whole; 1.7 in MDCs and 3.6 in LDCs (4.2 if China is excluded). These

Table 24.9
Population and Population Growth Rates of Selected Countries

Locality	Population Mid-1994 (millions)	Natural Increase (annual percent)	Doubling Time (years)
World	5,607.0	1.6	43
Slow Growth Countries:			
Estonia	1.5	−0.4	—
Hungary	10.3	−0.3	—
Bulgaria	8.4	−0.2	—
Russia	147.8	−0.2	—
Ukraine	51.5	−0.2	—
Germany	81.2	−0.1	—
Latvia	2.5	−0.1	—
Italy	57.2	0.0	2,310
Greece	10.4	0.1	1,155
Spain	39.2	0.1	630
Denmark	5.2	0.1	533
Belgium	10.1	0.2	330
Japan	125.0	0.3	267
United States	260.8	0.7	98
Rapid Growth Countries:			
Oman	1.9	4.9	14
Iraq	19.9	3.7	19
Solomon Islands	0.4	3.7	19
Syria	14.0	3.7	19
Iran	61.2	3.6	19
Togo (West Africa)	4.3	3.6	19
Comoros (East Africa)	0.5	3.5	20
Côte d'Ivoire (West Africa)	13.9	3.5	20
Niger	8.8	3.4	20
Yemen	12.9	3.4	20
Libya	5.1	3.4	21
Tanzania	29.8	3.4	21

Source: 1994 World Population Data Sheet. *Washington, DC: Population Reference Bureau., 1994.*

total fertility rates range from a low of 1.1 in San Marino to high of 7.6 in Yemen. Although population experts expect the TFR to slowly drop to 2.3 in the LDCs by the year 2025, that will still lead to a projected world population of 9 billion.[52]

As for forecasts on world population, the Population Reference Bureau, in their *1994 World*

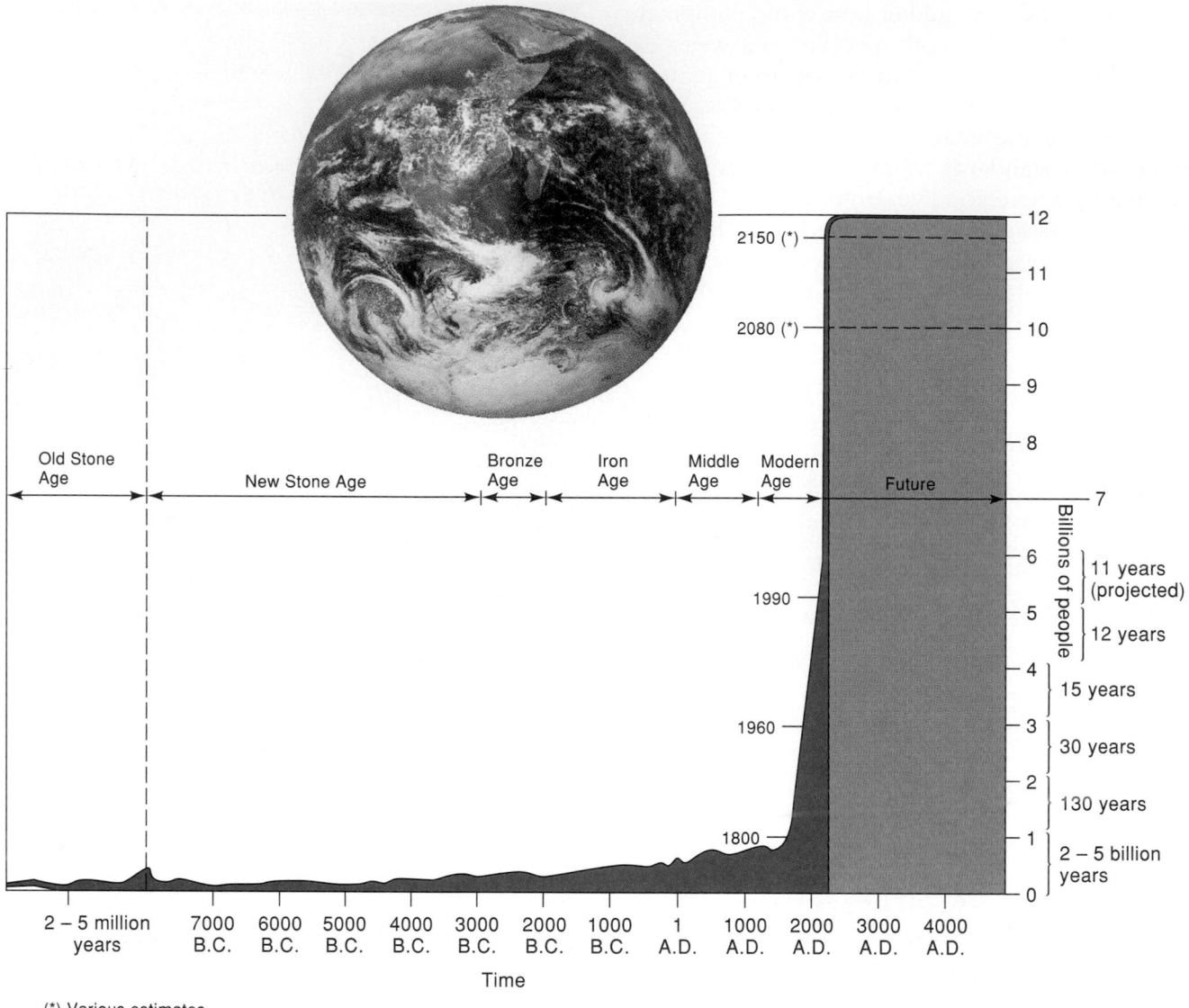

Old Stone Age · New Stone Age · Bronze Age · Iron Age · Middle Age · Modern Age · Future

2150 (*) — 12
2080 (*) — 10
1990 — 5
1960 — 3
1800 — 1

Billions of people

11 years (projected)
12 years
15 years
30 years
130 years
2 – 5 billion years

2 – 5 million years · 7000 B.C. · 6000 B.C. · 5000 B.C. · 4000 B.C. · 3000 B.C. · 2000 B.C. · 1000 B.C. · 1 A.D. · 1000 A.D. · 2000 A.D. · 3000 A.D. · 4000 A.D.

Time

(*) Various estimates

Figure 24.10
World Population Growth Through History

Source: McFalls, J. "Population: A Lively Introduction." Population Bulletin, p. 32 (October 1991).

Data Sheet estimate that by the year 2010, world population will stand at over 7.0 billion, and by 2025 at almost 8.4 billion.[53] Other organizations, such as the United Nations Population Fund (UNPF), have revised their figures somewhat upward. In 1980 the agency predicted that world population would stabilize at 10 billion people in about 100 years. Now UNPF estimates population will surpass 11.6 billion by year 2150. And this prediction is based on the assumption that LDCs can reduce their birth rate per mother, or TFR, now at 3.8, to 3.3 by the year 2000. If this expected drop in TFR is delayed until year 2010, the population will hit 12.5 billion by the next century.[54]

If the world population doubles over the next 100 years as predicted, today's problems seem trivial in comparison. In the 1960s, the idea of **zero population growth (ZPG)** was developed and considered as a viable solution to the rapid population growth. ZPG is a concept in which the number of births each year equals the number of deaths. This can be accomplished by families limiting themselves to no more than two offspring,

....

zero population growth (ZPG) the state in which the birth rate (plus immigration) equals the death rate (plus emigration) so that population is no longer increasing.

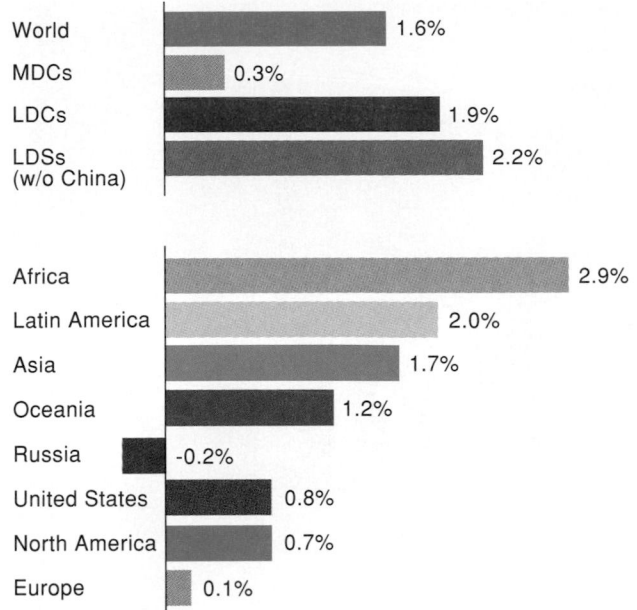

World	1.6%
MDCs	0.3%
LDCs	1.9%
LDSs (w/o China)	2.2%

Africa	2.9%
Latin America	2.0%
Asia	1.7%
Oceania	1.2%
Russia	-0.2%
United States	0.8%
North America	0.7%
Europe	0.1%

Figure 24.11
Average annual population change rate in various groups of countries in 1994. Population change rates in 1994 ranged from a growth rate of 5.0 percent in Gaza to a decline rate of −0.4 percent in Estonia.

Source: 1994 World Population Data Sheet. Washington, DC: Population Reference Bureau, 1994.

which replaces the two parents who produced them, or by countries introducing incentives such as tax advantages or subsidizing families with no more than two children. According to United Nations projections, the world will not reach ZPG until the years 2035–2100.[55]

PROVIDING FOR POPULATIONS

The burgeoning population of the world has critical needs for adequate goods and materials to maintain sustenance. Two essential needs are for adequate supplies of food and natural resources.

Food

Due to improved agricultural technologies and trade, overall world grain production increased 2.6-fold between 1950 and 1984, mostly due to increases in crop yields. During these years, per capita food production worldwide expanded by almost 40 percent. Yet, in a number of LDCs in Africa, Latin America, and Asia, the per capita food production has declined. In India alone, the per capita food production has declined 24 percent since 1983. Population growth has outstripped food pro-

duction in an area in which 2 billion of the world's 5.6 billion people live. They require food imports, mainly from the United States, Canada, Australia, Argentina, and France.

On average, people in the richest countries get 30–40 percent more calories than they need, and those in the poorest countries eat 10 percent less than they need.[56]

It is estimated that 25 percent of the world's population is undernourished. Of the 166 countries in the world, 133 are less developed, which means that they have to rely on the help of the 33 developed countries for their resources. In 43 of the less-developed countries, the average food production since 1950 has declined. This represents a decrease in food production for one out of every seven people. In Africa, the situation is even more bleak, with food production per person dropping 28 percent over the past 30 years, and decreases of another 30 percent are projected over the next 25 years.[57]

The Use of Nonrenewable Resources

Population numbers have a direct bearing on the supply of resources in the world. As the population increases, the use of natural resources also increases. Some of these resources are *perpetual,* since their sources are inexhaustible. Sunlight, for instance, is always in constant supply. Other resources, such as food, forests, grasslands, and animals, can be depleted and replaced; these are **renewable resources.** Other resources, or **nonrenewable resources,** exist in a fixed amount and are replaced very slowly, if at all. Fossil fuels, such as coal, oil, gas, and minerals are examples of nonrenewable resources.

While an increasing population uses more resources, an increasing standard of living further depletes resources. As the standard of living of a population rises, we can afford to buy more cars, live in larger homes, and purchase more consumer goods.

The United States, with 4.6 percent of the world's population, uses 20 percent of the world's energy, consumes 25 percent of the world's goods and services, and emits 22 percent of the carbon

renewable resources resources that can be depleted, but will be replaced through natural processes.

nonrenewable resources resources that, once depleted, will be replenished very slowly or not at all.

Undernourishment is a plague affecting many parts of the world. Food shortages are particularly devastating in many places in Africa.

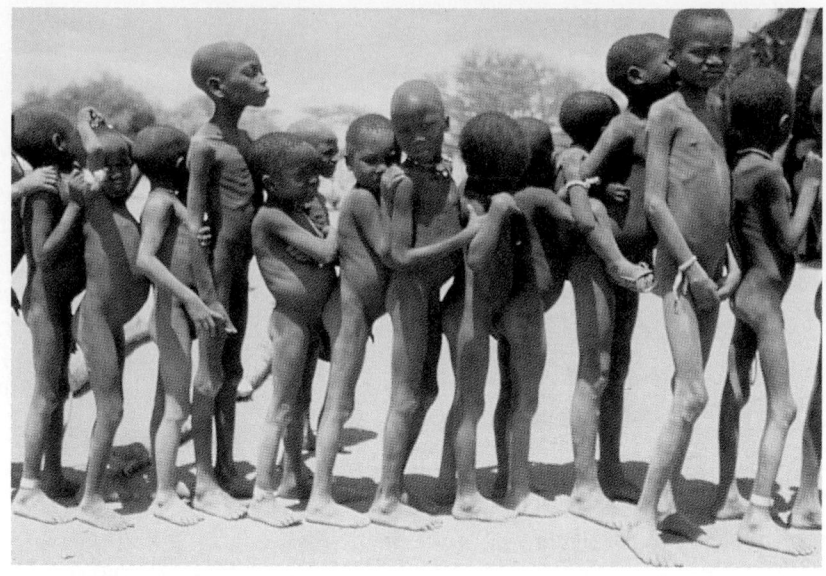

dioxide produced, a prime indicator of air pollution. By contrast, India, with 16.2 percent of the world's population, uses 3 percent of the world's energy, accounts for 1 percent of global goods and services, and emits 3 percent of the carbon dioxide produced.[57] Unless the overuse of nonrenewable resources by the developed countries is reversed, the less-developed countries will never realize their dreams of becoming self-sufficient.

CHECKPOINT

1. Discuss the world population increase during the year 1993.

2. Define the term *natural increase*.

3. Discuss the reasons why birth rates are dropping in some countries.

4. Explain the concept of zero population growth.

5. How does the population relate to food supplies?

6. Explain the contrast between renewable and nonrenewable resources.

A PERSONAL COMMITMENT

Your desire for environmental protection and health should lead you to action. You need to begin to take responsibility for sharing the earth's

wealth and making sure that its resources continue to flourish. Talking and reading about the environment cannot replace acting individually and collectively on what you know. If you are at the point of action, you should be prepared to endorse the Communication for Wellness: Your Commitment to Protecting the Health of the Environment.

CHECKPOINT

1. Discuss the responsibility of people in more-developed countries to preserve the environment.

2. List the things you can do to act both individually and collectively to combat environmental problems.

RESOURCES

Reading about environmental issues will keep you informed and up to date. Here are some titles of publications you may wish to borrow from your library or subscribe to:

Amicus Journal Natural Resources Defense Council, 122 East 42nd Street, New York, NY 10168

Audubon National Audubon Society, 950 Third Avenue, New York, NY 10022

Buzzworm P.O. Box 6853, Syracuse, NY 13217-7930

YOUR COMMITMENT TO PROTECTING THE HEALTH OF THE ENVIRONMENT

You can help protect the environment by being prepared to:

1. Evaluate your thinking about how the world works and sensitize yourself to the environment. You can compare the existing environment with what should be around your home, school, streets, or workplace.

2. Become ecologically informed. You should examine any throwaway thinking, and develop an ecological thinking.

3. Find a place or some piece of earth that you can become emotionally involved with, care for, and become prepared to defend.

4. Choose a simpler life-style, thereby reduce the use of resources and the production of wastes and pollution.

5. Reduce the number of "things" you have learned to depend upon. You can do this by:

- Becoming more self-reliant by reducing your dependence on commercial systems for water, energy, food, and livelihood.

- Starting to change your living patterns. Care for the environment begins at home.

- Acting locally while thinking globally. You can learn how to cooperate with others by becoming a part of environmental group activities in your neighborhood, at school, and in your town. Join a national environmental organization and be prepared to donate time and money.

- Helping to work on big pollution and environmental problems, largely through political action. Large-scale pollution is often the product of industry, government, or big agriculture.

- Starting a movement of awareness and action. Try to change the thinking and actions of one or two people close to you and then persuade them to change two others.

- Helping nurture, reassure, and understand people rather than threatening them or making them feel guilty. Be positive. There is plenty of work to be done and enough causes for all of us to contribute to.[a]

[a]Miller, R. "The Metal in Our Mettle." *FDA Consumer* December 1988–January 1989, pp. 24–27.

Environment Heldref Publications, 4000 Albemarle Street NW, Washington, DC 20016

Garbage: The Practical Journal for the Environment P.O. Box 56520, Boulder, CO 80321-6520

Greenpeace Magazine Greenpeace USA, 1436 U Street NW, Washington, DC 20009

National Wildlife National Wildlife Federation, 1400 16th Street NW, Washington, DC 20007

Nature 711 National Press Building, Washington, DC 20045

Sierra 730 Polk Street, San Francisco, CA 94108

State of the World Worldwatch Institute, 1776 Massachusetts Avenue NW, Washington, DC 20036 (published annually)

Worldwatch Worldwatch Institute, 1776 Massachusetts Avenue NW, Washington, DC 20036

You may also wish to join some local, state, or national organization devoted to sustaining the environment. Here are some organizations (and their addresses) you may decide to look into:

Cousteau Society 930 21st Street, Norfolk, VA 23517

Defenders of Wildlife 1244 19th Street NW, Washington, DC 20036

Greenpeace, USA, Inc. 1436 U Street NW, Suite 630, Washington, DC 20009

National Audubon Society 950 Third Avenue, New York, NY 10022

National Conservancy 1814 N. Lynn Street, Arlington, VA 22209

Population Reference Bureau 1875 Connecticut Avenue NW, Suite 520, Washington, DC 20009

Rainforest Action Network 300 Broadway, Suite 29A, San Francisco, CA 94133

Sierra Club 730 Polk Street, San Francisco, CA 94108, and 1408 C Street NE, Washington, DC 20002

Student Conservation Association, Inc. P.O. Box 550, Charlestown, NH 03603

Tree People 12601 Mulholland Drive, Beverly Hills, CA 90211

World Wildlife Fund 1250 24th Street NW, Suite 500, Washington, DC 20037

Zero Population Growth 1400 16th Street NW, 3rd Floor, Washington, DC 20036

SUMMARY

The environment dictates the availability of resources such as food, water, and air; it has much impact on us and we on it.

Ecology is the study of the relationship of organisms to their environment. Organisms exist in populations, ecosystems, and the biosphere. Non-living substances of the earth consist of simple chemicals, which operate in cycles; interfering with these cycles may lead to pollution.

Air pollution is the presence of harmful gases and particles in the air. Carbon oxides, nitrogen oxides, hydrocarbons, sulfur oxides, and ozone are common air pollutants. Photochemical smog results when air pollutants are trapped beneath a temperature inversion layer. High-altitude ozone protects us by screening out most ultraviolet radiation.

Water pollution is any change in fresh water that may adversely affect living organisms. Only 0.003 percent of the world's water is available for human and agricultural use. Pesticides and toxic metals are common sources of water pollution.

Waste disposal includes the disposal of solid wastes of all kinds, some of which are hazardous. Hazardous wastes can cause birth defects and cancer.

Radiation is the transmission of fast-moving energy particles. Radioactivity is radiation from unstable nuclei of atoms. Radioactivity comes from natural background and human-related sources. Of special concern are radioactive fallout, the operation of nuclear power plants, and the disposal of radioactive wastes.

Noise is unwanted sound, and can cause both physical and psychological reactions.

Population dynamics is a major environmental issue. World population continues to increase in great numbers, particularly in less-developed countries. Maintaining present population levels is called zero population growth. Food and natural resources are critical factors in providing for population needs.

Express your concern and take personal responsibility for the global welfare by becoming informed on environmental issues. Take steps to reduce your own unnecessary use of the world's resources and adding to its pollution problems by altering your life-style and working to persuade others to do likewise.

We all need to work together to preserve the earth's resources. Preserving the earth's health is an important goal in attaining and maintaining personal health.

REFERENCES

1. National Wildlife Federation. "20th Environmental Quality Index." *National Wildlife* (February/March 1988), 38–45.
2. Miller, G. *Living in the Environment.* 7th ed. Belmont, CA: Wadsworth, 1992.
3. Ibid.
4. Raven, P. *Environment.* New York: Saunders, 1993.
5. Miller, op. cit.
6. Uehling, M. "Missing the Deadline on Ozone." *National Wildlife* (October/November 1987), 34–37.
7. Raven, op. cit.
8. Miller, op. cit.
9. Ibid.
10. Consumer Reports, "Radon Detectors: How to Find Out If Your House Has a Radon Problem." *Consumer Reports* (July 1987).
11. U.S. Department of Health and Human Services. *The Health Consequences of Smoking.* Washington, DC: U.S. Department of Health and Human Services.
12. Miller, op. cit.
13. Ibid.
14. Raven, op. cit..
15. Miller, op. cit.
16. Ibid.
17. Farley, D. "Setting Safe Limits on Pesticide Residues." *FDA Consumer* (October 1988), 8–11.
18. Miller, op. cit.
19. Ibid.
20. National Academy of Sciences. *Regulating Pesticides in Foods: The Delaney Paradox.* Washington, DC: National Academy Press, 1987.
21. Environmental Protection Agency. *Pesticides Fact Book.* Washington, DC: Environmental Protection Agency, 1989.

22. Pimentel, D., and Levitan, L. "Pesticides: Amounts Applied and Amounts Reaching Pests." *Bioscience* 2 (1986), 86–91.
23. Miller, op. cit.
24. Greeley, A. "Getting the Lead Out." *FDA Consumer* (July–August 1991), 26–31.
25. Miller, R. "The Metal in Our Mettle." *FDA Consumer* (December 1988–January 1989), 24–27.
26. Clark, M. et al. "Interaction of Iron Deficiency and Leads and the Hematolytic Findings in Children with Lead Poisoning." *Pediatrics* 81 (1988), 247–254.
27. "The News on Lead." *University of California at Berkeley Wellness Newsletter* (November 1993), 4–6.
28. Science News. "Getting the Lead Out." *Science News* 132 (1987), 269.
29. Miller, op. cit.
30. Foulke, J. "Lead Threat Lessens, But Mugs Pose Problem." *FDA Consumer* (April 1993), 19–23.
31. Miller, op. cit.
32. Ibid.
33. Ibid.
34. Ibid.
35. Kaufman, D., and Franz, D. *Biosphere 2000*. New York: HarperCollins, 1993.
36. Miller, op. cit.
37. Ibid.
38. Ibid.
39. Kaufman and Franz, op. cit.
40. Miller, op. cit.
41. Ibid.
42. American Council on Science and Health. "Irradiated Foods." 1988. Available from the American Council on Science and Health, 1995 Broadway, New York, NY 10023-5860.
43. Rogan, A., and Glaros, G. "Food Irradiation: The Process and Implications for Dietitians." *Journal of the American Dietetic Association* 88 (1988), 833–838.
44. Williamson, C. "Irradiated Poultry. When?" *Food News for Consumers* (Winter 1993), 14.
45. Miller, op. cit.
46. Ibid.
47. Ibid.
48. Toufexis, A. "Now Hear This—If You Can." *Time* (5 August 1991), 50–51.
49. Miller, op. cit.
50. Tortora, G., and Grabowski, S. *Principles of Anatomy and Physiology,* 7th ed. New York: HarperCollins, 1993.
51. Miller, op. cit.
52. Ibid.
53. Haub, C., and Yanagishita, M. *1994 World Population Data Sheet of the Population Reference Bureau, Inc.* Washington, DC: Population Reference Bureau, 1994.
54. Linden, E. "Population: The Uninvited Guest." *Time* (1 June 1992), 54.
55. Haub, C. "Understanding Population Projections." *Population Bulletin* Vol. 43, No. 3 (April 1988).
56. Miller, op. cit.
57. Elmer-Dewitt, P. "Rich vs. Poor." *Time* (1 June 1992), 42–58.

SUGGESTED READINGS

Donahue, R. et al. *Soils and Their Management,* 5th ed. Petaluma, CA: Interprint, 1990.

Gordon, R., and Barbier, E. *After the Green Revolution: Sustainable Agriculture for Development.* East Haven, CT: Earthscan, 1990.

Jacobson, M. et al. *Safe Food: Eating Wisely in a Risky World.* Washington, DC: Living Planet Press, 1991.

Kaufman, D., and Franz, C. *Biosphere 2000.* New York: HarperCollins, 1993.

Matthews, J. *Greenhouse Warming: Negotiating a Global Regime.* Washington, DC: World Resources Institute, 1991.

Maybeck, M. et al. *Global Freshwater Quality.* Cambridge, MA: Basil Blackwell, 1990.

National Academy of Sciences. *Policy Implications of Greenhouse Warming.* Washington, DC: National Academy Press, 1991.

Population Reference Bureau: various publications. Membership: $25/yr students, $30/yr educators. Population Reference Bureau, 1875 Connecticut Avenue, NW, Suite 520, Washington, DC 20009.

Upton, A., and Graber, E. *Staying Healthy in a Risky Environment.* New York: Simon and Schuster, 1993.

GLOSSARY

abortifacient any substance or device used to cause an abortion.

abortion the termination of pregnancy before the fetus is viable.

absence seizures seizures characterized by brief loss of contact with the environment, eye and muscle fluttering, and sometimes, loss of muscle tone.

abstinence refraining from sexual intercourse.

accommodating behavior that is cooperative, but passive.

acetaldehyde an intermediate product in the metabolism of alcohol.

acetaminophen a synthetic drug with analgesic actions similar to aspirin.

acetic acid the acid in vinegar.

acetylcholine a chemical that plays an important role in the transmission of nerve impulses at synapses.

acid precipitation rain, snow, sleet, fog, or dew that contains higher than normal levels of sulfuric or nitric acid.

acquaintance rape a sexual assault in which the victim knows the assailant.

active carrier someone who has recovered from a disease, but still harbors the pathogen.

active immunity immunity that develops from exposure to an antigen and produces immune memory of that specific immune response.

active ingredient an ingredient responsible for the primary purpose of a drug preparation.

acupuncture a technique for treating certain painful conditions by passing long thin needles through the skin to specific points representing specific organs.

acute having a sudden onset and a short duration.

adaptive behavior behavior that enables a person to interact with his or her environment efficiently.

adenosine triphosphate (ATP) a substance found especially in muscle cells which, when split, releases stored energy.

adult-onset obesity obesity arising after adolescence.

adulterants inert or less-valuable substances used to dilute a product.

aerobic in the presence of oxygen; such exercise requires oxygen for continuous exertion.

aerobic exercise those continuous exercises involving major muscle groups requiring oxygen.

afterimages images that persist in the mind after their stimuli have ceased.

agar a culture medium providing a solid surface for the culture of microorganisms.

ageism stereotyping of and discrimination against people because they are old.

aggressive behavior attempting to accomplish our goals or fulfill our needs at the expense of others' rights, needs, or feelings.

aging the process of growing older; also defined as those series of cumulative, universal, progressive, intrinsic, and deleterious functional and structural changes that usually begin to manifest themselves at reproductive maturity and eventually culminate in death.

agoraphobia intense fear of places or situations from which it would be difficult or embarrassing to escape.

air pollution the buildup of chemical concentrations in the atmosphere to the point of causing harm to humans, other animals, vegetation, and materials such as metals and stone.

alarm reaction immediate response to a stressor, in which the body is prepared for emergency action.

alcoholic hallucinosis a form of alcohol withdrawal including hallucinations, nightmares, illusions, and misperceptions of reality.

alcoholic hepatitis inflammation of the liver produced by alcohol.

alcoholic neuropathy any disease of the nerves that is associated with heavy drinking.

alcoholism a disease characterized by strong psychological and, in severe cases, physiological dependency on alcohol and the inability to drink in moderation (loss of control).

alkaloid an alkaline (caustic) organic substance obtained from a plant.

allergen the substance causing an allergy.

allergy or **hypersensitivity** immune response against an otherwise harmless environmental substance.

allied health professionals health care professionals whose speciality areas are auxiliary to physicians and other health care professionals.

alpha-fetoprotein (AFP) screening a test measuring a substance produced by the fetal kidneys in the mother's blood.

altruism placing the well-being of others ahead of one's own; unselfishness.

Alzheimer's disease a degenerative brain disorder in which persons progressively lose the ability to read, write, talk, eat, and walk.

amenorrhea absence of menstrual periods.

amino acid a building block of protein.

amniocentesis obtaining amniotic fluid through surgical penetration of the abdomen to assist in the detection of birth defects.

amnion the innermost of the fetal membranes.

amniotic fluid the fluid contained in the amnion that protects the fetus from injury.

amphetamines a group of synthetically produced drugs that serve as nervous system stimulants.

anaerobic without oxygen; such exercise uses energy stored by the body for fast bursts of speed.

analgesic a drug that relieves pain.

anaphylaxis or **anaphylactic shock** a massive, potentially fatal allergic reaction.

androgynous combining male and female traits.

androgyny an openness to and acceptance of one's own feminine and masculine nature.

aneurysm   a ballooning out of the wall of a blood vessel due to a weakening of the wall by disease or other causes.

angina pectoris   chest pain resulting from the heart muscle receiving insufficient blood supply.

angioplasty   a procedure used to widen narrowed arteries.

anilingus   oral stimulation of the anal area.

anorexia nervosa   a disorder seen usually in teenage girls, involving self-starvation.

antacid   an agent that neutralizes acidity.

antagonism   one drug prevents or reduces the effect of another or two drugs mutually inhibit each other.

anti-inflammatory   a drug that reduces inflammation.

antibiotics   drugs produced by microorganisms and administered to fight bacteria and fungi.

antibodies or **immunoglobulins**   Y-shaped protein molecules produced by B lymphocytes to destroy or inactivate antigens.

antidiuretic   lessening urine secretion.

antigen   any substance that stimulates an immune response.

antihistamine   any drug that reduces mucus secretions by opposing the action of histamine, a body substance released from injured cells and that causes flushing of the skin, headaches, and lower blood pressure.

antimicrobial agents   drugs used to treat diseases caused by microorganisms.

antiperspirant   a substance that inhibits perspiration.

antipsychotics   drugs that produce emotional quieting and relative indifference to one's surroundings.

antipyretic   a drug that reduces fever.

anxiety   a vague feeling that something bad is about to happen.

aorta   the large artery that receives blood from the left ventricle and distributes it to the body.

aortic valve   the valve between the left ventricle and aorta.

aquifer   a layer of the earth's crust that contains groundwater.

areolae   the pigmented rings surrounding the nipples; areolae is the plural of areola.

arithmetic rate of drug breakdown   the same amount of a drug will be broken down in each equal time period.

arrhythmia   an abnormal heartbeat.

arteries   blood vessels that carry blood away from the heart to various parts of the body.

arterioles   small branches of arteries.

arteriosclerosis   hardening of the arteries.

arthritis   inflammation in one or more of a person's joints, usually accompanied by pain and, frequently, changes in structure.

artificial insemination   introducing sperm into the vagina or uterus by means other than intercourse.

artificial passive immunity   immunity resulting from the injection of antibodies.

artificial, or **human-related, radiation**   radiation arising as a result of human activities.

asbestos   a fibrous, incombustible natural mineral used in insulation material.

asbestosis   a chronic lung condition resulting from prolonged exposure to asbestos particles.

aspirin   acetylsalicylic acid; one of the most widely used analgesics and antipyretics.

assertive behavior   making our needs and desires known to others and, when necessary, defending our rights.

asthma   attacks of difficult breathing accompanied by wheezing and caused by spasm of the bronchioles or swelling of their lining.

asymptomatic   having no symptoms.

asymptomatic carrier   a person who harbors a pathogen without experiencing symptoms and is capable of transmitting it to other people.

atherosclerosis   a blood vessel disease in which the inner layers of artery walls become thick and irregular due to deposits of fat and cholesterol.

atria   the two upper chambers of the heart.

aura   a subjective sensation preceding an attack of some condition.

autoimmune disorder   a disorder arising from an immunologic response against a person's own tissue antigens.

autoimmune response   a self-destructive process in which a person's immune system attacks his or her own body.

autonomic nervous system   the portion of the nervous system that controls glands and involuntary muscles.

avoiding   behavior that is both passive and uncooperative.

B lymphocyte or **B cell**   lymphocyte processed by the bone marrow and capable of producing humoral immunity.

bacilli   rod-shaped bacteria.

balloon-laser welding   heating by laser of an artery, which has been widened by angioplasty, in order to stretch and weld the artery wall into a smooth surface.

barbiturates   a group of central nervous system depressant drugs derived from barbituric acid.

barrier methods   contraceptive methods that use a physical barrier to block the sperm from meeting the egg.

basal body temperature   the lowest body temperature of a healthy person during the time he or she is awake.

basal metabolic rate (BMR)   the measure of the number of calories the body needs for basal metabolism.

basal metabolism   the basic body functions that maintain life.

behavior modification   the systematic replacement of one set of behaviors for another.

behavior therapy   therapy based on the assumption that our actions are learned responses to stimuli and that new, more desirable, responses to the same stimuli can be learned.

behaviorism   a philosophy of psychological study holding that only observable behavior is a proper subject of psychological investigation.

benign   not cancerous.

bereavement   the state of having lost a loved one through death.

bicuspid (mitral) valve   the valve between the left atrium and left ventricle.

bilirubin   pigment from the breakdown of the hemoglobin in red blood cells.

bioelectrical impedance   a technique in which a weak electric current is run through the body to measure body composition.

bioequivalency   fact that the active ingredient(s) in a generic drug are identical to those in its comparable brand-name drug.

biofeedback a method of learning voluntary control over body functions that are usually involuntary, as a way of reducing stress.

biological aging aging of a person's anatomy and physiology in ways that affect a person's appearance and abilities, including the ability to survive.

biological therapy treatment of mental problems through biological methods such as medications.

biological value (BV) the measurement of a protein's efficiency in supporting the body's needs.

biopsy removal of a small piece of living tissue for microscopic examination.

biosphere all of the earth's ecosystems, collectively.

bipolar disorder (formerly manic depression) mood disorder characterized by extreme mood swings from deep depression to exaggerated joy.

birth control the regulation of conception, pregnancy, or birth by preventive devices or methods.

birth or **congenital defect** a defect present at the time of the birth of an individual.

bisexual a person who forms sexual relationships with people of either gender.

blackout period during which a person is drinking, but later will have no memory of that period.

blastocyst the young embryo when it consists of a fluid-filled ball of cells.

blood a complex mixture of fluid and cells that circulates through the body in the circulatory system.

blood alcohol level the percentage of alcohol circulating within one's blood.

blood-brain barrier a barrier membrane between the circulating blood and the brain that prevents some harmful substances from entering brain tissue.

blood count a count of red blood cells to white blood cells in whole blood.

blood pressure the force exerted by the blood against the artery walls.

blood typing the method used to determine the presence of certain proteins in blood.

blood vessels a network of tubes that carries blood throughout the body; the veins, arteries, and capillaries.

body composition the ratio of fat to fat-free (bone and muscle) body mass.

body mass index (BMI) indexing a person's weight to height by dividing the weight by the square of the height.

bonding the special emotional attachment that occurs between mother and newborn following birth.

bootlegger a person who manufactures or sells alcohol illegally.

bradycardia a slow heartbeat characterized by a pulse rate under 60 beats per minute.

brain death cessation of all brain function.

Braxton Hicks contractions intermittent painless uterine contractions that do not represent true labor pains.

breakthrough bleeding light vaginal bleeding between periods which may occur during use of progestin-containing pills.

breech birth when the fetal buttocks emerge first rather than the head.

bronchial carcinoma lung cancer.

bronchial pneumonia pneumonia that begins in the bronchi and can spread into the surrounding tissues.

Buerger's disease an inflammatory disease blocking the flow of blood through the arteries and veins of the extremities.

bulimia recurring binge-eating; also called **bulimarexia**.

bulimia nervosa recurring binge-eating followed by purging.

calculus an abnormal stonelike deposit, usually of mineral salts, somewhere in the body.

calendar methods the use of the calendar to calculate the onset and duration of the fertile, or safe, period each month in a woman.

caliper an instrument for measuring the thickness of materials.

calorie a unit of heat: a unit by which energy is measured.

cancer a group of diseases characterized by uncontrolled growth and spread of abnormal body cells.

candidiasis infection by the yeast, *Candida albicans*.

cannula a small tube used to withdraw the uterine lining.

capillary a microscopic blood vessel between an artery and a vein.

carbohydrate a group of chemical substances, including sugars and starches, that can be used efficiently as an energy source.

carboxyhemoglobin the compound formed by carbon monoxide and hemoglobin.

carcinogenic producing cancer.

carcinogens cancer-causing agents.

carcinoma a malignant tumor occurring in epithelial tissue.

cardiac arrest when the heart stops beating.

cardiopulmonary resuscitation (CPR) a combination of closed chest massage and mouth-to-mouth breathing used during a cardiac arrest to keep blood flowing to the heart muscle and brain.

cardiorespiratory endurance (CRE) or **aerobic capacity** the ability of the body to perform moderately strenuous activity over an extended period of time; also called cardiovascular endurance.

cardiovascular pertaining to the heart and blood vessels.

cardiovascular diseases (CVDs) diseases of the heart and blood vessels.

cardiovascular system the circulatory system, consisting of the heart and blood vessels.

cartilage a dense, firm tissue capable of resisting considerable pressure or tension.

cataract clouding or opacity of the lens within the eye.

catharsis release from guilt feelings.

catheter a tube passed through the body, often through a blood vessel, for injecting fluids into a body structure, such as the heart.

catheter atherectomy the use of a catheter rotating drill to shave off a plaque.

cavities (caries) gradual decay of a tooth.

celibacy abstinence or avoidance of sexual intercourse.

cell death death of individual body cells.

cell-mediated immunity the immune responses produced by T lymphocytes.

cell membrane or **plasma membrane** the delicate membrane, made of fat and protein, enclosing a cell and regulating the movement of all materials into and out of the cell.

cellulose a plant polysaccharide composed of glucose, indigestible by humans.

cerebral emboli blood clots formed in one part of the body and then carried by the bloodstream to the brain, where it blocks an artery.

cerebral hemorrhage the rupture of a diseased blood vessel in the brain.

cerebral thrombosis formation of a blood clot in an artery that supplies part of the brain.

cervical cap a small plastic or rubber contraceptive device which fits snugly over the cervix to serve as a barrier to sperm.

cervical effacement the shortening of the cervical canal.

cervix the neck of the uterus.

cesarean delivery delivery of a child through a surgical incision in the abdominal and uterine walls; also called cesarean section or C-section.

chain of infection series of events necessary to transmit disease from one host to another.

chancre the primary lesion of syphilis, an ulcer swarming with spirochetes.

chemical dependency the compulsive abuse of one or more drugs, despite the adverse consequences of this drug abuse.

chemotherapy the treatment of disease using drugs.

chiropractor the professional who treats health conditions by methods that include musculoskeletal manipulation.

Chlamydia unusually small bacteria that reproduce only in living host cells; have no ability to break down foods for energy.

chlorofluorocarbons (CFCs) propellants found in aerosol spray cans, industrial solvents, and styrofoam-type containers.

cholesterol a fat-derived sterol made in humans and animals and available in the diet.

chorion the outermost of the fetal membranes.

chorionic villi vascular projections from the chorion, or outermost fetal membrane.

chorionic villus sampling (CVS) the use of a catheter for removing a small sample of chorionic villi of the fetal membranes.

chromosomes structures in cells which contain genes.

chronic having a gradual onset and a long duration.

chronic bronchitis inflammation of the mucous membrane of the bronchial tubes.

chronic obstructive pulmonary disease (COPD) a group of respiratory disorders characterized by obstruction of the airflow in the lungs.

chronological age how long a person has lived.

chronological aging the passage of time since a person's birth.

cilia microscopic hairlike projections that clear pathogens from the lungs.

circumcision the surgical removal of part or all of the foreskin.

cirrhosis the replacement of functional liver cells by nonfunctional scar-like tissue.

clinical psychologist person who has special expertise in assessing psychological problems and treating people with emotional or behavioral problems by using psychological techniques.

clinical social workers people who have a masters (M.S.W.) or doctorate (D.S.W.) in social work and can counsel clients with emotional problems.

clitoris a small, sensitive structure near the front end of the vestibule.

coagulate to clot.

coarctation compression of the walls of a blood vessel.

coca paste an impure, cocaine-containing product made by pouring sulfuric acid over coca leaves.

cocaine hydrochloride the hydrochloride form of the alkaloid cocaine derived from the leaves of the coca shrub.

cocci spherical bacteria.

code of ethics a set of moral standards.

codependency the effects of chemical dependency on family members of a substance abuser.

coenzyme compounds that work with enzymes to promote the work of the enzyme; some vitamins are coenzymes.

coercive sex use of sex to exert power and maintain control.

cohabitation living together in a sexual relationship as unmarried persons.

coitus heterosexual intercourse referring to insertion of the penis into the vagina.

collaborating working together.

collateral circulation a system of smaller arteries that may open up and start to carry blood to a part of the heart when a coronary artery is blocked; also develops as a result of engaging in regular aerobic exercise.

colostrum a thin, yellow, milky fluid secreted by the breasts soon after delivery.

combustion burning.

commitment a pledge or assurance to stay true to a promise.

communicable disease one that is due to an infectious agent.

companionate love mature, predictable, and secure love.

competing when both partners are aggressively trying to fulfill their own needs, but cooperating little to ensure the need fulfillment of each other.

complete protein a protein containing all of the essential amino acids in proper balance.

complex partial seizures seizures characterized by a brief loss of contact with one's surroundings, mental confusion, staggering, and/or unintelligible sounds.

composting the accelerated breakdown of grass clippings and other organic solid wastes in the presence of bacteria to produce a humuslike product used as a soil conditioner.

compromising when a mutually acceptable solution to a conflict is found, but it only partially satisfies each person's needs.

conception the moment of fertilization of an ovum by a sperm.

congenital present at birth.

conflict any situation in which our wants, needs, or intentions are incompatible with the wants, needs, or intentions of another person.

congenital defect a defect present at the time of the birth of an individual.

congenital heart defect malformation of the heart or of its major blood vessels.

congenital immunity immunity resulting from antibodies crossing the placenta.

congestive heart failure the inability of the heart to pump out all the blood that returns to it.

constipation infrequent and difficult bowel movements.

contact lenses a small lens that fits over the cornea of the eye.

contagious capable of being passed from person to person.

continuum a progression of infinite degrees of some characteristic between two extremes.

contraception the prevention of conception.

contraceptive any technique, drug, or device that prevents conception.

control in an experiment, the standard against which observations or conclusions must be checked in order to establish their validity; for example, a person who or animal that has not been exposed to the treatment or condition being studied in the other people or animals.

convalescence the period of recovery after a disease.

convulsion sudden and repeated involuntary contraction of all of the body's muscles.

convulsive seizures repeated involuntary contraction of all of the body's muscles.

cool down continuation of exercise at a low intensity following a rigorous workout, to allow the body to adjust to a resting state.

cornea the clear, transparent front portion of the eye.

coronary artery bypass graft surgery surgery to improve the blood supply to the heart muscle.

coronary artery disease (CAD) an impeding of coronary blood flow to the heart; also know as **coronary heart disease (CHD).**

coronary occlusion an obstruction in a coronary artery.

coronary thrombosis formation of a blood clot in a coronary artery.

corpus luteum a yellow mass formed from an empty ovarian follicle after ovulation.

correlation a relationship between two variables.

cosmetic aging changes in outward appearance with advancing age.

cosmetics preparations for cleansing, beautifying, promoting attractiveness, or altering the appearance.

cough suppressant a drug that inhibits coughing.

courage the quality of mind or spirit that enables a person to face difficulty, danger, pain, or the unknown with firmness and without fear.

Cowper's glands paired glands located beneath the prostate gland on either side of the urethra that secrete preejaculatory fluid.

crack or **rock** freebased cocaine made by mixing cocaine hydrochloride, sodium bicarbonate (baking soda), and water.

cross-linkage formation of chemical bonds between the peptide units of proteins.

cross-tolerance an increased tolerance to one class of drugs following exposure to a different class.

crowning the first appearance of the fetal head in childbirth.

crucifers edible vegetables from the mustard plant family (Cruciferae).

cultural diversity people with a variety of histories, ideologies, traditions, values, life-styles, and languages living and interacting together.

culture all of the customs, beliefs, values, knowledge, and skills that are shared by a specific group of people.

cunnilingus oral stimulation of the female's genitals.

cyanotic having a blueness of skin caused by insufficient oxygen in the blood.

cystic fibrosis a hereditary disease causing production and accumulation of sticky mucus in the pancreas, lungs, and sweat glands.

cystitis inflammation of the urinary bladder, usually associated with infection.

daily value standard nutrient value developed by the FDA for use on food labels.

date rape a sexual assault that occurs on a date.

death the cessation of life.

decibel (db) unit used to measure the intensity, or loudness, of a sound.

decibel-A (dbA) a modified decibel scale.

decongestant drug agents that reduce congestion or swelling.

defense mechanisms unconscious psychological techniques we use to protect ourselves from uncomfortable feelings.

defibrillation use of electric currents to reestablish normal heart contraction rhythms.

delirium tremens a disorder including trembling and hallucinations; usually occurs during alcohol withdrawal.

denial keeping anxiety-producing realities out of one's conscious awareness.

dentifrice a powder or other substance for cleaning teeth.

dentist a medical practitioner specializing in the care of the teeth and gums.

deodorant a substance that masks or absorbs body odors.

deoxygenated without oxygen.

depersonalization the belief that you no longer exist, but are instead something inanimate or unreal.

depression a feeling of sadness and apathy.

designated driver the person who agrees to abstain from drinking and to drive the other members of the party home safely.

designer drugs hallucinogenic amphetamine derivatives.

detoxification process of removing the physiological effects of a drug from an addicted person.

diabetes a general term for diseases characterized by excessive urination.

diabetes mellitus a disorder of carbohydrate metabolism resulting in excessive sugar in the blood and sugar in the urine.

dialysis the process of circulating the blood through a machine to remove toxic materials, or by performing a fluid wash of the abdominal cavity, in cases of impaired kidney function.

diarrhea frequent passage of abnormally watery bowel movements.

diastole the part of the heart cycle when the heart is relaxed.

dietary fiber a food component that resists chemical digestion and provides bulk to keep material in the digestive tract moving.

dilation and curettage a first trimester abortion procedure in which the inner lining of the uterus is scraped.

dilation and evacuation a second trimester abortion procedure.

disaccharide descriptive term for a double sugar.

displacement transferring an emotion such as aggression, anger, or hostility from the person or situation with which it was originally associated to a new person or situation.

distillation condensation of a vapor that has been obtained from a liquid heated to its boiling point.

distress stress that has harmful effects.

diuretic a drug that speeds up body water loss through increasing the production of urine.

double-blind method experimentation in which neither the subject nor the evaluators know which subjects are in the control group.

drug any substance, other than a food, that modifies any function of the body.

drug resistance the ability of a pathogen to remain unharmed by a specific drug.

drunk driver a person driving under the influence of alcohol as defined according to the concentration of alcohol in the blood or exhaled air as determined by each respective state.

durable power of attorney for health care a document appointing a trusted person to make health care decisions should a person become incapacitated; such decisions might involve withdrawing or withholding treatment.

dysfunctional functioning with difficulty.

dysmenorrhea painful menstrual flow.

dyspareunia painful intercourse.

ecology the study of the interactions of living things with their environments.

economic aging age-related changes in a person's financial status.

ecosystem plants and animals and their nonliving environmental factors in a defined area.

ectopic pregnancy a fertilized egg implanted outside of the uterus.

edema swelling due to an abnormally large amount of fluid in body tissues.

ego in psychoanalytic theory, the conscious part of the mind.

ejaculation the sudden ejection of semen from the penis that occurs at the peak of sexual arousal; occurs in two stages, emission and expulsion.

ejaculatory duct the near end of the vas deferens that joins with the urethra, where sperm mixes with seminal vesicle fluid.

electrocoagulation thickening and closure of a tube by use of electric current.

electroencephalogram (EEG) a test that records the electrical activity of the brain.

electrolytes ionized salts in blood, tissue fluid, and cells.

embolism a blood clot that has moved and lodged in a blood vessel.

embryo the unborn child during the first eight weeks after conception.

emetics substances that produce vomiting.

emotional of or related to the emotions.

emotional intimacy an essential component of a sound relationship characterized by open communication and sharing of innermost feelings, needs, and desires.

emotions mental states that include three components: a characteristic feeling or subjective experience; a pattern of physiological arousal; and a pattern of overt expression.

emphysema a chronic pulmonary disease characterized by a breakdown of the alveolar walls, producing abnormally large air spaces that remain filled with air during expiration.

enabling any behavior that in any way allows or makes it easier for another person to continue substance abuse or other undesirable behavior.

endogenous originating within a cell or organism.

endometrial tissue the tissue located in the inner lining of the uterus.

endometriosis growth of endometrial tissue outside the uterus.

endorphin an endogenous opiate-like chemical.

endoscope a long tubular device with an optical system inserted through a small body opening for observing internal body parts or cavities.

enhancing interactions drug interactions in which the effects of one drug increase the effects of another.

enteric-coated any drug tablet or capsule that is coated with a special substance that will not dissolve until it reaches the small intestine.

enzyme a protein catalyst that speeds up the rate of a reaction without becoming a part of the process.

epidemiological relating to disease frequency and distribution.

epidemiologist scientist who studies the dynamics of disease frequency and distribution.

epididymis a tightly coiled tube alongside the testis that stores sperm.

episiotomy a surgical procedure in which the perineum is cut to facilitate childbirth.

erectile dysfunction (impotence) the inability to achieve or maintain an erection of sufficient firmness for coitus.

erectile tissue tissue that becomes firm when it fills with blood.

erogenous zones areas of the body that are especially sensitive to sexual stimulation.

erythrocytes red blood cells.

essential nutrients those nutrients a person *must* obtain from food, because the body cannot make them or make enough of them to satisfy its needs.

estrogen a hormone that stimulates development of the female reproductive tract and body characteristics.

ethics systems of moral values.

euphoria an exaggerated feeling of well-being or elation.

eustress stress that has beneficial effects.

euthanasia (1) dying easily or painlessly; or (2) the act of willfully ending life in someone with an incurable disease.

excitement, plateau, orgasmic, and **resolution** the cycle of four phases (stages) of the human sexual response.

exercise any muscular activity that maintains fitness.

exhaustion following prolonged high stress levels, the body's resistance to stressors is lost and illness or death occurs.

exhibitionism deriving sexual gratification from exposing the genitals or buttocks to unsuspecting and unconsenting strangers.

expectorant a drug that leads to the expulsion of mucus or phlegm from the throat or lungs.

external cue an environmental factor that prompts us to eat.

external locus of control believing that your life is under the control of other people or powers.

faith healing healing accomplished by supplication to a divine being or power without medical or chemical treatment.

fallopian tubes a pair of ducts that connect the ovaries to the uterus.

family planning the spacing, or the timing, of conception according to the wishes of the couple.

family practitioner a specialist in providing comprehensive medical care to the family unit.

family systems approach an approach to therapy that views a family as a system that seeks to maintain balance, with other family members altering their behavior in an attempt to compensate for the altered behavior of the chemically dependent person.

fat a lipid that is solid at room temperature.

fat-soluble dissolving in fat.

fat-soluble vitamins vitamins soluble in and absorbed into the body in fats.

Federal Trade Commission (FTC) the federal agency responsible for regulating false and misleading advertising and the selling of dangerous and ineffectual products.

fee-for-service a payment as the service is rendered; also called pay-as-you-go.

fellatio oral stimulation of the male's genitals.

female condom a pouch worn inside the vagina to serve as a barrier to sperm and to protect the woman against sexually transmitted disease transmission.

fermentation process in which yeast converts sugar into alcohol.

fertility awareness use of menstrual cycle charting with the use of barrier methods during the fertile days to avoid conception.

fertilization the union of the sperm cell nucleus with the ovum cell nucleus; also called conception.

fetal alcohol syndrome (FAS) (1) physical malformation to the embryo and fetus caused by intrauterine exposure to alcohol; or (2) a group of birth defects that occur in infants born to mothers who drink during their pregnancy.

fetishism the use of inanimate objects or body parts for sexual arousal.

fetus the developing child from the eighth week after conception until birth.

fibrillation rapid and uncontrolled contractions of individual heart muscle fibers.

fitness the general capacity to adapt and respond favorably to physical effort.

flexibility the ability to flex and extend each joint through its maximum range of motion.

fluoride a chemical element that is present in, or added to, water which helps reduce the rate of tooth decay.

flutter a tremulous, rapid movement of the heart.

follicle a small cavity in the ovary in which the ovum is located.

follicle-stimulating hormone (FSH) a gonadotropin that stimulates the ovary to produce a follicle in the female and sperm in the male.

food additives natural or synthetic substances that are added to processed foods to retard spoilage, provide missing nutrients, or to enhance flavor, color, or texture.

food allergy allergic reaction resulting from ingestion of foods to which a person has become sensitized.

Food and Drug Administration (FDA) the U.S. Department of Health and Human Services agency responsible for consumer protection.

food chain the sequential transfer of food energy from green plants to humans and other animals.

food exchange system lists of foods having the same number of calories and the same amounts of energy nutrients.

foreskin a loose fold of skin covering the glans.

formaldehyde a colorless, pungent, irritating gas commonly made by the oxidation of methyl alcohol.

free radicals highly reactive cell chemicals that are formed as by-products of normal chemical reactions within cells.

freebase cocaine that has been converted from the stable hydrochloride form to the less stable but more potent basic form.

frostbite the freezing or effect of freezing of body parts.

fungi primitive, spore-forming plantlike organisms.

gangrene death of tissue, usually due to insufficient blood supply.

gastroenteritis inflammation of the stomach and intestine.

gastrointestinal (GI) pertaining to the stomach and intestines.

gay a male who is primarily homosexual.

gender the biological state of being male or female.

gender dysphoria confusion over one's gender identity.

gender identity an individual's sense of being male or female.

gender role a person's masculine or feminine behavior and appearance, as viewed in context of cultural classification.

gender role identification how a person incorporates expected gender roles into his or her personality.

General Adaptation Syndrome the body's response to a stressor, made up of the stages of alarm, resistance, and exhaustion.

general internist a physician who practices internal medicine.

general practitioner (G.P.) a physician who has met the professional and legal requirements to provide general health care.

generic drug a prescription drug that has the same active ingredients as a brand-name drug; there may also be generic versions of nonprescription drugs.

genes basic units of heredity located on chromosomes.

geriatrics the branch of medicine that treats the conditions and diseases associated with aging and old age.

gerontology the study of aging.

gestalt shape or form.

gestalt therapy a theory of psychotherapy that rejects the analysis of emotions and behavior into discrete events of stimulus, perception, and response, but emphasizes awareness of the whole of a person's being.

gestational age the estimated age of a fetus as calculated from the first day of the last normal menstrual period; also called the menstrual age.

glans the head of the penis (in the male), and of the clitoris (in the female).

glaucoma excess pressure within the eye that can lead to blindness.

glucose a simple sugar sometimes known as blood sugar.

glycogen a polysaccharide composed of glucose, made in the body and stored in the liver and in muscles.

gonadotropin-releasing hormone (GnRH) hypothalamic hormone that acts on the pituitary gland.

gonadotropins hormones secreted by the pituitary gland that act on the gonads.

gonads male and female sex glands.

gonococcus the bacterium that causes gonorrhea.

gout hereditary metabolic disease characterized by acute attacks of arthritis caused by deposits of urate crystals in the joints.

grief the distress occurring as a result of any serious loss.

groundwater water that sinks into the soil where it may be stored for long periods.

group health insurance plan a policy that is written for a group of individuals at a uniform cost.

half-life (1) length of time it takes for a radioactive substance to lose one-half of its radioactivity; (2) the time needed for the breakdown of one-half of the amount of a drug remaining in the body.

hallucination a false sensory perception.

hallucinogens substances producing false sensory perceptions.

happiness a state of emotional well-being and contentment.

hashish resinous substance obtained from the flowers of *Cannabis* plants.

hazardous waste discarded solid, liquid, or gaseous wastes that threaten human health or the environment.

health as defined by the World Health Organization, a state of complete physical, mental, and social well-being.

health insurance a contract between an insurance company and a policyholder for the payment of health care costs.

health maintenance organization (HMO) an organization that provides a wide range of comprehensive health care services for a specified group at a fixed premium.

heart a muscular contractile organ.

heart block condition in which the conducting tissues of the heart fails to conduct impulses normally from the atrium to the ventricles. This causes altered rhythm of the heartbeat.

heart murmur a heart sound that may be caused by a leaking valve.

heart rate reserve (HRR) the difference between the maximal heart rate (MHR) and the resting heart rate (RHR).

heart transplant the transfer of a heart from one person to another.

heartburn return of the stomach's acid contents into the esophagus, causing a burning sensation.

heat cramps painful spasms of voluntary muscles in the arms, legs, and abdomen following a hard workout in a hot environment, without adequate fluid and salt intake.

heat exhaustion severe reaction to heat exposure.

heat stroke a severe and dangerous reaction to heat exposure which requires medical attention.

hemoglobin the oxygen-carrying pigment of the red blood cells.

hemorrhoids varicose (enlarged) veins in the rectal lining.

hepatitis inflammation of the liver.

histamine chemical released from injured cells to cause inflammation; also important in allergic reactions.

holistic relating to the philosophy that people function as complete units that cannot be reduced to the sum of their parts.

holographic will a handwritten and unwitnessed will.

homeopathy a system of disease treatment in which minute doses of a drug or remedy are administered, a large dose of which would in healthy persons produce symptoms of the disease; the theory that "like cures like."

homeostasis equilibrium of the internal environment of the body.

homosexuality sexual attraction primarily to people of one's own sex.

hospice a program or organization that provides care and support for dying people and their families.

host an organism that is infected by a parasite.

human chorionic gonadotropin (HCG) gonadotropic hormone produced by the tissues of the embryo and fetus.

Human Immunodeficiency Virus (HIV) the virus that causes AIDS.

human papilloma viruses the viruses that cause genital warts; some forms appear to cause cervical cancer.

humanism a philosophy of psychological study that emphasizes the whole person and the importance of each person's subjective experiences.

humanistic therapy therapy based on the belief that people will grow in constructive ways if they can be helped to explore and make use of their existing hidden potential.

humor the ability to laugh at ludicrous or ridiculous situations.

humoral immunity the immune responses produced by the release of antibodies by B lymphocytes.

hydrocarbons compounds containing carbon and hydrogen.

hydrogenate to add hydrogen to an unsaturated fat to make it more solid.

hydrostatic weighing underwater weighing technique in which the measure of body density, or weight, is compared with volume.

hymen a thin membrane that partially covers the vagina.

hyperarousal a sign of alcohol withdrawal characterized by symptoms including shaking, anxiety, and insomnia.

hyperplasia excessive proliferation of blood cells.

hypertension sustained high blood pressure.

hypnosis a psychological state, induced by a ritualistic procedure, in which the subject experiences changes in perception, memory, and behavior in response to suggestions by the hypnotist.

hypoglycemia low blood-sugar level.

hypothalamus a portion of the brain that regulates the pituitary gland and the autonomic nervous system, thereby controlling the stress response and sexual systems and processes.

hypothermia having a body temperature below normal.

hypothesis a tentative assumption made prior to experimental testing.

hysterectomy surgical removal of part or all of the uterus.

ibuprofen a synthetic drug with analgesic actions similar to aspirin.

id in psychoanalytic theory, the unconscious part of the human mind containing the libido and aggression.

identity one's concept of who he or she is.

immoral conduct that reduces self-esteem and self-worth, breaks down the capacity for communication, or results in exploitation.

immune memory memory of a specific immune response, allowing a rapid immune response upon repeated exposure to an antigen.

immunity (1) body defenses that act against specific pathogens; (2) state of being protected from a disease.

immunoglobulins Y-shaped protein molecules produced by B lymphocytes to destroy or inactivate antigens.

immunotherapy the production or enhancement of immunity in treating disease.

implantation embedding of the blastocyst into the uterine lining.

in situ in position, localized.

"I" statements expressions of your own feelings, emotions, or other responses.

in vitro fertilization (IVF) fertilization of the egg by sperm outside of the body.

incest sexual activity between persons too closely related to be allowed by law to marry.

incidence the frequency of occurrence of a disease over a period of time, usually a year, in relation to the size of the population in which it occurs.

incomplete protein a protein lacking one or more of the essential amino acids.

incubation period interval between infection and appearance of symptoms.

indigestion incomplete or imperfect digestion, usually accompanied by feelings of physical distress.

individual (family) health insurance plan a policy that is written for an individual or family at a particular cost.

induced abortion an abortion brought on intentionally.

infarct the dying of tissue.

infatuation an attraction based on similarity to an idealized partner.

infective dosage the number of pathogens necessary to overwhelm our body defenses and initiate an infection.

infertile inability or diminished ability to produce children.

inflammation tissue reaction to an injury including dilation and increased permeability of capillaries.

inhibin a hormone secreted by the gonads that inhibits FSH by the pituitary and GnRH release by the hypothalamus.

insomnia inability to sleep.

insulin a hormone produced by the pancreas and necessary for movement of sugar from the blood into the body cells.

insulin-dependent diabetes mellitus (IDDM) a form of diabetes mellitus in which regular injections of insulin are required to prevent death. Also known as Type I diabetes. Previously known as juvenile-onset diabetes.

interdependent two or more entities each being dependent upon the other(s).

interferons proteins released from virus-infected cells to protect healthy cells from viral damage.

internal locus of control having the feeling of being in control of your own life.

internal medicine the branch of medicine that treats diseases of the internal organs by nonsurgical means.

interstitial-cell-stimulating hormone (ICSH) a gonadotropin that stimulates the testes to secrete testosterone.

intervention a structured, confrontational technique used to help drug abusers overcome their rationalization and denial and accept the reality of their drug problems.

intrauterine device (IUD) a device placed inside the uterus and left there to interfere with the implantation of the fertilized egg.

intravenous into a vein.

invasive tending to spread into healthy tissue.

ionizing radiation radiation emitted by radioisotopes.

ischemia a diminished flow of blood to a tissue.

isokinetic contraction contraction in which the resistance matches the force throughout the full range of motion, resulting in the shortening of the muscle.

isometric contraction a contraction in which the force exerted by the muscle is equal to or less than the resistance, resulting in no shortening of the muscle.

isotonic contraction a contraction in which the force exerted by the muscle is greater than the resistance, shortening the muscle.

isotopes atoms which vary only in weight.

-itis suffix meaning inflammation of.

jaundice yellowing of the skin and whites of the eyes.

juvenile-onset obesity obesity arising in childhood and/or adolescence.

kilocalorie a unit of heat that is the equivalency of 1000 calories.

kosher the ritual fitness of food according to Jewish law.

kwashiorkor a disease resulting from protein deficiency in infants.

labia majora the outer lips covering the vaginal opening.

labia minora the inner lips covering the vaginal opening.

labor the act of giving birth; also called parturition.

laparoscopy the use of an endoscope for abdominal exploration.

lapses brief returns to drug use.

laser angioplasty surgery using a device that emits intense heat and power at close range by converting light into one small and extremely intense beam.

latent dormant or inactive.

laxative a substance that acts to loosen the bowels.

learned helplessness a feeling of lack of control over one's life; a condition in which previous inability to make changes in situations is transferred to other situations where changes could be made.

lens the transparent refracting body within the eye.

lesbian a female who is primarily homosexual.

lesion an area of damaged tissue; a wound or infection.

letting go breaking ties to earthly life so a person can die in peace.

leukemia uncontrolled growth of white blood cells.

leukocyte a white blood cell.

leukoplakia formation of white spots or patches on the mucous membrane of the tongue, gums, or cheeks common among users of smokeless tobacco; these are precancerous lesions that may become malignant.

leveling honest communication.

libido (1) in psychoanalytic theory, a basic energy directed at maximizing pleasure; (2) the sexual desire, also called the sex drive.

life expectancy the mean (average) longevity of a population.

ligation tying off.

lightening fetal descent into the pelvis; also called engagement.

lipid a group of chemical substances, including fats and oils, that contain carbon, hydrogen, and oxygen.

lipoprotein a cluster of lipids associated with a protein.

living will a document instructing one's physician to withdraw or withhold treatment under certain specified conditions.

lobar pneumonia pneumonia that affects one or more of the five lobes of the lungs, usually a primary infection.

local death death of a part of the body.

lochia a bloody uterine discharge following delivery.

locus of control one's sense of where the control over one's life lies; a person's perception of the amount of control he or she holds over his or her life.

logarithmic rate of drug breakdown the same *percentage* of the remaining drug is broken down during each equal time period.

longevity the duration of life of an individual.

loss of control the inability to drink in moderation.

love an intense feeling of affection characterized by a deliberate choice to act in the best interests of another person.

LSD lysergic acid diethylamide, a hallucinogenic derivative of an alkaloid in ergot fungus.

lumpectomy removing only a tumor and nearby tissue.

luteinizing hormone (LH) a gonadotropin that stimulates the ovary to release an ovum.

lymphocyte type of white blood cell involved in producing immunity.

lymphoma a malignant tumor occurring in the lymphatic system.

macrominerals minerals needed by the body in fairly large amounts.

macronutrients energy-producing and non-energy-producing nutrients such as fats, carbohydrates, proteins, sodium, and cholesterol needed by the body in greater amounts.

macrophages special white blood cells that patrol the inner surfaces of the lungs and destroy bacteria and other disease agents.

macula the area in the center of the eye's retina that functions as the eye's area of most acute or sharp vision.

macular degeneration irreversible destructive changes in the macula.

mainstream smoke smoke inhaled directly from a cigarette by its smoker.

major depression severe mood disorder in which a person experiences major depressive episodes.

malaise discomfort or uneasiness.

male condom a thin sheath worn over the erect penis to stop sperm from entering the vagina.

malignant cancerous.

mammogram x-ray of the breast.

marasmus a disease resulting from a caloric-protein deficiency, most often in young children.

marijuana the dried leaves and flowers of the hemp plant.

mastectomy removal of a breast.

masturbation stimulation of one's own genitals to derive sexual pleasure.

maximal heart rate (MHR) theoretical maximum rate at which your heart can beat for your age.

Medicaid state programs of public health care assistance provided to people who are unable to afford medical expenses.

medical physician a trained and licensed practitioner of medical arts.

Medicare the hospital insurance system and the supplemental medical insurance for the elderly under Social Security.

meditation a method of producing a relaxed state of consciousness by focusing one's thoughts.

megadosing taking concentrations above those recommended by the RDA.

melanoma a form of skin cancer in which there is a darkening of the skin.

memory cells B or T cells that retain the memory of a specific immune response.

menarche the first menstrual period of a female during puberty.

menopause the period that marks the permanent cessation of menstrual activity.

menstrual cycle the monthly reproductive cycle in women that begins with the menstruation.

menstrual extraction suctioned removal of the uterine lining just before the next menstrual period.

menstruation the monthly shedding and discharge of endometrial tissue and blood from the uterus.

mental of or related to the mind.

mescaline an amphetamine-like hallucinogenic compound contained in the peyote cactus.

metabolism the sum total of all the chemical reactions that occur in the body.

metabolite a product of metabolism.

metastasis the spread of disease from one organ or body part to another.

methaqualone a powerful sedative drug.

microbes or **microorganisms** microscopic living things.

micronutrients non-energy-producing nutrients, such as vitamins and minerals, needed by the body in lesser amounts.

migraine periodic headache attacks often accompanied by visual disturbances and nausea.

millirem (mrem)   one one-thousandth of a rem.

mineral   a naturally occurring inorganic substance.

minilaparotomy   a tiny surgical opening of the abdomen.

miscarriage   a natural termination of the embryo or fetus before it is capable of living outside the uterus; a spontaneous abortion.

monoclonal antibodies   antibodies made outside the body by cultures of antibody-forming cells.

monogamous   usually defined as having one sexual partner at a time or as being married to one person at a time. We define a mutually monogamous relationship as one in which, over an extended period of time, two persons engage in sexual activity only with each other.

monogamy   an exclusive sexual involvement with only one partner at a time.

monosaccharide   a descriptive term for a single-unit sugar.

monounsaturated fatty acid   a fatty acid with one point of unsaturation.

mons veneris   fatty, hair-covered pad over the female's pubic bone.

moral   conduct that enhances growth, builds trust, and helps a person reach his or her potential.

moral values   values that guide us in our conduct with and treatment of other people.

morula   the young embryo, which consists of a solid mass of cells.

mourning   the culturally sanctioned expression of grief.

multiple sclerosis   progressive degeneration of the myelin sheaths.

muscular endurance   the ability to repeat a particular action or hold a particular position for an extended time.

muscular strength   the ability to exert maximum force, usually in a single exertion.

mutation   an inheritable change in a gene; mutations are the source of new genes.

myelin sheath   a fatlike covering over the fibers of some of the neurons of the brain and spinal cord.

myocardial infarction (MI)   the damaging or death of an area of the heart muscle.

myocardium   the muscular wall of the heart.

myotonia   tensing of muscles.

narcotic   a drug that can relieve pain and cause sleep.

narcotic-antagonist   a drug that prevents or reverses the action of a narcotic (opiate).

natural family planning (NFP)   use of menstrual cycle charting and the postponing of intercourse during the fertile days to avoid conception.

natural passive immunity   immunity resulting from antibodies that are passed from a mother to her baby, across the placenta and in breastfeeding.

natural, or background, radiation   radiation arising in the natural environment.

naturopathy   a therapeutic system that does not use drugs or therapy, but employs natural forces such as light, heat, air, water, and massage.

near-death experience   when a person is resuscitated and survives after his or her pulse and breathing have stopped.

necrosis or **gangrene**   death of an area of tissue surrounded by healthy tissue.

neonatal   the first six weeks after birth.

neurological   pertaining to the nervous system.

neurotransmitter   a chemical released from one brain cell to stimulate or inhibit another brain cell.

nicotine   a poisonous alkaloid found in tobacco leaves.

nits   eggs of lice.

nocturnal emission   an involuntary orgasm that occurs during sleep, usually associated with an erotic dream; also called a "wet dream."

noise   unwanted sound.

nomogram   a graph representing the relationship between numerical variables.

non-insulin-dependent diabetes mellitus (NIDDM)   a form of diabetes mellitus in which there is sufficient insulin present, but cells become less sensitive to it. Also known as Type II diabetes. Previously known as adult (mature)-onset diabetes.

nonessential nutrients   nutrients that may come from the foods a person eats, or be made by the body, in sufficient amounts to satisfy its needs.

nonprofit or voluntary hospitals   hospitals that are publicly owned and are operated as nonprofit institutions.

nonrenewable resources   resources that, once depleted, will be replenished very slowly or not at all.

normal aging   the gradual, inevitable changes that occur over time and that can be observed in all animal species.

nurse   a medical professional who provides patient care ranging from simple health care tasks to expert professional techniques.

nutrient density   a measure of the nutrients a food provides relative to the energy it provides. The more nutrients and the fewer the calories, the higher the nutrient density.

nutrients   substances needed by the body to maintain life.

nutrition   the process of absorbing and using food substances for growth, repair, and maintenance of the body.

obesity   excess storage of fat.

occlusion   the closure of a passage.

oil   a lipid that is liquid at room temperature.

oncogene   a gene that has the ability to transform a normal cell into a cancerous one.

oncology   the branch of medicine dealing with tumors.

ophthalmologist   a physician who specializes in the treatment of refractory disorders and diseases of the eye; also called an oculist.

opiates   opium and its natural and synthetic derivatives.

opioids   opium-like substances.

optician   a person who makes optical appliances.

optometrist   a nonphysician who is trained to examine the eyes for refractory disorders.

oral contraceptive   a contraceptive hormone taken orally.

organic   carbon-containing compounds.

organism   any living thing.

orgasm   the highly pleasurable body response that occurs at the climax of sexual arousal as the result of the sudden release of neuromuscular tension.

orgasmic platform   the narrowing of the vagina entrance during sexual excitement.

osteoarthritis   gradual destruction of the cartilage of a joint and overgrowth of bone in the joint.

osteopathic physician a trained and licensed practitioner of osteopathic medicine.

osteoporosis increased porosity of bone resulting from excessive calcium loss, seen most often in elderly women.

ova (eggs) female sex cells; ova is the plural of ovum.

ovaries female sex glands.

over-the-counter (OTC) drugs nonprescription drugs.

overweight any weight above table weight, some specify 10–20 percent above.

ovulation the periodic release of an ovum (egg) from the ovary.

oxygenate to supply with oxygen.

ozone a three-atom type of oxygen formed when an atom of oxygen reacts with oxygen already in the atmosphere.

pacemaker a small mass of nerve tissue in the wall of the right atrium that produces electrical impulses that cause the heart to contract.

pancreas a gland located behind the stomach and connected by a duct to the small intestine. The gland produces both pancreatic juice to assist in food digestion and insulin to assist cells in blood sugar absorption.

panderer one who recruits prostitutes.

panic severe, disabling anxiety.

panic disorder severe, disabling anxiety.

paraphrasing restating what someone has said, putting the message into one's own words.

parasitic worms multicellular true animals that draw nourishment from living hosts such as humans.

parasympathetic nervous system the branch of the autonomic nervous system that acts to restore and conserve energy.

paresis paralysis and mental deterioration caused by degeneration of the brain and spinal cord in late syphilis.

particulate matter solid particles or liquid droplets suspended or carried in the air.

passionate love early, idealistic, noncritical love; infatuation.

passive-aggressive a personality behavior characterized by both excessive passivity and aggressiveness.

passive behavior denying our own needs and rights by failing to express our true feelings and desires.

passive immunity short-term immunity that results from receiving preformed antibodies.

passive smoke exposure to smoke from other people's cigarettes; also called second-hand or sidestream smoke.

patent ductus arteriosus a persistent pathway between the main pulmonary artery and the aorta of the newborn.

pathogen disease-causing organism.

pathological aging aging marked by the presence of diseases that result from unhealthful living habits.

pectin a plant polysaccharide composed of glucose, indigestible by humans.

pediatrician a specialist in the treatment of children's diseases.

pedophilia a type of child sexual abuse in which there is sexual contact between an adult and a child.

pelvic inflammatory disease (PID) a severe infection of the abdominal cavity which, if left untreated, carries the risk of death.

penile implant a mechanical device inserted within the penis in order to aid in erection.

penis an external male genital organ through which urine and semen pass.

perceptual distorter a substance that distorts sensory perceptions.

peripheral nerve any nerve supplying the outer part of the body.

persistent vegetative state (PVS) chronic wakefulness without awareness.

personality the overall response of a person to his or her environment.

pesticide any chemical used to kill plant or animal pests.

phagocytes white blood cells that are capable of phagocytosis.

phagocytosis engulfing of solid particles by a cell.

pharmacist a professional trained to formulate and dispense drugs; a druggist.

pharmacology the study of drugs and their origin, nature, properties, and effects upon living organisms.

phencyclidine (PCP) an anesthetic formerly used in veterinary (and briefly in human) medicine.

photochemical smog a complex mixture of air pollutants produced in the atmosphere by the reaction of hydrocarbons and nitrogen oxides under the influence of sunlight.

pimp one who "manages" the prostitute's time and money.

pituitary gland a small gland, attached to the base of the brain, that produces various hormones controlling other glands, including the testes and ovaries.

placebo an inert substance.

placenta a spongy structure in the uterus through which the fetus obtains nourishment.

plaque a deposit of fatty substances in the inner lining of the artery wall.

plasma the liquid portion of the blood.

platelets blood cells that aid in blood clotting.

pneumonia inflammation of the lungs.

podiatrist a medical practitioner who treats foot conditions.

pollution a change in the physical, chemical, or biological characteristics of the air, water, or soil that can affect the health, survival, or activities of humans or other living organisms in a harmful way.

polydrug abuse the simultaneous abuse of more than one drug.

polysaccharide many monosaccharides linked together.

polyunsaturated fatty acid a fatty acid with two or more points of unsaturation.

populations groups of individuals of the same species living in the same geographical area.

pornography the graphic depiction of erotic behavior with the intent of stimulating sexual arousal.

portal of entry where the pathogen enters its new host.

portal of exit the avenue by which pathogens leave the body of an infected host.

positive reinforcement any stimulus that increases the probability that a behavior will occur.

postpartum following childbirth.

postpartum depression an emotional low that may follow the birth of a child.

potentiation when a drug enhances a certain effect of another drug, but does not have that effect by itself.

preejaculatory fluid sticky fluid secreted prior to ejaculation, and which may contain sperm.

preferred provider organization (PPO) an arrangment whereby a third-party payer contracts with a group of physicians who furnish services at lower-than-usual fees in return for prompt payment and certain volume of patients.

premature ejaculation early, or involuntary, ejaculation with such frequency that a couple's sexual enjoyment is adversely affected.

premenstrual syndrome (PMS) the physical discomfort and emotional mood swings that some women experience before menstruation.

prenatal before birth.

prepaid health insurance health insurance, which for a predetermined amount of money, meets all of the medical needs of members.

presbycusis impairment of hearing with advancing age.

presbyopia loss of ability to focus on close objects due to loss of elasticity of the lens of the eye.

prevalence the number of cases of a disease present in a specified population at a given time.

primary care basic, or general, care given at the person's first contact with the health care system.

primary infection an infection that develops in healthy tissue.

prions infectious particles consisting of protein only.

problem drinkers those whose drinking causes interpersonal, family, or work problems.

problem drinking drinking that causes problems in any area of a person's life or problems for other people.

proctosigmoidoscopy visual examination of the rectum and sigmoid (lower) colon by use of an instrument (sigmoidoscope).

prodromal period the initial stage of a disease.

progesterone a hormone that prepares the uterus for pregnancy and causes the breasts to enlarge in preparation for breastfeeding.

programmed aging theories attribute aging to built-in mechanisms acting to ensure the finite lives of organisms.

progressive overload an increase in muscular strength by the progressive increase, over time, in the demands placed on a muscle.

Prohibition a period in the United States from 1920 to 1933 during which all alcohol sales were outlawed.

projection attributing one's unacceptable characteristics, behaviors, or urges to others.

prophylactically for prevention.

proprietary hospitals hospitals whose operations are intended to make a profit.

prostaglandins a group of substances produced by the body that affects the contraction of the uterus.

prostate gland a gland that surrounds the neck of the bladder and urethra, and that secretes a fluid portion of semen.

prosthesis an artificial organ or body part.

prostitution engaging in sexual activity in exchange for money or gifts.

protein a compound composed of carbon, hydrogen, oxygen, and nitrogen arranged as a strand of amino acids.

protozoa microscopic, single-celled animal-like organisms.

psilocin and **psilocybin** two hallucinogenic chemicals produced by mushrooms.

psychedelic a substance producing a mental state of great calm and intensely pleasurable perception.

psychiatrist a physician who has taken further training to specialize in mental disorders.

psychoactive drugs drugs that affect moods, emotions, perceptions, and behavior and may be used specifically for their mind-altering effects.

psychoanalyst therapist who uses intense exploration of the patient's unconscious mind in order to bring repressed conflicts up to consciousness.

psychoanalytic theory the theory that assumes that unconscious forces influence human behavior.

psychodynamic therapies therapies that assume that unconscious forces influence human behavior.

psychological aging age-related changes in how people think and act.

psychomotor physical activity associated with mental processes.

psychoneuroimmunology the study of the relationships that exist among the mind, nervous system, the hormonal system, and the immune system.

psychopharmacology the science of drugs that affect emotional states and behavior.

psychosomatic pertaining to the relationship of the mind and the body.

psychotherapy treatment of emotional disorders using psychological, rather than biological methods.

psychotic affected by psychosis—severe personality disintegration and loss of contact with reality.

psychotomimetic mimicking a psychosis.

puberty the period of time during which a person becomes functionally capable of reproduction.

public hospitals hospitals that are owned and operated by some level of federal, state, county, or local government.

pulmonary valve the valve between the right ventricle and pulmonary artery.

pulse the rythmic throbbings of the arterial walls.

quackery the practice of pretending to have knowledge or skill in medicine.

radiation transmission of energy through matter and space in the form of fast-moving particles.

radioactive capable of giving off radiation.

radioisotopes radioactive isotopes.

radon a radioactive gas.

random assignment experimentation in which each person has an equal chance of being assigned to either the experimental or the control group.

rape forcing a person to have unwanted sex.

rationalization making up socially acceptable excuses for our behavior rather than exposing the true reasons.

reaction formation masking an unacceptable or distressing trait by assuming an opposite attitude or behavior.

rebound effect the development of effects opposite to those of the drug as a drug is eliminated from the body.

receptor site a special protein on the surface or within a cell with which a drug, neurotransmitter, or hormone interacts.

recombination   any process that produces new combinations of existing genes.

Recommended Dietary Allowance (RDA)   nutrient intakes suggested for the maintenance of health in people in the United States.

rectum   lower part of the large intestine.

refractory disorder   inability to focus the eyes or to perceive images correctly.

refractory period   the period immediately following ejaculation, during which males are unable to experience further orgasms.

regression   retreating to a more immature form of behavior during times of stress.

relapse   recurrence of a disease after apparent recovery.

rem   roentgen equivalent in humans.

remission   a decrease in or abatement of the symptoms of a disease.

renewable resources   resources that can be depleted, but will be replaced through natural processes.

replication   the process of reproduction.

repression   a process by which unacceptable thoughts, memories, desires, or motives are excluded from consciousness and left to operate in the unconscious mind.

reservoir   the source of a pathogen.

resistance   (1) a sustainable level of stress in which the resistance to stressors increases; (2) the nonspecific defenses against disease; (3) the ability of a pathogen to survive in the presence of an antimicrobial drug.

resource recovery   salvaging usable metals, paper, and glass from solid waste and selling them to manufacturing industries for recycling or reuse.

resting heart rate (RHR)   the heart rate when the body is at rest.

retina   the nerve-containing innermost layer of the eye, which receives the images formed by the lens.

Reye's Syndrome   an acute condition affecting the brain and liver; seen in children after a serious virus infection.

Rh factor   a protein found in red blood cells.

rheumatic fever   an infectious disease that inflames the inner lining of the heart and causes rheumatic heart disease.

rheumatic heart disease   damage done to the heart, particularly the heart valves, by one or more attacks of rheumatic fever.

rheumatoid arthritis   an autoimmune disorder marked by severe inflammation of the joints and sometimes other organs.

rhinorrhea   thin watery discharge from the nose.

rickettsia   unusually small bacteria that reproduce only in living host cells; most are carried by insects or ticks.

salicylate   any form of salicylic acid, the active ingredient in aspirin.

salicylism   toxic condition caused by an overdose of salicylic acid.

sarcoma   a malignant tumor occurring in connective tissue.

schizophrenia   mental disorder characterized by severe disruptions in thinking, perception, and emotions, in which people are out of touch with reality.

scrotum   thin, loose pouch of skin that contains the testes.

secondary care   medical care provided by another physician upon referral by a patient's primary care physician.

secondary infection   one that develops in tissue damaged by a primary infection.

sedation   state of being calmed.

sedative-hypnotic drugs   drugs that depress the central nervous system.

self-actualization   making full use of your abilities and working toward achieving your full potential as a human being.

self-care   health care we can provide to ourselves.

self-concept   the way we perceive ourselves as functioning human beings.

self-esteem   one's subjective sense of personal worth.

self-transcendence   the ability to rise above your own self.

semen   a grayish-white, sticky mixture of sperm and seminal fluid discharged from the urethra of the male during ejaculation.

seminal vesicles   glands that produce fluid that activates sperm and increases their capacity to swim.

seminiferous tubules   highly coiled tubules in the testes that produce sperm.

senescence   the phase of old age toward the end of the lifespan in which functional deterioration of the body leads to an increased probability of death.

senility   the physical and mental deterioration which is associated with advanced biological aging.

sensate focus exercises   a series of touching exercises designed to teach nonverbal communication and to reduce anxiety about achieving an erection.

septum   the partition between the right and left sides of the heart.

serum   plasma minus its coagulating proteins.

set-point   a concept that there is a point at which the body's weight is set.

sexual arousal   the activation of reflexes involving the sex organs and the nervous system.

sexual dysfunction   a sexual disorder that interferes with a full or complete sexual response cycle.

sexual fantasy   any daydream of a sexual nature.

sexual harassment   unwelcome sexual advances, requests for sexual favors, or other visual, verbal, or physical conduct of a sexual nature.

sexual orientation   an individual's attraction to persons of the same, opposite, or both sexes.

sexual paraphilia   a sexual disorder in which sexual arousal and response is pleasurable, yet whose object and/or aim deviates from the norm.

sexual sadomasochism   variant sexual behavior in which inflicting pain (sadism) and submitting to pain (masochism) occur simultaneously.

sexual values   a sexual code of ethics that determines how our sexuality is expressed.

sexually transmitted diseases (STDs)   diseases that are commonly transmitted through sexual contact.

shock wave lithotripsy   crushing of a calculus in the bladder or urethra by the use of high intensity sound waves.

sinsemilla   "without seeds," marijuana produced from unfertilized female plants.

skinfold thickness test   a method for determining the thickness of fat beneath the skin; also called the fatfold test.

smog   see *photochemical smog.*

social aging   age-related changes in the interactions people have with each other.

social drinkers   those who drink only in a social context.

solid wastes   any unwanted or discarded material that is not a liquid or a gas.

sound   any identifiable noise.

sperm   male sex cell.

sphygmomanometer   an instrument for measuring blood pressure.

spirilla   spiral bacteria.

spirochetes   long, slender, coiled bacteria.

sputum   the material expelled by coughing or clearing the throat.

starch   a plant polysaccharide composed of many units of saccharide.

statutory rape   sexual intercourse between an adult and a minor who are not married to each other.

stem cell   immature lymphocyte.

stenosis   constricting or narrowing of a heart valve or blood vessel.

sterilization   the surgical interruption of the male or female reproductive tracts, preventing the passage of sex cells, and thus fertilization.

stillbirth   birth of a dead fetus which, if born alive, would have been capable of living outside the uterus.

stimulant   any drug that increases functional activity.

stochastic aging theories   also called error theories, relate aging to external forces that damage cells until they can no longer function adequately.

stress   a group of bodywide, non-specific defense responses induced by any of a number of stressors.

stressor   any situation or event that elicits the stress response.

stroke   a cerebrovascular accident in which the blood supply to part of the brain is interrupted through rupture or blockage of a blood vessel supplying the brain.

sublimation   redirecting socially unacceptable urges into socially acceptable behavior.

subliminal seduction   a method of using sexual suggestions below the threshold of consciousness to sell products.

subluxation   a partial or incomplete dislocation of the vertebrae.

sucrose   a double sugar known as table sugar.

suction lipectomy   removal of fatty tissues.

sudden cardiac death   death that occurs unexpectedly and instantaneously, or shortly after the onset of symptoms.

sudden infant death syndrome (SIDS)   the completely unexpected and unexplained death of an apparently well infant.

sun protection factor (SPF)   measurement of the ability of a sunscreen product to prevent sunburn.

sunscreen   a substance used to protect the skin from UV rays.

superego   in psychoanalytic theory, our conscience or our sense of right and wrong.

suppository   a semisolid substance containing spermicide that is introduced into the vagina, where it dissolves.

suppression   consciously avoiding thinking about something that would cause stress or anxiety.

surface water   precipitation that does not filter into the ground, but becomes runoff into rivers, streams, and lakes.

surfactant   a secretion produced inside the fetal lungs that makes breathing by the newborn easier.

susceptible   having little resistance to a disease.

sympathetic nervous system   the branch of the autonomic nervous system that prepares the body for emergency action.

sympathomimetic   a drug that mimics the effects of the sympathetic nervous system.

synapse   the junction between two neurons.

syndrome   a group of signs and symptoms that collectively characterize a particular disease or condition.

synergism   when two drugs produce effects that are more powerful than the sum of the effects of each drug if taken individually.

synesthesia   when the stimulus of one sense (such as hearing) produces the perception of another sense (such as smell).

systemic   pertaining to a whole body rather than to one of its parts.

systemic lupus erythematosus (SLE)   an autoimmune disease affecting the joints, skin, kidneys, and other body systems.

systole   the part of the heart cycle when the heart is in contraction.

T lymphocyte or **T cell**   lymphocyte processed by the thymus and capable of producing cell-mediated immunity.

tachycardia   an abnormally rapid heartbeat characterized by a pulse rate over 100 beats per minute.

target training zone   the rate at which the heart is beating to get the maximum aerobic effect.

tars   thick, black, sticky materials produced when tobacco is burned.

teratogens   environmental agents that cause congenital malformations by affecting the embryo or fetus.

term birth   the duration of a normal pregnancy.

testes   male sex glands.

testosterone   a male sex hormone produced primarily in the testes.

thanatology   the study of death.

THC   tetrahydrocannabinol, the active ingredient in marijuana.

thermal inversion layer   a layer of air trapped under a layer of less-dense warm air, thus reversing the usual situation.

thrombosis   formation of blood clots.

thrombus   a blood clot which forms inside a blood vessel.

tissue fluid   fluid which bathes body cells.

tolerance   the body's ability to adjust to increasing levels of a drug.

tonic-clonic convulsive episodes, accompanied by loss of consciousness and falling.

toxemia a condition during pregnancy in which poisonous body wastes are retained by the body.

toxic pertaining to or caused by a poison.

toxins poisons produced by bacteria.

toxoid modified bacterial toxin used as a vaccine.

trace minerals minerals needed by the body in minute amounts.

trachoma a severe eye infection that can lead to blindness.

training effect beneficial changes your body makes to aerobic exercise of sufficient intensity, duration, and frequency.

training intensity (TI) how hard a person must train to achieve a given level of cardiorespiratory endurance.

tranquilizers or **antianxiety drugs** drugs with sedative and antianxiety effects, also used as muscle relaxants and anticonvulsants.

transient ischemic attack (TIA) a temporary strokelike event that lasts for only a short time and is caused by a temporarily blocked blood vessel.

transmission transfer of a pathogen to a new host.

transplacental across the placenta.

transsexual an individual with a persistent sense of discomfort with his or her biological gender.

transvestism deriving sexual pleasure from dressing in the clothing of the other sex.

tricuspid valve the heart valve between the right atrium and right ventricle.

triglyceride the major class of dietary lipids containing three fatty acids.

trimester of pregnancy a third of pregnancy, or approximately 13 weeks.

troposphere the innermost layer of the atmosphere.

tubercle the characteristic lesion caused by the tubercle bacillus.

tuberculosis an infectious disease caused by the tubercle bacillus.

tumor or **neoplasm** a mass of new tissue that grows without serving any useful function.

ulcer an open lesion (sore).

ultrasound examination taking a picture of a developing fetus using sound waves.

ultraviolet radiation (UV) rays beyond visible light at the violet end of the spectrum.

umbilical cord a cordlike attachment containing blood vessels that connects the fetus with the placenta.

underweight any weight more than 10 percent below desirable weight.

urates salts of uric acid, normally present in the urine.

urethra duct for the discharge of urine from the bladder and the carrying of semen.

uterus a muscular, pear-shaped reproductive organ in which the embryo and fetus develop.

vaccine preparation of one or more antigens used to stimulate the development of active immunity.

vacuum aspiration the removal of a fetus by suction.

vagina a tubular organ that forms a passageway between the vestibule and the uterus.

vaginal diaphragm a shallow, dome-shaped device that is positioned inside the vagina over the cervix to serve as a barrier to sperm.

vaginal spermicide a chemical agent applied in the vagina that kills or immobilizes sperm.

vaginismus involuntary spasm of the lower vaginal muscles when penetration by the penis is attempted.

vaginitis inflammation of the vagina.

values the principles or standards by which we assign worth.

varicose distended, swollen veins.

vas deferens a tube that carries sperm upward from each epididymis to the ejaculatory duct..

vasectomy the surgical closing of the vas deferens to prevent conception.

vasocongestion the filling of the genitals and breasts with blood during sexual arousal.

vasoconstrictive causing blood vessels to constrict.

vector insect or similar carrier of a pathogen.

vegan a person who excludes all animal derived food from his or her diet; pure, or total, vegetarian.

vegetarian a general term for a person who prefers plant food products to animal products.

vein any blood vessel that carries blood from various parts of the body back to the heart.

ventricles the two lower chambers of the heart.

ventricular premature contractions an occasional abnormal impulse between normal impulses delivered by nerve cells ourside the pacemaker.

venule a small branch of a vein.

very-low-calorie diet diet plans that provide from 400 to 800 calories a day, a protein intake about two times the RDA, with no fat and little carbohydrate.

vestibule an area between the labia minora.

viable capable of living.

viroids infectious particles consisting of nucleic acid (RNA) only, with no protein.

virulence degree of disease-causing ability.

viruses infectious particles consisting of nucleic acid (either DNA or RNA) and protein and, in some cases, an outer envelope of protein and fat.

vitamins organic compounds vital to body function.

volatile easily vaporized or evaporated.

voyeurism deriving sexual gratification from secretly viewing people disrobing, nude, or engaging in sexual activity.

vulva the external genitals of the female.

walking pneumonia mild form of pneumonia, usually caused by *Mycoplasma pneumoniae*.

warm-up exercises performed immediately before physical activity to prepare the body for rigorous exercise.

water pollution any physical or chemical change in surface or groundwater that can adversely affect living organisms.

water-soluble vitamins vitamins soluble in water.

wellness the constant and deliberate effort to stay healthy and achieve the highest potential for well-being. It is a lifestyle that emphasizes such health-promoting behaviors as eating a healthful diet, avoiding harmful substances, enjoying regular exercise, and cultivating self-esteem.

withdrawal the removal of the penis from the vagina prior to ejaculation as a method of controlling conception; also called coitus interruptus.

withdrawal syndrome or **abstinence syndrome** a group of symptoms that occur when a drug that causes physiological dependence is no longer taken.

xanthine chemical substance in the alkaloid family with stimulant properties; an example is caffeine.

"you statements" statements that judge another's behavior and place responsibility for your emotions on that other person.

zero population growth (ZPG) the state in which the birth rate (plus immigration) equals the death rate (plus emigration) so that population is no longer increasing.

zoophilia obtaining sexual arousal through sexual contact with animals; also known as bestiality.

zygote the fertilized ovum.

CREDITS

PHOTOS

Unless otherwise acknowledged, all photographs are the property of HarperCollins.

Unit Openers: Unit 1 **1** © Benn/Stock, Boston. Unit 2 **49** Herwig/Stock, Boston. Unit 3 **109** © Bachmann/ PhotoEdit. Unit 4 **253** © Weinrebe/Stock, Boston. Unit 5 **369** © 1992 Mannheim/Stock South. Unit 6 **429** © Hutchings/PhotoEdit. Unit 7 **547** © Daemmrich/ The Image Works. Unit 8 **697** Daemmrich/The Image Works.

Chapter 1 **2** © Vincent/PhotoEdit; **4** Brueghel, Madrid, Prado/Art Resource, NY; **7** Rogers/Stock, Boston; **11** Erika Stone; **19** © Herwig/Picture Cube; **22** Newman/ PhotoEdit; **23** Daemmrich/Stock, Boston.

Chapter 2 **26** © Gianetti/Stock, Boston; **29** © Newman/PhotoEdit; **32** © Angier/Stock, Boston; **33** © Freeman/PhotoEdit; **34** © Young-Wolff/PhotoEdit; **35** © Siteman/Stock, Boston; **37** © Sidney/PhotoEdit; **43** © McCarthy/Picture Cube; **49** © Kingston/Picture Cube.

Chapter 3 **53** (top left) Anna Zukerman/PhotoEdit; (top middle) Deborah Davis/PhotoEdit, (top right) Erika Stone, (bottom left) PhotoEdit, (bottom middle) Myrleen Ferguson/PhotoEdit, (bottom right) © Robert Brenner/ PhotoEdit, **57** Clayton/Stock South; **62** Tony Freeman/ PhotoEdit; **64** © Young-Wolff/PhotoEdit; **65** Jean-Claude LeJeune; **66** Holland/Stock, Boston; **68** Norma Morrison; **70** Tony Freeman/PhotoEdit.

Chapter 4 **74** © MacDonald/Picture Cube; **77** © Freeman/PhotoEdit; **82** AP/Wide World; **86** © David R. Frazier; **92** (top left) © Davis/PhotoEdit, (top right) Richard Hutchings/PhotoEdit, (bottom left) Myrleen Ferguson/PhotoEdit, (bottom right) © 1990 McCarthy/ Stock South; **97** © Brenner/PhotoEdit; **109** © Bachmann/PhotoEdit.

Chapter 5 **110** Newman/PhotoEdit; **114** (top) © Ferguson/PhotoEdit, (bottom) © Ferguson/PhotoEdit; **115** © 1992 Ulrike Welsch; **117** © 1983 Ulrike Welsch;

126 © Palmer/Picture Cube; **129** © Richards/PhotoEdit; **131** © 1992 Farley/Monkmeyer; **132** © Coletti/Picture Cube; **134** © Sidney/PhotoEdit.

Chapter 6 **140** © Hill, Jr./Stock, Boston; **146** © Conklin/ PhotoEdit; **152** © Phillips/Photo Researchers; **165** © Druskis/Stock, Boston; **169** © Bachmann/Stock, Boston; **171** © Griffin/The Image Works.

Chapter 7 **178** © Esbin-Anderson/The Image Works; **185** © Freeman/PhotoEdit; **189** (top) © Joel Gordon, (bottom) © Joel Gordon; **195** (bottom) © Newman/ PhotoEdit; **200** © Newman/PhotoEdit.

Chapter 8 **212** © Austen/Stock, Boston; **217** © David Phillips/Photo Researchers; **222** CEDRI, (bottom right) Petit Format Nestle Science Source/Photo Researchers; **226** Etra/PhotoEdit; **229** (all) Reprinted with permission of Ann Streissguth. From Streissguth, A. P., Aase, J. M., Clarren, S. K., Randels, S. P., LaDue, R.A., Smith, D.F. (1991). Fetal Alcohol Syndrome in Adolescents and Adults. *Journal of the American Medical Association* 265 (15): 1961–1967; **233** Courtesy Kelly Mountain; **237** (all) Erika Stone; **238** Nettis/Stock, Boston; **239** Erika Stone; **247** (top) © Brenner/PhotoEdit, (bottom) © Dwyer/Stock, Boston.

Chapter 9 **254** © 1992 McCarthy/Stock South; **258** Migdale/Stock, Boston; **266** © B&B Photos/Custom Medical Stock; **274** © Ogust/The Image Works.

Chapter 10 **296** © McCarthy/PhotoEdit; **301** (top) Yoav Levy/Phototake, (bottom) Scott, Foresman; **317** © Thompson/Picture Cube; **322** Erika Stone.

Chapter 11 **330** Bachmann/Stock South; **334** © 1989 Mark Hunt Backdrops/Light Source Stock; **338** Norma Morrison; **340** © 1992 Ulrike Welsch; **348** © Vincent/ PhotoEdit; **350** © Daemmrich/The Image Works; **351** © 1991 Hangarter/Picture Cube; **361** © 1994 Schaefer/ Picture Cube.

Chapter 12 **370** © Greenberg/Picture Cube; **378** © Etra/ PhotoEdit; **380** Bruce Curtis/Peter Arnold, Inc.; **382** © Freeman/PhotoEdit; **388** © 1990 Aron/PhotoEdit; **392** ©

Freeman/PhotoEdit; **394** Lawrence Migdale; **397** Susan Wilson/Decisive Moment.

Chapter 13 **402** © Hutchings/PhotoEdit; **406** Morgan/Science Source Library/Photo Researchers; **407** Charles Harbutt/Actuality Inc.; **412** © Mulvehill; **416** © Siluk/The Image Works; **417** Alan Oddie/PhotoEdit; **420** John Regan/Decisive Moment; **422** Oscar Palmquist/Lightwave.

Chapter 14 **430** © MacDonald/Picture Cube; **433** (left) Custom Medical Stock Photo, (right) © Katz/Stock South; **436** © Walker/Picture Cube; **440** © Newman/PhotoEdit; **441** Lawrence Migdale; **443** Brown/Stock, Boston; **446** © Sidney/The Image Works; **447** Larry Mulvehill/Photo Researchers; **452** Joseph Nettis/Photo Researchers.

Chapter 15 **460** © Roth/Picture Cube; **466** Tim Malyon/Science Photo Library/Photo Researchers; **473** © Tony Freeman/PhotoEdit; **474** Tony Freeman/PhotoEdit; **475** Courtesy U.S. Department of Justice, Drug Enforcement Administration; **478** Custom Medical Stock; **479** Courtesy U.S. Department of Justice, Drug Enforcement Administration; **487** Scott Camazine/Photo Researchers; **489** Tony Freeman/PhotoEdit.

Chapter 16 **494** McQueen/Stock, Boston; **499** © 1989 Edrington/The Image Works; **503** © Gordon T. Hewlett 1972 ; **504** Tony Freeman/PhotoEdit; **506** © Stephen McBrady/PhotoEdit; **507** Richard Hutchings/Photo Researchers; **509** © 1993 Denny/PhotoEdit; **510** © Michael Newman/PhotoEdit; **511** Edward Lettau/Photo Researchers; **512** John Radcliffe Hospital/Science Photo Library/Photo Researchers; **514** © Barnes/PhotoEdit.

Chapter 17 **518** © Hutchings/PhotoEdit; **523** © Beck/Picture Cube; **528** © Bob Daemmrich/The Image Works; **530** William H. Mullins/Photo Researchers; **531** Ann Streissguthy, The University of Washington; **532** Robert Brenner/PhotoEdit; **537** Tony Freeman/PhotoEdit; **539** (top left) © 1990 Brown/Picture Cube, (top right) © 1992 Ulrike Welsch, (bottom left) © Craig/Picture Cube, (bottom right) © Newman/PhotoEdit; **541** © 1990 Hawkins/Stock South.

Chapter 18 **548** © Hill/The Image Works; **554** © 1973 Noble Proctor/Photo Researchers; **555** Custom Medical Stock Photo; **557** (top left) © Greco/The Image Works, (top middle) Barbara Rios/Photo Researchers, (top right) Coco McCoy/Rainbow, (bottom left) C.W. Brown/Photo Researchers, (bottom middle) Frederick Beortgia/Photo Researchers, (bottom right) Dan McCoy/Rainbow; **564** © Bob Daemmrich/The Image Works; **566** Joyce Photographics/Photo Researchers; **573** Hank Morgan/Science Source/Photo Researchers; **574** © Mulvehill/The Image Works; **579** Lowell Georgia/Science Source/Photo Researchers.

Chapter 19 **584** © Hill/The Image Works; **593** Sygma; **595** © Newman/PhotoEdit; **598** (left) National Institutes of Health, (right) © John Wilson/Photo Researchers; **600** (left) © 1993 Custom Medical Stock Photo, (right) National Institutes of Health; **603** (top left) © 1991 National Medical Slide/Custom Medical Stock, (bottom right) National Institutes of Health; **605** (top left) National Institutes of Health, (bottom right) National Institutes of Health; **608** Rotker/Photo Researchers; **609** Photo Researchers; **610** © Callaghan/Phototake.

Chapter 20 **616** © Daemrich/The Image Works; **624** (top and bottom) Rotker/Phototake; **629** Stevie Grand/SPL/Photo Researchers; **630** Don and Pat Valenti/Taurus Photos, Inc.; **636** (left) Custom Medical Stock Photo, (right) John Eads; **647** © Haramaty Mula/Phototake NYC; **648** © Seitz/Photo Researchers; **649** Simon Fraser/Helam General/Science Photo Library/Photo Researchers.

Chapter 21 **652** © 1993 Gupton/Stock, Boston; **655** (left and right) Cecil H. Fox/Science Source/Photo Researchers; **661** Hank Morgan/Rainbow; **662** (top) © Overton/Phototake, (bottom) © Rotker/Phototake; **664** Science Photo Library/Photo Researchers; **668** Louisa Preston/Photo Researchers; **675** Paul Light/Lightwave; **683** © Daemmrich/The Image Works.

Chapter 22 **698** © McCarthy/PhotoEdit; **703** © Frisch/Stock, Boston; **707** Joseph Nettis/Photo Researchers; **712** © 1993 Denny/PhotoEdit; **713** Michael Gadomski/Photo Researchers; **715** Linda Moore/Rainbow; **716** © Yoav Levy/Phototake NYC.

Chapter 23 **730** © Oddie/PhotoEdit; **734** Walsh/Picture Cube; **736** Will & Deni McIntyre/Photo Researchers; **739** © MacDonald/Picture Cube; **742** © Newman/PhotoEdit; **744** Morgan/Photo Researchers.

Chapter 24 **756** Yurka; **759** Karen Herian/Lightwave; **772** John Chason/Gamma/Liaison; **778** © Paul Conklin/PhotoEdit; **786** (top) Will McIntyre/Photo Researchers, (bottom) Darryl Baird/Lightwave; **792** W. Campbell/Sygma.

TEXT AND ILLUSTRATIONS

Table 1.2 From *Medical World News*, July 1993. Reprinted by permission of Miller Freeman Publications, Inc.

Feature 2.2 From *Your Perfect Right: A Guide to Assertive Living,* 6th ed. Copyright © 1990 by Robert E. Alberti and Michael L. Emmons. Reprinted by permission of Impact Publishers, Inc., P. O. Box 1094, San Luis Obispo, CA 93405. Further reproduction prohibited.

Chapter 11 In Your Hands: A Summary of Your Fitness from *Your Guide to Getting Fit,* 2nd ed. by I. Kusinitz and M. Fine. Copyright © 1991 by Mayfield Publishing Company. Reprinted by permission of Mayfield Publishing Company.

Fig. 12.1 "Interactions Among Types of Aging" adapted from *Human Aging* by DiGiovanna & Augustine, 1994, p. 8. Reprinted by permission of McGraw-Hill, Inc.

Feature 12.6 From "Labors of Love" by John Wood from *Modern Maturity,* Aug./Sept., 1987. Copyright © 1987 American Association of Retired Persons. Reprinted by permission of Modern Maturity.

Feature 17.5 "Am I an Alcoholic?" from "Detecting Alcoholism, the CAGE Questionnaire" *JAMA* 252, No. 14, 1984, pp. 1905–07. Copyright © 1984 American Medical Association. Reprinted by permission.

Fig. 20.5 "Adapted from "The Formation of Plaques in Atherosclerosis" from *Understanding Nutrition,* 6th ed. by E. Whitney & S. Rolfes, p. 557. Copyright © 1993 by West Publishing Company. All rights reserved. Reprinted by permission of the authors.

Fig. 20.9 Adapted from *Principles of Anatomy and Physiology,* 7th ed. by G. J. Tortora & S. R. Grabowski, p. 619. Copyright © 1993 by Biological Sciences Textbooks, Inc., A & P Textbooks, Inc., and Sandra Reynolds Grabowski. HarperCollins College Publishers.

Fig. 20.11 Adapted from *Principles of Anatomy and Physiology,* 7th ed. by G. J. Tortora & S. R. Grabowski, p. 618. Copyright © 1993 by Biological Sciences Textbooks, Inc., A & P Textbooks, Inc., and Sandra Reynolds Grabowski. HarperCollins College Publishers.

Table 20.3 "Food for a Healthy Heart" from *Understanding Nutrition,* 6th ed. by E. Whitney & S. Rolfes. Copyright © 1993 by West Publishing Company. All rights reserved. Reprinted by permission of the authors.

Feature 20.1 "What to Do If You Suspect a Heart Attack" from *Heart and Stroke Facts,* p. 18. Copyright © 1992, 1993 American Heart Association. Reprinted by permission.

Feature 20.2 From *Women and Heart Disease* by Edward Diethrich, M.D. Copyright © 1992 by Edward B. Diethrich, M.D. Reprinted by permission of Times Books, a division of Random House, Inc.

Chapter 20 Communication for Wellness: How to Make Your Arteries Younger (or Older) than They Are, from *Berkeley Wellness Letter,* June 1987. Copyright © 1987 Health Letter Associates. Reprinted by permission of the University of California at Berkeley Wellness Letter.

Chapter 20 In Your Hands: Taking Your Measure of Heart Disease Risk, from *Health Risks* by Dr. Elliott Howard. Copyright © 1986 Elliott Howard. Reprinted by permission.

Fig. 21.11 "Incorrect and Correct Pelvic Alignment" from *Fitness & Wellness,* 2nd ed. by Werner W. K. Hoeger and Sharon A. Hoeger. Copyright © 1993 Morton Publishing Co. Reprinted by permission.

Figure 21.12 "Your Back and How to Care For It." All rights reserved. Reprinted by permission of Schering Corporation, Kenilworth, NJ.

Feature 21.1 "Cancer Survival" from *Cancer Facts and Figures,* 1993. Reprinted by permission of American Cancer Society, Inc.

Table 21.1 "Information on Some Major Cancers" from *Cancer Facts and Figures,* 1993. Reprinted by permission of American Cancer Society, Inc.

Table 21.2 "Cancer Survival Rates" from *Cancer Facts and Figures,* 1993. Reprinted by permission of American Cancer Society, Inc.

Table 21.6 "Tests For Early Detection of Cancer" from *Cancer Facts and Figures,* 1993. Reprinted by permission of American Cancer Society, Inc.

Chapter 21 Communication for Wellness: Coping with Cancer from *The American Cancer Society Cancer Book* by Arthur I. Holleb. Copyright © 1986 by The American Cancer Society. Reprinted by permission of Doubleday, a division of Bantam Doubleday Dell Publishing Group, Inc.

Fig. 22.3 "Assault On The Skin" from *Time,* July 23, 1990. Copyright © 1990 Time Inc. Reprinted by permission.

Table 22.3 "Caffeine in Some Common Drinks and Drugs" adapted from "The Daily Dose" from *Berkeley Wellness Letter,* July 1988. Copyright © 1988 Health Letter Associates. Reprinted by permission of the University of California at Berkeley Wellness Letter.

Feature 23.4 "Take Charge of Your Medical Records" from *Berkeley Wellness Letter,* November 1993. Copyright © 1993 Health Letter Associates. Reprinted by permission of the University of California at Berkeley Wellness Letter.

Fig. 24.3 "What Is Ozone?" from *Los Angeles Times,* Apr. 23, 1991. Copyright © 1991 Los Angeles Times. Reprinted by permission.

Fig. 24.5 "Annual Deaths" adapted from *Living in the Environment,* 7th ed. by G. Miller. Copyright © 1992 Wadsworth Publishing Co. Reprinted by permission.

INDEX